W 8/22
W 1/16
W 11/17 PLC 16th    JY - - '74
W 5/19

# The Lupus Encyclopedia

A Johns Hopkins Press Health Book

Donald E. Thomas, Jr.
MD, FACP, FACR

# *The* Lupus
# ENCYCLOPEDIA

*A Comprehensive
Guide for Patients
and Families*

JOHNS HOPKINS UNIVERSITY PRESS    BALTIMORE

*Note to the reader.* This book is not meant to substitute for medical care of people who have lupus, and treatment should not be based solely on its contents. Instead, treatment must be developed in a dialogue between the individual and his or her physician. This book has been written to help with that dialogue. The author and publisher are not responsible for any adverse consequences resulting from the use of information in this book.

*Drug dosage.* The author and publisher have made reasonable efforts to determine that selection and dosage of drugs discussed in this text conform to the practices of the general medical community. The medications described do not necessarily have specific approval by the U.S. Food and Drug Administration for use in the diseases and dosages for which they are recommended. In view of ongoing research, changes in governmental regulations, and the constant flow of information relating to drug therapy and drug reactions, the reader is urged to check the package insert of each drug for any change in indications and dosage and for warnings in precautions. This is particularly important when the recommended agent is a new and/or infrequently used drug.

© 2014 Johns Hopkins University Press
All rights reserved. Published 2014
Printed in the United States of America on acid-free paper
9 8 7 6 5 4 3 2 1

Johns Hopkins University Press
2715 North Charles Street
Baltimore, Maryland 21218-4363
www.press.jhu.edu

Library of Congress Cataloging-in-Publication Data

Thomas, Donald E., Jr., 1961–
 The lupus encyclopedia : a comprehensive guide for patients and families / Donald E. Thomas, Jr., M.D., FACP, FACR.
   pages cm. — (A Johns Hopkins Press health book)
 Includes bibliographical references and index.
 ISBN 978-1-4214-0983-2 (hardcover : alk. paper) — ISBN 1-4214-0983-6 (hardcover : alk. paper) — ISBN 978-1-4214-0984-9 (pbk. : alk. paper) — ISBN 1-4214-0984-4 (pbk. : alk. paper) — ISBN 978-1-4214-0985-6 (electronic) — ISBN 1-4214-0985-2 (electronic) 1. Systemic lupus erythematosus—Encyclopedias. I. Title.
 RC924.5.L85T46 2013
 616.7'72003—dc23

                                                                              2012042648

A catalog record for this book is available from the British Library.

Figures 1.1, 10.1, 11.1, 12.1, 12.2, 13.1, 14.1, 16.1, 17.1, 21.1, 21.2, 24.1, 24.2, 26.1, 27.1, 28.1–28.3, 30.1, 30.2, 33.1, 37.1–37.3, and 38.1 and those on pages 255, 568, 570, and 572 are by Jacqueline Schaffer.

*Special discounts are available for bulk purchases of this book. For more information, please contact Special Sales at 410-516-6936 or specialsales@press.jhu.edu.*

Johns Hopkins University Press uses environmentally friendly book materials, including recycled text paper that is composed of at least 30 percent post-consumer waste, whenever possible.

To my parents, Donald and Nancy Thomas, who worked very hard all their lives in very difficult, demanding jobs in factories. The many hours that they spent working double shifts so their family of six children could benefit in the end are priceless; I will never be able to repay them for their sacrifices. It is because of these sacrifices that I am able to live the American Dream. I am lucky to have them as my parents.

To my grandparents, L. Ross and Laura Thomas. Ever since I was a small child, they told me I could do whatever I put my mind to. When I thought I was stupid, they told me I was smart. A big turning point in my life was in the fifth grade; I was in the remedial reading class due to problems during my fourth-grade year. They urged me to strive beyond my preconceived abilities. Taking on their challenge, I memorized a long poem about a pirate. I got up in front of the class and recited it by heart without missing a line. My teacher, Mrs. Wine, took me by the hand, led me to the "smart" reading classroom, and told me that that was where I belonged. How empowering an event that was. I never looked back. In fact, I have made it a point throughout my life to encourage others who are not performing up to their abilities to do the same in their lives. My grandma almost died of asthma when I was young. I told her that I was going to become a doctor to help people like her, and that is what I have done. I wish my grandparents were alive today to see what I am doing. I know that they are looking down on me from heaven with a smile. Thanks, Grandma and Grandpa, your memory lives on.

To one of my best friends in high school, Gordon Blue, his parents (Ruth and Carlos), and all the Blue sisters. When I was in college, I ran out of money and had to drop out of school at a critical point in my education. When I had nowhere else to turn, the Blue family took me into their home. They knew I wanted to become a doctor and they wanted to help me. Living with them in the Houston area gave me the chance to work, get back on my feet, and finish college. By fortune, it facilitated my ability to be accepted to and attend one of the best medical schools in the United States, Baylor College of Medicine. The Blues are my second family and I am indebted to them for extending to me their hand and love.

To my Bengal cat, Adam; my African grey parrot, Timmy; my Coton de Tulear dog, Citeaux; and my newest puppy, Musette. They can be my biggest fans and supporters. I would be so exhausted and worn out from writing on many a weekday night and long weekend, yet their unconditional love and snuggling would always revive me, renew me with energy, and replace my tired frown with a smile!

Most importantly, I dedicate this to those stricken with lupus who have succumbed to the disease and its complications. I will never forget the teenager who died of severe lupus in our county hospital many years ago because she and her family could not afford proper healthcare. By the time I saw her, it was too late. I will never forget how she told me she was not going to live and how I grieved alongside her loving mother. I hope our healthcare system will continue to improve so that people do not have to die from this disease simply because they come from families with little money. To my neighbor Tim's mother: I never knew her, but he talks about how she died of lupus and its complications during a time when therapies were not nearly as good as they are today. I dedicate this book to all lupus patients who have not survived the fight. I hope that the current research and new therapies for lupus will prevent the deaths of lupus patients in the not too distant future. I know this book can give to you, the reader, the knowledge and wisdom that can protect you from a similar fate. Keep reading on.

# CONTENTS

FIGURES

## PHOTOGRAPHS

How do you understand, much less solve, a problem like lupus? Even a quick scan through the pages of this book will tell you that you are about to undergo a crash course in medicine, including nearly every medical specialty. How do you grasp such a complex disease, one that can involve every system in the body? Lupus was first recognized as a disease of the skin in the mid-nineteenth century, but the systemic nature of the disease was not appreciated until the 1940s. It took practically the entire twentieth century to complete the list of primary clinical and laboratory manifestations of the disease and the conditions that occur along with lupus.

Where does such a clinically variable disease start? Definitely not from just a single point. This book guides you through many factors that contribute to the expression of the disease. The first is genes. As researchers advance in their understanding of the nature of the human genome, they believe that dozens of genes may be involved.

Another factor is environmental influences, including drugs, toxins (people who have lupus should never smoke, as this book stresses several times), and radiation. Science is now shedding light on how the environment influences gene expression. As there is nothing that we can do about the nature of the genes that our parents "chose" to give us, there is hope that, not too far in the future, we can control how genes are expressed.

Then comes the factor of hormones. Hormones clearly play a role because most of the people who have lupus are women. Still, we do not know how exactly hormones instruct the immune system to go awry against itself, and most of the studies so far are circular, without any useful insights into this mechanism.

Next come the factors that interfere with the function of the immune system. Simply put, the immune system loses its supervisory skills and fails to control self-destructive elements. But this failure comes along with an inherent limitation to fend off infections. This book teaches how infections remain among the main causes of death and how proper vigilance and prompt treatment of infections prevent days spent in the hospital and prolong a good life for patients.

From my perspective it seems that each person who has lupus starts from a different point and follows a unique set of pathways in developing lupus. Many of the pathways overlap, and as Dr. Thomas reports in this book, people who have lupus all have in common auto-antibodies, immune complexes, and cells with reactivity against their own elements. Something that I would like to add is that each organ that becomes involved offers its own special mooring facilities.

My experience was similar to that shared by Dr. Thomas in his preface. I was assigned to participate in the care of a 24-year-old woman when I was a senior in medical school. She had fevers, chest pain, and swollen joints and legs. Systemic lupus erythematosus was on the top of the list of possibilities, and the subsequently discovered presence of antinuclear antibodies, anemia, and low platelet and lymphocyte counts helped seal the diagnosis. The treatments in those days were not nearly as good as they are today, and we had to depend on giving her large doses of prednisone, which unfortunately gave her a whole set of other problems in addition to her lupus. Her face is still vivid in my memory. At the time, she was engaged to be married and wanted to live a normal life. Her anxious and inquisitive eyes have continued to ask me, "Will you find a cure for me?" Now, decades later, doctors can diagnose patients with the disease faster, treat them more effectively, minimize drug-related side effects, and take better and faster care of infections and other conditions linked to lupus. Doctors can promise a normal and lengthy life to most people who have systemic lupus but cannot be complacent without positively answering the proverbial "Are we there yet?"

During the last half-century, intense study of the immune system granted us a better understanding of how the immune system develops, how it does its job, and how it malfunctions in people who have autoimmune diseases and in particular systemic lupus erythematosus. Clinical investigators and the pharmaceutical industry alike have taken advantage of this knowledge and have tried to develop novel drugs to better control lupus. As you will learn, the last time the FDA approved a drug for lupus, prior to the recent approval of Benlysta, was in the late 1950s. Fair to say that the approved use of steroids and anti-malarials, both with clear ability to control the immune system, should not subtract from the value of cyclophosphamide and mycophenolic acid (CellCept) in treating people who have lupus nephritis. The approval of Benlysta was welcomed with great fanfare despite the fact that its effect was slow to come and the trials somehow did not include enough of those who suffer more from the disease.

There has been much discussion among lupus experts addressing the question of why doctors do not have more new drugs for lupus patients. Many new biologic drugs have seen the light of approval at the FDA courts for rheumatoid arthritis, which is a closely related cousin to lupus. There is no one correct answer. Common arguments used include the clinical diversity of the disease, the lack of tools to measure disease activity with sufficient fidelity, and the inherent difficulty in designing proper clinical trials. Notwithstanding the reasons for the failure to enlist more approved drugs for lupus, doctors become dependent on using therapies that are not FDA-approved to treat systemic lupus.

Dr. Thomas and I met for the first time when he was a fellow in rheumatology and I was a young attending physician at the Walter Reed Hospital in Washington, DC. He and I share a strong interest in understanding the nature of the disease and the top-notch care of patients who have lupus. Walter Reed allowed us to take care of the interests of the patients without ever needing to be concerned about the cost and the ability of the patients to afford care. Lupus is a demanding partner in the life of the patient, and you will soon learn that prompt diagnosis, close care by specialists, tight control of medications and their side effects, and tenacious efforts to control comorbidity (infections, cardiovascular disease, and cancer) make all the difference in the world.

Doctors are continuously pressed to shorten their encounter with their patients while the documentation component of patient care looms continuously larger. And this could be fine in the wisdom of the regulators should the doctors deal with simple, self-limited, one-dimensional diseases. Obviously, the Procrustean (one fits all) approach is damning to patients who have lupus and their doctors. The doctors have little time to go over the many dimensions of the disease that each patient brings to each office visit and no time to educate them properly. Doctors who care deeply about their patients know very well that it is the patients who take charge of their diseases who fare the best. They come to the office prepared, and it is their doctors' duty to educate them further. They bring knowledge acquired from the internet (usually unfiltered and noncritical), and their doctors are pressed to transfer scientific knowledge to properly fill in the gaps. It is incumbent upon the healers to translate the medical information to the patients so patients can maximize the earned benefit. In these encounters much is lost in the translation that compromises the welfare of the patient.

Dr. Thomas might well have majored in classics, as he does a beautiful job in translating all Greek- and Latin-infested medical jargon into clear English (his writing is the Orwellian clean windowpane). Patients want to be educated and *The Lupus Encyclopedia* will provide them with tools to fight the Wolf of the American writer Flannery O'Connor (chapter 20). People who have lupus and their primary care doctors will find in this book all the information they need—and the information is not lost in translation!

GEORGE C. TSOKOS, MD
Professor of Medicine, Harvard Medical School
Chief, Division of Rheumatology
Beth Israel Deaconess Medical Center
Boston, Massachusetts

Keep reading this preface! I suspect that most modern readers in our fast-paced, social networking world do not read the preface to a book. They would rather just dive right in. But if you or someone you care about has lupus, the information and advice in this preface could be lifesaving.

Did you know that . . .

cigarette smoking decreases the effectiveness of the most important therapy used to treat lupus?

eating alfalfa sprouts and mung bean sprouts can make lupus worse?

eating foods such as walnuts, olive oil, and flax seed may potentially be helpful in lupus?

taking Echinacea (an herb used to "treat" colds) can make lupus worse?

any source of ultraviolet light, including indoor lighting, makes lupus worse?

the newer, environmentally friendly home light bulbs (compact fluorescent bulbs) give off more ultraviolet light than the older incandescent light bulbs and can make lupus more active?

you are exposed to less ultraviolet light from the sun if you drive with your car windows up as opposed to driving with them down?

memory problems and fatigue are very common in people who have lupus, and there are ways to look for their causes and therefore potentially help decrease their severity?

most people who have systemic lupus erythematosus will live a long, normal life, especially if they know the right things to do to keep their lupus under control?

if someone who has systemic lupus dies, it more commonly is due to a heart attack, stroke, or infection instead of the lupus itself?

broken bones from osteoporosis are potentially deadly (a silent killer), are common in lupus, and are preventable?

annoying dry mouth, dry eyes, or dry skin may be important clues for an under-recognized complication of lupus called Sjögren's syndrome?

20% of people who have lupus will have severe pain, profound fatigue, and trouble with memory due to a condition called fibromyalgia?

if you take medicines to calm down the acidity of your stomach, then you should be taking a specific type of calcium supplement?

I have had a special interest in lupus for more than twenty years after I saw a young woman ravaged by severe kidney disease from lupus, and I witnessed the troubling complications that she had experienced from high doses of steroids. I felt a sense of sadness and helplessness in caring for this young person who should have been living her dreams and aspirations instead of spending days at a time in a hospital bed. I asked, "Why does the immune system of a person who has lupus decide to attack the very body to which it belongs? What can we do to keep lupus from damaging the body and give people their lives back?" Those questions drove me to become a rheumatologist (the specialist who most commonly treats lupus).

Over the years, I realized that there were many things that a person who has lupus needs to do in order to do well. Lupus is an immensely complex disease, so there were too many things to teach a person who has lupus during the brief time allotted at doctor appointments. Therefore, I came up with a list of "do's and do not's" that I called the Lupus Secrets. I named them "secrets" not because doctors and nurses are trying to hide them from patients but because, even though they were very important measures that all lupus patients needed to do to stay healthy, most patients did not know about them. Doctors and nurses as healthcare providers need to focus so much on the physical examination, lab test results, and medicines that they often do not have the time to discuss these other important aspects of lupus care. Yet knowing and practicing these lesser-known facts can make the difference between living a good quality of life with lupus or letting the lupus control one's life. Therefore, over the years I have given the Lupus Secrets to my patients as an easy-to-read, concise, important handout. I have amended the handout over the years based on the latest medical information. I have reproduced it in chapter 44 of this book. People who have lupus and want to be in more control of it should practice these "secrets."

It is much easier to practice these measures if you know why they are important in the first place. Therefore, this book goes into detail about why they are important, as well as giving out practical advice on how to incorporate these strategies into your daily life. For example, most people who have lupus know it is important not to be out in the sun. Yet it is important to learn how to decrease ultraviolet exposure from sources other than just the sun; chapter 38 explains these important concepts thoroughly.

During my career, I have been saddened when I have seen people who have lupus not do well or, even worse, die. Most of these cases were completely preventable. I do not mean to minimize how severe and devastating this disease can be because it can be deadly. Yet most people who I have witnessed die from their systemic lupus did not receive adequate treatment. One was a young woman who had no access to adequate healthcare, which reflects many of the inadequacies of the current healthcare system. Her situation was truly a sad event for me to witness. Most of the others were due to the patients themselves deciding not to take the advice of their physicians. Instead, they decided to rely on herbs and natural therapies. Others were afraid of the side effects of the medicines their doctors were recommending. If these people could have been more educated in what lupus is, what causes it, what happens when it is treated versus when it is not, and how to put the potential side effects of medicines into perspective, then maybe they would have accepted treatment, lived much longer, and had a much better quality of life.

I can understand why some people are afraid to take medicines. When pharmacists hand them a piece of paper along with their prescriptions that says "this medicine may cause hepatitis, kidney failure, cancer, and even death," it has to make them think twice before taking these medications. As a physician, I know how infrequent these side effects occur in reality compared to how much more often the medicines help people who have lupus. Therefore, I have put this information into easier to understand terms so that patients can learn what the potential side effects of the medicines are, how often they actually occur, how to look out for side effects, and even how to prevent them in the first place.

Other problems from lupus are not directly due to the overactive immune system. These additional problems include such things as heart attacks, infections, cancer, broken bones from osteoporosis, fatigue, memory problems, and many more. Instead of simply listing these problems in this book, I explain them in detail. More importantly, I give practical advice on what to do about them. For example, if you have lupus, have trouble getting out of bed, and have no energy, what is going on and what can you do? The sections of this book on fatigue, sleep problems, fibromyalgia, and depression give you very practical advice on things you can try out yourself to try to feel better. Often, at a doctor's visit, the physician does not have the time to go through all of these very important possibilities and solutions. In this book, they are right at your fingertips. You can let your doctor work on looking for things such as low blood counts, lupus activity, kidney problems, thyroid problems, and the like while you work on looking at these other potential causes and treatments.

## How to Use This Book

One thing that I have been very impressed about in my patients who have lupus is the research many of them have done to learn about lupus. While many people only want to know the basics and straightforward instructions, others want to know all the medical facts about their problems, including the meaning of all their abnormal lab results. Therefore, I wrote this book with both groups in mind. Much of the information is written in a basic, easy-to-understand format in nonmedical terms so that most people can understand the medical aspects of the disorder and the proper things to do well. In addition, I give complex medical terms with explanations as well. I want people who have lupus to be able to look up the actual medical terminology that their doctors use, so that they can understand in more depth about what is going on. Therefore, I do not apologize for some of the highly technical aspects of the book. You can skip over these parts of the book and stick to the more practical and easy-to-read sections if you wish.

The book is divided into five main parts. Part I explains in detail what lupus is. It discusses what causes it, what other immune disorders are associated with it, and what labs diagnose the disease and as well as which are used to follow lupus disease activity. The chapters in part II go into detail about how the immune system of the person who has lupus can attack different parts of the body. This part of the book is divided into chapters based on different organ systems of the body. Part III is devoted to other complications of lupus that are not directly due to the immune system but occur for other reasons in people who have lupus. These problems include osteoporosis and fibromyalgia. Part IV discusses the various treatments for lupus. Finally, part V covers practical matters, such as talking to your doctor, how to have a successful pregnancy, health insurance and affordable healthcare, and disability. The final chapter in this part of the book reproduces my Lupus Secrets checklist.

I recommend that the reader consider performing the following steps in order. This will increase your chances of learning the most useful, important information first, and you will derive as much benefit as possible from this book.

*Step 1: Start practicing the Lupus Secrets right away.* Copy the Lupus Secrets in chapter 44 and read it over on a regular basis. Work on practicing all these measures on a regular basis. Once a habit on the list becomes a natural and constant part of your life, you can put a checkmark next to it. Your goal is to make all of them regular habits and have checkmarks next to all the recommendations. At first, do these things even if you do not understand completely why it is so important to do. As you read more about lupus in this book, the purposes behind these recommendations will become clear and help to make these practices part of your lifestyle. If you would like a quicker reason or explanation, each recommendation lists those sections of the book that discuss the information in detail.

*Step 2: Read the following chapters.* These particular chapters give essential information that make it easier to understand what lupus is and why it is important to do many of the things that your doctor recommends that you do:

Chapter 1 explains what lupus is and how your doctors diagnosed it. This information is especially important because it makes it easier for you to communicate to health professionals and doctors about exactly what type of lupus you have and what problems it causes you.

Chapter 3 discusses the causes of lupus. Everyone wants to know why they have it, and this gives the latest information about these causes. In addition, some of these causes are controllable. In other words, you can actually make changes in your life to decrease the severity of lupus by knowing what things can actually cause it or make it worse.

Chapter 4 is an exhaustive list of labs used in lupus. Do not read this chapter from start to finish. Instead, read the first part of the chapter up until just after where it explains how to collect a urine sample adequately for your doctor. All patients who have systemic lupus should be providing urine samples regularly to their doctors to make sure that the lupus is not affecting the kidneys. If someone collects a urine sample incorrectly, it is possible for the skin around the genital area to contaminate the urine with skin cells, proteins, fluid, and bacteria. Contamination can potentially cause incorrect diagnoses of urinary tract infections and possible kidney inflammation when these may not be the problems at all. Collecting a proper sample can prevent misdiagnosis and keep you from having to return to the doctor's office to give a better sample.

If you have noticed dry mouth, dry eyes, dry skin, or have dry vaginal problems, read chapter 14. Many people who have lupus have no idea that these problems may be due to Sjögren's syndrome because of their lupus. It is important to address these problems to prevent avoidable medical issues.

Chapters 19 and 20 list the factors that can cause some people who have lupus to have more severe disease and what can cause them to die. While many of these things are uncontrollable (such as age and gender), many things are controllable. Knowing what these conditions are can make the difference between doing well and not doing well.

Chapter 21 is devoted to the number one cause of death in people who have lupus: cardiovascular disease complications from heart attacks, strokes, and blood clots. Knowing what measures you can take to decrease your risk of developing these problems is essential to living longer.

Chapter 22 is about infections. Many people overlook this essential topic. Infections are the second most common cause of death in people who have lupus. It is in your power to prevent many infections from occurring in the first place. If an infection does occur, this chapter tells you what to look out for and what measures you need to take to have it treated. Knowing and practicing the information in this chapter and in chapter 21 is empowering.

Chapter 23 is all about cancer. Fortunately, cancer runs a distant four (compared to heart disease, infections, and the lupus itself) as a cause of death in people who have lupus. Nonetheless, some cancers do occur more commonly in people who have lupus, and there are things you can do to prevent them from occurring.

Chapter 24 discusses osteoporosis, which occurs more commonly in people who have lupus. It contains practical advice on how to prevent it from occurring and how to treat it if it does occur. Do not skip this chapter. There are very good reasons that doctors call osteoporosis a "silent killer," yet it is completely avoidable. In addition, there is a lot of media hype surrounding the medications used to treat osteoporosis, causing untoward fear of these medicines. This chapter speaks to those concerns and puts them into proper perspective.

Chapters 26 and 31 should be read by people who must take steroids for their lupus. These chapters give detailed information about steroids as well as practical advice on how to prevent side effects from these important medicines.

Chapter 29 talks about therapies in general and explains some important principles in the treatment of lupus. It discusses how to evaluate the potential for side effects from medications, and gives information on how to take and manage medications properly.

Chapter 30 covers the anti-malarial medications, such as Plaquenil (hydroxychloroquine,) which all people who have systemic lupus should be taking.

Chapter 38 is one of the most important chapters in this book. Treating lupus is not just about taking pills. People who have lupus should be doing many things besides taking medications that are essential in doing well with lupus. This chapter deserves to be read more than once.

Chapter 40 covers subjects that are often missing in books aimed at specific diseases. Knowing how to navigate your doctor's office and how to communicate effectively with your doctor and his or her staff can go a long way in your doing well. This chapter takes some of the mystery out of how to effectively deal with your doctor.

*Step 3: Get a copy of your records, notes, labs, x-rays, and other results.* This is the point where you can delve into exactly how your doctors diagnosed your lupus and how you are doing. You should keep these records yourself anyway, just in case you need them for future reference or if you need to give them to other doctors. You may have to pay a fee to have them copied, as doing this can create a lot of work for the staff at your doctor's office, but the information provided can be invaluable. Look up any term, word, or diagnosis that is in your notes in the index at the end of this book, and it will direct you to the parts of the book that discuss subjects specific to your lupus. I have tried to be as complete as possible, so most problems from lupus are found in this book. If there is anything in your records not listed in this book, then you can discuss it with your doctor. Look at your lab results. Again, you can look up various labs listed in the index to find specific discussions. Chapter 4 is dedicated to labs. This is an exhaustive chapter and is primarily to be used as a reference tool to help you understand better what lab results may or may not mean.

*Step 4: Skim chapters that sound interesting to you; read in detail those that pertain to your particular situation and interests.* There is a lot of information, facts, historical accounts, and related healthcare concerns in this book. Whenever a new situation occurs with your lupus, or if a new test is ordered, look it up in the index to investigate it further.

*Step 5: Consult the Patient Resources at the end of the book if you want help with your lupus.* Many helpful resources are available to help people who have lupus. This includes patient support groups, financial assistance, and other books on lupus.

*Step 6: Check in to my official Facebook page at www.facebook.com/LupusEncyclopedia and follow me on Twitter @lupusencyclopedia to find out the latest news about lupus.* Medical knowledge and lupus treatments are constantly changing. What doctors know about lupus and how they treat lupus today will be different within a few years after this book is published, and a revision with these additions will be needed. Until then, I will keep you updated on the website.

*Step 7: If you have any comments or recommendations, please email me at lupusencyclopedia@gmail.com and let me know what you would like to see in a future revision of this book.* As you can tell from the beginning of this preface, I am committed to helping people who have lupus, and want to do so in the best ways possible. When I write a revision to this book in a few years, I want it to be better and improved. This book is for you, the reader, and I want to make sure I am not forgetting anything you feel is important. If I have missed any topics, or if I have made any comments in this book that you do not understand or that you do not think are correct or appropriate, I would like to know. I will take all comments and recommendations very seriously. Please be brief in your email, and please do not relate any personal information. I cannot give any medical advice about anyone's medical problems. Only a doctor who has done a thorough evaluation can do this.

Thank you, and I wish you the best in life and health.

In August 2009, I received a phone call from Jacqueline Wehmueller in the middle of a very busy day at work in my rheumatology practice. I did not know who she was, so she introduced herself as the executive editor for consumer health at the Johns Hopkins University Press. She wanted to know if I would be interested in writing an educational book about lupus directed toward patients. She had heard and read some of the educational material from my work with the Lupus Foundation and felt that I was a good candidate for such a challenge. I love educating and teaching, but it had never crossed my mind to write a book. Although the prospect filled me with a lot of anxiety (because I was worried about doing a good job), I accepted her invitation. The rest is history, and writing this book took up almost all of my spare time during the next three and a half years. I am indebted to Jackie for giving me this opportunity. In addition, she has been invaluable in leading me by the hand as a novice writer. Her recommendations and her expert editing make me appear a much better writer than I innately am. I also wish to thank Sara Cleary, editorial assistant at JHUP, who constantly gave me great advice and guidance for many of the technical aspects in writing this book. I greatly appreciate the hard work put into the illustrations by Jacqueline Schaffer. She shared my interest in making complex immunologic topics easier to understand, and I think that she did an amazing job for such a difficult subject. I cannot forget Maria denBoer, my copy editor. For those who do not know what a copy editor is (I sure did not know before writing the book), think of your college English teacher commenting on, grading, and correcting the grammatical mistakes in your entire book. I hope I got at least a C initially. Thankfully she made many corrections, and it is, I hope, now closer to an A!

Delving into the history of lupus was very interesting and presented its own challenges in terms of context and interpretation. I wish to thank Dr. Darrel W. Amundsen, professor emeritus of Classics, Western Washington University, for his very helpful interpretation of the healing of the bishop of Liège from lupus as depicted in the *Miracles of St. Martin* (see introduction to chapter 1). In addition, Sharon Farmer, professor of history at the University of California Santa Barbara, provided invaluable recommendations on how to procure a copy of the illustration of the healing of the bishop. She also gave me practical advice on the potential problems with the dates provided in older books on these historical matters.

I could not have become a proficient rheumatologist, helping patients who have lupus, if it were not for my mentors. My first rheumatology mentor was Steven Older,

MD. He taught me rheumatology while I was an internal medicine resident at Brooke Army Medical Center in San Antonio, Texas. He introduced me to the young person with lupus mentioned in the preface who sparked my interest in lupus and rheumatology. Dr. Older taught me good habits, such as keeping thorough records and notes on my patients; I continue to practice those habits to this day. Other excellent physician-teachers include Gregory Dennis, MD, and Gary Klipple, MD, who were the chiefs of the Rheumatology Service at Walter Reed Army Medical Center during my fellowship training. Dr. Dennis and Dr. Klipple offered me the opportunity to enter their rheumatology program; they were unswerving in their expectations for thoroughness, and it paid off. Dr. William Gilliland and Dr. Scott Vogelgesang gave me everyday instruction during my training, and often had to put up with my keeping them in the clinic very late on Fridays. I always wanted to be very thorough with my patients, and that often meant their spending longer amounts of time with me than normal, getting home late to their families.

I have had the privilege of working with many excellent nurses and other medical professionals over the years. In particular, I owe Betsy Mewshaw, RN, a big thank you. During my rheumatology fellowship, she was instrumental in teaching me the value of going beyond the minimum expectations in helping patients. She showed me the value of educating patients properly. She taught me how important it is to look at the patient as a whole, and include the family in important medical care discussions. Today, my office walls are lined with numerous patient education pamphlets as an ongoing legacy of what Betsy taught me to do.

I was fortunate enough to work under the guidance of George Tsokos, MD, in his laboratory for a year. Dr. Tsokos is one of the leaders in lupus research, and he taught me many things about some of the causes of lupus at a very detailed immune system level. Although I realized during that year that I liked taking care of patients more than working with white blood cells in a laboratory, that experience proved to me how difficult and challenging it is to conduct proper research in the field of lupus. John Klippel, MD, current president of the Arthritis Foundation, was my teacher while I worked on the rheumatology ward at the National Institutes of Health. He impressed me with how down-to-earth and humble even some of the most famous dignitaries in rheumatology can be. He was never afraid to say "I don't know" to a question about a rheumatologic problem, proving the point that there is so much that doctors still do not know and that they need to learn more about many issues involving the care of patients.

This project has truly taken a lot of time during the past few years. It would have been impossible without the help and support of my private practice medical director, Jonathan Adelson, MD, and our office manager, Barbara Taylor. They allowed me to cut back on my clinic responsibilities during critical periods of deadlines in completing the book and supplied me with an immense amount of essential staff help in the preparation of the manuscript.

Many people reviewed sections of the manuscript and gave me very helpful recommendations and comments that I took seriously and used to change parts of the manuscript into more readable and useful forms that nonmedical people could understand and appreciate better. These include Gary O'Connor, Barbara Taylor, Brittany Taylor, Khristian Jones, Amanda Nelson, Anthony DeBartolo, and many of my patients.

The best teachers about lupus have been my patients. I am indebted to all of them over the years. Every patient who has lupus is different, and they all taught me something valuable, about not only lupus but about life in general. I learned from them that lupus does not always follow the rules, even those presented in the best lupus textbooks. Before I set out to write the book, I asked my patients what they would want in a book about lupus, what they liked in current books available, and what was missing so I could add it to this one. I received a ton of useful advice and I put their recommendations into print. Many of my patients reviewed parts of the manuscript and gave me advice on making useful changes. Others allowed me to photograph them to include helpful images in the book. Therefore, I especially wish to thank my patients PA, SA, A A-P, NB, DC, LC, SD, CF, AH, CH, CJ, EJ, LJ, TJ, CL, AM, DM, KM, LM, MM, NM, PM, TM, EP, KP, CR, JR, RW, CS, DS, SS, HT, TW, and others for this additional help.

I also want to thank Penny Fletcher, previous president and CEO of the Lupus Foundation of America DC/MD/VA chapter, and her wonderful staff. I worked with Penny for many years at the Lupus Foundation and through the years she has allowed me many opportunities to get involved with her, the medical staff, and, most importantly, the patients in many different aspects. Her guidance on patient education has been very helpful. In addition, Penny Fletcher, Jessica Gilbart (the current president and CEO), the board of directors, Arthur Weinstein, MD and other members of the Medical Scientific Advisory Council have turned the DC/MD/VA chapter into one of the premier leaders in patient education and advocacy for lupus. Their expertise and devotion to people who have lupus is unsurpassed and appreciated.

Last, and definitely not least, I owe a great deal of thanks, love, and appreciation to my partner Gary. Much of my spare time outside of work has been spent preparing for, researching, and writing this book. That left very little time for things we usually enjoy doing such as going to movies, eating out, and visiting friends and family. He has been incredibly supportive and understanding. He also helped me a lot in preparing the manuscript by reading and editing many of the chapters, interpreting some of the German and Latin texts used in my research, and spending hours of his time with the mundane task of proofreading the alphabetization and inclusion of medical definitions for the index of this work. His keen eye for detail as a lawyer was incredibly helpful.

Just as important as thanking those who have helped me is to also mention those who have not helped me, in the context of disclosing potential bias. I have been a speaker regarding systemic lupus and about the use of Benlysta for the pharmaceutical company GlaxoSmithKline and was reimbursed for those talks. They played no role in any of the contents of this book.

# PART I

# Definitions, Causes, and Diagnosis of Autoimmune Disease

# What Is Lupus and How Is It Diagnosed?

## How Lupus Got Its Name: Beginning with a Catholic Bishop in the Middle Ages

How did "lupus," the Latin word for "wolf," come to be associated with a disease that now affects 1.4 million Americans (about 300,000 of whom have the systemic form)? Medical historians have identified several possibilities, but the fact is that we do not know with 100% certainty. We do know that people have used "lupus" to describe a disease since the Middle Ages.

Possibly the first recorded use of the word "lupus" to identify a disease was in AD 855, when Herbernus (also called Hebernus), the archbishop of Tours, France, wrote in his *Miracles of St. Martin* a passage that began "Episcopus Leodici, Hildricus nomine, vir morum honestate laudabilis, occulto Dei judicio morbo, qui vulgo lupus dicitur." The English translation of the passage reads:

> The bishop of Leodicum [now known as Liège in Belgium], Hildricus by name, and a man praiseworthy for the uprightness of his morals, was, by a secret judgment of God, pitiably, or rather extraordinarily, troubled with a disease that is popularly called lupus. Moreover, he was especially afflicted in the buttocks. Therefore, it was misery to behold [him]. In fact, so severely was the strength of the illness raging, consuming, nibbling away at, devouring the man's flesh . . . the deeply rooted disease, though sometimes feeding on the outside, nevertheless was more intimately consuming his internal matter.

Hildricus was miraculously cured of the disease after spending seven days and nights at the shrine of Saint Martin in Tours. "Lupus" described a disease that ate away not only the flesh but also the "internal matter." Of special note, although the written account for this miracle is dated AD 855, the original author most likely wrote it between AD 1140 and AD 1185. (It was common for medieval scribes to cite incorrect authors or dates in their texts.) The figure on the following page is a sixteenth-century woodcutting depicting the healing of the bishop of Liège of his lupus by Saint Martin and Saint Brice.

There is also physical evidence that lupus is an ancient disease. The oldest evidence of a lupus-like disease is the mummy of a 14-year-old girl who died in AD 890 in Peru. Her remains are at the Regional Museum of Ica in southern Peru. Examination of the mummy shows evidence of hair loss, leathery skin, lung disease, and inflamma-

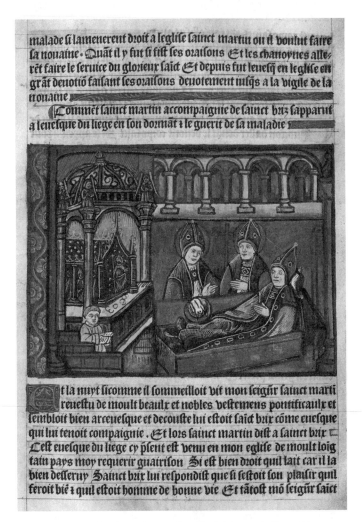

malade si lamenerent droit a leglise sainct martin ou il voulut faire
sa nouaine · Quât il y fut si fist ses oraisons Et les chanoynes alle-
rêt faire le seruice du gloneur saict Et depuis fut leuesq en leglise en
grât deuotiô faisant ses oraisons deuotement iusqs a la vigile de la
nouaine

Commêt sainct martin accompaignie de sainct briz sapparut
a leuesque du liege en son dormât & le guerit de sa maladie

t la nuyt sicomme il sommeilloit vit mon seignr saintt marti
reuestu de moult beaulx et nobles vestemens pontificaulx et
sembloit bien arceuesque et decouste lui estoit saict briz cône euesque
qui lui tenoit compaignie . Et lors sainct martin dist a sainct briz
Cest euesque du liege cy psent est venu en mon eglise de moult loig
tain pays moy requerir guairison Si est bien droit quil lait car il la
bien desseruy Sainct briz lui respondist que si sestoit son plaisir quil
feroit biê & quil estoit homme de bonne vie Et tâtost mô seignr saict

Saint Martin and Saint Brice curing the bishop of Liège of lupus
From *La Vie et les Miracles de Monseigneur Saint Martin*, L1 v, 1496.

tion around the heart (pericarditis). These are the types of problems that can occur in
someone who has severe systemic lupus (which this book is about). Subsequent studies of the kidneys, heart, skin, and lungs showed microscopic changes consistent with
what we would expect to see in lupus.

Rogerius Frugardi (also called Roger Frugard) was a famous physician from the
twelfth century in Italy. He originally wrote (and was edited by Roland of Parma in the
thirteenth century) "in partibus extremis ut in pedibus cruribus et coxis dicitur lupus," referring to ulcerating sores on the legs and calling the affliction lupus. The dermatologist Moritz Kaposi wrote that the sixteenth-century Italian physician Giovanni
Manardo stated that the sores of lupus appear "as if a hungry wolf eats his own flesh."
Lupus was mainly associated with ulcerations of the legs for centuries after that, un-

4

til 1684, when John Dolaeus, a physician in what is now Germany, described lupus closer to our modern understanding of the disease as a destructive process attacking the face. At the turn of the nineteenth century, Robert Willan, a British dermatologist, also described destructive lesions of the face and called the disease lupus. After Willan's description, doctors used the term "lupus" to describe skin diseases that mainly caused destructive lesions of the face. These sores of lupus probably encompassed a variety of diseases, including discoid lupus, tuberculosis, leprosy, cancer, and sarcoidosis.

Today "lupus" can refer to three different and unrelated diseases of the skin. "Lupus pernio" refers to a disease called sarcoidosis, "lupus vulgaris" to the infection tuberculosis, and "lupus erythematosus" to the disease that this book is about. Before modern medicine was able to differentiate between these, the term "lupus" probably included all three of these diseases. When a destructive skin disease, most often affecting the face, is due to lupus erythematosus, we call this chronic cutaneous lupus (see chapter 8).

We will probably never completely know the exact, true origins of the term "lupus." What we do know is a great deal about the disease that we now call lupus erythematosus. This chapter describes the disease lupus erythematosus and provides details about how it is diagnosed.

····

What is the disease that we call lupus? In understanding lupus, it is helpful to look at what lupus is not. Lupus is not a cancer, such as breast cancer or leukemia. Nor is it a contagious disease, like chickenpox or the flu. A person who has lupus cannot spread it to another person.

Lupus is an autoimmune disease. "Auto-" comes from the Greek word for "self," and "-immune" refers to the immune system of the body, the system that protects against disease. There are many autoimmune diseases or disorders where the immune system of the body attacks the body itself. To understand autoimmune diseases such as lupus (where the immune system works abnormally), we have to understand how the immune system normally works.

The immune system is the part of the body that usually protects us from foreign or bad things in the body. ("Foreign" in this context refers to substances that are not normally found in the body.) The immune system is composed largely of the white blood cells (leukocytes). White blood cells are different from the other blood cells, the red blood cells (erythrocytes) and the platelets (thrombocytes). Lymph nodes are another important part of the immune system. Lymph nodes are small, ball-shaped bodies linked by lymph vessels in the body, and are located in areas such as the neck, armpits, and groin. The leukocytes can travel to and from the blood along these lymph vessels to the lymph nodes, which are collections of many other important immune-related cells.

The lymph nodes are a meeting place for immune cells to communicate with each other when the body encounters infection, allergens (substances we may be allergic to), and anything else that stimulates immune system activities. You may have noticed that your lymph nodes swell when you have an infection. If you have a strep throat (due to a bacterial infection in the back of the mouth, throat, and tonsils), for example, the lymph nodes in the front of your neck may become swollen and tender. This occurs because the lymph nodes fill up with numerous white blood cells that are attacking the bacteria in the throat. The skin, intestines, and spleen (a small organ located in the left upper part of the abdomen, under the ribcage) are other important components of the immune system.

The primary job of white blood cells is to act like guards of the body. Whenever the white blood cells encounter something that does not belong in the body, they identify it as being potentially bad. It could be an infection invading the body, foreign chemicals (such as some medicines), allergens (like the skin dander from a cat or pollen from a flower), or even something abnormal made within the body itself, such as cancer cells. The white blood cells can recognize these invaders by their chemical structure and notice that they are things that are not normally found in the body.

The invaders can be foreign molecules (such as the part of penicillin to which some people are allergic) or foreign proteins (such as can be found in the cell wall of a bacterium) that are not normally found in the body. The white blood cells identify these proteins by using molecules called antibodies. Antibodies are an important part of the immune system. Antibodies recognize and attach to proteins called antigens by combining with them like a key (the antigen) fitting into a lock (the antibody).

The body's ability to recognize these invaders is amazing. There are millions of potential antigen molecules, and each one has its own unique shape. Therefore, the immune system has to try to make up millions of different-shaped antibodies to correspond to the millions of potentially different shaped antigen molecules that we might possibly encounter.

What happens when the antigens meet the immune system? When white blood cells first encounter these invading foreign antigens, they will communicate with other white blood cells and let them know that foreign invaders are present. These white blood cells release chemical messages that the other white blood cells recognize. These chemical messages, called cytokines, ask the other white blood cells to act in a particular way. As these foreigners invade, the cytokines will signal other white blood cells to come to the invaded area and defend the body from attack.

The white blood cells can attack the invaders in several ways. One of the most common is for the white blood cells to swallow the invaders, in a process called phagocytosis. ("Phago-" means "eat" and "-cytosis" refers to cells.) The white blood cells swallow the invaders and then use very strong chemicals and enzymes to digest them.

In mild infections, the immune system gets rid of the bad germs without our even knowing it. Exposure to mild infections occurs daily as germs and other foreign substances repeatedly try to cause us harm. This is a good example of the immune system working perfectly. It protects us without our even realizing it.

The immune system is complex and difficult to describe. Figure 1.1 attempts to simplify how one part of the immune system works. It illustrates how the immune system responds to poison ivy. Poison ivy is a good example to use because most people can easily visualize the inflammation and damage that occurs (itchy, red, swollen skin) after coming in contact with poison ivy. Discussing the effects of poison ivy is a good introduction to how the immune system can cause inflammation and damage when it reacts to other things such as infections. This is a helpful stepping-stone to understanding how the immune system can cause problems in people who have lupus.

In people who are sensitive to poison ivy, the immune system assumes it is protect-

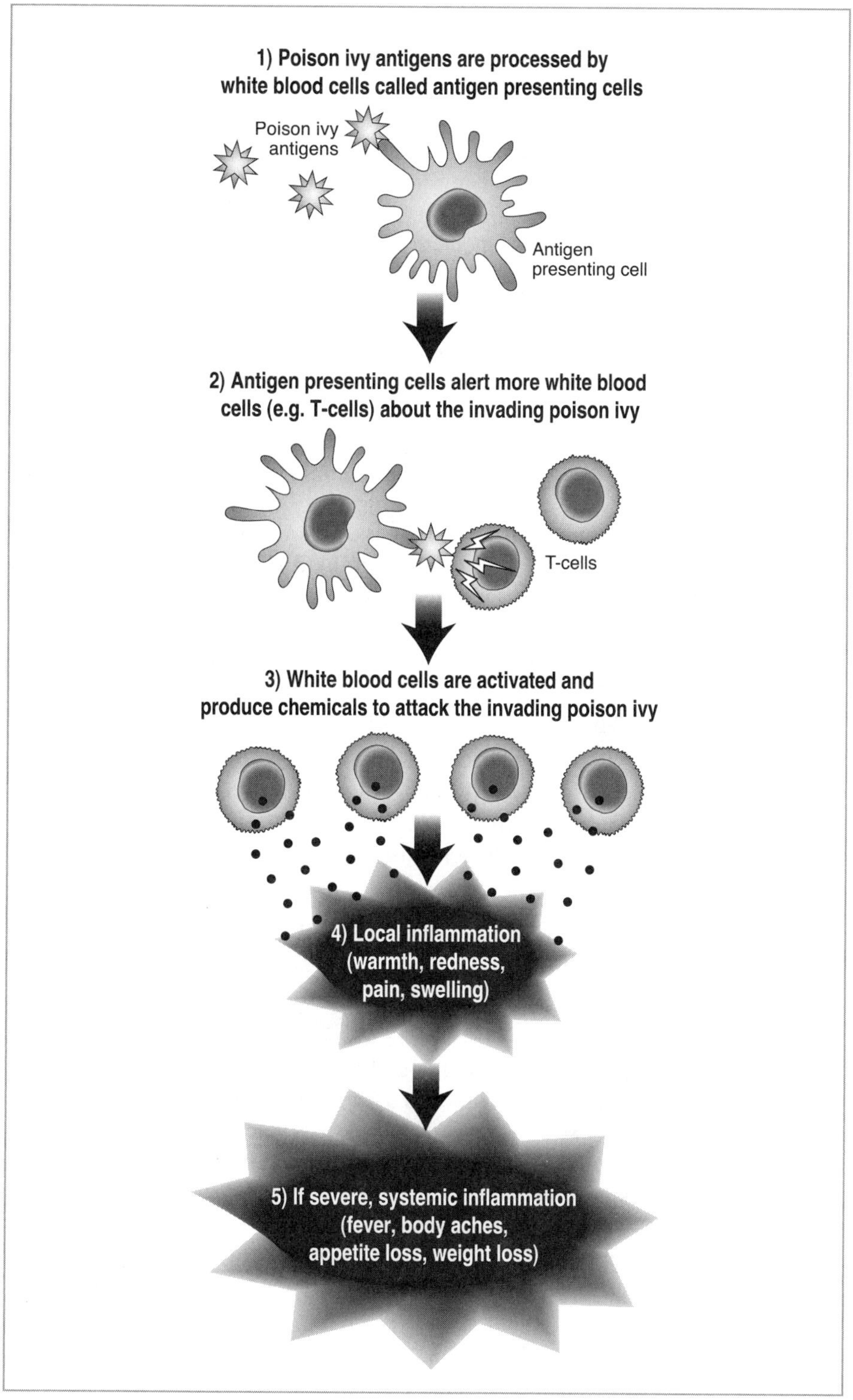

Figure I.I  How the immune system causes inflammation when trying to protect us

ing the body against the poison ivy; it considers the oils of the poison ivy plant to be an invading and dangerous substance. In the process of trying to protect the body, it actually causes inflammation, which can damage parts of the body. In the case of poison ivy, these problems are temporary and only involve parts of the skin. The immune system in people who have systemic lupus causes inflammation and damage in multiple parts of the body.

How does the immune system respond to poison ivy?

1. The poison ivy first comes in contact with white blood cells of the immune system called antigen-presenting cells, which recognize small, molecular parts of the poison ivy called antigens. These antigens are unique to poison ivy and help the antigen-presenting cells identify them as such. Many different cells (such as antigen-presenting cells) play important roles in the immune system. Just think of them as workers with different names in an organization where they are trying to get a job done. The immune system is the larger organization that is attempting to protect the body. Each worker in the immune system (such as the antigen-presenting cells) has a different job to do, or may have many different roles in the organization. The job description of antigen-presenting cells is to be the initial identifiers of "invaders" (such as poison ivy, viruses, fungi, bacteria, and even cancer cells) and then to tell other members of the immune system to go on the offensive against these invaders. (This initial step is similar to what occurs in the person who has systemic lupus after sunlight or other sources of ultraviolet light damage the person's skin cells.) When poison ivy touches the skin, antigen-presenting cells identify the oils of the plant as being "bad" and initiate this process.

2. The antigen-presenting cells travel through channels called lymph vessels to lymph nodes, where they communicate with other white blood cells called T-lymphocytes (or T-cells for short) by showing these foreign antigens to them.

3. These T-cells tell other white blood cells to come and attack.

4. The entire army of alerted members of the immune system travels to the area of skin that was exposed to the poison ivy and attacks the invading poison ivy oils. These white blood cells then release even more chemicals that cause the blood vessels of the skin to swell and leak. This allows even more white blood cells to come to the area and enter the affected skin. This swelling and leaking of the blood vessels causes redness, warmth, and swelling of the skin to occur. In fact, some of the swelling with fluid produces painful blisters. The white blood cells release irritating chemicals (in their attempts to protect us) that actually irritate the nerves and skin, causing pain and itching. Thus, the person suffers from red, warm, swollen, itchy skin that also has oozing blisters. Although the immune system is trying to protect us from the poison ivy, it actually ends up making us miserable. These problems of redness, warmth, swelling, and discomfort (or itching) are common things that occur with inflammation in the body.

5. When inflammation caused by the immune system is strong and intense enough, it can even affect the entire body, adding fever, body aches, loss of appetite, and weight loss to the picture. These complications of inflammation can occur with systemic

infections (such as those caused by viruses and bacteria), cancers, and diseases such as systemic lupus.

The above example explains what happens when the immune system responds to poison ivy. A similar chain of events takes place when someone allergic to cat dander or plant pollen encounters those substances, but they occur in other parts of the body (such as the eyes, nose, and lungs) and cause slightly different problems (such as sneezing, itchy eyes, and coughing).

The immune system can be defective in other ways besides allergic reactions. Sometimes the immune system underperforms. For example, when the human immunodeficiency virus (HIV) infects someone, the virus over time destroys T-cells. Without T-cells, the person infected with HIV cannot properly fight off certain types of infections and will likely die from a severe infection due to AIDS (acquired immunodeficiency syndrome) if not treated. This type of immune system problem is an immunodeficiency disease. The immune system is deficient (or lacking) in some way and stops protecting the person from foreign intruders and even from cancer cells. Because of this, people who have HIV get certain cancers more commonly than other people do.

On the opposite end of the spectrum of immunodeficiency disorders (like HIV infection) are the autoimmune diseases where the immune system overperforms, attacking the body itself. Recall how molecules can act like antigens when interacting with the immune system. They combine with the antibodies of the immune system like a lock and key. The immune system's antibodies identify the antigens as being foreign, in other words, not part of one's own body, and cause the immune system to attack them.

All of the molecules and proteins in the body can also act as antigens and potentially interact with the antibodies of the immune system. During infancy, the immune system learns that our own antigens are part of ourselves and eventually comes to ignore these antigens and not attack them. In people who have autoimmune diseases, however, something goes very wrong at some point. The immune system "forgets" that certain antigens in the body actually do belong there. In the person who develops rheumatoid arthritis (an autoimmune disease), for example, the immune system somehow no longer recognizes the normal antigens of the joints as being part of the body and begins to attack the joints. This ends up causing inflammation, similar to that described earlier in the poison ivy example, but it occurs within the joints. The immune system in the person with rheumatoid arthritis attacks the joints, causing inflammation with warmth, swelling, pain, and sometimes redness. Without proper treatment, the person who has rheumatoid arthritis develops crippling of the joints along with pain and swelling.

There are many different autoimmune diseases. For example, juvenile diabetes is actually an autoimmune disease where the immune system does not recognize the cells in the pancreas that make insulin as being a normal part of the body, so the immune system attacks and destroys these cells. That person is then unable to make insulin, which is required to keep glucose (sugar) levels under control and, therefore, must inject himself or herself with insulin for the rest of his or her life. Another example would be autoimmune thyroid diseases. One of the most common is Hashimoto's thyroiditis, which occurs when the immune system attacks the cells of the thyroid and over time causes the gland to stop making enough thyroid hormones. Thyroid hormones are an important part of the metabolism and normal levels are essential for the body to function correctly. This resulting lack of thyroid hormones requires the person to take a thyroid supplement for the rest of her or his life. This is one of the most common autoimmune disorders, affecting up to 10% to 15% of the population at some time in their lives.

Juvenile-onset diabetes and Hashimoto's thyroiditis are examples of organ-specific autoimmune disorders. An organ, such as the thyroid gland, pancreas, skin, or stomach, is a highly specialized body structure. This group of autoimmune diseases occurs when the immune system attacks just one type of organ in the body (the thyroid with Hashimoto's and the pancreas in juvenile-onset diabetes). There are numerous examples of organ-specific autoimmune diseases. Graves' disease attacks the thyroid, causing overactivity. Pernicious anemia attacks the stomach cells that absorb vitamin B-12, causing vitamin B-12 deficiency, which in turn can lead to nerve and blood count problems. Addison's disease attacks the adrenal glands, which sit on top of the kidneys. Vitiligo attacks pigment-producing cells of the skin, causing white patches. Autoimmune hepatitis causes inflammation of the liver. Myasthenia gravis produces antibodies that react with muscle cells, causing muscle weakness. Multiple sclerosis attacks the coating of the nerves of the brain and spinal cord.

While some autoimmune diseases only affect one organ, others can affect multiple organs of the body and are called systemic autoimmune diseases. The musculoskeletal system would be an example of an organ system, made up of multiple organs, such as the bones, muscles, ligaments, tendons, and bursas. The most common systemic autoimmune disease is rheumatoid arthritis. This occurs when the immune system attacks the lining of the joints and tendons in the musculoskeletal system. This causes multiple areas of joint pain, swelling, and stiffness, and over time can cause crippling joint deformities. The immune system can also attack the skin, causing lumps (called rheumatoid nodules) under the skin; it can attack the lining of the lungs or heart, causing pleurisy, fluid buildup, and chest pain. It can also attack the lungs, causing scarring and shortness of breath. "Systemic" describes its ability to affect multiple organs and systems of the body. Other common terms used by doctors which mean the same as "systemic autoimmune disease" include "connective tissue disease" and "collagen vascular disease." Other systemic autoimmune diseases include disorders such as scleroderma (which causes thickening of the skin), Sjögren's syndrome (which causes dry mouth and dry eyes), polymyositis and dermatomyositis (which cause muscle weakness), vasculitis (which causes inflammation of blood vessels), as well as systemic lupus erythematosus, which is the subject of this book. All of these diseases commonly cause joint pain (called arthralgia) or overt inflammation of the joints (called arthritis). That is why rheumatologists ("arthritis doctors") became the experts in diagnosing and treating these diseases.

Systemic lupus erythematosus, SLE for short, is the classic example of a systemic autoimmune disease. SLE can potentially affect any system and organ of the body. The immune system in people who have SLE is overactive. It thinks that different parts of the body do not belong in the body and therefore attacks them. The areas of the body it can attack differ from person to person, so people who have SLE can have a wide range of manifestations. For example, in many people who have SLE, the immune system attacks the cells that line the joints or tendons, thinking that these normal body parts are foreign. The white blood cells attack them, just as they would an invading bacteria or foreign chemical like poison ivy. This in turn causes pain and sometimes swelling, warmth, and redness of the joints (the signs of inflammation discussed earlier). Most people who have SLE have joint pain or arthritis at some point during their illness, and about half have it at the onset.

One of the hallmarks of SLE is that it stimulates the production of many different types of antibodies, especially antinuclear antibodies. B-cells of the immune system produce the antibodies used in fighting off foreign invaders in the body (such as bacteria, viruses, etc.). Normally, the immune system learns not to make antibodies against the body itself. However, in SLE, it begins to do just that. The immune system of the person who has SLE does not believe that some molecules (antigens) of the body's own cells belong there. It actually begins to produce antibodies against these antigens, especially those within the nucleus of the cells. The nucleus is the part of the cell where the DNA (genetic code) is contained. We are actually able to check for these antibodies against nuclear antigens by a blood test called an antinuclear antibody test, or ANA test for short. Almost all people who have SLE are positive for this particular test. This is very valuable because if someone has some problems that the doctor thinks could potentially be due to SLE, she or he can order an ANA blood test. If it comes back normal or negative, the person most likely does not have SLE, and the doctor has to consider other possible diagnoses.

Here is a very good question to ask: "If all of these systemic diseases can affect multiple organ systems, and all of them can cause arthritis, how do you know it is SLE instead of one of the other diseases?" Simply put, each systemic autoimmune disease has certain characteristics that set it apart from the others. For example, with SLE, sometimes the lupus can attack the skin, causing a scarring, oval-shaped rash on the face or scalp called discoid lupus. A biopsy of the rash can confirm the diagnosis of lupus. This particular rash can occur as a part of SLE but not the other systemic autoimmune diseases. Some people who have lupus develop a butterfly-shaped rash on the face, called a malar rash. This red rash occurs on the cheeks (the malar area) and the nose.

SLE can cause a lowering of the number of platelets, or it can sometimes cause a rare type of anemia (a low red blood cell count) called autoimmune hemolytic anemia. These blood cell problems do not typically occur with the other systemic autoimmune disorders.

SLE can also affect the kidneys, causing an inflammation called glomerulonephritis, or nephritis for short. The doctor may order a kidney biopsy if nephritis is a possibility. A biopsy is a medical procedure where the doctor removes a tiny piece of tissue (in this case the kidney) and then examines it under a microscope. (See chapter 12 for more details on kidney biopsies.) The way that the biopsied tissue appears under the microscope can actually confirm the diagnosis of lupus in some people. The kidney tissue from a person who has lupus nephritis looks very different compared to kidney tissue from those who have other autoimmune diseases.

Certain blood tests can also be very helpful. As mentioned previously, almost all individuals who have SLE are positive for the ANA test, but many people who have other autoimmune diseases are also positive for this particular blood test. However, other blood tests are sometimes positive in people who have SLE, but rarely in those who have other diseases. These tests include anti-Smith, anti-double-stranded DNA (anti-ds DNA), and anti-ribosomal-P antibodies. Therefore, a positive anti-Smith, anti-ds DNA, or anti-ribosomal-P antibody test can be very helpful in making a diagnosis of SLE. Chapter 4 discusses these tests in more detail. If someone appears to have a systemic autoimmune disease and is positive for antinuclear antibodies, but also has other lupus-specific problems going on (such as discoid lupus, a low platelet count, autoimmune hemolytic anemia, inflammation of the kidneys, or a positive anti-Smith or anti-ds DNA), then the chances of that person having SLE are greatly increased.

In summary, SLE is a systemic autoimmune disease (where the immune system thinks that multiple parts of the body do not belong there) and causes the production of antinuclear antibodies as a hallmark of the disease. The immune system then attacks these different areas of the body. There are some problems that may occur in a person who has lupus that set it apart from some of the other systemic autoimmune diseases (such as rheumatoid arthritis, scleroderma, and Sjögren's syndrome), such as a low platelet count, autoimmune hemolytic anemia, discoid lupus, a butterfly (malar) rash, and a positive anti-Smith antibody or anti-DNA antibody. As discussed below, distinguishing SLE from other autoimmune disorders can be very challenging. Some people with symptoms will need to see several specialists to get a definitive diagnosis.

So far, I have been discussing systemic lupus, in which the immune system can attack any part of the body. Once it becomes symptomatic, this form of lupus generally lasts for the rest of the person's life and usually requires lifelong treatment with medications. Systemic lupus is the primary form of lupus that this book addresses, but other types of lupus include drug-induced lupus, cutaneous lupus, and neonatal lupus (table 1.1).

*Drug-Induced Lupus.* Some medicines can evoke a reaction in the immune system, causing it to become overactive; they actually cause a systemic-type of lupus, which is usually less severe. Most people who have drug-induced lupus will experience joint pain or arthritis. Many of them will develop other problems, such as inflammation around the lining of the heart or lungs, causing chest pain (called pleurisy). Some individuals will get a rash. There are some differences between SLE and drug-induced lupus. For example, drug-induced lupus affects men and women equally. This is quite different from SLE, where women represent approximately 90% of all people who have SLE. Drug-induced lupus affects more white people than black people, while SLE is more common in blacks. In addition, the average age of people affected by drug-induced lupus is about 60 years old, while the average age for the onset of SLE is 20 to 30 years old. All individuals who have drug-induced lupus are ANA positive, and most are positive for a blood test called anti-histone antibody as well.

**Table 1.1** Types of Lupus

Systemic lupus erythematosus

Drug-induced lupus

Cutaneous lupus

Neonatal lupus

When the person who has drug-induced lupus stops taking the offending medicine, the lupus goes away. This is in sharp contrast to SLE, which is a lifelong disorder. The majority of reported cases of drug-induced lupus have occurred with procainamide, hydralazine, isoniazid, and methyldopa. Fortunately, doctors do not prescribe these medications very often anymore. Note that the vast majority of people who take these medicines will never develop lupus.

Although these drugs may cause drug-induced lupus, most of them would rarely cause someone who has SLE to have a flare of the disease. For example, if a person who has SLE has high blood pressure it is acceptable for the doctor to treat him or her with hydralazine. This is perfectly fine to do, as it would be rare for hydralazine to worsen disease activity in someone who has lupus. Another example would be a woman who has SLE who has recurrent seizures. It would be appropriate for her doctor to put her on an anti-epileptic medicine such as Dilantin (phenytoin) even though it can potentially cause drug-induced lupus.

One important caveat is that people who have SLE should generally not take the sulfa antibiotic trimethoprim-sulfamethoxazole (more commonly known by the brand name Septra or Bactrim). Doctors treat many common infections, such as urinary tract infections, with trimethoprim-sulfamethoxazole. This antibiotic has a high potential for causing lupus flares or other types of drug reactions in people who have lupus. Therefore, most rheumatologists agree that their patients who have lupus should avoid it and take other antibiotics instead. In fact, I recommend that my patients actually list it as one of their allergies so that they do not forget to inform other doctors. Even with this warning, I have had several patients who have SLE go to the emergency room, get diagnosed with a UTI, are prescribed Septra or Bactrim (they forgot to list these as potential allergies), and then show up in my office with a bad flare of their SLE.

*Cutaneous Lupus.* Cutaneous lupus occurs when lupus causes inflammation of the skin ("cutaneous" is a medical term referring to the skin). There are several types of cutaneous lupus. Each type may occur as a part of systemic lupus; however, the majority of people who have cutaneous lupus do not develop the systemic form. The two forms of cutaneous lupus that may occur by themselves are chronic cutaneous lupus and subacute cutaneous lupus. Chronic cutaneous lupus is the most prevalent form of skin involvement from lupus, and discoid lupus is the most common type of chronic cutaneous lupus. The term "discoid" refers to the disk, oval, or round shapes of the individual areas of rash. It most commonly occurs on the head, especially on the scalp, on the cheeks, and in the ears. If it involves the scalp, it can cause areas of irreversible hair loss due to its causing permanent damage to the skin and hair follicles. It can also cause light and dark areas by permanently scarring the skin. Fortunately, only about 10% of people who have discoid lupus will also develop SLE. On the other hand, about 25% of those who have SLE also have discoid lupus.

Subacute cutaneous lupus is the other type of skin lupus that can occur by itself in the absence of systemic lupus. Small red, scaly, or ring-shaped areas appear, usually on the back, chest, arms, and face. They get worse with sun exposure and enlarge if not treated quickly. However, unlike discoid lupus, they usually do not cause permanent damage to the skin or irreversible hair loss. They may leave some slight pigment changes, but not as severe as in discoid lupus. About 50% of people who have subacute cutaneous lupus may also develop SLE. I discuss both of these forms of cutaneous lupus in more detail in chapter 8.

*Neonatal Lupus.* "Neonatal" is the medical term for newborn. This form of lupus may occur when the mother has certain antibodies, especially anti-SSA and anti-SSB antibodies, in her blood. These antibodies can cross the placenta and enter the fetus's bloodstream; they then may attack the baby's tissues, causing inflammation or damage. There are two main forms of neonatal lupus. The first occurs when the antibodies attack the electrical conduction system of the fetus's developing heart. The electrical system of the heart is essential for the heart to work correctly, causing it to pump blood to the rest of the body. Doctors try to diagnose this form of neonatal lupus as early as possible to try to treat it. However, sometimes even treatment will not correct the problem. In this case, the baby may need a pacemaker put in immediately after birth to keep the heart beating. Unfortunately, this is a permanent problem requiring life-long use of a pacemaker.

The other form of neonatal lupus occurs when antibodies from the mother enter the fetus and attack the baby's skin cells, causing a red lupus rash that becomes apparent at birth or soon after exposure to light. Since these antibodies persist in the baby's circulation for only six to eight months, the rash resolves by at least 8 months of age and is not a permanent problem.

## How Is Systemic Lupus Erythematosus Diagnosed?

Sometimes, diagnosing SLE is difficult. At other times, the diagnosis of SLE can be straightforward and easy to make. Unfortunately, more times than not, a person who has SLE may have seen many different doctors, including several rheumatologists (doctors who specialize in diagnosing lupus), over a period of many years before a definite diagnosis is made.

This difficulty in diagnosing SLE is due to several factors. At the outset, SLE may start very gradually, only causing a couple of mild problems at first; additional problems develop slowly over time. In many, if not most people who have SLE, it can be impossible to pinpoint exactly when the disease began. The immune system may initially cause minor problems that the person does not notice, and there may not be any definitive blood test abnormalities to help identify the problem as SLE. The immune system may initially just cause one problem at a time. For example, it may at first cause some nonspecific fatigue and achiness for a few weeks. Then a few months later, it may cause the fingers to turn pale when the cold winter weather arrives. The individual affected may feel this is a nuisance if these episodes are mild and just brush them off. Then the person may feel well for a year or so before developing swollen, painful joints. During this initial stage, the person who has SLE may realize that something is wrong, but it may be impossible for a doctor to be able to determine whether the symptoms are due to SLE or something else. Doctors will often use the term "undifferentiated connective tissue disease," "undifferentiated collagen vascular disease," or a "lupus-like disease" to describe these slow-onset cases of lupus.

SLE can also attack virtually any part of the body. When it does, the doctor must consider all diseases that can do the same thing. For example, some infections like parvovirus, hepatitis C, and Lyme disease can cause arthritis, fatigue, rash, and many of the same blood abnormalities that SLE causes. A person who has one of these infections can have a positive antinuclear antibody test, just as people who have lupus can have a positive ANA. This can cause some difficulty in discriminating between disorders such as infection and lupus. Other disorders such as fibromyalgia, chronic fatigue syndrome, anxiety disorder, and depression may cause fatigue, joint pain, and muscle pain just like SLE can. Many autoimmune diseases such as multiple sclerosis, rheumatoid arthritis, and autoimmune thyroid disease may also cause many of the same symptoms as lupus and can even result in many of the same blood test findings such as a positive antinuclear antibody test. The number of diseases that can cause problems similar to what we see in lupus is large. It includes the above disorders as well as cancer, liver diseases, lung diseases, kidney diseases, and many more.

Making a diagnosis of SLE involves putting all of the pieces of the puzzle together. The doctor combines results from the history, the physical examination, the blood and urine tests, and other medical test results. Then the doctor has to consider all of the diseases that can potentially cause each of the problems present and eliminate those that do not make sense or are unlikely to explain all of the abnormalities. The doctor determines that the affected person has systemic lupus erythematosus if nothing else fits and the cluster of problems is consistent with a diagnosis of SLE.

The task of the doctor in evaluating a person who possibly has SLE can be very challenging when factoring in all these considerations. In fact, a person may need to see several specialists to evaluate the problem. The initial step in the evaluation process is for the physician to take a thorough history and to perform a physical examination. During this process, the doctor will ask the person whether she is having any symptoms. Symptoms are what the individual has been actually feeling or noticing herself; she should describe them to the doctor in her own words. For example, the doctor may ask the person if she has ever developed a rash (not just sunburn) on the arms and face after sun exposure, or has had any sores on the roof of the mouth, or whether her fingers ever turn white or blue when exposed to the cold. It is common for people who have SLE to experience these problems. Just as importantly, the doctor will question the individual to see if she may have symptoms that might suggest diseases other than lupus. For example, the doctor may ask her if she started to feel unwell after exposure to a child with fifth disease or if she works in a daycare center. If so, then parvovirus infection is a possibility because it can cause problems very similar to those experienced with lupus.

After asking for symptoms in the history portion of the evaluation, the doctor will usually perform a thorough physical examination, searching for clues as to whether the person may have any evidence of lupus or of other diseases that can mimic lupus. The doctor will look at the skin to see if there are any lupus rashes. He will examine the mouth and nose to see if there are any ulcers. He will listen to the lungs for possible inflammation or fluid and to the heart to see if there are abnormal heart sounds or murmurs. He will examine the joints to see if there is any inflammation and will search for possible clues in many other parts of the body.

After the history is taken and a physical exam is performed, it is essential that testing be done, especially blood and urine tests. The most important initial test is the antinuclear antibody test (ANA for short). The reason this is so important is that virtually every person who has SLE will be positive for this test. If the test is negative, then SLE is highly unlikely, and it is very important to consider other diagnoses. If the ANA test is positive, the workup does not stop there. As noted above, most diseases that cause systemic inflammation, such as infections, cancers, and other systemic autoimmune diseases, may also cause positive ANA tests. Autoimmune disorders that are not systemic, such as thyroid disease and multiple sclerosis, can also cause positive ANA tests. The doctor will therefore consider ordering additional tests to look for these other possibilities.

To complicate the matter even further, about 15% of people who do not have infection or autoimmune disease are positive for ANA. With many people being positive for ANA, and many other diseases also causing a positive ANA test, the vast majority of people who have a positive ANA do not even have SLE at all, but have something else going on.

If the ANA test is positive, the doctor will order additional tests looking for the possibility of SLE. A complete blood count can detect a low white blood cell count, a low platelet count, or autoimmune hemolytic anemia, which can all occur in SLE. A urine sample can see if there is any evidence of inflammation of the kidneys, called glomerulonephritis (or nephritis for short). Liver function blood tests can see if there is any evidence of liver inflammation, and a kidney function blood test called serum creatinine can see if there is a problem with kidney function. Of course, if any of these tests are abnormal, the doctor also must consider other diseases that can look like SLE and cause the same problems. For example, if the liver function tests are elevated, the doctor must figure out whether the person could have other liver problems, such as viral hepatitis C infection, hepatitis B, or autoimmune hepatitis. Like SLE, these particular diseases can also cause joint pain, rashes, and a positive ANA.

The physician will also order other blood tests that look more closely at the immune system. Some antibody tests are specific for SLE. In other words, when these particular antibody blood tests are positive, it is much more likely that the person has SLE instead of some other disease. These antibodies include anti-double-stranded DNA, anti-Smith, and anti-ribosomal-P antibodies. However, even these "specific" antibodies are not 100% accurate, and a doctor cannot diagnose systemic lupus based on the results of any isolated antibody test result.

Doctors may also need to order non-blood medical tests to work up the possibility of SLE. A chest x-ray can check to see if there is any fluid around the lungs, which can occur when lupus causes inflammation of the lining of the lungs. A chest x-ray can also check to see if there is any inflammation or scarring of the lungs, which may also happen with SLE. The chest x-ray can also potentially find other diseases that can mimic SLE. For example, another disease called sarcoidosis (which can also cause rashes, arthritis, low blood counts, and fatigue) can cause large swellings of lymph glands that the doctor may see on the chest x-ray and help make the diagnosis of sarcoidosis. An ECG (short for electrocardiogram) can look to see if there is evidence of inflammation around the heart due to SLE. An echocardiogram, which is an ultrasound of the heart, can check to see if there is fluid around the heart from SLE.

Doctors sometimes need to order a biopsy. For example, if the doctor sees evidence of inflammation in the kidneys (such as protein or some cells in the urine sample), she or he may need to order a biopsy of the kidney to see whether it is due to SLE or a different disease. A biopsy of the skin can also be helpful to see if a rash is being caused by SLE. Out of all the tests for SLE, these biopsies are the most specific and most helpful in making an accurate diagnosis of SLE in some people.

With the exception of a kidney or skin biopsy, the vast majority of these symptoms, physical exam findings, and medical test abnormalities are not enough by themselves to make a diagnosis of SLE. Due to the difficulty in making a diagnosis and trying to increase the reliability of a diagnosis of SLE for research purposes, the American College of Rheumatology (ACR) devised a set of classification criteria in 1982. An international group of doctors who specialize in lupus revised and improved these criteria in 2009. These criteria help doctors make a diagnosis of SLE so that primarily people who have SLE are included in research studies that investigate treatments and disease characteristics of SLE. The ACR is a professional medical organization made up of doctors, other health providers, and scientists from all over the world. It is a leader in advocating research and education for all forms of musculoskeletal disorders (diseases that affect the muscles, bones, joints, ligaments, and tendons), including the systemic autoimmune diseases. Although doctors originally developed these criteria to use in research, many doctors also find them useful in diagnosing SLE in clinical practice. Other than making a definite diagnosis of SLE by a kidney biopsy (which is the most accurate diagnostic test we have), the ACR classification criteria is the best tool available to doctors to help guide them in making a diagnosis of SLE. No other diagnostic test or clinically useful diagnostic definition exists. Non-physicians can also use these criteria to help them understand SLE and some of its most common problems.

These criteria for SLE can be satisfied if a person has lupus nephritis (proven by a kidney biopsy) and a positive ANA or anti-double-stranded DNA test. Otherwise, doctors can classify someone as having SLE if the person has four out of seventeen possible criteria.

These criteria are divided into two major sections. The first are the "clinical criteria," and the second are the "immunologic criteria." A person must have at least one criterion from each of these two sections counted in his or her total of four or more criteria. The criteria are as follows.

## Clinical Criteria

1. *Acute or Subacute Cutaneous Lupus.* "Cutaneous" refers to the skin, so cutaneous lupus occurs when lupus affects the skin. There are numerous ways that lupus can affect the skin. However, three major groups occur only in people who have lupus: acute cutaneous lupus, subacute cutaneous lupus, and chronic cutaneous lupus. This first criterion includes only the first two groups.

a. *Acute cutaneous lupus* includes the classic malar (or butterfly) rash as well as a more generalized rash. Doctors use the word "acute" to refer to a disorder that has lasted for only a short time. The rash of acute cutaneous lupus may last a few hours, a few weeks, or sometimes longer. It usually does not cause permanent skin damage. It is also quite sensitive to ultraviolet light, becoming more prominent with sun exposure. The malar rash is a red rash that occurs on the cheeks (also called the malar eminences, and hence the name "malar rash") and the nose. "Butterfly rash" also describes this problem because it occurs over the bridge of the nose and on the cheeks. The red nose looks like the body of a butterfly, and the red rash on the cheeks looks like the wings of a butterfly. The nasolabial folds (the deep, depressed lines that extend from the sides of the nose down to the sides of the lips) are usually not involved. The reason for this is that ultraviolet light rays strike most prominently on the top of the nose and cheeks, causing inflammation in lupus, but they do not contact this crease as intensely. If the nasolabial folds are greatly involved, then the doctor must consider other possible causes for the rash. The physician must also be very careful in that there are other more common red rashes of the face that can look like the lupus malar rash. Rosacea and seborrheic dermatitis can especially mimic the red face of lupus. There may be some other reason for a positive ANA and joint pain. A more generalized rash can also occur in acute cutaneous lupus. This form causes multiple red spots all over the body, but especially on the light-exposed areas. Generalized acute cutaneous lupus especially affects the face, the V-line of the upper chest, the upper back, and the tops of the arms and hands.

b. *Subacute cutaneous lupus* is a red rash that tends to last longer than acute cutaneous lupus and looks like either scaly, red areas or ring-shaped areas (connected circles) most commonly occurring on the arms, hands, chest, back, and abdomen. Sunlight causes it to be more prevalent. This rash can sometimes leave areas of pigment change (light or dark) when it heals and the redness disappears.

2. *Chronic Cutaneous Lupus Erythematosus.* This group of lupus rashes tends to last for a long time (i.e., are "chronic"), and unfortunately can cause permanent scarring to the skin when they heal. The most common form of chronic cutaneous lupus is discoid lupus. As mentioned before, the vast majority of people who have discoid lupus have it by itself, yet 10% of them will have it due to systemic lupus. On the other hand, about 25% of individuals who have SLE also have discoid lupus as a part of their SLE. These rashes are typically round (like a disk) or oval-shaped as their name implies. They are often scaly, reddish-colored blotches that most commonly occur on the neck, face, scalp, or outer parts of the ears. Unfortunately, as they enlarge they cause irreversible color changes (darker and lighter) as well as hair loss. A skin biopsy can determine if it is discoid lupus or not. Chapter 8 goes into more detail about other forms of chronic cutaneous lupus.

3. *Oral and Nasal Ulcers.* These are open sores occurring inside the mouth, inside the nose, or at the back of the throat. Often these are painless, and the person does not even know they are there. This is one of the reasons the rheumatologist usually examines a person's mouth and nose. The most common area for them to occur is on the roof of the mouth on the hard palate area.

4. *Non-Scarring Alopecia.* "Alopecia" is the medical term for hair loss. "Non-scarring alopecia" refers to thinning of the hair that is not necessarily permanent. There can be thinning of the hair diffusely, but often it occurs most prominently at the front edges of the hairline. The hair can be fragile, breaking easily, causing the hair strands to be shorter than normal. When lupus is treated, the hair usually grows back.

5. *Inflammatory Synovitis.* The synovium is the tissue that lines most of the joints of the body. Doctors call inflammation of the synovium synovitis (synonymous with inflammatory arthritis). To satisfy this criterion, there needs to be inflammation in at least two joints. There has to be evidence of joint line tenderness with morning stiffness

or inflammatory swelling (which feels rubbery in consistency) of the joints. Just having joint pain (called arthralgia) does not count for this criterion. Non-inflammatory arthritis also does not count. For example, a joint with degenerative arthritis (which is a non-inflammatory arthritis) causes bony swelling instead of soft tissue swelling. Although this form of arthritis causes joint pain and swelling as well, it is incorrect to use it as a criterion for lupus, which causes a completely different type of arthritis.

6. *Serositis.* The serosa is a very thin tissue that covers the outside of the heart, lungs, and abdominal cavity. Lubricating fluid located in the serosa allows the heart, lungs, and abdominal contents to glide smoothly under the overlying tissues without friction. Serositis occurs when inflammation affects the serosa and causes pain during movement of the involved structures.

a. *Pericarditis* is the term used when serositis occurs around the heart. Persons with pericarditis may have chest pain that worsens on taking a breath (called pleuritic chest pain) or chest pain when they try to lie down. The physician may pick it up on physical exam by hearing something called a rub when she or he listens to the heart with a stethoscope. This sound occurs when the inflamed tissues rub roughly (instead of smoothly) against each other as the heart beats. An echocardiogram (a type of ultrasound of the heart) or an ECG, which looks at the electrical activity of the heart, may also diagnose it.

b. *Pleuritis* occurs when serositis occurs around the lungs. The person with pleuritis often has chest pain that worsens with deep breathing (called pleuritic chest pain). The doctor can diagnose pleuritis when he or she hears the inflamed lung serosa rubbing roughly over each other through a stethoscope (a rub). Fluid buildup within the serosal lining of the lung can also show up on a chest x-ray.

c. *Peritonitis* is the term used by doctors when serositis occurs in the lining of the inner wall of the abdomen. It is not nearly as common as pericarditis and pleuritis. It causes abdominal pain that worsens with movement, so the person tends to try not to move very much and tightens the abdominal muscles to lessen the pain. The pain is usually aggravated when the doctor gently pushes anywhere on the abdomen during the physical examination, and then worsens when he or she quickly releases his or her hand off the abdomen (called rebound tenderness).

7. *Renal Disorder.* "Renal" refers to the kidneys, and about 40% of people who have SLE will develop inflammation of the kidneys, called glomerulonephritis (or nephritis for short). The earliest way to pick it up is by examining a urine sample. If there is an elevated amount of protein, red or white blood cells, or a clump of cells called a cellular cast in the urine, then the person may have nephritis due to SLE. The doctor will usually want to get a kidney biopsy to make sure the nephritis is due to SLE instead of another kidney disease.

8. *Neurological Disorder.* SLE can affect any part of the nervous system (brain, spinal cord, and nerves) in many different ways. SLE may lead to problems with seizures (also known as epilepsy). Seizures occur when the nerves of the brain are overactive, causing the arms and legs to jerk uncontrollably, hallucinations, or a multitude of other uncontrollable events. The person can be either awake or unconscious during these episodes. Another nerve disorder used for this criterion is psychosis. The person who

has psychosis may hallucinate, speak incoherently (not making sense to those around her or him), or exhibit abnormal behavior. This can be a very scary thing for loved ones to see, while the person who has psychosis may not realize there is anything unusual at all. Mononeuritis multiplex occurs when multiple nerves of the body are inflamed or damaged, causing multiple areas of numbness and/or weakness in the arms and legs. Myelitis is an inflammation of the spinal cord that can cause loss of sensation and paralysis in the legs. Peripheral and cranial neuropathies can cause numbness or weakness anywhere in the body, while cerebritis (inflammation of the cerebrum or brain) can cause acute confusion. Chapter 13 goes into detail about the potential neurologic problems caused by SLE.

9. *Hemolytic Anemia*. Anemia occurs when there is a decreased number of red blood cells, which transport oxygen to the cells of the body. Doctors diagnose anemia by finding a low hemoglobin count or hematocrit in the CBC (complete blood cell count). People who have SLE can have anemia due to many potential causes. Autoimmune hemolytic anemia is the only type of anemia used as a criterion to diagnose SLE. This occurs when the immune system attacks and destroys the red blood cells. The bone marrow works very hard at trying to replace the destroyed red blood cells, producing a large number of immature red blood cells, called reticulocytes, and releasing them into the bloodstream. Finding an elevated number of reticulocytes in the blood helps the doctor make this diagnosis.

10. *Leukopenia or Lymphopenia*. Leukopenia describes a decrease ("-penia" is the Greek term for "a deficiency of") in the white blood cells (leukocytes). Lymphocytes are a type of white blood cell, and lymphopenia occurs when the number of lymphocytes is lower than normal. A CBC can check for these low white blood cell counts to help diagnose SLE.

11. *Thrombocytopenia*. Thrombocytes (also called platelets) are cell fragments carried around in the bloodstream and are important for clotting. Platelets clump together and prevent people from bleeding too much. Thrombocytopenia occurs when the number of thrombocytes is lower than normal. Thrombocytopenia in people who have SLE usually does not cause any problems, but occasionally it can be severe enough to cause bruising and bleeding.

Immunologic Criteria

1. *Antinuclear Antibody (ANA)*. The ANA test is the hallmark blood test for SLE. In fact, the current blood test for ANA (when performed by a laboratory method called immunofluorescence) is so good that it would be rare to have SLE and to have this blood test be persistently negative. If the ANA is negative, then the physician needs to consider a different diagnosis for the patient. See chapter 4 for more details.

2. *Anti-ds DNA*. This test detects antibodies directed at double-stranded DNA, which is the genetic code found within the nuclei of cells. It is important to differentiate this from anti-ss DNA (anti-single-stranded DNA), which is very nonspecific for lupus (it can be seen in many other disorders) and is not part of the criteria. Not only is this particular blood test helpful in diagnosing SLE, it can also be useful in following the

treatment of the disease in some people (being higher during periods of increased disease activity and lower or normal when they are doing well).

3. *Anti-Smith*. The anti-Smith is a very specific blood test. It is rare to find a positive result in people who do not have SLE (see chapter 4).

4. *Antiphospholipid Antibodies*. Antiphospholipid antibodies include lupus anticoagulant, anticardiolipin antibodies, and anti-beta-2 glycoprotein I. They may cause false positive tests for syphilis. These particular antibodies can be associated with recurrent blood clots and miscarriages in some people who have SLE. Chapters 4, 9, 11, 18, 21, and 41 go into detail about the problems that these antibodies can potentially cause.

5. *Low Complements*. Complements are very important parts of the immune system. Their levels can both rise and fall during periods of lupus inflammation. Elevated levels are common with many diseases that cause inflammation, while low levels are not very common. In SLE, the complement levels can be decreased in some individuals either due to their being used up too quickly by the overactive immune system or due to a genetic deficiency in that particular complement (and this genetic deficiency actually causes the person to have SLE). Specifically, the physician is looking for low levels of C3, C4, or CH50 complements on the blood tests to satisfy this criterion.

6. *Direct Coombs' Antibody*. The Coombs' antibody can potentially attack red blood cells. Sometimes it can cause hemolytic anemia, described in the "Clinical Criteria" section. If a person has autoimmune hemolytic anemia, the Coombs' antibody cannot count as a criterion because it would be redundant.

· · · ·

If a physician believes that a person possibly has lupus, and the person's symptoms and signs satisfy four or more of the above criteria, then the person likely has SLE. However, this is not foolproof. For example, a person who has rheumatoid arthritis (RA) could have inflammatory arthritis, pleurisy due to her RA, a low white blood cell count (which can happen with RA), and a positive ANA (which occurs in 30% of people who have RA). If one were to go strictly by the above criteria, this person could be incorrectly diagnosed with SLE because she is positive for four criteria. However, it is up to a good doctor to try to figure out whether this person has SLE or RA. The doctor probably needs to order additional tests or may need to follow the person over time before determining if the diagnosis is absolutely SLE or RA. Sometimes it may be impossible, even for the best rheumatologists, to be able to tell the difference for sure. This illustrates one example of how these criteria are not perfect. Someone can even have SLE, yet only have two or three of the criteria.

The more criteria a person has, the more likely it is that the person has SLE. For example, if someone has an increased amount of protein in the urine, inflammatory arthritis, seizures, thrombocytopenia (low platelet cell count), photosensitive rash, pleurisy, and painless ulcers on the roof of the mouth, and is ANA positive (i.e., has eight criteria), that person more than likely has SLE. It would be very unlikely that something else would be causing all of these problems in the same individual. However, it is not impossible. It takes a thorough evaluation by a doctor experienced at diagnosing SLE to be certain of the diagnosis.

Rheumatologists are the physicians who most commonly diagnose and treat people who have lupus. They typically do a three-year internal medicine or pediatrics residency during which they are taught some of the basics of diagnosing SLE, and then they spend an additional two to three years in a rheumatology fellowship learning the intricacies of diagnosing and managing SLE (as well as many other musculoskeletal disorders). Even after all that training, they continue to learn the subtleties as well as potential pitfalls of making the diagnosis of SLE by caring for many patients over many years of practice. Experienced rheumatologists learn that diagnosing SLE is much more complex than just using the classification research criteria presented above. However, understanding these criteria can make it easier for the non-rheumatologist to begin to understand how doctors diagnose SLE.

## An Important Recommendation

Diagnosing SLE can be difficult. Someone can have a mistaken diagnosis of systemic lupus. This most commonly occurs when a doctor who is not experienced in diagnosing lupus finds a positive ANA test in someone who is having medical problems. In this case, the positive ANA test may be due to something other than SLE. An inaccurate diagnosis may be due to the inexperience of the physician, or it may be due to the difficulty in making the correct diagnosis when there are so many other diseases that can mimic SLE. For example, a doctor may diagnose someone as having SLE if the person has a positive ANA test, Raynaud's phenomenon, flushing of the face, and joint pain. Over time, a different disorder, such as scleroderma, may become evident as the cause of the symptoms.

When a rheumatologist evaluates someone diagnosed with SLE by a previous doctor, he or she should first confirm that the diagnosis is correct. The doctor will take a thorough history, perform a physical examination, and run appropriate laboratory tests as mentioned above. A person who has SLE that is under good control on medication can actually have a negative ANA test, making it virtually impossible for the new doctor to confirm the diagnosis of SLE. About 20% of people with SLE will become negative for ANA with treatment. Seeing a negative ANA will cause a new rheumatologist to become very skeptical about the diagnosis of SLE. People who have SLE can help themselves and their new doctor by keeping a copy of their records, especially those showing how their initial doctor confirmed a diagnosis of lupus. Patients may see new doctors for any number of reasons: a doctor retires or moves away, a patient moves, the patient's insurance coverage changes and forces her or him to switch to another rheumatologist, or the patient wishes to obtain a second opinion or becomes uncomfortable with his or her current doctor.

Obtain and keep copies of the initial notes, labs, biopsy results, x-rays, and consultation notes that helped your initial doctor make the diagnosis of SLE. Store these records permanently at home. You can give copies to any new doctors whom you may see in the future. Some people do not keep their medical records because they think that old records are easy to obtain. This is not necessarily true, however, because doctors are required to store old records for only a certain period of time. It is an especially difficult situation for a person who has mild SLE. If the doctor diagnosed the person with SLE many years previously, there is a good chance that those records are not available anymore. Find out and make notes about which criteria you specifically satisfied that led your doctor to make the diagnosis of SLE.

One real-life example illustrates how this information can be helpful. A patient of mine who had classic SLE moved to Chicago because of her job. I forgot to give her copies of my notes and lab results before she went. Her new rheumatologist was skeptical about the diagnosis because her ANA test was negative (which can happen when someone's lupus is under good control with treatment). The new doctor stopped her lupus therapies. Predictably, her disease flared up and her labs became abnormal again. My patient would have had a smooth transition in care without any suffering if she had had a copy of her old records to give to her new rheumatologist.

### KEY POINTS TO REMEMBER

1. Systemic lupus erythematosus is a systemic autoimmune disease. It is due to the immune system of a person being overactive and attacking multiple areas of the body. One of the hallmarks of SLE is that it produces antibodies directed at different parts of the body.

2. SLE is not contagious (in other words, it cannot be spread to other people), nor is it a cancer.

3. Virtually everyone who has SLE is positive for a blood test called antinuclear antibody when performed by a laboratory method called immunofluorescence. However, ANA is also positive in other autoimmune diseases, infections, cancers, and some inflammatory diseases. In addition, about 20% of people without any of these diseases are also positive for ANA in small amounts.

4. There are four main types of lupus: systemic lupus erythematosus, drug-induced lupus, cutaneous lupus, and neonatal lupus.

5. SLE is a great imitator, mimicking many other diseases. Therefore, the doctor must consider many other diagnoses when evaluating a person who may possibly have lupus.

6. SLE can sometimes come on gradually over time. This can make it potentially difficult to diagnose. A doctor may not correctly diagnose SLE until after the person has seen many different doctors over months or years.

7. Doctors use the 2009 revision of the American College of Rheumatology's classification criteria to classify someone as having SLE if he or she has four out of seventeen criteria. The more criteria someone has, the stronger the chances of having SLE. However, some people can have SLE even though they have only two or three criteria.

8. Keep copies of the labs, biopsies, and initial doctors' notes that led to your diagnosis of SLE in a safe, permanent place at home so any new doctors you see can review the work done by your previous doctors.

# The Other Systemic Autoimmune Diseases

## The Accidental "Pocket" Discovery of Systemic Autoimmune Diseases

Some important discoveries in medicine occur by pure accident coupled with keen observation. For example, in 1928, Sir Alexander Fleming studied the bacteria *Staphylococcus* and noticed that a mold had grown in one of his Petri dishes, causing the surrounding bacteria to die. He identified the mold as *Penicillium* and named the substance produced by this *Penicillium* "penicillin." This discovery forever changed the course of history by providing a treatment for infections for the first time, saving millions of lives over the decades since Fleming's discovery. Although an accident led to the discovery, it took an observant and intelligent individual to notice the abnormality and pursue it as something potentially useful.

Something similar happened with lupus. Dr. Malcolm Hargraves was a hematologist (a blood disease expert) who had a special interest in performing and interpreting bone marrow biopsies. In February 1946, he examined the bone marrow from a boy who had an unexplained disease. Hargraves knew only that the boy had severe pain and temperature and color changes in his arms and legs. He noted some unusual cells in the bone marrow, where it appeared that the cells had swallowed (a process called phagocytosis) an unusual substance. The boy's dermatologist told Dr. Hargraves that he believed the boy probably had systemic lupus erythematosus.

Over the next two days, the dermatologist sent two patients who had definite SLE to Dr. Hargraves. Dr. Hargraves performed bone marrow biopsies on them and confirmed that they had the same unusual cells in their bone marrows as did the boy. Dr. Hargraves studied more people who had SLE in the same way. Another doctor in his lab, Dr. Robert Morton, was able to show that these cells from people who had SLE were white blood cells that were engulfing and digesting the nuclei of other cells of the body. They named these cells "LE cells" because they were found in people who had lupus erythematosus. Dr. Hargraves subsequently noted that he had seen similar cells in two other children in 1943 and 1945, and that these children, too, had unexplained systemic diseases, possibly also SLE. Hargraves published his findings in January 1948, but without reaching definite conclusions about why these cells occurred in people who had lupus.

Dr. Hargraves stated that his published paper on the LE cell "opened Pandora's box." He was flooded with special requests from other doctors and scientists interested in this unusual observation in people who had SLE. Before this time, the cause of SLE was totally unknown, and its diagnosis was very difficult to make until people were already very ill with the disease. In fact, the most common way doctors diagnosed SLE was during an autopsy after the person had already died from it. Pursuing information that could lead to earlier diagnosis and could help define what caused the disease was a high priority for doctors with a special interest in lupus. The doctors who tried to reproduce Dr. Hargraves's results told him that they were not seeing the same cells in their patients who had lupus. Dr. Hargraves noted that these doctors were examining the bone marrow biopsies right away, after the completion of the procedures. When he did the studies this way, he did not see these LE cells, either. He then recalled that the first time he noted the cells from one of the children was when there was a delay in looking at the biopsy. He had to transport the specimen from the procedure room to his laboratory to study it. In that sample, he just saw a few of these cells. The second time, the patient was in a hospital a block away from his laboratory, so even more time passed before he could examine the biopsy, and he had noted more of these cells than in the first. The third time he had noted these LE cells was in a biopsy specimen from a patient who was at St. Mary's Hospital in Rochester, about half an hour's walk from his lab. He stuck the specimen in its glass tube into his pocket, and quite a bit of time passed before he could examine it. This third specimen contained a large number of the LE cells. This suggested that something was occurring while the specimens were outside of the body, causing these LE cells to increase in number, but that whatever was happening was not happening within the bone marrow of patients while it was still in their bodies.

The doctors were not finding these LE cells in the fresh bone marrow of people with SLE, but in samples that sat for a while. This caused the doctors to suspect that there may be something in the blood of people with lupus causing the phenomenon. The next step was to take plasma (the clear liquid portion of blood) from some people who had SLE and incubate it with bone marrow cells from people who did not have SLE. Examining these bone marrow biopsies under the microscope showed, in the blood of people who did not have SLE, their own white blood cells swallowing and digesting their own cells. In other words, they also showed LE cells, even though the people did not have lupus. This proved there was something in the fluid part of the blood of people who had lupus that caused the white blood cells to phagocytize and digest the nuclei of other cells. For the first time ever, doctors were witnessing the phenomenon of autoimmunity, where the immune system was actually causing the white blood cells to attack their own cells.

Performing bone marrow and blood exams on people suspected of having SLE and looking for these LE cells subsequently became an important way to diagnose the disease more accurately and earlier than ever before. In fact, Dr. Edmund Dubois, who ran the largest lupus clinic in the world, in Los Angeles, noted that during the years 1948 and 1949 he only diagnosed eleven cases of SLE. However, he diagnosed forty-four cases from 1950 to 1951, with the aid of the LE cell test. Researchers believed that this marked increase in new diagnoses of lupus was due to their ability to diagnose it much earlier and more accurately.

Performing this lab test to look for LE cells was time intensive and complex, however. Scientists and doctors interested in lupus searched for ways to simplify it. Later research showed that the immune systems of people who had SLE antibodies in their blood were directed toward proteins from their own cells (therefore called auto-antibodies), especially toward the central part of their cells called the nucleus (hence, antinuclear antibodies). Recall from chapter 1 that antibodies are very important proteins of the immune system that normally recognize invading foreign proteins (called antigens). In people who have autoimmune diseases, these antibodies (or auto-antibodies) can attach to the normal protein antigens found within their own bodies. These auto-antibodies in people who had lupus caused their own immune system to attack cells in their own bodies. These auto-antibodies would attach to the nuclei of cells in the bone marrow specimen in the lab, and then white blood cells from the blood would recognize the auto-antibodies on these cells and engulf them. They would think they were foreign invaders, not realizing they were attacking parts of their own body.

The white blood cells that swallowed up other cells from the bone marrow (because of these auto-antibodies) were what researchers were seeing under the microscope. Specifically, the immune system was directing auto-antibodies toward the nucleus; the researchers therefore called them antinuclear antibodies, or ANA for short. In 1957 the ANA test was born and was soon the lab test of choice to diagnose SLE because it was much easier to perform. A positive ANA test was even more common among people who had SLE than an abnormal LE cell test. With the ANA test doctors could diagnose the disease even more easily and at much earlier stages compared to the LE cell test. These tests paved the way for doctors to understand lupus as being an autoimmune disease, where the immune system (the white blood cells and antibodies) was attacking the body of the individual. Evidence supporting the concept of autoimmune diseases was born.

Although doctors mainly saw the LE cell test in people who had SLE, they recognized that the ANA test was positive in many related diseases. "Collagen vascular diseases" or "connective tissue diseases" became the collective name for these diseases, which have some similar microscopic tissue characteristics. In addition, this group of diseases causes similar problems, such as arthritis. With the discovery that SLE was most likely a multisystem autoimmune disease, it held to reason that these other collagen vascular diseases were also systemic autoimmune diseases, as well. Since each of them can cause very similar symptoms and some of the same blood test abnormalities, it can be easy to confuse them in the same individual. It is also possible for one individual to have more than one systemic autoimmune disease, adding to the confusion (called overlap syndrome). In addition, a person may develop characteristics of a connective tissue disease—for example, the person may have an inflammatory arthritis and a positive ANA test—yet not fall neatly into one diagnosis (such as SLE). Rheumatologists often diagnose these people as having an "undifferentiated connective tissue disease." The purpose of this chapter is to make it easier to understand systemic autoimmune diseases. What are their similarities and differences? And why is it important to distinguish between them?

· · · ·

SLE is one of the systemic autoimmune diseases. This group of diseases shares some common problems and can sometimes be difficult to differentiate from each other. More than one type can even occur together within the same person. Therefore, it is important for the person who has SLE to understand these possibilities.

To add to the confusion, different doctors use different terms to describe these diseases. Although "systemic autoimmune disease" is the term used in this book, other rheumatologists may use the term "collagen vascular disease" or "connective tissue disease" to refer to the exact same thing. This can be puzzling, but it can be helpful to understand why these different terms exist for the same set of disorders.

In 1942, Dr. Paul Klemperer and his co-workers first used the term "collagen diseases" to describe SLE and scleroderma. These two disorders had similar characteristics. When tissue from patients who had the two disorders was examined under the microscope; there were similar abnormalities within the connective tissues and collagen. Klemperer and his co-workers called these diseases "systemic diseases of connective tissues" and "systemic collagen diseases." Connective tissues are the substances found outside of the cells of the body and that bind them together. Collagen is the primary protein that makes up the connective tissues of the body. Subsequently, Klemperer and his co-workers added other diseases to this group, including dermatomyositis and vasculitis. In 1947, Dr. Arnold Rich also noted that these diseases affected the blood vessels of the body. He dubbed them "collagen-vascular diseases" to reflect the involvement of the blood vessels (vascular) in addition to the collagen of the connective tissues. Eventually researchers discovered that these diseases were actually autoimmune diseases that attacked multiple organ systems and hence were able to group them together as "systemic autoimmune diseases." Currently, any of these terms are useful in describing this group of diseases (listed in table 2.1).

## Common Features of Systemic Autoimmune Diseases

All systemic autoimmune diseases are due to the immune system attacking multiple organs and systems of the body. They may very well share some of the same genes that cause them as well. It is not out of the ordinary for these diseases to occur in members of the same family (such as having an aunt who has Sjögren's syndrome and a mother who has rheumatoid arthritis when you have SLE). This demonstrates that some of the same genes must cause some of the same diseases. However, why one person would develop one disease and another person in the family would develop a different one

**Table 2.1** Systemic Autoimmune Diseases

Systemic lupus erythematosus

Sjögren's syndrome

Rheumatoid arthritis

Systemic sclerosis (scleroderma)

Polymyositis and dermatomyositis

Vasculitis

Mixed connective tissue disease

Systemic autoimmune diseases are also known as collagen vascular diseases or connective tissue diseases.

**Table 2.2** Similar Problems Caused by Systemic Autoimmune Diseases

Arthritis and joint pain

Raynaud's phenomenon

Eye problems: scleritis, episcleritis, conjunctivitis, uveitis

Lung problems: pleuritis, interstitial lung disease

Pericarditis

Peripheral neuropathy

Reddish-colored or bruised-appearing rash

Blood count problems: anemia of chronic disease and leukopenia

Positive ANA, anti-RNP, anti-SSA, and RF

is unknown. It is not too surprising, then, that these diseases can cause similar problems in different people. Table 2.2 lists problems common to many of these systemic autoimmune diseases. Fortunately, there are treatments to control these problems in the vast majority of people affected by them.

For example, all of these disorders can cause inflammation of the joints, leading to arthritis. In fact, this is one of the most commonly shared problems and is the primary reason we consider rheumatologists (also known as arthritis doctors) to be the experts when it comes to diagnosing and treating these diseases.

All of them can also cause Raynaud's phenomenon. This is when the fingers or toes turn blue or white with exposure to cold or with stress. Similarly, they can all affect the eyes, which contain a great deal of collagen and connective tissue making up the sclera (the whites of the eyes), the conjunctiva (the clear coating covering the sclera), the iris (the colored part of the eye), and the uvea (the middle tissue layer of the eye). Therefore, they can all cause inflammation of parts of the eye (scleritis, episcleritis, conjunctivitis, iritis, and uveitis). Sometimes people who have these diseases will develop red, painful eyes and/or blurred vision as one of their very first problems.

Autoimmune diseases can cause inflammation of the lungs (pneumonitis) that can appear similar to infectious pneumonia (coughing, fever, and an abnormal chest x-ray). However, the problem is due to the immune system (instead of an infection) attacking the lungs. Therefore, the person's health does not improve with antibiotic treatment. The term "pleura" refers to the lining around the lungs. If inflammation from these autoimmune diseases affects the pleura of the lungs, doctors call it pleuritis (or pleurisy). Pleurisy causes the person to feel chest pain when breathing in. Interstitial lung disease, or pulmonary fibrosis, occurs when the connective tissue of the lung is attacked, causing scarring. This can in turn lead to shortness of breath and/or coughing. All of these systemic autoimmune diseases can cause any of these lung problems.

Systemic autoimmune diseases may affect the heart as well, most commonly causing inflammation of the pericardium, the lining of the heart (called pericarditis). Like pleurisy, pericarditis can cause chest pain when a person is breathing in or lying down.

Autoimmune disorders can also cause nerve damage, resulting in numbness, tingling, burning pain, or even weakness in the arms and legs due to a condition called peripheral neuropathy. These diseases can even produce enough inflammation through-out the body that the bone marrow makes a decreased number of red blood cells, causing anemia of inflammation (more commonly called anemia of chronic disease). A few of these disorders, especially rheumatoid arthritis, Sjögren's syndrome, and SLE, may also cause a low white blood cell count (leukopenia). Inflammation of the skin can also occur with many of these diseases, causing nonspecific rashes that may appear as reddish-colored or bruised-appearing areas.

To make things even more confusing, all of these diseases can also cause blood tests of the immune system to be positive or abnormal. For example, all of them can cause a positive antinuclear antibody (ANA), anti-RNP, anti-SSA, or rheumatoid factor (RF). See chapter 4 for more details on these tests.

## Undifferentiated Connective Tissue Disease

Before we look at each of the systemic autoimmune diseases in more detail, it is helpful to understand undifferentiated connective tissue disease (UCTD). Some doctors use "lupus-like disease," "incomplete lupus," "latent lupus," "probable lupus," or "undif-ferentiated collagen vascular disease," but all of these terms are similar in meaning.

UCTD is a common diagnosis for patients of rheumatologists. In fact, more people have UCTD than have SLE. If diagnosed with UCTD, you are not alone; 10% to 20% of all referrals to major medical center rheumatologists (such as at Johns Hopkins Hos-pital and the Mayo Clinic) initially have an undifferentiated connective tissue disease. Sometimes a systemic autoimmune disease will occur in a person, yet come on slowly and cause very nonspecific problems at first (such as those listed in table 2.2) along with abnormal lab tests (such as a positive ANA and/or RF). Rheumatoid factor is a type of antibody produced by the immune system that occurs in about 80% of people who have rheumatoid arthritis. That is why it ended up with the name "rheumatoid factor." However, all of the systemic autoimmune diseases can also cause a positive RF test. For example, 30% of people who have SLE are positive for RF. Because of this, doctors can sometimes incorrectly diagnose a person who has SLE (with a positive ANA and RF) with rheumatoid arthritis if arthritis was the predominant problem when the dis-ease first appeared.

If any of the problems listed in table 2.2 occur in the absence of a specific mani-festation of one of these autoimmune diseases, then it may be impossible to know for sure which disease the person may have (such as the person who has SLE who initially only had arthritis and was both ANA and RF positive). Another example would be if someone begins to have problems with her or his fingers turning white and blue with exposure to cold (Raynaud's), joint pain without actually having inflammatory arthri-tis, and anemia, and is positive for ANA. This person could end up having any of the disorders listed in table 2.1. It may take some time to watch and see what happens be-fore knowing exactly which systemic autoimmune disease the person has. The doctor will do a lot of testing (antibody blood tests, urine test, x-rays, etc.) to see if anything specific is occurring that could help make a definite diagnosis, but this is not always possible. The rheumatologist may only know that something is causing a systemic problem with inflammation and that it is most likely one of these autoimmune dis-eases but cannot be sure which one it is.

Another possibility is that the person's symptoms may not be due to one of these diseases at all. For example, some infections, such as parvovirus, can cause many of the same problems (arthritis, anemia, rash, and a positive ANA and/or RF), and look exactly like a systemic autoimmune disease. So the doctor will usually also look for these other possibilities. However, blood tests are often not available to detect viral infections. In these circumstances, doctors may opt to wait and see if the problems just go away on their own. That should happen with most viral infections.

As far as what happens with UCTD, there are several possibilities. One is that the condition could just go away on its own. In fact, one study showed that about one-third of people diagnosed with UCTD had no disease at all after following them over a ten-year period. Most likely, it was an infection causing the problems, which then went away after the body fought off the infection and the immune system eventually calmed down. Another possibility is that the condition could actually be one of the systemic autoimmune diseases (see table 2.1), and it may take some time before the rheumatologist knows which one it is. Some studies suggest that this occurs in approximately one-third of people who have UCTD. Other studies have shown that about 10% to 15% of people who have UCTD develop SLE by five years after the initial diagnosis of UCTD. Factors that seem to increase the chances of developing SLE include being young (teenage years and twenties); having hair loss, pleurisy, or discoid lupus; or being positive for Coombs', double-stranded DNA, or Smith antibodies.

The other possibility is that UCTD may never get worse, nor evolve into anything definitive. This actually occurs in most people diagnosed as having UCTD. In this case, the diagnosis for the person would continue to be UCTD. Not having a definite diagnosis can be frustrating to people, who may feel like they are in limbo. However, the long-term prognosis (in other words, how they will do over the long run) is usually better with UCTD compared to full-blown SLE or one of the other diseases over time.

Although UCTD can cause many unanswered questions on the part of the person who has it, it does not prevent it from being treatable. The reason for this is that the problems caused by the different systemic autoimmune diseases are usually treated the same, no matter which one is causing that particular problem. For example, blood pressure medicines are useful in treating Raynaud's phenomenon (they dilate and open up the arteries to the fingers and toes, increasing the blood flow to these appendages). Anti-inflammatory medicines and medicines that calm down the immune system may be useful for inflammatory arthritis, eye inflammation, or pleurisy. Methotrexate (see chapter 32) is useful in treating inflammatory arthritis. It is very exciting to see recent studies showing that the use of the anti-malarial hydroxychloroquine (see chapter 30) not only treats UCTD successfully, but also may decrease the chances of it progressing to full-blown SLE in many individuals.

## Sjögren's Syndrome

Sjögren's (pronounced SHŌ-grĭnz) syndrome is probably the most common systemic autoimmune disease, affecting 2% to 4% of women during their lifetime. It is estimated that one out of every seventy Americans has Sjögren's syndrome. In this disorder, the immune system primarily attacks the glands of the body that secrete fluids (called exocrine glands). Most commonly it affects the lacrimal glands, which secrete tears, causing dry eyes, and the salivary glands, which secrete saliva, causing a dry mouth. However, it can also affect other exocrine glands of the body, causing dryness of the skin, ears, nose, and vagina as well.

As with SLE, most people who have Sjögren's syndrome are women. In fact, 90% to 95% of people who have Sjögren's syndrome are women. They typically present to their doctor complaining of these problems in middle age. Sjögren's syndrome is usually a very slowly progressive disease that at first produces mild dryness but then gradually worsens over time. A woman may find herself having blurred vision, having a feeling of grittiness in the eyes, having to carry water with her to try to keep her mouth moistened, and having dry, itchy skin, especially in the colder months of the year.

The classical presentation of dryness and being positive for ANA, anti-SSA, anti-SSB, and/or RF (see chapter 4 for more details on these labs) is usually enough to make a diagnosis of Sjögren's. However, sometimes the doctor will order a minor salivary gland biopsy to confirm the diagnosis. Inside the lips just underneath the moist skin, there are numerous tiny salivary glands. The doctor can numb the lip with an anesthetic, make a small incision, and remove a few of these glands. The doctor can then look at these glands with a microscope to see if there is inflammation from Sjögren's syndrome. This is a simple procedure easily done in a doctor's office, not requiring admission to a hospital.

Sjögren's syndrome may occur by itself (called primary Sjögren's syndrome) or it may occur in conjunction with one of the other systemic autoimmune diseases (called secondary Sjögren's syndrome). Approximately 30% of those who have SLE will also develop Sjögren's syndrome. Chapter 14 discusses Sjögren's syndrome in people who have lupus in detail. People who have primary Sjögren's syndrome are at an increased risk of developing a particular type of cancer of the lymph glands called lymphoma. People who have the primary form of Sjögren's syndrome are about forty-four times more susceptible to developing this type of cancer compared to people who do not. Between 10% and 15% of them may develop lymphoma over time. This type of cancer usually causes persistently enlarged lymph glands (such as in the neck, armpits, or groin), as well as fevers, weight loss, and night sweats. Therefore, it is very important for people who have Sjögren's syndrome to see their doctor if they note persistently swollen glands in these areas.

## Rheumatoid Arthritis

Rheumatoid arthritis (RA) is the most well-known systemic autoimmune disease, affecting about 1% of the population. As with SLE and Sjögren's syndrome, it affects more women than men; there are two to three women who have RA for every man who has RA. Rheumatoid arthritis is a systemic autoimmune disease, which comes as a surprise to many people who visualize it as just arthritis. RA can affect many different organs of the body other than the joints, including the lungs, heart, skin, liver, and kidneys. Its primary target, though, is the tissue lining the joints and tendons called the synovium. RA causes this synovial lining to become inflamed and thick. The inflammation associated with this thickened synovium attacks and destroys the cartilage (cushioning of the joints) and the nearby bones. This in turn can cause crippling deformities that can be quite devastating. Fortunately, therapies these days are much improved and most people are able to get into remission or at least prevent the deformities from happening by using the newer medications for RA. Since RA and SLE can both cause an inflammatory arthritis and similar abnormal lab tests (ANA and RF), it can sometimes be difficult to tell if someone has SLE or RA early in the course of the illness. One clue that can be helpful is if the doctor sees erosions on x-rays of the joints. Erosions are areas of the bone that have been "eaten away" by the arthritis, causing permanent damage. These erosions are uncommon in the arthritis of SLE. In addition, a blood test called CCP antibody (see chapter 4) is much more common in RA than in SLE and can be helpful in distinguishing between the two disorders. RA and SLE can occasionally occur in the same person. Rheumatologists sometimes call this "rhupus."

## Scleroderma

Scleroderma, or "systemic sclerosis," is a systemic autoimmune disorder that has a predilection for causing scarring and thickening of the tissues of the body, especially the skin. "Sclero-" comes from the Greek word for "hard" and "-derma" means "skin." This disease essentially causes the skin to thicken, especially on the hands, fingers, and face. It causes similar problems in other areas of the body, especially the blood vessels. In fact, almost everyone who has scleroderma will have Raynaud's phenomenon. Sometimes the scleroderma can affect the muscles of the intestinal tract, causing problems with persistent heartburn, constipation, and inefficient absorption of nutrients. Scarring of the lungs (interstitial fibrosis or interstitial lung disease), pulmonary hypertension (increased blood pressure in the arteries of the lungs), and kidney disease can occur in people who have scleroderma and need to be looked for diligently. Scleroderma can occasionally occur in individuals who have SLE as an overlap syndrome (discussed below).

## Polymyositis and Dermatomyositis

People who have SLE can develop myositis (inflammation of the muscles), which causes muscle achiness and muscle weakness. However, it can also occur as a systemic autoimmune disease called polymyositis. Individuals who have this disease will develop weakness mainly in the muscles of the upper arms, neck, and upper legs, causing difficulty raising the arms up (such as to brush one's hair) and standing up from a chair without using the hands to push oneself up and out of the chair. Most people with polymyositis have no pain, but occasionally it can cause muscle discomfort as well. Dermatomyositis occurs when in addition to inflammation of the muscles causing weakness, inflammation of the skin also develops, causing red-, purple-, or pink-colored rashes.

Doctors diagnose these diseases by finding muscle weakness on the physical examination followed by the discovery of elevated muscle enzymes on blood tests (e.g., CPK, aldolase, LDH, AST, and ALT levels, as discussed in chapter 4). Doctors often do an EMG (electromyogram) test to check for abnormal electrical activity of the muscles, followed by a muscle biopsy. This disease is very important to diagnose and treat as soon as possible, as the muscle weakness can progress to the point where the person develops dangerous problems with weakness of the muscles that aid in breathing.

People who have dermatomyositis have an increased risk of developing cancer. The reason for this is unknown. This may occur before the doctor makes the diagnosis or any time afterward, and it can occur in any part of the body. Therefore, the physician of a patient who has dermatomyositis will usually take a thorough history and do a complete physical examination followed by appropriate screening tests for cancer. (Of special note, we generally do not see this increase in cancer in children who have dermatomyositis.) In addition, as with the other systemic autoimmune diseases, people who have polymyositis and dermatomyositis may have additional problems, such as Raynaud's phenomenon, interstitial lung disease, or arthritis.

## Vasculitis

Vasculitis means inflammation of blood vessels. There are many types of vasculitis, which are named depending on the types of problems they cause, the parts of the body they affect, the types of blood tests that are positive, and biopsy results. These diseases cause problems depending on which parts of the body the affected blood vessels involve. When blood vessels become inflamed from vasculitis, there is decreased blood flow to that particular part of the body (and therefore less oxygen and nutrients), causing damage to the tissues. The blood vessels can also leak out blood and fluids, causing swelling and bruising of the affected area. One of the most common types of vasculitis is called leukocytoclastic vasculitis, which occurs when the small blood vessels of the skin are affected, resulting in numerous small bruised areas on the skin, especially on the lower legs. Other areas of the body commonly involved include the lungs, nerves, and kidneys. Some vasculitides (plural for vasculitis) may be detected with a blood test called ANCA (anti-neutrophil cytoplasmic antibody, discussed in chapter 4). This includes polyangiitis with granulomatosis, previously called Wegener's granulomatosis (which can affect the kidneys, lungs, and sinuses), and microscopic polyarteritis nodosa (which often affects the lungs and kidneys).

Henoch-Schönlein purpura is a vasculitis found primarily in children. It usually affects the small blood vessels of the skin, causing small bruised areas, especially on the lower legs. It can also affect blood vessels of the intestinal tract (causing bloody feces and abdominal pain) as well as of the kidneys.

Giant cell arteritis (also called temporal arteritis) occurs in older people. It affects the arteries of the head and neck and usually causes headaches. If it affects the main artery going to the eye, it can cause the abrupt onset of permanent blindness. It is diagnosed by obtaining a biopsy of a superficial artery, just underneath the skin, located at the temple (hence the name temporal arteritis). Treatment with steroids not only alleviates the headaches, but also prevents the loss of vision. Giant cell arteritis can also be associated with a very painful disease of the muscles and joints called polymyalgia rheumatica, which responds amazingly well to treatment with steroids.

These are just a few of the named types of vasculitis. Describing the others in more detail are beyond the scope of this book. All of the systemic autoimmune diseases, including SLE, can also cause vasculitis.

## Overlap Syndrome

It is possible for anyone who has any of the above-mentioned systemic autoimmune diseases to have more than one. "Overlap syndrome" is the term for this occurrence. Having Sjögren's syndrome along with another disorder is one of the most common overlap syndromes. People who have SLE may develop some of these other systemic autoimmune diseases as an overlap syndrome as well, especially Sjögren's syndrome. About one-third of people who have SLE will have an additional systemic autoimmune disease. If someone who has SLE also develops rheumatoid arthritis, some physicians will call this overlap syndrome "rhupus," combining the terms "rheumatoid arthritis" and "lupus" into one word.

## Mixed Connective Tissue Disease

Mixed connective tissue disease (MCTD) is a systemic autoimmune disease where features of several different systemic autoimmune diseases occur in the same person, who will have a high RNP antibody (see chapter 4). In fact, RNP antibody is found in all people who have MCTD. However, many people who have SLE are also positive for RNP antibody and do not have MCTD. Some laboratories will include an explanation on the lab report stating that the positive RNP antibody is indicative of MCTD, but this is not true in most cases. Your rheumatologist can figure out whether you have MCTD, SLE, or even both if you are positive for RNP antibody.

The vast majority of people who have MCTD have Raynaud's phenomenon. The other most common problems include inflammatory arthritis, muscle pain and/or weakness, and swollen fingers. Over time MCTD will evolve into more of an SLE-like disease in some people, while in other individuals it will act more like scleroderma. It is very important for doctors to evaluate and follow these patients closely to make sure they do not develop a complication called pulmonary hypertension (see chapter 10).

Simply being positive for RNP antibody does not mean that someone has MCTD. About 30% to 40% of people who have SLE are positive for RNP antibody. Those who are positive for RNP have an increased chance of having the same problems as people who have MCTD, especially Raynaud's phenomenon. Sometimes a person can develop problems most suggestive of MCTD, such as inflammatory arthritis and Raynaud's phenomenon along with a high positive RNP antibody. That person may fulfill classification criteria for MCTD but not for SLE. Then over time, she or he may develop other problems that are classic for SLE, making SLE a better fit for his or her diagnosis. This can become confusing for the person involved, who receives different diagnoses over time.

MCTD is often confused with UCTD (undifferentiated connective tissue disease, discussed above). Some people could be incorrectly diagnosed with MCTD while they really have UCTD, and vice versa. Doctors who are not rheumatologists generally make these mistakes, but occasionally some rheumatologists use these terms interchangeably by mistake as well. The distinction between the two is important, however, because people who have UCTD will often have a better long-term outcome in terms of their health and complications from the disorder. Some people who have UCTD will actually have all their symptoms and problems go away over time or the disease remains mild and does not progress. Those who have MCTD more typically have chronic disease that lasts all their lives and must be treated and followed closely. In addition, over time, some people who have MCTD will evolve to fulfill criteria for two or more of the connective tissue diseases and their doctors could consider them to have a type of overlap syndrome.

## To Make Things Even More Confusing . . .

Although physicians like to try to divide patients up neatly into one diagnosis or another, there really is a lot of overlap between them. In fact, what we call SLE is probably not one particular disease at all, but most likely many different diseases that we are just not able to differentiate using currently available medical tests. For example, how can one say that the person who has SLE with recurrent blood clots, a low platelet count, and pleurisy really has the exact same disease as the person who has SLE with inflammatory arthritis, a butterfly rash, and hair loss? In fact, many experts feel that even rheumatoid arthritis is most likely a group of different diseases that we are not able to distinguish at this time. Furthermore, as seen above, many of these diseases share similar problems, and these problems and lab test results can fluctuate over time, which can cause some controversy with diagnosis in any particular person. One rheumatologist may feel that the individual has SLE, while another may feel that person has UCTD, while still another may feel he or she has MCTD.

It is important to try to fit a person into one disease category or another mainly because certain potential problems are more common in some of these diseases compared to others. For example, doctors must follow people who have SLE closely to ensure they do not develop inflammation of the kidneys (nephritis), which occurs in 40% to 50% of patients. Doctors treating people who have MCTD and scleroderma need to monitor them closely to make sure they do not develop pulmonary hypertension, a condition that is more common with these diseases. People who have RA need to have their arthritis brought into complete remission to ensure that they do not develop permanent joint damage or deformities. On the other hand, it may be fine to allow people who have SLE to have some mild, tolerable joint discomforts without increasing their immunosuppressant medications. A person who has Sjögren's syndrome needs to be carefully monitored if she develops persistently swollen lymph glands because it could potentially be due to lymphoma (a cancer of the lymph glands).

In addition, it is not necessary to pigeonhole someone exactly into one diagnosis to treat it. Doctors often treat the same problems similarly, no matter which connective tissue disease a person has. For example, treatment for inflammatory arthritis includes NSAIDs, hydroxychloroquine, methotrexate, and steroids no matter if that person has RA, SLE, UCTD, scleroderma, Sjögren's syndrome, or MCTD.

It can be understandably frustrating as a patient to have a diagnosis such as UCTD and feel like you are in limbo or do not have a real diagnosis at all. On the other hand, it can be frustrating to keep hearing over time that you have a different diagnosis by different rheumatologists. Unfortunately, a lot of this has to do with doctors' limitations in diagnosing patients, but nonetheless, it does not prevent doctors from treating patients and taking proper care of them.

Due to these difficulties with diagnosis, it is never a bad idea to get a second opinion from another rheumatologist, especially since the diagnosis and treatments for these disorders can have important long-term consequences. Most rheumatologists, including myself, feel more than happy to have patients see another rheumatologist for a second opinion. Never feel guilty or badly for wanting to do so. If you do decide to get a second opinion, make sure that you get copies of all lab and test results to show to the new doctor as that will greatly simplify the second-opinion process. It could be quite expensive to have all the tests needlessly repeated, or the second doctor could miss certain important clues to your diagnosis if you do not do this. If you get a negative reaction from a doctor due to your wanting a second opinion, then it is probably better to change doctors anyway because no doctor is 100% infallible.

## KEY POINTS TO REMEMBER

1. The systemic autoimmune diseases are a group of diseases where the immune system attacks parts of the person's own body. SLE is one example of these diseases.

2. Other terms used interchangeably for systemic autoimmune disease include "collagen vascular disease" and "connective tissue disease."

3. All of these diseases can cause similar problems, which include Raynaud's phenomenon, interstitial lung disease, inflammatory arthritis, inflammation of the eyes, and rashes.

4. All of these diseases can cause similar blood test abnormalities, which include positive ANA, positive RNP, positive SSA, positive RF, elevated ESR, elevated CRP, and anemia, making these particular blood tests nonspecific in diagnosing any particular systemic autoimmune disease.

5. When someone has evidence of a systemic autoimmune disease but only has problems found in all of these diseases, and this person does not fulfill diagnostic criteria for any particular disease, then doctors may label that person as having an undifferentiated connective tissue disease, or UCTD for short (sometimes also called lupus-like disease, latent lupus, and even probable-lupus).

6. A UCTD may over time evolve into one of the definite systemic autoimmune diseases (such as SLE or RA), or it may remain UCTD, or it may even go away spontaneously.

7. People who have SLE can also have any of the other systemic autoimmune diseases (called an overlap syndrome).

8. Mixed connective tissue disease (MCTD) and undifferentiated connective tissue disease (UCTD) are not the same disorders. Even doctors commonly mistakenly interchange these terms.

9. Consider getting a second opinion from another rheumatologist if you are at all uncomfortable with your diagnosis. Make sure to provide copies of all your workup results to the doctor doing the second opinion.

# What Causes Lupus?

## Why Are Most People Who Have Lupus Women?

There is a rare disorder in men called Klinefelter's syndrome. To understand what Klinefelter's syndrome is, we need to look at why boys are born as boys and girls are born as girls. The way we become who we are as individuals is due to genes. These are the individual, tiny parts of the DNA. Each gene is responsible for giving us certain attributes, such as blue or brown eyes, or darker or lighter colored skin. Many genes connect to each other to form a very long piece of material called DNA, which in turn combines with other molecular structures into chromosomes. These chromosomes are located inside the nuclei of most cells of the body. Each cell of the human body normally has forty-six chromosomes existing as twenty-three pairs. One chromosome of each pair comes from the mother and one comes from the father. One of these chromosome pairs is composed of the sex chromosomes. There are two types of sex chromosomes, either Y or X. A woman has two X-chromosomes (one from her mother and one from her father); a man has an X-chromosome and a Y-chromosome paired together (the X came from his mother and the Y came from his father). Being either XX or XY, with rare exceptions, determines whether a person is born as a female or as a male, respectively.

However, not all things in nature happen perfectly. Sometimes even the sex chromosomes do not transfer perfectly from one generation to the next generation. One example is the genetic disorder called Klinefelter's syndrome. This occurs when a baby receives an extra X-chromosome and is born as a baby identified as a boy. Most commonly, this occurs when a baby receives two X-chromosomes plus one Y-chromosome (XXY instead of the usual XY), but other variations may also occur, such as receiving three X-chromosomes and one Y-chromosome. This occurs in one out of one thousand boys born, so it is more common than people realize. Boys who have Klinefelter's syndrome tend to be taller than normal, do not have much body hair, have broad hips and narrow shoulders, have smaller than normal testicles, and are infertile. So why would I bring this up in a book about SLE? It is because men who have Klinefelter's syndrome are sixteen times more likely to develop SLE than other men are.

There is another genetic disorder called Turner's syndrome. This occurs when a girl is born with just one X-chromosome instead of the normal pair of two X-chromosomes. Girls who have Turner's syndrome are infertile, have extra skin on the neck (called a webbed neck) and misshaped elbows, and are shorter than normal. Interestingly, they have a lower chance of developing SLE than other females.

Because men who have Klinefelter's syndrome have an increased risk for developing SLE by having an extra X-chromosome, and women who have Turner's syndrome are less likely to develop SLE by having one less X-chromosome, there is something about the X- and Y-chromosomes themselves or the sex hormones involved in SLE. About 90% of all people who have SLE are women. Why does this occur? This chapter goes deeper into the complex issues surrounding the causes and triggers of systemic lupus erythematosus and answers these and other questions about the mysteries of the causes of lupus.

. . . .

We do not know all of the causes of lupus, which are complex and still under intense investigation. Figuring out what causes lupus is the only way we can possibly develop a cure for it. What does not cause lupus is also important. It is not contagious; you cannot give it to someone else or catch it from someone else (other than by inheriting the genes from your parents). It is not a cancer or malignancy.

Our current understanding of what causes lupus consists of numerous factors that can affect the immune system. These factors include genetics, the environment, and gender. You have to be born with the genes in the first place for the disease to develop. Therefore, we can partially consider the disease genetic. However, the vast majority of people who are born with the genes will never develop lupus. It appears that the more predisposing factors you have, the higher the chances you have of developing lupus (figure 3.1). For example, if you are a male born with just a few genes from one parent, have never smoked cigarettes, and have not exposed yourself to the sun excessively, you have a lower chance of developing lupus. However, if you are a female who has inherited multiple genes from your father and mother, have smoked cigarettes, and have exposed yourself frequently to the sun, then you have a higher chance of developing lupus.

When people are diagnosed with a chronic disease, they often feel guilty and blame themselves. These are unfounded, detrimental thoughts. If you have lupus, it is not your fault! You have no control over what genes you were born with, so please erase those guilty thoughts out of your mind if you have been blaming yourself in any way about having lupus. Instead, harness your mental energy and thoughts to focus on learning as much as you can about lupus so that you can empower yourself to deal with it to the best of your abilities.

## Genetic Predisposition

Genes are a set of instructions for the body for everything that makes us who we are as individuals. It is the genes we get from our mothers and fathers that determine if we are born with blue eyes or brown hair, if we get dimples or a big nose, and even if we are destined to be geniuses or not. Collections of genes bind together to form what we call DNA and chromosomes that are located in the central nucleus of every cell of the body.

Genes certainly play an important role in the inheritance of certain diseases. For example, sickle cell anemia affects about one out of every 625 African Americans. It is due to the hemoglobin (the oxygen-carrying protein found in red blood cells) having an abnormal shape, which in turn disfigures the red blood cells into being sickle-

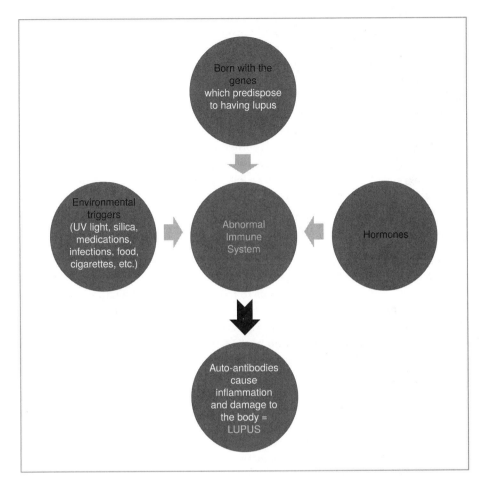

**Figure 3.1** The causes of lupus

shaped instead of being round. These deformed red blood cells are destroyed in the blood system too quickly and this can cause low red blood cell counts (anemia). A person must be born with two sickle cell genes to get the disease; one must come from the mother and one from the father. If you get both, then unfortunately you will definitely get sickle cell disease. If you only inherit one gene, then you have what is called sickle cell trait, which does not cause the severe problems that full-blown sickle cell disease does. If a person who has the sickle cell trait has children with someone else who has sickle cell trait, then 25% of their children will develop full-blown sickle cell disease.

The genetics of developing lupus are much more complicated as there appear to be many genes that can cause lupus, and most people who are born with these genes do not ever develop lupus. The evidence for genes playing an important role in causing the disease is substantive. Lupus tends to be more common in some ethnic and racial groups compared to others. For example, according to the Lupus Foundation of America, Inc., lupus occurs in one out of 700 Caucasian American women between the ages of 15 and 64 years old; however, it occurs in one out of 254 African American women of the same ages. Multiple studies from other countries have reproduced these racial differences as well. It appears that certain ethnic groups, such as those of African, Asian, and Hispanic descent, have a higher number of people affected by lupus than others. The best explanation for this would be the genetics passed down from one generation to the next.

Another clue to the importance of genetics in people who develop lupus is how often it occurs in twins. Identical twins are born with the same genes (hence the term "identical") from both their father and mother. This is the reason they look and sound almost exactly alike. When an identical twin has SLE, there is approximately a 25% chance that the other twin will also develop SLE. This illustrates that there is more going on to cause lupus other than just having the genes. If being born with the genes that cause lupus were the only important reason, then 100% of identical twins who have the genes for lupus would develop lupus. As a comparison, when one looks at fraternal (or non-identical) twins, the chance of both twins developing lupus is much less. Fraternal twins do not obtain the exact same genes from each parent. They can even be male and female. Their genetic makeup differences are similar to those of siblings who are born at different times to the same mother and father. In fraternal twins, if one twin develops lupus the chances of the other twin developing SLE are 2%—much less than in identical twins. However, this is still markedly higher than for people who do not have a sibling who has SLE. In fact, if someone has a sibling who has SLE, that person has a thirty times higher chance for developing SLE compared to someone who does not.

Therefore, there are other factors at play (such as environmental triggers and hormones), which I discuss further below. This is why we prefer to say that when someone is born with the genes that can cause lupus, it is a "genetic predisposition." In other words, being born with these lupus genes increases the chances that that person could develop SLE, or "predisposes" that person to developing SLE, but they do not guarantee that it will happen.

We have known for some time that some people who have SLE have identifiable abnormalities of their immune systems that appear to play an important role in their developing the disease. One of these problems involves the complement system. Your rheumatologist will usually check a blood test called complement levels, particularly the third and fourth complement levels (called C3 and C4), each time you get labs done. Complements (which I discuss as well in chapters 1 and 4) are very important proteins that play an integral role in the immune system. C3 and C4 levels will sometimes decrease when the immune system is particularly active in someone who has SLE. If someone is born with a deficiency in some of these complement factors (especially C2 and C4) they have an increased risk of having SLE. These particular individuals can be identified by finding very low levels of these complements on laboratory testing that persist even when their disease improves with treatment. These complement deficiencies are most likely due to a person being born with certain abnormal genes, which in turn makes this particular part of the immune system act abnormally.

The genes that cause lupus do not necessarily only lead to lupus, but can also potentially cause other autoimmune disorders as well, which complicates the genetic question. People who have lupus are more likely to have other family members who have other autoimmune diseases, such as rheumatoid arthritis, scleroderma, and autoimmune thyroid disease (as well as many other types of autoimmune disorders).

Currently, this is a very exciting time in our understanding of human genes. In 1990, the National Institutes of Health in coordination with the U.S. Department of Energy set out to identify all genes found in humans. Thirteen years later, they finally identified and stored 22,400 genes in computer databases for doctors and scientists to work with. This was only the beginning of the work. Now many scientists and physicians are looking at these genes closely to see which ones may be the causes of certain diseases, hoping that this will lead to potentially important treatments and cures in the future. Thus far, doctors have identified more than thirty genes that definitely appear to play a role in the development of SLE. Each of these genes increases the appearance of abnormalities in the immune system. Many people who have SLE are born with more than one of these genes, and it appears that the more genes you inherit, the higher the chances of developing the disease. At present, we are not at the point of being able to test individuals for these genes. In the future, this could happen, especially if we are able to use the information to cure or prevent the disease. There is even the possibility of developing vaccinations for people who inherit these genes to prevent lupus from occurring in the first place.

### "If I have lupus, what are the chances my children will develop lupus?"

So what are the chances of your children developing SLE if you have the disease? Lupus patients commonly ask their rheumatologists this question. The exact chances of one's children developing lupus are unknown. Some experts believe that if a mother has SLE, her daughters have as much as a 10% chance of developing SLE while only 2% of her sons will develop it. The lupus experts at the Lupus Clinic at Johns Hopkins Hospital think that if a mother has SLE the chances of her having a child with the disease is only about 2% overall. However, the answer to this question involves much more than just assigning a number. It all depends on genetics. In some families with numerous lupus genes the chances of having a child who will develop lupus may be very high, while in another family with very few lupus genes it may be very low.

Is it necessary to test for SLE in children of parents who have the disease? Most rheumatologists recommend not doing so. About 25% of children born to women who have SLE will be ANA positive (the screening test for lupus), yet the vast majority of them will never develop SLE. This knowledge would most likely cause unnecessary anxiety in these particular children over their lifetimes. Also, there is no way to prevent them from developing the disease if they are predisposed to it. In addition, are we going to recommend that each of them see a doctor repeatedly during their lives to see if they develop the disease or not? That could turn into quite a time-consuming and expensive alternative. Another problem occurs in those who are not ANA positive. Being negative for ANA at any particular time does not mean that one will not develop SLE at some time in the future. Children who are not ANA positive could potentially develop the false hope that they may never develop SLE.

Currently, most rheumatologists recommend that the children of parents who have SLE learn what the symptoms of SLE are. If any of these symptoms ever occur, then they should see their physician for appropriate testing. Something that the children of parents who have SLE should consider doing to decrease their risk of developing

**Table 3.1** How the Children of People Who Have SLE Can Try to Prevent Lupus

- Avoid the sun, tanning, tanning booths, laying out at the beach
- Wear sunscreen every day no matter what season it is
- Do not take sulfa antibiotics
- Do not eat mung bean sprouts or alfalfa sprouts
- Eat a diet rich in omega-3 fatty acids (flaxseed, coldwater fish, walnuts)
- Include olive oil in your diet
- Have your vitamin D level checked; take a supplement regularly if it is low
- Do not smoke cigarettes
- Avoid the herbal supplement Echinacea

lupus would be to avoid things that can trigger SLE (table 3.1). There are no studies to prove that taking these precautions decreases the risk for developing lupus. However, practicing these measures may theoretically help.

## Environmental Triggers

Most people who are born with the genes that can cause lupus never develop the disease. As with most autoimmune diseases, doctors believe that something in the environment has to interact with the immune system in these genetically predisposed individuals in a particular way for the disease to occur. Lupus appears to have several possible triggers.

## Epigenetics

Anyone who reads a lot about lupus is bound to run across the term "epigenetics" so I briefly discuss the term here. Previously in this chapter I talked about how the genes that we are born with can cause a person to develop lupus. The term "genetics" refers to the study of these genes. Our genes are made up of molecules of DNA. However, these molecules of DNA are not isolated and pure. Constant chemical reactions occur with them throughout our entire lives, and they react with numerous other important bodily and environmental compounds. These reactions and interactions can change how the DNA actually functions. Related changes (epigenetic) can also occur to other important genetic-related substances inside of our cells as well. These changes can last the entire life of a person and can even be passed down to subsequent generations. Although many of these changes can be important to us, some can be detrimental, such as those that can occur and cause a person to develop lupus. As an example, many genes that cause lupus do not cause a person to actually develop lupus unless they become abnormal or activated through the process of epigenetics. This can occur due to something in the environment causing a change to occur in the genetic DNA. This process is considered an epigenetic process and can be caused by any of the environmental factors discussed in this section. Environmental influences on our DNA, through the process of epigenetics, are felt to be a major reason identical twins do not always develop lupus even though they both have the exact same genes. One of them could have had something occur (such as a viral infection, smoking, or too much sunlight exposure) to alter his DNA through this process of epigenetics. This is a new area of research and is quite complex, but appears promising in allowing us to better understand how lupus occurs.

## Ultraviolet Light (UVB and UVA-2)

In 1888, the first description of sun exposure causing lupus appeared in a medical journal. In that article, a famous dermatologist named Jonathan Hutchinson mentioned what he called "sunblain" (a medical term that is not used anymore). He described it as a "condition of inflammation, which is excited by exposure of the part—tip of nose, ears, or cheek, or possibly even the hands—to the direct influence of a scorching sun." Dr. Hutchinson also noted that "whatever ensues from influences of this kind, should it become chronic, is almost sure to take the form of lupus erythematosus."

For decades, we have known about the influence of the sun in causing lupus. Someone developing her first symptoms shortly after a very sunny vacation is not out of the ordinary. This is due to the influence of just a small part of the light spectrum called ultraviolet light. Ultraviolet light is so named because its wavelength frequency is higher ("ultra" is Latin for "beyond") than that of the color violet, and it is not visible to humans. The colors of the visible rainbow can be recalled by using the mnemonic ROY G. BIV, which stands for red, orange, yellow, green, blue, indigo, and violet (see figure 38.1). These colors of visible light are ones that human eyes can detect. The color violet is the visible color with the highest wavelength frequency. The wavelength frequency of ultraviolet light is greater than the visible color of violet and is just below that of x-rays. UV light is capable of causing chemical reactions. There are three bands of UV light: UVA, UVB, and UVC rays. In addition, UVA light is further broken down into UVA-1 and UVA-2 spectrums. It appears that UVA-2 and UVB rays are the most important ones in lupus. The sun is the major source of UVA and UVB rays. However, indoor lighting also emits UVA and UVB light. UVC light does not make it through the atmosphere so it is not a factor for people who have lupus; UVA-1 light may actually be beneficial to them (see chapter 37).

UVA-2 and UVB rays damage the cells of the skin and are the reason that sunburns, skin aging, and skin cancer occur. In people who are born with the genetic predisposition to develop SLE, these UV rays continuously interact with the cells of the skin, which in turn release their internal contents into the blood and tissues of the body, exposing them to the immune system. This interaction of ultraviolet light with the cells of the skin occurs constantly, even with the lower amounts of ultraviolet light given off by indoor lighting. These cells damaged by the UV light subsequently release their contents, including those found in their nuclei. These nuclear proteins (also called nuclear antigens) are particularly responsible for interacting with the immune system of a person who has lupus (especially with the famous antinuclear antibodies of lupus), encouraging it to become more active and cause inflammation and damage to various parts of the body. Current evidence suggests that this increased activation of the immune system not only causes the rashes of lupus (such as the butterfly rash or a sun-sensitive rash), but also occurs in other parts of the body, causing other problems, such as arthritis, pleurisy, and kidney damage. This is why it is important that all people who have lupus protect themselves from UV light as detailed in chapter 38.

## Silica

Silica is a mineral found in quartz, sand, rocks, and soil. There have been numerous studies implicating the exposure to silica and the later development of lupus as well as other autoimmune diseases, such as rheumatoid arthritis, scleroderma, and inflammatory diseases of the lungs. Increased exposure to silica can occur in various occupations, including mining, highway construction/repair, stone masonry, bricklaying, foundry work, dry cleaning, working with pottery and ceramics, working with computer wafers, and janitorial work. In addition, silica can cause lupus in laboratory animals, especially mice with a predisposition to developing lupus. Laboratory studies show that silica also has direct effects on the immune system.

## Medications

As discussed in chapter 1 under drug-induced lupus, medications can cause lupus. The first report of a drug causing a lupus-like disease was in 1954, when a report suggested that a 44-year-old woman developed very low blood cell counts after receiving a blood pressure medicine called hydralazine (also called Apresoline). Numerous drugs have since been implicated, but the vast majority of these cases have involved just a few drugs, such as hydralazine, methyldopa (also used to treat high blood pressure), procainamide (used to treat heart rhythm problems), and isoniazid (used to treat tuberculosis). Researchers have not fully been able to determine the reason these medications cause lupus. Fortunately, this form of lupus disappears when the drug is withdrawn. One medication deserves special attention, and that is the sulfa antibiotic prescribed under the names Bactrim and Septra. A large percentage of people who have lupus will have a flare of their disease or develop an allergic reaction when taking this antibiotic. Therefore, many lupus experts recommend that people who have lupus never take this antibiotic.

The latter part of this chapter discusses the role of sex hormones, such as estrogen, in causing lupus or making it worse. Therefore, it makes sense to wonder if SLE may occur more often or worsen in women who take estrogen-containing medications. Recent studies suggest that birth control pills containing small doses of estrogen may not cause lupus more often, or make SLE worse in someone who already has it. Therefore, most lupus experts agree that birth control pills are probably fine for women who have lupus to take, but it is probably best to take one that has a low estrogen dose. After menopause, some women take estrogen-containing medications to decrease the effects of menopause such as hot flashes. These contain higher amounts of estrogen and appear to increase mild lupus flares; therefore, it is probably best to avoid them. Anywhere from 30% to 50% of women who have SLE are positive for antiphospholipid antibodies (see chapters 4 and 9), which can cause dangerous blood clots. Anyone who is positive for these antibodies should avoid hormonal medications containing estrogen.

## Infections

SLE may first develop during or soon after a flu-like illness or viral syndrome. When a person contracts the flu or a viral infection, the body produces increased antibodies specifically targeting the infecting virus. These antibodies help the immune system fight the virus to aid the body in getting rid of the infection. These antibodies usually last the rest of the person's life to fight off another invasion if the same virus infects the person again in the future. Doctors are able to determine if a particular virus infected someone in the past by looking for these antibodies in the blood. Some studies have shown that a higher number of people who have lupus are positive for antibodies to some viruses compared to people who do not have lupus, thus suggesting that these viral infections may possibly play a role in the development of SLE.

Epstein Barr virus (EBV) in particular may be a possible trigger or cause of lupus. EBV is the virus that causes mononucleosis (commonly called mono). In a 1972 study, children with lupus had higher levels of EBV antibodies in their blood compared to children who did not have lupus. EBV has been the most studied infection in lupus causation. Several studies have shown an increased association between having high levels of EBV antibodies in the blood and developing SLE at some point after the EBV infection. However, it has not yet been 100% proven that EBV definitely triggers lupus.

There have also been reports of people who have lupus having actual parts of viruses in their body tissues. Researchers have found larger amounts of EBV, parvovirus, cytomegalovirus (CMV), and herpes virus particles in the bodies of people who have lupus compared to people who do not have lupus. This provides direct evidence that a viral infection may possibly have played a role in their developing SLE. There have even been case reports in the medical literature of people developing SLE or lupus-like diseases after other infections, such as CMV and parvovirus. In fact, parvovirus infection can cause an illness that can look exactly like lupus but disappears over time. In my own practice, I have two patients who developed classic SLE after having well-documented parvovirus infections. Their lupus continues to persist many years after they contracted the initial infection.

## Food

There have been case reports of alfalfa sprout ingestion causing the onset of SLE. Alfalfa and mung bean sprouts contain high levels of L-canavanine, an amino acid protein that stimulates the immune system. In one study, researchers fed macaque monkeys a diet high in alfalfa and other L-canavanine-containing products. More than half of the monkeys ingesting these products developed lupus problems such as kidney inflammation and autoimmune hemolytic anemia and had increased amounts of ANA and anti-DNA levels as well as lowered levels of complement (immune problems commonly seen in SLE). Therefore, it is probably prudent for people who have SLE to avoid alfalfa and mung bean sprouts.

Some doctors recommend that people who have lupus not ingest garlic since it may theoretically increase the activity of the immune system. However, there really is no evidence that eating garlic causes lupus in humans. In fact, there is some evidence that garlic may actually have some anti-inflammatory properties.

## Vitamin D Deficiency

Vitamin D is a very important hormone manufactured by the cells of the skin. It is most commonly associated with its role in maintaining normal calcium levels in the body and keeping the bones strong. However, vitamin D is also important for proper immune system function. The lack of vitamin D has been associated with an increased chance of having some autoimmune diseases, such as systemic lupus erythematosus, antiphospholipid antibody syndrome (discussed in chapter 9), juvenile diabetes, multiple sclerosis, and rheumatoid arthritis. In addition, people who have increased skin pigmentation (such as people of African and Hispanic descent) have lower levels of vitamin D since the skin pigment melanin prevents ultraviolet light from penetrating the skin. The skin has difficulty manufacturing enough vitamin D as a result. These ethnic groups tend to have lower levels of vitamin D than lighter-skinned groups such as Caucasians. A 2012 study showed that when light-skinned people who had SLE developed low vitamin D levels in winter months they were more likely to have flares of their lupus compared to when their vitamin D levels increased in months that had a lot of sunshine. This finding is interesting because we usually associate more sun exposure to lupus flares (due to the increase in UV light). This adds to the evidence of needing adequate vitamin D levels to have a better working immune system.

Most people who have SLE have low levels of vitamin D and should take a vitamin D supplement regularly. Several studies have shown that people who have more severe lupus tend to have lower levels of vitamin D compared to those who have milder disease. In fact, a 2012 study even showed that vitamin D levels could potentially be used to monitor lupus disease activity like other blood tests that track SLE, such as anti-ds DNA levels. Vitamin D deficiency has to be entertained as a possible cause or trigger for lupus to develop in someone who is born with the genes predisposing to lupus.

## Cigarette Smoking

In 1980, a report published findings of a 25-year-old lab technician who came into regular contact with a chemical called hydrazine. She developed an illness very similar to SLE, with sun sensitivity, fatigue, joint pain, and a red rash on the face. Tobacco contains hydrazine. In fact, multiple studies have shown an increased risk of developing systemic lupus, cutaneous lupus, and other autoimmune diseases, such as rheumatoid arthritis, due to smoking tobacco. A 2010 study showed that people who currently smoke cigarettes had a higher chance of developing SLE compared to people who do not smoke and people who had previously stopped smoking. Tobacco also contains numerous other toxins, such as cadmium and insecticides, which can potentially be associated with an increased risk of developing autoimmune diseases as well.

## Other Environmental Triggers

Pesticides may also increase the risk for developing SLE; however, studies are inconclusive. The Women's Health Initiative (a large, ongoing study of women looking at multiple health issues) showed an increased risk for autoimmune diseases (including lupus) in women who used and mixed insecticides compared to women who did not. This risk was highest in women routinely exposed to these pesticides.

In 2003, researchers reported that a group of chemicals called phthalates caused the immune systems of lupus-susceptible mice to become more active and produce higher amounts of anti-ds DNA (a very important lupus auto-antibody; see chapter 4). Other researchers have since then reproduced these results. This is of concern because phthalates are used in so many products in our society. There is a legitimate concern that these products could potentially increase the occurrence and activity of autoimmune disorders such as SLE. At this time, there are no studies addressing this in people who have SLE, but doctors and scientists are investigating this possibility. In the meantime, there is not enough evidence for doctors to warn their patients to avoid these substances; doing so would be incredibly difficult since they are present in so many common items. If a person who has SLE wishes to minimize her exposure to phthalates, she would have to try to use as much naturally occurring products (especially plant-based) as possible and avoid manufactured plastics, cosmetics, paints, rubber, toys, paints, and cleaners. Looking for the words "phthalate-free" on cosmetic products and "VOC-free" in paints is a good place to start. You can use glass products instead of plastic, eat fresh and frozen foods instead of canned foods, and avoid fabric softeners (dryer sheets and liquids) as well as many air fresheners. Another common source for phthalates for people who have lupus is enteric-coated pills. An enteric coating delays the release of a medicine into the intestinal system. Enteric-coated capsules and tablets can decrease problems with stomach upset, but they are high in phthalates.

Vaccines have rarely been associated with developing SLE. The medical literature contains only a small number of reports. However, in my own practice, I do have one patient who developed SLE immediately after receiving the vaccine against yellow fever. Therefore, I am convinced it can happen, although it is fortunately rare. The medical term used to describe this sort of reaction is "autoimmune syndrome induced by adjuvant" (ASIA for short). "Adjuvant" is the medical word meaning "a substance that can cause the immune system to become more active when exposed to it." Examples of adjuvants that can stimulate the immune system include vaccines, silicone, and infections.

Echinacea is an herbal supplement, which people sometimes take to help with colds and the flu. Echinacea can increase the activity of the immune system. Since lupus is a disease where the immune system is already overactive, Echinacea therapy is not advised for people who have the disease. In Europe, where herbal medications have had a long history of acceptance as therapy for medical illness, Echinacea even carries a warning suggesting that it should not be taken by people who have autoimmune diseases. In fact, the Lupus Center at Johns Hopkins Hospital has reported that some of their SLE patients have developed severe lupus flares while taking Echinacea.

Some doctors have also recommended that people who have autoimmune diseases not take melatonin. This is based on the theory that melatonin may increase activity of the immune system. However, there is no concrete evidence to make this recommendation. Most importantly, there have been no studies on people who have lupus using melatonin. Several studies in mice that have lupus have shown that female mice receiving treatment with melatonin actually developed less inflammation, less auto-antibody production, and less kidney inflammation from their SLE. One study using melatonin in people who had a related autoimmune disease, rheumatoid arthritis, showed that melatonin had no bad or good effects on the disease. However, a couple of studies on male mice given melatonin did show increased amounts of inflammation. Therefore, there is not enough evidence to conclude that taking melatonin can cause lupus or not, nor can doctors recommend that women who have SLE not take it. To be prudent, however, it may be best for men who have SLE to avoid it.

Another potential cause of SLE flaring in some people is stress. There are only a few studies showing this possibility. Most rheumatologists would agree that stress appears to increase disease activity in their lupus patients and therefore probably does have an effect on the immune system.

Working with solvents may also trigger lupus to become more active. Exposure to solvents may occur in various jobs, including working with paints, nail polish, or dyes and processing film. In fact, trichloroethylene, a commonly used industrial solvent, can have significant effects on the immune system and studies show that it accelerates the onset of lupus in mice. However, so far, the link between lupus in humans and solvent exposure is weak at best.

## Why Do Women Get Lupus More Often Than Men?

As previously mentioned, about 90% of people who have lupus are women. Possible factors include the effects of hormones on the immune system, the presence of genes that cause lupus occurring on the X-chromosome (the female sex chromosome), and a phenomenon called microchimerism (explained below).

### Hormonal Influences on the Immune System

There is quite a bit of evidence pointing to the effects of sex hormones on the immune system. Although SLE can occur at any age (the youngest reported patient was 6 weeks old, excluding cases of neonatal lupus), it is most common for SLE to develop in adolescent girls and women who are menstruating (and therefore have a significant amount of estrogen-related hormones). The number of women who develop SLE during childbearing years far outweighs the number of men who develop SLE in this same age range. However, in children (before the onset of puberty) and in older adults (after menopause) the difference between the numbers of females and males who develop lupus is not nearly as dramatic. The influence of sex hormones would seem to be the most likely explanation for this difference.

It is not out of the ordinary for women who have SLE to notice an increase in their lupus symptoms, such as arthritis pain, just before and during menstruation. Lupus has a tendency to become more active during the hormonal changes of pregnancy or soon after delivery in approximately 25% of women. Women who begin menstruation at an earlier age than average appear to have an increased risk of developing SLE. Women who take high-estrogen birth control pills and postmenopausal women who take estrogen also have an increased chance of developing SLE. In addition, there have been reports of lupus developing in women who take fertility hormones.

Some studies have shown that there are abnormal levels of sex hormones in both women and men who have SLE. Women who have active SLE have lower levels of the male sex hormones (androgens), while some men with SLE have lower testosterone (the male hormone) and higher estrogen levels (female hormones).

It should not be surprising, then, that sex hormones have important interactions with the immune system. Mice exposed to female hormones such as estrogen have an increased chance of developing SLE, while exposure to the male hormone testosterone decreases the chances of developing it. Human studies have also demonstrated that female hormones such as estrogen and prolactin cause increased inflammation and stimulate various portions of the immune system.

## Genes on the X-Chromosome

Earlier in this chapter, I discussed how being born with certain genes that cause lupus may lead to the development of SLE later in life. An additional important discovery has shown that some of the gene abnormalities predisposing a person to SLE are located on the female X-chromosome. One pair of inherited chromosomes, the sex chromosomes, determines whether we are born male or female. The X-chromosome is the female chromosome and the Y-chromosome is the male chromosome. We get one sex chromosome from our mother and one from our father. If someone gets two X-chromosomes, then the person develops into a female; if someone gets an X-chromosome (from the mother) and a Y-chromosome (from the father), then the child develops (with rare exceptions) into a male.

Some of the genes that cause lupus, including IRAK1, TLR7, and MECP2, have been located on the X-chromosome. Since women have two X-chromosomes and men only have one, women are twice as likely as men to inherit these particular lupus-causing genes. Normally, one of the X-chromosomes in women becomes inactive. However, in some women who have SLE, it appears that this does not always occur. This increases the chances that the lupus genes on their extra X-chromosome will become active.

## Microchimerism

The chimera is a fire-breathing female monster in Greek mythology. Her head and body are that of a lion, the head and neck of a goat are present in her midsection, and her tail consists of the body and head of a snake. Science has borrowed the word "chimera" to mean an animal that is composed of cells coming from two different and separate animals, yet occurring in the same individual. One example of a real-life chimera is the angler fish, found deep within the oceans. The male is one hundred times smaller than the female and attaches himself to a female by biting her and then digesting the tissues around the bite. The female angler fish's body gradually absorbs the body of the male. While his organs are absorbed into hers, his testicles mature and enlarge, ensuring a lifelong supply of sperm to fertilize her eggs throughout the duration of her life.

A form of chimerism occurs in humans as well. The placenta is the organ that separates an unborn fetus's body from the body of its mother. It acts as a barrier to keep unwanted materials from the mother from entering the baby's body while also protecting the mother by not allowing certain materials to pass from the fetus into her body. The placenta does allow important nutrients, hormones, and oxygen to pass from the mother to her fetus, while waste products can pass from the fetus to the mother's blood supply for subsequent disposal. However, this barrier is not perfect. Some of the cells of the unborn baby may accidently pass into the mother's blood. This results in microchimerism ("micro-" meaning small)— some cells of her child persist in the mother's body on a microscopic level. This may also work in reverse: some of the mother's cells may pass into the baby and persist there throughout the baby's lifespan. It is much more common for fetal cells to enter the mother, than vice versa. Normally, the immune system would consider these cells as being foreign and attack them to protect the person from this invasion. However, in some people, the immune system is not able get rid of these microchimeric cells and they persist. In some cases, this may eventually end up causing an abnormal immune response. This has been shown to be a possible cause of the autoimmune disease scleroderma. In a 2001 study a woman who had lupus had male cells containing XY-chromosomes (presumably from one of her previously born sons) present in the lupus-affected organs of her body. Interestingly, the tissues of her body not attacked by lupus inflammation did not have these cells present. Another study found that the kidneys of women affected by lupus nephritis (inflammation of the kidneys) contained male chimeric cells twice as often as kidneys not affected with lupus nephritis. This is an important focus for future research.

### KEY POINTS TO REMEMBER

1. As with other autoimmune diseases, SLE occurs in people who are born with the genes that predispose them to getting the disease. In other words, they get these genes from their parents, but having these genes alone does not necessarily mean they will develop SLE.

2. Numerous genes can cause SLE. The more of these genes someone is born with, the higher the chances that person has of developing SLE.

3. Some ethnic groups, such as African Americans, have an increased risk of developing SLE because they harbor more lupus-causing genes.

4. Certain environmental triggers may interact with these genes to turn them on and cause SLE to occur. These possible triggers include sun exposure, occupational exposure to silica (such as working with pottery and ceramics), some medications, infections (such as Epstein Barr virus and parvovirus), eating alfalfa sprouts, having low vitamin D levels, and smoking tobacco.

5. Women are much more likely to develop SLE compared to men due to the influence of sex hormones on the immune system and the presence of some genes that can cause SLE being located on the X-chromosome.

6. Microchimerism occurs when fetal cells pass through the placenta and persist in the mother's body. It is an interesting but unproven cause of SLE and other autoimmune diseases.

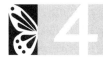

# The Meaning of All Those Test Results

### What Does Syphilis Have to Do with Lupus?

Syphilis, which is a sexually transmitted disease, does not cause lupus, nor is lupus in any way related to syphilis infection. However, the story of syphilis and the story of systemic lupus erythematosus do have interesting, intersecting paths.

From the 1500s to the 1900s, syphilis was one of the most devastating diseases in the world. Syphilis is an infectious disease that spreads by sexual contact. In its more advanced stages, it can kill the infected person by damaging the brain, spinal cord, heart, and aorta (the large blood vessel coming out of the heart). Doctors discovered the bacterium that causes syphilis, *Treponema pallidum*, in 1905. Soon after the identification of *T. pallidum*, they began to look for a way to diagnose syphilis more accurately and at earlier stages.

August Paul von Wassermann was a physician and scientist specializing in bacteria at the Robert Koch Institute of Infectious Diseases in Berlin, Germany, at the turn of the twentieth century. He had an interest in developing tests to diagnose infectious diseases. He and a German dermatologist, Albert Neisser, found that when blood serum (the clear yellow part of blood with the blood cells removed) of people who had syphilis was added to a mixture of beef heart extract, animal blood serum, and red blood cells, the blood cells would clump together (precipitate). They noted that the serum from people who had more severe infections formed the largest amounts of precipitate. This observation became the basis for developing the first available lab test for syphilis. They reported their findings in 1906, and doctors named the exam the Wassermann test, after its primary developer.

Although the test would become invaluable in detecting syphilis at an earlier and more treatable stage, doctors soon noted that people who had syphilis were not the only ones with a positive Wassermann test. In fact, in 1910, just four years after its discovery, a doctor reported the case of a person who had lupus who had a positive Wassermann test for syphilis, but did not have any signs of syphilis. In medical terminology, a "false positive test" means that someone is positive for a particular medical test but does not actually have the disease. After 1910, doctors noted that people who had lupus with a false positive syphilis test were not uncommon. Better tests for syphilis, such as the VDRL and RPR tests, have replaced the Wassermann test; false positive tests occur in approximately 30% of people who have SLE.

Having syphilis has always carried a very negative connotation since it is a sexually transmitted disease. Unfortunately, over the past century, many people who had SLE were wrongly accused of having syphilis because SLE causes false positive syphilis tests, and this subjected them to undue hardship and discrimination. For example, Dr. John Haserick, a physician in Ohio, described a 25-year-old unmarried woman who tested positive for syphilis in 1941 during her premarital examination (at that time, syphilis testing was required before getting married). She denied any previous sexual encounters, but nonetheless her marriage was postponed, undoubtedly by her upset fiancé. She later became a recluse. Doctors gave her 101 drug injections for the "treatment" of syphilis from 1942 through 1944. Doctors at the Cleveland Clinic followed her; a thorough exam showed that she was indeed a virgin. She became ill in 1948 with fevers, fatigue, and abdominal cramps. She later died at her home in 1949 after suffering from jaundice, kidney disease, and serositis due to SLE. Who knows how many other unfortunate people have suffered over the years when lupus caused a false positive syphilis test?

The Medical Clinic of the Johns Hopkins University and Hospital in Baltimore, Maryland, began to follow a group of patients who had false positive syphilis tests in the 1930s through the 1950s and noted that 6.7% of their 210 patients with false positive syphilis tests had definite SLE. They reported their findings in 1955 and described the characteristics of some of these SLE patients. Looking back at that paper, it is interesting that they noted recurrent blood clots, called deep venous thrombosis, in a couple of patients. At that time, doctors considered blood clots "an uncommon manifestation of SLE." In addition, one of these patients also had migraine headaches and low platelet counts. Another patient had recurrent miscarriages and eventually had a stroke. Recurrent blood clots, migraine headaches, low platelet counts, recurrent miscarriages, and strokes are now recognized as being part of a complication of SLE called the antiphospholipid syndrome (discussed in chapters 9, 18, and 41), which can occur in some people who have SLE who have a false positive RPR or VDRL syphilis test.

Recall that in chapter 1 I discussed how a false positive syphilis test helps diagnose people who have SLE. Now you can see how it may help identify those who may be at increased risk for particular problems, such as developing blood clots or having recurrent miscarriages due to the antiphospholipid syndrome. People newly diagnosed with SLE soon realize that it is essential to have blood and urine tests done on a regular basis to monitor their illness. The number of individual tests performed can be daunting, and your doctor will most likely not have the time to go over the results of all these tests at every visit. I think it is important for you to be able to understand what the results of many of these tests may or may not mean to have a better understanding of how you are doing. The purpose of this chapter is to give you some of the details about these test results.

One word of caution: the interpretation of any test result depends on what is going on in a particular person. Books written for laypersons such as this cannot go into all the detail that is required to interpret test results accurately in the same way that your doctor can or that a medical textbook can do. You should use this book as a guide to help you understand your own test results, but your physician should be the final authority in interpreting what your test results mean in your particular case.

. . . .

This chapter explains the tests that doctors use to diagnose and follow the course of SLE. It can be helpful for people who have lupus to understand what their test results may or may not mean. Some lab results can be important in pointing out potential problems they may face with their lupus, while other abnormalities may not be important at all. This chapter begins with those tests that doctors use most often to follow people with lupus on a regular basis. It then covers those tests that doctors usually use initially during the workup of a person who has lupus or whenever particular problems come up over time. Every laboratory has different normal values for lab tests; therefore, I do not discuss what is considered normal for most of the lab tests. The normal values for any particular test usually appear on the lab results. In addition, I do not cover every section of a test, but only the parts that are most important for people who have SLE to understand in relation to their disease.

Some lab tests are performed primarily to help make the diagnosis of SLE (table 4.1) and to make sure that other disorders mimicking SLE are not present. These include tests such as antinuclear antibody (ANA), anti-Smith antibody, rheumatoid factor (RF), and cyclic citrullinated peptide antibody (all discussed below). In fact, doctors use the vast majority of the tests listed below under "Immunological Tests" for initial diagnostic purposes instead of for following disease activity. Doctors use other labs frequently to monitor disease activity and to see how SLE is responding to treatment (table 4.2). These include the urinalysis, complete blood cell count (CBC), C3 and C4 complement levels, chemistry panel, and anti-double-stranded DNA (anti-ds DNA) levels. Doctors also use some tests to follow the effects of medications for treating SLE to ensure that they cause no side effects. These most commonly include a CBC, chemistry panel, and urinalysis.

You do not need to read this chapter from beginning to end unless you are motivated to do so and driven to learn as much as you can. You should read the section on how to collect a urine sample properly, because people who have SLE usually need to give urine samples regularly. Other than that, you should use this chapter as a reference source. Whenever you notice any abnormal labs, look them up in this chapter so that you can get a good sense of what the results may or may not mean. You can usually tell if any of your labs are abnormal if you see "high" or "low" printed next to a lab in your lab results. You can also tell by comparing them to the expected normal values that appear under the label "reference range" or "normal." You can use the index at the back of this book to find where a particular test is located in this chapter more quickly. This chapter has several sections, covering urine tests (urinalysis, urine protein-to-creatinine ratio, and the twenty-four-hour urine test) and blood tests (metabolic panel, complete blood cell counts, miscellaneous tests, and immunological tests).

You may also want to consider asking your doctor what antibodies were positive during the workup of your lupus and look them up under the "Immunological Tests" section at the end of this chapter. This could give you some additional clues as to what kinds of problems you may or may not be at increased risk for with your SLE. Different laboratories often have slightly different names for the same tests. I have included alternate names for tests in parentheses after test names.

**Table 4.1** Lab Tests Most Helpful in Making a Diagnosis of SLE

| Test | How It Is Helpful |
|---|---|
| Urinalysis | Presence of cellular casts, elevated protein, or increased RBCs or WBCs could mean inflammation of kidneys (nephritis) |
| Complete blood count (CBC) | |
| WBCs | May be decreased in SLE |
| Hemoglobin | May be decreased in SLE |
| Platelets | May be decreased in SLE |
| Lymphocyte count | May be decreased in SLE |
| Antinuclear antibody | Positive in almost all people who have SLE |
| Anti-ds DNA antibody | Positive in 40% to 80% of people who have SLE; increased risk of kidney inflammation (nephritis); may fluctuate with disease activity; not commonly found in people who do not have SLE |
| Anti-Smith antibody | Positive in 15% to 30% of people who have SLE; rare in people who do not have SLE |
| Antiphospholipid antibodies (lupus anticoagulant, anticardiolipin antibodies, anti-beta-2 glyco-protein I, and false positive tests for syphilis, e.g., RPR and VDRL) | Present in about 50% of people who have SLE; increases risk for blood clots and miscarriages |
| C3, C4, and CH50 complement levels | May be decreased in people who have SLE; may fluctuate with disease activity; low C3 or C4 may be due to a genetic deficiency in complement causing SLE |
| Coombs' antibody | May be positive in people who have SLE; increases risk of hemolytic anemia (see explanation later in this chapter) |
| Ribosomal-P antibody | Only found in people who have SLE |

## The Tests Performed on Urine

### Urinalysis

*How to Do It.* You urinate into a cup provided by the laboratory. If the doctor is going to use the sample to look for a possible infection, then she or he will order a urine culture and will ask you to urinate into a sterile cup with a lid on top of it. In this case, it is important to make sure that the specimen has not been contaminated by bacteria from sources other than the bladder and kidneys. For example, bacteria from the fingers or from the skin surrounding the urethra (the tube through which urine flows out of the body) could potentially contaminate the specimen if not collected correctly. There can even be bacteria inside the urethra itself, which could also contaminate the urine sample as well. Therefore, the doctor will ask you to obtain a "clean catch midstream" sample of urine. To do this, you first wash your hands. Then carefully remove the lid from the cup (making sure not to touch the inside of the cup or the inside of the lid) and lay the lid with the inside section facing up. Place the cup on an easy-to-reach surface. Then you pull apart the labia if you are female or retract the foreskin if you are a male with one hand. Using your other hand, you wipe the urethra three times with three sterile wipes (front to back if you are a female). Continue to keep the labia or foreskin retracted with one hand and grab the cup with the other hand. You then urinate the first couple of seconds into the toilet (this gets rid of any bacteria that may have been in the urethra), and then you urinate into the cup to the fill line. It is important

Table 4.2  Lab Tests Most Helpful in Following Disease Activity in SLE

| Test | How It Is Helpful |
| --- | --- |
| Urinalysis | Presence of cellular casts, elevated protein, or or increased RBCs or WBCs could mean inflammation of kidneys (nephritis). These should improve during successful treatment of nephritis. |
| Random urine protein/ creatinine | Elevated level could mean kidney inflammation (nephritis). This level should decrease with successful treatment. |
| Complete blood cell count (CBC) | |
| WBC | May be decreased when SLE is active. |
| Hemoglobin | May be decreased when SLE is active; often improves when SLE responds to treatment. Doctor should rule out causes other than SLE (such as iron deficiency). |
| Platelets | May be decreased when SLE is active; should improve when SLE responds to treatment. |
| Lymphocyte count | May be decreased in SLE. |
| Anti-ds DNA antibody | May increase during increased SLE activity and decrease with successful treatment. Does not change with disease activity in some people. |
| C3, C4 complement levels | May decrease during increased SLE activity and improve with successful treatment. Levels do not change with disease activity in some people. |

that you empty the last part of your urine into the toilet again (which is the reason for the term "midstream"). You should immediately put the lid securely on the cup, making sure not to touch the inside of the lid or cup. If the doctor will not be doing a urine culture, you do not have to use a sterile cup. You should follow this same procedure if your doctor requests a regular urine sample without a culture added. You will probably get a non-sterile cup without a lid. Just make sure not to touch anywhere inside the cup with your fingers when you collect the urine sample.

*How to Find It on Your Lab Results Slip.* Look for "urinalysis," "macroscopic urinalysis," and/or "microscopic urinalysis."

*What It Looks For.* The urinalysis usually has two major parts. The first part (called the macroscopic urinalysis by some labs) uses a thin slip of test paper called a dipstick. The lab technician dips it into the urine and then takes it out and observes it. The dipstick has multiple small sections that change color to signify a particular result. These include color, character (such as clear), specific gravity, pH, urine protein, urine glucose, urine ketones, occult blood, urobilinogen, urine bilirubin, leukoesterase, and nitrite. I discuss only protein, urine glucose, occult blood, leukoesterase, and nitrite, as these are often the most important to evaluate when assessing a person who has SLE.

The second major part of the urinalysis is the microscopic urinalysis. Doctors do not always order this test since it requires substantially more work in the laboratory and is not always necessary for purposes of diagnosis. The laboratory technician places a drop of urine on a slide and evaluates it under the microscope (hence "microscopic") to see if there are any increased numbers of cells (red blood cells, white blood cells, or epithelial cells) or other materials, such as bacteria, yeast, crystals, or casts.

Doctors primarily use urinalysis in SLE patients to see if there is any evidence of nephritis (inflammation of the kidneys). They also use it to monitor patients with known nephritis to see how they are responding to therapy. In addition, the test can potentially pick up other problems, such as urinary tract infections, kidney stones, side effects of medicines, or cancer of the kidneys or bladder.

## Urine Macroscopic Exam

*Urine Protein.* There are several ways to measure urine protein. The most common one is the dipstick method. I discuss this test here. Normally, very little protein passes through the kidneys into the urine. The result is reported as either negative, trace (or 10 mg/dl), 1+ (30 mg/dl), 2+ (100 mg/dl), 3+ (300 mg/dl), or 4+ (> 2,000 mg/dl). A normal result would be either "negative" or "trace." A result of 1+ may or may not be important, but 2+ or higher usually means that something is causing too much protein in the urine.

Your doctor may order a urine protein-to-creatinine ratio. This test gives a more accurate measurement of how much protein is leaking into the urine to see if there is truly a problem going on. Doctors can also follow it over time to see if a patient who has known kidney disease improves or worsens. For example, a person with "trace" or "negative" on the dipstick urinalysis could have this test done to see if the result is actually abnormal or not. If the protein-to-creatinine ratio is normal, then the urine protein result is normal. If the result is above the upper limits of the normal range, then there is too much protein in the urine. (You will see "creatinine" many times in this chapter in the discussion of the kidney tests. To learn about what creatinine is, look under "Creatinine" in the section "The Tests Performed on Blood" later in this chapter.)

If there is an excessive amount of protein in the urine (called proteinuria), then your physician will most likely investigate this further to find out the cause. He may order a twenty-four-hour urine collection or even a kidney biopsy to see if there is any evidence of lupus nephritis.

The vast majority of people who have lupus nephritis have an elevated amount of urine protein. This is the primary reason doctors routinely check the urine of patients who have SLE during office visits. Besides lupus nephritis, there are other potential causes of excessive protein in the urine. One would be an increased amount of blood in the urine because red blood cells contain a lot of protein. Sometimes medications taken by people who have lupus can also cause proteinuria, such as non-steroidal anti-inflammatory drugs (like ibuprofen and naproxen). Or a person could have another type of kidney problem such as kidney disease due to diabetes or high blood pressure. Increased urine protein can also be due to a urinary tract infection.

There are also some benign causes of increased urine protein. For example, it can increase after exercise, due to fever, or during pregnancy. False positives can also occur; this is best for your doctor to figure out.

*Urine Glucose.* Glucose generally does not pass into the urine unless the blood glucose levels are greater than 180 mg/dL. This mainly occurs in people who have diabetes and is particularly of concern in lupus patients who take steroids such as prednisone as they are at increased risk of developing diabetes.

*Blood (Occult Blood).* This is a screening test for blood, but it is not highly specific and false positives can occur. If it is positive it is usually followed up by a microscopic exam, where the lab technician will examine the urine under a microscope to see if there are truly too many red blood cells in the urine or not. This result appears in the "urine microscopic exam" section. Blood in the urine can be due to menstruation, urinary tract infections, or kidney stones. However, other possible causes include lupus nephritis, other causes of kidney disease, and even cancer of the kidneys or bladder, so further evaluation is always important.

*Leukoesterase.* This is a screening test to see if there may be an increase in white blood cells in the urine. It does this by measuring an enzyme called leukoesterase that white blood cells secrete. If the level of this enzyme is elevated, a microscopic exam is often done to see if there is truly an increase in white blood cells or not. Elevated leukoesterase levels could be due to a urinary tract infection, which is the most common cause. Leukoesterase can also be elevated in other conditions, such as lupus nephritis and other kidney diseases. If mucus or cells from the surrounding skin contaminate the urine, which can occur with improper cleaning prior to sample collection, there could also be a false positive.

*Nitrite.* The test for nitrite can be positive if there are bacteria in the urine, which can be either due to a urinary tract infection or due to contamination from improper cleaning when collecting the urine sample.

### Urine Microscopic Exam

*RBC (Red Blood Cells).* An elevation of red blood cells in the urine can be due to menstruation (blood getting into the urine by contamination from the surrounding vaginal tissues), urinary tract infection, or kidney stones. Lupus nephritis, other kidney diseases, and kidney or bladder cancer can also cause an increase; any increase in RBCs is a reason for further investigation.

*WBC (White Blood Cells).* An elevation of white blood cells in the urine can be due to a urinary tract infection (UTI), lupus nephritis, or other kidney diseases. It can also be due to contamination from surrounding tissues if not cleaned properly when collecting the urine sample.

*Squamous Epithelial Cells.* If there is an increase in squamous epithelial cells, this usually means that the patient did not clean the skin properly and it contaminated the urine sample. This can result in falsely elevated RBC, WBC, and bacteria counts in the sample.

*Bacteria.* Bacteria should not be present in a properly collected specimen of urine. If there is an increased number of squamous epithelial cells, then the specimen collection was not performed properly, and the contamination by skin and bacteria that surrounds the urethra makes the results of the urinalysis untrustworthy. In fact, contamination due to improperly collected urine is the most common cause of bacteria in a urine sample and is not clinically important. If there is truly an increased amount of bacteria (not due to contamination), it may or may not mean that you have a urinary tract infection (UTI). If you have symptoms of a urinary tract infection, such as pain while urinating, discomfort in the lower part of the abdomen, increased frequency in urinating, the urge to urinate more than usual, or back pain with fever, then you most likely have a UTI and should be placed on antibiotic therapy. "Asymptomatic bacteriuria" is the term used to describe the presence of bacteria in the urine without these symptoms. Doctors usually do not treat it, because it is common for women to have some bacteria in their urinary tract—this usually does not cause an actual infection. In addition, giving antibiotics in this instance increases the chances of causing bacteria to become resistant to antibiotics. However, it is better to treat people who have asymptomatic bacteriuria if they are pregnant or if they are going to undergo bladder, kidney, or other urinary tract surgeries. Many physicians treat their patients who are immunosuppressed if they have asymptomatic bacteriuria as they may be at greater risk of developing an actual UTI. So a doctor may treat SLE patients who are on medications such as methotrexate, prednisone, mycophenolate, and azathioprine with antibiotics if they have bacteria in their urine but do not have symptoms of a UTI.

*Casts.* The kidneys have a large number of tiny tubes, called tubules, through which urine flows before it goes into the ureters (which are the larger tubes that connect the kidneys to the bladder). Sometimes urine can clump up in these tiny tubules, then break free and flow into the ureters along with the rest of the urine. The term for these microscopic cigar-shaped (or cylindrical) clumps is "casts." Appearance under the microscope determines the type of cast. Hyaline casts are common and are not indicative of a kidney disease. However, red cell casts, white cell casts, epithelial casts, fatty casts, granular casts, waxy casts, and broad casts can all be present in people who have various forms of kidney disease, including lupus nephritis.

## Urine Protein-to-Creatinine Ratio (Protein/G Creat, Protein/Creat Ratio)

*How Doctors Do It.* The urine sample for the urine protein-to-creatinine ratio test goes through a machine that measures the concentration of protein and creatinine, and then divides the protein by the creatinine to obtain the ratio. This gives a good estimation as to whether the kidneys are secreting too much protein or not and by how much. It is much more accurate than the protein measured on the dipstick. The higher the number above normal, the more protein is being filtered through the kidneys daily.

*What It Looks For.* This test checks to see whether there is too much protein being filtered through the kidneys. Many rheumatologists order this test for SLE patients at most, if not all, office visits to make sure that they do not have nephritis. The results of the protein concentration (labeled as protein, urine) and creatinine concentration (labeled as creatinine, urine) appear separately. These two values are not helpful by themselves as they can vary greatly depending on whether you may have been drinking a lot of fluids that day (the urine will be diluted) or may have been a little dehydrated (the urine will be concentrated). Only pay attention to the results of the actual protein-to-creatinine ratio result. Sometimes the ratio does not appear on the lab slip and your physician must calculate it.

The causes of an increased protein-to-creatinine ratio are the same as for macroscopic urine protein previously discussed. It is especially very helpful to follow people who have kidney disease over time to see if they are responding to treatment or not.

## Twenty-Four-Hour Urine

*How to Do It.* You must collect a twenty-four-hour urine properly and meticulously. If done correctly, it is the most accurate way to measure how much protein is leaking through the kidneys. You should choose a day when you can most easily collect all of your urine as you must collect every drop of urine during a twenty-four-hour period. Choosing a day when you can stay home all day tends to be the best way to ensure this. On the morning of your collection, you should empty your first urine void into the toilet, and mark down the time when you do this. Then collect every drop of urine for the rest of the day. Store the plastic jug as directed by your laboratory (either at room temperature or in the refrigerator). If you have a bowel movement, you must also collect the urine that comes at the same time. Try not to allow any feces into the urine jug, but if this happens, leave them in the urine jug and do not try to remove them. When you get up the following morning, try to urinate into the jug within ten minutes of the time you marked down the day before. For example, if you marked down 6:55 AM, you should collect the last sample between 6:45 AM and 7:05 AM. If you need to urinate an hour or so before that time, collect that urine; then drink a full glass of water or more to ensure you can urinate within ten minutes of the marked time. If you need to urinate within twenty minutes of that time, try to hold it until it is time to do so. Try to return the jug to the laboratory within a day or two of the collection, the sooner the better. Also, if you have a creatinine clearance ordered, you will need to give a sample of blood at the same time you drop off your urine collection.

### Twenty-Four-Hour Urine Protein

*What It Looks For.* This is the most accurate way to measure how much protein is being filtered through the kidneys. It is valuable in trying to classify what type of kidney disease the person has, and can be very helpful in following how someone responds to treatment.

### Twenty-Four-Hour Urine Creatinine Clearance

*What It Looks For.* This is a way of measuring how well the kidneys are actually functioning (or how well the kidneys are filtering wastes out of the blood on a daily basis). The medical term for measuring kidney function is the "glomerular filtration rate" (GFR). Calculating the creatinine clearance on a twenty-four-hour urine collection is one way to measure kidney function (or GFR) in a routine clinical setting. The GFR can also be estimated (eGFR) by measuring the serum creatinine in the blood, which I discuss later in this chapter. The higher the creatinine clearance result, the better the kidneys are functioning. For example, a creatinine clearance (or GFR) of greater than 90 mL/min is considered normal. Anything less than 90 mL/min signifies that the kidneys are not functioning correctly. Complete kidney failure, also called end-stage renal disease, occurs when the level is below 10 mL/min to 15 mL/min. Dialysis is then required to filter wastes out from the blood mechanically. The twenty-four-hour urine creatinine clearance is very useful in seeing if someone has any degree of kidney failure, and also in determining how well a person who has kidney disease is responding to treatment.

## The Tests Performed on Blood

### Metabolic Panel (Chemistry Panel, BMP, or CMP)

*How Doctors Do It.* A lab technician draws blood from a vein and places it in a red top tube that has a vacuum in it (called a Vacutainer). It includes multiple tests that give your doctor important information about the kidneys, liver, electrolytes, blood sugar, acidity, and protein levels. I list only those tests that I feel are most important for people who have SLE.

*Glucose.* Glucose is a very important sugar used by the body for energy. However, too high of a glucose level may indicate a disease called diabetes mellitus. This is of particular concern in people who have SLE for a couple of reasons. First, many people who have SLE are treated with steroids such as prednisone that can cause diabetes or worsen existing diabetes. Second, people who have SLE are at increased risk of developing heart attacks, hardening of the arteries, and strokes. Having diabetes can cause these processes to occur at an even earlier age compared to someone who does not have diabetes. If the glucose level is normal, there is nothing to worry about. If it is increased, you should have blood drawn again after fasting for eight hours because the glucose may be artificially elevated if you consumed any food or beverage before the test. If asked to fast for your labs, you should not eat or drink anything, except water, for about eight hours. A common recommendation is not to consume anything except water after having dinner or supper the night before, then getting your labs done first thing the following morning.

The glucose level can be useful for making a diagnosis of diabetes. Currently, a person is considered to have diabetes if the fasting glucose level is 126 mg/dL or higher. A person is considered to have impaired fasting glucose (also called non-diabetic hyperglycemia and borderline diabetes) if the level is 100 mg/dL to 125 mg/dL. In addition, your doctor can diagnose diabetes if the glucose level is 200 mg/dL or higher even if you were not fasting because even after eating, it is not normal for the glucose to get that high. Since glucose tests can fluctuate a lot from day to day, the American Diabetes Association recommends that doctors confirm the test as abnormal on two different days before a making a diagnosis of diabetes. If you are diagnosed with diabetes, it is imperative that you work very closely with your primary care provider or a diabetes expert (called an endocrinologist) on diet, exercise, and medications as indicated to get your diabetes under the best control possible to decrease your risk of complications.

*BUN (Blood Urea Nitrogen).* Urea nitrogen is a waste product of the body, and it can be elevated due to its not being excreted from the body properly due to kidney disease, dehydration, the use of fluid pills (diuretics), congestive heart failure, or severe liver disease. However, it can also be elevated simply from eating a high-protein diet, after trauma, or even from taking steroids like prednisone. Therefore, by itself, it is not really a very useful test. It is most helpful if it is used in combination with creatinine and eGFR (estimated glomerular filtration rate), discussed below. If there is decreased kidney function, then it is best to use the BUN-to-creatinine ratio discussed below instead of the BUN by itself.

*Creatinine (Serum Creatinine or Scr).* Creatinine is a waste product that comes from the muscles in the body and from meat we ingest, after which the kidneys excrete it into the urine. If the kidneys do not function normally, then the level of creatinine will increase in the blood. Measuring the level of creatinine in the blood is therefore one of the easiest ways to estimate how well the kidneys are functioning. If it is too high, then the person's kidneys are not working normally at filtering wastes from the blood and the person may have kidney disease or other potential problems, such as dehydration, heart failure, or liver failure. The person may be on diuretics. Measuring creatinine by itself is not an accurate way for determining kidney function. Creatinine levels can vary due to things such as how muscular the person is, age, race, and gender. To try to correct for some of these variables, it is better to use the estimated glomerular filtration (eGFR) discussed below instead of relying on the creatinine level by itself.

*BUN-to-Creatinine Ratio (BUN:Scr).* The BUN can be helpful in a person who has decreased kidney function (as determined by the eGFR, discussed below). It is most useful when assessed in relation to the serum creatinine level—the term for this is the "BUN-to-creatinine ratio." Normally, this ratio should be less than 20:1. If someone has decreased kidney function (as determined by an elevated eGFR), and if the BUN-to-creatinine ratio is greater than 20:1, there could be certain factors that are decreasing blood flow to the kidneys, such as dehydration, the use of diuretics ("fluid pills"), congestive heart failure, or severe liver disease. Another possibility for an increase in this ratio is if the person has significantly decreased muscle mass. This scenario is particularly common in people as they get older.

*eGFR.* The medical term for measuring kidney function is "glomerular filtration rate" or "GFR." Your doctor can make a close estimate by taking the serum creatinine and using it in a mathematical equation that includes age, gender, and race. It is therefore more accurate than just using the serum creatinine by itself. It certainly is not perfect, and can be inaccurate in some people, such as those who are obese or who are of Asian descent. The eGFR should be 60 mL/min or greater. If it is less than 60 mL/min, then the kidneys are not properly filtering the blood, and there may possibly be some kidney damage. GFR is very important to ensure there is no evidence of kidney damage, which can occur due to many possibilities, including lupus nephritis. In addition, some medicines, such as non-steroidal anti-inflammatory drugs, which are used to treat pain, should not be used in people who do not have normal kidney function. If the eGFR is less than 60 mL/min for three months or longer, then that person has chronic kidney disease. If the eGFR is less than 15 mL/min, then she has kidney failure and may need dialysis.

*Albumin.* Albumin is an important protein that the liver manufactures, and it is the main protein found in the blood. Most of the time, this blood test is not very helpful. Studies have shown that many times it can be lower than normal and be of no clinical significance. Chronic inflammation can cause decreased albumin levels and is therefore a common reason for low albumin levels in people who have SLE. However, a markedly low albumin level could also be due to severe liver disease (due to the liver not being able to make enough albumin), severe kidney disease (where too much albumin leaks out of the blood and into the urine), or severe malnutrition. Doctors recommend that people who take a medication called methotrexate have their albumin levels monitored regularly along with the ALT level to make sure that they do not have any liver problems from the methotrexate (in which case the albumin level could be low). A high albumin level is usually due to dehydration.

*AST (SGOT).* AST (SGOT), along with alkaline phosphatase, ALT, and bilirubin, are grouped under the term "liver function tests." AST is an enzyme found in multiple parts of the body, especially the liver, muscles, the heart, the pancreas, and red blood cells. Lower than normal levels in the blood are not significant. Elevated levels can potentially be due to multiple reasons, including liver problems, muscle disease, heart problems, and hemolytic anemia. AST along with ALT are important blood tests often used to monitor for any potential liver problems. AST is clinically significant when elevated in conjunction with an elevated ALT level. These tests are especially helpful in monitoring people who are on certain medications that can potentially affect the liver, such as methotrexate, azathioprine, leflunomide, and non-steroidal anti-inflammatory drugs. Mild elevations are often tolerated, but values that are two to three times over the upper limits of normal usually require a change in therapy (such as lowering the dose of the medicine or stopping it). Another compounding issue is that problems with muscle can also cause elevated AST and ALT levels. Therefore, a doctor will often order muscle enzyme tests, such as CPK and aldolase, if AST and ALT are elevated to see if they are coming from the muscles instead of from the liver. It is not uncommon to have mildly elevated AST levels without a definite cause when the ALT is normal.

*Alkaline Phosphatase.* This is another enzyme also found in many parts of the body. However, cells of the bones and liver produce the largest amounts in the body. Slightly elevated levels are very common and usually are not clinically important. However, if the level is very high, doctors can order additional blood tests to figure out if the elevation is coming from the bones or from the liver. Possible causes of liver alkaline phosphatase elevations include medication effects, gallstones, other liver problems such as fatty liver, and even cancer of the liver or pancreas. Causes of bone elevations include vitamin D deficiency, bone injury, Paget's disease of the bone, as well as other bone problems.

*ALT (SGPT).* As mentioned above under AST, this test is often used in conjunction with the AST to determine whether there are any problems with the liver or muscles.

*Bilirubin, Total.* Your body produces bilirubin when the body breaks down the red blood cells when they reach the end of their useful lifespan. The liver secretes bilirubin into bile and excretes the bile via the gallbladder into the intestines where it eventually leaves the body mixed with the feces. If there is a liver problem that prevents this excretion of the bile, then the blood bilirubin level may increase. If it becomes very high, then bilirubin will cause a yellowish coloration of the skin and whites of the eyes (called jaundice). However, there are other causes of elevated bilirubin levels. One example is hemolytic anemia, which can occur in some people who have lupus. Hemolytic anemia is due to the destruction of an excessive number of red blood cells by the immune system of the body. This causes an excessive release of hemoglobin into the blood, which is then converted into bilirubin.

## Complete Blood Cell Count (CBC)

*How Doctors Do It.* A lab technician will draw blood from a vein and place it into a purple top tube that has a vacuum in it (called a Vacutainer). A CBC is composed of multiple tests that give your doctor important information about your blood counts. I list only those tests that I feel are most important for people who have SLE.

There are three major types of blood cells: white blood cells, red blood cells, and platelets. All three of these can be affected by SLE or by the medications used to treat SLE, and therefore are usually monitored regularly.

*White Blood Cells (WBC).* The medical term for white blood cells is "leukocytes." A lower than normal level of WBCs is called leukopenia. Leukopenia is one of the problems that can happen in SLE and is one of the American College of Rheumatology's classification criteria for SLE (see chapter 1). In addition to helping make a diagnosis of SLE, the WBC level can also potentially fluctuate with disease activity in some people who have SLE. A dropping white blood cell count could mean that there is more lupus activity, or it could also be a sign of other problems, such as a side effect from a medication. If a person who has SLE has a low white blood cell count as a part of SLE, occasionally it can improve with treatment; however, most patients' white blood cell counts do not improve significantly.

One of the most important reasons for following the white blood cell count is to ensure that a person is not developing a side effect from a medication. For example, many of the medicines used to treat SLE, such as methotrexate, azathioprine, mycophenolate, and rarely hydroxychloroquine, can cause the white blood cell count to drop. If the level becomes too low, then there is an increased risk for infections. If the WBC count is lower due to a medicine, often the doctor will lower the dose of the offending medicine, or even stop it to try to prevent an infection. An elevated white blood cell count in people who have SLE is most commonly due either to the effects of steroids (such as prednisone) or due to infection.

The WBC count includes the quantity of all white blood cells. However, there are actually several different types of white blood cells. The CBC also measures these. They include neutrophils (also called granulocytes), lymphocytes, monocytes, basophils, and eosinophils. The first two are the more important ones that doctors follow in their SLE patients and I discuss them below.

*Hemoglobin (HGB or Hb).* Hemoglobin is a protein found in red blood cells. It is very important in carrying oxygen to the cells and tissues of the body by way of the bloodstream. The laboratory measures its concentration in the blood and reports it as the hemoglobin. The term for a lower-than-normal hemoglobin amount is "anemia." In general, doctors consider hemoglobin values lower than 13 g/dL to 14 g/dL in men and below 12 g/dL in women as anemia. However, these values do vary slightly depending on a number of factors—such as the laboratory, age, race, and whether the person is a smoker or lives at high altitudes. Mild anemia is very common in people who have SLE and generally is not treated. However, occasionally severe anemia may occur, which means that the cells of the body are not getting enough oxygen, which can cause fatigue, shortness of breath, and heart palpitations. There are many potential causes of anemia in people who have SLE and a discussion of this is in chapter 9. Higher than normal hemoglobin levels are generally not a concern in those who have SLE, and is most common in those who smoke cigarettes.

*Hematocrit (HCT, "crit").* Another way to check for and monitor anemia is the hematocrit, which measures the proportion of blood volume that is composed of red blood cells. Generally, doctors consider levels of less than 41% in men and less than 36% in women to be anemia. However, the hemoglobin measurement tends to be more accurate overall compared to the hematocrit. Therefore, I tend to prefer using the hemoglobin in assessing for anemia. However, there are physicians who use the hematocrit instead.

*MCV.* MCV stands for mean corpuscular volume, and is a measurement of the average size of the red blood cells. It is most useful in trying to figure out the cause of anemia. For example, a low MCV could be due to a deficiency in iron or possibly to a genetic cause of anemia (such as thalassemia, a blood disorder in which the body produces an abnormal form of hemoglobin). A high MCV, meaning that the red blood cells are on average larger than normal, could possibly be due to vitamin B-12 deficiency, folic acid deficiency, a response to medications such as methotrexate, low thyroid hormone (hypothyroidism), or excessive consumption of alcohol. The most common causes of anemia in people who have SLE are anemia of chronic disease (where the MCV is usually normal or less commonly lower than normal) due to inflammation, and iron deficiency anemia (where the MCV is lower than normal). Iron deficiency is common because many SLE patients are women who are still menstruating and therefore losing iron when they bleed with their menstrual cycles.

*Platelet Count.* Platelets (also called thrombocytes) are technically not really cells at all. True cells have a nucleus that contains DNA, the genetic code. Platelets are actually highly specialized fragments of cells and do not contain nuclei. They are very important for clotting, and keep us from bleeding. SLE can occasionally cause the platelet count to be lower than normal (called thrombocytopenia), and is one of the American College of Rheumatology's classification criteria for SLE (see chapter 1). The normal platelet count is generally about 140 $10^3/\mu L$ or higher. However, it is rare to have an actual bleeding problem due to low platelets unless the number is less than 30 X $10^3/\mu L$. Therefore, doctors tolerate values as low as 50 X $10^3/\mu L$ before considering therapy to try to raise the platelet count. The platelet count can be elevated due to various reasons, which include infections, other causes of inflammation, and iron deficiency anemia.

*Neutrophils (Absolute Neutrophil Count).* Neutrophils are white blood cells that are very important for fighting infections, especially bacteria. Some people who have SLE can have a low neutrophil count (called neutropenia) due to their lupus. Some medicines used to treat lupus can also affect the neutrophil count. If the neutrophil count becomes too low due to a medication, then it places the person at increased risk for infection, and the doctor may lower the dose of the medicine or stop it completely.

*Lymphocytes (Absolute Lymphocyte Count).* Lymphocytes are another type of WBC and include B-cells and T-cells that are very important components of the immune system. They identify foreign invaders of the body by recognizing their foreign proteins, called antigens (discussed in chapter 1), and help alert the rest of the immune system to fend them off. B-cells produce the antibodies of the immune system. Antibodies identify and attach to molecules called antigens (this helps the immune system identify foreign substances invading the body). The number of lymphocytes is commonly lower than normal in people who have SLE (called lymphopenia). In fact, it is the most commonly decreased white blood cell in lupus. It may or may not improve with treatment. Lymphopenia is also one of the American College of Rheumatology's classification criteria for SLE (see chapter 1).

## Miscellaneous Labs

*Aldolase.* Aldolase is an enzyme that appears in all cells of the body. However, the highest amounts are in muscles, the brain, and the liver. The test is mainly used in people who have SLE to determine if they have inflammation of the muscles (called myositis), in which case the level would be increased. Doctors use it along with other "muscle enzymes" such as CPK, LDH, myoglobin, AST, and ALT for this purpose. Doctors also use it to follow the treatment of myositis. If treatment is bringing the muscle inflammation under control, then the aldolase level should decrease over time.

*ALKPHOS.* See Alkaline Phosphatase under Metabolic Panel

*Calcitriol (1, 25 di-OH Vitamin D).* See Vitamin D, 1, 25-Dihydroxy

*Creatine Kinase (Creatine Phosphokinase, CK, and CPK).* Creatine kinase is an enzyme found in highest amounts in the major muscles of the body. Doctors consider it the most useful blood test to see if people who have SLE have myositis (inflammation of the muscles). People who have myositis typically have weakness of their arms and legs, have difficulty raising their arms up above their head, and have trouble standing up from a chair without using their hands and arms to help themselves up. In people who have myositis, the CPK level is usually elevated along with other muscle enzymes, such as aldolase, LDH, myoglobin, AST, and ALT. If someone does have myositis, it is helpful to follow the CPK with treatment as the CPK level should decrease if the treatment is working. CPK is also found in the heart and the brain, so it can also be elevated in people who have had a heart attack or a stroke. The amount of CPK in the blood is directly proportional to the amount of muscle in the body. Therefore, it is not unusual for muscular people or athletes to have a higher than normal CPK level and have nothing wrong with them.

*Creatine Phosphokinase.* See Creatine Kinase

*Creatinine, Urine.* See Urine Protein-to-Creatinine Ratio under Urine Tests

*Erythrocyte Sedimentation Rate (Sedimentation Rate, Sed Rate; ESR, Westergren).* The erythrocyte sedimentation rate is a test doctors most commonly use to check for inflammation. Most people who have active SLE have an elevated ESR; however, many do not. Some SLE patients who have no active disease can also have an elevated ESR for no apparent reason. It is most helpful to use in people who develop an elevated ESR during times of disease activity and a normal ESR during periods of good disease control. ESR can be elevated due to reasons other than inflammation, such as anemia, older age, being female, and being pregnant.

*ESR.* See Erythrocyte Sedimentation Rate

*Folate, Hemolysate (Folate, Serum; Folate, Plasma; Folic Acid).* Serum folate levels can vary a lot based on recent dietary intake and not reflect the body's actual folate level. Serum folate levels are not as accurate in detecting deficiencies in folate compared to RBC folate levels; therefore, doctors usually use RBC folate levels instead. See Folate, RBC for more information.

*Folate, RBC.* Folate is another term for vitamin B-9. Leafy, green vegetables, fruits, and fortified grains and cereals are primary sources of folate. A deficiency in folate can cause a type of anemia where the red blood cells become larger than normal (called megaloblastic anemia). Therefore, doctors most commonly check it in people who have anemia. The cause is usually a diet deficient in folic acid–rich foods or alcoholism. However, in people who have SLE, a medication used to treat SLE called methotrexate may also cause it. Doctors treat it by having patients increase the dietary intake of foods rich in folic acid and take folic acid supplements. Folic acid deficiency can also cause a type of congenital abnormality called a neural tube defect, and therefore doctors recommend that pregnant women take the supplement as well.

*Folate, Serum.* See Folate, Hemolysate

THE MEANING OF ALL THOSE TEST RESULTS

*Haptoglobin.* Haptoglobin is a protein that binds to hemoglobin when destroyed red blood cells release their hemoglobin into the blood. The red blood cells could become damaged either because they are too old, are not needed anymore, or due to a condition called hemolytic anemia. Hemolytic anemia is an autoimmune form of anemia where the immune system attacks the red blood cells and destroys them. It occurs in approximately 10% of people with SLE and is one of the American College of Rheumatology's classification criteria for SLE (see chapter 1). With excessive destruction of red blood cells (hemolysis) due to hemolytic anemia, a larger than normal amount of hemoglobin is released into the bloodstream and binds to haptoglobin. Therefore, there is a smaller amount of measurable free haptoglobin. Typically, the haptoglobin level is very low and may be undetectable during periods of significant hemolytic anemia. This is the main reason doctors measure haptoglobin levels in SLE patients. However, the liver makes haptoglobin, and will produce extra haptoglobin during periods of increased body inflammation. Therefore, people who have SLE may have an elevated haptoglobin level during periods of more intense disease activity due to increased systemic inflammation.

*Hemoglobin $A_{1c}$ (Glycated Hemoglobin, Hemoglobin $A_1$, Hb $A_1$, and Hb A1c).* Hemoglobin $A_{1c}$ is a blood test used in the diagnosis and monitoring of diabetes. This is important to consider in some people who have SLE because steroids used to treat lupus can sometimes cause or worsen diabetes. Doctors regularly measure glucose (sugar) levels in the blood of lupus patients; however, glucose levels can fluctuate greatly depending on the amount of sugar present in a recent meal. Hemoglobin $A_{1c}$ is a measure of the average amount of glucose in the body over the preceding several months and does not vary due to recent changes in diet. Normally, the hemoglobin $A_{1c}$ level should be less than 6.0%. Doctors can diagnose diabetes if the hemoglobin $A_{1c}$ level is 6.5% or higher on two separate occasions.

*Parathyroid Hormone, Intact (Parathyroid Hormone, PTH).* The parathyroid glands are four very tiny glands that sit behind the much larger thyroid gland just below the Adam's apple in the neck. The parathyroid glands secrete PTH to help regulate how much calcium we have in our bodies. It stimulates the bones to release calcium into the bloodstream, the kidneys to hold on to calcium instead of secreting it into the urine, and the kidneys to make more active vitamin D, which in turn increases the absorption of calcium from the intestines. Low PTH levels are not common in people who have SLE.

High PTH levels can occur due to many possible reasons. One of the most common is vitamin D deficiency. Regular sun exposure is the primary source of vitamin D because the skin produces vitamin D in response to ultraviolet-B light. However, doctors ask lupus patients to stay out of the sun and to use sunscreen regularly because ultraviolet light causes lupus to become more active. Therefore, a high percentage of people who have lupus are deficient in vitamin D. More parathyroid hormone is produced during periods of vitamin D deficiency to try to make the kidneys produce more active vitamin D as well as to cause the release of more calcium from the bones to maintain normal blood calcium levels. If someone is vitamin D deficient and the doctor treats him or her with vitamin D supplements, the PTH level should lower as the vitamin D levels improve.

The PTH can be elevated in people who have lupus kidney disease. One complication of these elevated PTH levels due to kidney disease is that PTH continues to cause the release of more calcium from the bones until they become brittle (a condition called osteomalacia). Often kidney doctors (nephrologists) will use various therapies in kidney disease patients who have high PTH levels to lower those levels and to decrease the risk of brittle bones.

Another common cause of elevated PTH levels is a condition called primary hyperparathyroidism where an enlarged parathyroid gland is secreting too much PTH on its own. Sometimes doctors must remove the enlarged parathyroid gland surgically. This condition does not occur more often in people who have lupus compared to people who do not have lupus.

*Protein, Urine.* See Urine Protein-to-Creatinine Ratio under Urine Tests

*PTH.* See Parathyroid Hormone

*Reticulocyte Count.* Reticulocytes are immature red blood cells released regularly from the bone marrow; they then mature in the bloodstream. When there is destruction of too many red blood cells, as in hemolytic anemia, the bone marrow responds by releasing more reticulocytes into the bloodstream to take the place of the destroyed red blood cells. Therefore, a very high reticulocyte count can be useful in diagnosing hemolytic anemia in people who have SLE. Other forms of anemia, such as anemia of chronic disease, iron deficiency anemia, vitamin B-12 deficiency, or folic acid deficiency, do not cause as much of an increase in reticulocytes because the bone marrow has difficulty making more red blood cells because of these deficiencies and inflammation.

*Sedimentation Rate.* See Erythrocyte Sedimentation Rate

*Synovial Fluid Nucleated Cells (Synovial Fluid Polymorphonuclear Cells).* The synovial fluid is the fluid that occurs in the joints of the body. The joints are the hinges between bones that allow us to move. Some examples are the hips, knees, ankles, shoulders, and elbows. If someone develops inflammation of a joint (called arthritis), sometimes the joint will produce an excessive amount of fluid. It can be helpful for the doctor to remove the fluid to help the joint feel better. The doctor may send a sample to the lab for analysis to help figure out what is causing the arthritis. SLE can cause an inflammatory arthritis. Since inflammation involves white blood cells, the synovial fluid of joints affected by an inflammatory arthritis typically has an elevated white blood cell count (or synovial fluid nucleated cell count). This value is 2,000 cells/mL or higher when there is an inflammatory arthritis. Sometimes people who have lupus can have an arthritis not related to their lupus, such as osteoarthritis, which is a non-inflammatory arthritis due to aging or trauma. Its synovial fluid cell count should be less than 2,000 cells/mL. Therefore, in people who have both SLE and osteoarthritis, this lab test can be helpful in figuring out whether a swollen, painful joint is due to increased lupus activity or whether it is due to the unrelated osteoarthritis. Some people who have SLE can have severe kidney disease that may cause increased fluid to build up in the body, including the joints (a condition called nephrotic syndrome). This does not occur very often, but when it does, the joints can swell due to this excessive fluid. The synovial fluid cell count in this case would also be less than 2,000 cells/mL.

*Thiopurine Methyltransferase Activity (TPMT).* Doctors often obtain this test in people before prescribing azathioprine (Imuran). Azathioprine is an immunosuppressant commonly used to treat some people who have lupus. The body relies on an enzyme called thiopurine methyltransferase to break the medication down in the body (metabolize it). Approximately 11% of people make a lower than normal amount of TPMT, and therefore are at higher risk for side effects from azathioprine, such as bone marrow suppression (causing low blood cell counts) and liver damage. This test can be very helpful before a patient starts taking azathioprine to see if she or he is a good candidate for taking the medication. If the level is lower than normal, then a lower dose of azathioprine should be used (or not at all) and blood counts and liver enzymes should be monitored more closely.

*Thyroid-Stimulating Hormone (Thyrotropin; TSH, 3rd Generation).* The hypothalamus produces the thyroid-stimulating hormone and the pituitary gland releases it in the brain, where it enters the bloodstream; it then interacts with the thyroid gland in the neck and causes it to release thyroid hormones. TSH is the most sensitive and useful test in detecting an underactive thyroid (called hypothyroidism) or an overactive thyroid (called hyperthyroidism). About 10% of people who have SLE will have an abnormal functioning thyroid gland due to autoimmune thyroid disease; therefore, doctors commonly monitor TSH in people who have SLE. If TSH is abnormal, a doctor can then order other thyroid function tests (such as T3 and T4 levels) to determine whether the cause of the thyroid dysfunction is a problem with the thyroid gland itself or whether it is due to the brain releasing an abnormal amount of TSH. However, doctors should not rely solely on T3 and T4 levels, because they can be artificially elevated or decreased due to differences in proteins in the blood. The most common cause of an elevated TSH level is hypothyroidism due to Hashimoto's disease (an autoimmune thyroid disease). A decreased TSH level could be due to an overactive thyroid gland, also called hyperthyroidism (Graves' disease is one possible autoimmune cause of this). The TSH level is also very useful in monitoring treatment. For example, if a patient treated for hypothyroidism due to Hashimoto's disease has an elevated TSH level, then that person needs to be on a higher dose of thyroid hormone supplement medicine. If the same patient were to have a lower than normal TSH level, then she or he needs to be on a lower dose of thyroid supplement medication.

*TSH, 3rd Generation.* See Thyroid-Stimulating Hormone

*Vitamin B-12 (Cobalamin, B-12).* Doctors measure vitamin B-12 levels in people who have anemia or nerve problems because vitamin B-12 deficiency can cause both types of disorders. People who have SLE can potentially develop anemia (low red blood cell counts) and nerve problems, but it is always important to rule out other possible causes such as vitamin B-12 deficiency when these occur. The term for the anemia associated with vitamin B-12 deficiency is megaloblastic anemia (megaloblastic means that the red blood cells are larger than normal [recognized as an elevated MCV on the CBC]). Nerve damage from vitamin B-12 deficiency can cause tingling of the legs, muscle weakness, difficulty walking, memory loss, and irritability. Vitamin B-12 deficiency can also contribute to osteoporosis where the bones become more fragile with less calcium density in them. The most common reason for vitamin B-12 deficiency is decreased absorption due to disorders such as pernicious anemia, alcoholism, Sjögren's syndrome, gastritis, *Heliobacter pylori* infection, or having had gastric bypass surgery. Pernicious anemia is actually an autoimmune disorder where the immune system attacks the cells that are responsible for absorbing vitamin B-12 in the stomach. The elderly are at particularly increased risk for vitamin B-12 deficiency. Vitamin B-12 deficiency is rarely caused by a diet deficient in vitamin B-12, but it can be seen in vegetarians (since meat is the primary dietary source of vitamin B-12) or in pregnant women if they do not eat enough meat products or other vitamin B-12-rich foods. Low vitamin B-12 levels are easily treated by oral vitamin B-12 supplements, vitamin B-12 shots, or a nasal spray containing vitamin B-12. Sometimes lifelong therapy is required if the reason for the deficiency is not reversible (such as with pernicious anemia). If the vitamin B-12 level is borderline or low normal, someone can still possibly have a deficiency. In this case, the doctor may order a methylmalonic acid level and a homocysteine level, both of which would be elevated in vitamin B-12 deficiency. Elevated vitamin B-12 levels are usually of no great concern.

*Vitamin D, 1, 25-Dihydroxy (Calcitriol; 1, 25 di-OH Vitamin D).* Calcitriol is the most active form of vitamin D. The kidneys produce it from calcidiol (vitamin D, 25-hydroxy). However, it does not last very long in the bloodstream and is not reliable when monitoring for most vitamin D problems. See Vitamin D, 25-Hydroxy.

*Vitamin D, 25-Hydroxy (Calcidiol, 25-Hydroxycalciferol, 25-OH-D).* This is the most useful blood test for diagnosing and monitoring vitamin D problems. Unfortunately, most people who have SLE are deficient in vitamin D. In fact, this often occurs even before they are treated for their lupus, and can become worse due to their being instructed to avoid the sun and use sunscreen regularly (since sun exposure is the major source of vitamin D). Vitamin D deficiency causes brittle bones (called osteomalacia in adults and rickets in children), but has also been associated with other potential problems, such as increased risks for cancer, death from heart attacks and strokes, and asthma in children. The "normal" value for vitamin D can vary from lab to lab; however, doctors generally agree that, for levels less than 20 ng/mL, treatment with vitamin D supplements is appropriate.

*Vitamin D, 25-Hydroxy, D2 (Vitamin D 25-OH D2, Ergocalciferol).* This is not a useful test in monitoring or diagnosing vitamin D levels. See Vitamin D, 25-Hydroxy.

*Vitamin D, 25-Hydroxy, D3 (Vitamin D 25-OH D3, Cholecalciferol).* This is not a useful test in monitoring or diagnosing vitamin D levels. See Vitamin D, 25-Hydroxy.

## Immunological Tests

These tests do not usually appear on a laboratory results sheet under "Immunological Tests," but rather under their individual names. In addition, various laboratories will have different names listed on the lab results. For example, one lab may label an anti-double-stranded DNA test result as "dsDNA Antibody," while another may label it as "Anti-ds DNA." To simplify the list that follows, if a test name can be used with or without the "anti-" prefix I include it without the prefix. In other words, if your lab test shows that you have a positive "anti-Sm antibody," look under "Sm antibody." Synonyms for lab tests appear in parentheses after each lab term. Your doctor can order numerous possible immunologic tests. This list is not meant to be exhaustive, but it does include some of the most commonly ordered tests for SLE patients or patients whose doctors suspect they may have SLE. The laboratory performs all of these tests on blood samples.

*Antinuclear Antibody (ANA, FANA).* This test is the hallmark, or the "holy grail" of sorts, of detecting SLE as it is rarely negative in people who have SLE when tested by the immunofluorescence assay (IFA) lab method on HEp-2 cells (explained below). Since it is such an important test, I am describing this test in more detail than the others are. Its presence in a person fulfills one of the American College of Rheumatology's classification criteria for SLE (see chapter 1). If the test is negative, an SLE diagnosis is questionable. Although people who have lupus have different problems and organ system involvement, this is the common thread uniting almost all of them. People who have SLE can rarely be negative for ANA, but they are positive for other antibodies such as anti-ds DNA or anti-SSA or have SLE because of a genetic deficiency in complement levels.

The nucleus is the center structure of the cells of the body. It occurs within a fatty membrane and contains the genetic DNA and numerous other molecules responsible for carrying out very important cellular functions. People who have SLE make antibodies that aim at various proteins/antigens found within the nucleus (including the DNA itself). Antinuclear antibodies, in fact, represent a multitude of different antibodies instead of just one antibody. Many of these are actually found in people who do not have SLE (approximately 15% of people are positive for ANA), yet some are specific for various diseases (such as anti-Smith and anti-ribosomal-P antibodies being specific for SLE). In addition, multiple other disorders, such as other autoimmune diseases, liver disease, infections, and cancers, or taking certain medicines can cause positive ANAs. In fact, the vast majority of people who are ANA positive actually do not have lupus at all. That is why this test should not be called the "lupus test." When someone is positive for ANA, it is important to conduct other tests, including those measuring other antibodies, which are more specific for various diseases. This helps determine whether the person has lupus, has another disease, is taking a medication known to cause a positive ANA, or (most commonly) that the ANA is not associated with any disease at all.

There are generally two different methods for testing for antinuclear antibodies. The first is actually performed by various techniques lumped together as "solid phase immunoassays," including a testing method called a multiplex assay. Many laboratories and insurance companies adopt these methods because they are relatively inexpensive (they can be conducted on numerous blood samples at the same time) and less time-consuming. This recent trend is unfortunate as there are many false positives and false negatives with this method. While a truly positive antinuclear antibody test performed by the immunofluorescence assay (IFA) method, discussed below, represents up to 150 different possible antibodies, the multiplex assays only detect 8 to 10. In fact, up to 35% of people who have SLE test negative using this method. The way to spot this method on your own lab slip is to look for the words "ANA-D," "ANA Direct," "Antinuclear Antibodies Direct," "ANAchoice (tm) Screen," or "ANA Screen," followed by a simple numerical result not containing a colon, as well as the words "negative," "positive," or "equivocal," and without including a pattern (as described under IFA, below). The American College of Rheumatology recommends that doctors not order this test due to its inaccuracy and especially because of its propensity for missing the diagnosis of SLE and other rheumatic diseases. If you feel you may have SLE and have had this test performed on you, and it comes back negative, you should ask your physician to redraw your labs and ask specifically for an "ANA, IFA" instead.

The second lab method for looking for ANAs is the IFA (immunofluorescence assay). This is the gold standard for screening for possible SLE. As mentioned, it can detect up to 150 different antibodies directed toward protein antigens inside the cells of the body. With the currently used laboratory methods on HEp-2 cells, it is rare to have SLE and to be negative for ANA with this method of testing. So what are HEp-2 cells? "HEp-2" stands for Human Epithelial" cells and refers to cells that came from the epithelial tissues of the larynx of a 46-year-old man who had throat cancer in 1946. Since 1946, they have been grown and reproduced continuously in cultures in laboratories around the world. Although this person was incredibly unfortunate to have this cancer, the vast majority of people who have SLE worldwide are indebted to him for helping to make their diagnosis of lupus possible.

This test is performed by applying the person's serum (the clear liquid portion of blood separated from the blood cells) to some HEp-2 cells on a microscope slide. If antinuclear antibodies are present in the person's blood, they will bind to protein antigens on the HEp-2 cells. The lab technician then adds liquid containing specially treated antibodies called immunoglobulins. Each immunoglobulin contains a glowing chemical that makes it fluoresce under certain lights. These immunoglobulins attach to the ends of antibodies. So if there are antinuclear antibodies from the person's blood attaching to the antigens of the nucleus on the HEp-2 cells, these glowing immunoglobulins will attach to those antibodies. When the lab technician looks at the HEp-2 cells under the microscope, if she or he sees a yellowish-green glow on the cells, it means the ANA test is positive. If the cells do not glow, then the ANA test is negative. However, there is more to the test than this.

If the ANA is positive, the lab technician will dilute the person's serum down with an equal amount of another solution in multiple steps; the test is repeated using more diluted amounts each time. When the lab technician adds an equal amount of the diluting solution to the serum, the result is a 1:1 mix (or titer). When the lab technician mixes another equal sample of dilution solution, it is a 1:2 titer. The test is repeated this way until the fluorescent glow is no longer visible. The last titer in which the lab technician sees fluorescent glowing is the final titer result. The more dilutions that can be made (and therefore, the higher the titer number), the higher the concentration of antinuclear antibodies present in the person's bloodstream. Most labs consider a titer of 1:40 or greater to be a positive ANA. The higher the titer, the greater the chances are of that particular ANA result being associated with a disease such as SLE. For example, a person who has an ANA of greater than 1:1280 is much more likely to have an autoimmune disorder or systemic inflammatory disease (such as SLE) than is a person who has an ANA of 1:160.

72

There is another part of the test as well. The glowing ANA antibodies can form different patterns. These patterns can provide clues as to what types of antibodies may be causing the positive ANA. From a practical standpoint, these patterns usually contribute little to diagnosing the patient, but I discuss them since they appear in the lab results. By far the two most common patterns are diffuse (also called homogenous) and speckled. They appear under the microscope just like they sound. The diffuse pattern looks like a solid sheet of fluorescent green, while the speckled pattern has many little dots. These are the most common patterns seen in people who do not have SLE. These two patterns also appear with auto-antibodies commonly seen in SLE, with DNA and histone antibodies causing the diffuse pattern and Smith, RNP, SSA, and SSB antibodies causing the speckled pattern. Since these two patterns are the most common, and they are seen in both people who do not have SLE and those who have SLE, the reported pattern is usually not very helpful except in a minority of cases. For example, another pattern, called the nucleolar pattern, is more commonly seen in people who have diffuse scleroderma (also called systemic sclerosis). The centromere pattern is due to centromere antibodies that are commonly seen in the CREST (which stands for Calcium deposits, Raynaud's phenomenon, Esophageal dysmotility, Sclerodactyly, and Telangiectasias) form of scleroderma, but they can also be seen in some people who have SLE as well. There are also rarer and less helpful patterns. From a practical standpoint, though, the pattern reported is usually not that helpful.

Once a person who has SLE is ANA positive, the doctor does not ever need to check the test again. ANA levels do not reliably fluctuate with disease activity, so they are not helpful in following people who have lupus. About 20% of people who have SLE will develop a negative ANA during treatment. This can cause potential problems for patients when they see a new rheumatologist because of insurance changes or due to moving to a different area. I have had several SLE patients who were under excellent control seen by new rheumatologists elsewhere. When their antibodies were negative, the doctors stopped their medicines and told them that they did not have SLE. Unfortunately, all of them flared up again, including one unfortunate individual who had a stroke and developed kidney disease as the result. That is why it is important for patients to keep records of their initial lab results and doctor's notes, as mentioned in chapter 1, so that they can present this information to new doctors and keep this from happening to them.

There are a couple of additional important points regarding the ANA test. First, many people have a positive ANA without it being associated with any disease at all, including SLE. Most studies show that anywhere from 10% to 20% of all people considered "normal" are positive for antinuclear antibodies. In addition, as discussed in chapter 1, ANA can be positive due to many other diseases and even from medications. Therefore, further testing is always required in someone who is positive for ANA if that person is suspected of possibly having SLE.

*ß-2 Glycoprotein I Antibodies (Beta-2 Glycoprotein I Antibodies, Anti-ß-2 Glycoprotein I, and ß-2 GPI).* ß-2 GPI is one of the phospholipids to which anticardiolipin antibodies bind. Antiphospholipid antibodies appear in approximately 30% to 45% of people who have SLE. People who are positive for these antibodies are at increased risk for blood clots and miscarriages. The presence of ß-2 GPI in a person also fulfills one of the American College of Rheumatology's classification criteria for SLE (see chapter 1; also see cardiolipin antibodies).

*Beta-2 Glycoprotein I Antibody.* See ß-2 Glycoprotein I Antibodies

*C3.* See Complement C3

*C4.* See Complement C4

*Cardiolipin Antibodies (Anticardiolipin Antibodies, ACA, ACLA).* Cardiolipin is a fatty molecule (called a phospholipid) that was originally discovered in animal hearts in the 1940s. "Cardio-" comes from the Greek word for "heart." Cardiolipin antibodies are antibodies that target phospholipids called cardiolipin, and are therefore included under a group of antibodies called the antiphospholipid antibodies. In other words, anticardiolipin antibodies are one type of antiphospholipid antibody along with lupus anticoagulant, beta-2 glycoprotein I antibody, and antiphosphatidyl serine antibody. Antiphospholipid antibodies can also cause false positive syphilis tests in people who have SLE. About 55 percent of people who have SLE are positive for ACAs, but the percentage varies from 17% to 87% depending on the test method and the study population. They appear as IgG, IgM, or IgA anticardiolipin antibodies. Antiphospholipid antibodies can occasionally cause strokes, blood clots in the legs (called deep venous thrombosis), blood clots in the lungs (called pulmonary embolism), blood clots in the arteries of the heart leading to heart attacks, or blood clots in the placenta resulting in miscarriages. People who are positive for antiphospholipid antibodies and have blood clots or recurrent miscarriages have what is termed the "antiphospholipid syndrome" (see chapters 9 and 18). Over time, approximately 50% of SLE patients who have antiphospholipid antibodies (such as ACAs) may get blood clots or have recurrent miscarriages. High levels of IgG ACAs tend to be most associated with these blood clots; however, they can also occur with elevated levels of IgM and IgA ACAs. A positive IgM ACA may also increase the risk of developing hemolytic anemia. The presence of ACA in a person fulfills one of the American College of Rheumatology's classification criteria for SLE (see chapter 1).

*CCP Antibodies.* See Cyclic Citrullinated Peptide Antibodies

*Centromere Antibody (Anticentromere Antibody, ACA).* Centromere antibodies are more commonly found in people who have a systemic autoimmune disease called systemic sclerosis (scleroderma), especially a form called systemic sclerosis with limited cutaneous involvement, or CREST syndrome. However, they can also appear in people who have SLE. One recent study found 2% of people who have SLE were positive for ACA; however, they did not have any evidence of scleroderma. Therefore, centromere antibodies most likely do not have any special significance in people with SLE.

*CH50.* Complements are components of a complex group of important proteins in the immune system that work together with antibodies and white blood cells to attack and destroy invading organisms such as bacteria. CH50 is a blood test that measures how well nine of those complement proteins are working together. The CH50 level can decrease in some people who have active SLE and in fact is one of the American College of Rheumatology's classification criteria for SLE (see chapter 1).

*Chromatin Antibody (Anti-Chromatin Antibody).* Chromatin refers to the complex of DNA and other proteins that form chromosomes inside the nuclei of cells. About 70% of people who have SLE are positive for these antibodies, and they appear more commonly in SLE than in other systemic autoimmune diseases. People who have SLE who are positive for chromatin antibody are at increased risk for developing lupus kidney disease compared to those who are not positive for it. However, about 40% of people who have SLE who are positive for these antibodies do not have kidney disease. In addition, as with anti-histone antibodies, people who have drug-induced lupus also have an increased chance of being positive for chromatin antibodies.

*Complement C2 (Complement Component C2).* Complements are components of a complex group of important proteins in the immune system that work together with antibodies and white blood cells to attack and destroy invading organisms such as bacteria. Doctors generally do not follow C2 levels in monitoring SLE patients, but may request them to see if there is a deficiency in C2 levels (which can be genetic). Hereditary deficiency in C2 complement can cause SLE.

*Complement C3 (Complement Component C3).* Complements are components of a complex group of important proteins in the immune system that work together with antibodies and white blood cells to attack and destroy invading organisms such as bacteria. C3 complement levels can increase due to any cause of inflammation (including SLE). When it is elevated, it is usually not a very useful finding to follow. However, other people who have SLE will develop decreased C3 complement levels due to it being "consumed" during the immune activation process. In these individuals, if their C3 level consistently drops during times of disease flare and improves during times of disease control, it can be very helpful to monitor. It is especially useful in following some people who have lupus kidney disease. Some people who have lupus always have a low C3 level that does not fluctuate very much with disease activity; in those individuals, it is not very helpful to follow the blood test.

It is routine practice for doctors to follow both C3 and C4 levels together as potential markers of lupus disease activity. In addition, the presence of a low C3 level in a person fulfills one of the American College of Rheumatology's classification criteria for SLE (see chapter 1).

*Complement C4 (Complement Component C4).* Complements are components of a complex group of important proteins in the immune system that work together with antibodies and white blood cells to attack and destroy invading organisms such as bacteria. C4 complement levels can increase due to any cause of inflammation (including SLE). In this situation, it is usually not a very useful finding to follow. However, some people who have SLE will develop decreased C4 complement levels due to it being "consumed" during the immune activation process. In these individuals, if their C4 level consistently drops during times of disease flare and improves during times of disease control, it can be very helpful to follow. It is especially useful in some people who have lupus kidney disease. Some people always have a low C4 level that does not fluctuate very much with disease activity. In those patients, it is not very helpful to follow the blood test. Some people who have SLE are born with a genetic deficiency of

C4 and are unable to manufacture very much of it. They usually have a low level of C4 whether their lupus is active or not.

It is routine practice for doctors to follow both C3 and C4 levels together as potential markers of lupus disease activity. In addition, the presence of a low C4 level in a person fulfills one of the American College of Rheumatology's classification criteria for SLE (see chapter 1).

*Coombs', Direct (Coombs' Antibody, Coombs' Test).* Coombs' antibodies are antibodies that attach to red blood cells and may cause the immune system to damage them and remove them from circulation faster than normal. These damaged red blood cells "break open" and the spleen removes them from circulation, leading to a low red blood cell count. This causes a type of anemia called hemolytic anemia. Sometimes this form of anemia in people who have SLE can be severe. When a person who has SLE has anemia, Coombs' antibody can be one of tests ordered to try to find out if the anemia is due to hemolytic anemia or not. However, Coombs' antibodies are also very common in people who have SLE who do not have hemolytic anemia, occurring in approximately 65% of patients. Therefore, other tests are usually done as well (such as bilirubin, haptoglobin, and a reticulocyte count) to see if there is actually any evidence for hemolytic anemia if the Coombs' test is positive. In addition, the presence of a direct Coombs' antibody in a person fulfills one of the American College of Rheumatology's classification criteria for SLE (see chapter 1).

*C-Reactive Protein (CRP).* C-reactive protein is a protein that can increase due to inflammation and therefore is sometimes elevated when SLE is active. However, these elevated levels are usually mild. CRP can also be elevated in people who are at increased risk of having heart attacks, and people who have SLE are at increased risk of developing heart attacks at a younger age than others do. The exact reason for this is unknown at this time, and most cardiologists do not recommend following CRP as a marker for heart disease. CRP levels in general are not that useful to follow in people who have SLE except in the case where the doctor is trying to figure out whether a sick SLE patient is having a bad flare of SLE or whether he or she may have an infection. In that case, if the CRP is extremely high, then the patient may be more likely to have an active infection going on. However, the opposite is not true. A normal or slightly elevated CRP level does not rule out the possibility of an infection. In addition, all people who have SLE who have very high CRP levels do not always have an infection. Sometimes this elevated CRP appears in people who are having a flare of their SLE, especially if it is one complicated by serositis (such as pleurisy or pericarditis; see chapters 10 and 11), lung inflammation, or arthritis.

*Cryoglobulins.* "Cryo-" comes from the Greek word for "cold" and refers to a type of molecule of the immune system (called immunoglobulins) that clump together or precipitate when the blood becomes cooler. These tend to be found in higher amounts in people who have SLE and increase with disease activity. People who are positive for cryoglobulins tend to have an increased chance of having lupus kidney involvement (nephritis).

*Cyclic Citrullinated Peptide Antibodies (Anti-CCP Antibody, CCP IgG Antibodies, CCP Antibody).* Doctors most commonly use the CCP antibody to diagnose rheumatoid arthritis. However, 8% to 25% of people who have SLE are also CCP positive (depending on the testing method used and the patient population). People who have SLE who are positive for CCP antibody are more likely to have arthritis than those who are CCP negative. In addition, people who have SLE who have arthritis and who are CCP antibody positive are at increased risk of developing joint deformities and having evidence of erosions on x-ray. Erosions are areas where the inflammation from arthritis has eaten away part of the bone next to the joint. These findings are more typical of rheumatoid arthritis than of lupus arthritis, and may therefore actually represent an overlap of SLE and rheumatoid arthritis occurring in the same person.

*Dilute Russell's Viper Venom Test.* See Lupus Anticoagulant

*DNA (Single-Stranded) Antibodies (Anti-ss DNA, ss-DNA Antibodies).* DNA, or deoxyribonucleic acid, is the genetic code contained in the nuclei of the cells of the body. It is composed of two strands of proteins twisted around each other like a braid. This is how DNA normally exists in the cells and the term for this is "double-stranded DNA." If the two strands are separate, the term for each strand is "single-stranded" DNA. Antibodies that are directed to just the single strands (i.e., anti-single-stranded DNA) are very nonspecific. Although they appear in 70% of people who have SLE, they also appear in many other disorders, including non-rheumatologic conditions.

*dsDNA Antibody (Anti-ds DNA Antibody, Anti-Double-Stranded DNA Antibody, DNA (DS) AB, Anti-Native DNA).* DNA (deoxyribonucleic acid) is the genetic code contained in the nuclei of the cells of the body. It is composed of two strands of proteins twisted around each other like a braid. This is how DNA normally exists in the cells, and it is called double-stranded DNA or native DNA. Antibodies directed toward this DNA structure appear in 40% to 80% of people who have SLE (depending on the laboratory method and the patient population studied). Its presence causes a diffuse (or homogenous) pattern of ANA by IFA method. It is a fairly specific blood test for SLE (meaning that a positive test is not common in people who do not have SLE). In fact, the detection of these antibodies in a person fulfills one of the American College of Rheumatology's classification criteria for SLE (see chapter 1). In addition to helping diagnose SLE, it can also be useful in managing and following the treatment of lupus because the level of anti-ds DNA will fluctuate with disease activity in some people. In other words, during a disease flare of SLE it may increase, and during periods of disease inactivity (either spontaneously or due to treatment) it may normalize or decrease in value. However, this is not true of all people. Some people will have elevated anti-ds DNA levels that do not fluctuate with disease activity. It usually takes some time following the person for the doctor to determine its usefulness. In addition, people who are positive for anti-ds DNA are at increased risk of having lupus kidney disease or vasculitis as a part of their disease. Vasculitis is a condition where there is inflammation of the blood vessels, which can damage different parts of the body such as the skin. However, just as with the majority of tests used in SLE, these possibilities are less than perfect. There are people who are anti-ds DNA positive who do not have SLE, and there are certainly people who have SLE who are positive for anti-ds DNA and yet never develop kidney disease or vasculitis. When this test is positive, however, it helps the physician pay closer attention to these possibilities.

*ENA (Extractable Nuclear Antibodies).* See Extractable Nuclear Antibodies

*Endomysial Antibody (IgA Endomysial Assay, EMA).* IgA endomysial antibodies are useful in helping to diagnose an autoimmune disease called celiac disease, which causes difficulty with absorption of nutrients in the intestines. This antibody rarely appears in people who have SLE. However, they are at increased risk of having celiac disease compared to people who do not have SLE. If a person who has SLE has symptoms suggestive of celiac disease, a positive EMA can help in making the diagnosis. See also Tissue Transglutaminase Antibody.

*Extractable Nuclear Antibodies (Anti-ENA, Antiextractable Nuclear Antibodies, and ENA).* These are antibodies directed at the antigens of proteins found in the "extract" of cells. There are many different proteins/antigens in this "extract," and therefore numerous different potential antibodies directed toward them. Collectively, these antibodies help make up the antinuclear antibodies (ANA); a positive ANA test is usually required to make a diagnosis of SLE. When someone is positive for ANA, the next step is often to see if one can identify any individual antibodies that are more specific for any particular disease and that may be responsible for the positive ANA test. Although, technically, these ENAs include a number of antibodies—such as anti-RNP, anti-Smith, anti-SSA, anti-SSB, anti-Jo 1, and anti-Scl 70 antibodies—many laboratories mainly use this term for anti-RNP and anti-Smith antibodies. See RNP Antibody and Smith Antibody.

*Fluorescent Treponemal Antibody Absorption Test (Treponema Pallidum Antibodies, FTA-Ab, FTA-ABS).* This test is done to establish whether a person has syphilis or not. The screening tests for syphilis (which is a sexually transmitted disease) are usually the RPR and VDRL tests. If either of these is positive, it is mandatory to conduct a more specific test for syphilis since false positives can occur with RPR and VDRL. The FTA-ABS is one of those confirmatory tests. If someone is positive for RPR or VDRL, yet negative for the FTA-ABS, then that person has a false positive syphilis test. SLE is one of the conditions that can cause a false positive syphilis test, and, in fact, its presence in a person fulfills one of the American College of Rheumatology's classification criteria for SLE (see chapter 1). In addition, an antiphospholipid antibody may be the cause of a false positive syphilis test in SLE. In this case, the person may be at increased risk of developing blood clots and other complications, such as recurrent miscarriages (discussed in detail in chapters 9 and 18). However, even this test is not 100% foolproof, as there are people who have SLE who can also have a false positive FTA-ABS test, and other confirmatory tests for syphilis need to be utilized (such as the *Treponema pallidum* particle agglutination test).

*Gliadin Antibody (Anti-Gliadin Antibody, Gliadin Antibody Profile).* Anti-gliadin antibody is often used to help diagnose an autoimmune disorder called celiac disease, which causes the intestines not to absorb nutrients correctly. However, about 23% of people who have SLE are positive for anti-gliadin antibodies without having celiac disease. In fact, a positive gliadin antibody in people who have SLE is not clinically useful. See also Endomysial Antibody and Tissue Transglutaminase Antibody.

*H2a/H2b Antibody.* See Histone Antibodies

*H3 Antibody.* See Histone Antibodies

*H4 Antibody.* See Histone Antibodies

*Histone Antibodies (Anti-Histone Antibodies, H2a/H2b Antibody, H3 Antibody, and H4 Antibody).* Histones are protein complexes that are associated with DNA in the nuclei of the cells; together, histones and DNA make up the chromosomes. Antibodies directed at histones are common in SLE, occurring in 50% to 70% of people who have the disease. Its presence causes a diffuse (homogenous) pattern ANA by the IFA method. They also appear in other systemic autoimmune diseases, such as rheumatoid arthritis and scleroderma. However, they are most useful in diagnosing drug-induced lupus (see chapter 1). The presence of histone antibodies in a person who has SLE is not particularly useful.

*La Antibody (Anti-La).* See SSB.

*Lupus Anticoagulant (Dilute Russell's Viper Venom Test, PTT-LA with Reflex to Hexagonal Phase Return, dRVVT with Mixing Study, LAC, dRVVT, Kaolin Clot Time).* Lupus anticoagulant is considered one of the antiphospholipid antibodies along with anticardiolipin antibody, beta-2 glycoprotein I antibody, and antiphosphatidyl serine antibody. Antiphospholipid antibodies can also cause false positive syphilis tests in people who have SLE. Together, they can also appear in people who have antiphospholipid syndrome, which can cause recurrent blood clots, miscarriages, and other problems. Approximately 30% of people who have SLE are positive for LAC, and approximately half of them may develop blood clots over time. In addition, its presence in a person fulfills one of the American College of Rheumatology's classification criteria for SLE (see chapter 1).

The term "lupus anticoagulant" is confusing because a coagulant is a substance that causes increased clotting of the blood (i.e., causes blood clots). When a substance coagulates, it becomes thicker. An anticoagulant does just the opposite (i.e., it causes blood to thin out and cause excessive bleeding). Yet people who have lupus anticoagulant are actually at increased risk of blood clots instead of excessive bleeding. This term comes from how the antibodies work. There is a clotting blood test called partial thromboplastin time (or PTT for short). Generally, people who have a higher than normal PTT test bleed too easily. However, in the 1940s and 1950s doctors noted that some people who had lupus had abnormally increased coagulation tests such as the PTT. However, these individuals did not bleed easily as one would expect; instead, they were later found to have an increased chance of having blood clots. This has to do with the fact that the antibodies responsible for lupus anticoagulant do not actually cause increased bleeding. Instead, they interfere with how the PTT test is done, giving artificially increased results while not truly interfering with the ability of the blood to clot.

Another interesting thing about this test is that one of the most common ways to detect these antibodies is by using the venom from the Russell's viper, which is found in India. This snake's venom is the fifth most poisonous of all snake venoms in the world, and it kills more humans yearly than any other snake in the world. The venom causes the blood of its victim to clot. The lab technician mixes a dilute amount of venom with the serum from a lupus patient's blood in a test tube and adds a small amount of phospholipid. Normally, the blood should clot within a certain amount of time. The venom has to have phospholipids present to cause clotting. If the person has antiphospholipid antibodies (called lupus anticoagulant in this case) present, these lupus anticoagulant antiphospholipid antibodies bind to the phospholipids and prevent the venom from interacting with them. Clotting takes longer than expected, making the test positive for the lupus anticoagulant.

*Microsomal Antibody (Antithyroid Microsomal Antibody).* See Anti-Thyroid Peroxidase Antibody

*Phosphatidyl Serine Antibody (Antiphosphatidylserine Antibody).* This is also one of the antiphospholipid antibodies as described in detail under cardiolipin antibodies above. They appear in approximately one-third of people who have SLE.

*PTT-LA with Reflex to Hexagonal Phase Return.* See Lupus Anticoagulant

*Rapid Plasma Reagin Test (Nontreponemal Test, Serologic Test for Syphilis, RPR, STS).* RPR is a screening test for syphilis, a sexually transmitted disease. However, it is possible to be positive for this test yet not have syphilis. If the RPR is positive, a doctor must do a confirmatory test for syphilis, such as the fluorescent treponemal absorption antibody test or the *Treponema pallidum* particle agglutination test. If either of these tests is negative, then the person does not have syphilis, but instead has a false positive syphilis test. Anywhere from 15% to 30% of people who have SLE have a false positive syphilis test. False positive syphilis tests result from a type of antiphospholipid antibody that may cause recurrent blood clots or miscarriages (the antiphospholipid syndrome). In addition, the presence of a false positive syphilis test in a person fulfills one of the American College of Rheumatology's classification criteria for SLE (see chapter 1).

*RF, RF IgA, RF IgG, or RF IgM.* See Rheumatoid Factor

*Rheumatoid Arthritis Factor.* See Rheumatoid Factor

*Rheumatoid Factor (Rheumatoid Arthritis Factor, RA Factor, RA Latex Turbid, RA Latex, RF Titer, RF, RF IgA, RF IgG, and RF IgM).* Immunoglobulins are important proteins of the immune system that identify foreign proteins, or antigens, and protect the body from them. Rheumatoid factor is an immunoglobulin that attaches to other immunoglobulins. Rheumatoid factor may play an important role in the normal immune system in helping to clear away and remove unwanted immunoglobulins. Therefore, many people are positive for RF. Doctors most commonly use rheumatoid factor to help in the diagnosis of rheumatoid arthritis (RA) because approximately 80% of people who have rheumatoid arthritis have higher than normal levels of RF. However, elevated levels of RF exist in people who have many diseases that cause inflammation, such as infections, cancers, liver diseases, lung diseases, and other autoimmune disorders such as SLE. In fact, approximately one-third of people who have SLE are positive for RF. Some people who have SLE are found to be RF positive when their doctor is initially working up their condition while trying to figure out whether they have SLE, rheumatoid arthritis, or some other reason for having joint pain. Additionally, some people who have SLE can also have rheumatoid arthritis (called an overlap syndrome, or sometimes "rhupus" specifically referring to a combination of rheumatoid arthritis and lupus in the same individual). In those cases, RF often is positive because the person has rheumatoid arthritis in addition to having systemic lupus. Other than that, RF is not particularly helpful in monitoring people who have SLE as it does not consistently predict any special complications in lupus and has not been helpful in monitoring the disease.

*Ribosomal-P Antibody (Anti-P).* Ribosomal-P antibodies are one of the most specific blood tests to help in the diagnosis of SLE. In other words, if someone is positive for ribosomal-P antibodies, she or he probably has SLE as it rarely, if ever, appears in people who do not have lupus or people who have other systemic autoimmune diseases. About 20% of people who have SLE are positive for these antibodies, but it may be as high as 40% to 50% in Asians and in children who have SLE. People who are positive for this antibody are at increased risk of developing inflammation of the liver due to their lupus (lupus hepatitis) compared to lupus patients who are negative for the antibody. However, most people who test positive for this antibody do not develop hepatitis. Other complications of lupus that may increase in people who are positive for this antibody include lupus skin disease and kidney inflammation. Initial studies on ribosomal-P antibodies in the early 1990s suggested a strong association with developing severe depression and psychosis (hallucinations, delusional thoughts, and disorientation). Recent studies have suggested an increased but weak association with these problems. In other words, slightly more people with SLE who have severe depression and psychosis may be positive for ribosomal-P antibody compared to other people who have SLE, but most people who are positive for ribosomal-P antibody do not develop severe depression or psychosis. A 2012 study showed an increased risk of anxiety disorder (discussed in chapter 13) in children who have SLE who are positive for ribosomal-P antibodies.

*RNP Antibody (Anti-Ribonucleic Protein, Anti-RNP, and Anti-Sm/RNP).* Anti-RNP is often included as one of the extractable nuclear antibodies by some laboratories. It appears in 30% to 40% of people who have SLE. Its presence causes a speckled pattern ANA by the IFA method. People who have SLE who are positive for RNP antibody often have Raynaud's phenomenon (Raynaud's is discussed in chapter 11). They also have an increased chance of having esophageal dysmotility causing difficulty with swallowing. Myocarditis (see chapter 11) and pulmonary hypertension (see chapter 10) may also occur more often in those who are RNP positive. RNP antibodies are not very specific for any particular disease. They can appear in people who have SLE, rheumatoid arthritis, Raynaud's phenomenon, and scleroderma. It is most useful in diagnosing a systemic autoimmune disease called mixed connective tissue disease (see chapter 2) where it appears in high amounts. It does not fluctuate consistently with disease activity, and therefore is not helpful in following how SLE responds to therapy.

*Ro Antibody (Anti-Ro).* See SSA

*RPR.* See Rapid Plasma Reagin Test

*Scl-70 Antibody.* See Scleroderma Antibody

*Scleroderma Antibody (Anti-Scleroderma 70 Antibody, Topoisomerase I Antibody, and Anti-Scl 70).* This antibody most commonly appears in a condition called scleroderma (also called systemic sclerosis). Scleroderma is a systemic autoimmune disease that can cause thickening of the skin. It also tends to be associated with an increased risk for having scarring of the lungs, called interstitial lung disease. People who have SLE are typically not positive for this antibody unless they have an overlap syndrome with scleroderma (see chapter 2).

*Sm Antibody.* See Smith Antibody

*Smith Antibody (Anti-Smith Antibody, Anti-Sm, and Sm Antibody).* The anti-Smith antibody is included in the extractable nuclear antibodies along with anti-RNP antibodies. Anywhere from 15% to 30% of people who have SLE are positive for the anti-Smith antibody. Its presence causes a speckled pattern ANA by the IFA method. It usually occurs along with anti-RNP. In other words, if anti-Sm is positive, anti-RNP is usually positive. Doctors first reported the anti-Smith antibody in an aspiring actress named Stephanie Smith. After a diagnosis of SLE in 1959, she died of the disease in 1969 at 22 years of age. The antibody was named after her. The most important thing about anti-Smith antibody is that it is very specific for SLE; it rarely appears in individuals who do not have lupus or have other diseases. It is so specific for people who have lupus that it is included in the American College of Rheumatologist's classification criteria for systemic lupus (see chapter 1). One influence on its presence is race—it is more common in blacks than it is in whites. There is no clear proof that it fluctuates with disease activity; therefore, this test is useful only for diagnosing lupus, and not in following how lupus responds to therapy.

*SSA (Anti-Sjögren's Syndrome A, Sjögren's Anti-SS-A, Anti-SSA, Ro Antibody).* Anti-SSA and anti-SSB antibodies were first discovered in 1961 in people who had Sjögren's syndrome, which is a systemic autoimmune disorder that causes dry eyes and dry mouth. The medical terms for them are "Sjögren's syndrome-A" and "Sjögren's syndrome-B" antibodies (or SSA and SSB for short). Then, in 1969, another lab described antibodies in people who had lupus and named them anti-Ro and anti-La, with "Ro" and "La" being the first two letters of the last names of the lupus patients in whom the antibodies were initially found. Researchers later showed that anti-SSA was the same as anti-Ro, and that anti-SSB was the same as anti-La. These terms are now interchangeable, with anti-SSA meaning the same thing as anti-Ro and anti-SSB meaning the same thing as anti-La.

Anti-SSA is more commonly found than anti-SSB, seen in anywhere from 20% to 60% of people who have SLE depending on the patient population and the laboratory method used to detect the antibodies. Anywhere from 75% to 95% of people who have Sjögren's syndrome are positive for this antibody as well. However, anti-SSA can appear in other autoimmune disorders, such as rheumatoid arthritis, scleroderma, and polymyositis. It can also appear in people who do not have any known associated disease. People who have SLE who are anti-SSA positive have an increased risk of developing rashes with sun exposure (especially subacute cutaneous lupus), inflammation of the lungs (pneumonitis), inflammation of the liver (hepatitis), inflammation of the pancreas (pancreatitis), inflammation of the heart (myocarditis), low platelet counts (thrombocytopenia), and low lymphocyte counts (lymphopenia). In addition, although it is rare, many people who have SLE, but who are negative for ANA, are found to be anti-SSA positive.

One of the most important potential problems is that this antibody is able to cross through the placenta and enter the fetus of a woman who is positive for this antibody. These antibodies can potentially cause tissue damage in the heart or skin of a baby (called neonatal lupus) whose mother is anti-SSA positive (see chapters 1, 18, and 41). Fortunately, this occurs in only about one out of fifty mothers who are positive for anti-SSA.

*SSB (Anti-Sjögren's Syndrome B, Sjögren's Anti-SS-B, Anti-SSB, and La Antibody).* Anti-SSB antibodies usually appear in people who are also positive for anti-SSA antibodies. It is detectable in 15% to 25% of people who have SLE, and in 40% to 60% of people who have Sjögren's syndrome. Its presence causes a speckled pattern ANA by the IFA method. It is unusual to be positive for anti-SSB without also being positive for anti-SSA antibody. People who have SLE who are positive for both anti-SSA and anti-SSB antibodies are less likely to develop lupus kidney disease. Women who are positive for anti-SSB antibodies and get pregnant are at slight risk of having a child with neonatal lupus. In addition, people who have SLE who are positive for anti-SSB antibodies are at high risk of developing Sjögren's syndrome over time.

*ss-DNA Antibodies.* See DNA (Single-Stranded) Antibodies

*Thyroglobulin Antibody.* See Thyroid Antithyroglobulin Antibody

*Thyroid Antithyroglobulin Antibody (Antithyroglobulin Antibody, Thyroglobulin Antibody, and TgAb).* Approximately 10% of people who have SLE will also have autoimmune thyroid disease. TgAb is especially found in high levels in a thyroid disorder called Hashimoto's thyroiditis, but can appear in other autoimmune thyroid diseases such as Graves' disease.

*Thyroid Microsomal Antibody (Antimicrosomal Antibody, Microsomal Antibody, and Anti-Thyroid Peroxidase Antibody).* See Thyroid Peroxidase Antibody

*Thyroid Peroxidase Antibody (Thyroperoxidase Antibody, TPO Antibody, and TPOAb).* About 10% of people who have SLE will also have autoimmune thyroid disease. Thyroid peroxidase antibody especially appears in high levels in a thyroid disorder called Hashimoto's thyroiditis, but can also appear in other autoimmune thyroid diseases such as Graves' disease.

*Thyroid Stimulating Hormone Receptor Antibody.* See Thyrotropin Receptor Antibody

*Thyrotropin Receptor Antibody (Thyroid Stimulating Hormone Receptor Antibody, TSH Receptor Antibody, Thyrotropin-Binding Inhibitory Immunoglobulin, TSH Receptor-Binding Inhibitory Immunoglobulin, TRAb, and TBII).* Approximately 10% of people who have SLE will also have autoimmune thyroid involvement as well. Thyrotropin receptor antibody appears in people who have an autoimmune thyroid condition called Graves' disease, which causes an overactive thyroid (hyperthyroidism) and an enlarged thyroid gland (goiter).

*Tissue Transglutaminase Antibody (Anti-Tissue Transglutaminase, Anti-tTG).* Tissue transglutaminase antibodies are useful in diagnosing an autoimmune disease called celiac disease, which causes difficulty with the absorption of nutrients from the intestines. Anti-tTG antibodies can be either IgG (immunoglobulin G) or IgA (immunoglobulin A). It is the IgA form that is highly specific for celiac disease. This antibody rarely appears in people who have SLE. People who have SLE are at increased risk of having celiac disease compared to the normal population. If a person who has SLE has symptoms suggestive of celiac disease, a positive IgA Anti-tTG can help in making the diagnosis of celiac disease. See also Endomysial Antibody.

*Topoisomerase I Antibody.* See Scleroderma Antibody

*TPMT.* See Thiopurine Methyltransferase Activity

*Treponema Pallidum Antibodies.* See Fluorescent Treponemal Antibody Absorption Test and *Treponema Pallidum* Particle Agglutination Test

*Treponema Pallidum Particle Agglutination Test (TPPA).* This is another confirmatory test for syphilis (also see Fluorescent Treponemal Antibody Absorption Test). Since people with SLE can have false positive RPR and VDRL syphilis tests, it is important to follow these up with a TPPA or FTA ABS. If the initial positive RPR or VDRL has a negative TPPA, then that person has a false positive test for syphilis as a part of lupus. If the TPPA is positive, then that means that the person was infected with syphilis at some time in the past and needs evaluation and possibly treatment if not done so before.

*VDRL.* See Venereal Disease Research Laboratory Test

*Venereal Disease Research Laboratory Test (VDRL).* This is another screening test used to diagnose syphilis (see also Rapid Plasma Reagin Test). Anywhere from 15% to 30% of people who have SLE will be positive for this test due to antiphospholipid antibodies and not due to being infected with syphilis. The term for this is a "false positive syphilis test." A doctor should do a follow-up test, such as a *Treponema pallidum* particle agglutination test or a fluorescent treponemal antibody absorption test, to see if the person truly has been infected by syphilis before or whether the positive VDRL is a false positive test result due to their SLE.

### KEY POINTS TO REMEMBER

1. People who have SLE need to know how to collect a urine sample properly because one is usually required at most office visits.

2. People who have SLE should have labs done regularly to monitor for potential lupus problems affecting blood counts, the liver, and the kidneys. The most common labs performed regularly include a complete blood cell count, metabolic chemistry panel, urinalysis, random urine protein/creatinine, C3 complement, C4 complement, and anti-ds DNA level.

3. Many people who have lupus also need labs drawn regularly to ensure that no side effects occur from medications.

4. A doctor may request testing for a large number of antibodies if she or he suspects that the patient has a diseases that can mimic lupus. Other than anti-ds DNA, doctors do not usually repeat these tests because most antibody levels do not fluctuate with disease activity.

5. It can be useful to know what antibodies you are positive for to understand how your doctor diagnosed lupus and potentially what problems from SLE you are at increased risk of developing.

# PART II

# How Lupus Affects the Body

# How SLE Directly Affects the Body

## First Description of Lupus as a Systemic Disease

For many centuries, lupus was described as a disease affecting the skin. It was not until the nineteenth century that Dr. Moritz Kaposi, a famous dermatologist (skin doctor), outlined the systemic effects of lupus. Dr. Kaposi was born in Hungary but attended medical school in Vienna, Austria, where he spent the rest of his career as a physician. You may recognize his name, as he was the first to describe a type of skin cancer called Kaposi's sarcoma that occurred among middle-aged men. Today Kaposi's sarcoma is most commonly found in HIV-infected people who develop AIDS.

In 1875, Dr. Kaposi was the first to describe lupus affecting more than just the skin. In his book, he describes patients with lupus as having "oedematous, tubercular, painful swelling, of the consistence of firm dough, affecting the skin and the tissues around the joints." This described perfectly the arthritis that affects most people who have SLE. He goes on to say, "Aching, boring, deep-seated pains in the bones . . . Severe pains in the large joints frequently occur in the course of the disease." In the same textbook, he goes on to describe lupus also causing lymph gland swelling, fever, loss of energy, pneumonia, and irregular menstrual cycles. He also mentions how some patients will have symptoms that come and go, or as doctors commonly describe as "waxing and waning." He goes on to discuss how some patients will only have discoid lupus (lupus that affects the skin) without ever developing the systemic form, yet how they must relate to one another since patients with SLE can also develop the discoid form of lupus. Dr. Kaposi's close study of his patients and his descriptions of the systemic form opened the door for physicians to become aware of their relationship.

This book discusses the problems of SLE in two large sections. Part II (this section) covers those problems that are directly due to the immune system attacking the body (the direct autoimmune problems). Part III highlights problems that occur in people who have lupus due to other reasons. Part II (chapters 5–20) deals with the direct effects of SLE and goes into detail about how SLE can affect the body when the immune system attacks various parts of the body. Some problems and complications of SLE, though, occur indirectly because of permanent damage to the body from previous periods of inflammation or from drugs used to treat SLE. There are other problems (such as fibromyalgia) for which we do not have a definite explanation as to why they occur more often in people with lupus, which I also discuss. All of these are dealt with in part III (chapters 21–28) and include things such as infections, heart attacks, strokes, osteoporosis, and fibromyalgia.

The reason for separating these problems into these two sections is that most problems that are directly due to the immune system attacking the body (found in part II) respond to medications that target the immune system. The problems found in part III (problems that are not directly due to the immune system attacking the body) must be treated and dealt with in ways other than with medicines that target the immune system. For example, about 20% of people who have SLE will also have severe pain and fatigue due to a disorder called fibromyalgia. However, fibromyalgia is not directly due to the immune system attacking the body, and therefore does not respond to immune system therapies such as steroids. Instead, treatment includes medicines that normalize chemical imbalances of the pain nerves of the body (such as antidepressants and anti-seizure medicines). This chapter serves as an introduction to how SLE can affect the body in general. It lists patient characteristics (such as certain labs, age, gender, etc.) that rheumatologists note that may increase the chances for lupus causing certain problems in certain individuals, and discusses the topics of flares and clinical quiescence.

．．．．

SLE can affect the body in many different ways. Chapters 5 to 20 focus on the direct effects of SLE on the immune system, which cause inflammation and damage to different parts of the body resulting in arthritis, rashes, kidney disease, and low blood counts.

The problems and symptoms of lupus vary greatly from person to person. Sometimes a person newly diagnosed will say, "I can't have lupus because I don't have the butterfly rash and joint pain." But lupus affects everyone differently. No rhyme or reason explains why some problems will occur in one person and very different problems in another person. Sometimes we have clues. For example, a person who is anti-SSA positive (anti-SSA antibody is one of the antibodies that can be seen in the blood tests of some people who have lupus) has an increased chance of getting rashes with sun exposure, as well as dry mouth and eyes. A person who has a high positive anti-ds DNA and low C3 and C4 complements in her or his blood tests (see chapter 4) has an increased chance of developing inflammation of the kidneys (nephritis). Ethnicity, gender, and even income also play a role (see chapter 19). For example, people who have lower incomes, children, and men who have SLE have a higher chance of having more severe lupus, which includes kidney disease (nephritis). However, it is also not uncommon for a person to be anti-SSA positive and never develop a skin rash or to have elevated anti-ds DNA with low complement levels and never develop nephritis. Some abnormalities even appear to be protective. For example, people who are positive for anti-SSB antibodies have a lower chance of developing lupus nephritis. Table 5.1 lists some clues that can sometimes predict what potential complications of lupus can occur in a particular person. Rheumatologists look carefully for these potential problems in people who have these abnormal lab tests or who fit these particular demographics (such as age, sex, and race). Just because you are positive for a particular blood test does *not* necessarily mean you will end up with that particular associated lupus problem. You may want to ask your rheumatologist what antibodies and lupus blood tests you are positive for so you can understand some of the variables that he or she is monitoring *for you.*

**Table 5.1**  Some Predictors of Possible Problems in SLE

| Lab Finding or Demographic | SLE Problem |
| --- | --- |
| Tests that identify antiphospholipid antibodies (beta-2 glycoprotein I antibody, lupus anticoagulant, cardiolipin antibodies, false positive syphilis tests, antiphosphatidyl serine antibodies) | Blood clots, strokes, heart attacks, low platelet counts, hemolytic anemia, livedo reticularis rash, kidney involvement (blood clots), memory problems, miscarriages |
| Chromatin antibody | Kidney disease in 60% of people |
| Low C3 and C4 complement | Kidney disease (nephritis) |
| Coombs' antibody | Autoimmune hemolytic anemia |
| Cryoglobulins | Kidney disease, vasculitis |
| CCP antibody | Aggressive arthritis, rheumatoid arthritis (rhupus) |
| Double-stranded-DNA antibody | Kidney disease, inflammation of blood vessels (vasculitis) |
| Ribosomal P antibody | Liver, kidney, and skin disease; anxiety, depression, psychosis |
| RNP antibody | Raynaud's phenomenon, esophageal dysmotility, pulmonary hypertension, myocarditis |
| SS-A (Ro) antibody | Sun-sensitive rash, Sjögren's syndrome, lung inflammation, low platelet counts, myocarditis, pancreatitis, hepatitis, subacute cutaneous lupus; neonatal lupus |
| SS-B (La) antibody | Sjögren's syndrome, neonatal lupus; but less likely to have kidney disease |
| African American race | Kidney and brain disease, pleurisy, discoid lupus |
| Men | Possibly overall more severe disease compared to women |
| Children | More major organ (especially kidneys) disease than adults |
| Elderly | Less severe inflammation than in younger adults. Less low blood counts, Raynaud's, hair loss, butterfly rash, sun-sensitive rashes, and less kidney and brain involvement than younger adults. However, permanent damage occurs more easily in the aging organs. Higher chances of Sjögren's syndrome, pleurisy, lung disease, and arthritis. |

Again, recognize that none of these is set in stone. For example, there are elderly people who have severe lupus with kidney disease; most African Americans do not develop brain inflammation or kidney disease; most women who have lupus who are anti-SSA positive do not deliver a baby with neonatal lupus. These are simply problems that are more likely to occur in these particular individuals.

The symptoms and problems of lupus can occur for a long time before it is even possible to make a diagnosis of SLE. Certainly, some people will have an abrupt onset of SLE. A previously healthy person can become ill with definite SLE very quickly with many problems. There are others, though, who will develop a mild problem here and there, over time gradually adding problems until the doctor is able to make a correct diagnosis. This can sometimes take years.

This is a good time to mention the concept of "flares" patients will hear mentioned quite often in reading about lupus or from their own doctor or other patients. A flare is when someone has either a worsening of lupus problems, or a problem that was under good control then comes back, or a new problem occurs that was not present before. The Lupus Foundation of America (LFA) has come up with a formal definition of a lupus flare: "A flare is a measurable increase in disease activity in one or more organ systems involving new or worse clinical signs and symptoms and or laboratory measurements. It must be considered clinically significant by the assessor and usually there would be at least consideration of a change or an increase in treatment." For example, if person who has SLE is doing perfectly fine one day, then the next day develops a low-grade fever and some open sores on the roof of her mouth, she is said to be having a flare of her SLE. Another example would be someone who has arthritis in the knuckles from her lupus, but it does not bother her very much (in other words, she has mild, persistent arthritis). If her knuckles start to become more swollen and painful, she is having a flare of her SLE since the arthritis is getting worse than it normally is.

The formal statement from the Lupus Foundation of America helps to define what a flare is when doing research in lupus patients. However, it can be useful outside a research setting as well. For example, lab results can help define a flare in addition to the person's description of how she or he is feeling. If you are having a flare of your lupus, such as having sores in your mouth, it is imperative to see your doctor for evaluation. It is a good idea to have your doctor check your lupus labs to make sure something more serious is not going on with any internal organs such as the kidneys or liver or with your blood counts. Although someone may have recurrent mild flares that do not require any treatment changes, sometimes lupus may cause more severe problems (such as inflammation of the kidneys) that may not be apparent unless you get the proper blood and urine tests done to look for this possibility. Your doctor may need to consider adjusting your medications and treatment regimen if you are having a flare.

It is always a good idea to determine why you may be having the flare. Often, flares occur for no good reason. A 2012 study from Johns Hopkins showed that arthritis and lupus affecting the skin were more apt to flare during spring and summer when there is presumably more UV light exposure from the sun. Lupus nephritis (kidney inflammation) was also more common in the summer months. Serositis occurred more often in the fall, leading the authors to speculate the possibility of infections increasing this problem. Note that this study was performed in Maryland and so the findings do not necessarily apply to other parts of the country, but it does bring up some interesting results regarding the impact of the sun and possibly of infections causing flares in lupus.

Some common causes of flares include not being diligent with wearing sunscreen, not avoiding ultraviolet light as carefully as you should, not taking your medications regularly, or even smoking cigarettes. If you can identify a potential cause for the flare, then it will help you learn to work on that particular aspect of your medical care and try harder to keep it from happening again. Some things are more difficult to control, however. For example, increased stress can precipitate a flare. Controlling stress may be difficult to do, especially when some things (such as increased pressure at work) may be less in your control. Table 38.8 lists some practical things you can do to decrease stress by making life less hectic. Of course, there are factors over which you have no control at all, such as the hormone fluctuations that occur during menstrual cycles. However, it is always a good idea to try to find correctible factors that account for a flare and work on them if you can.

Although many people who have SLE will have the same pattern of problems from their lupus recurrently, SLE can cause new problems at any time. A rheumatologist would consider the occurrence of a new problem (based on symptoms or a new abnormal lab test) as a flare. For example, if someone always has low complement levels and a high anti-ds DNA level but the urine samples are always normal, then that person is stable and can be said to be doing well (i.e., does not have a flare). However, if this same person then develops a lot of protein in the urine due to an onset of lupus nephritis, her rheumatologist would consider this a flare of her lupus. Therefore, it is important for you as a lupus patient to be on the lookout for a recurrence of symptoms you have had previously with your lupus because if they occur you may be having a flare and need to contact your doctor. It is just as important to learn what other problems can occur in lupus.

Not everyone who has SLE develops recurrent flares. Many respond so well to treatment that their symptoms and problems come under control and never or rarely recur. Doctors describe this as being "clinically quiescent" or "in remission." Quiescent means that something is in a state of dormancy or inactivity. If someone who has SLE is "clinically quiescent," this means that their disease has been calmed down sufficiently with the current medications. Being clinically quiescent does not mean that the lupus is gone, however; it simply means that it is under good control under the current medication regimen. Therefore, it is very important that someone who is clinically quiescent continue to take his or her medications and see the doctor regularly to ensure that the SLE stays under good control. Unfortunately, too many people who have SLE stop taking their medicines and seeing their doctors when they start to feel well and are "clinically quiescent." This sometimes occurs because the person is in denial about having lupus as a lifelong disease. Usually she or he shows back up in a rheumatologist's office later with a flare. Sometimes these flares can be severe and even life threatening.

The rest of part II is devoted to the wide range of problems that systemic lupus causes in the body. The following chapter discusses symptoms, such as weight loss, fevers, and fatigue (called constitutional symptoms), and the other chapters discuss each organ system separately, including the specific medical tests that doctors order to diagnose these different problems. SLE can cause an amazing number of potential problems in the body. This book discusses both common and uncommon problems. However, it is beyond the scope of this book to discuss the rarest complications of SLE. If this book does not discuss a particular problem that your lupus is causing, please ask your doctor to direct you to other sources of information.

### KEY POINTS TO REMEMBER

1. SLE can cause numerous problems in the body that differ from person to person.

2. Some problems are directly due to inflammation (such as nephritis and arthritis). Rheumatologists often use anti-inflammatory and immunomodulating medicines to treat these lupus problems. The following chapters of part II discuss these in detail.

3. Other problems (such as fibromyalgia and osteoporosis) seen commonly in people who have SLE are not directly due to the inflammation of lupus. They may be due to medications, long-term damage from SLE, or other reasons. Doctors treat these problems with therapies other than immunomodulating medicines. The chapters in part III cover these complications of lupus.

4. Blood abnormalities, age, gender, or ethnicity may increase the chances of developing certain problems from SLE (table 5.1).

5. SLE can have periods of being quiet (clinical quiescence) and periods of increased activity (called flares). It is important to see your doctor during flares to ensure that other problems (such as nephritis) are not occurring.

6. Do not stop taking your medications when you are feeling well. You will put yourself at risk for a potential flare that can sometimes be severe and even life threatening.

# Constitutional Symptoms

## Lupus and Your "Constitution"

A person's overall general health (both physical and mental) is sometimes referred to as her or his "constitution." Doctors use the term "constitutional symptoms" to refer to how someone feels overall when ill. These potential constitutional problems include weight loss, fever, and fatigue. These are very nonspecific symptoms; that is, they can occur with many diseases that can affect the whole body, such as infections (like the flu), cancer, and systemic diseases such as SLE. Most people who have SLE develop constitutional symptoms at some point; however, some never do. They can occur any time the disease is active, or they can occur due to problems other than from lupus. This chapter discusses these issues in detail.

## Fatigue

Fatigue is a general loss of energy that includes both physical and mental exhaustion. Mild fatigue may affect people only when they are trying to do something active; they then feel better with rest. Severe fatigue causes problems even when someone is resting. Fatigue is one of the most common problems in people who have SLE, affecting 80% to 100% of them. Many rheumatologists and their patients consider fatigue to be one of SLE's most frustrating symptoms. It can sometimes be difficult to find a reason for the fatigue, and it can be very difficult to treat. Fatigue is sometimes a direct result of the systemic inflammation due to active SLE. If so, it usually responds well to treatment with medications that calm the immune system, such as steroids, Plaquenil (hydroxychloroquine), or methotrexate.

Fatigue may be due to many other problems. Depression, fibromyalgia, stress, sleep disorders, anemia, hypothyroidism, poor lifestyle habits, and medication side effects can all cause fatigue. Therefore, when a person who has SLE continues to have significant fatigue when the SLE appears to be well controlled, the physician must consider these other possible causes and treat them appropriately. If you have significant fatigue, ask your doctor to check you for these other problems. Consider taking some home surveys like the ones for depression (table 13.4), anxiety disorder (table 13.2), obstructive sleep apnea (table 6.3), and fibromyalgia (first section of chapter 27). A high score may indicate that you have one of these disorders that commonly cause fatigue in lupus patients. Lupus experts have found that the most common reasons for having significant fatigue when the lupus is not active are fibromyalgia (see chapter 27) and depression (see chapter 13), so these two problems should especially be considered as possible causes. Another common cause of fatigue is adrenal insufficiency (see chapter 26) if it occurs while the dose of steroids are being decreased (called steroid withdrawal). If you notice that you are becoming more fatigued as your steroid dose decreases, read chapter 26 and discuss this possibility with your doctor.

Symptoms that feel similar to fatigue but are different include weakness and drowsiness. Weakness relates to the actual loss of muscle strength. Examples would include difficulty raising your arms up to brush your hair because the muscles feel weak (as opposed to painful) or difficulty standing up from a chair due to weakness in the muscles of your legs. If weakness (instead of fatigue) is present, then problems with the muscles, nerves, or joints may be possible causes. Drowsiness, such as falling asleep easily during the daytime, can sometimes signal a problem with sleep such as sleep apnea. Of course, you can have fatigue in combination with weakness and/or drowsiness, in which case it can be very difficult to separate these symptoms. Being able to identify which symptoms you actually have can greatly assist your doctor in reaching a correct diagnosis of what is wrong and how to approach it to get you better.

## How to Treat Fatigue

There are some things that you can do to try to improve your energy level (table 6.1). It is important to realize that fatigue rarely has a simple cure. For example, patients often ask what vitamin they should take, or if they can have a vitamin B-12 shot to help them with energy. However, it is rare for vitamins to help unless the person actually has a significant vitamin deficiency. If you have significant fatigue, do everything listed in table 6.1 to identify possible causes as well as to try to feel better.

Sometimes fatigue can be a consequence of inadequate sleep. Problems with sleep include not getting enough hours of sleep, having difficulty falling asleep, or waking up in the middle of the night and being unable to get back to sleep. Some people can also have a sleep disorder, such as obstructive sleep apnea, and not realize it. When your mind and body do not get good quality sleep, you are bound to be drowsy, sleepy, or fatigued in the daytime. Difficulty with memory, poor coping skills, depression, and obesity are all health problems tied into lack of sleep. You need to ensure you are getting adequate sleep at night. Most sleep experts recommend eight hours of restful sleep for most people. Unfortunately, today's fast-paced lifestyle means that a large percentage of people do not get enough sleep. If you do not get eight hours of full sleep at night and do not feel well rested when you get up, then you need to work on your sleep habits, or "sleep hygiene" (table 6.2).

Read table 6.2 several times and commit yourself to ensuring that you follow everything listed there if you are experiencing fatigue and sleeping problems. Many people sabotage their sleep by unconsciously getting into regular habits that disrupt the sleep cycle.

A common cause of fatigue in people who have SLE is a sleep disorder called obstructive sleep apnea. This is a condition where the soft tissues of the neck cause the breathing passages to narrow while someone sleeps and leads to restless sleep. Some common symptoms of sleep apnea are daytime fatigue, falling asleep easily while at rest (such as while watching TV), snoring, having difficulty concentrating, being moody, and waking up with a headache or dry mouth. It is more common in people

**Table 6.1**  How to Help Decrease Your Fatigue and Increase Your Energy Level

- See your doctor to look for possible specific causes of fatigue.
- Take the home surveys on obstructive sleep apnea (table 6.3), anxiety disorder (table 13.2), depression (table 13.4), and fibromyalgia (chapter 27). Let your doctor know if you score high on any of these tests.
- Work on sleep hygiene techniques (table 6.2).
- Take DHEA up to 200 mg a day if your lupus is active and if approved by your doctor.
- Take vitamin D supplements if your vitamin D level is low.
- Go on a low-calorie or low-carbohydrate diet to lose weight if you are overweight.
- Consider trying an antidepressant if any depression symptoms exist (such as insomnia, difficulty concentrating, moodiness, loss of interest in doing activities, loss of libido or sexual interest, if you have decreased doing social activities, or if you have feelings of guilt or low self-worth).
- Learn your limits; pace yourself.
- Educate family, friends, co-workers, and employers about your condition and how it affects you.
- Learn to ask for help when you need it.
- On bad fatigue days, do not do more than one important activity. You can try to do more on better days.
- Identify stressors in your life. Work with a mental health professional if needed.
- Learn to decrease stress in your life (table 38.8).
- Exercise regularly (consider something "fun" such as Wii Fit, mentioned in the text).

who are overweight and who have a larger than normal neck size. High percentages of people who have SLE are obese and therefore at increased risk of having sleep apnea. In addition, studies show that doctors under-diagnose sleep apnea in women (90% of SLE patients are women); in other words, a large percentage of women who have sleep apnea do not know they have it. Not only can sleep apnea cause fatigue, but it also increases the risk of heart disease and high blood pressure if left untreated. There are numerous ways to treat sleep apnea, including weight loss and wearing a mouth guard to position the mouth properly while sleeping. Many people need to wear a mask placed over the nose or mouth while they sleep that forces air into the lungs to keep them breathing correctly. The most commonly used device is a CPAP (Continuous Positive Airway Pressure) machine. In some cases, surgery is performed to remove excessive tissue within the throat, allowing the person to breathe properly. Whatever the treatment consists of, it can make a big difference in energy levels and the quality of life in those who have sleep apnea.

The STOP questionnaire is a simple questionnaire you can take to determine if you may have obstructive sleep apnea (table 6.3). STOP stands for Snoring, Tired, Ob-

**Table 6.2** Sleep Hygiene Techniques

- Maintain a regular sleep schedule; get up and go to bed the same time daily even on non-work days and holidays.

- Reduce stress in your life.

- Get exposure to light first thing in the morning to set your biological clock. Consider using a non-UV source of light exposure such as the Philips goLITE.

- Exercise daily; mornings and afternoons are best. Don't exercise right before bedtime.

- Avoid naps late in the afternoon or evening.

- Finish eating two to three hours before bed; a light snack is fine, but avoid foods containing sugar as it can stimulate the mind and interfere with falling asleep.

- Limit fluids before bed to keep from getting up to urinate throughout the night.

- Avoid caffeine six hours before bed.

- Do not smoke; if you do, don't smoke for two hours before bed; nicotine is a stimulant.

- Avoid alcohol two to five hours before bed; alcohol disrupts the sleep cycle.

- Avoid medicines that are stimulating (ask your doctor).

- Avoid stimulating mind activities for a few hours before bed (reading technical articles, listing tasks to do, trouble-shooting, paying bills, etc.).

- Have a hot bath one to two hours before bed; it raises your body temperature and you will get sleepy as your temperature decreases again afterward.

- Keep indoor lighting low for a few hours before bed.

- Establish a regular, relaxing bedtime regimen (aroma therapy, drink warm milk, read, listen to soft music, meditate, pray, do relaxation/breathing exercises).

- Ensure your sleeping environment is quiet and comfortable (comfortable mattress and pillows; white noise like a fan; pleasant, light smells).

- If pets ever wake you, keep them outside of the bedroom.

- Use the bedroom only for sleep and sex; never eat, read, or watch TV in bed.

- Never keep a TV, computer, or work materials in your bedroom.

- Go to bed only when sleepy.

- If you can't go to sleep within fifteen to twenty minutes in bed, go to another room and read something boring under low light, meditate, pray, listen to soft music, or do relaxation/breathing exercises until sleepy.

- If you have dry mouth problems, use a mouth lubricant such as Biotene Mouth Spray before you go to bed.

served, and Pressure. If you answer "yes" to 2 or more of the 4 questions, then you have an increased risk for having sleep apnea. If you do not answer "yes" to 2 or more of the questions, also ask yourself if your body mass index (BMI) is over 30 (see table 21.2), you are over 50, or your neck circumference is 16 inches or larger if you are a woman (or 17 inches or larger if you are a man). If you answer "yes" to any of these questions, then sleep apnea should be considered a possible cause of your fatigue and you should let your doctor know. Obstructive sleep apnea is easy to diagnose with a sleep study at a sleep center (often located at hospitals).

Another therapy that may be of benefit is DHEA. DHEA is a steroid hormone called dehydroepiandrosterone and many people who have SLE have lower than normal levels. Some studies have shown that DHEA may help increase a sense of well-being and decrease fatigue levels in people who have mild to moderate disease activity when they take 200 mg a day. However, acne and increased hair growth are potential side effects; therefore, it is best to consult your doctor before taking it. If your doctor tells you that your lupus is under good control, then DHEA will most likely not help with fatigue, as a 2010 study reported. You can obtain DHEA over the counter without a prescription, but you have to be careful because many off-the-shelf products do not have the correct amounts of DHEA since the FDA does not provide quality controls on over-the-counter supplements. It is best to get a prescription from your doctor and have a compounding pharmacist provide a high-quality product for you instead.

A couple of studies have suggested that vitamin D deficiency may be associated with fatigue in SLE patients. A 2010 study showed that when doctors prescribed vitamin D supplements to lupus patients who had low vitamin D levels, energy levels increased. A 2012 study failed to show any relationship between vitamin D levels and people who have SLE; however, this was a small study of only twenty-four women. The role of vitamin D and energy level is therefore not completely certain. However, most people who have SLE are deficient in vitamin D and should be on a supplement as discussed in chapters 3 and 38.

Losing weight through dieting can also improve energy levels. This point is intuitive to physicians. Countless times doctors see patients with lupus proclaim improvements in energy and their sense of well-being simply after losing weight through lifestyle changes such as diet and exercise. Yet, a 2012 study in the journal *Lupus* was able to demonstrate this improvement scientifically. Women who had SLE had signifi-

---

**Table 6.3** STOP Questionnaire for Obstructive Sleep Apnea

---

Do you *S*nore loudly (louder than talking or loud enough for people to hear through closed doors)?

Do you often feel *T*ired, fatigued, or sleepy during the daytime?

Have you ever had anyone *O*bserve you stop breathing while you sleep?

Are you being treated or have you received treatment for high blood *P*ressure?

If you answer "yes" to two or more of the above, then you should have a sleep study done to make sure you do not have obstructive sleep apnea.

---

cant improvements of their fatigue after losing weight over a six-week period. Half the women used a low-carbohydrate diet and the other half used a standard low-calorie diet. The amount of weight lost and the amount of energy increase were similar in the two groups.

Two of the most common causes of fatigue in people who have lupus are depression and fibromyalgia (see chapters 13 and 27). These two conditions are related and are due to an imbalance of chemicals in the nerves of the body that are involved with mood, sleep, energy levels, memory, and pain. Treatment for both includes medications that attempt to normalize these chemical imbalances, most often antidepressants. If you have significant fatigue, then you should take the home surveys on depression and fibromyalgia. If you score high on these questionnaires, ask your doctor if you have either of these conditions and have them treated. Studies also suggest that a significant number of people who have unexplained fatigue can improve with the use of antidepressants even if they do not have full-blown depression. Since most antidepressants are generally safe, some experts recommend their use in people who have fatigue if a definite reason for the fatigue is not apparent. They feel that the potential benefits of a medication (i.e., having less fatigue) outweigh the potential risk for side effects from these medicines.

Doctors cannot overemphasize the importance of regular exercise to treat fatigue. Many of the problems that can contribute to fatigue in lupus (such as depression, fibromyalgia, sleep apnea, and insomnia) improve with regular exercise. However, this can be one of the most difficult things for some people to do. It can appear counterintuitive to force yourself to move and exercise more when your body is telling you not to. Numerous studies have shown that exercise is important in dealing with fatigue. One study used Nintendo's Wii Fit, an interactive exercise program that you can plug into your television. Fifteen sedentary (i.e., non-exercising) women who had SLE who were experiencing moderate to severe fatigue exercised using Wii Fit three days a week for thirty minutes at a time. At the end of ten weeks, they had significant reductions in their fatigue levels. This is not an advertisement for Wii Fit, but it is a good illustration of how nonathletic lupus patients with life-altering fatigue can become motivated and improve their energy levels after exercising regularly.

Sometimes there can be a dramatic improvement in energy levels with the treatment of lupus or another medical problem, such as sleep apnea, poor sleep habits, untreated hypothyroidism (an underactive thyroid), anemia, or infection. Unfortunately, a significant proportion of people who have fatigue do not have one easily identifiable cause, and these are the most difficult cases to treat. Often a combination of problems is occurring, such as insomnia, depression, anxiety, stress, or fibromyalgia that are contributing to the fatigue problem. It is imperative that these individuals strictly adhere to the sleep hygiene habit recommendations, rest when they need to, and consider therapies such as DHEA, vitamin D, or antidepressants. Often in these cases, the fatigue can persist. The therapies mentioned can help at least to decrease the severity of the fatigue. Doctors often feel powerless helping these patients, who live each day with a loss of energy and have great difficulty being able to do simple daily tasks. I hope that we will be able to find better solutions in the future for this very difficult problem in lupus, and I hope that the previous section gives you some tools to use in the meantime.

## Fever

Many people think that 98.6°F is the normal body temperature. It actually varies quite a bit from person to person, ranging from 96.0°F to 100.8°F when taken orally (with the thermometer placed under the tongue), and varies based on the time of day. Body temperature is usually lowest at 6:00 AM and is highest at 6:00 PM. You have a fever if your oral temperature in the early morning is greater than 98.9°F and if your late afternoon temperature is greater than 99.9°F. Of people who have SLE, 50% to 60% will develop fevers from their lupus. Fever due to inflammation from SLE generally responds well to acetaminophen (Tylenol), non-steroidal anti-inflammatory drugs (NSAIDs) such as ibuprofen or naproxen, and steroids. However, you should never automatically blame a fever on lupus. It is very important to consider infection as a possible cause because people who have SLE are at increased risk for developing infections. Infections in people who have lupus may need treatment other than medicines that decrease the fever. People who have SLE, who have a fever, especially if they are on immunosuppressant medicines like prednisone, should always see their primary care physicians right away to make sure it is not an infection. It can be a potential mistake to wait and see if the fever resolves on its own. Certainly, fevers due to minor infections, such as colds, are common, and may not require antibiotics; however, it is better to leave this determination up to a healthcare provider. The reason is that infection is one of the leading causes of death in lupus patients and most often occurs when people do not take symptoms such as having a fever seriously.

## Weight Loss

Weight loss due to lupus occurs in about 25% of people who have the disease. It can be a result of decreased appetite, but can also be due to the increased use of calories by the body due to fever and the systemic inflammation associated with untreated SLE. Weight loss can also occur from involvement of the intestinal tract in people who have lupus, such as gastroesophageal reflux, causing reduced caloric intake. Chapters 15 and 28 discuss these problems in more detail. When weight loss is due to the systemic inflammation from SLE, it generally can be reversed with treatment of the disease (such as using steroids as well as other therapies such as hydroxychloroquine or Plaquenil).

However, other things can also cause weight loss, including certain medications, such as hydroxychloroquine and azathioprine, which can sometimes cause a loss of appetite and subsequent weight loss as a side effect. Other conditions that can potentially cause loss of weight in people who have lupus include depression, an overactive thyroid (called hyperthyroidism), malabsorption of calories (such as from celiac sprue or gluten hypersensitivity, as discussed in chapter 15), and even cancer. Therefore, if a person who has SLE has weight loss and the lupus appears to be calm, doctors must consider other possible causes.

1. "Constitutional" symptoms (fever, fatigue, and weight loss) occur commonly in SLE but may be due to other disorders as well.

2. If you have a fever, it is very important to see your doctor right away. Although fevers occur with SLE, you must consider infection first.

3. Fatigue is one of the most common and bothersome problems in people who have SLE.

4. If fatigue is due to inflammation from lupus, energy levels should improve when the lupus is treated with steroids and other medicines such as Plaquenil that calm down the immune system.

5. There are other problems to consider as causes of fatigue, such as abnormal thyroid hormone levels, liver problems, kidney problems, and anemia. The doctor can check for these with blood and urine tests.

6. If these tests are all unremarkable, then you need to consider other possibilities as the cause of fatigue. Take the tests for depression (table 13.4), anxiety disorder (table 13.2), obstructive sleep apnea (table 6.3), and fibromyalgia (the first section of chapter 27). If you score high on any of these tests, let your doctor know for proper evaluation and treatment.

7. If you have significant fatigue, make sure to follow the advice in table 6.1 and work hard on improving your sleep hygiene (table 6.2).

8. Problems other than SLE can cause weight loss, including depression, gastrointestinal issues, overactive thyroid, and malabsorption (such as celiac disease). Even hydroxychloroquine (the medicine most commonly used to treat SLE) can cause weight loss.

# The Musculoskeletal System

## Rheumatism

People often use the term "rheumatism" to refer to any type of body aches and pains. The origins of the term are ancient, going back to the Roman physician Galen of Pergamum, who lived in the second century AD. Like many physicians of his time, he believed that medical illnesses were due to the imbalance of fluids in the body called humors. One of these humors was phlegm, also known as mucus (the other three humors were blood, yellow bile, and black bile). Galen observed that when someone was sick with a respiratory illness (such as pneumonia or the flu), the person would often have body and joint pain as well. The sick person might produce a lot of phlegm, coughing up sputum (a type of phlegm), and have a runny nose (another type of phlegm). Galen thought that the overproduction of phlegm could also "flow" inward inside the body and into the joints (similar to flowing out of the body from the nose and lungs). "Rheuma-" comes from the Greek word for "flow." This inward "flow" (or "rheuma") of phlegm into the joints could cause pain, swelling, and stiffness. Therefore, he coined the word "rheumatismos" to refer to illnesses consisting of body aches and pains, including arthritis.

The term "rheumatism" became more popular after the French physician William de Baillou provided the first modern description of arthritis in the early 1600s. In fact, he borrowed the term "rheumatismos" from Galen. The word for the doctors who would become experts in treating arthritis would eventually be "rheumatologists," or the experts at treating "rheumatism." Today doctors consider "rheumatism" to be a very nonspecific term (i.e., a term that can refer to several different things instead of one specific thing). Primarily nonmedical people use it to refer to any type of body ache or pain. It no longer has any specific medical meaning. However, the term for doctors who treat these "rheumatism" conditions is still "rheumatologists."

Approximately 90% of people who have SLE have joint or muscle pain at some point due to their lupus. Since the musculoskeletal system is the most common part of the body to be affected by SLE (causing aches and pains or "rheumatism"), rheumatologists became the specialists dedicated to the diagnosis and management of SLE patients. In fact, arthritis can occur with all of the systemic autoimmune diseases (rheumatoid arthritis, scleroderma, Sjögren's syndrome, polymyositis, and vasculitis). Therefore, the rheumatologist generally takes care of all these disorders.

The musculoskeletal system is responsible for allowing you to move. It includes the muscles (hence "musculo-"), bones (hence "skeletal"), and joints. The joints are the hinges between the bones that allow us to move. The bones of people who have SLE can develop problems such as osteoporosis (fragile bones that can break or fracture) and avascular necrosis (where a section of bone dies). However, these are usually not due to the inflammation of lupus itself and therefore are discussed in part III.

This chapter goes into more detail about how SLE can affect various parts of the musculoskeletal system.

## Arthralgias and Myalgias

Arthralgias are pains in the joints, and myalgias are pains in the muscles. The ending "-algia" comes from the Greek word for "pain." These pains will often be termed "polyarthralgias" and "polymyalgias" as well ("poly-" means "many"). Between 90% and 95% of people who have SLE will have muscle and/or joint pain as a part of their lupus. These, along with fatigue, are the most common symptoms that SLE patients have. Experiencing arthralgias and myalgias does not necessarily mean that there is actual arthritis (actual inflammation or damage in the joints) or muscle inflammation. The doctor may or may not see any evidence of inflammation on examination. Just having joint and muscle pain without actual joint inflammation is not used as part of the classification criteria for SLE (as discussed in chapter 1) because this type of pain is very common in many other conditions. If the pain is due to the systemic inflammation of lupus, then it usually responds well to treatment of the lupus with medicines such as acetaminophen, non-steroidal anti-inflammatory drugs (NSAIDs), and steroids. However, arthralgias and myalgias can sometimes be due to other problems, such as depression, fibromyalgia, hypothyroidism, and sleep apnea. Therefore, the doctor must consider and treat these other possibilities if joint and muscle pains persist when the SLE itself appears to be calm.

## Arthritis

About 50% of people who have SLE will develop actual inflammation of the joints—the medical term for this is "arthritis." As discussed in chapter 1, inflammatory arthritis is one of the classification criteria in diagnosing SLE. An arthritis diagnosis is appropriate if the physician finds evidence of joint inflammation, such as swelling and decreased range of motion on physical examination. Usually, joint x-rays are normal in lupus arthritis. They are more useful in making sure there are no other reasons for the joint pain. Many rheumatologists are also now using ultrasound (also known as sonogram ["sono-" means "sound"]) to help diagnose inflammation in the joints of people who have systemic lupus. The ultrasound machine can use a special technique called "power Doppler." The doctor can actually view the tissues of the joints and surrounding structures and determine whether there is any active inflammation or not. The rheumatologist can do the ultrasound in the office. It can be helpful for the doctor to be able to tell whether the pain is due to active inflammation or not. The arthritis of lupus can affect just a few joints or many joints. Sometimes there may be some stiffness in the joints in the morning when the person first wakes up, but it is usually brief. If there is severe stiffness that lasts for more than an hour in the morning, then the doctor may consider the possibility of rheumatoid arthritis in addition to SLE. The pain of lupus arthritis is often more severe relative to the amount of swelling that the doctor finds on the physical examination. In fact, lupus arthritis pain can be one of the most disabling problems in some people.

Another important clue to lupus being the cause of arthritis is which joints are painful. Lupus arthritis most commonly affects the knees, elbows, wrists, knuckles, and middle joints of the fingers. When a person who has SLE develops pain in the neck, shoulder muscles, back, and sides of the hips, then something other than SLE is usually the cause. Possible causes of pain in these areas include bursitis, tendonitis, degenerative arthritis, and especially fibromyalgia. In fact, approximately 20% of people who have SLE also have fibromyalgia (see chapter 27). Doctors treat fibromyalgia very differently than the arthritis of lupus. In addition, lupus does not typically cause "pain all over," which is more commonly due to something else such as fibromyalgia or depression. Your rheumatologist is the best person to help sort out exactly what is causing your pain to establish the best way to treat it.

Fortunately, the arthritis of lupus is usually not crippling or deforming. This is in contrast to the related autoimmune disorder, rheumatoid arthritis, which causes crippling arthritis if not treated. Rheumatologists treat lupus arthritis with NSAIDs, steroids, and hydroxychloroquine. Sometimes doctors need to prescribe stronger medicines such as methotrexate, mycophenolate, azathioprine, leflunomide, cyclosporine A, and biologic drugs such as rituximab (Rituxan) and belimumab (Benlysta). Two additional biologic medications that are FDA-approved to treat rheumatoid arthritis, abatacept (Orencia) and tocilizumab (Actemra), may also be helpful in people who fail the previously listed medications. I discuss all of these in detail in later chapters. Since the arthritis of lupus is usually not crippling or deforming, the goal of treatment is usually to decrease the pain, stiffness, and swelling to acceptable levels. This contrasts with the treatment of rheumatoid arthritis where complete remission of all inflammation is the goal.

Some people with the arthritis of lupus develop joint deformities where the joints become abnormally bent. In fact, there is one particular type of deforming arthritis in lupus, called Jaccoud's (pronounced yah-COOZ) arthropathy. Jaccoud's arthropathy causes deformities that the doctor can straighten out on physical exam, but that revert back to the deformed shape after the doctor releases the affected appendage. Unfortunately, when Jaccoud's deformities occur, they are permanent. The goal of treatment of Jaccoud's arthropathy is to get the arthritis inflammation completely into remission with medications (just as in rheumatoid arthritis) to try to prevent it from worsening in the future.

Another potential problem is that some people who have SLE will also have rheumatoid arthritis. Rheumatologists sometimes call this combination of diseases "rhupus." These patients will typically have a lot of joint swelling on examination, morning stiffness lasting an hour or longer, and evidence of joint and bone damage on x-rays (called erosions), and are often positive for RF and/or CCP antibodies in their blood work (see chapter 4). Rheumatologists usually treat the arthritis of "rhupus" aggressively with medications to get the arthritis into remission and try to prevent deformities from developing.

If a patient just has achy joints (arthralgias) without having actual inflammation of the joints (arthritis), doctors usually prescribe pain relievers for treatment. These include acetaminophen (Tylenol), NSAIDs (such as ibuprofen and naproxen), or other analgesics such as tramadol (Ultram and Ultracet).

A very important part of the treatment regimen of people who have arthritis and arthralgias is exercise. Due to the discomfort that may occur in SLE, many people are not able to be as active as they were before they developed lupus. They can lose muscle mass, strength, and joint flexibility, preventing them from doing activities as they normally should. This can lead to deconditioning of the muscles of the body and cause even more aches and pains to develop. This becomes a vicious cycle where the pain leads to less activity, less activity causes loss of function and more pain, and so on. Numerous studies show that people who have arthritis who force themselves to exercise regularly actually have less pain overall, develop more muscle mass, are able to do more activities, and have a better quality of life. Not only does exercise help with pain and function, but it has other benefits such as keeping weight under better control, decreasing the chances of developing strokes and heart attacks (see chapter 21), and helping with mood in people who have problems with depression. Regular exercise should be a very important component in the treatment of all people who have SLE.

### KEY POINTS TO REMEMBER

1. Arthritis exists when there is actual inflammation of the joints (as determined by your doctor on physical examination).

2. Arthralgias refer to pain in the joints that may or may not be due to actual inflammation or damage in the joints (i.e., arthritis).

3. Arthritis (but not arthralgias) is included as one of the American College of Rheumatology's classification criteria used to diagnose SLE.

4. Arthralgias in SLE may be due to the lupus, but can also be caused by other possible problems, such as fibromyalgia and depression.

5. The arthritis of SLE rarely causes permanent joint damage and deformities.

6. In people who have joint deformities, joint damage on x-rays, or rhupus, the goal is to try to get the arthritis into remission using medications. Remission means that there is no evidence of inflammation on physical examination and minimal to no discomfort and morning stiffness.

7. Joint x-rays are usually normal in people who have SLE.

8. Doctors usually treat lupus arthritis with NSAIDs, steroids, and hydroxychloroquine. Stronger immunosuppressants (such as methotrexate, mycophenolate, or azathioprine) may be necessary if the pain or inflammation is severe. Leflunomide is FDA approved to treat rheumatoid arthritis and is another alternative treatment. Some people will require biologic medications, such as rituximab or belimumab.

9. Arthralgias (joint pain) without actual inflammation (arthritis) are treated with pain relievers such as acetaminophen (Tylenol), NSAIDs (such as ibuprofen and naproxen), or other analgesics such as tramadol (Ultram and Ultracet), but not the stronger immunosuppressant medicines.

10. Regular exercise is very important for all people who have arthralgias and arthritis.

## Tendonitis

Tendonitis is also common in SLE. The tendons are sinewy, inelastic fibrous tissue that connect the muscles to the bones. When muscles contract to move parts of the body, it is the tougher tendons that enable them to move the much stronger bones. The tendons in unison with the muscles and joints of the body allow us to be able to move and do all the activities we are able to enjoy doing. Just as lupus can cause inflammation of the joints, it can also cause inflammation of the tendons (tendonitis). Tendonitis usually causes pain around and between the joints of the body. Sometimes there can be swelling as well. Some examples of tendonitis that can occur in SLE include rotator cuff tendonitis (at the shoulder), epicondylitis at the elbow (commonly called tennis elbow and golfer's elbow), flexor tenosynovitis in the palm of the hand (also called trigger finger), Achilles' tendonitis (back of the ankle), and plantar fasciitis (bottom of the heel).

Just as with arthritis, the tendonitis of SLE is treated with NSAIDs, steroids, and hydroxychloroquine (Plaquenil), while stronger medications such as methotrexate are used for difficult cases. Resting the tendon to allow the body to heal it is one of the most important things to learn to do. If you have tendonitis, it is very important to abide strictly by the joint protection measures listed in tables 7.2 and 7.3. Injections with a corticosteroid (cortisone injections) is also one of the safest and quickest ways to treat tendonitis. Using an ice pack as needed can also help to decrease the severity of pain from tendonitis.

## Myositis

Myositis refers to inflammation of the muscles caused by a direct attack by the immune system; it can occur in 10% of people who have SLE. This inflammation may cause muscle weakness. In fact, although there can be some achiness in the muscles (called myalgias), actual muscle weakness is the more common symptom. In fact, although many people who have SLE may develop myalgias to some degree, most do not actually have myositis. Myositis usually affects the muscles closest to the shoulders, hips, and thighs. Therefore, some people have difficulty raising their arms to brush their hair or difficulty standing up from a chair without using their hands to push themselves up due to the weakness of these particular muscle groups. The physician may find these muscles to be weak on examination and find an elevation in muscle enzymes in the blood work (such as CPK, aldolase, LDH, and AST levels; see chapter 4). Often there is enough evidence from these diagnostic findings to warrant treatment, but sometimes more specialized tests are required.

One of these tests is an electromyogram (EMG for short). This test, done in a doctor's office or a hospital, measures the electrical activity of the muscles. It is not a very comfortable test because a technician inserts tiny needles into the muscles to measure their electrical activity when the person is resting as well as when the technician instructs her or him to move the muscles. A doctor usually does not order this test unless he or she thinks it is important in making a correct diagnosis. Usually, a doctor will order a nerve conduction study at the same time as the EMG to determine whether there is evidence of nerve involvement from lupus causing the muscle weakness. The technician applies sticky electrodes to the skin, causing a tiny electrical shock to occur between the electrodes to see how well the nerves respond. This test is also uncomfortable because of the electrical shocks, but again, can provide very important information regarding the health of the nerves.

If the doctor suspects myositis, he or she can also order magnetic resonance imaging (MRI) of the muscles to see if there is any evidence of inflammation. MRI is a special type of imaging usually done with the person lying down on a table, then entering a narrow tube where magnetic waves help take pictures of the body. Since this procedure does not use radiation, there is no risk of developing cancer from the study. Sometimes MRIs are not helpful if there is significant metal in the body, and they can be dangerous if someone has a pacemaker or other implanted electronic device. Therefore, alert the technician or doctor if these scenarios apply to you. In addition, people who are claustrophobic often have difficulty getting through the test since the person has to go into a very narrow tube and hears very loud noises from the machine. If you are claustrophobic, you may want to ask your doctor for medication to calm your nerves before having the test, or have it done in a special MRI machine called an "open MRI," which does not enclose a person in a tight tube and is easier for people who have claustrophobia to tolerate. However, normal MRIs provide results that are of higher quality and accuracy.

If there is still the possibility of myositis or if the doctor needs to consider other options after the above tests, a muscle biopsy may be required. A "biopsy" is the medical term for when the doctor takes a small piece of tissue from the body for examination under a microscope. A doctor most commonly takes a muscle biopsy from the large muscle in front of the thigh or from the deltoid muscle at the top of the arm. In a biopsy, usually performed as an outpatient procedure, a surgeon numbs the area with an anesthetic and then makes a cut in the skin down to the muscle (an incision); a piece of the muscle is removed and sent to the laboratory. The doctor then closes the incision with sutures.

If myositis occurs in people who have lupus, doctors usually treat it with steroids. Sometimes they also use immunosuppressant drugs, such as methotrexate, azathioprine, mycophenolate, or intravenous immunoglobulin (IVIG for short). However, if a person just has achy muscles (myalgias) without having actual inflammation of the muscles (myositis), they are treated with pain relievers, such as acetaminophen (Tylenol), NSAIDs (such as ibuprofen and naproxen), or other analgesics such as tramadol (Ultram and Ultracet).

Just as with arthritis and arthralgias, regular exercise is very important for people who have myositis or myalgias. Regular strengthening exercises, in particular, are very important for people who have developed actual muscle weakness from their myositis. It can be beneficial to see a physical therapist to learn which exercises are most helpful in strengthening the affected muscles.

Problems other than myositis and nerve damage can cause muscle weakness in people who have lupus (and is the reason why all these different types of studies are often necessary). For example, steroids (the medications used to treat myositis) can potentially produce muscle damage and weakness by causing the muscle fibers to become smaller and weaker (muscle atrophy). This type of muscle problem usually does not cause an elevation in muscle enzymes, and a muscle biopsy will show smaller than normal muscle fibers without any inflammation. It is very important for a doctor to sort this out because the treatment for lupus myositis is to use steroids or increase the dose of steroids, while the treatment of steroid-induced muscle weakness (called steroid myopathy) is to decrease the dose of steroids. Other potential causes of muscle weakness include other drugs (such as anti-malarials) and metabolic problems such as diabetes, hyperthyroidism, and hypothyroidism.

**KEY POINTS TO REMEMBER**

1. Myositis means "inflammation of the muscles."

2. Myositis is usually painless, but occasionally muscle pain may also occur.

3. Weakness, especially of the upper arms (causing difficulty raising the arms) and the hips (causing difficulty standing up from a chair), is the most common symptom.

4. Some people who have myositis are diagnosed with an overlap syndrome with polymyositis (see chapter 2) when they have myositis with their SLE.

5. Myositis is diagnosed by finding muscle weakness on physical examination and elevated muscle enzymes in the blood (CPK, aldolase, LDH, and AST levels).

6. Sometimes, EMG tests and muscle biopsies are necessary to make the diagnosis.

7. Doctors usually treat myositis with steroids. Sometimes stronger immunosuppressants are necessary. Doctors sometimes use IVIG and rituximab as well.

8. Other causes of muscle problems, such as steroid side effects or thyroid problems, should be ruled out in people who have myositis and myalgias.

9. Myalgias (achy muscles) without actual inflammation (myositis) are treated with pain relievers such as acetaminophen (Tylenol), NSAIDs (such as ibuprofen and naproxen), or other analgesics such as tramadol (Ultram and Ultracet).

10. All lupus patients who have myositis or myalgias should exercise regularly.

## How to Treat Your Pain

Since the vast majority of people who have SLE will get aches and pains due to their lupus, it is very important to learn how to control them. There are things you can do on your own without relying completely on prescription medicines to gain control (table 7.1). Some people who have SLE have to take numerous medications to treat their lupus while at the same time avoiding side effects from those medicines. They would rather learn how to decrease their pain through measures other than taking additional prescription medicines.

**Table 7.1** How to Decrease Aches and Pains from Lupus

Protect involved joints (tables 7.2 and 7.3)

Exercise

    Range of motion and stretching

    Low-impact aerobic exercise

    Strengthening exercise

Over-the-counter medicines

Other modalities

    Heat and ice

    Meditation and prayer

    Yoga

    Biofeedback

    Acupuncture

    Stress reduction

## Joint Protection

One of the most important things in dealing with pain, and one of the least known, is called joint protection. When you rest a painful joint or tendon, you help to decrease inflammation, damage, and degeneration. These techniques should be used for all arthritides (the plural of arthritis). Whenever you develop pain in any part of your body, practice the following general joint protection measures as well as the joint protection recommendations for that particular part of the body. Overuse of a joint, incorrect use of a joint, and improper posture all contribute to injury and pain. Learning how to avoid these can go a long way in decreasing additional pain and injury. If you do it quickly enough in cases such as overuse tendonitis and arthritis, you can even stop the pain and may not need to see your physician.

*General Principles of Joint Protection.* Whenever pain persists, it is important to consider the possibility that you may be overstressing your joints and tendons. Think carefully about what you do at your job, at home, and while engaging in sports that may be aggravating your condition. For example, a person may keep getting wrist pain and then realize that this seems to occur most often the day after she crochets, one of her favorite hobbies. Repetitive tasks such as crocheting are some of the most common contributors to joint and tendon damage. Some of the most common causes of repetitive use tendon injury today are using computers and texting on cell phones. Therefore, it is important to identify activities that are exacerbating your joint pain and to do them less and for shorter periods. Another example would be the mother who keeps getting severe pain at the base of her thumb and then realizes that this often happens when she picks up her baby. Having to hold the thumb back while holding a baby can put a lot of stress on the tendons that move the thumb, so severe tendonitis can result. Learning to pick up and hold a baby in such a way that it does not stress those particular tendons can make a big difference in relieving the inflammation and pain. Using a wrist splint to help rest those tendons can also be very helpful.

Personality assessment is also important. The person who is a compulsive worker and perfectionist may have the attitude of "I'm going to finish this job if it kills me." This type of person needs to learn to respect her aches and pains, pay attention to what her body is telling her, and recognize this potentially self-destructive behavior. People who feel that they must do everything or that they are the only one who will get something done right can be particularly guilty of this. For example, a mother may insist that the house stay clean and organized in a certain way (after all, this is what her husband and children expect). Even though she may have severe arthritis pain, she pushes herself to clean everything to meet her own expectations, thereby causing her body more damage and pain. At the same time, her resentment toward her loved ones builds, and she ends up feeling that they do not care enough to help her. It becomes a vicious cycle where the pain, mental frustration, stress, and resentment continue to worsen over time. This not only damages the person's joints, but her relationships with the ones she loves. It can be very important to learn how to change your expectations, how not to be such a perfectionist, and realize that there is more than one way to live or work in a certain environment (such as how clean the house has to be). Learning to avoid certain tasks can be just as important as learning to perform a task in a manner that puts less stress on the joints. Table 7.2 lists some general joint protection techniques, while table 7.3 offers joint protection advice for various parts of the body.

## Exercise

Regular exercise is important for people who have SLE because it may help prevent strokes and heart attacks and it helps keep weight under control. It is also important for people who have arthritis since it improves function, preserves the joints, and decreases pain. Recommended exercises may vary depending on the exact problem as well as what parts of the body are affected. For example, the person who has myositis

**Table 7.2** General Joint Protection Techniques

- Respect pain; pain should warn you to decrease or avoid certain activities.
- Balance work and rest.
- Maintain strength and range of motion (see the subsequent sections on exercise).
- Decrease effort during tasks when using the painful part of your body.
- Simplify work tasks.
- Avoid any body position that causes pain, unnatural postures, or deformity.
- Use stronger, larger joints whenever possible.
- Avoid staying in one position for too long.
- Avoid activities that cannot be interrupted such as standing in long lines, carrying a package for a long distance, or going to public places (such as banks, grocery stores) during peak customer times.

**Table 7.3** Joint Protection Techniques for Specific Parts of the Body

*Head and neck:* You can use these techniques for neck pain, neck and head injuries, temporomandibular joint syndrome (TMJ for short), "pinched nerves" in the neck, and tension headaches

- Avoid sitting or standing in one place for more than thirty minutes at one time. Long periods of sitting can induce more neck strain than lifting heavy objects.

- Take frequent breaks during tasks in which your body does not move (e.g., while knitting, typing, etc.). Include tasks that allow your body greater movement (such as getting up and sweeping the floor for a few minutes after fifteen minutes of computer work).

- Align your head, neck, and trunk during rest and activities.

- Avoid stressful head positions (e.g., lying on a sofa with your head propped up, falling asleep in a chair and allowing your head to drop forward, or using more than one pillow to sleep on).

- Align your entire trunk, chest, and head on a slanted wedge or a very large pillow while watching television or reading in a reclining position. Proper body alignment decreases muscle strain and spasms.

- Elevate the entire mattress or the head of the bed if it is necessary for you to sleep with your head elevated. In other words, do not rely on pillows to do this.

- Sleep on your side or back, keeping your arms below chest level.

- Clenching the jaw can cause muscle spasms in the neck; use relaxation techniques or a bite spacer that you can get from your dentist.

- Store heavy items that you use daily no higher than the shoulders and no lower than the knees.

- Use a stepstool when lifting heavy items from shelves higher than the shoulders.

- Avoid the "birdwatcher's neck" that involves jutting the head forward as if watching birds through field glasses (such as what you get if staring at a computer screen that is positioned too high).

- Be conscious of stressful head positions when you concentrate, drive, or are tense.

- Use headsets or a speakerphone for prolonged or frequent telephone use.

- Place your computer screen at eye level and use a "document holder," "copyholder," or "book holder" to place work at eye level next to the screen.

- Use an adjustable chair and vary the height of the seat frequently during prolonged sitting.

- Maintain the proper hand-to-eye work or reading distance of sixteen inches.

- Position your body and work materials in such a way that your neck remains straight during activities.

- Use plastic goggles or eyeglasses with plastic lenses when playing sports.

Joint Protection Techniques (*continued*)

- Wear a safety helmet when cycling.

- Vary swim strokes and head position during swimming and water exercise. When diving, be certain that pools are of proper depth.

*Back and hips* (for the hips, also use the measures used for the knees, below)

- Strengthen and use the abdominal muscles that support your back. Learn to do crunches that do not strain your back. Get advice from your physician, ask an exercise instructor, or ask for a physical therapy consult to learn how.

- Perform trunk and hamstring flexibility exercises regularly.

- Do a regular strengthening and stretching program for abdominal and back muscles. It is best to do all these exercises first thing in the morning right after you get out of bed.

- Attain and maintain an ideal body weight.

- Avoid prolonged periods of sitting or standing. Use active sitting techniques such as "wiggling the pelvis" and rocking to activate and relax the pelvic muscles. Break up seated tasks, such as deskwork and card games, by standing and moving around for a few minutes every fifteen to thirty minutes.

- When standing for prolonged periods, place one foot on a higher surface (stool, brick, phone book) for a while and then alternate.

- Wear supportive cushion-soled shoes when standing or walking on concrete surfaces.

- Use proper rest and sleep positions. As an example, sleeping on your side with your legs slightly bent and a pillow between your knees or on your back with your knees and feet elevated with a cushion or pillow relieves stress on your back. Do not sleep on your stomach. If this proves difficult, placing a tennis ball in a pocket sewn onto the front of a T-shirt is a simple method to produce pressure and awaken you if you roll on your stomach. You should keep your arms below your shoulders.

- To release a painful "locked back," lie on your back and elevate your legs to the 90/90 position (hips and knees both bent at 90 degrees). Rest your lower legs on a chair or piano stool.

- Turn your body while moving your feet in alignment so that your toes point in the direction you are facing.

- To move objects at your side, rotate your entire body by moving your feet.

- When lifting an object, bend your knees, keeping your back straight. Use the palms of your hands or your forearm, instead of one hand, to pick up and carry an object.

- To lift large or heavy objects, move the object to your chest, lift it with your arms, and use your thigh muscles for strength. Hold the object close and centered in front of you.

- When lifting children and pets, be prepared for sudden shifts of weight. Do not carry a child on your side. Carry small children using a front or back harness pack.

Joint Protection Techniques (*continued*)

- For a sore "tail-bone" (coccyx), protect the point of tenderness at the tip. Sit on a foam cushion three inches thick and the size of the seat cushion. Cut a three-inch circle out of the cushion center for pressure relief. Place the cushion under your tailbone whenever you sit or do exercises on the floor.

- A leg length discrepancy of more than a half inch can cause back pain. Try a corrective insert to raise your shorter leg, and determine if pain is improved.

- Use cruise control when driving long distances.

- Do not carry a large wallet in a back pocket. Check for pressure placed on the pelvic bones by a wallet, tight belt, or constricting jeans that can squeeze nerves in the pelvis or groin.

- Always bend at the knees (keeping your back straight), not at the waist, even when you pick up something light off the floor such as a penny.

- Use a stepstool to reach overhead objects.

- Do trunk-stretching and leg-stretching warm-up exercises before sporting activities.

*Shoulders*

- Prevent cumulative movement damage by frequently interrupting repetitive tasks such as washing windows, vacuuming, and working on an assembly line. Take a mini-break and change position every twenty to forty minutes. Keep your elbows close to your body. Change the angle of shoulder motion when possible.

- Sleep with your arms below the level of your chest.

- If using crutches, adjust them properly to about two inches below the armpits. Carry weight on your ribs and hands, not under your arms. A forearm cane may be preferred.

- Rise from a chair by pushing off with your thigh muscles, not your hands.

- Take frequent breaks when working with your arms overhead.

- To grasp an object at your side or that is behind you, turn your entire body and face the object.

- Use assistance devices such as extended handles on combs, hairbrushes, toothbrushes, utensils, and dustpan handles; use a small cart for carrying things.

- Get rid of that large, heavy purse. Remove all items from your purse that you do not use on a regular basis. Get out of thinking that you have to carry everything "just in case."

- Use your far arm and hand across the front of your body to reach a car seat belt.

- A swivel or wheeled chair may be useful when tasks done from a seated position are in various locations.

- Keep your hands below the 3 o'clock and 9 o'clock position on the wheel when driving. If possible, use a steering wheel that tilts.

- Swimming: Strengthen and maintain shoulder muscles with proper exercises.

Joint Protection Techniques (*continued*)

- Tennis: Learn the proper serving and stroke techniques. Respect pain, avoid overuse, use frequent rest breaks. Relax your grip between strokes. Maintain shoulder strength through exercise; be aware of proper posture and positioning of joints.

- Weight lifting: Use proper lifting techniques. Consider getting assistance from a personal trainer or physical therapist to learn proper techniques if you are uncertain.

- Cycling: Avoid falling onto an outstretched arm. Learn to fall by pulling your arm in and rolling onto your shoulder.

- Golfing: Perform conditioning exercises year-round to avoid shoulder injuries. Learn proper swing and impact. Consider seeing a professional golf instructor to learn proper techniques if you are unsure. You may need to learn to move with less full strokes if you have significant tendonitis or arthritis of the shoulders. There should be no discomfort during your swing.

*Elbows and forearms*

- Avoid pressure and impact to the elbow.

- Do not contact any firm surface with your elbow when sitting.

- Use your abdominal muscles to help roll over when getting out of bed.

- Do not push off with your elbow against a hard surface when changing body position.

- Use relaxation techniques focused on your hands and arms to protect your forearm muscles.

- Recognize and avoid repetitive hand-clenching or excessive hard gripping. Wear stretch gloves with the seams to the outside for nighttime hand-clenching.

- Avoid forced gripping or twisting. Use kitchen aids such as jar openers, enlarged grips on utensils, or power tools. Look for items such as OXO Good Grips.

- Take periodic breaks and alternate tasks during manual activities.

- Use a light, two-handed grip when shaking hands repeatedly.

- Avoid prolonged use of tools requiring twist/force motions.

- Hold tools with a relaxed grip. Use foam or plastic pipe insulation (sold at hardware stores) on tool handles.

- Take frequent short breaks.

- Do not lean directly on your elbows; stabilize with your forearms.

- Change to a better work position or use elbow pads for protection.

- Use proper grip and play techniques with golf clubs, racquets, bats, or other pieces of sports equipment. Consult a pro for grip problems.

- Use elbow-protective equipment when playing hockey, roller-blading, or skating.

- Use stretch, strengthening, and relaxation exercises to condition the tissues that surround the elbow. Consider seeing a physical therapist to learn these exercises.

Joint Protection Techniques (*continued*)

*Hands*

- Recognize and avoid repetitive hand-clenching or excessive hard gripping. Wear stretch gloves with the seams to the outside for nighttime hand-clenching.

- Avoid forced gripping or twisting. Use kitchen aids such as jar openers, enlarged grips on utensils, or power tools. Look for items such as OXO Good Grips.

- When stirring food, hold the utensil with your thumb on top (as if you were stabbing a block of ice with an ice pick) and stir with shoulder motions.

- Avoid hanging a purse strap over your wrist or carrying heavy suitcases.

- Do not lean on your hands while standing by a table.

- Open jars by putting pressure on the top with your palm and twisting from the shoulder instead of by gripping the lid with your fingers.

- Pad the handles on utensils, tools, and the steering wheel with pipe insulation.

- Use assistance devices such as special faucet turners/levers, button hooks, elastic shoelaces, door openers, loop scissors, self-opening scissors, luggage carriers, mitt potholders, rubber jar lid openers, and an electric toothbrush.

- Wear stretch gloves while driving.

- Take periodic breaks and alternate tasks during manual activities.

- Use a light, two-handed grip when shaking hands repeatedly.

- Avoid prolonged use of tools requiring twist/force motions.

- Hold tools with a relaxed grip. Use foam or plastic pipe insulation (sold at hardware stores) on tool handles.

- Enlarge the handles of work tools; a two-and-one-quarter-inch diameter is optimum for most people.

- Texturize handle surfaces to provide an easier hold with less squeezing.

- Interrupt repetitive tasks (e.g., typing, peeling vegetables, knitting, and playing cards) with short breaks.

- Interrupt lengthy writing sessions by stopping for one to two minutes every ten minutes.

- Rest your hands flat and open instead of tight fisted.

- Use stronger, larger joints such as your shoulders whenever possible.

- Use your palms and forearms to carry heavy objects.

- Push, slide, or roll objects instead of lifting them.

- Use pencil grips and pad the stapler.

- Keep your hands off chairs when standing up from a sitting position.

Joint Protection Techniques (*continued*)

- Bend and straighten (wiggle) your fingers and wrists often.

- Grasp objects with your hand and all your fingers. Use both hands as much as possible when lifting heavy objects.

- Use real tools, not your thumbs, to pinch and push in your daily job activities. Use pliers for hard-to-remove Velcro fasteners.

- Power tools (e.g., screwdrivers and drills) are often preferable and easier to use than manual tools.

- Avoid uncomfortable hand positions.

- Keep your hand and wrist extended for work activities. Adapt tools with handles designed so that your wrist is straight.

- Use a wrist rest while working on a keyboard. Use a mouse pad that has a cushioned wrist rest with it.

- Use an appropriate tool to hit or move objects.

- Fit the handles of vibrating tools with shock absorbers or rubber, or wear gloves with gel inserts. Avoid strong vibrations and vibrations lasting longer than an hour at a time.

- Wear an appropriate splint or brace for rest and activity if joints are painful. Ask your doctor to refer you to an occupational therapist to get a proper splint if you have difficulty finding one.

- Ask your doctor to send you to an occupational therapist about work-induced and housework-induced problems, splinting, and modifying or adapting tools and equipment.

- Use proper grip size for racquet sports and golf. Golfers with arthritis should try using cushion grips and the baseball grip style (i.e., no locking fingers). Relax your grip until just before ball impact. Consult a pro for grip advice.

- Use a bowling ball with five finger holes. Have the edges of the holes beveled or smoothed out instead of being sharp.

*Knees and hips* (for the hips, also use the protection measures used for the back)

- Strengthen your thigh muscles (quadriceps and hamstrings) to protect your knees.

- If stair-climbing causes or increases knee pain, limit the activity and strengthen your thigh muscles until the pain subsides.

- Avoid deep-knee bending; use reach tools to pick up items from the floor.

- Avoid kneeling. If it is customary to kneel at church, remember that kneeling is not required to pray and it is bad for the knees.

- Straighten your knees or stand up at least every thirty minutes during prolonged periods of sitting to relieve pressure and stretch tight muscles. This is especially important during long car and plane trips.

- Short, brisk walks will increase leg circulation and exercise muscles.

Joint Protection Techniques (*continued*)

- Buy shoes with no heels and with shock-absorbing soles, and check them often for signs of wear. Wear shoes with good arch supports. Do not wear women's high heel shoes or flats without good arches.

- Use your thigh muscles to rise from a chair.

- Use a mechanic's or gardener's stool when working on the floor or on the ground. Sit with your legs apart and reach forward to perform tasks such as gardening or scrubbing floors.

- Use protective kneepads if you must work on hands and knees.

- Consider raised or container gardening to reduce stress and effort.

- Consider assistance devices such as elevated seats with armrests, raised toilet seats, shower bench, extended shoehorns, long-handled reachers, bathtub grab bars, and walking aids such as a cane or walker if needed.

- Stationary biking provides safe, low-impact exercise. Adjust the seat height so that your knees bend slightly at the low point of the down stroke, and no more than 90 degrees flexed on the upstroke. Increase resistance gradually. Consider a recumbent bike if you have a bad back.

- Perform a regular stretching program for the muscles of your upper and lower legs. Tight muscles can contribute to knee problems. Consider asking your doctor to send you to a physical therapist to learn proper stretching techniques.

- Treat knee injuries promptly with the RICE techniques (Rest, Ice, Compression, and Elevation). Seek medical attention if pain and instability persist.

- Engage in exercise and sports activities on a regular basis instead of occasional weekend participation. Include warm-up and cool-down activities as well as appropriate stretching in your routine. Consider asking your doctor to refer you to a physical therapist to learn proper exercise techniques.

- Consider doing water exercise classes designed for people with arthritis several days a week.

- Modify or avoid knee-twisting dance steps or exercises.

- Avoid sitting with a leg folded under.

*Feet and ankles*

- Choose footwear with comfort, support, and utility in mind. Do not wear shoes that cause pain or fatigue. Get professional advice when necessary. Appropriate shoes will provide support and comfort for the weight-bearing foot with room for the toes to extend fully and to broaden out during weight bearing. Do not wear shoes tapered or pointed at the toes (i.e., wear shoes with a squared "toe box"). Proper fit should be determined by having the foot size measured while standing not sitting. You should wear cushioned soles with shock-absorbing material. Wear shoes with a good arch support. Do not wear women's high heel shoes or flats. Do not wear sandals or flip flops, or go bare foot.

Joint Protection Techniques (*continued*)

- Loose-jointed people should be particularly careful to protect the ankles and feet. Sprains and strains can increase instability.

- Orthotic inserts can provide needed support and positioning assistance. Consult an experienced professional about the choice of an orthotic, whether having it custom made or obtaining it over the counter. Use orthotics in sports shoes and everyday shoes.

- Maintain an appropriate weight to reduce stress on your feet and ankles.

- Running shoes, walking shoes, or aerobics shoes are more supportive and comfortable for the flexible or arthritic foot. Good running shoes and arch supports are important.

- Use a metatarsal pad or bar to relieve pressure or pain at the forefoot.

- Treat ankle sprains promptly with RICE techniques (Rest, Ice, Compression, and Elevation). Seek medical advice if swelling and pain do not subside.

- Use footwear that is designed for the sport you are playing.

- Keep your feet meticulously clean and dry, especially between your toes.

- Look for blisters and pressure sores. Change your shoes or get professional advice if these signs of stress develop.

- Avoid chemical agents or cutting to remove calluses; they have formed for a reason. Find out what that reason is and fix it.

- Cut your toenails straight across and regularly.

- Plan ahead to avoid excessive walking when your feet are painful.

- Run on dirt or track surfaces; avoid running on concrete or asphalt.

should be doing different exercises than someone who has hip arthritis who in turn should be doing slightly different exercises than someone who has hip bursitis. It is best to ask your doctor for advice regarding specific exercises or consider asking him or her to send you to a physical therapist for proper assessment and instruction. I discuss some basics however on what general types of exercises you should do regularly. The broad categories of exercise are range-of-motion, stretching, aerobic, and strengthening exercises. A good, well-balanced exercise program should include each of these categories. If you have significant arthritis in weight-bearing joints (feet, knees, and hips) or the back; then water exercise classes are a good choice. All four categories of exercise are easily performed in water while putting less stress on the joints.

*Range-of-Motion and Stretching Exercises.* The range of motion of a joint refers to how far a joint can move in all directions. Over time, arthritis and pain can cause a loss of range of motion and therefore a loss of proper function. Maintaining range of motion as much as possible is very important. You should move painful joints through their full range of motion every day. Use the hand of the opposite side of the body to move the painful joint gently as far as it can go without causing pain. Repeat this in every direction in which that joint can move.

You can do stretching exercises at the same time that you do range-of-motion exercises. They should be a regular part of the exercise regimen either before or after aerobic or strengthening exercises. Stretching helps to keep the joints, muscles, and ligaments limber and flexible. You can do numerous stretching exercises. You can find them in exercise books or on the internet, or learn about them from a physical therapist or exercise instructor. It is important to concentrate on staying relaxed while stretching. Each joint or muscle that is stretched should be held at a point where a feeling of stretching is felt without pain. If it is painful, then you should relax the stretch slightly. You should hold the stretch for fifteen to thirty seconds; breathe deeply and slowly to help relax your muscles.

*Aerobic Exercises.* Another term for aerobic exercises is "endurance exercises." Aerobic exercises work large muscle groups continuously to keep the heart rate elevated. Examples include brisk walking, stationary bicycling, high- and low-impact aerobic exercises, swimming, dancing, walking on a treadmill, and using an elliptical exercise machine. Studies show that aerobic exercise decreases pain in people who have arthritis, helps with weight loss, lessens stress and depression, improves muscle strength and function, helps control diabetes and high blood pressure, helps to prevent heart attacks and strokes, and increases lifespan. You should exercise to the point where you are breathing harder than normal but are still able to speak in full sentences. It can also be very helpful to exercise strenuously enough to reach your target heart rate (which depends on your age). You can ask your doctor what target heart rate he or she recommends. It is also easy to find target heart rate calculators on the internet such as at the Mayo Clinic's site, www.mayoclinic.com/health/target-heart-rate/SM00083. It is best to do some sort of aerobic exercise for twenty to forty-five minutes four to five days a week. However, when first starting an exercise regimen it is very important to begin very slowly to avoid injuring joints, tendons, and muscles that are probably not used to exercising. Start with five to ten minutes of very light exercise and slowly build up to the recommended final goal.

*Strengthening Exercises.* When you have pain or arthritis, the muscles around the painful joints begin to weaken, tighten up, and get smaller ("atrophy" in medical terms). This becomes a vicious cycle because the muscle becomes dysfunctional which in turn causes even more pain and disability. Regular strengthening exercises are vital in maintaining the strength of the muscles to increase function and improve or retain a good quality of life. If you are healthy then it can be easy to go to a gym and learn what exercises to do from a personal trainer or gym staff member. Consider getting exercise equipment to use at home as well. If you have more significant health problems, especially if you have arthritis and joint pain, it would be better to get your doctor's advice or ask for a referral to a physical therapist who can teach you what exercises to do on your own. Today a variety of exercise classes exist in the community designed specifically for people with arthritis. Attending these classes can be educational and good for your health, and they can add a positive social aspect when you exercise along with people who have similar problems.

## Over-the-Counter Medicines

There are medications that are available over the counter that you can safely use to help control pain. While this chapter provides recommendations regarding when and how to use them, it is also very important that you read the package instructions thoroughly. Also, check with your doctor first to make sure a given medication is safe to use in light of any other medical problems you may have, and to ensure it is safe to use with your other medications. Never take any over-the-counter medicines without doing this first; otherwise, there is always the potential risk for drug interactions.

*Acetaminophen (Tylenol, Numerous Other Brand Names).* Acetaminophen is one of the safest pain relievers. It is the drug of choice to treat osteoarthritis (also called degenerative joint disease).

*Generic available*: Yes.

*How acetaminophen works*: Not fully understood.

*What benefits to expect from acetaminophen*: Can decrease the severity of aches and pains and fever.

*How acetaminophen is taken*: The maximum recommended daily dose is 4,000 mg a day (table 7.4). If significant pain relief does not occur by taking it on an as needed basis, then you should try taking it regularly around the clock instead of just as needed. It can take up to a week to get the full effect when taken this way. This would be the equivalent of taking 500 mg tablets (Tylenol Extra Strength) two tablets at a time four times a day.

Acetaminophen can help decrease pain in combination with NSAIDs, as they appear to decrease pain through different mechanisms. Therefore, acetaminophen can help decrease pain more if you are already taking an NSAID. It is generally safe to take along with an NSAID as well. See the following section about NSAIDs.

*Alcohol/food/herbal interactions with acetaminophen*: People who have had a history of excessive alcohol intake or alcoholism should not take acetaminophen unless their doctor makes sure that their liver functions properly. Do not drink more than two servings of alcohol a day while taking acetaminophen. One serving is the equivalent of 8 ounces of beer, 5 ounces of wine, or a shot of hard liquor. Women of lower body weight should probably restrict their alcohol intake to one serving a day or less when taking acetaminophen.

Acetaminophen is absorbed best when taken on an empty stomach.

St. John's wort can decrease absorption. Avoid Echinacea, kava, willow, and meadowsweet, which may increase the risks for liver and kidney problems with acetaminophen.

**Table 7.4**  Dosing of Acetaminophen (Tylenol)

| | |
|---|---|
| acetaminophen 650 mg (Tylenol Arthritis) | 2 tablets 3 times a day |
| acetaminophen 500 mg (Tylenol Extra Strength) | 2 tablets 4 times a day |
| acetaminophen 325 mg (Tylenol Regular Strength) | 3 tablets 4 times a day |

*Potential side effects of acetaminophen*: Significant side effects from acetaminophen (table 7.5) are minimal as long as you do not take a higher dose than normal and as long as you do not drink too much alcohol. It is the safest systemic pain medicine available. Since some prescription pain medicines (especially opioids) also contain acetaminophen, it is very important to make sure you are not taking too much acetaminophen. Always check with your doctor if you are taking any pain medicines before purchasing anything over the counter.

*What needs to be monitored while taking acetaminophen*: Nothing.

*Reasons not to take acetaminophen (contraindications or precautions)*:

- If you have liver disease, have had hepatitis, or have drunk alcohol excessively in the past, ask your doctor before taking acetaminophen.

- If you drink more than two servings of alcohol in any twenty-four-hour period, check with your doctor before taking acetaminophen.

- Check with your doctor first to make sure you are not taking any prescription medicines that contain acetaminophen, as you may need to decrease your dose of acetaminophen.

- Check with your doctor if you have kidney disease, as you may need to take less acetaminophen per day.

*While taking acetaminophen*: Contact your doctor immediately if you develop jaundice (yellow skin and whites of eyes).

*Pregnancy and breast-feeding while taking acetaminophen*: May increase the risk of asthma in a newborn baby. May increase the risk of patent ductus arteriosus if taken during the third trimester. Probably safe to take in small amounts during the first two trimesters. It is best to check with your obstetrician before taking acetaminophen.

Although small amounts of acetaminophen enter breast milk, the American College of Pediatrics has stated that it is "compatible" to take acetaminophen while breast-feeding.

*Geriatric use of acetaminophen*: No dose adjustments needed unless there is significant chronic kidney disease.

**Table 7.5** Potential Side Effects of Acetaminophen (Tylenol)

| | Incidence | Side Effect Therapy |
|---|---|---|
| **Nuisance side effects** | | |
| Rash | Rare | Stop taking medicine. |
| **Serious side effects** | | |
| Liver failure when taking more than 4,000 mg a day or if drinking too much alcohol | Rare | Seek medical attention immediately if you try to overdose on the medicine. |

**Table 7.6**  Over-the-Counter NSAIDs

aspirin (Ascriptin, Bayer, Ecotrin)

ibuprofen (Advil, Midol, Motrin, Nurofen)

naproxen (Aleve)

*Non-Steroidal Anti-Inflammatory Drugs.* Non-steroidal anti-inflammatory drugs (NSAIDs for short) are the largest group of medications used for aches and pains, and many brands are available over the counter (table 7.6). It is very important to make sure that you are not taking any prescription NSAIDs before you consider taking an over-the-counter NSAID (see chapter 36). However, it is generally safe to take an NSAID along with acetaminophen to help in decreasing pain.

*Generic available*: Yes.

*How NSAIDs work*: NSAIDs are weak anti-inflammatory medications. In other words, they appear to decrease inflammation albeit only slightly. They inhibit an enzyme in the body, causing less production of chemical substances called prostaglandins. Prostaglandins are important in causing inflammation, but they also have significant roles in keeping the body healthy (such as protecting the stomach, stabilizing blood pressure, regulating kidney function, helping the platelets work normally, and many others). Because most NSAIDs decrease the production of many different types of prostaglandins (good and bad), not only can they help with pain and inflammation but they can also cause side effects (such as stomach ulcers, high blood pressure, kidney failure, bleeding, and many others).

The low-dose NSAIDs obtained over the counter probably have minimal, if any, anti-inflammatory effects. Instead, they have analgesic (pain-relieving) properties that are noticeable when they are taken as needed and in smaller doses. The analgesic effects tend to parallel the dose. In other words, high doses tend to decrease pain more than lower doses. For simple pain relief, it is better to take the lowest dose needed to decrease the potential of side effects, which are more apt to occur at higher doses. However, to help with inflammation (the anti-inflammatory effects of NSAIDs), you need to take them at higher, prescription-strength doses on a regular basis.

Not all NSAIDs work in everyone. One NSAID may work very well in one person, and not at all in another. Therefore, if you try one NSAID (Aleve or naproxen, for example), and it does not help, then you should try taking a different form (such as Advil or ibuprofen).

*What benefits to expect from NSAIDs*: Decreased pain and fever.

*How NSAIDs are taken*: The over-the-counter forms are in pill, capsule, liquid, and topical forms. Follow the instructions, as dosing depends on which medication is used.

If you take a daily aspirin to prevent heart attacks and strokes, check with your doctor before taking NSAIDs, as the combination increases the risk for ulcers. If your doctor allows you to take them together, make sure to take the aspirin first thing in the morning, and wait at least two hours before you take either naproxen or ibuprofen;

otherwise, the NSAID will negate the blood-thinning properties of the aspirin. You want the aspirin to thin the blood to prevent heart attacks and strokes.

*Alcohol/food/herbal interactions with NSAIDs*: Avoid alcohol with NSAIDs as it can increase the risk for developing stomach ulcers.

You should take NSAIDs with food to decrease stomach upset.

Avoid alfalfa, anise, bilberry, bladderwrack, bromelain, cat's claw, celery, chamomile, coleus, cordyceps, dong quai, evening primrose, fenugreek, feverfew, garlic, ginger, ginkgo biloba, ginseng (American, Panax, and Siberian), grape seed, green tea, guggul, horse chestnut seed, horseradish, licorice, meadowsweet, motherwort, prickly ash, red clover, reishi, SAMe (S-adenosylmethionine), sweet clover, tamarind, turmeric, and white willow. All of these have additional anti-platelet activity increasing the risk of bleeding.

*Potential side effects of NSAIDs*: By far the most common side effects of NSAIDs are their effects on the stomach (table 7.7). They cause numerous potential problems ranging from heartburn, bloating, and diarrhea/constipation to outright ulcers. Most people who get a bleeding ulcer from NSAIDs have no warning (i.e., no stomach upset or pain) probably due to the decrease in pain that NSAIDs produce. They can also cause other problems, such as elevated blood pressure, swelling of the ankles (called edema), and decreased kidney function. Most people should not take an over-the-counter NSAID without checking with a physician first to make sure it is safe for them.

*What needs to be monitored while taking NSAIDs*:

- Blood tests for kidney function, liver function tests, and blood counts

- Blood pressure

*Reasons not to take NSAIDs (contraindications or precautions)*:

- Decreased kidney function

- Severe liver disease

- Blood pressure is not well controlled

- You have had congestive heart failure

- Active stomach ulcer

- Upcoming surgery (so that you do not bleed too much during surgery)

- If you have had severe allergic reactions to other NSAIDs or aspirin products

- Aspirin sensitivity, which includes nasal polyps and asthma due to aspirin

- Check with your doctor first especially if you have high blood pressure, diabetes, heart problems, or a history of stroke or heart attacks, or if you are on blood thinners (such as Plavix, Coumadin, or heparin)

*While taking NSAIDs*:

- Contact your physician immediately if you throw up blood, develop abdominal pain, have bright red blood in your feces, or develop black tarry feces. These could be warning signs of a bleeding ulcer. Remember, though, that most people have no preceding stomach upset or pain from a bleeding ulcer due to NSAIDs.

**Table 7.7** Potential Side Effects of NSAIDs

| | Incidence | Side Effect Therapy |
|---|---|---|
| **Nuisance side effects** | | |
| Heartburn, nausea, and stomach pain | Common | Take with food, or discuss with your doctor to either try a different NSAID or take a medicine to decrease stomach acidity. |
| Cramping or diarrhea | Common | Take with food, reduce dosage, or switch to a different NSAID. |
| Fluid retention, ankle-swelling (edema), weight gain | Common | Decrease sodium salt intake, stop NSAID, see doctor. |
| Headache, drowsiness, dizziness, difficulty concentrating | Common | Try a different NSAID. |
| Increased bleeding and bruising | Common | Usually no treatment or stop NSAID. |
| Ringing in the ears or decreased hearing | Common | Discontinue NSAID. |
| Elevated liver enzyme blood tests | Common | Usually minimal problems. Your doctor may continue NSAID, decrease dose, or change to a different NSAID. |
| Rash | Uncommon | Discontinue NSAID. |
| **Serious side effects** | | |
| Elevated blood pressure | Common | Stop NSAID, lower dose, or change to a different NSAID. |
| Gastritis, esophagitis, stomach ulcers | Uncommon | Stop NSAID and take medicine to decrease stomach acidity. |
| Bleeding ulcers (bloody stools, vomit blood, or have black tarry stools) | Uncommon | Seek medical attention immediately. Discontinue NSAID and take medicine to decrease stomach acidity. |
| Decreased kidney function | Uncommon | Discontinue NSAID. |
| Hepatitis (liver inflammation and damage) | Rare | Stop NSAID. |
| Decreased blood counts | Rare | Discontinue NSAID. |

Side effect incidence key (these are approximations as they can vary widely study to study): rare < 1% occurrence; uncommon 1%–5% occurrence; common > 5% occurrence

- Contact your doctor if you develop heartburn, diarrhea, constipation, rash, elevated blood pressure, shortness of breath, yellowish-colored whites of the eyes (jaundice), or swelling of the ankles.

- If you have any dental procedure or surgery scheduled, you will need to stop the NSAID beforehand.

- Inform your doctor about all your prescribed and over-the-counter medicines before she or he prescribes you medication for pain. It is important to make sure you are not taking two different NSAIDs at the same time.

- Let your doctor know before he or she prescribes you anything to ensure that there are no drug interactions.

- Do not take two or more NSAIDs. The only exception is if your doctor gives you approval to take an NSAID with low-dose aspirin (used to prevent heart attacks and strokes). Make sure to ask your doctor to consider giving you a drug to decrease acidity of the stomach if you take aspirin plus another NSAID to prevent stomach ulcers.

*Pregnancy and breast-feeding while taking NSAIDs*: It is reassuring that a 2012 report showed no increased risks of major fetal malformation from NSAIDs. This study looked at a total of 109,544 pregnancies between 1998 and 2009 of which 5,267 women were taking NSAIDs.

If you have trouble getting pregnant (infertility), consider not taking NSAIDs, which may decrease fertility. There was a 2011 report from Canada that suggested that NSAIDs might increase the risk for miscarriage if taken during the first twenty weeks of pregnancy. However, an editorial about the study criticized the findings and pointed out some important flaws. Until known for sure, if you do not absolutely need to take an NSAID during the first twenty weeks, it is probably best not to do so.

NSAIDs should not be taken at week 30 of pregnancy or later to prevent a problem called patent ductus arteriosus (a problem where a very important blood vessel does not close properly in the baby's heart and lung circulation). Many doctors recommend not taking NSAIDs during the third trimester entirely.

Naproxen (Aleve) is not recommended during breast-feeding. Ibuprofen (Advil, Motrin, and Nuprin) appears in breast milk, but the American Academy of Pediatrics has approved it as being "compatible" with breast-feeding.

*Geriatric use of NSAIDs*: Older people have a much higher chance for side effects such as elevated blood pressure, ulcers, kidney failure, heart failure, and heart attacks from NSAIDs and should not take them unless approved by their physician.

*Capsaicin Topical Therapies (Zostrix, Capzacin)*.
  *Generic available*: Yes.
  *How capsaicin works*: Capsaicin is the active ingredient found in chili peppers of the genus *Capsicum* (where capsaicin gets its name). When applied to the skin, it causes the nerves that sense pain to release a chemical called substance P. Substance P is important for transmitting pain impulses to the brain. The continuous release of substance P from the nerves due to capsaicin eventually causes the nerves to become deficient in substance P. Due to this action, capsaicin initially causes a burning sensation, but over time, decreases pain in the area.

*What benefits to expect from capsaicin*: Decreased severity of pain when used regularly on the same area. It takes two to four weeks of regular usage three to four times a day to obtain significant pain relief.

*How to take capsaicin*: You apply capsaicin to the skin overlying the painful joint. You must use it at least three times a day, preferably four times a day, on a regular basis. If you use it less than three times a day, or for less than two weeks, you will get minimal pain relief benefits. It does cause a burning sensation, so you should be very careful not to touch sensitive areas such as the mouth, eyes, nose, or genitals with the fingers used to apply the cream. Using products with special applicators, using gloves to apply the cream, or washing your hands with soap and water thoroughly after using it can be helpful in preventing this. In addition, you should not rub it into the skin, which can intensify the burning discomfort; just apply it lightly to the skin. The burning intensity decreases over time.

*Alcohol/food/herbal interactions with capsaicin*: No precautions.

*Potential side effects of capsaicin*: Listed in table 7.8.

*What needs to be monitored while taking capsaicin*: Nothing.

*Reasons not to take capsaicin (contraindications or precautions)*: Do not use on any rash or open sore.

*While taking capsaicin*:

- Do not apply heat or a bandage over the area.

- Avoid direct sun exposure to skin surface.

*Pregnancy and breast-feeding while taking capsaicin*: There is no evidence of human risk during pregnancy, but check with your doctor before using capsaicin.

Excretion in milk is unknown. Check with your doctor.

*Geriatric use of capsaicin*: No special precautions needed.

**Table 7.8** Potential Side Effects of Capsaicin

|  | *Incidence* | *Side Effect Therapy* |
|---|---|---|
| **Nuisance side effects** | | |
| Burning discomfort of the skin | Almost everyone | Gradually decreases over time. Minimize by not rubbing into the skin, apply lightly, use regularly not just as needed. Do not apply a heating pad on top of skin where applied. Do not apply on lupus rash. |
| **Serious side effects** | | |
| Severe burning if it contacts sensitive surfaces (eyes, lips, nose, genitals) | Common | Flush with soap and cold water. Seek medical attention for eye exposure. |

## Other Modalities

You and your doctor can consider numerous other modalities to try to reduce pain such as acupuncture, massage therapy, yoga, or tai chi. There is a discussion of these in chapter 39.

### KEY POINTS TO REMEMBER

1. Make sure to learn the joint protection techniques listed in tables 7.2 and 7.3 to prevent injury to the joints and tendons and to help decrease your pain.

2. Exercise regularly with a combination of range-of-motion, stretching, aerobic, and strengthening exercises. Consider asking your doctor for a physical therapy consult to learn how to exercise properly.

3. If you have significant arthritis of the back, hips, knees, or feet, consider participating regularly in water exercise classes designed for people with arthritis.

4. Acetaminophen (Tylenol) is the safest medicine to take for pain, but be careful if you drink excessive amounts of alcohol or have liver problems. Make sure you do not take too much acetaminophen if any of your pain medicines also contain acetaminophen.

5. Over-the-counter NSAIDs include naproxen and ibuprofen. They have many potential side effects and drug interactions. Always ask your doctor before taking them.

6. If you take an NSAID and also need to take aspirin daily (to prevent heart attacks and strokes), take the NSAID at least two hours after you take the aspirin so it does not interfere with how the aspirin works.

7. Consider asking your doctor for a medicine to lower stomach acidity to decrease the chances of developing ulcers while taking an NSAID.

8. Capsaicin cream is one of the safest over-the-counter therapies for joint pain, but you must use it regularly three to four times a day to decrease pain. One of the key ingredients is chili peppers, so you have to be careful not to get it in your eyes or on other mucous membranes (nose, mouth, genitals, etc.).

9. See chapter 39 for other methods of treating pain, such as acupuncture and massage.

# Skin and Mucous Membranes

## The Largest Organ of the Body

The skin is the largest organ of the body, weighing six pounds in the average person. It can be thought of as the bag keeping your internal organs in place, but it serves many other functions as well—including keeping your temperature stable, absorbing moisture and gases, excreting waste minerals and moisture, keeping too much water from evaporating from the body, and acting as a means for you to touch and feel your environment. It is an important barrier against the outside world (such as bacteria and viruses) and actually contains an important part of the immune system (such as antigen-presenting cells mentioned in chapter 1). Of course, skin is also very important in terms of how each person looks and is recognized by others.

Areas where the skin enters the body and becomes lubricated—such as the inside of the mouth, nose, vagina, and anus—are called mucous membranes. More than 80% of people who have SLE will have involvement of the skin or the mucous membranes of the mouth or nose. After joints, the skin and mucous membranes are the next most commonly involved parts of the body in SLE. Although these problems are rarely life threatening, the impact can be tremendous when it comes to your appearance and the potential problems it can cause with self-esteem. There are many different ways that lupus can affect the skin and mucous membranes and this chapter goes into more detail about them. It also covers hair and nails since they can also be affected by lupus.

· · · ·

Two types of skin problems occur with SLE—those that are specific for lupus (in other words, they are only seen in lupus patients) and those that are seen with lupus patients but also in other disorders as well. The lupus-specific rashes are termed "cutaneous lupus" ("cutaneous" means "skin") and are divided into acute cutaneous lupus, subacute cutaneous lupus, and chronic cutaneous lupus (table 8.1). Any of the specific cutaneous lupus rashes fulfill classification criteria for the diagnosis of SLE, as discussed in chapter 1.

## Lupus-Specific Rashes

Doctors usually diagnose lupus rashes by the way they appear on physical examination. However, sometimes a skin biopsy is necessary to know for sure. A skin biopsy is a very simple procedure performed in a doctor's office on an outpatient basis. The doc-

**Table 8.1** Types of Cutaneous Lupus (Lupus-Specific Rashes)

Acute cutaneous lupus erythematosus (ACLE)

    Butterfly (also malar) rash

    Sun-sensitive (also photosensitive rash and polymorphous light eruption) ACLE

    Generalized ACLE

Subacute cutaneous lupus erythematosus (SCLE)

    Papulosquamous (also called psoriasiform) SCLE

    Annular (also called polycyclic) SCLE

Chronic cutaneous lupus erythematosus

    Discoid lupus erythematosus (DLE)

        Localized DLE

        Generalized DLE

    Lupus panniculitis (also called lupus profundus)

    Lupus erythematosus tumidus

    Chilblains lupus

    Hypertrophic (also hyperkeratotic and verrucous) DLE

tor anesthetizes the skin, snips out a small piece of skin, and sews up the area with either sutures (surgical thread) or suture adhesive tape. The doctor then sends the skin sample to a laboratory for examination under a microscope. Sometimes in order to make a proper diagnosis, the doctor may need to order a special type of biopsy study called immunofluorescence. This is where the pathologist (the doctor who examines biopsies under the microscope) performs a special type of examination looking for the deposit of lupus antibodies between the upper (epidermal) and lower (dermal) skin layers.

## Acute Cutaneous Lupus Erythematosus

There are several forms of acute cutaneous lupus erythematosus (ACLE) ("acute" means "lasting for a short time") and all of these occur in the context of SLE. They do not occur in people who do not have SLE. They include a butterfly rash, a sun-sensitive rash, and a generalized acute cutaneous lupus rash. All of these are sensitive to ultraviolet light and therefore can increase with exposure to light and sun. They usually have a similar appearance, with a reddish or pinkish discoloration of the skin that becomes more prominent with sun exposure. They may cause a warm sensation to the skin, but usually are neither itchy nor painful. These rashes may persist for days to weeks, especially after significant sun exposure, but can also be fleeting, lasting only a few hours. Fortunately, when these rashes resolve with treatment, they do not cause permanent scarring of the skin. However, occasionally they may leave some dark-colored areas, or what doctors call "post-inflammatory hyperpigmentation." This occurs more often in dark-skinned individuals. This is a response of the skin to the inflammation caused by an increase in the amount of melanin (dark pigmentation of the skin) within the cells of the skin.

A butterfly rash (photograph 8.1) is a reddish- or pink-colored rash occurring on the parts of the face exposed more to the sun (the cheeks and bridge of the nose). If someone were to draw an outline around the rash, the redness of the cheeks would look like the wings of a butterfly and the rash on the bridge of the nose would look like its body. Other terms for this are "malar rash" and "malar erythema" ("malar" refers to the cheek area, while "erythema" means "redness"). Up to 60% of SLE patients will develop a butterfly, or malar, rash. Not all red faces in people who have lupus, however, are due to the malar rash of lupus. Other possibilities that sometimes have to be considered include acne rosacea (adult-onset acne), seborrheic dermatitis (which is a type of scaly skin inflammation), and even the use of steroids (which can cause a red face). Therefore, it sometimes takes the help of a skin doctor (dermatologist) to help correctly diagnose and treat this type of problem in people who have lupus.

Another form of acute cutaneous lupus is a sun-sensitive rash, also called a photosensitive rash, produced from exposure to light. This causes a reddish-colored rash to occur mainly on those parts of the body that are exposed to light, such as the cheeks, forehead, chin, lips, ears, upper back and chest areas, and top parts of the hands and forearms. On the hands, this type of rash frequently causes a red rash between the joints of the fingers (instead of directly over the joints) as well as a reddish discoloration of the skin next to the fingernails. This form of ACLE occurs in up to 69% of patients.

A generalized acute cutaneous rash is very similar to a photosensitive rash, but a reddish rash also occurs on parts of the skin covered with clothing. This form of rash (as well as the photosensitive rash) especially seems to occur in people who are particularly sick with their SLE, often with fever, joint pain, and other problems going on as well. Doctors will often call this type of rash a "maculopapular rash"—macules are small red blotches that you cannot feel when you run your hand over them, while

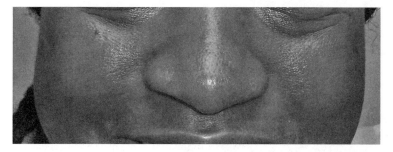

**Photo 8.1** Malar erythema in a person who has SLE. There is pinkish discoloration on the cheeks. Most people who have a malar rash will have a mild pink discoloration (as in this person), while others may have a more intense and more easily noted red rash.

papules are red splotches that are raised above the skin's surface—because it is a combination of both of these lesions over a large area of the skin. Although not common, occasionally this type of acute cutaneous lupus rash can also cause blisters to form on the skin. This typically happens in people who are sick with severe lupus.

### Subacute Cutaneous Lupus

Subacute cutaneous lupus erythematosus (SCLE) occurs in two forms. One appears as red, scaly patches, almost like psoriasis, and is called either psoriasiform SCLE or papulosquamous SCLE (both referring to the same thing). The other form of SCLE appears as reddish-colored rings of rash called annular or polycyclic SCLE (photograph 8.2). One potential importance of distinguishing the two forms is that people who have the annular (polycyclic) form of SCLE appear to have milder SLE and are less likely to get kidney or brain involvement.

SCLE always worsens with exposure to light, and, in fact, there is even a case in the medical literature of it occurring from exposure to a photocopier machine. Many people who have subacute cutaneous lupus are positive for anti-SSA antibodies (discussed in chapter 4), and the rash can occasionally be caused or made worse by some medications. For example, some blood pressure medicines (such as diuretics, calcium channel blockers, beta-blockers, and ACE inhibitors) can cause this rash. Therefore, if a person started any of these medicines even years before the rash, it is usually a good idea to stop the medication and see if the rash disappears. Unfortunately, when it heals, this type of rash can cause permanent discoloration to the skin as areas of light- and dark-colored splotches.

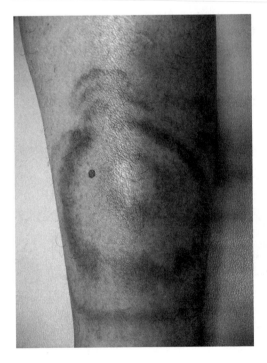

Photo 8.2 Subacute cutaneous lupus erythematosus, annular form on the lower leg, an unusual location. Note that most people who have subacute cutaneous lupus do not have rashes that are annular to the point of looking like a "bull's eye" as in this individual. More often they appear as smaller areas of ring-shaped lesions (as in the annular form) or scaly, red patches (as in the papulosquamous form).

While all people who have acute cutaneous lupus also have systemic lupus, only 50% of people who have SCLE also develop SLE. In addition, the severity of the systemic lupus overall tends to be milder compared to SLE patients who do not have subacute cutaneous lupus. Although SLE overall appears to be less severe in people who have SCLE, sometimes severe SLE can occur (as with brain and kidney involvement), but it more commonly occurs in those with the papulosquamous (or psoriasiform) type of SCLE.

## Chronic Cutaneous Lupus

Chronic cutaneous lupus erythematosus (CCLE) is more common than the cutaneous lupus forms described above. There are several different types of CCLE. All of them tend to occur for a long time and often leave permanent scarring and color changes to the skin in the areas in which they occur.

By far the most common form of CCLE is discoid lupus erythematosus (DLE). In fact, DLE is a very common rash seen by dermatologists (skin doctors) with most DLE patients only having the skin problem and never developing the systemic form of lupus. The question always arises about the chances of developing the systemic form of lupus once you have developed the discoid form. Although some medical experts have said that only 10% of DLE patients will go on to develop SLE, this figure may be too low. A recent report from Sweden showed that women who had DLE had a 20% chance of developing SLE within three years after the first diagnosis of discoid lupus. It is called discoid because the rash occurs in the shape of small round or disc-shaped areas. It usually begins as small, reddish bumps. The red area then spreads outward, but in the middle of the area where the bumps initially appeared there will be a scarred area of skin with permanent loss of hair and pigment changes to the skin (photograph 8.3). DLE occurs most commonly on the face and neck area. When lesions occur on the scalp, they unfortunately can cause areas of permanent hair loss. This form of permanent hair loss is termed "scarring alopecia" ("alopecia" means "hair loss"). DLE often occurs on the ears. The person who has it may not notice anything unusual except that the skin just outside the ear canals tends to be scaly. Due to the disfiguring and scarring that this type of lupus can potentially cause, it is important to have it examined and treated by a doctor as fast as possible to decrease the possibility of permanent skin damage. About 20% of people who have systemic lupus will develop DLE as part of their lupus at some point in time.

There are two forms of DLE: localized DLE and generalized DLE. People who have localized DLE have the rash only on the head and neck area, while those who have generalized DLE also have it on other parts of the body. One important reason for this distinction is that people who have the localized form tend to have a less severe form of SLE with less kidney disease and other severe organ involvement compared to those who have generalized DLE.

Another form of CCLE is lupus profundus (also called lupus panniculitis). This form of CCLE appears as firm, tender areas under the skin, especially on the upper arm and thigh areas. It causes inflammation of the fat underneath the skin ("panniculitis" means "inflammation of fat"). Often there are no skin changes at all. At other times, there may be a discoid lupus-like rash on the surface of the skin with pink, dark, and/or light color changes (photograph 8.4). Sometimes lupus panniculitis can be quite

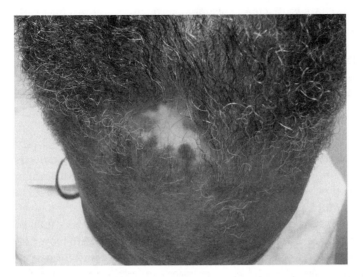

**Photo 8.3** Discoid lupus erythematosus with scarring alopecia on the scalp of a person who has SLE. Note the round or disc shape with a central area of permanent loss of hair (called scarring alopecia) and pigment change. The lighter (pinkish) tinge reflects that there is some active inflammation occurring and it can potentially grow larger.

painful, unlike most other rashes seen with lupus, which do not cause discomfort. Often these rashes are accompanied by classic DLE lesions. If left untreated, they can cause the loss of tissue (especially fat) under the skin, leaving permanent areas of indentation in the skin.

Lupus erythematosus tumidus ("tumidus" means "swollen") is another form of CCLE. Skin lesions are pink or purple in color, and often appear on sun-exposed areas. Tumid lupus tends to respond to treatment with steroids and anti-malarials such as hydroxychloroquine (Plaquenil).

Chilblains lupus skin lesions are reddish-colored areas on the fingers or toes due to inflammation caused by exposure to cold. In fact, "chil-" comes from the word "chill" and "-blain" means "an inflammatory swelling or blister." Chilblains lupus especially can often be painful and itchy. Chilblains lupus can also be called "pernio." Do not be confused by the words "lupus pernio." The term "lupus pernio" is more appropriate for a type of rash that is due to a totally different and separate disease called sarcoidosis.

Hypertrophic DLE is another form of CCLE. Other terms for it are "hyperkeratotic DLE" and "verrucous DLE." Covering the DLE sores is much-thickened skin that looks wart-like in appearance. In fact, "verrucous" is the medical term for "wart." This form of DLE is quite rare.

The treatment for the specific lupus rashes varies depending on their severity. If they are mild and cover a small area, then topical cortisone or tacrolimus cream may be used. Injections of cortisone into localized rashes can be especially helpful for some cases of chronic cutaneous lupus. If the rash is more extensive, then systemic medications such as anti-malarials, azathioprine, steroids, thalidomide, acetretin, or possibly mycophenolic acid may be necessary. It is most common for doctors to prescribe the anti-malarial medication hydroxychloroquine (Plaquenil) to treat the rashes of lupus. However, if hydroxychloroquine is not effective, they will often add quinacrine or stop hydroxychloroquine and change it to chloroquine (discussed in chapter 30).

If blisters occur as part of the lupus rash, then a medication called Dapsone (which is also used to treat leprosy) may be useful. All people who have cutaneous lupus should avoid being out in the sun and use sunscreen daily on all areas of the body that are exposed to light (see chapter 38). If the rash has left some post-inflammatory hyperpigmentation (dark-colored areas) a dermatologist may be able to help by prescribing lightening creams to help decrease the amount of dark pigmentation left by the rash.

**KEY POINTS TO REMEMBER**

1. Lupus-specific rashes only occur in people who have lupus.

2. Usually lupus-specific rashes are easy to diagnose by their appearance on physical exam, but sometimes a skin biopsy is necessary.

3. All lupus-specific rashes worsen with UV light exposure. Although all lupus patients should protect themselves from UV light, those who get these rashes should be extra careful. See chapter 38.

4. All people who have acute cutaneous lupus have the systemic form of lupus (SLE), but the vast majority of those who have chronic cutaneous lupus (such as discoid lupus) do not have the systemic form.

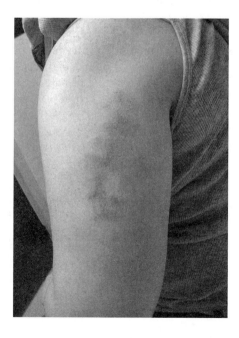

**Photo 8.4** Lupus profundus (lupus panniculitis) on the upper arm of a person who has SLE. What makes lupus profundus (panniculitis) easier to identify is the deep, firm swelling that you can feel underneath the skin where the inflammation of fat is occurring.

5. Medications can sometimes cause subacute cutaneous lupus, especially some blood pressure medicines. If you develop this type of rash and you recently started a new medicine, let your doctor know because he or she should consider stopping it and seeing if the rash disappears.

6. Chronic cutaneous lupus (such as discoid lupus) can cause permanent scarring, pigment changes, and hair loss. If it flares (with redness, increased size of lesions, or tenderness), contact your doctor for treatment. The faster it is treated, the less likelihood there is of permanent damage.

7. Treatment includes anti-malarials such as hydroxychloroquine. Some people who have particularly severe rashes may require stronger drugs such as steroids and other immunosuppressant medicines. For chronic cutaneous lupus (such as discoid lupus) cortisone injections and creams can be very helpful.

## Lupus Nonspecific Rashes

Systemic lupus can cause problems with the skin in ways that are not specific to lupus (table 8.2). In other words, these problems can occur in conditions other than lupus.

### Mucosal Ulcers and Mucositis

Ulcers are open sores where the overlying skin has eroded away, leaving tissue beneath the skin surface exposed. These can occur in the mucosa of people who have SLE. The mucosae (plural of mucosa) are lubricated skin surfaces such as the areas found inside the mouth, nose, and vagina. Mucosal ulcers in the mouth are also sometimes called aphthous ulcers; however, most people who have aphthous ulcers do not have lupus (i.e., there are many potential causes of aphthous ulcers. Having mucosal ulcers in the mouth or nose is one of the classification criteria to diagnose SLE, as discussed in chapter 1. Up to 45% of people who have SLE will develop oral or nasal ulcers. Oral ulcers can occur anywhere inside the mouth, but most commonly appear on the roof of the mouth. They are usually painless, but occasionally can be painful. Another term used for mucosal ulcers, especially when there is widespread inflammation, is "mucositis." Sometimes these sores can spread to the lips as well. This primarily occurs in people who become very sick with their SLE when it is affecting other major organs (such as the kidneys) and is often accompanied by fever. The most common cause of sores on the lips (often called canker sores, fever blisters, or cold sores in laypersons' terms) is infection from the herpes simplex virus in which case it tends to recur throughout the person's life. Seeing your doctor for antiviral medications may help to decrease the severity of these outbreaks.

Nasal ulcers typically occur on the septum (the wall dividing the right and left nostrils) or on the mucosal skin covering the thick center cartilage of the nose. These can be painful. Vaginal ulcers are rare, only occurring in 1% to 2% of SLE patients.

Medicines used by doctors to control SLE such as steroid pills (such as prednisone and methylprednisolone) and anti-malarials (such as Plaquenil) usually help to decrease the severity of these mucositis outbreaks. However, sometimes using local applications of steroids can be useful. For example, a steroid (called triamcinolone) in a

**Table 8.2** Nonspecific Rashes Seen in People Who Have SLE

Oral, nasal, and vaginal mucosa ulcers

Alopecia (hair loss)

Cutaneous vasculitis

    Palpable purpura

    Urticarial vasculitis

    Ulcers

Livedo reticularis

Telangiectasias

Palmar erythema

Erythromelalgia

Bullous lupus

Urticaria (hives) and angioedema

Cutaneous mucinosis

Subcutaneous nodules

Calcinosis cutis

Nail changes

Skin color changes

    Vitiligo

    Post-inflammatory hyperpigmentation

    Anti-malarial-induced hyperpigmentation

    Quinacrine-induced yellow skin coloration

special thick compound called Orabase can be applied to ulcers in the mouth. If this is done as soon as they occur and then used every few hours, it can cause the sores to heal faster than usual. For particularly painful oral ulcers, an anesthetic (benzocaine) in Orabase can decrease the discomfort. Likewise, steroid nasal sprays can be used for nasal ulcers and mild steroid creams can be used for vaginal ulcers. All of these can be prescribed by a physician.

## Alopecia

There are two major forms of alopecia, or hair loss, which can occur in people who have SLE. I described the first form, scarring alopecia, briefly in the section on DLE (see photograph 8.3). Scarring alopecia is an area of permanent hair loss usually due to DLE. It is best to treat it aggressively and quickly to prevent permanent hair loss. Cortisone creams and cortisone injections can be helpful, but most people benefit most from systemic medications such as hydroxychloroquine.

The other form of alopecia is non-scarring alopecia (photograph 8.5). Another common term for it is "lupus hair." This form of alopecia is the most commonly occurring nonspecific skin problem found in people who have SLE. It consists of thinning of the hair; the strands of hair are often fragile and break easily leaving short strands of hair often described as stubby in appearance. Non-scarring alopecia can occur diffusely throughout the scalp, but has a tendency to be most prominent at the front hairline. This type of hair loss is due to the hair follicles resting during periods of increased lupus disease activity (called telogen effluvium), presumably to save energy and calories in the body for more important functions than growing hair. This condition is usually reversible and the hair grows back when treatment brings the SLE under control. Non-scarring alopecia is another criterion used in the classification criteria in diagnosing SLE, as discussed in chapter 1.

People who have either scarring or non-scarring alopecia should avoid and protect themselves from ultraviolet light, as discussed in chapter 38. You should wear a hat whenever you are outside and use sunscreen every day on all exposed areas of the skin.

Another cause of non-scarring alopecia that can occur in people who have SLE is alopecia areata. Alopecia areata is actually another autoimmune disorder where the im-

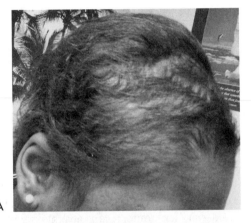

A

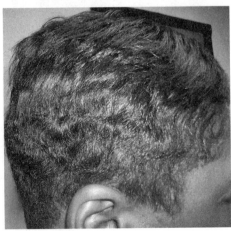

B

Photo 8.5 Non-scarring alopecia in a person who has SLE, before (A) and after (B) treatment. This individual developed non-scarring alopecia during a flare of lupus nephritis. Notice how the hair loss is most prevalent at the front part of the scalp (A). She would wear a headscarf to cover her head. After treatment with a combination of mycophenolate and prednisone in addition to her hydroxychloroquine, the person's hair grew in to the point where it could be styled (B).

mune system attacks the hair follicles and causes the hair loss. Typically, small areas of hair loss occur. Within these areas, there may be some hairs that are much shorter than normal; this is often described as "exclamation point hairs" when discovered on physical examination.

There can be other causes of hair loss in lupus patients, however. For example, thyroid disorders and stress can sometimes cause hair loss (both of which are reversible). Medications such as steroids, methotrexate, leflunomide, and cyclophosphamide can also cause hair loss. Fortunately, after people stop taking the offending medications, the hair grows back. In addition, both women and men can develop hair loss related to aging and genetics, which a doctor should always consider when hair does not grow back normally after treating the SLE adequately and after ruling out other causes.

## Cutaneous Vasculitis

"Vasculitis" means "inflammation of the blood vessels." Vasculitis can occur in any of the blood vessels of the body in people who have SLE. When vasculitis occurs, there may be decreased blood flow to the particular area of the body that the blood vessels supply, which can cause pain and damage to the tissues. The blood vessels can also leak, causing swelling and bleeding into the surrounding tissues. When vasculitis occurs in the blood vessels of the skin, it can appear in many different forms. Palpable purpura is the most common form. Your doctor may also call it leukocytoclastic vasculitis. This usually occurs on the lower legs and looks like a bunch of tiny areas of bruising ("purpura" is one of the medical terms for "bruising"), and "palpable" means that the bruised areas are slightly raised so they can be felt when you run your fingers over the bruised areas. This condition occurs due to tiny amounts of blood leaking from the inflamed blood vessels beneath the skin surface. Often the ankles swell due to the leaking of fluid from the inflamed blood vessels into the tissues of the ankles and legs.

When cutaneous vasculitis causes palpable purpura, it usually does not cause much of a problem beyond the cosmetic appearance and occasional swelling. However, on rare occasions, cutaneous vasculitis can be severe, causing large areas of painful dead skin to develop and lead to open ulcers. These most commonly occur on the legs and treatment requires high doses of steroids and strong immunosuppressant medicines.

Urticarial vasculitis is a less common form of vasculitis seen in people who have lupus. The areas of vasculitis look similar to hives (the medical term for hives is "urticaria"). The skin lesions of urticarial vasculitis are typically slightly raised areas of skin that are tender to the touch. When they heal, they often leave pigment changes on the skin. Usually a skin biopsy is required to diagnose urticarial vasculitis accurately.

Doctors usually check SLE patients who develop vasculitis for substances in the blood called cryoglobulins. "Cryo-" comes from the Greek word for "cold," while "globulins" refer to antibodies. These particular antibodies precipitate and clump together with cooler temperatures. "Precipitation" is a scientific term meaning that a substance in a liquid solidifies; for example, if you warm up a pan of water and pour in a bunch of salt, the salt dissolves in the water. When the water then cools down in the refrigerator, salt begins precipitating out of the water as salt crystals on the edges of the pan. What happens in people who have cryoglobulinemia (cryoglobulins in their blood) is that the cryoglobulins can clump together and precipitate in parts of the body that are cooler than other parts. This may occur in the cooler skin of the legs, causing bruised appearing areas and inflammation of the blood vessels (vasculitis). Doctors treat this condition with high doses of steroids along with immunosuppressants. Sometimes doctors have to use a special type of treatment called plasmapheresis, which removes the cryoglobulins from the blood. (See photograph 8.8 to see one of the effects of cryoglobulins in an SLE patient [a condition called erythromelalgia]).

Sometimes vasculitis of the skin can occur along with vasculitis in other organs of the body such as the kidneys. Therefore, if you develop the symptoms of vasculitis, it is important to see your doctor immediately to make sure this is not the case. Most of the time, cutaneous vasculitis occurs by itself, without involvement of internal organs, but it is important that your doctor checks you thoroughly, especially the first time it happens.

*Livedo Reticularis.* Livedo reticularis (photograph 8.6) is a form of rash due to decreased blood flow in small blood vessels beneath the skin. It appears as net-like areas of reddish or purplish discoloration, especially on the arms and legs. It rarely causes any significant problems, usually does not cause permanent scarring, and can increase during periods of stress and exposure to cold. People who have livedo reticularis sometimes (but not always) are positive for antiphospholipid antibodies (see chapters 4 and 9).

*Telangiectasias.* Telangiectasias (photograph 8.7) are areas of tiny, dilated blood vessels under the skin that sometimes are blanchable, meaning that if you press on them they will temporarily lose their reddish or purplish coloration due to the blood being squeezed out of the blood vessels. However, the coloration quickly returns when the

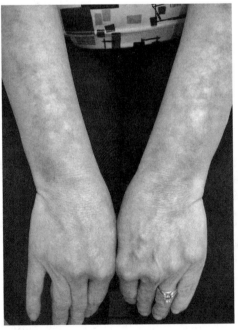

**Photo 8.6** Livedo reticularis on the arms of a person who has SLE.

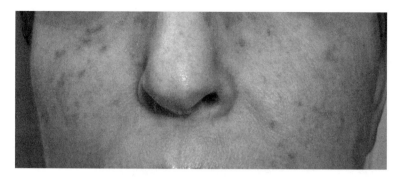

**Photo 8.7** Telangiectasias on the cheeks of a person who has SLE overlap with scleroderma. What makes these red marks different from other red rashes seen with SLE is that they occur below the skin surface, do not cause any bumps that can be felt, and if you apply pressure with your finger to one of the red splotches, the red color temporarily goes away because the blood is squeezed out of the underlying dilated blood vessels under the skin, then the redness returns as the vessels fill up with blood again.

blood refills the blood vessels. They most commonly occur on the hands, around the fingernails, on the face and lips, and even inside the mouth and on the tongue.

*Periungual Erythema.* "Peri-" comes from the Greek for "around" while "-unguis" is Greek for "nail." If dilated blood vessels under the skin (similar to telangiectasias) occur in the skin next to the finger nails (also called the nail fold), that area of skin can appear redder than normal. In fact, some doctors will describe these alternatively as periungual telangiectasias. Similarly, dilated blood vessels can also occur on the edges of the eyelids causing them to appear reddish as well. Antiphospholipid antibodies (see chapter 4) are more common in people who have these findings. Similar to telangiectasias, these dilated blood vessels are usually permanent and do not improve.

*Palmar Erythema.* Reddish discoloration of the palms occurs in approximately 4% of people who have SLE due to increased blood flow in the blood vessels of the skin of the palms. If the reddish color is net-like in appearance (as in livedo reticularis), it could be due to antiphospholipid antibodies. It is rarely a major problem and is not treated.

*Erythromelalgia.* Erythromelalgia (photograph 8.8) refers to when the hands and/or feet become intensely red, hot, and painful due to dilated or inflamed blood vessels. The affected extremities usually feel better with cold and worse with warmth. This is just the opposite of people who have Raynaud's phenomenon and whose hands and feet feel better with heat and worse with cold. I have had several SLE patients who developed erythromelalgia. Two of them behaved the same way due to the discomfort of this particular problem. When I entered the exam room, these patients were standing at the sink running cold water over their hands to help them feel better. Both were visibly miserable from the severity of the pain. Both responded well to high doses of steroids and aspirin-type medicines. Fortunately, this lupus complication is rare.

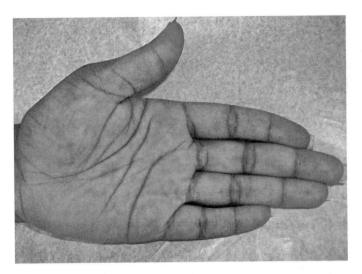

**Photo 8.8** Erythromelalgia in a person who has SLE. Note the splotches on the palm and fingers. She had very painful palms that felt worse with warmth and better when she would stick her hands under cold water. Blood tests showed her to be positive for cryoglobulins. This resolved with treatment with steroids and mycophenolate for her nephritis (kidney inflammation).

*Bullous Lupus.* "Bullous" is the medical term referring to fluid-filled blisters on the skin. Several types of bullous skin disorders can occur in people who have SLE, and often a skin biopsy is necessary to identify which type a person has. Doctors sometimes use the terms "lupus pemphigus," "vesiculobullous annular subacute cutaneous lupus," and even "bullous discoid lupus" when they describe these blistering type rashes if they are directly due to lupus (which can be proven by the biopsy result), while reserving other terms when they are not specific for lupus patients. Examples of bullous rashes that can occur in people who have lupus but may be due to a disorder other than lupus include dermatitis herpetiformis (often seen in celiac disease), epidermolysis bullosa acquisita, bullous pemphigoid, pemphigus erythematosus, and porphyria cutanea tarda. These conditions are due to the immune system attacking the parts of the skin that connect the outer and inner layers of the skin (except for porphyria cutanea tarda, which is not an autoimmune process). When inflammation occurs due to this autoimmune attack, the layers will separate and fill up with fluid. This form of cutaneous lupus, bullous lupus, does not respond well to many drugs used to treat lupus such as steroids, azathioprine, mycophenolate, or methotrexate. Dapsone (which is also used to treat leprosy) is a commonly used medication to treat these blistering conditions.

*Urticaria and Angioedema.* "Urticaria" is the medical term for "hives." Urticaria commonly occurs when a person is exposed to something to which he or she is allergic. For example, when someone allergic to cats is exposed to one he or she may develop itchy raised areas or bumps (hives; also called welts). Urticaria can also occur in people who have SLE due to inflammation caused by lupus itself. The hives often get worse with sun exposure, just like other forms of cutaneous lupus.

A related problem is angioedema. Urticaria occurs due to inflammation and swelling in the skin itself, while angioedema is due to inflammation causing swelling of the tissues deeper than the skin. This can especially occur on the face, particularly around the eyes or on the lips. The swollen areas may or may not be uncomfortable or tender. Both urticaria and angioedema typically improve when the systemic inflammation of SLE is treated (such as with steroids).

*Cutaneous Mucinosis.* Cutaneous mucinosis is rare in SLE. It is due to the deposition of mucin in the skin. Mucin is a lubricating substance that your mucous membranes (such as the ones inside your mouth) typically secrete. Doctors do not know why it deposits in small collections under the skin of some SLE patients. It typically appears as small areas of purplish bumps. A skin biopsy is usually required to diagnose it. I have only had one patient who had this with her SLE, and the bumps got smaller when her lupus was treated but never completely disappeared. Fortunately, they were very small and did not cause any major cosmetic problems.

*Subcutaneous Nodules.* Subcutaneous nodules are firm, round, rubbery feeling lumps that may occur under the skin in 5% to 10% of people who have SLE. They appear most commonly on the fingers, but can also occur on the feet, arms, and legs. They are very similar to the skin nodules that appear in people who have rheumatoid arthritis. In fact, most SLE patients who have subcutaneous nodules have an arthritis that is very similar to rheumatoid arthritis with significant swelling and stiffness in their joints, and they are often positive for rheumatoid factor in blood tests. This seems to occur more commonly in people who have an overlap of SLE and rheumatoid arthritis (often called "rhupus" for short). Sometimes the nodules get smaller when doctors treat SLE systemically with drugs such as steroids and methotrexate, but not always. If they are uncomfortable or large, cortisone injections usually help to decrease their size and the resulting discomfort.

*Calcinosis Cutis.* Calcium deposits can occur under the skin in some people who have SLE. They appear as hard lumps under the skin, often pale in color in dark-skinned individuals. Doctors diagnose this condition from x-rays (the deposits appear as bony-looking structures). Fortunately, calcinosis cutis is not very common in SLE patients. There are some rare reports of these calcified areas occurring extensively under the skin of people with SLE, but this is more common in another systemic autoimmune disease called dermatomyositis. Unfortunately, therapies other than surgical removal do not seem to help very much with this condition.

*Nail Changes.* Quite a few changes can occur with the fingernails and toenails in people who have lupus. They may develop hard lines or ridges on the surface of their nails; the edges of the nails may lift off the underlying skin at the end of the nails; indentations or pits may occur as well as areas of unusual dark or reddish discoloration. These changes do not necessarily improve with treatment of the SLE.

*Skin Color Changes.* Some medical conditions primarily cause skin color changes. One such condition is vitiligo, which causes light-colored areas to occur on the skin (photograph 8.9). These can be either small or large, and can occur on any part of the body. There may be just a few small areas involved, or a large percentage of the skin can be involved in more extreme cases. There is usually a sharp demarcation between the patches of lighter color and the surrounding areas of normal skin coloration. They tend to become more prominent during summertime if the surrounding skin becomes tanner (although people who have lupus should use sunscreen regularly and not develop a tan). Like lupus, vitiligo is an autoimmune disease. The immune system attacks the cells of the skin that produce melanin, which gives pigmentation to the skin. Other than causing some cosmetic concerns in some people, it is not a dangerous condition, and there is no treatment for it.

After cutaneous lupus inflammation resolves, sometimes the cells of the skin will produce more pigment (melanin) in those areas. This can unfortunately be a permanent problem, causing dark patches of skin to appear especially on the cheeks, forehead, nose, and ears. Lightening creams are sometimes prescribed with strict sun avoidance. You should see a dermatologist to help with this problem.

One of the potential long-term side effects of using anti-malarial medications such as hydroxychloroquine (Plaquenil), chloroquine, and quinacrine is the development of dark-colored patches on the skin (photograph 8.10). They often appear brown, black, or black and blue and tend to develop on the legs, especially around the shins. However, they can happen anywhere on the body; involvement of the neck is especially common. The coloration may decrease when the dose of the medicine decreases. Since anti-malarial medicines are the safest medications to treat SLE, it is preferable to continue the medicine and put up with the skin discoloration instead of risk a lupus flare if you stop taking the medicine. However, if you discontinue the medicine, the skin color can improve.

Quinacrine can cause an unusual yellowish discoloration of the skin and whites of the eyes. This occurs in about 25% of people who take it. The yellow tint does improve after the dose of the medicine is decreased or after the person stops taking it.

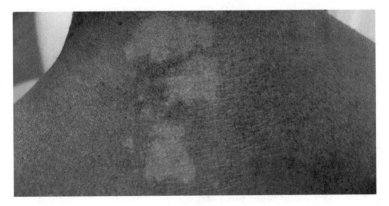

**Photo 8.9** Vitiligo on the upper back of a woman of African descent who has SLE.

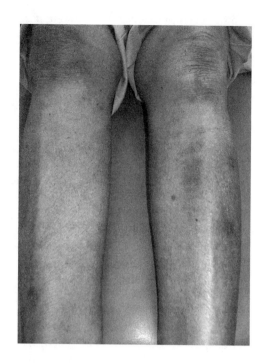

Photo 8.10 Dark patches of skin due to Plaquenil in a woman who has SLE.

## General Skin Care Advice

If you avoid ultraviolet light (see chapter 38), use sunscreen religiously every day, never smoke cigarettes, and stay well hydrated by drinking plenty of water daily, you will win the majority of the battle as far as having healthy, good-looking skin. However, if you have cutaneous lupus and have skin pigment changes, hair loss, or excessive hair growth (which can happen with some medicines), a dermatologist's help can be invaluable. You should see a dermatologist in addition to your rheumatologist to assist in your care since they might know the most helpful strategies. Dermatologists are also experts when it comes to which creams and lotions to use. For example, although doctors often prescribe cortisone creams for actively inflamed lupus rashes, if these creams are used on areas of skin that are not actively inflamed, you can actually cause permanent harm by causing thinning of the skin, acne, and excessive amounts of blood vessels becoming visible under the skin.

Covermark and Dermablend both have multiple products that can be used over skin changes due to lupus to improve the skin's cosmetic appearance. Another advantage of these products is that they also contain sunscreen. Interestingly, using a green-tinged primer for foundation makeup can decrease the redness of lupus rashes such as from telangiectasias, steroid-induced facial redness, and the butterfly rash of lupus. Examples of green primers include Smashbox brand Photo Finish Color Correcting Foundation Primer, Adjust, and Make Up For Ever HD Microperfecting Primer (green shade). Other popular makers of green primer include Bodyography, L'Orea, and Pur Minerals, No. 7. Only a small amount of these green primers should be used, but they can significantly decrease the amount of skin redness. Since hair loss can occur with lupus, many women who have SLE also rely on the use of hats and wigs. I am often amazed at how real today's wigs can be. It is not uncommon for me to examine one of my patients very closely to see how her lupus is doing and then be surprised that she is wearing a wig that I mistook as her actual hair.

My patients often ask me if they should get a tattoo or not. People who have SLE should not get tattoos for several reasons. Although many tattoo artists are professionals and pride themselves in using proper sterile technique, infections can and do occur. These infections include hepatitis B, hepatitis C, *Staphylococcus aureus*, endocarditis (heart infection), and HIV. If someone is on a medication that suppresses the immune system, the occurrence of one of these infections could be potentially deadly. If people are not on an immunosuppressant medicine at the time of getting the tattoo, but they acquire a chronic infection from it such as hepatitis B or hepatitis C, this would greatly decrease the number of medications that could be safely used for their lupus in the future if their lupus were to worsen. In addition, some people who have lupus have actually developed cutaneous lupus at the tattoo site because of the tattoo itself.

## KEY POINTS TO REMEMBER

1. Nonspecific rashes may occur in people who have SLE related to the autoimmune disease, but they can also occur in other disorders as well.

2. Ulcers in the mouth and nose are one of the most common cutaneous (skin) manifestations of SLE. They are usually painless but occasionally can be painful. Steroid creams can be helpful.

3. Non-scarring alopecia improves and the hair grows back when treatment brings lupus under better control, but your doctor should consider other possible causes, such as hypothyroidism, steroid use, stress, aging, or genetics.

4. You should show any skin problem to your doctor so she or he can determine whether it is due to SLE or an unrelated problem.

5. If you begin to develop dark areas of skin in areas not previously affected by lupus rashes (especially the shins), let your doctor know as it may be due to hydroxychloroquine (Plaquenil).

6. Consider seeing a dermatologist regularly in addition to your rheumatologist to ensure that you are getting the best skin care advice possible.

7. The use of cosmetics (especially green tinted primer to hide redness), hats, and wigs can be very helpful in covering up some of the aesthetic problems from lupus.

8. Tattoos need to be avoided by all people who have SLE; they increase the risks of infection and cutaneous lupus.

# Blood and Lymph Systems

## Hughes Syndrome and "Sticky Blood"

You cannot talk about lupus and not talk about blood. The two are intricately entwined. The immune system, with its army of white blood cells, is the culprit for causing the disorder in the first place, and the white blood cells travel through the blood and lymph systems. SLE requires the drawing of blood for testing because this is where the antibodies are found that help a doctor make the diagnosis. Most people who have SLE, but not all, will also have low blood counts of one type of another that can help doctors make the diagnosis, and occasionally can cause problems such as bleeding (if they have low platelet counts) or fatigue (if they have low red blood cell counts, or what is called anemia). These low blood counts will be discussed in detail in this chapter.

One of the most intriguing aspects of lupus is the antiphospholipid antibody syndrome, first mentioned in chapter 4. This problem is important for people who have SLE because anywhere from one-third to one-half of them will be positive for these particular antibodies.

To understand this problem, it is important to know details about the blood and lymph systems first. For example, there are blood tests that show how well the blood clots or coagulates. One of these tests is the partial thromboplastin time (or PTT for short). If someone has a problem with bleeding too much then it can sometimes be helpful to check this PTT test because there are some diseases (like the famous bleeding disease called hemophilia) where the PTT test is longer than normal due to the person having a genetic disorder in which important clotting proteins are missing. The blood from these people does not clot (or coagulate) well, and they bleed too easily. Therefore, a longer than normal PTT level is usually a sign of a bleeding disorder. These particular bleeding disorders can be diagnosed in the laboratory by adding these missing proteins to a sample of blood from a person who has a high PTT level and who bleeds easily. Adding the correct missing clotting protein to the person's blood sample causes the specimen to clot properly. The cause of the bleeding disorder is established by determining which protein he or she is missing.

Beginning in 1948, doctors discovered that some lupus patients also had these long PTT (coagulation) levels, but when clotting proteins were added to their blood samples in the laboratory, the patients' blood surprisingly did not clot properly. It was determined that they had some sort of inhibitor or antibody inhibiting their PTT (coagulation) test. The term "anticoagulant" was coined to describe these inhibitors or proteins that were prolonging the PTT test results in these patients. Doctors initially thought that these anticoagulants could possibly cause these people who had SLE to bleed more easily.

However, systemic lupus does not always follow the rules of logic. In 1951, Dr. Allyn Ley and colleagues from Cornell University in New York reported a young man who had developed a blood clot in his leg and had an elevated PTT level (just the opposite of what should happen). A report in 1954 showed this anticoagulant was also present in a woman who had recurrent miscarriages. Then in 1963, Dr. E. J. Walter Bowie and his team of doctors at the Mayo Clinic in Minnesota (the birthplace of the LE cell as described in the first section of chapter 2) reported on a group of SLE patients who were positive for these anticoagulants. However, the surprising thing was that instead of having excessive bleeding, these patients were having problems with the blood being too thick and causing increased blood clots—again, just the opposite of what should have been happening. By 1972, enough of these clotting problems had been noted in patients with this abnormal blood test that it was finally called lupus anticoagulant. From that point on, doctors and medical students have been stuck with having to learn that this blood test actually does just the opposite of what it should theoretically do ("anticoagulant" should mean, "the opposite of clotting" or "increased bleeding," but these patients actually clot too easily).

In 1983, Dr. G. R. V. Hughes presented his now famous article linking numerous problems with these lupus anticoagulants. He noted that not only did they appear in patients who had blood clots, but also in people with low blood counts, neurological problems, strokes, heart attacks, a rash called livedo reticularis (discussed in chapter 8), and other abnormal blood tests such as false positive syphilis tests and anticardiolipin antibodies. All of these antibodies (including the lupus anticoagulant, which is an antibody) had the same thing in common. They were all directed toward a fat-containing molecule, called phospholipid, which is found on all cell surfaces. The problem of having these antiphospholipid antibodies along with recurrent blood clots or recurrent miscarriages was subsequently named after Dr. Hughes as "Hughes' syndrome" or what is now more commonly called "antiphospholipid syndrome." Due to its causing the blood to clot easier, some people even call it "sticky blood" disease.

Fortunately, doctors are able to prevent these problems from occurring by advising their patients to use blood thinners such as aspirin. This chapter goes into detail about the problems that SLE can cause in the blood cells and lymph nodes as well as blood clotting problems (i.e., antiphospholipid syndrome).

••••

Abnormalities of the blood cells and lymph nodes are some of the most common problems seen in people who have SLE. There are three different types of blood cells—white blood cells, red blood cells, and platelets—and the levels of all three types can drop in people who have SLE. Production of the blood cells begins primarily in the bone marrow, which is contained in the middle of the bones, especially the largest ones, such as those of the arms, legs, pelvis, and spine. The bone marrow is constantly churning out new white and red blood cells, as well as platelets, to take the place of cells in the blood that have already done their job and are removed by organs such as the spleen. A blood test called the complete blood cell count (or CBC for short), as discussed in chapter 4, can actually count the numbers of each of these blood cells. These numbers can help doctors figure out what is happening in the blood as well as in the bone marrow. This is the reason that doctors order a CBC for SLE patients whenever they order blood work. There are also components of the blood that are important for clotting and bleeding that SLE can affect.

The lymph system is a complex connection of channels called lymphatic vessels that attach to round or oval rubbery swellings called lymph nodes. The spleen, a large organ found in the upper left part of the abdomen, can also be considered part of the lymphatic system. The lymphatic system is a very important part of the immune system; therefore, it is not surprising that SLE can affect it, as well.

An important characteristic of the blood is its ability to clot. When you get a cut, the platelets and numerous important proteins adhere to the cut blood vessels. These platelets and special proteins clog up the cut blood vessels and stop the bleeding. As we just learned, some people have antibodies called antiphospholipid antibodies that actually make their blood thicker than normal. This can cause blood clots to form in the blood vessels of the body, causing problems such as strokes. The medical term for this is the "antiphospholipid antibody syndrome."

## Problems with White Blood Cells

White blood cells are called leukocytes (also spelled leucocytes)—"leuko-" coming from the Greek word for "white," and "-cyte" from the Greek word for "cell." These are very important cells of the body that are the guards and soldiers of the immune system. They are the cells responsible for identifying and fighting bacteria, viruses, and other invading foreign organisms and objects (even things such as splinters) when they enter the body. SLE can sometimes cause the white blood cell count to be lower than normal. This is called leukopenia—"penia" coming from the Greek word meaning "decreased, less, or a lack of something." There are several types of white blood cells, each with their own special function in protecting the body. The most important types of white blood cells in regard to SLE are the neutrophils and the lymphocytes. Neutrophils are especially important for fighting off bacterial infections, while lymphocytes play numerous roles, including fighting off viral infections and ensuring proper overall immune system function. The medical term for a decrease in neutrophils is "neutropenia," while the term for a decrease in the lymphocytes is "lymphopenia." By the way, to add to the confusion, neutrophils are also called granulocytes, and therefore the term for lower than normal levels is "granulocytopenia," which means the same thing as neutropenia. Lymphopenia is more common in people who have SLE, occurring in as many as 90% of them.

Since white blood cells are so important in fighting off infections, low blood counts should cause infections. However, this does not seem to be the case. Although people who have SLE have an overall increased risk for developing infections, this risk does not seem to be related necessarily to the low white blood cell counts. One 2011 study suggests that having a low neutrophil count (neutropenia) may increase the risk of having an infection of the vaginal area (vulvovaginitis); however, this possibility needs to be confirmed in future follow-up studies.

Doctors usually do not treat the low white blood cell count in SLE patients since it usually does not cause any outright medical problems. In addition, low white blood cell counts do not seem to improve much with SLE treatment in most patients. On the other hand, steroids such as prednisone usually cause the white blood cell count to increase, but this also occurs in people who have normal white blood cell counts after treatment with steroids. One advantage of measuring the white blood cell count is that it can help make a diagnosis of SLE in some patients. It can also be helpful in monitoring the course and degree of disease activity in people who have lupus as blood counts can decrease during periods of increased disease activity. Finally, a white blood count is helpful in monitoring for potential drug side effects.

Sometimes a doctor can link low blood counts directly to recurrent infections, but this is very uncommon. In my practice, I have a patient who had severe neutropenia due to SLE, and she had recurrent boils (skin infections). She developed nephritis (kidney inflammation), so I had to treat her with a strong immunosuppressant drug called mycophenolate (CellCept and Myfortic). I was quite cautious because I was aware that this could possibly cause her white blood count to get even worse or increase her risk for infections even more. However, it was a pleasant surprise when her white blood cell count actually improved from the effect of the mycophenolate and her skin infections completely disappeared. This is just one example of how complicated SLE can be. Certainly, I was hoping that this would happen since, if I could control her SLE better with mycophenolate, then theoretically, the white blood cell count might improve, but this was not a certainty and researchers have never really studied this. Whenever doctors treat patients with any medication, they always try to treat them in the safest possible way without causing harm. In this instance, I could not be 100% sure I was doing the correct thing. Fortunately, it was the right thing to do, and both her kidneys and blood counts improved with the therapy.

Sometimes a low white blood cell count can be due to the drugs used to treat SLE. In fact, almost all of the medications used to treat SLE (except for steroids) can potentially cause low white blood cell counts. This can present a problem when the doctor sees a patient's white blood cell count go lower than normal, or lower than what the patient's blood cell count usually is.

Occasionally, but not often, a biopsy of the bone marrow is necessary to help determine what the problem is. The decision to get a bone marrow biopsy is usually made by a blood specialist called a hematologist. The bone marrow is the tissue inside of the bones that produces most of the blood cells. Sometimes a doctor has to do a bone marrow biopsy if he or she is not sure why the blood counts are abnormal. This may be necessary for problems of not only the white blood cells but also red blood cells and platelets. Doctors usually do bone marrow biopsies on an outpatient basis in their offices. The most common location of the biopsy is the hard bone of the pelvis. The doctor injects local anesthesia into the area of the biopsy. She or he then inserts a biopsy needle through this numbed-up area into the bone, and removes a piece of the bone. Since it is very difficult to anesthetize the bone itself, there usually is some discomfort associated with the procedure. The doctor then sends the biopsy to the lab for evaluation under a microscope by a doctor called a pathologist to determine the problem. It can take several days to several weeks to get the results of the biopsy back.

1. Low white blood cell counts (leukopenia) are very common in people who have SLE.

2. Low numbers of lymphocytes (lymphopenia) are more common than low numbers of neutrophils (neutropenia or granulocytopenia).

3. Although white blood cells are very important for fighting off infections, most of the time their numbers are not low enough to cause recurrent infections.

4. Medications used to treat SLE often do not improve the numbers of white blood cells.

5. Sometimes medications used to treat SLE (such as methotrexate, azathioprine, mycophenolate, and cyclophosphamide) may lower the white blood cell count, requiring the dose of the medicine to be lowered or for it to be stopped.

## Problems with Red Blood Cells

The medical term for the red blood cells is "erythrocytes." "Erythro-" comes from the Greek word for "red." The job of the erythrocyte is to carry hemoglobin, a protein that distributes oxygen to all the cells of the body and is essential for all body functions. A decreased amount of erythrocytes is called anemia. A doctor diagnoses anemia by finding a low hemoglobin level and a low hematocrit on the complete blood count (CBC) blood test (see chapter 4 for more details). Since having enough red blood cells is essential for carrying oxygen throughout the body, having anemia can potentially cause all sorts of problems. Mild anemia (the hemoglobin is greater than 11 mg/dl) usually causes no problems at all. However, the farther the hemoglobin drops below this number, the greater the chances of it causing problems. How quickly the anemia occurs is also significant. For example, someone who has had anemia for a very long time could be considered to have severe anemia on the blood tests, yet not feel bad at all since her or his body most likely has become used to being anemic and has learned to compensate for the anemia in other ways. On the other hand, someone may develop a mild anemia very quickly, such as losing blood from a stomach ulcer, for example, and feel extremely fatigued even though the anemia is mild. Symptoms of anemia may include feeling tired and short of breath with exertion. In people who have severe anemia, or in people who have heart or lung problems who become anemic, more severe symptoms may occur, such as chest pain, shortness of breath at rest, light-headedness, and even feeling faint.

There are numerous reasons people become anemic, including people who have SLE. It is very important to figure out exactly why someone is anemic because the treatment of the anemia completely depends on its cause. That is why a doctor usually asks a patient to come in for more blood work (anemia workup) when he or she finds that the person is anemic. I discuss the more common reasons for anemia in SLE below in order of relative frequency.

## Anemia of Chronic Disease

Anemia of chronic disease is the most common anemia seen in people who have SLE. Another term for this is "anemia of inflammation" and it is due to the systemic inflammation of SLE that causes the bone marrow to produce less red blood cells than normal. Doctors usually diagnose it by observing normal-sized red blood cells on the CBC with a normal MCV (called normochromic anemia). MCV stands for "mean corpuscular volume" and it measures the volume (or size) of the red blood cells. Less commonly, the MCV may be lower than normal (called microcytic anemia) in anemia of chronic disease. Usually iron studies are necessary to diagnose this type of anemia. On the iron studies, the serum iron level may be normal or lower than normal. The most helpful results of iron studies in diagnosing anemia of chronic disease are a normal to high ferritin level and decreased total iron binding capacity (TIBC). However, sometimes it can be difficult to tell the difference between anemia due to iron deficiency and anemia of chronic disease. In this instance, the doctor may have the patient take iron supplements to see if iron levels improve (supplements would cause levels to improve if there is iron deficiency, but not if it is anemia of chronic disease). In very difficult cases, a bone marrow biopsy may be necessary, as discussed in the section on white blood cell counts. In anemia of chronic disease there will be normal amounts of iron present in the bone marrow biopsy; iron levels will be low if the person has iron deficiency.

Anemia of chronic disease generally improves as the SLE improves overall. Occasionally it may not improve very much, or it may cause some of the problems noted above (such as fatigue and shortness of breath). In these cases, a group of medications called erythropoietins (such as Aranesp, Epogen, and Procrit) can be useful in bringing the red blood cell count up and helping the person feel better. These medications are given by injection in a doctor's office.

## Iron Deficiency Anemia

Iron is a mineral and is a very important component of the oxygen-carrying hemoglobin found in the red blood cells. People who do not have enough iron in their bodies cannot make enough hemoglobin for red blood cells and therefore become anemic. The most common reason for becoming iron deficient is blood loss since the hemoglobin-containing red blood cells contain a large amount of the body's iron. By far the most common cause of blood loss is menstruation. Since SLE usually occurs in women of childbearing age, they often have iron deficiency anemia simply from losing blood during their monthly menstrual cycles. The second most common reason is bleeding from somewhere in the gastrointestinal tract. For example, ulcers in the stomach may slowly leak blood. Polyps, which are stalks of abnormal tissue inside of the intestines, may also bleed. More importantly, colon cancer can slowly leak blood and cause iron deficiency anemia. A less common cause of iron deficiency is malabsorption where someone does not absorb iron normally from his or her food. The term for one malabsorption problem that may occur is "celiac sprue" or "gluten hypersensitivity." This is a problem where gluten (which is in certain grain products such as wheat) causes an allergic type of reaction inside the intestines, causing them not to absorb many nutrients properly. The treatment for this is to avoid foods that have gluten.

Iron deficiency anemia most commonly causes the red blood cells to be smaller than normal, called microcytic anemia. The MCV test on the CBC is smaller than normal in microcytic anemia. Iron studies in iron deficiency anemia usually show a decreased serum iron level, a low ferritin level, and an elevated TIBC.

In addition to causing the usual symptoms of anemia such as fatigue, iron deficiency can sometimes cause a condition called pica. "Pica" is the medical term describing craving and eating substances that do not have nutritional benefits. For example, people who have iron deficiency may develop a craving to eat clay or more commonly, a craving to eat ice (the term for this is "pagophagia"). Exactly why they develop this particular craving is not entirely understood.

The treatment for iron deficiency is to take iron supplements, which can be purchased over the counter. Iron absorbs best when taken on an empty stomach because acid helps with absorption better. Therefore, it is best to take an iron supplement that has vitamin C in it (which increases stomach acidity) and to take it on an empty stomach. If someone who has iron deficiency has difficulty increasing the iron levels or blood counts by taking iron pills, sometimes iron may need to be given in IV (intravenous) fluids administered in a doctor's office.

Since iron deficiency can sometimes be due to bleeding somewhere in the intestinal tract, a doctor may perform an endoscopy where a fiberoptic scope is inserted either through the mouth to look into the esophagus and stomach (called an esophagogastroduodenoscopy, or EGD for short) or through the anus to look into the colon (called a colonoscopy). These procedures are usually recommended for anyone who has any symptoms that point to potential problems in the gastrointestinal tract, such as nausea, stomach upset, stomach pain, diarrhea, constipation, or blood in the feces. They are also indicated if there are nonspecific symptoms such as unexplained weight loss. Someone who develops iron deficiency and does not have menstrual cycles should always get a thorough gastrointestinal workup, including endoscopies, if there is no other reason for bleeding (such as recent surgery or trauma).

## Autoimmune Hemolytic Anemia

When the immune system attacks and destroys the red blood cells directly, it causes autoimmune hemolytic anemia. This is the only type of anemia that is one of the classification criteria to diagnose SLE, as discussed in chapter 1, and it may occur in up to 10% of people who have SLE. Typical blood work findings for this type of anemia include a decreased haptoglobin level, an elevated reticulocyte count, increased LDH and bilirubin levels, and a positive Coombs' antibody (see chapter 4 for more details on these tests). In addition, the doctor may examine the blood under the microscope to help in diagnosis.

If autoimmune hemolytic anemia occurs along with a low platelet count, this is called Evan's syndrome. A small percentage of people who develop Evan's syndrome can subsequently develop SLE after which it is realized that the anemia and thrombocytopenia were due to SLE the entire time.

This type of anemia is not nearly as common as anemia of chronic disease or iron deficiency anemia, but it is usually more severe when it does occur. Severe autoimmune hemolytic anemia requires treatment with high doses of steroids and other immunosuppressant medications such as azathioprine, mycophenolate, cyclosporine, and cyclophosphamide. Rituximab (Rituxan), belimumab (Benlysta), and IVIG (intravenous immunoglobulin) therapy have also been used with success.

## Anemia due to Renal Insufficiency

Anemia is common in people whose kidneys do not work normally. When there is a decrease in kidney function, it is called renal insufficiency ("renal" means "kidney") or chronic kidney disease. Doctors diagnose renal insufficiency by finding a lower than normal estimated glomerular filtration rate (eGFR) on blood work, or a decreased creatinine clearance on a twenty-four-hour urine sample (see chapter 4 for more details). Renal insufficiency means that the kidneys are not as effective at removing toxic substances from the blood compared to the kidneys of people without kidney problems. The most common causes of renal insufficiency are diabetes, high blood pressure, and aging. People who have SLE may have kidneys that do not function normally. In addition, 40% to 50% of SLE patients will develop inflammation of the kidneys (called nephritis), which can also cause decreased kidney function. Therefore, many SLE patients have chronic kidney disease. The kidneys secrete an important hormone called erythropoietin, which goes into the bloodstream and to the bone marrow. Erythropoietin stimulates the bone marrow to make red blood cells. When someone develops kidney disease, there is often a decreased amount of erythropoietin produced. Subsequently the bone marrow starts to make fewer red blood cells, which causes anemia.

If the hemoglobin level on the blood tests is 11 g/dL or higher, it is not appropriate to treat this type of anemia. However, if it is less than that, especially if problems such as fatigue are present, then erythropoietin medications such as Aranesp, Procrit, or Epogen may be beneficial. These medications are injected in a doctor's office.

## Vitamin B-12 Deficiency

Vitamin B-12 is very important for the formation of blood cells and for the proper functioning of nerves. When there is a deficiency of vitamin B-12 in the body, it is possible for anemia and nerve damage to occur. The red blood cells usually are larger than normal (called macrocytic anemia), leading to an elevated MCV on the CBC test (see chapter 4). Subsequent blood tests show either a low vitamin B-12 level or an elevated methylmalonic acid level. Prompt treatment is necessary to prevent significant nerve damage. One potential cause of vitamin B-12 deficiency is an autoimmune disorder called pernicious anemia, which is due to the immune system attacking the parietal cells in the stomach or to a substance called intrinsic factor that the parietal cells secrete. Vitamin B-12 absorption partly relies on binding to intrinsic factor to be absorbed in the small intestine. So in pernicious anemia, which causes a reduction in intrinsic factor, there is decreased absorption of vitamin B-12, causing low body levels of vitamin B-12. Doctors usually diagnose it by finding gastric parietal cell antibodies or intrinsic factor antibodies in a patient's blood tests. Although vitamin B-12 deficiency does not occur more commonly in people who have lupus than in other people, it is important for the doctor to consider since anemia is so common in people who have lupus and the doctor should look for all potential causes, other than just the lupus.

Other causes of vitamin B-12 deficiency include having a condition called atrophic gastritis (which is more common in older people), eating a vegetarian diet, alcoholism, or having malabsorption problems (such as what can happen after gastric bypass surgery). Some medications can also cause vitamin B-12 deficiency, especially those used to decrease the acidity of the stomach, such as proton pump inhibitors like omeprazole (Prilosec). The diabetic medicine metformin can also cause decreased absorption of vitamin B-12.

Most people who have vitamin B-12 deficiency, even those who have pernicious anemia, do well by taking over-the-counter vitamin B-12 (also called cyanocobalamin) 1,000 mcg to 2,000 mcg each day. However, there are some people who still do not normalize their blood levels with this regimen; they may require either injections of vitamin B-12, which can be given in the doctor's office or by the person at home (after he or she is taught how to do it) or use of a nasal spray called Nascobal once a week.

## Folic Acid Deficiency

Folic acid (also known as folate) deficiency is most commonly due to either a poor diet lacking in green, leafy vegetables or drinking too much alcohol. Just like vitamin B-12 deficiency, it also causes macrocytic anemia, with larger than normal red blood cells on the CBC test and an elevated MCV level. The best way to diagnose it is to find a low red blood cell folic acid level in the blood. It is usually easy to treat by taking a folic acid supplement every day and by decreasing alcohol consumption. Although folic acid deficiency does not occur more commonly in people who have lupus than in other people, it is important for the doctor to consider since anemia is so common in people who have lupus and the doctor should look for all potential causes, other than just the lupus.

## Anemia due to Medications

Many of the immunosuppressant medicines that doctors use to treat SLE, such as methotrexate, mycophenolate, azathioprine, and cyclophosphamide can also cause anemia. They do so by affecting the bone marrow and causing it to produce fewer red blood cells than normal.

### KEY POINTS TO REMEMBER

1. Doctors diagnose anemia by finding a low hemoglobin level or a low hematocrit on the CBC.

2. The specific cause of anemia must be determined to know how to treat it.

3. Mild anemia (hemoglobin above 10 mg/dL) usually does not cause any problems and may not need to be treated.

4. Possible symptoms of anemia include fatigue, shortness of breath, lightheadedness, chest pain, and heart palpitations. Iron deficiency can cause a craving to eat ice (pagophagia).

5. The most common anemias in people who have SLE are iron deficiency anemia (the treatment for this is iron supplements) and anemia of chronic disease (the treatment for this is management of the lupus itself).

6. Autoimmune hemolytic anemia is due to the immune system attacking the red blood cells and destroying them. It can be severe and the treatment for it is high doses of steroids and immunosuppressant drugs. It is the only type of anemia that is one of the classification criteria for diagnosing SLE (see chapter 1).

7. Deficiencies of vitamin B-12 and folic acid can cause a macrocytic (larger than normal red blood cells) anemia and are treated with vitamin supplements.

8. A doctor can treat anemia due to kidney disease and anemia of chronic disease with injections of erythropoietin medications such as Aranesp and Procrit.

## Problems with Platelets

### Low Platelet Counts (Thrombocytopenia)

Platelets are the third type of cellular component found in the blood. However, although many people call platelets one of the three types of blood cells, they actually are not cells at all, but parts of cells. Cells, by definition, must have a nucleus, which contains the genetic DNA material. However, platelets do not contain DNA. They come from cells in the bone marrow called megakaryocytes, and are actually tiny pieces of these megakaryocytes that are released into the bloodstream. In the bloodstream, the term for these tiny pieces of cells is "platelets," or "thrombocytes." "Thrombo-" comes from the Greek word meaning "clot," and refers to the function of platelets, which is to cause the blood to clot. Platelets are very important because if a blood vessel gets cut or leaks, the job of the platelets is to stick together in clumps, form a clot, and stop the bleeding.

Just as with the white blood cells and the red blood cells, the immune system in the person who has SLE can attack the platelets and cause them to decrease in number. Normally, there are approximately 140,000 or more platelets per microliter of blood in the CBC test (depending on which lab is used). If this count is lower than normal, then the term for it is "thrombocytopenia." A low platelet count can potentially cause someone to bleed and bruise more easily than normal if there are not enough thrombocytes to clot and stop bleeding. However, platelets are usually very effective and can still function normally in most SLE patients who have low platelet counts. Most people do not have bleeding problems unless the platelet count drops below 25,000/μL. However, there is the possibility of bleeding more than you should with trauma or surgery if your platelet count is less than 50,000/μL, and many doctors begin to treat patients with medications if the platelet count gets below that number. Thrombocytopenia occurs in anywhere from 10% to 25% of people who have SLE. High doses of steroids plus immunosuppressants such as azathioprine, mycophenolate, cyclosporine, or cyclophosphamide are often used. Rituximab (Rituxan), belimumab (Benlysta), and IVIG are also used.

There are other potential therapies as well, such as a hormone medicine called Danazol or a biologic intravenous medicine called rituximab. Sometimes medications may not help reverse severely low platelet levels, and people may need to have their spleen removed surgically. The spleen is a large, important organ of the immune system found in the upper left side of the abdomen; it removes platelets from circulation that have been attacked by the immune system in people who have SLE.

Another potential cause of thrombocytopenia in people who have lupus is the antiphospholipid antibody syndrome (explained in more detail later in this chapter). This syndrome causes blood clots to form. Some people who have this syndrome have low platelet counts. Doctors believe that this occurs due to the platelets being used up in tiny areas of increased clotting in the body.

Some people can develop thrombocytopenia before they develop SLE. When thrombocytopenia occurs alone and doctors figure out that it is due to an autoimmune reason, they call it immune thrombocytopenic purpura or idiopathic thrombocytopenic purpura (ITP for short). The term "idiopathic" means that doctors do not know the exact cause of a problem. ITP can be caused by many different conditions, with SLE only being one of them. About 10% of people who have ITP will go on to develop SLE during their lives. Recall that in chapter 1 I discussed that SLE can sometimes start with just one problem at a time and can occasionally take months to years before it fully manifests itself. This can sometimes be the case with ITP where the ITP may occur many years before SLE becomes apparent. After SLE is diagnosed, it becomes clear that the low platelet counts were actually due to SLE the entire time. If ITP occurs along with autoimmune hemolytic anemia, it is called Evan's syndrome. Similar to ITP, Evan's syndrome can occasionally evolve over time into SLE.

## Thrombotic Thrombocytopenic Purpura

Thrombotic thrombocytopenic purpura (TTP) is a severe but rare potential complication of SLE. "Thrombotic" means that there is an increased amount of blood clotting going on in the body; "thrombocytopenic" means that the platelet count is lower than normal; and "purpura" is the medical term for "bruising." Why is there more clotting when the number of platelets is lower than normal? In the person who has TTP, the clotting system of the blood is overactive, most commonly due to an infection, which uses up the blood's platelets in the clots (and therefore they decrease in number). These numerous clots in the body decrease blood flow to the essential organs of the body and can cause kidney failure, neurologic problems such as seizures and confusion, a type of anemia called microangiopathic hemolytic anemia, and fever. Unfortunately, without treatment, this condition is 100% fatal. However, high doses of steroids and a type of treatment called plasmapheresis greatly increase the chances of the person recovering from this problem.

### KEY POINTS TO REMEMBER

1. The most common causes of thrombocytopenia in SLE are usually either the immune system attacking and decreasing the number of platelets or a condition called the antiphospholipid antibody syndrome.

2. Bleeding problems usually do not occur until the platelet count drops below 50,000/μL, so often doctors do not use stronger medicines unless the number decreases even more.

3. Removal of the spleen may be necessary in severe, resistant cases.

4. Thrombotic thrombocytopenic purpura is a rare cause of low platelet counts and is always life threatening when it occurs, requiring high doses of steroids and plasmapheresis.

## Monoclonal Gammopathy

Monoclonal gammopathy occurs in about 5% of people who have systemic lupus. It is helpful to review a little bit about the immune system when trying to understand what monoclonal gammopathy is.

Plasma cells are a certain type of white blood cell (specifically B-cells or B-lymphocytes) that produce immunoglobulins or antibodies (a kind of protein). In the immune system, these antibodies are normally directed toward potential invaders of the body to maintain health. Plasma cells make numerous types of immunoglobulins. Any one particular plasma cell makes only one particular type of immunoglobulin. These many types of plasma cells in turn produce different types of immunoglobulins in sufficient quantities to fight off the many different invading organisms (like bacteria and viruses). The immune system carefully regulates the plasma cells, making sure that no one type of plasma cell gets out of control and ends up reproducing too many similar plasma cells of its own kind. If the immune system loses control over one of these plasma cells, it may start to divide and multiply too much, making too many of its own kind. These excessive plasma cells end up producing an unhealthy amount of their own particular immunoglobulin.

Most immunoglobulins can also be classified medically as being a type of "gamma globulin." Gamma globulins are proteins in the blood that are heavier than all other proteins when measured on a laboratory test called a serum protein electrophoresis. "-Opathy" comes from the Greek word meaning "abnormality"; therefore, "gammopathy" is used to denote an abnormal production of gamma globulins, especially immunoglobulins or antibodies, by the plasma cells of the immune system. A large number of the same type of plasma cell (all making the same immunoglobulin or gamma globulin) can be considered a clone of that one particular type of plasma cell. The term "monoclonal" means "one clone" of a particular plasma cell, all making the same gamma globulin. Therefore, putting it all together, the term for a bunch of the same type of plasma cells making too much of the same immunoglobulin (or gamma globulin) is "monoclonal gammopathy." The problem with monoclonal gammopathy is that if these plasma cells become too uncontrolled and multiply too quickly they can potentially begin to displace normal cells of the body, a condition commonly known as cancer or malignancy. Specifically, the term for a cancer due to monoclonal gammopathy is "multiple myeloma," which laypersons often call a type of "bone cancer" because it especially is prone to invading the bones of the body causing them to stop producing proper amounts of normal blood cells. The bones also fracture and break. It can be a very deadly type of cancer.

Monoclonal gammopathies progress to become cancer in only a few people. If people who do not have lupus have monoclonal gammopathy (but not cancer, such as multiple myeloma), they are said to have "monoclonal gammopathy of undetermined significance" (or MGUS for short). It can be hard to tell which people who have an MGUS will progress to develop actual cancer and that is why "undetermined significance" is part of the term. Only about 1% of people who have an MGUS will develop multiple myeloma. However, multiple myeloma can be such a devastating cancer that it is very important that these people be followed closely by their doctor to try to catch it early if it does occur so that proper treatment can be given.

Although 1% of people who have MGUS every year develop multiple myeloma, this may occur less often in people who have SLE and MGUS. Recall from chapter 1 that people who have lupus make too many antibodies against the body due to the plasma cells being overactive. Therefore, it is not surprising that some of these plasma cells may produce too many of their own selves, causing monoclonal gammopathy, which the doctor can pick up on blood tests. The reason that monoclonal gammopathy occurs in lupus is due to the overactive immune system and may be a totally different situation compared to other people who develop MGUS as a stepping stone to developing full-blown multiple myeloma. A study in 2007 from Canada showed that none of their studied lupus patients who had MGUS developed multiple myeloma over an average of eight years, so this is reassuring. However, since multiple myeloma can be so devastating doctors need to carefully monitor blood tests over time to ensure that this does not happen.

The bottom line is that monoclonal gammopathy in lupus refers to the abnormal production of too much of one type of gamma globulin by the plasma cells of the immune system. Your doctor may call it monoclonal gammopathy or monoclonal gammopathy of undetermined significance (MGUS). There is very little chance that it will progress to multiple myeloma, but this is not 100% certain. It most likely is not anything to worry about in the larger scheme of things, but your doctor will monitor your blood work over time to ensure nothing bad (progression to multiple myeloma) occurs.

## Problems with Lymph Nodes

The lymph nodes (often called lymph glands by many people) are small, oval-shaped, rubbery tissue connected to each other by lymphatic channels. They are important collections of specialized white blood cells. Circulating white blood cells travel to them during periods of stimulation of the immune system. For example, if you get a strep infection in your throat, the white blood cells that identify the infecting bacteria will go to the lymph nodes in your neck to communicate with other white blood cells about this attack, and cause even more white blood cells to go to the throat to kill the bacteria. The number of white blood cells that end up filling up the lymph nodes can become enormous, causing your lymph nodes to swell up and become tender or uncomfortable (often noted as "swollen glands"). The medical term for swelling of the lymph nodes is "lymphadenopathy." Since SLE is due to the immune system becoming more active, it should not be surprising that lymphadenopathy is common in people who have the disease. Anywhere from 40% to 50% of SLE patients will have lymphadenopathy with swollen lymph nodes often noticeable in the neck, armpits, and groin. In some people, the lymph nodes swell during flares of their lupus, but sometimes they can remain slightly swollen even when the lupus appears to be well controlled.

Sometimes the cause of swollen lymph nodes can be other problems such as infection and cancer, especially a type of cancer called lymphoma. If infection causes lymphadenopathy, there is usually a fever as well. Therefore, if you get a fever, you should see your doctor right away and make sure you do not have an infection. SLE patients have a three to five times increased chance of developing the type of lymph cell cancer called lymphoma. If you develop particularly large lymph nodes, your doctor may get a biopsy to determine whether this is due to your lupus or to lymphoma. If lymph nodes are an inch or larger, are not tender, and do not go away with treatment with steroids or antibiotics, then it is usually a good idea to have them biopsied. If you are over 40 years old, if you have an enlarged spleen, or if the lymph node swelling occurs behind or just above the collar bone (clavicle), then a biopsy is indicated to rule out lymphoma.

## Problems with the Spleen

The spleen is an organ found in the left upper part of the abdomen, underneath the ribs. It is an important part of the immune system because it removes things that have been tagged for removal by antibodies. In up to 45% of people who have SLE, the spleen may become enlarged. Often the liver will also be enlarged as well. Your doctor may find this on physical examination or by accident when he or she does an ultrasound study or CT scan of the abdomen for other reasons. The medical term for an enlarged spleen is "splenomegaly" and usually it is not a problem in most SLE patients.

A rare finding in SLE is a condition called functional asplenia. This term is basically used to describe a spleen that does not function, putting the person at high risk for certain infections, especially from pneumococcal and salmonella. Prior to availability of the pneumococcal vaccine, most people who had SLE who developed pneumococcal infection died from sepsis. Doctors can suspect this condition based on some findings that can be seen under the microscope when a complete blood cell count is performed and confirmed using a nuclear medicine test called a liver-spleen scan (also called a liver-spleen scintigraphy). People who have lupus who have functional asplenia absolutely need to get vaccinated against pneumococcus (called a Pneumovax; see chapter 22) to prevent severe infection.

### KEY POINTS TO REMEMBER

1. Enlarged lymph nodes (lymphadenopathy) and an enlarged spleen (splenomegaly) are common in people who have SLE, but rarely cause problems. Many people use the term "swollen glands" for lymphadenopathy.

2. Sometimes a lymph node biopsy is required if lymph nodes remain enlarged, to make sure there is no evidence of a type of cancer of the lymphatic system called lymphoma.

## Antiphospholipid Syndrome

Between 30% and 50% of people who have SLE will be positive for a particular type of antibody called antiphospholipid antibodies. These antibodies include anticardiolipin antibodies, lupus anticoagulant, beta-2 glycoprotein I antibodies, and antiphosphatidylserine antibodies. Antiphospholipid antibodies can also be identified by the appearance of false serologic tests for syphilis (false positive RPR or VDRL) in the blood work. These antibodies are explained in more detail in chapter 4. The presence of these antibodies can potentially cause increased clotting. Approximately 50% of people who have these antibodies can develop increased clotting problems over time if not treated. These problems include blood clots in the legs called deep venous thrombosis (DVT), blood clots in the lungs called pulmonary embolus (PE), blood clots in the arteries of the brain causing a stroke, blood clots in the spinal cord causing paralysis due to transverse myelitis, and even blood clots in the arteries of the heart causing a heart attack. In addition, women who have these antibodies and become pregnant are at increased risk of having complications such as a miscarriage due to blood clots forming in the placenta (the organ that connects the fetus to the mother in the uterus). The rash known as livedo reticularis, as described previously, can occur due to tiny blood clots in the small blood vessels of the skin, and the platelet count can even become lower than normal due to platelets being used up in the body due to this increased clotting problem. Small clots can also occur on the valves of the heart (called valvular heart disease or Libman-Sacks endocarditis), causing difficulty with blood traveling normally through the heart. Many rheumatologists ask their patients who have these antibodies to take a low dose of aspirin every day to try to prevent blood clots from forming. The different types of problems that blood clots can cause due to the antiphospholipid syndrome are discussed next, followed by how they are treated.

### Deep Venous Thrombosis

"Thrombus" is the medical word for "blood clot." Deep venous thrombosis (DVT) occurs when a blood clot forms in one of the deep veins of the arms or legs. It is much more common in the legs than it is in the arms. Often the person will notice constant pain and swelling in one leg, which is sometimes associated with redness and warmth, especially over the calf. This problem is considered a medical emergency because if the blood clot breaks loose from the blood vessel wall, it can travel up to the lungs, causing a pulmonary embolism, which can be deadly. Anyone who has symptoms should go immediately to the emergency room, where doctors will usually do an ultrasound of the leg. An ultrasound is a medical imaging study where gel is placed on the skin; a plastic instrument called a probe or transducer is then placed on top of the gel. It can then take pictures deep under the skin to see if there is any sign of a blood clot.

### Pulmonary Embolus

"Pulmonary" refers to the lungs, and an "embolus" is a blood clot that travels through the bloodstream. If an embolus travels to the bloodstream of the lungs, the medical term is a "pulmonary embolus" (PE). The most common source of a PE is deep venous thrombosis. Unfortunately, this is a potentially deadly problem. If the embolus is large enough it can block significant blood flow to the lungs, causing the person not to be able to get enough oxygen into the blood from the lungs. Someone with a PE usually has shortness of breath and/or chest pains. A doctor can diagnose it by a combination of tests, including an electrocardiogram (ECG), blood tests such as the D-dimer test, and chest x-rays. However, a better type of x-ray is necessary to know for sure. One of the best x-ray studies is the spiral CT (also called CT pulmonary angiography), which is a special type of CT scan of the chest. In places that do not have this test available, then a type of x-ray called a V/Q (ventilation/perfusion) scan is necessary.

## Cerebrovascular Accident

If a blood clot occurs in one of the arteries of the brain, there is blood flow loss to that part of the brain, causing part of the brain to die. The term for this is a "cerebrovascular accident" (CVA), or more commonly a "stroke." You can think of it as a "heart attack of the brain." Sometimes a blood clot in the brain can be temporary, causing symptoms that are brief and that completely go away. This is termed a "transient ischemic attack" (TIA)—"transient" means "lasting for a short time"—or "mini-stroke" in layperson's terms. Although the outcome of a TIA is much better than the permanent problems seen in a CVA, it is nonetheless still a very important matter because anyone who has had a TIA is at high risk of developing a full-blown CVA at some point in the future.

The symptoms of a CVA depend completely on which part of the brain it affects. These can include difficulty talking, numbness, weakness, a droopy face, blurred vision, loss of vision, headache, and the inability to move normally.

A doctor may suspect that a person has had a CVA if a physical examination shows compatible signs. Imaging studies of the brain such as a CT scan or MRI can confirm the diagnosis. Strokes can occur for other reasons in people who have SLE and these will be discussed further in chapter 21.

## Transverse Myelitis

Transverse myelitis occurs when there is damage to part of the spinal cord. The cause may be inflammation from SLE, but more commonly the cause is a clotted artery due to the antiphospholipid syndrome. This is a devastating complication because it usually causes permanent paralysis in the legs and often does not improve with treatment. I have only had one patient with this complication. It affected the spinal cord of the neck and caused her to develop paralysis, incoordination, and the loss of sensation. Miraculously, she regained all of her strength after being treated with high doses of steroids and a strong immunosuppressant drug called cyclophosphamide.

## Myocardial Infarction

A myocardial infarction (or MI for short), which is more commonly known as a heart attack, occurs when a blood clot occurs in an artery of the heart (called a coronary artery) and causes part of the heart muscle to die. The most common symptom of an MI is chest pain, often described as a severe pressure in the chest, which often radiates into (i.e., spreads to) the arm or neck. Sometimes nausea or shortness of breath can be a predominant symptom. A doctor may diagnose an MI by finding typical abnormalities on an electrocardiogram, along with blood tests that measure enzymes released from the heart muscle due to the damage from the MI. Myocardial infarctions due to antiphospholipid antibodies are not very common. However, MIs due to other problems associated with SLE are the number one cause of death in lupus patients in the United States. Therefore, it is very important to learn how to prevent them. Chapter 21 discusses this subject in detail.

### Recurrent Miscarriages

The placenta is the organ that connects the fetus to the uterus of the mother. Some women who have antiphospholipid antibodies will develop blood clots in the placenta, which can later lead to the loss of blood flow to the fetus and cause a miscarriage. This can happen at any time during pregnancy. In a woman who has recurrent miscarriages early in pregnancy, or has had even just one second- or third-trimester miscarriage, it is always important that doctors check for this potential cause. Giving these women blood thinners during pregnancy greatly increases the chances of their having a successful pregnancy.

. . . .

If any of these problems occur in a person who is positive for any antiphospholipid antibodies, he or she is said to have the antiphospholipid syndrome (APS or APLS for short). The problem with people who develop any of these problems is that they are at high risk for them recurring if not treated appropriately. In fact, they tend to develop the same types of problems repeatedly if untreated. For example, someone who has APS who develops a stroke is more likely to develop another stroke instead of a DVT. Most people who have had blood clots or recurrent miscarriages due to APS are placed on blood thinners such as warfarin (Coumadin), heparin through an IV when in the hospital, or self-injectable heparin such as Lovenox. Anyone who has had a blood clot from APS leading to a stroke, DVT, PE, or heart attack usually needs to take the blood thinner, usually warfarin, for the rest of her or his life. People who take warfarin must get a blood test called a PT INR (prothrombin international normalized ratio) at regular intervals to make sure that their warfarin is at the correct dose. The normal PT INR level is about 1.0. The higher it is from 1.0, the "thinner" the blood is due to the warfarin. Usually the doctor tries to keep the PT INR somewhere between 2.0 and 3.0 for most patients depending on their particular situation. For patients who have particularly severe antiphospholipid antibody syndrome (such as having multiple blood clots or who have had a heart attack), a higher PT INR level of 3.0 to 4.0 may be recommended. If the blood is too thin (too high of a PT INR) due to the warfarin, then the person is at risk of bleeding too much and the dose has to be lowered. If the PT INR level is too low (and therefore the person is at risk of forming blood clots), then the doctor must increase the dose. Most people who have APS who take a blood thinner regularly have a much lower chance of developing problems with recurrent blood clots. However, they are at increased risk of bleeding due to their medication and need to take necessary safeguards against this possibility as directed by their doctor.

A woman who develops miscarriages due to APS will generally give herself heparin shots during and right after pregnancy to try to have a normal pregnancy. Doctors often recommend taking a low dose of aspirin every day in addition to the heparin to keep the blood thin. By doing this, most women who have APS are able to have a successful pregnancy.

It is essential that people taking warfarin learn as much as they can about what substances can interfere with its working properly. For example, foods that have vitamin K in them (e.g., many green vegetables) will keep it from working correctly. Therefore, the person on warfarin has to learn how to keep their vitamin K levels stable (taking into consideration food and vitamin supplements) because any change in the amount of vitamin K intake can greatly affect how the warfarin is working, causing potential drastic changes in the PT INR levels. These types of changes may require modification in the dose of warfarin. It is also best that the person on warfarin not smoke cigarettes or drink alcohol since these practices also affect how warfarin works in the body. Many medications will either increase or decrease the effects of warfarin, so a doctor should follow up any new medicines or changes in doses with a blood PT INR level to make sure that adjustment of the warfarin dose is not necessary. People on warfarin must have their PT INR checked on a frequent basis.

The medication hydroxychloroquine (Plaquenil) may have some benefits in people who have APS. Studies show that hydroxychloroquine may possibly decrease the risk of clotting and may decrease the production of these antibodies in lupus patients.

A particularly severe type of antiphospholipid antibody syndrome deserves special mention and that is the condition of catastrophic antiphospholipid syndrome. In this rare complication, blood clots are occurring in the person who has APS in multiple areas of the body causing multiple organs to fail. These people are very sick and usually end up in an intensive care unit in the hospital. For severe cases such as this, and for people who have APS who are not responding to the normal therapies outlined above, more aggressive treatments using high doses of steroids, IVIG (see chapter 35), apheresis (see chapter 35), and additional strong medications such as cyclophosphamide and rituximab (Rituxan) may be needed.

Not all people who have APS have SLE. In fact, about 50% have what is termed "primary antiphospholipid syndrome," meaning that they have the autoimmune APS problem without associated SLE.

### KEY POINTS TO REMEMBER

1. Between one-third and one-half of people who have SLE are positive for antiphospholipid antibodies, cardiolipin antibody, lupus anticoagulant, beta-2 glycoprotein I antibody, and phosphatidyl serine antibody. Antiphospholipid antibodies can also potentially cause a person who has lupus to have a false positive blood test for syphilis.

2. Up to 50% of people who have these antibodies may develop blood clots or have miscarriages during pregnancy since these antibodies can potentially cause increased clotting of the blood.

3. If you are positive for any of the antiphospholipid antibodies, consider taking low-dose aspirin (such as 81 mg a day) to help prevent these blood clots.

4. People who do have blood clots usually need to be on blood thinners such as warfarin, aspirin, and heparin for the rest of their lives.

5. People who continue to have recurrent blood clots on standard therapy or people who develop the rare condition called catastrophic antiphospholipid syndrome may require high doses of steroids, apheresis, IVIG, cyclophosphamide, or rituximab (Rituxan).

6. The treatment for women who have had miscarriages due to APS is usually heparin and aspirin during pregnancy to try to have a successful pregnancy.

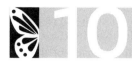

# The Respiratory System

## Breathing

The respiratory system, also called the pulmonary system ("pulmonary" means "lung"), begins at the nose and mouth where we breathe air in and out, continues down the major windpipe called the trachea, which branches out into smaller windpipes called bronchi, and then ends up in the lungs. The last part of the lungs reached by air that we breathe in are tiny, microscopic sacs called alveoli that have incredibly thin walls lined with tiny blood vessels called capillaries (see magnified view in figure 10.1). Oxygen is absorbed from the air we breathe in through the alveolar walls and into the capillaries and then dissolves in the bloodstream. The blood entering the lungs by way of the pulmonary arteries is bluish in color since it lacks oxygen. When more oxygen is absorbed into these blood vessels at the level of the alveolar sacs, the oxygen binds to hemoglobin in the red blood cells, causing the blood to become reddish in color. At the same time that oxygen is being absorbed, gases that the body does not need (most importantly, carbon dioxide) are released from these tiny blood vessels in the walls of the alveoli into the air so you can exhale them out of your body. Systemic lupus can potentially affect any of these structures, causing difficulties with breathing and this chapter focuses on these problems.

••••

Although SLE can affect any part of the respiratory system, the primary area that is involved is the lower respiratory system (figure 10.1), at the level of the alveoli and interstitium, the blood vessels of the lungs, and the pleural lining of the lungs. About 50% of people who have SLE will develop involvement of the respiratory system.

## Pleuritis (Pleurisy)

The term for the tissue lining the lungs is the "pleura." It consists of two very thin layers of smooth, lubricated membranes. One envelops the lungs, while the other layer attaches to the inside of the muscles and ribs around the lungs. Between these two layers is a light coating of fluid. Its purpose is to act like a lubricant when the lungs expand when breathing in and deflate when breathing out. This allows the lungs to glide smoothly under the rib cage when you breathe. A similar type of lining also exists around the heart (called the pericardium) and around the abdominal contents (called the peritoneum). The medical term for these linings (pleura, pericardium, and peritoneum) is "serosa." SLE can cause inflammation of the serosa and the medical term for this is "serositis" ("-itis" means "inflammation of"). In fact, it occurs so frequently in people who have SLE that it is included in the diagnostic criteria for SLE (see chapter 1). When serositis occurs in the pleura, the medical term is "pleuritis" (also known as pleurisy). Similarly, the medical term is "pericarditis" when it occurs in the pericardium around the heart, and "peritonitis" when it occurs in the peritoneal lining around the abdominal contents.

Serositis from SLE causes similar symptoms in these three areas. Healthy serosa allow the lungs, heart, and abdominal organs to move smoothly and effortlessly. When there is inflammation of this lining, an increased amount of fluid and numerous white blood cells enter the lining's space. The lubricating fluid loses its smoothness and the layers rubbing against each other become roughened during this inflammatory process. This mainly causes pain when moving that particular organ. Therefore, when pleuritis occurs, there is pain when the person tries to breathe in and out as the two roughened, now inflamed, surfaces rub against each other. This makes breathing painful and difficult. Sometimes the pain can be excruciating. It can occur anywhere in the chest area. Normally people are not conscious of their breathing, but with pleuritis, every breath is noticeable because of the pain.

When chest pain that worsens with breathing develops, the medical term is "pleuritic chest pain." People who have pleurisy or pericarditis due to lupus often develop pleuritic-type chest pain. However, any painful process involving chest wall structures important in breathing can cause a similar type of chest pain. These other possibili-

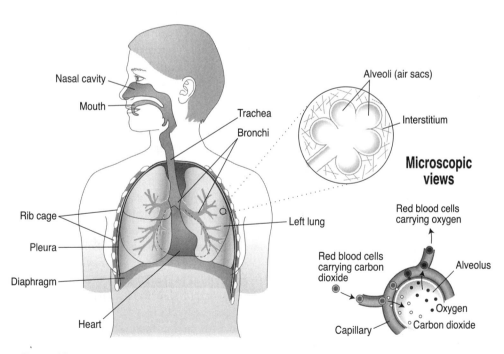

**Figure 10.1** The respiratory system

ties include broken ribs, inflammation of the ribs (called costochondritis), or other painful muscle problems such as fibromyalgia. A doctor must consider these other causes when evaluating someone who has chest pain that worsens while breathing (i.e., pleuritic chest pain).

To sort out these possibilities, the doctor usually has to conduct other tests. The doctor will listen to the lungs and heart. He or she may hear a "rub," which is caused by the friction of the layers of the inflamed pleura or pericardium rubbing over each other (it sounds like two pieces of sandpaper being rubbed against each other). Usually with serositis, the erythrocyte sedimentation rate, or ESR (an inflammatory blood test explained in more detail in chapter 4), is highly elevated. If the ESR is normal, then other causes of the chest pain are more likely. The doctor often orders a chest x-ray to see if there is a collection of fluid in the pleura around the lungs. Although with pleuritis the amount of extra fluid that occurs is often very small, sometimes there can be a large amount, causing what is called a pleural effusion (an "effusion" is a medical term meaning "a collection of fluid"). This pleural effusion may be large enough to be visible on the chest x-ray. The doctor may also order an ECG (electrocardiogram). This does not help in diagnosing pleuritis, but the ECG results might be abnormal, which may be helpful in diagnosing pericarditis, which can also cause pleuritic chest pain.

Pleuritis (pleurisy) is fairly common in people who have SLE, occurring in 40% to 50% of them at some point in life. This makes it the most common lung problem seen in people who have SLE. However, many people have it but never notice it. We know this because autopsies performed on people who had SLE show that up to 90% have evidence of inflammation of the pleura. Although pleurisy can be very painful and can cause shortness of breath, it rarely causes significant damage since it occurs outside the lungs and not in the lungs themselves.

Sometimes if there is a pleural effusion, a doctor can drain the fluid. The term for this procedure is a "thoracentesis." The doctor numbs up the chest wall muscles and skin, then inserts a needle through the numbed-up area until it reaches the fluid. The doctor then draws the fluid out. A laboratory analysis of the fluid can be helpful in determining the cause of the pleural effusion. This rarely is necessary in people who have lupus, but is most useful if it is the first time the person has had a pleural effusion and its cause is unknown. The reason for evaluating the fluid is that many disorders can potentially cause a pleural effusion, and the doctors must consider all these possibilities. Other systemic autoimmune diseases (like rheumatoid arthritis), infections, cancer, and kidney or liver failure can all cause fluid buildup in the pleura. The pleural fluid will have different laboratory characteristics depending on the cause. If the person has a particularly large pleural effusion, it can cause difficulty breathing. In this case, the doctor should do a thoracentesis to help the person breathe easier.

The treatment for pleuritis is usually anti-inflammatory medicines. For mild cases, non-steroidal anti-inflammatory drugs (NSAIDs) such as ibuprofen may be used. In more severe cases (where the person has severe pain or if a large pleural effusion is present) steroids may be necessary. Recurrent cases of pleuritis usually respond well to hydroxychloroquine, but sometimes stronger medications such as methotrexate, azathioprine, mycophenolate, rituximab (Rituxan), belimumab (Benlysta), or abatacept (Orencia) are necessary. Severe, life-threatening cases of pleuritis (which can be associated with large pleural effusions) may require the use of cyclophosphamide.

1. Pleuritis (also called pleurisy) is the most common lung problem seen in people who have SLE.

2. Most of the time pleuritis causes no symptoms or problems.

3. The most common symptoms include pleuritic chest pain (pain with breathing), cough, and shortness of breath.

4. The initial treatments for pleuritis are NSAIDs, steroids, and/or hydroxychloroquine (Plaquenil).

5. More resistant or severe cases may require stronger medicines such as methotrexate, azathioprine, mycophenolate, rituximab (Rituxan), belimumab (Benlysta), or abatacept (Orencia).

6. If there is a lot of fluid around the lungs due to the pleuritis (called a pleural effusion), then it may need to be drained by a procedure called thoracentesis.

## Pneumonitis

"Pneumonitis" is the term for any form of inflammation of the lungs. In fact, pneumonia due to infection is a type of pneumonitis. Lupus can attack the lungs in some people, causing inflammation that can behave like pneumonia. It typically causes a cough, fever, chest pain, and sometimes shortness of breath if it is severe. It can be so similar to pneumonia that hospitals admit some people who have SLE, diagnose them with pneumonia, and treat them with antibiotics when in fact they have inflammation from their lupus instead of an infection. Further testing would have shown significant scarring and inflammation of the lungs.

Lupus pneumonitis occurs when the immune system attacks the alveoli and/or interstitium of the lungs (see magnified view in figure 10.1). Each bout of inflammation causes symptoms similar to those of pneumonia, such as cough, shortness of breath, chest pain, and fever. After it resolves, it may leave permanent scarring and damage to the lungs. If this permanent damage is mild, the person may not have any problems at all. However, if it is severe, the person may end up having breathing problems. Fortunately, pneumonitis only occurs in 3% to 10% of people who have SLE.

Often doctors order a chest x-ray when someone has an unexplained cough. In a person with pneumonitis due to lupus, this x-ray will show something that doctors call an infiltrate (fluid collecting in either the interstitium or alveoli of the lungs). The alveoli are the very tiny air sacs of the lungs where the exchange of oxygen and carbon dioxide takes place. The interstitium is the connective tissue that supports the alveoli and holds them together. When an infiltrate appears on the chest x-ray, the doctor cannot be certain if it is due to infectious pneumonia or something else such as lupus pneumonitis because they look the same on x-ray. Therefore, the doctor usually prescribes antibiotics for the person who has lupus (in addition to treating the lupus) just in case it is an infection.

A doctor may order other tests in the person suspected of having lupus pneumonitis. This usually occurs when, after treatment for "pneumonia," the person does not improve as expected. One of these tests is a chest CT scan. The doctor will order a special CT scan called a high-resolution CT scan, which is better able to determine what is happening in the lungs. A CT scan uses quite a bit more radiation than a chest x-ray and for that reason doctors do not order it very often. In the person who has lupus pneumonitis, the CT scan may show scar tissue in the interstitium due to previous damage. It may also show what the radiologist may describe as a "ground-glass appearance," which is exactly what it sounds like—the CT image looks like ground glass. This finding sometimes means there is fluid in the alveoli due to inflammation of the alveoli (called alveolitis). Alveolitis is a classic finding in lupus pneumonitis, but it also occurs in other conditions such as infectious pneumonia or congestive heart failure, so it is not specific for lupus pneumonitis. Therefore, other tests, such as a bronchoscopy, may be necessary. Bronchoscopy refers to the insertion of a fiberoptic scope into the windpipe (usually through the nose after sedation to make the person comfortable) and then down into the trachea and bronchi to look into the lungs. At this point, the doctor can take pictures, collect fluid to send for cultures and other lab tests, and even take a biopsy to help try to establish what is causing the problem. Under the microscope, a biopsy from a person who has lupus pneumonitis shows a lot of inflammation of the lung tissue. These findings do not appear only in SLE, but when seen in a person who has lupus, it is sufficient for a diagnosis of lupus pneumonitis. The importance of the biopsy is to make sure there is not another reason for the lung problem, such as infection, cancer, or other problems such as vasculitis (discussed in chapter 2).

If the above tests cannot establish the diagnosis, then an open lung biopsy may be necessary. With an open lung biopsy, the surgeon cuts into the chest wall and removes a small piece of lung tissue (the biopsy) for examination under a microscope. Doctors usually reserve this biopsy for people who have especially severe symptoms or in whom proper treatment depends on what the results show. For example, treating lupus pneumonitis requires medicines that suppress the immune system (and can make infection worse), whereas a lung infection is treated with antibiotics. Therefore, obtaining a correct diagnosis is very important. Out of all the tests described above, the lung biopsy is the most specific. In other words, it is the test that has the highest likelihood of telling the doctors exactly what the problem is. However, it is also the test that has the most potential complications, so it is performed only if doctors believe that it is absolutely necessary.

Most commonly, doctors make the diagnosis of lupus pneumonitis in two particular cases. The first is the person who has recurrent bouts of "pneumonia" that never resolve completely with antibiotics and then the doctor eventually diagnoses the person with SLE. After treatment for SLE, these bouts of pneumonia stop occurring. In hindsight, doctors assume that these were most likely bouts of pneumonitis due to SLE instead of infectious pneumonia. The other most common scenario is the person who receives treatment for "pneumonia" with antibiotics but does not get better. She then gets a chest x-ray and CT scan, both of which show an infiltrate in the lungs. A doctor who specializes in the lungs, called a pulmonologist, performs a bronchoscopy. The doctor sends fluid from the bronchoscopy to the lab and it shows no evidence of infection (pneumonia). After additional workup to search for other causes of pneumonitis, including blood work, urinalysis, and possibly even an open lung biopsy, the doctor may diagnose SLE with pneumonitis.

Some medications for treatment of lupus, such as methotrexate and azathioprine, can actually cause pneumonitis. Stopping these medications is very important in this case.

Lupus pneumonitis usually requires high doses of steroids either through an IV or by mouth to decrease the inflammation. In addition, a doctor usually needs to prescribe a strong immunosuppressant medicine such as azathioprine, mycophenolate, or cyclophosphamide to help with the treatment, to help to decrease the dose of steroids, and to try to prevent it from recurring.

Unfortunately, if not diagnosed and treated, lupus pneumonitis has a high mortality rate. A medical report from the 1970s showed that 50% of people who had lupus pneumonitis died from this particular problem. Currently, with better diagnostic tests and treatments, the prognosis appears to be much better. I have personally cared for quite a few people with lupus pneumonitis, and fortunately, none of them has died from this complication.

### KEY POINTS TO REMEMBER

1. Lupus pneumonitis occurs when lupus causes inflammation of the lung tissue.

2. The symptoms of lupus pneumonitis are similar to those of infectious pneumonitis—such as cough, fever, shortness of breath, and chest pain.

3. Chest x-rays and CT scans for infectious pneumonia and lupus pneumonitis appear similar, so often the person needs treatment for both possibilities (both antibiotics and immunosuppressants).

4. Some medicines for treatment of lupus (such as methotrexate and azathioprine) can sometimes also cause inflammation of the lungs. The doctor sometimes needs to stop these medications if he or she is not sure whether they are contributing to the lung problem.

5. A high-resolution CT scan can be useful to see if lupus pneumonitis is active, as it will appear like "ground glass." This indicates that immunosuppressant medicines may be necessary.

6. When lupus pneumonitis heals, it usually leaves some scar tissue or interstitial lung disease.

7. Lupus pneumonitis once had a high mortality rate. People do much better today as long as doctors identify and treat the condition quickly and aggressively, but it can still be very dangerous.

## Interstitial Lung Disease (Pulmonary Fibrosis)

The interstitium is the connective tissue that supports the alveoli and the small airway passages in the lungs (see magnified view in figure 10.1). When this interstitium (or interstitial tissue) becomes scarred, the condition is called interstitial lung disease (or ILD for short) or pulmonary fibrosis (both terms are used interchangeably). Scarring in the body occurs as a response to injury or inflammation. Often the body will form an excessive amount of connective tissue and collagen after trying to heal areas affected by inflammation. Just think of the scar left after you get a cut on your skin. A similar process can occur in the interstitium of the lung after injury or inflammation, such as after inflammation due to lupus. This scar tissue is not very flexible (again, think of that tough scar left on your skin after a big cut), so the lungs in the person who has ILD become less elastic, causing more difficulty breathing. In addition, blood vessels (which are necessary for proper oxygen uptake from the air) cannot go through this scar tissue; it can also compress the alveolar air sacs (which are essential for proper gas exchange). All of these factors can cause problems with inadequate absorption of oxygen and exhalation of carbon dioxide, which in turn leads to breathing problems. The person who has ILD will thus often have shortness of breath and a cough.

After pleuritis, ILD is the second most common lung problem seen in lupus, occurring in 10% to 20% of people who have SLE. There are a few common scenarios for ILD to occur in people who have lupus. The first would be the person who has recurrent bouts of pneumonitis. Each bout of pneumonitis can cause permanent scarring of the lungs (or ILD). Another scenario is the person who gradually develops a cough and/or shortness of breath. The symptoms may be mild and persistent, or they may gradually worsen over time, causing the person to see the doctor to determine the cause. The final common scenario is the person who feels fine and has no breathing problems at all, but the doctor will hear something abnormal on physical examination when he or she listens to the lungs or will see evidence of interstitial lung disease on a chest x-ray or PFTs (pulmonary function tests). The reason the person may not have any symptoms is most likely due to the inflammation and scarring occurring very mildly and slowly over time. Although there is some damage to the lungs, it most likely occurred so slowly that the person's body was able to compensate for this loss of lung tissue.

Diagnosing ILD begins with a physical exam by the doctor. Often a doctor can hear changes in lung sounds with a stethoscope. A common description for this is "Velcro crackles" because they resemble the sound a Velcro strap makes when someone pulls it apart. ILD in SLE typically affects the base of the lungs, so these crackles are usually most prominent there when the doctor listens to the person's breathing.

A chest x-ray usually, but not always, shows scarring of the interstitium of the lungs. The radiologist (a doctor who examines x-rays) may describe these as "increased interstitial markings" or "interstitial infiltrates." Often the doctor will order a high-resolution CT of the chest, which shows the type and pattern of the lung changes. It is especially helpful to determine if there is actual active inflammation, which may show up as a "ground glass" appearance, or if there is scarring of the interstitial tissue. This can be useful in determining whether high doses of steroids or strong immunosuppressant medicines are indicated.

Pulmonary function tests (PFTs for short) are usually required. These tests are conducted in a pulmonary or respiratory lab at a hospital or in the office of a lung specialist. PFTs in the person who has ILD will usually show a couple of abnormalities. The interpreting physician will usually note this as a "restrictive pattern" or "restrictive lung disease" along with an indication of whether there is mild, moderate, or severe involvement. A restrictive pattern means that the lungs do not expand normally, which is due to the inelastic nature of the scar tissue due to ILD. ILD is only one cause of restrictive lung disease. A more common cause is obesity (being overweight causes difficultly in taking a full breath). There is another part of the PFTs that is very helpful in determining the cause of the restrictive pattern—this is the "Diffusion capacity of the Lung for Carbon monoxide," or DLCO for short. In this test, the person conducting the test asks the patient to breathe in air containing a very small amount of carbon monoxide and hold it for ten seconds. Then the amount of carbon monoxide breathed back out is measured. The better the lungs are at absorbing gases, the less carbon monoxide they will exhale (due to it being absorbed through the walls of the alveolar sacs and into the blood vessels in the walls of the alveolar sacs). If there is any disease causing problems with either the alveolar sacs (such as pneumonitis or other diseases like emphysema) or the blood vessels (such as pulmonary hypertension, described below) or both (as in ILD), then the DLCO will be lower than normal. If the DLCO is lower than normal, the interpreting doctor will describe it as "decreased diffusion capacity" along with an indication of the severity—mild, moderate, or severe. If the restrictive pattern is due to obesity, and the lungs are normal, then the diffusion capacity, or DLCO, will be normal. The numerical results of the restrictive pattern and the DLCO can also be very helpful in monitoring how the ILD does over time. For example, if there is some reversible inflammation in the lungs, after treatment with medicines for SLE, then the DLCO and restrictive pattern may improve when the patient takes the PFTs again. If the ILD was due to permanent scarring with no active inflammation, or if the medicines for the SLE are not helping the lungs, then the numbers may stay the same or even worsen when the patient repeats the PFTs. Therefore, the PFTs can be a good way to monitor treatment.

When a doctor sees a person who has ILD, one of the first things he or she tries to determine is whether the ILD is due to permanent scarring (which does not improve with medicines) or whether there is active inflammation. If there is active inflammation, then steroids and other immunosuppressant medications (such as azathioprine, mycophenolate, belimumab, or cyclophosphamide) may be helpful in decreasing the inflammation. This treatment can potentially prevent the lung condition from worsening or even make the lungs better. One way to figure this out is to see "ground glass" changes on the high-resolution CT scan, which can sometimes indicate active inflammation of the alveoli (also called alveolitis). The other test that can be done to determine if there is active inflammation in the lungs is a bronchoscopy (discussed above under the section on pneumonitis), where fluid can be obtained from the lungs and examined for inflammation. Another way to determine if there is active inflammation is by the doctor administering a trial of steroids to see if studies such as the pulmonary function tests (PFTs) or x-rays improve with the steroid treatment. This trial of steroids is purely an experiment. In other words, the doctor cannot be entirely sure that there is active inflammation. The only way to determine it (if there is not "ground glass" on the CT scan or there are not bronchoscopy fluid results) may be to treat the person with steroids and then retest the person after treatment (with PFTs, chest x-ray, and/or another CT scan) to see if the treatment improved the person's condition.

If interstitial lung disease is felt to be active with inflammation, the treatment is similar to the medications described in the previous section on pneumonitis. The TNF inhibitor infliximab (see chapter 33) has also been suggested as a treatment for difficult to treat cases by a panel of European lupus experts.

Fortunately, ILD usually does not lead to respiratory failure (like severe emphysema, asthma, or acute pneumonitis). However, it certainly can potentially cause many problems. Although some people never have any symptoms at all, others may have varying degrees of breathing problems and coughing. The breathing problems usually cause shortness of breath with activities and may limit how much activity, exertion, and exercise the affected person may do. ILD may cause significant limitations in the person's quality of life.

The person who has ILD should take some important precautions. First, smoking cigarettes will make it worse. Although no one who has lupus should smoke (as discussed in detail in chapter 38), it is even more important for the person who has ILD. Smoking cigarettes can cause the ILD to get worse and increases the chances of getting severe lung infections. Many people who have SLE can have problems with their esophagus (the tube connecting the mouth to the stomach). One such problem is gastroesophageal reflux disease (GERD for short), where stomach contents back up into the esophagus (usually causing heartburn). Another problem is esophageal dysmotility (described in chapter 15), where the muscles do not work normally in pushing food down into the stomach. The problem with these two conditions is that acidic contents from the stomach can travel from the stomach up the esophagus while the person is lying down or sleeping, then drip back into the trachea (or windpipe), then go down into the lungs where this acidic fluid can cause even more lung damage or worsening of the ILD. So it is very important that the person who has GERD (or esophageal dysmotility) and ILD be extra vigilant in taking antacid medication every day, as well as in keeping her or his GERD under control (see table 15.1).

As mentioned in the preceding section on pneumonitis, some medications such as methotrexate and azathioprine may cause inflammation of the lungs. Sometimes the doctor needs to stop these medications if she or he is not sure whether they are contributing to the lung problem or not.

The lungs are constantly under attack from germs that we breathe in every day. Usually normally functioning lungs and normal immune systems are very good at protecting people from these germs. However, people who have ILD due to lupus are particularly at increased risk for lung infections, such as pneumonia, since their lungs do not function normally and they also have an immune system that is not capable of protecting them as well as it should. It is therefore very important to do everything possible to prevent lung infections. Although most, if not all, people who have SLE should get a flu shot each fall and a Pneumovax (vaccination against pneumococcal pneumonia, discussed in chapter 22) at least once during their life, it is even more important for people who have ILD.

### KEY POINTS TO REMEMBER

1. Interstitial lung disease (also called pulmonary fibrosis) is a common problem in people who have SLE.

2. ILD is due to permanent scarring in the lungs.

3. A doctor can diagnose ILD with chest x-ray, PFTs, and a CT scan of the chest. Occasionally other studies, such as bronchoscopy and lung biopsy, may be necessary to rule out other possible problems.

4. Most people who have ILD do well with proper treatment.

5. Sometimes ILD can cause problems such as shortness of breath and it can sometimes progress and worsen over time.

6. If ILD is worsening (presumably due to pneumonitis), then steroids and strong immunosuppressants such as azathioprine, mycophenolate, cyclophosphamide, rituximab (Rituxan), or infliximab (Remicade) may be necessary.

7. If a person has GERD and ILD, it is very important to treat the GERD aggressively (see table 15.1) because it can exacerbate ILD.

8. People who have ILD should never smoke cigarettes.

9. Some medicines used to treat lupus (such as methotrexate and azathioprine) can sometimes cause inflammation of the lungs. Therefore, the doctor may need to stop them if she or he is not sure whether they are contributing to the lung problem.

10. Everyone who has ILD due to lupus should get a yearly influenza vaccination and should get a vaccination against pneumococcus (called Pneumovax) once or twice in their life.

## Pulmonary Hemorrhage

"Hemorrhage" is the medical term for "bleeding." Therefore, "pulmonary hemorrhage" means "bleeding in the lungs." Similar terms used to describe this lung problem include "diffuse alveolar hemorrhage" and "hemorrhagic alveolitis." This does not mean the same thing as coughing up blood (medically known as "hemoptysis"). In fact, coughing up blood is usually due to lung problems other than pulmonary hemorrhage. Pulmonary hemorrhage occurs when there is severe inflammation and damage in the alveolar air sacs, causing blood to leak into these sacs. The symptoms are usually similar to those of acute lupus pneumonitis—fever, cough, and shortness of breath (the same symptoms, by the way, that occur with infectious pneumonia). Although SLE is one of the causes of pulmonary hemorrhage, it can also occur in other systemic autoimmune diseases (especially in vasculitis) as well as from infections or due to some medications. When it occurs in SLE, about half of the time there is blood in the sputum (spit), but the rest of the time there is not. Usually the person with pulmonary hemorrhage becomes sick quickly. Most people end up on a machine called a ventilator to help them breathe. Since pulmonary hemorrhage can act very similar to infectious pneumonia, doctors place most people on antibiotics (just in case it is an infection). Usually, a doctor will note that lupus is active in other parts of the body as well. In fact, close to 100% of people who have alveolar hemorrhage also have inflammation of the kidneys (called nephritis). The test results are very similar to those of people who have lupus pneumonitis and people who have an actual infection (pneumonia). "Fluffy" alveolar infiltrates usually appear on the chest x-ray. Since it is almost impossible to tell whether the lupus patient has pulmonary hemorrhage, lupus pneumonitis, or a severe infection, often a bronchoscopy is necessary (as discussed above in the section on pneumonitis). A doctor can obtain samples of fluid from the lungs for examination in the laboratory under the microscope and also order cultures to see if there is infection. These tests can help the doctor figure out which problem is occurring. In the person who has pulmonary hemorrhage, there will be an excessive amount of blood in the fluid. In addition, observing something called hemosiderin within the white blood cells will provide evidence that these white blood cells have been "cleaning up the blood" (hemosiderin is a molecule containing iron and is broken down from red blood cells).

It is important to rule out infection (because then the doctor knows that antibiotics are not the correct way to treat the person). It is also important to determine whether the person has lupus pneumonitis or pulmonary hemorrhage. The reason is that the mortality rate for pulmonary hemorrhage is very high and the patient requires even more aggressive treatment than that used for pneumonitis. If extra blood and hemosiderin appear in the fluid from the lungs from the bronchoscopy, then the doctor can be confident that the person has a pulmonary hemorrhage. In addition to the high doses of steroids (which the person probably is already getting by this point), the doctor will also usually treat her or him with a very strong immunosuppressant medicine called cyclophosphamide, and will often use a blood filtering treatment called apheresis or plasmapheresis (both discussed in detail in chapter 35). The use of rituximab (Rituxan) also appears to be promising in treating this disorder as well.

Fortunately, with modern medicine, the prognosis for people with pulmonary hemorrhage appears to be improving. Studies from the early 1990s and earlier showed that 75% to 90% of people died from this complication. Most recent studies show that up to three out of four afflicted patients survive the episode (although one recent study from Mexico only showed a 32% survival rate). Fortunately, the treatments for alveolar hemorrhage are improving over time. It is unknown how people who have had an episode of pulmonary hemorrhage do in the future after the incident. I do not know of any long-term studies addressing this question. Nonetheless, the people who have SLE who have suffered a pulmonary hemorrhage have severe SLE and should have aggressive therapy with very close monitoring by their doctors for the rest of their lives. The patient and doctor should take any flare of lupus seriously and treat it accordingly.

### KEY POINTS TO REMEMBER

1. The term for bleeding into the lungs due to severe inflammation of the lungs from lupus is "pulmonary hemorrhage."

2. Pulmonary hemorrhage is a rare but severe complication from SLE. It can have a high mortality rate even with proper treatment.

3. Most of the symptoms pulmonary hemorrhage causes are similar to those of pneumonia (cough, fever, and shortness of breath), but sometimes there can be blood in the coughed-up sputum or phlegm.

4. The treatment for pulmonary hemorrhage is high doses of steroids and the very strong immunosuppressant cyclophosphamide, along with a special treatment called apheresis or plasmapheresis.

## Pulmonary Embolism

I discussed pulmonary embolism (PE) in the section on antiphospholipid syndrome (APS or APLS for short) in chapter 9. Most SLE patients who have PE develop it due to antiphospholipid antibodies that cause increased clotting. The cause of PE is usually a blood clot occurring in one of the large veins of the leg (called a deep venous thrombosis or DVT) that becomes detached and travels to the lungs where the clot clogs a vein. Embolus and thrombosis are both types of blood clots. A thrombus is a blood clot that occurs right where it first formed. An embolus is a blood clot that ends up in a vein or artery after it travels there from somewhere else. A PE blocks blood flow to a section of the lung. The problems and symptoms the person develops depend on how large the blood clot is, and how large and essential the clogged vein is in providing blood flow to the lungs. Shortness of breath and chest pain are the most common symptoms. Sometimes, but not always, the person may also have had discomfort and swelling in a leg, especially the calf area. If the clot is especially large, then the problem with shortness of breath can be great and even potentially life threatening. Up to 10% of SLE patients may develop a PE during their lifetime.

Doctors usually diagnose PE by either a V/Q (ventilation/perfusion) scan or spiral CT, and less commonly with an angiogram (as explained in the previous section on APS). It requires treatment with blood thinners, usually starting with an injectable blood thinner called heparin. If the PE is particularly severe and causes extremely low oxygen levels, heart failure, or low blood pressure, then sometimes surgery to remove the blood clot (called embolectomy) or the use of a strong blood clot dissolver may be needed. After the patient stabilizes in the hospital on heparin, then the doctor will add a blood thinner in pill form called warfarin (Coumadin) to take the place of the heparin. If the PE is determined to be due to APS, then usually the person will remain on a blood thinner for the rest of his or her life. The reason for this is that studies show that when people develop a blood clot due to APS, they have a high chance of developing the same type of blood clot again in the future.

**KEY POINTS TO REMEMBER**

1. Pulmonary embolism is a blood clot in the arteries of the lungs that usually originates from a blood clot in the leg.

2. PE can cause problems such as shortness of breath, chest pain, and fever.

3. Severe cases can be deadly.

4. The cause is usually antiphospholipid antibodies in people who have SLE (see chapter 9).

5. The treatment for PE is blood thinners such as heparin and warfarin (Coumadin). People who have antiphospholipid antibodies usually need to take blood thinners for the rest of their lives.

## Pulmonary Hypertension

The medical term "hypertension" means "high blood pressure." Pulmonary hypertension (PH for short) specifically refers to a problem where the blood pressure within the pulmonary arteries is higher than normal. It is much less common than the everyday hypertension that many people have. The pulmonary artery is the major artery (blood vessel) that carries blood away from the heart to the lungs. The pulmonary artery then branches off into many smaller pulmonary arteries. Their purpose is to carry blood to the lungs so that oxygen can enter the bloodstream from the lungs and then the oxygen-rich blood travels throughout the body. About 10% of people who have SLE have higher than normal blood pressure in the pulmonary arteries. It is unknown exactly why this occurs. However, it appears that it is more common in people who are positive for antiphospholipid antibodies. Therefore, the formation of blood clots may play a role. Autopsies show that the pulmonary artery walls are thicker and more scarred than normal, but there is usually no active inflammation. In addition to antiphospholipid antibodies increasing this risk, Raynaud's phenomenon (where the fingers turn white or blue with exposure to cold) and RNP antibodies increase the chances of developing PH. Many people who have mild PH do not have any symptoms or problems from their pulmonary hypertension, but it can progress and worsen over time, so it is important to monitor it closely. People who have moderate to severe PH may have problems with shortness of breath, chest pain, dry cough, fatigue, heart palpitations, light-headedness, and swelling of the ankles. Severe PH has a high mortality rate, causing problems with oxygen supply to the body, heart failure, and blood clots in the lungs. For that reason, it is a very important complication of lupus for doctors to identify and treat.

On physical exam, the doctor may suspect pulmonary hypertension if the second heart sound is louder than normal. When the doctor listens to the heart with the stethoscope, he or she listens for the typical "lub-dub" sounds. The second heart sound is the "dub" portion and occurs when the pulmonic and tricuspid heart valves close. The pulmonary valve is the valve between the right side of the heart (the right ventricle to be exact) and the pulmonary artery. Since pulmonary hypertension causes elevated blood pressure in the pulmonary artery, when the pulmonary valve closes, the high blood pressure in the pulmonary artery causes the valve to close harder than normal, causing a louder than normal sound.

If a doctor suspects that someone has pulmonary hypertension (such as having a loud second heart sound on examination or shortness of breath or chest pains) the doctor will usually send the patient for additional tests such as echocardiogram and PFTs. An echocardiogram is an ultrasound (also called a sonogram or ultrasonography) of the heart. For this test, the technician applies some gel to the chest, and then places a plastic, blunt instrument called a probe (or transducer) on the gel. This probe sends sound waves into the body, where they bounce off the internal organs of the body and back into the probe, where a computer forms a picture by reading these sound waves (or ultrasounds). A doctor can use an echocardiogram to look for all kinds of problems with the heart, including excessive fluid around the heart, blood clots in the heart, infection, problems with the valves, and problems with the heart muscle itself. When looking for the possibility of pulmonary hypertension, the technician will calculate the pulmonary artery systolic pressure (PASP). A normal PASP is 30 mm of mercury or less. A pressure greater than 30 mm of mercury is *possibly* elevated. An echocardiogram can only estimate the pressure. Some people can have pulmonary hypertension and yet still have a normal PASP on echocardiogram, while others may appear to have an elevated PASP yet actually have normal pressures. Due to these inaccuracies, tests that are more accurate are often needed, such as a cardiac catheterization as described below.

PFTs can also be helpful. People who have pulmonary hypertension usually have a decreased DLCO on PFTs and the description on the PFTs is "decreased diffusion capacity." In fact, a low DLCO is often the very first abnormality to show up in a person who has mild pulmonary hypertension (in other words, in someone with a normal echocardiogram and who feels perfectly fine with no shortness of breath).

If a doctor suspects pulmonary hypertension after doing the previously mentioned tests, the next step is usually to do a right-sided cardiac catheterization. This is a special test where the doctor places a long, thin tube (a catheter) into a large vein, in the neck, the wrist, or the groin after anesthetizing the area with a numbing medication. The doctor carefully threads the catheter through the large vein until it enters the right side of the heart. The doctor can actually measure exactly what the blood pressures are in the right side of the heart and in the pulmonary artery. This is the best way to establish whether someone has pulmonary hypertension or not, and how severe it is.

In mild cases of PH, no treatment may be necessary, but the doctor will monitor the tests (especially the echocardiogram and PFTs) on a regular basis to ensure it does not get worse. Another common test is a six-minute walk test. During the six-minute walk test, people being tested walk as far as they can for six minutes to monitor if they get short of breath or not. The six-minute walk test is a reliable, easy test that correlates with the severity of pulmonary hypertension quite well.

In moderate to severe cases of PH where there is difficulty breathing, medications are prescribed to relax the pulmonary arteries and lower the pulmonary blood pressure. Pulmonary hypertension once had a high mortality rate. Since the recent arrival of medications specifically to treat pulmonary hypertension, this has changed. The lifespans and qualities of life of people who have pulmonary hypertension have increased substantially with the use of these medications. The wide variety of medications used is beyond the scope of this book. Other therapies commonly used include oxygen, blood thinners such as warfarin, diuretics (fluid pills), and exercise.

## KEY POINTS TO REMEMBER

1. Pulmonary hypertension occurs when the blood pressure in the arteries of the lungs is higher than normal.

2. A doctor diagnoses PH with an echocardiogram and often a right-sided cardiac catheterization.

3. Mild PH may not cause any symptoms at all and may not need treatment. It may just be monitored using echocardiogram, six-minute walk testing, and PFT tests at regular intervals to ensure it does not worsen.

4. In moderate to severe cases, PH can cause shortness of breath and chest pain, and over time it may cause heart failure and blood clots in the lungs.

5. The doctor may treat PH with medicines that relax the arteries of the lungs.

## Shrinking Lung Syndrome

Shrinking lung syndrome is a rare complication in SLE. There are only eight cases in the medical literature, so we really do not know very much about it. People who have shrinking lung syndrome have shortness of breath and pleuritic chest pain (pain worsened when they try to breathe). Chest x-rays show that the diaphragm (the muscle at the base of the lungs that helps us breathe) is higher up in the chest than normal. Lung studies on these patients have been contradictory, with some showing that the diaphragm does not work normally while others suggesting that it does. The cause of this disorder is unknown. Steroids such as prednisone seem to ease the condition.

### KEY POINTS TO REMEMBER

1. Shrinking lung syndrome due to SLE is a very rare complication of lupus.

2. The cause of this syndrome is unknown.

3. The syndrome causes shortness of breath.

4. The doctor diagnoses the syndrome with chest x-rays and PFTs.

5. The treatment for this condition is steroids.

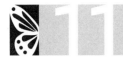

# The Heart and Blood Vessels

## 100,000 Miles of Blood Vessels

The heart is the muscular organ in the chest that is about the size of both fists placed together and is responsible for circulating blood throughout the body. One drop of blood only takes about 20 seconds to leave the heart, go through the circulation, then return to the heart. The heart pumps approximately 2,000 gallons of blood per day and beats about 100,000 times a day. That would be about 280,000,000 times in an 80-year lifespan. That is a lot of work for one muscle and shows how specialized of an organ it is. The blood vessels of the body through which it pumps the blood would measure around 100,000 miles in length if you were to lay all of them out in one line. That line would go around the equator four times! This chapter deals with how SLE may affect the heart and blood vessels.

• • • •

The heart (figure 11.1A) consists of four chambers (two large ventricles and two smaller atria) that fill up with blood, and two sides—a right side and a left side. The illustration's right and left sides are oriented as if you were looking directly at the heart through the front chest of a person with the heart's left side on your right. Each atrium (atrium is the singular form of atria) allows blood to flow into its corresponding ventricle by way of a small hole covered by a valve that can open and close. The heart's valves are one-way valves (when working properly) that allow blood to only flow in one direction (from the atria to the ventricles). Blood initially arrives at the heart by way of very large veins (the superior vena cava from the upper body and the inferior vena cava from the lower body [located on the left side of the diagram]). These empty blood (from which the body has already extracted most of the oxygen) into the right atrium. Both the right and the left atria squeeze at the same time and this causes the blood in the right atrium to travel through the hole covered by a valve (the tricuspid valve) into the right ventricle. Then the two ventricles (left and right) also squeeze at the same time. This causes the tricuspid valve to close and pushes blood through another valve called the pulmonary valve. The pulmonary valve directs the blood into the pulmonary artery, which is the large blood vessel that carries this oxygen-void blood into the lungs.

The blood that enters the pulmonary artery then travels to progressively smaller pulmonary arteries and arterioles until it reaches the tiniest blood vessels (called capillaries). The capillaries are in the walls of the tiny alveolar air sacs (see figure 10.1) so that oxygen is absorbed into the blood (which causes the now bluish-colored blood to

A

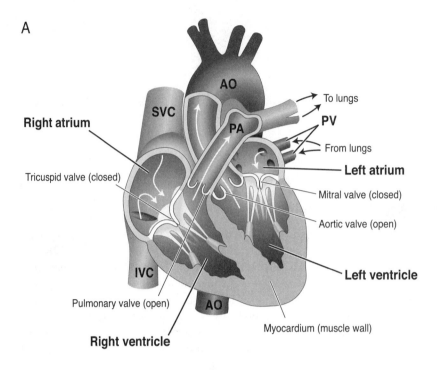

Right atrium

SVC

AO

To lungs

PA

PV

From lungs

Tricuspid valve (closed)

Left atrium

Mitral valve (closed)

Aortic valve (open)

IVC

Left ventricle

Pulmonary valve (open)

AO

Right ventricle

Myocardium (muscle wall)

B

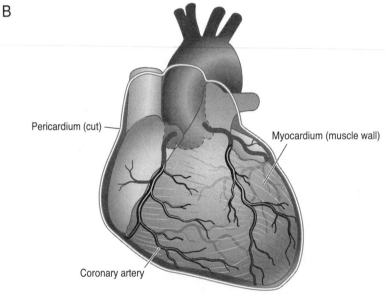

Pericardium (cut)

Myocardium (muscle wall)

Coronary artery

**Figure 11.1** The heart. (Abbreviations: IVC, inferior vena cava; SVC, superior vena cava; AO, aorta; PA, pulmonary artery; PV, pulmonary veins)

turn red with the oxygen) and gases not needed by the body (such as carbon dioxide) are excreted. The medical term "vein" denotes a blood vessel that leads to the heart (such as the superior and inferior vena cava mentioned earlier, which lead to the right atrium of the heart). "Artery" is the term used to denote a blood vessel that carries blood away from the heart (such as the pulmonary artery that carries blood from the right ventricle to the lungs).

The oxygen-rich blood in the tiny capillaries of the lungs then travels to larger and larger blood vessels called pulmonary veins, the largest of which empties it into the left atrium. Again, the left and the right atrium squeeze at the same time, causing blood to flow from the left atrium through a hole linked to the left ventricle, which has another one-way valve called the mitral valve. Then, when the right and left ventricles squeeze, the blood in the left ventricle flows out of the heart through the last valve called the aortic valve and into the largest artery of the body (called the aorta) from which blood pumps throughout the entire body. During the squeezing of the ventricles to force blood out of the heart, the mitral valve closes so that blood does not flow backward into the left atrium. This closing of the mitral valve (along with the tricuspid valve) causes the first heart sound, or the "lub" part of the "lub-dub." The second part of the "lub-dub" heart sounds occurs when the large right and left ventricles relax. During this relaxation, the pulmonary valve (which leads from the right ventricle into the pulmonary artery) and the aortic valve (leading from the left ventricle to the aorta) close and together make a sound responsible for the "dub." The doctor often can tell if there is a problem with the heart if these heart sounds are abnormal when he or she listens to the heart with a stethoscope.

After the blood flows from the heart to the large aorta, the aorta divides into progressively smaller blood vessels (called arteries). The arteries divide into even smaller ones (called arterioles) and finally into tiny blood vessels (capillaries). It is from the capillaries that the cells of the body absorb the oxygen as well as nutrients from the blood to function properly. The cells of the body also release waste products into the capillaries and the blood carries them away for proper disposal. The blood in the capillaries then flows into slightly larger blood vessels (venules) and then into larger blood vessels (veins). The veins of the body contain blood from which most of the oxygen has been absorbed by the cells of the body, and thus appear bluish in color underneath the skin.

Lupus can cause inflammation and affect the heart and the blood vessels. This chapter discusses these problems.

## Pericarditis

"Peri-" comes from the Greek word for "around," "enclosing," or "surrounding," while "cardio" refers to the heart and "-itis" means "inflammation." The pericardium (figure 11.1B) is the sac of tissue that envelops the heart and is one of the serosa of the body (see the section on pleuritis in chapter 10 to read more about the serosa and serositis). There is normally a small amount of lubricating fluid between the heart and the pericardium. It allows the atria and ventricles to contract easily in a confined area of the chest (i.e., in the pericardial sac). Just as with pleuritis, SLE causes inflammation in the pericardium and the medical term for this is "pericarditis" (a type of serositis). As with pleuritis, it is one of the American College of Rheumatology's classification criteria for diagnosing SLE. It is very common in SLE patients, with up to 60% having evidence of pericarditis at the time of autopsy. However, only about 25% actually develop symptoms of pericarditis, meaning that most people do not develop any significant problems from it. Just as pleuritis is the most common lung problem in SLE, pericarditis is the most common heart problem directly related to SLE. While pericarditis is the most common problem of the heart that is directly due to lupus inflammation, coronary artery disease (due to blocked arteries) is the number one heart problem overall. However, coronary artery disease is due to factors other than just lupus, as discussed in more detail in chapter 21.

As with pleuritis, inflammation from lupus pericarditis can cause the pericardium to produce more fluid than normal, causing excessive fluid to accumulate in the pericardial sac (the space between the heart muscle and the pericardium). This fluid is normally slippery and slick, but with the inflammation from lupus, the number of white blood cells increases in the fluid, and other inflammation-induced changes can cause this fluid to lose its lubricating effects. This combination of events causes the most common symptom of pericarditis, which is pleuritic chest pain (chest pain worsened with breathing). The chest pain of pericarditis can occur anywhere in the chest, but people most commonly describe it as underneath or just to the left of the breastbone (the sternum). Sometimes, this chest pain is worse when the person lies on her back, causing great difficulty with sleeping. If the fluid accumulates enough, a condition called cardiac tamponade can occur, causing difficulty with the heart pumping blood effectively, low blood pressure, a fast heart rate, and shortness of breath. This can be a life-threatening situation. However, as mentioned, most people who have pleural inflammation from lupus notice no problems at all, and doctors diagnose it by accident or not at all.

The doctor may be able to hear signs of pericarditis on physical exam when he listens to the heart. Typically, doctors describe this as a pericardial rub, where there is a sound like two pieces of sandpaper rubbing against each other with each heartbeat. However, this can come and go, so usually the doctor does not hear anything abnormal. Doctors often order an ECG (electrocardiogram). A technician or doctor performs this by placing sticky electrodes on multiple areas on the chest, as well as on the arms and legs. These electrodes are able to sense the electrical activity of the heart and display it in graph form printed on a piece of paper.

Usually the ECG is sufficient for making a diagnosis of pericarditis. However, sometimes an echocardiogram is performed to look for possible fluid around the heart and to make sure there are no other heart problems. On echocardiogram, usually an increased amount of pericardial fluid is observed around the heart.

The usual treatment for pericarditis is the use of non-steroidal anti-inflammatory drugs (NSAIDs, like ibuprofen) and moderate to high doses of steroids (depending on how severe it is). In most cases, the anti-malarial hydroxychloroquine is sufficient in controlling the inflammation, but occasionally stronger immunosuppressants such as methotrexate, azathioprine, mycophenolate, or belimumab may be needed. If there is a lot of fluid causing difficulty with the heart pumping blood properly (cardiac tamponade), the fluid has to be drained from the pericardial sac (called a pericardiocentesis). This is usually performed in an operating room and a piece of the pericardial tissue is removed, creating a pericardial window to allow excess fluid to leak out of the sac so it does not accumulate.

A minority of people can develop a complication called constrictive pericarditis. This occurs when the pericardial sac becomes permanently thickened and does not allow the heart to expand and contract normally, causing difficulty pumping blood correctly. Doctors sometimes need to perform a pericardiectomy to treat constrictive pericarditis. During this procedure the pericardial sac is removed surgically to allow the heart to pump normally again. The heart can then usually work well even without the pericardium.

The vast majority of the time, though, pericarditis is either no problem at all, or is controllable with medications. It rarely causes any permanent heart problems (such as constrictive pericarditis).

### KEY POINTS TO REMEMBER

1. Pericarditis is the most common heart problem seen in people who have SLE.

2. Most people do not have any problems or symptoms from pericarditis.

3. When pericarditis does cause problems, it is most often in the form of pleuritic chest pain (pain that worsens with breathing), often exacerbated by lying down. Shortness of breath may also occur.

4. Doctors usually diagnose pericarditis using an ECG and/or echocardiogram (ultra-sound of the heart).

5. The treatment is usually steroids and/or NSAIDs and Plaquenil.

6. More severe or resistant cases may require stronger immunosuppressant medicines, such as mycophenolate, azathioprine, methotrexate, or belimumab.

7. If a large amount of fluid builds up, causing difficulties with the heart working properly, then surgery to drain the fluid (pericardiocentesis) and/or cutting a small hole in the pericardium (pericardial window) or even removing the pericardium completely (pericardiectomy) may be required.

## Myocarditis and Cardiomyopathy

"Myo-" is the Greek word for "muscle" and "-carditis" means "inflammation of the heart." The heart is one huge muscle called the myocardium (see figures 11.1A and 11.1B) whose sole function is to pump blood through the body. Myocarditis occurs when SLE causes direct inflammation of the heart muscle. Over time, the body may be able to heal the inflammation, but often will leave permanent scar tissue (a condition called fibrosis). When there is either active inflammation or fibrosis of the heart muscle, the heart may not be able to squeeze normally and may have difficulty pumping blood correctly. This can cause shortness of breath, chest pain, and a rapid heart rate. When it is severe, fluid may back up in the lungs and collect in the ankles (called edema), causing the ankles to become swollen. Congestive heart failure occurs when the heart is unable to pump blood efficiently and fluid builds up in the body. Fortunately, only 5% to 10% of SLE patients will develop myocarditis that actually causes any significant problems, even though autopsy studies show that 40% to 70% of SLE patients have had some degree of myocarditis at some point in their lives. Therefore, just as with pericarditis, most of the time the inflammation is not severe enough to cause notable problems or the diagnosis is missed by the doctors. It appears that being African American, having myositis (discussed in chapter 7), and being positive for anti-RNP or anti-SSA antibodies may be risk factors for developing myocarditis.

The results of an ECG may first suggest the diagnosis of myocarditis, where there may be some nonspecific ECG abnormalities, or a chest x-ray may suggest that the heart is larger than normal. The echocardiogram is the best noninvasive test used to make this diagnosis, as the echocardiogram will show that the heart muscle does not contract or squeeze normally.

A doctor would usually perform a cardiac catheterization in most patients to ensure that blocked arteries are not the cause of the cardiac muscle not working properly. The doctor injects a dye into the heart and into the blood vessels that feed the heart muscle (called the coronary arteries) so that a video can show how well the heart works, how well it squeezes blood, and if there are any blocked arteries. In addition, the cardiologist can see if the heart valves are performing correctly. If the cause of myocarditis is not evident from the visual inspection of the heart and blood vessels, the doctor performing the procedure (usually a heart doctor called a cardiologist) can take a small biopsy from inside the heart. Examination of the biopsy specimen under the microscope can help determine what is causing the myocarditis. In fact, rarely, the most common medicine used to treat lupus, hydroxychloroquine, can lead to myocarditis. A biopsy is the best way to tell whether the myocarditis is coming from the hydroxychloroquine or from the lupus itself.

Doctors may use the term "cardiomyopathy" instead of "myocarditis." In many cases, this is a more accurate term. The ending "-pathy" comes from the Greek word for "suffering" or "disease." "Cardiomyopathy" literally means "a disease of the heart muscle." The only way to tell whether someone actually has active inflammation of the heart (or myocarditis) would be to obtain a biopsy and see the actual inflammation under the microscope. However, most patients do not undergo a biopsy and the doctor diagnoses it based on an abnormal echocardiogram and/or cardiac catheterization. In this instance, it can be impossible to tell whether there is still active inflammation going on (myocarditis) or whether there is permanent scarring (fibrosis) of the cardiac muscle as the cause of the cardiomyopathy. Therefore, the diagnosis of cardiomyopathy, instead of myocarditis, would be more accurate in most patients. In addition, there are numerous potential causes of cardiomyopathy, including blocked coronary arteries (called coronary artery disease), high blood pressure, medications, viral infections, heart valve problems, and congenital/genetic problems. It is up to the team of physicians (including the rheumatologist and the cardiologist) to sort these possible issues out. However, in cardiomyopathy due to lupus, one can assume that at some point in the past active inflammation from myocarditis had occurred in the lupus patient diagnosed with a cardiomyopathy (after other causes such as high blood pressure, heart valve problems, or blocked coronary arteries have been ruled out by the doctors).

A recent test has emerged that appears to be able to better diagnose active inflammation of the heart (myocarditis) compared to other heart problems such as non-inflammatory cardiomyopathy. The test is called a cardiac MRI that has the benefits of not being invasive and does not use radiation. It should become more widely available in the near future to help diagnose lupus myocarditis more accurately to help with very important treatment decisions. It may very well help doctors diagnose myocarditis in SLE more often and at earlier stages compared to when they had to rely on biopsies alone.

Just as with many other severe lupus problems, the treatment for lupus myocarditis is high doses of steroids. Sometimes stronger immunosuppressants such as methotrexate, azathioprine, mycophenolate, belimumab, or cyclophosphamide may be necessary. Recent studies also suggest that IVIG (intravenous immune globulin) may be useful as well. If there is actual congestive heart failure due to severe heart muscle damage, then heart medications—to help the heart beat better (such as digoxin), control blood pressure, and remove excessive fluid (diuretics)—may be used as well.

### KEY POINTS TO REMEMBER

1. Cardiomyopathy refers to any damage to the heart muscle.

2. Although lupus can cause cardiomyopathy, a doctor must consider other causes, such as coronary artery disease, hypertension, diabetes, heart valve problems, and congenital disorders.

3. Usually an echocardiogram and a cardiac catheterization are necessary to diagnose cardiomyopathy.

4. A cardiac MRI can be helpful in diagnosing active inflammation of the heart muscle (myocarditis).

5. Severe cases of cardiomyopathy and myocarditis may lead to congestive heart failure, causing fluid to accumulate in the lungs and ankles and causing shortness of breath and chest pain.

6. If there is active inflammation of the heart (myocarditis) from SLE, then doctors use steroids and strong immunosuppressants such as azathioprine, methotrexate, mycophenolate, belimumab, or cyclophosphamide.

## Valvular Heart Disease

There are four valves in the heart that act as one-way valves between different sections of the heart and the arteries that carry blood out of the heart. They include the tricuspid valve (between the right atrium and the right ventricle), the pulmonary valve (between the right ventricle and the pulmonary artery), the mitral valve (between the left atrium and the left ventricle), and the aortic valve (between the left ventricle and the aorta). When these valves function normally, they help keep the blood flowing and pumping in the correct direction in the heart and throughout the rest of the body.

However, occasionally there can be problems with the valves. Valvular stenosis occurs when the valve opening becomes tighter and smaller than normal. This makes it harder for the blood to get through the opening. The heart muscle often has to work harder at squeezing the blood through. This can cause the heart muscle to enlarge, which is not a good thing. In addition, the chamber of the heart trying to squeeze blood through this valve may gradually get larger and larger over time. Another potential problem is valvular insufficiency (also called valvular regurgitation). This is when the one-way action of the valve stops working correctly, and blood begins to leak backward through the valve instead of going in the correct direction. This can also cause the heart muscle and heart chambers to get larger than normal. Most people who have valvular heart disease (VHD for short) have mild problems; in fact, most do not notice any problems at all. However, sometimes chest pain, shortness of breath, heart palpitations, cough, light-headedness, and even congestive heart failure may occur.

A doctor can often detect valvular stenosis and regurgitation (insufficiency) when he or she listens to the heart with a stethoscope. Blood that is being forcefully squeezed through a stenotic valve or blood that flows backward through a malfunctioning valve typically causes certain sounds that doctors call murmurs. The next step is to get an echocardiogram, which can show if there is an abnormality of a heart valve or not, as well as determine how severe it is. Studies show that VHD occurs more commonly in lupus patients than in people who do not have lupus. Fortunately, most of the time, these abnormalities are mild and require no specific therapy.

A 2011 study from McGill University in Quebec, Canada, looked at 217 of their SLE patients. They found that one-third of the patients had mitral valve abnormalities while only 4% had aortic insufficiency. Interestingly, very few of these patients had a heart murmur on physical examination. None of them had Libman-Sacks endocarditis (probably reflecting the better treatment of lupus these days). The vast majority of these patients had no significant problems from their valvular heart disease. The doctors at McGill University plan on following these patients closely over time to see if their valve problems worsen or not, which will be invaluable to our knowledge about valvular heart disease and SLE.

Valvular heart disease in people with SLE can occasionally be more substantial, causing the symptoms described in the preceding paragraph. In this instance, a cardiac catheterization may be necessary to get a better handle on how severe the situation is. Medications to help the heart and blood pressure may be necessary. In addition, if the VHD is more than just mild, the cardiologist may want to do an echocardiogram on a regular basis (such as once a year or so) to ensure it does not worsen over time. If severe enough, surgery may be necessary to replace the valve, but, fortunately, this is rare.

Another problem that can occur with the valves of the heart is Libman-Sacks endocarditis. "Endo-" is the Greek term for "inside." The endocardium is the tissue that lines the inside of the heart chambers and the valves of the heart. Endocarditis specifically refers to inflammation or infection involving the valves of the heart. In 1923, Dr. Emanuel Libman and Dr. Benjamin Sacks described an unusual type of endocarditis in patients who had systemic lupus that was unrelated to infection (which is the most common cause of endocarditis in people who do not have lupus). They described wart-like (verrucous) growths on the valves of the heart in lupus patients. This has been termed Libman-Sacks endocarditis (also verrucous endocarditis) after the doctors who first described it. The growths are composed of cellular debris, a small amount of inflamed tissue, and blood clots. Later studies have shown that most patients are positive for antiphospholipid antibodies, which therefore may be the cause of these abnormalities. Although they usually cause no problems, occasionally one of these growths can break away from the valve and travel through the body (called an embolus) where it can eventually block off a blood vessel somewhere else in the body. If this occurs in the brain, it can cause a stroke. Rarely, multiple tiny pieces can break off, causing problems with the kidneys and brain or rashes that look like vasculitis. If the growths are large enough, the heart valve may develop valvular regurgitation. In mild cases, the doctor would most likely monitor the severity of the valve over time, using an echocardiogram regularly. If the endocarditis becomes severe, then surgery may be required.

Another potential problem with VHD, especially Libman-Sacks endocarditis, is that the valves may be at increased risk of becoming infected (called subacute bacterial endocarditis) which can be very dangerous. This most commonly occurs after dental procedures, when bacteria from the mouth enter the bloodstream and subsequently land on the valves of the heart, causing a severe infection. Fortunately, this complication is rare. Previously, many rheumatologists recommended that their SLE patients receive antibiotics prior to dental procedures to prevent this from occurring. However, the more recent guidelines and recommendations from the American Heart Association in 2007 do not recommend that doctors give antibiotics to most people who have SLE even if they have VHD. The only ones who should be given antibiotics are those who have had surgery on their heart valves or those who have had infectious endocarditis in the past.

### KEY POINTS TO REMEMBER

1. SLE can affect any of the four heart valves.

2. Doctors diagnose valvular heart disease by echocardiogram and sometimes by cardiac catheterization.

3. Libman-Sacks endocarditis, also called verrucous endocarditis, is usually associated with antiphospholipid antibodies, sometimes requiring treatment with blood thinners.

4. The medical terms for a leaky valve are "valvular regurgitation" and "valvular insufficiency."

5. "Stenosis" is the medical term for a damaged valve that has a smaller opening than normal.

6. About one-third of people who have SLE may have valvular heart disease on echocardiogram studies, yet it most often is mild and not causing any problems noticeable to the person who has it.

7. More severe cases may cause shortness of breath, chest pain, and light-headedness. They require treatment with medicines to help the heart and blood pressure.

8. If a person has a severely damaged valve or has had surgery on one, she may need to take antibiotics around the time of dental procedures to prevent a heart valve infection called subacute bacterial endocarditis.

9. Severe heart valve problems may require valve replacement surgery.

## Conduction Abnormalities

An electrical system that lies within the heart muscle intricately orchestrates the way that the heart beats properly to pump blood into the lungs and throughout the body. The medical term for this complex system is the "cardiac electrical conduction system" and the term for any problems with it is "conduction abnormalities." If the electrical activity within the heart muscle is abnormal, this could potentially cause problems with the heart muscle squeezing properly. The atria and ventricles may not squeeze blood in the proper pattern or order, or they may contract too quickly or too slowly. A doctor diagnoses conduction system abnormalities by ECG (see the description of the ECG in the section on pericarditis). Although older studies suggested that up to 74% of SLE patients had conduction abnormalities, recent studies show that between 10% and 32% of patients show evidence of such problems on ECG. These electrical conduction problems may be due to previous bouts of myocarditis, but problems not directly related to the lupus, such as coronary artery disease or thyroid disease, can also cause it. Fortunately, the vast majority of the time these are minor problems (such as first- and second-degree heart block, right bundle branch block, and left bundle branch block) that never require treatment. However, occasionally someone may have a severe conduction problem (such as third-degree heart block, atrial fibrillation, or atrial flutter) that may cause shortness of breath, heart palpitations, chest pain, and fainting. In these situations, medicines or interventions to help the electrical system work more efficiently may be necessary. Severe cases may require the insertion of a pacemaker.

### KEY POINTS TO REMEMBER

1. Most cardiac conduction abnormalities in people who have SLE are mild, do not cause problems, and are picked up on ECG.

2. More severe types of conduction abnormalities (such as third-degree heart block, atrial fibrillation, or atrial flutter) may cause shortness of breath, heart palpitations, light-headedness, and chest pain.

3. In severe cases, medicines, heart interventions, or even a pacemaker may be required for treatment.

## Vasculitis

"Vasculitis" is the medical term meaning "inflammation of blood vessels." When vasculitis occurs in a blood vessel, it causes decreased blood flow through the vessel and the leakage of fluid out of the blood vessel. The decreased blood flow can cause the tissues that rely on that blood vessel to get an inadequate amount of oxygen and nourishment from the blood, leading to pain and even tissue death. The leakage of fluid out of the blood vessel and into the surrounding tissues can cause swelling. Some organs of the body have numerous blood vessels coming from different directions to provide several routes of blood supply to the same tissues. The medical term for this is "collateral blood supply." If vasculitis occurs in one section of the blood vessels and not the other, then the tissues will still get adequate oxygen and nourishment and the vasculitis may not cause any notable problems thanks to this collateral blood supply.

Vasculitis can occur in any organ of the body in people who have SLE but it is more common in some areas than others. The skin is by far the most commonly affected area and the medical term for this is "cutaneous vasculitis." (There is a detailed discussion in chapter 8.) Vasculitis is much less common in other parts of the body, but can occur in the back of the eye (retinal vasculitis) and in the gastrointestinal tract (mesenteric vasculitis). There is a discussion of these conditions in chapter 15 (the gastrointestinal tract) and chapter 16 (the eyes). Rarely, vasculitis can occur in the kidneys, liver, and nerves. A biopsy is sometimes required for a doctor to diagnose it correctly. The doctor can also order an angiogram. This is a special type of x-ray where a radiologist injects dye in the vein that shows up on x-rays of the veins and arteries. Vasculitis appears as areas of constrictions and dilatations of the blood vessels. People who have vasculitis of the internal organs (such as the kidneys and the liver) and nerves are usually very sick and require high doses of steroids, along with strong immunosuppressant medicines such as azathioprine, mycophenolate, or cyclophosphamide.

The vasculitis in SLE can occasionally be due to abnormal proteins called cryoglobulins (see photograph 8.8). The doctor diagnoses this with a blood test that can measure cryoglobulins in the blood. If present, then a special form of treatment called apheresis (or plasmapheresis) may be necessary to filter the cryoglobulins out of the person's blood.

### KEY POINTS TO REMEMBER

1. "Vasculitis" is the term for inflammation of the blood vessels.

2. The organ of the body that lupus vasculitis most commonly affects is the skin (see chapter 8).

3. Cryoglobulins are sometimes involved in vasculitis. These are immune system proteins that clump together in cooler parts of the body.

4. If severe enough, vasculitis can cause decreased blood flow to the affected organ, leading to pain and tissue death. It can also cause fluid to leak out of the blood vessels causing swelling of the tissues involved.

5. Mild cases involving the skin may not require any treatment, but more severe cases (especially if they affect the internal organs) may require steroids or stronger immunosuppressant medicines such as azathioprine, methotrexate, mycophenolate, or cyclophosphamide.

## Raynaud's Phenomenon

Raynaud's phenomenon (RP for short) is the most common problem that occurs in the cardiovascular system of people who have SLE, appearing in approximately one-third of them. RP causes the fingers and/or toes to become pale and/or dark purple (photograph 11.1) with exposure to cold, which is sometimes followed by reddish coloration after rewarming. Sometimes the fingers may become painful or have a tingling sensation during the event. The person who has RP may be so sensitive to cold that it can occur while she or he is shopping in the refrigerated section of the grocery store or is holding a cold drink. In some people, stressful events can also cause Raynaud's phenomenon. Raynaud's phenomenon is named after the French physician Maurice Raynaud who first described Raynaud's phenomenon in a young woman in 1862.

RP is due to the arteries of the hands and feet having a smaller than normal inner channel through which blood flows. This occurs when lupus causes the walls of the arteries to be thicker than normal (figure 11.2). Whenever anyone is exposed to cold temperatures, the nerves of the skin, blood vessels, and brain sense the colder temperature and then send chemical messages along the nervous system to the arteries of the skin, hands, and feet, telling them to constrict to keep as much warm blood as possible away from the skin, fingers, and toes. This helps to prevent the body from losing vital warmth through the skin, and to keep the blood and inner part of the body with the vital organs (like the brain, kidneys, and heart) at the correct warm body temperature. In the vast majority of people, this chain of events just causes the skin to feel cooler than normal. However, in the person who has RP (who has smaller than normal

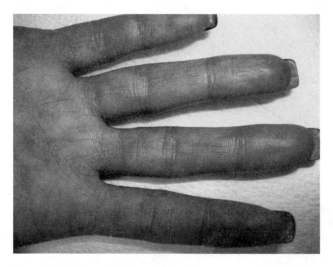

Photo II.I  Raynaud's phenomenon in a person who has SLE. Sometimes an attack of Raynaud's may affect one finger at a time, as is the case in this photograph showing discoloration of the pinky of a woman as she sits in a cold examination room, or it may affect all the fingers in others.

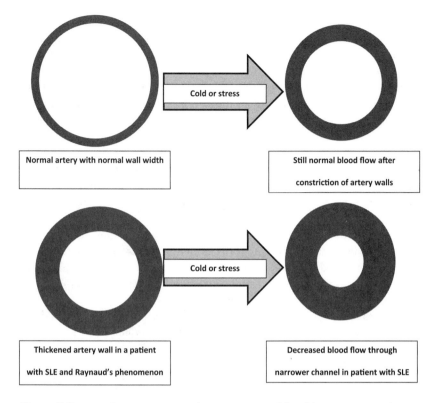

**Figure II.2** Normal artery compared to SLE artery with cold exposure causing Raynaud's phenomenon in some people who have SLE

blood flow channels) the flow of blood is restricted so much that there is less blood flow to the fingers and toes. They become colder than normal. Since there is less blood flow, the fingers and toes (and sometimes the ears and nose) may become pale. Then as the tissues and cells use up the oxygen and release more carbon dioxide into the blood, this causes the normally red blood to become blue or purple. With rewarming, there may be a reddish coloration as more fresh red blood flows in.

In some cases, after repetitive episodes of RP, the tissues of the fingertips may not have enough nutrients and oxygen to remain normal. Over time, the fleshy parts of the fingertips (on the palm side) may lose tissue and become tapered and thin instead of staying plump. In more severe cases of RP, blood flow may be so restricted during the episodes that the tissues on the fingertips may actually die due to the lack of nutrients and oxygen. This can potentially cause open sores to develop. These can be very painful and are prone to infection if not treated properly. Trauma to the fingertips, even minimal trauma, appears to increase the possibility of this happening.

The thickened blood vessel walls that cause RP are usually a result of previous inflammation and are a permanent problem. Therefore, RP usually does not get better over time and does not improve with the use of anti-inflammatory medicines such as steroids and immunosuppressant medicines. RP also usually does not vary between lupus flares and remissions.

It is very important for people who have RP to keep the core body temperature warm. Table 11.1 lists suggestions for lifestyle approaches for treating the symptoms of RP. While using mittens or gloves helps to keep the hands warm, it does not keep the core body temperature warm. It is also very important to wear a hat because a large percentage of body heat is lost through the head. Mittens can be more helpful than gloves, allowing the fingers to be next to each other. Biofeedback can also be useful. It trains the brain to learn to keep the blood vessels more relaxed and open. Relaxed blood vessels cause the hands and feet to be warmer, which decreases the severity of the RP attacks. The biofeedback therapist attaches temperature sensors to the fingers and toes to teach the brain how to warm them up. I have actually done this myself. I was amazed at my mind's ability to raise the temperature of my hands and feet in this manner.

Some migraine medicines, such as sumatriptan and ergotamine, cause the blood vessels of the body to constrict and can make RP worse. A patient may need to avoid taking them during times when RP is active. Other medicines that also exacerbate RP include decongestants (used for colds and allergies), amphetamine-like diet pills, and diet supplements containing ephedra. Foods and beverages containing caffeine can also make RP worse, and patients should avoid them.

Allowing mild Raynaud's attacks to occur is acceptable as long as they are not painful, fairly easy to control, and do not cause the loss of tissue in the fingertips or open sores. However, if the attacks are not mild, then medications may be necessary. These

**Table 11.1** Non-Medicine Ways to Treat Raynaud's Phenomenon

- Avoid cold places.
- Wear layers of clothing in cool temperatures.
- Wear mittens, which are preferable to gloves.
- Wear heavy wool stockings.
- Wear a hat in cool temperatures.
- Keep hand warmers in your pockets (available at stores that sell hunting equipment).
- Wear battery-heated gloves (make sure they are a high-quality brand).
- To stop a Raynaud's attack, rub your hands together, run them under warm water, put them under your armpits, or whirl your arms around like a windmill to increase blood flow to your hands.
- Avoid vibrating tools, which can worsen Raynaud's.
- Do not smoke cigarettes (nicotine constricts blood vessels).
- Avoid caffeine (caffeine constricts blood vessels).
- Avoid taking decongestants, amphetamine-like diet pills, and herbs containing ephedra (all of these constrict blood vessels).
- Protect your fingertips to prevent sores from occurring.

medicines help to relax the artery walls and allow more blood to flow to the fingers and toes. A group of medicines used to treat high blood pressure called calcium channel blockers, especially nifedipine (Procardia), seem to be particularly helpful in many people. However, a doctor may also use other calcium channel blockers such as amlodipine (Norvasc) or diltiazem (Cardizem). Other blood pressure medicines—including reserpine, prazosin, hydralazine, minoxidil, and losartan—can also be helpful. Studies show that the antidepressant fluoxetine (Prozac) is helpful in some people. Nitroglycerin, which doctors most commonly use to dilate the heart blood vessels for heart angina, comes in the form of pills, cream, and patches. Bosentan (Tracleer) is FDA approved to treat pulmonary hypertension, but can also help RP. Doctors use sildenafil (Viagra and Revatio) most often for men to help achieve erections. It works by dilating the blood vessels of the penis. However, it also can work well for Raynaud's attacks by dilating the blood vessels in the fingers and toes. Researchers first developed all of these medicines to treat other disorders (hypertension, depression, angina, pulmonary hypertension, and even erectile dysfunction) but they can work equally well for RP. Patients often react with surprise when prescribed some of these medicines (especially Prozac and Viagra), and it sometimes requires an explanation of why the doctor is prescribing them for their RP. Some people may also benefit from taking a low dose of aspirin daily (81 mg). This can help thin out the blood and may decrease the severity of the RP attacks.

For particularly severe, resistant cases of RP, measures that are more drastic may be necessary, such as a sympathectomy—a surgical procedure in which a surgeon cuts the sympathetic nerves to the hands. In addition, a doctor can inject an anesthetic around the nerves (called a sympathetic nerve block) to keep them from causing the constriction of the blood vessels.

### KEY POINTS TO REMEMBER

1. Raynaud's phenomenon is a common problem in people who have SLE, causing the fingers and/or toes to become cold, pale, and/or purple colored with cool temperatures and/or stress exposure.

2. Raynaud's is due to permanent thickening of the walls of the arteries instead of active inflammation. Therefore, it does not fluctuate with lupus disease activity and does not usually improve when SLE is under good control.

3. It is important to follow the suggestions in table 11.1 to try to keep the core body temperature warm and keep the body's blood vessels relaxed to help keep the Raynaud's attacks from being too severe.

4. Medicines may be required to relax the blood vessels in some cases. Some medicines were originally developed to treat other disorders (such as hypertension, depression, angina, pulmonary hypertension, or erectile dysfunction).

5. Biofeedback is a special technique for Raynaud's phenomenon that trains the mind to relax the blood vessels and warm up the hands and feet.

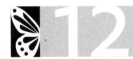

# The Urinary System

## Why You Need to Give a Urine Sample So Often

Caring for the urinary system, particularly the kidneys, is a priority of care and is the primary reason rheumatologists have their patients come in regularly for blood tests and urine samples, even when they feel perfectly fine. Between 40% and 50% of people who have SLE will have inflammation of the kidneys (also called nephritis) at some point in their lives. Nephritis is more common in younger people who have SLE, affecting approximately two-thirds of children. It varies by ethnicity, affecting two-thirds of African Americans yet only about 20% of Caucasians. People who have SLE of lower income tend to develop lupus nephritis more often than people with higher incomes. Asian SLE patients can have their urinary bladder affected by lupus cystitis, but this is very rare in the United States. This chapter goes into much more detail about this very important system of the body, which is so often a target of SLE.

. . . .

The urinary system (figure 12.1) begins with the kidneys, which are large organs located in the back of the abdomen around the level of the lower ribcage. True to their namesake, they are similar to kidney beans in shape. Their function is to filter out toxins and waste products from the blood so that they can be excreted in the urine. Blood arrives at the kidneys by way of the renal arteries, which then branch out (top of figure 12.2) to become smaller and smaller until they enter the actual filtering portion of the kidneys called the nephrons (bottom of figure 12.2); there are more than a million nephrons in each kidney. The nephron is composed of a glomerulus that filters most waste products from the blood. This waste product then flows into the nephron's tubule where processes that are more intricate occur to ensure that the proper amounts of fluids, minerals, and waste products are either excreted into the urine or reabsorbed into the bloodstream. The urine formed in each nephron's tubule then flows into a larger collecting duct that eventually carries the urine to the larger ureter of that particular kidney. Each kidney has one ureter that sends the urine into the urinary bladder (see figure 12.1), which is a muscular collecting organ for the urine. As it slowly becomes full with the urine, the muscular walls expand, letting the person know that it is time to urinate. The muscular wall of the urinary bladder squeezes the urine into one large tube (called the urethra), that allows the urine to leave the body.

SLE primarily causes problems in the kidneys in the glomeruli where the filtering of blood takes place. Although the urinary system includes four major structures—the

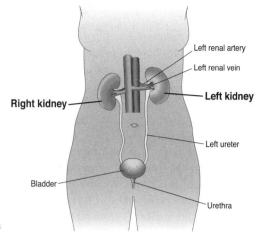

**Figure 12.1** (*right*) The urinary system

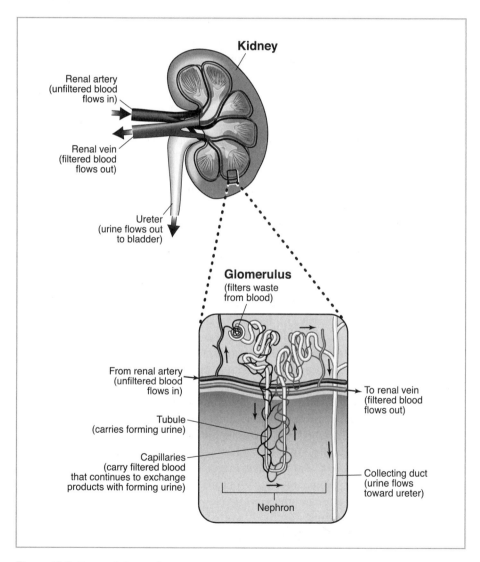

**Figure 12.2** Parts of the nephron

kidneys, the ureters, the urinary bladder, and the urethra—SLE affects the kidneys most. The urinary bladder is rarely involved—when it is, the medical term is "lupus cystitis"—while the ureters and urethra are not involved.

## Kidneys

Significant inflammation of the kidneys from lupus occurs in 40% to 50% of patients at some point in life. The medical terms for this are "lupus nephritis" and "lupus glomerulonephritis," which are generally interchangeable terms. The primary reason that doctors recommend that patients see them every few months for blood and urine testing, even when they are feeling fine, is because of lupus nephritis. In undeveloped countries where modern healthcare is not as accessible, lupus nephritis continues to be the primary cause of death. In developed countries, such as the United States, most people who develop lupus nephritis do very well on therapy. When doctors can identify it at the earliest stages (with urine and blood tests), therapies generally have excellent results. In my own patients, over the past twenty years, I have never had a lupus nephritis patient require dialysis who was compliant with recommended follow-up visits and treatments. Although 50% to 60% of people who have systemic lupus will never develop any significant problems from kidney involvement, it is actually more common than once thought. A 2012 study did kidney biopsies on SLE patients who had no evidence of kidney involvement in their urine or blood work. Fifty-eight percent of them showed some inflammation occurring in the kidneys due to lupus. Therefore, even if the usual blood and kidney tests suggest patients are doing well, they still have a high chance of the lupus being active in the kidneys, and they are at risk of this becoming worse if not monitored closely. Sometimes it can be difficult to convince someone who is doing well to continue to come in regularly for lab work. If she realizes that the lupus can be active, even when she feels perfectly fine and the labs are normal, but that she can do well if the doctor picks problems up early, it may provide the motivation she needs to stick to her rheumatologist's follow-up recommendations. I do not advocate that all lupus patients get a kidney biopsy. There is no evidence that mild kidney inflammation (i.e., there is active kidney inflammation on biopsy, but the urine test is normal) should be treated aggressively. The person's current medication, such as hydroxychloroquine (Plaquenil), is probably an adequate treatment.

SLE affects the kidneys primarily by causing the deposition of immune complexes from the blood in the filtering glomeruli. Immune complexes are important byproducts of the immune system formed by various immune molecules binding together. When the antibodies attach to antigens (as discussed in chapter 1) like a key in a lock, that antibody-antigen combination is an immune complex. The formation of immune complexes is a normal occurrence in everyone. In people who have SLE, the immune system can make abnormal types of immune complexes in large numbers, leading to inflammation and damage in various parts of the body. Lupus antibodies (such as anti-ds DNA) attach to the antibodies' target antigens (ds DNA in this example), along with various complement molecules in a person who has lupus and can then get trapped (deposited) in large numbers in the blood vessels of the kidneys. It appears that anti-ds DNA is the primary antibody contributing to kidney damage in most patients. The lupus patient's immune system produces these immune complexes (which incorporate anti-ds DNA antibodies) and causes inflammation. Particular molecules of the immune system called complements (such as C3 and C4 complement; see chapter 4) are depleted in the process. In many people who have lupus nephritis, anti-ds DNA levels may rise and C3 and C4 complements may decrease, reflecting this process. Rheumatologists frequently order these blood tests on a regular basis in lupus patients, looking for possible early signs of lupus nephritis. In some people who have SLE, the rheumatologist may see increasing anti-ds DNA levels in the blood (reflecting the increased number of anti-ds DNA immune complexes) as well as decreasing levels of C3 and C4 complements (since these molecules are being used up in the lupus inflammatory process producing these immune complexes). This can alert the doctor to pay closer attention because there may be an increased chance of the SLE flaring, possibly with associated kidney disease.

There are several different sections of the glomerulus that lupus can affect, in various degrees of severity. These variables determine how severe the disease is and how it should be treated. A kidney biopsy (discussed below) is the only way to know exactly what is happening and how to treat it. A kidney biopsy showing lupus nephritis is so specific for SLE that it is the only manifestation of SLE in the American College of Rheumatology's classification criteria that can clinch the diagnosis of SLE even if there is nothing else going on.

The glomeruli are very important for filtering waste products into the urine. However, when there is inflammation, other important parts of the blood can also leak into the urine. For example, there are many important proteins in the blood, especially albumin, which perform numerous essential functions in the body. When lupus nephritis occurs, an increased amount of protein (including albumin) leaks into the urine and is detectable in the urine sample tests (see chapter 4). In fact, the vast majority of people who have significant lupus nephritis have increased levels of protein in the urine (called proteinuria) and this is the main reason the doctor asks for a urine specimen at each office visit. In addition to protein, red and white blood cells can also leak into the urine, and finding more of these blood cells in the urine sample can also reflect the possibility of lupus nephritis. Sometimes these extra blood products (proteins and blood cells) collect into clumps called casts while they are inside the microscopic-size urinary tubules and the kidneys excrete them into the urine. These urinary casts are another abnormality that the doctor will look for. Casts are only visible under the microscope and do not generally cause any color changes to the urine.

As with inflammation occurring in any part of the body from SLE, the amount of inflammation in the kidneys can vary from mild to severe. If it is mild, then there may be just a small amount of extra protein in the urine (proteinuria) and nothing else. However, if there is severe inflammation occurring in most of the nephrons and glomeruli of both kidneys, then kidney function may be compromised, causing a backup of dangerous waste products in the blood and body (they are not being properly eliminated in the urine). Doctors determine how well the kidneys are functioning by using blood tests that look for blood urea nitrogen (BUN for short), serum creatinine (sCr), and estimated glomerular filtration rate (eGFR). There is a detailed explanation of these tests in chapter 4. The serum creatinine is the more important number. The higher the sCr is, the poorer the kidney function is. However, kidney function depends on other variables, such as age, sex, and race. These variables, along with the sCr, are part of a calculation of a number reflecting kidney function—the term for this is the "estimated glomerular filtration rate" (eGFR for short). This number is even more accurate than the sCr for measuring kidney function. Sometimes doctors will order a twenty-four-hour collection of urine to also measure the kidney function and the amount of protein loss, as discussed in chapter 4. Since all SLE patients must provide urine samples on a regular basis, I would encourage all SLE patients reading this book to read chapter 4 on how to properly obtain a urine sample. This will ensure that you do it correctly and decrease the chances of inaccurate results.

The kidneys do more than just filter waste products out of the blood. They also have other very important functions. For example, they secrete a hormone called erythropoietin, which travels through the blood and then to the bone marrow, where it signals the bone marrow to make more red blood cells. When a significant amount of inflammation and/or damage occurs in the kidneys, the kidneys make less erythropoietin and therefore fewer red blood cells form, causing anemia. In severe cases of anemia, symptoms include fatigue, shortness of breath, and paleness.

The kidneys also play an integral part in helping to maintain normal blood pressure. If enough inflammation or damage occurs, then the person's blood pressure can become elevated.

The kidneys play an important role in the regulation of electrolytes, such as potassium and calcium. With worsening damage, potassium levels can increase and calcium levels can decrease. The doctor usually monitors these levels closely. Vitamin D, which the skin normally manufactures due to activation by ultraviolet light from the sun, transforms in the kidneys into a more important form that the body utilizes better. With worsening kidney problems, the kidneys produce less functional vitamin D. This reduced production of vitamin D, along with the lower levels of calcium in the blood (due to the kidney disease), can cause the parathyroid glands (located in the neck behind the thyroid gland) to make more parathyroid hormone (PTH for short), causing a condition called hyperparathyroidism. These elevated levels of PTH cause the bones to lose additional calcium, which can cause them to become fragile and more liable to fracture.

With mild lupus nephritis or early in the disease process, the person who has lupus nephritis feels perfectly fine. In fact, this is the best time to diagnose it because it is easier to treat at this stage. This is the reason the doctor checks the urine and blood work regularly. Most of the symptoms of lupus nephritis occur when the inflammation is severe or if significant permanent damage has occurred, causing a major loss of kidney function. However, it takes a large decrease in kidney function before most people feel like something is wrong. Most of the symptoms of severe lupus nephritis are nonspecific and relate to the backup of waste products in the blood, as well as other complications, such as anemia and elevated blood pressure. Common symptoms include a vague sense of not feeling well, fatigue, headaches, nausea, and upset stomach. When lupus nephritis is more severe, it can cause shortness of breath, chest pain, and itchy skin.

One common symptom in people who have lupus nephritis is edema. This occurs when extra fluid leaks out of the blood vessels of the body. The effects of gravity then cause this fluid to collect into the parts of the body that are closest to the ground. Since people are usually sitting and standing most of the day, they will develop swelling of the ankles and feet due to this fluid collecting in these areas. It usually gets worse throughout the day. When affected people lie down at night, the fluid redistributes to the rest of the body. Then when they get up in the morning, the fluid accumulation is less in the ankles than when they went to bed. Edema can occur due to two main reasons. First, proteins (especially albumin) are required in the blood to hold the liquid part of the blood inside the blood vessels. If enough protein is lost in the urine (reflected by a larger amount of protein on the urine tests and a low albumin level on the blood tests), there is an insufficient amount to maintain fluids inside the blood vessels and edema occurs. The amount of edema depends on how much protein is being lost in the urine and the lower amount of albumin in the blood. In addition, when kidney function worsens, the ability of the kidneys to regulate the amount of salt (sodium) and water retained in the body changes, and often the body retains too much water and sodium, causing an increase in edema.

In the early stages of lupus nephritis, it is possible to significantly decrease or stop the inflammation. However, if it is left untreated, permanent scarring of the kidneys may occur causing the kidneys not to work properly and even fail to the point where the person needs dialysis. The goal of the rheumatologist who cares for SLE patients is to try to catch lupus nephritis at the earliest and most treatable stages before permanent kidney damage develops.

In summary, the vast majority of patients have no symptoms. If a person is losing a lot of protein in the urine (which can occasionally occur early in the disease), then swelling of the ankles may occur. This typically is most notable toward the end of the day and less notable when the person first gets out of bed. In more severe cases of lupus nephritis, fatigue, shortness of breath, nausea, chest pain, and itchy skin may occur.

Lupus nephritis does not cause "kidney pain." It is common for patients to become afraid of possibly having lupus nephritis because their lower back (area of the kidneys) hurts. However, lupus nephritis does not cause this. The most common cause of these symptoms are lower back strain due to problems unrelated to lupus—such as being overweight, osteoarthritis of the back, or straining the back while lifting. Other kidney problems may cause pain in this area—including severe kidney infection (which will usually also cause high fever, chills, and increased urinary frequency), and kidney stones (which are usually incredibly painful and require treatment in the emergency room). The most dangerous (but least common) cause would be kidney cancer. The latter usually also causes blood in the urine in a urine sample and requires an ultrasound or CT scan to diagnose.

Physical examination by the doctor usually does not show any abnormalities at all. However, in more severe cases, the blood pressure may be elevated and ankle edema may be present.

The blood and urine tests are essential in determining if lupus nephritis is occurring. As mentioned above, there is an increased amount of protein in the urine, and occasionally there may be an increased number of red and white blood cells and even urinary casts. If lupus nephritis is severe enough, the sCr is elevated (along with a corresponding lowered eGFR), indicating that the kidneys have enough inflammation or damage to alter how well they are filtering the blood. If a large amount of protein is leaking, then the blood level of albumin will be low (in which case there is usually edema present on physical exam as well). If the kidney function is decreased enough, or if the SLE is causing enough inflammation, there may also be a lower hemoglobin level than usual (i.e., anemia).

When the doctor finds abnormalities indicating that something is wrong with the kidneys, he or she tries to determine if something other than SLE may be causing the problem. For example, a woman who is menstruating can have an increased amount of blood and protein in the urine. Urinary tract infection also can increase urine protein, red blood cells, and white blood cells, so the doctor usually orders a urine culture to rule out this possibility. Some medications, especially non-steroidal anti-inflammatory drugs (NSAIDs such as ibuprofen and naproxen), can also cause kidney problems. The doctor usually stops any NSAIDs and reevaluates the kidney tests after stopping them to see if the test results improve when the patient is off the medicine. In addition, the doctor may order an ultrasound of the kidneys just to make sure there are no kidney stones or other problems.

When other options have been ruled out (i.e., menstrual blood, infection, NSAIDs, etc.), then the next test of choice is a kidney biopsy. This is very important because it is the only way to see exactly what is happening with the kidneys. For example, many people who have SLE have other medical problems such as diabetes and hypertension, which are the most common causes of kidney disease in the United States. Sometimes the only way to establish the cause (e.g., SLE, diabetes, hypertension, etc.) is to obtain a kidney biopsy. As mentioned previously, a biopsy refers to removal of a small amount of tissue of the body that is then examined under a microscope. A kidney biopsy is usually an outpatient procedure. Most commonly, an interventional radiologist (an x-ray doctor who specializes in doing biopsies under x-ray) performs the biopsy. He or she usually uses a CT scan x-ray or an ultrasound to figure out the best spot to do the biopsy. The doctor injects numbing medication with a needle into the tissues of the back to make the procedure more comfortable, and then inserts a very thin needle through the numbed up area until it enters the kidney to obtain a small piece. Usually several pieces are obtained to ensure that enough kidney tissue is present to be studied accurately under the microscope. This is usually a very safe procedure, with the patient being able to go home shortly after the biopsy. However, bleeding at the biopsy site is a possible complication. This can cause abdominal pain or blood in the urine. In this case, the doctor may admit the person to the hospital for observation after finishing the biopsy. It is important to stop all medicines that can cause bleeding (such as aspirin, NSAIDs, warfarin, and Plavix) before the procedure. Your doctor should advise you on when to stop these medicines. Infection is also a possible complication and can cause pain and fevers. Again, these are very uncommon problems from the biopsy but are important to consider.

The doctor doing the biopsy then sends the specimen to a lab that specializes in reading kidney biopsies. The kidney pieces are prepared in multiple ways so that they can be studied using various microscope techniques, including looking at them under an electron microscope as well as looking for the presence of antibodies causing a reaction in the kidneys (using a special test called immunofluorescence staining). All of these tests usually take quite a while to be done. It can take anywhere from one to three weeks to get all of the tests fully completed depending on which lab they are sent to.

One reason for doing the biopsy is to make sure that the person does not have a kidney problem due to something other than lupus. For example, if medications, diabetes, or high blood pressure are the cause of the kidney problem, this can be determined with the biopsy, and the treatment would be vastly different (stopping the offending medicine or controlling blood pressure better) than using strong immunosuppressants for lupus nephritis.

If the biopsy does show lupus nephritis, it is important to establish how lupus is affecting the kidneys. Sometimes it can be such a mild inflammation that no treatment is necessary, and other times it can be so severe that very high doses of steroids and very strong immunosuppressants such as cyclophosphamide may be required. In addition, the biopsy can show whether there is a lot of active inflammation (often labeled as an activity index), which means that treatment with strong immunosuppressant medicines can potentially help. It can also show if there is so much irreversible, permanent scarring of the kidneys (often reported as a chronicity index on the biopsy report) that it would not be worth using potentially dangerous strong immunosuppressants because most of the kidney is already destroyed and that preparations should be made for dialysis instead.

The kidney biopsy can show the various ways that lupus is affecting the kidneys. There are currently two different methods of reporting these results. The initial method from 1982 is from the World Health Organization (WHO) and is called the WHO classification. The International Society of Nephrology (ISN) and the Renal Pathology Society (RPS) designed the more recent method (abbreviated as the ISN/RPS classification). Although the latter goes into much more subtle detail than the WHO classification, fortunately, they both contain the same major designations.

Each classification method includes six different major possibilities and each uses a roman numeral (I–VI) to designate it. For example, if a biopsy ends up showing lupus membranous nephritis (discussed below), the biopsy report would read "WHO Class V lupus nephritis." If the pathologist (a doctor who specializes in reading biopsies) prefers the more recent classification, the same biopsy would read "ISN/RPS Class V lupus nephritis" along with some additional subdivisions added to this class. However, the doctor would interpret both as showing membranous nephritis. Since the treatment of lupus nephritis depends on the actual biopsy result, I separate the biopsy result possibilities in the following lupus nephritis section. If you have had a kidney biopsy for lupus nephritis, it is important for you to know what your actual result showed, and you can use this section to understand your results better. In addition, all patients need to get a copy of their kidney biopsy result and keep it with their own personal health records at home for possible future use if needed (table 12.1).

## Classification of Lupus Nephritis

*WHO Class I (or ISN/RPS Class I)*. The term for this in the WHO classification is "nil disease" ("nil" coming from the Latin word for "nothing" or meaning "a quantity of no importance") and "minimal mesangial lupus nephritis" in the ISN/RPS classification. This result shows that there is some deposition of immune complexes in the kidneys but without any significant inflammation. Class I lupus nephritis usually does not progress over time and usually does not need any treatment. This is by far the best diagnosis (other than a completely normal biopsy result).

**Table 12.1** Lupus Nephritis Biopsy Classifications

| WHO Class | WHO Name | ISN/RPS Class | ISN/RPS Name | Treatment |
|-----------|----------|---------------|--------------|-----------|
| I | Nil disease | I | Minimal mesangial lupus nephritis | None |
| II | Mesangial or purely mesangial disease | II | Mesangial proliferative lupus nephritis | Usually none needed unless it worsens |
| III | Focal segmental proliferative glomerulonephritis | III | Focal lupus nephritis | Steroids and immunosuppressants |
| IV | Diffuse segmental proliferative glomerulonephritis | IV | Diffuse lupus nephritis | Steroids and immunosuppressants |
| V | Membranous glomerulonephritis | V | Membranous lupus nephritis | Steroids and immunosuppressants |
| VI | Advanced sclerosing glomerulonephritis | VI | Advanced sclerosing lupus nephritis | None. Possibly prepare for dialysis |

*WHO Class II (or ISN/RPS Class II).* The terms for this are "purely mesangial disease" in the WHO classification and "mesangial proliferative lupus nephritis" in the ISN/RPS classification. The mesangium is the thin layer of tissue that supports the glomerular blood vessels. When lupus inflammation occurs mostly in this area and there is no significant inflammation in other parts of the kidney, then the medical term is "mesangial nephritis," which is a mild form of lupus nephritis. Most patients require no treatment at all and it usually does not progress or worsen. However, occasionally a patient with Class II lupus nephritis can progress to a more severe type of lupus nephritis over time, usually requiring another biopsy and treatment based on the results. Patients who have mesangial nephritis do not have any symptoms from the kidney problem.

*WHO Class III (or ISN/RPS Class III).* The terms for this are "focal segmental proliferative glomerulonephritis" in the WHO classification and "focal lupus nephritis" in the ISN/RPS classification. This is the first of the significant lupus nephritis problems. Focal means that less than half of the glomeruli on the kidney biopsy are involved with significant lupus nephritis. It is basically a milder version of Class IV lupus nephritis. Sometimes Class III lupus nephritis can be mild with absolutely no symptoms at all, cause just a little bit of protein in the urine, and have normal kidney function. However, on the other end of the spectrum, it can also be severe, causing fatigue, anemia, edema, high blood pressure, lots of protein in the urine, and even decreased kidney function. Due to the chances for worsening and kidney failure if not treated, it usually requires treatment with high doses of steroids as well as a strong immunosuppressant such as azathioprine, mycophenolate, or, in severe situations, cyclophosphamide.

*WHO Class IV (or ISN/RPS Class IV).* Terms for this are "diffuse proliferative glomerulonephritis" in the WHO classification and "diffuse lupus nephritis" in the ISN/RPS classification ("diffuse" meaning that more than half of the glomeruli on the kidney biopsy have significant lupus nephritis). This is the most aggressive form of lupus nephritis in that most patients will go on to kidney failure and need dialysis if not treated promptly and aggressively. It requires high doses of steroids and either mycophenolate or cyclophosphamide. Most patients are fatigued, do not feel well, and may have significant anemia and edema. Many patients have high blood pressure, requiring treatment with blood pressure medicines, and many have decreased kidney function. If the kidney function deterioration is severe, dialysis may be necessary to filter the blood. However, if a doctor catches it quickly enough and treats it aggressively, and kidney function improves with treatment, dialysis may be stopped.

*WHO Class V (or ISN/RPS Class V).* Terms for this are "membranous glomerulonephritis" in the WHO classification and "membranous lupus nephritis" in the ISN/RPS classification. Up to this point, advancing from Class I to Class IV has resulted in the higher numbers, indicating more severe kidney involvement. This is not the case for Class V membranous nephritis. Membranous nephritis mainly occurs in a slightly different section of the glomerulus than the previous types. It is less likely to worsen to the point of complete kidney failure than Classes III and IV (yet, about 30% do need dialysis over the long term if not treated). However, it can potentially cause many problems. The reason is that typically it causes the kidneys to lose a lot of protein. Sometimes the amount of protein lost can be enormous and causes a condition called the nephrotic syndrome, in which the protein loss is so large that the blood albumin level is low, edema is present, and the cholesterol level is high. Occasionally the amount of protein loss can be so massive that large amounts of fluid may leak from the blood vessels of the body, causing severe edema throughout the entire body, even around the eyes. The treatment of the resulting edema can sometimes be very difficult due to this massive loss of protein and usually requires large doses of diuretics (fluid pills). Although the nephrotic syndrome more commonly occurs in membranous nephritis, it also can occur, but less often, in Class IV lupus nephritis and even less often in Class III lupus nephritis.

One particularly unusual complication, which appears in people who have membranous nephritis, is renal vein thrombosis. This occurs when the nephrotic syndrome causes the loss of certain proteins of the clotting system (particularly those that decrease clotting), causing the blood to clot more easily. A blood clot will often occur in the large veins leading out of the kidneys (the renal veins), causing back or flank pain and worsening kidney function. The doctor needs to treat it with blood thinners.

Just as in Class III and IV lupus nephritis, high doses of steroids and immunosuppressant medicines are used. However, the treatment is not as standardized as that of the other two classes. There are several reasons for this. First, it is not as common overall as Class III and IV lupus nephritis. Since there are a larger number of people who have Class III and IV lupus nephritis, it has been easier to conduct larger and more extensive studies to establish the best treatment for these other two forms. In addition, Class III and IV lupus nephritis uniformly progresses to kidney failure rapidly without prompt and aggressive treatment. However, a large number of people who have membranous lupus nephritis will not worsen over time, or if they do, this may occur slowly. Most lupus nephritis experts agree that doctors should use steroids along with immunosuppressant medicines in most patients. In addition to azathioprine, mycophenolate, and cyclophosphamide mentioned previously, cyclosporine-A is another immunosuppressant that may be used.

*WHO Class VI (or ISN/RPS Class VI).* Terms for this are "advanced sclerosing glomerulonephritis" in the WHO classification and "advanced sclerosing lupus nephritis" in the ISN/RPS classification. Another term that doctors will often use when describing patients' kidney findings in this category is "glomerulosclerosis." As with any area of the body affected by lupus inflammation, if treatment does not control the inflammation quickly enough, or if the inflammation is severe enough, then the kidney heals with scar tissue (similar to how the body heals a skin cut with scar tissue). This scar tissue takes the place of normal functioning kidney tissue. The more scar tissue, the less normally functioning kidney remains to be able to filter the blood properly. Class III, IV, and V lupus nephritis can all have some scar tissue in the biopsy and vary in degree. When a doctor sees this, she or he will often note it in a chronicity index. The higher the chronicity index, the more scarring there is and the less likely that medications will be helpful. At the extreme end, if there are more than 90% of the scarred glomeruli (also called sclerosed) on the biopsy, it is labeled as Class VI or advanced sclerosing nephritis. This biopsy result means that very little else can be done because there is very little inflammation left to treat. Unfortunately, the person with this result will have to manage it with blood pressure medicines as needed and diet and prepare to undergo dialysis.

····

As you can see from the above descriptions, doctors generally treat Class III, IV, and V lupus nephritis with high doses of steroids and immunosuppressant medications. Your doctor may recommend that you get high doses of steroids, usually methylprednisolone (Solumedrol), through an IV for one to three days followed by high doses of oral steroids, usually prednisone or methylprednisolone. Studies show that using high doses of intravenous steroids initially increases the chances for the kidney inflammation to go into remission sooner. IV steroids also help the physician taper the doses of oral steroids sooner, therefore decreasing the chances for side effects. The doctor may especially consider doing this if the patient has moderate to severe kidney disease (basing it on a combination of the lab results, blood pressure, and kidney biopsy results).

As far as which immunosuppressant medicine to use, the doctor will usually base his or her decision on how severe the kidney inflammation is as well as on the person's race. Doctors usually treat the most severe cases with IV cyclophosphamide. This is a very strong chemotherapy medication that has been used to treat lupus nephritis for decades. It has been the most studied medication for lupus nephritis and has been the most effective, providing most patients with excellent results over a long period after their treatment compared to other medications. For example, if a person has Class IV lupus nephritis (one of the worst types on biopsy), high blood pressure (which is a bad sign), and decreased kidney function (low eGFR on the blood tests), most rheumatologists and nephrologists would use IV cyclophosphamide if there are no contraindications (reasons for not using it) and if the kidneys were not too permanently scarred. This regimen, along with high doses of IV steroids, would have the best chances of improving the patient's condition and even of possibly achieving remission. Doctors most commonly give IV cyclophosphamide once a month for about six months. After that, the doctor may continue it for a while but give it every three months, or the doctor may switch to a different medication, such as mycophenolate or azathioprine. Another way of using IV cyclophosphamide is the Euro-Lupus regimen where a lower dose is given every two weeks for only six doses, then switching over to a different medication (such as azathioprine or mycophenolate). However, this latter regimen has primarily been studied in women of European ancestry and should probably be reserved for that particular population. In fact, a 2010 Puerto Rican study demonstrated that this Euro-Lupus regimen was not as effective in their SLE patients compared to the standard, higher-dose monthly regimen. IV cyclophosphamide has many potential side effects, as discussed in chapter 32, so the doctor must carefully weigh the pros and cons of the treatment against what would happen without the treatment.

When cyclophosphamide is switched over to a different medication after the kidney disease is brought under better control, doctors call the medicine that is switched to "maintenance therapy." Many experts prefer using mycophenolate over azathioprine for maintenance therapy. In a 2012 study Mary Anne Dooley, MD, and a renowned panel of worldwide lupus experts showed that the use of mycophenolate worked better than azathioprine and more patients actually tolerated mycophenolate better. A primary reason to consider azathioprine over mycophenolate would be cost issues, as explained later in this chapter.

For less severe cases of lupus nephritis, often mycophenolate (CellCept and Myfortic) is used. Studies show that it is as effective as cyclophosphamide in many people who have Class III and IV lupus nephritis, and probably is overall safer than using IV cyclophosphamide. At least it usually does not cause infertility and hair loss is much less common compared to what occurs with the use of cyclophosphamide. The patient takes mycophenolate in pill form. (There is a more detailed discussion in chapter 32.) Although studies show that it is probably as effective as cyclophosphamide in many people who have lupus nephritis, there have not been studies of patients who have the most severe forms of nephritis. That is the reason that doctors still use IV cyclophosphamide in those cases.

Doctors must consider some interesting ethnicity situations as well when it comes to treating lupus nephritis. For example, African Americans and Hispanic patients appear to do better with mycophenolate compared to how they do on azathioprine, so it is becoming a more popular choice with doctors in treating these ethnic groups. In addition, some African Americans appear not to do as well on IV cyclophosphamide overall compared to how Caucasian patients do. Therefore, if an African American patient is on IV cyclophosphamide and does not improve within a few months, the doctor will switch that patient to mycophenolate instead in the hopes that she or he will do better. People of African ancestry also appear to require higher doses of mycophenolate compared to those of European ancestry. This probably reflects differences in metabolism and absorption of the medicine.

If a patient has milder lupus nephritis, and especially if that patient is Caucasian, then azathioprine may be used, which is another immunosuppressant medicine also explained in more detail in chapter 32. One reason for this is that many people who have milder disease do well and can go into remission on azathioprine. In addition, doctors have used azathioprine for decades and thus, many rheumatologists and nephrologists are more comfortable prescribing it instead of mycophenolate, which is a newer medication. Another very important point about azathioprine concerns the cost. If someone has no insurance, or a type of insurance where she or he pays a percentage of the cost of the medication, then cost can become a major issue. For example, according to www.drugstore.com in January 2013, the cost of one-month supply of azathioprine at 150 mg a day dosing was $84, while an equivalent monthly supply of mycophenolate mofetil (the generic equivalent of CellCept) at 3,000 mg a day (which generally is comparable to 150 mg a day of azathioprine) was $780 per month. Mycophenolate sodium (Myfortic) is even more expensive at $949 per month for 6 tablets a day.

Another medication sometimes used to treat lupus nephritis is cyclosporine A, also discussed in chapter 32. Doctors use it primarily for Class V nephritis. However, the doctor must monitor it more frequently than the other medications and therefore doctors do not use it as often as they used to.

Generally, the prescribing physician chooses one of these medications, and monitors the patient very closely, often every two to four weeks initially. If there is an excellent response—with decreasing protein in the urine, improving blood pressure, and improving kidney function on blood tests within the first few months—this is a very good sign. Studies suggest that if a patient responds in the first few months, he or she has a much better chance of having an excellent long-term outcome and a good chance of going into remission using that particular medication. One parameter has shown that if the amount of protein in the urine decreases by more than 25% within the first eight weeks then that person has an excellent chance of having an overall good response to that particular medication. However, not everyone is so lucky. It is not always possible to choose the best medication the first time around. If a doctor does not see improvement within the first few months, then she or he may change the medication to one of the other medications. In addition, it is not uncommon to repeat the high doses of IV steroids again when the medicine is changed.

If the person does not respond to a second immunosuppressant medicine, then the doctor may try a third immunosuppressant. This may be one of the ones I mentioned above, or one of the newer medications. Rituximab (discussed in chapter 33) and the newest medicine used for lupus, belimumab (chapter 34), have both shown promising results in some people who have lupus nephritis. A special word about belimumab (Benlysta)—it may be confusing to some patients when they may read that it was not studied in patients with kidney disease. This statement is not accurate at all. Many patients in the studies did have lupus nephritis. Only patients who had the most severe forms of kidney disease were not studied. In fact, a 2012 report in the journal *Lupus* showed that there were significant improvements in patients who had lupus nephritis who participated in the belimumab clinical studies. In 2012, a European consensus report by a group of lupus experts also suggested the possibility of using TNF inhibitors (see chapter 33). This group of biologic medications probably needs more study before being widely implemented in the treatment of lupus nephritis.

All people who have lupus nephritis still need to take hydroxychloroquine (Plaquenil) along with the stronger immunosuppressant medicines listed above. Studies show that people who have lupus nephritis generally do better if they take Plaquenil as part of their regimen compared to only taking the stronger medications.

The treatment of lupus nephritis is complex. It does not simply involve prescribing steroids and immunosuppressant medicines. Many other problems can occur in a person who has lupus nephritis, such as proteinuria (protein in the urine), anemia, abnormal electrolytes, low vitamin D levels, and edema, and they must be addressed as well.

Most people who have proteinuria are placed on one of two different types of blood pressure medicines, called angiotensin converting enzyme inhibitors (ACE inhibitors for short) or angiotensin receptor blockers (ARBs for short). The currently used medicines are listed in table 12.2. Doctors use these medicines even in patients who have normal blood pressures. The reason they are used is that the protein that leaks out of the kidneys due to lupus nephritis can damage the kidneys. ACE inhibitors and ARBs both can decrease this leakage of protein from the kidneys. They can help keep the kidneys healthier and may even keep them functioning better. However, they can occasionally cause side effects, such as cough, light-headedness, and dizziness. The ACE inhibitors in particular can sometimes cause a nagging, dry cough. If any of these side effects occur, you should let your doctor know so that he or she can try a different medicine. For example, the ARBs are less likely to cause a cough than the ACE inhibitors. Your doctor will also monitor your potassium level because the ARBs and ACE inhibitors can sometimes increase the amount of potassium in the blood. He or she will also monitor your kidney function (the sCr and eGFR) in your blood work because these medications can sometimes cause the kidney function to decrease due to decreased blood flow to the kidneys. This latter side effect is easily reversible by decreasing the dose of the medicine.

It is extremely important to control blood pressure in people who have lupus nephritis. If the blood pressure is elevated, this can cause further damage to the kidneys and blood vessels of the body, which can increase the risks for heart attacks and stroke. Doctors recommend keeping the blood pressure less than 130/80 in people who have active lupus nephritis who have increased protein in the urine. If the protein level is normal, than a goal of less than 140/90 is recommended.

In addition to treating the high blood pressure, it is imperative that high cholesterol be treated as well. Although diet alone may be adequate in people who have high cholesterol by itself, people who have lupus nephritis and high cholesterol problems should generally take a cholesterol-lowering medication. Most experts recommend a medicine that is in the statin category as the drug of choice.

The anemia caused by lupus nephritis is not due to a lack of iron, so taking iron supplements alone does not help. It is due to the decreased production of the hormone erythropoietin, as mentioned previously. It does not cause any significant problems in most people who have lupus nephritis, but occasionally it can cause fatigue. In addition, if the hemoglobin level is particularly low, it can also be associated with heart problems and difficulties with memory and thinking. If fatigue or memory problems occur, or if the hemoglobin is below a certain level (usually target hemoglobin is between 10 g/dL and 12 g/dL), then the anemia can be treated with injections of either darbepoetin alfa (Aranesp) or epoetin alfa (Epogen or Procrit).

**Table 12.2** ACE Inhibitors and ARBs Used in Lupus Nephritis

| ACE Inhibitors | ARBs |
|---|---|
| benazepril (Lotensin) | candesartan (Atacard) |
| captopril (Capoten) | irbesartan (Avapro) |
| enalapril (Vasotec) | losartan (Cozaar) |
| fosinopril (Monopril) | telmisartan (Micardis) |
| lisinopril (Prinivil, Zestril) | valsartan (Diovan) |
| moexipril (Univasc) | |
| perindopril (Aceon) | |
| quinapril (Accupril) | |
| ramipril (Altace) | |
| trandolapril (Mavik) | |

Sometimes people who have lupus nephritis need to take extra potassium, calcium, or vitamin D supplements, depending on the results of their blood tests. Although kidney disease, ARBs, and ACE inhibitors can increase potassium levels, sometimes a doctor needs to use diuretics (fluid pills) such as furosemide (Lasix). Furosemide commonly decreases potassium levels, requiring the use of a potassium supplement. Diet can be beneficial depending on the circumstances. Diet recommendations are quite complex and vary according to the degree of kidney damage, proteinuria, edema, and so on and are best prescribed by a kidney doctor (called a nephrologist), sometimes with the help of a dietician.

If significant edema occurs, you can treat it by elevating your feet and legs when you sit and lie down. Compression stockings are tight stockings that you can buy from pharmacies and medical supply stores. If you wear these soon after getting up in the morning, they can decrease the amount of swelling in the legs. Sometimes people take medications to decrease the amount of fluid. Doctors call these "fluid pills" and "diuretics." However, diuretics can sometimes cause problems with kidney function, as well as electrolyte imbalances such as low or high potassium or calcium levels, so doctors usually follow patients closely with blood tests.

There are other kidney problems that occur in SLE patients due to lupus, but they are much less common. For example, people who have antiphospholipid antibodies may have multiple tiny blood clots in the blood vessels of the kidneys (which are visible on a kidney biopsy). In this situation, blood thinners such as warfarin would be the treatment of choice. I discussed thrombotic thrombocytopenic purpura (TTP) in the platelet section of chapter 9. This can also cause multiple tiny blood clots in the kidneys as well as kidney failure. Rarely, vasculitis (inflammation of the blood vessels) may also occur (also diagnosed on kidney biopsy). The treatment for this condition is similar to that for the more severe forms of lupus nephritis, using high doses of steroids and immunosuppressant medicines, such as azathioprine, mycophenolate, or cyclophosphamide.

If the kidneys completely stop working, the medical term is "end-stage renal disease" (or ESRD for short). This occurs when the eGFR on blood testing or the creatinine clearance on the twenty-four-hour urine test is below 15 ml/min. At this point, the kidneys are no longer able to filter harmful blood products out of the blood and secrete them into the urine. When this occurs, dialysis is necessary. In dialysis, a machine filters harmful substances that the kidneys would normally take care of out of the blood. There are two forms of dialysis. One is hemodialysis—where the person goes to a dialysis unit and a needle with tubing is inserted into the person's arm so that a dialysis machine can filter the blood. Most people who have ESRD usually do this about three times a week. The other form of dialysis is peritoneal dialysis—a machine connected to tubing goes into the person's peritoneal cavity (which surrounds the abdomen) to filter the blood. The advantage of peritoneal dialysis is the patient can do it at home but must do it more often than hemodialysis. This latter form of dialysis may be less effective in SLE. Patients on hemodialysis seem to have better control of their SLE, most likely due to the dialysis removing harmful antibodies from the blood. In fact, many people with lupus are able to get off steroids when they are on hemodialysis.

SLE patients appear to do as well with a kidney transplant as other people who get transplants and do not have SLE, in that their body does not reject the kidney any more often than kidney transplant patients who do not have SLE. The best type of kidney to transplant is one from a family member with a blood type similar to that of the person with SLE. Otherwise, a properly matched kidney from a cadaver or live non-related donor may also be used. People who have SLE who have undergone a kidney transplant usually do not have a recurrence of lupus nephritis in the transplanted kidney. Although the SLE patients accept the new kidney as often as people who do not have lupus, they unfortunately have a higher long-term death rate compared to non-lupus patients who get kidney transplants. A 2011 study showed that ten years after a kidney transplant, 85% of non-lupus patients were alive, while only 71% of SLE patients were still alive. The primary cause of death in the lupus patients are heart-related conditions, such as heart attacks, with 67% of the lupus patients dying due to a heart-related condition, while only 40% of the non-lupus patients died from heart complications. This illustrates the importance of preventing heart disease in people who have SLE (see chapter 21 for more details).

## Urinary Bladder

SLE rarely affects the bladder. However, an entity called lupus cystitis can rarely occur in Asian women who have SLE, particularly in Japan and China. It is very rare in the United States. Common symptoms include increased frequency in urination as well as having a feeling of urgency to urinate (symptoms that are similar to those caused by a bladder infection). In addition, most patients also have inflammation of the gastrointestinal tract, and develop abdominal pain, nausea, and vomiting. In fact, some people have the abdominal symptoms with no urinary tract symptoms at all, which may make it more difficult to reach a correct diagnosis. Doctors diagnose it by a procedure called a cystoscopy. A urinary tract surgery specialist (a urologist) inserts a tiny fiberoptic scope into the urethra. He or she can look into the bladder and obtain a tiny biopsy, which may show inflammation of the bladder wall from lupus with examination under the microscope. The treatment for this is steroids and immunosuppressant drugs.

## KEY POINTS TO REMEMBER

1. African Americans and Hispanics are especially at high risk for lupus nephritis.

2. Lupus nephritis does not cause any unusual symptoms until after significant damage has already occurred.

3. It is important to have blood and urine tests to look for the possibility of lupus nephritis regularly when you are feeling well to try to identify lupus nephritis at its earliest stages so that treatments can be more successful.

4. If you do get a kidney biopsy, make sure to keep a permanent copy for your personal records. Keep it safe at all times because it may come in very handy if you have to get a new doctor in the future (such as if you move or change insurance companies).

5. Make sure that your blood pressure remains below 130/80 if you have proteinuria (less than 140/90 is sufficient if your urine protein level is normal). If it is higher, see your doctor to get it lowered (usually using medicines) to help protect your kidneys.

6. If you have an increased amount of protein in your urine, make sure your doctor is treating you with an ACEI or an ARB (listed in table 12.2).

7. Treatment of lupus nephritis can be quite complex, often requiring multiple medications to control the immune system as well as treat electrolyte disorders, high blood pressure, proteinuria, edema, high cholesterol, and anemia, and to prevent side effects from the medicines (such as using medicines to prevent osteoporosis from the steroids).

8. With early, aggressive treatment, most people who have lupus nephritis do well and do not develop end-stage renal disease, which requires dialysis treatment.

9. Patients who have kidney problems should never take NSAIDs (such as ibuprofen and naproxen).

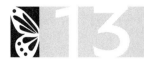

# The Nervous System

## The Nerves

The nervous system is one of the most complex systems in the body. It is responsible for how we think, love, and hate; our personalities; our ability to move our muscles; our senses of feeling, smelling, tasting, hearing, and seeing; our ability to stand and walk; and the regulation of our blood pressure and our heartbeats. All these functions are regulated by cells called nerves that are connected to each other and send messages to each other via tiny amounts of chemical messengers called neurotransmitters as well as electrical activity traveling up and down the nerves to transmit messages. This chapter discusses how SLE can affect this vitally important system of the body.

....

The nervous system can be divided into the central nervous system (CNS), composed of the brain and spinal cord, and the peripheral nervous system, which encompasses the nerves that lead to and from the CNS to the rest of the body (figure 13.1). Lupus involvement of the nervous system is so complex and complicated that in 1999 the American College of Rheumatology (ACR) devised a classification system to help doctors describe their patients in similar ways to standardize treatment and research. The ACR lists them as neuropsychiatric syndromes ("neuro-" referring to the nerves and "psychiatric" referring to psychiatric conditions) and divides them into nineteen different types that are further separated into those that affect the central nervous system and those that affect the peripheral nervous system. It is important to include psychiatric conditions (such as depression, anxiety disorder, and schizophrenia) because they are disorders caused by an abnormality of the nerves of the brain. The ACR neuropsychiatric syndromes are listed in table 13.1. I use this system to organize this chapter because it is good for patients to understand how lupus doctors think and how they classify certain problems that occur in lupus. I also make an exception to my explanation in chapter 5 about the organization of this part of the book (part II). I mentioned there that I would list lupus problems that are directly due to the immune system affecting organs in part II and complications of lupus due to other problems in part III. The ACR includes both types in this system, so I do so in this chapter as well. Some examples of neuropsychiatric syndromes that may occur due to problems other than the direct influence of the immune system causing inflammation include headaches, anxiety, cognitive dysfunction (memory problems), and mood disorders.

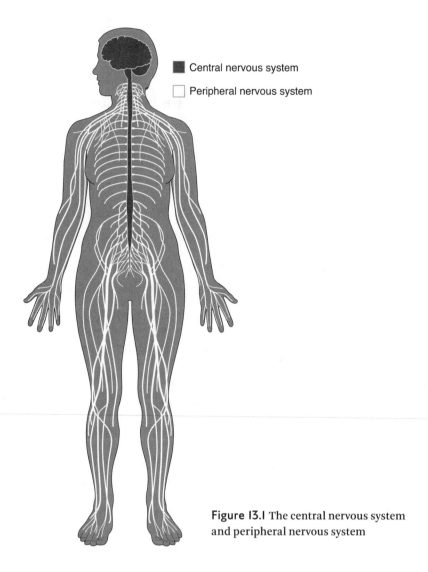

Central nervous system

Peripheral nervous system

**Figure 13.1** The central nervous system and peripheral nervous system

## Central Nervous System

### Aseptic Meningitis

The meninges are the tissues and membranes that envelop the brain and spinal cord. When there is inflammation of the meninges, it is called meningitis. Meningitis typically causes headaches, fever, stiffness of the neck, and intolerance of light shining in the eyes. When severe, it can cause difficulty with thinking. It may be difficult to keep the hips and knees straightened out while lying down, and patients may find it more comfortable to keep the hips and knees bent. On physical examination, the classic finding is nuchal rigidity ("nuchal" refers to the neck). The doctor will try to push the person's head down toward the chest, but this causes increased neck pain and muscle spasms.

The most important thing with meningitis is to make sure that it is not due to a bacterial or other type of infection because this can be deadly if not identified and treated immediately. For this reason, the person with suspected meningitis will be started immediately on antibiotics (just in case there is an infection) and a spinal tap (also called a lumbar puncture) is performed. A lumbar puncture is done by the doctor numbing up the lower back with some anesthetic (usually lidocaine) using a very thin needle. Then a larger needle is inserted through the numbed-up area until it reaches the spinal canal within the spine to collect some of the cerebrospinal fluid for examination. It is rare to have significant complications from a lumbar puncture. Bleeding and infection are possible, as with most invasive medical procedures, but are fortunately rare. The spinal cord itself ends a few levels up from where the lumbar puncture is performed, so spinal cord injury should not be possible. This is important to know because many people are fearful of getting a lumbar puncture due to their concern about possible spinal cord injury.

**Table 13.1** ACR Neuropsychiatric Syndromes Observed in SLE

Central nervous system

    Aseptic meningitis

    Cerebrovascular disease

    Demyelinating syndrome

    Headache (including migraine and pseudotumor cerebri)

    Movement disorder

    Myelopathy

    Seizure disorders

    Acute confusional state

    Anxiety disorder

    Cognitive dysfunction

    Mood disorder

    Psychosis

Peripheral nervous system

    Acute inflammatory demyelinating polyradiculoneuropathy

        (Guillain-Barré syndrome)

    Autonomic disorder

    Mononeuropathy, single/multiplex

    Neuropathy, cranial

    Plexopathy

    Polyneuropathy

The fluid, called the cerebrospinal fluid (or CSF for short), is then sent to the lab where the number of white blood cells is counted; this count can help differentiate different types of brain and spinal cord problems. Tests for other diseases such as Lyme disease, viral infections, and fungal infections are also done. The fluid is examined under the microscope to look for bacterial infection, and a culture is also done to exclude infection or to identify specific bacteria and microorganisms. Infections can usually be diagnosed quickly from the tests, especially the Gram stain. However, sometimes the doctor has to wait for the results of cultures, which can take several days. A culture is performed by placing some of the fluid in various lab containers that contain food (agar) that different bacteria and microorganisms can grow on. It is important to keep the person on antibiotics "just in case" until the results are complete. As you will learn later in this book, infections are one of the most common causes of death in people who have lupus, so it is very important to be careful and make sure there is no infection in cases such as this.

If the CSF shows an increased number of white blood cells, this means that there is inflammation occurring around the brain and/or spinal cord. This helps to confirm a diagnosis of meningitis. If no bacteria or other microorganisms are found on the Gram stain, cultures, and other tests, then the meningitis is called aseptic meningitis ("a-" means "not" and "septic" means "infectious"). That means that there is inflammation of the meninges, but it is not due to a bacterial infection. It still may not be due to lupus though. For example, many types of viruses can cause aseptic meningitis. Fortunately, the vast majority of these are mild infections that resolve on their own. Another common cause of aseptic meningitis in people who have SLE is the use of non-steroidal anti-inflammatory drugs (NSAIDs) such as ibuprofen and naproxen. It is not known why, but people who have lupus are at increased risk of developing this particular side effect from NSAIDs. Therefore, if a person who has lupus develops meningitis, in addition to being treated with antibiotics (in case of bacterial infection), it is important that any NSAIDs be discontinued. Fortunately, this cause of meningitis resolves when the NSAID is stopped. The drugs azathioprine (Imuran) and intravenous immunoglobulin (IVIG for short) may also rarely cause aseptic meningitis in people who have lupus.

If all the above potential causes have been ruled out as causes of the meningitis, then it is presumed that the aseptic meningitis is directly due to inflammation from SLE. In that case, the doctor will usually treat it with high doses of steroids. This appears to be a rare manifestation of SLE. Usually the meningitis is due to either medications (such as NSAIDs) or an infection.

## KEY POINTS TO REMEMBER

1. Headache, fever, difficulty tolerating light in the eyes, and a stiff neck are common symptoms of meningitis.

2. Bacterial meningitis is potentially deadly, so usually patients are treated with antibiotics and a lumbar puncture is performed to send CSF to the lab for cultures.

3. NSAIDs such as ibuprofen and naproxen can cause aseptic meningitis in people who have SLE. It resolves when the NSAID is stopped.

4. Lupus aseptic meningitis is treated with steroids.

## Cerebrovascular Disease

Cerebrovascular disease refers to problems related to the blood vessels of the brain ("cerebro-" meaning "brain" and "-vascular" referring to blood vessels). This occurs in up to 18% of people who have SLE. The primary result of cerebrovascular disease is what is called a cerebrovascular accident (or CVA for short). A CVA is called a stroke in layperson's terms. It can be thought of as a "heart attack of the brain." It is due to a decrease or lack of blood supply to a section of the brain, which causes damage to that particular part of the brain and can potentially cause a part of the brain to die. Which problems occur all depends on what part of the brain is affected. For example, if the CVA affects the part of the brain responsible for movement of the right leg and arm, then the person may develop a sudden onset of weakness on the right side of the body. Other common symptoms include the sudden onset of numbness on one side of the body, difficulty speaking, difficulty with balance, and loss of vision. Sometimes a sudden, severe headache may occur. Since a stroke is potentially deadly but can be treated effectively if done so quickly, it is very important for anyone having the sudden onset of any of these symptoms to seek medical care immediately.

If stroke symptoms occur but then resolve on their own, it is called a transient ischemic attack, or TIA for short. This is sometimes called a "mini-stroke" in layperson's terms. If someone has a TIA, she or he is at high risk of developing a full-blown CVA in the future. Immediate medical attention is required as with a CVA.

People who have SLE are twice as likely to develop CVAs and TIAs compared to people who do not have SLE. In fact, cerebrovascular disease, along with heart attacks and other vascular problems, are among the top three causes of death in people who have SLE. In fact, after the first few years of an SLE diagnosis, the most common cause of death in lupus patients are vascular complications such as strokes and heart attacks. Therefore, it is vitally important that people who have SLE do everything possible to decrease their chances of developing these problems. This is explained in more detail in chapter 21. This includes maintaining proper body weight; exercising regularly; not smoking; eating a proper diet; and ensuring that blood pressure, sugar levels, and cholesterol levels are kept under control.

There are several different ways that CVAs and TIAs may occur in people who have SLE. Many medical tests are required to determine the cause so that proper treatment can be administered. If physicians administer a type of blood thinner (called thrombolytic therapy) quickly enough, there is the possibility of reversing the stroke and preventing permanent brain injury. The best results occur when this treatment is provided within ninety minutes of the first onset of symptoms, but can be helpful if given up to four and a half hours of onset. Usually a CT scan (a series of x-ray views) of the brain will be performed to make sure there is no bleeding in the brain before the medicine is given. With thrombolytic therapy, more than one-third of people who have had a stroke will fully recover.

After this acute stage, one of the most important things is to determine what caused the stroke. This helps the doctor decide on the best way to treat the person and prevent additional strokes in the future.

One potential cause of strokes in people who have SLE is the antiphospholipid syndrome (APS), as discussed in chapter 9. Anywhere between one-third and one-half of SLE patients are positive for tests caused by antiphospholipid antibodies, including anticardiolipin antibody, lupus anticoagulant, beta-2 glycoprotein antibody, false positive syphilis test, and anti-phosphatidylserine antibody (discussed in chapters 4 and 9). These antibodies can sometimes cause the blood to clot more easily than normal and can lead to blood clots (called thromboses) in the arteries and veins of the body. If clots occur in the arteries of the brain, they can cause a TIA or CVA. Unfortunately, once someone has developed a TIA or CVA from the antiphospholipid syndrome, they are at high risk of developing additional strokes in the future. APS is treated with blood thinners such as warfarin, clopidogrel (Plavix), and aspirin. Usually, it is recommended that people who have APS take these for the rest of their lives.

People who have SLE can also have a stroke due to vasculitis, which is an inflammation of the blood vessels. The inflammation of an artery causes decreased blood flow to the brain, as well as leakage of blood into the brain. An angiogram may be performed. This is an x-ray of the arteries that allows the blood vessels to be visualized. An alternative test would be a magnetic resonance angiogram (MRA for short), which is similar but done with an MRI machine. With vasculitis, these studies may show intermittent areas of narrowing and dilatations (called beading by the radiologist) in the arteries in the brain or an area of artery ballooning (called an aneurysm). If vasculitis is suspected, it is treated with high doses of steroids and other immunosuppressants, such as azathioprine, mycophenolate, or cyclophosphamide. The term "CNS vasculitis" is used much too loosely by many doctors. Studies show that true vasculitis of the blood vessels of the brain due to lupus is a very rare occurrence. This has been shown in autopsy studies of patients who have died from neuropsychiatric lupus.

Bleeding into the brain can also cause a CVA or TIA. This can be seen in people who have very low platelet counts (thrombocytopenia) due to lupus. Its treatment is dependent on using therapies to manage SLE and increase the platelet count. In emergency bleeding situations such as this, doctors can give platelet transfusions to raise the platelet count. If the person is taking blood thinners such as aspirin, warfarin (Coumadin), or clopidogrel (Plavix), a stroke could occur because of bleeding into the brain due to the medicine. The stroke would most likely not be due to the lupus itself. Stopping the offending medication is the first line of therapy. In the case of warfarin, vitamin K and transfusions containing clotting factors can be given to reverse the effects of the warfarin.

Thrombotic thrombocytopenic purpura (TTP) can also cause CVAs and TIAs by causing numerous small blood clots in the arteries of the brain. Its diagnosis and treatment are discussed in chapter 9.

Hardening of the arteries can cause strokes. The medical term for hardening of the arteries is "atherosclerosis" or "arteriosclerosis" (these two terms are often used interchangeably). Hardening of the arteries occurs over time and is the primary cause of heart attacks and strokes in people as they get older. It is the number one cause of death in the United States. When atherosclerosis occurs in the arteries of the brain, blood flow decreases to parts of the brain, causing a stroke. People who have SLE can develop hardening of the arteries at a younger age than people who do not have SLE. The term "accelerated atherosclerosis" or "accelerated arteriosclerosis" is sometimes used to refer to this fact. The reasons why this process may develop faster in people who have SLE is further discussed in chapter 21. Atherosclerosis is prevented by not smoking, controlling blood pressure and diabetes, lowering cholesterol, and adhering to a proper diet and maintaining a healthy weight.

Another potential cause of stroke is an embolus. An embolus is a blood clot that travels through the bloodstream. There are several common places for an embolus to originate from, including the carotid arteries, the aorta, and the heart. Vascular studies such as an ultrasound, an MRA, and an echocardiogram can be done to search for sources of emboli. If an embolic source is identified, treatment is directed at whatever caused the embolus. If it is due to arteriosclerosis or atherosclerosis, then a substance called plaque will be found on the inside of the arteries. Plaque is a buildup of cholesterol mixed with clotted blood that can loosen and travel to the brain, causing a stroke. If it is due to arteriosclerosis, it is treated as discussed in the preceding paragraph. If there is severe narrowing of the carotid arteries, surgery may be needed to clear them. If Libman-Sacks endocarditis is diagnosed (discussed in chapter 11), antiphospholipid antibodies are often present. In this case, treatment includes blood thinners such as warfarin.

### KEY POINTS TO REMEMBER

1. A cerebrovascular accident (also called a stroke) can be thought of as a "heart attack of the brain" where blood flow decreases to part of the brain, causing permanent damage.

2. Common symptoms of a CVA include abrupt-onset weakness, numbness, difficulty walking or speaking, and loss of vision.

3. If a person develops symptoms of a CVA, but then they resolve on their own, it is called a transient ischemia attack or a mini-stroke.

4. If symptoms of a CVA occur, it is important to seek medical attention immediately because quick treatment can prevent permanent brain damage.

5. CVAs, along with heart attacks, are among the top causes of death in people who have SLE, so it is very important to control weight, blood pressure, diabetes, and cholesterol levels and not smoke to prevent them.

6. Sometimes CVA and TIA can be due to the antiphospholipid antibody syndrome. In this case, lifelong treatment with blood thinners such as warfarin (Coumadin) is needed.

7. If the CVA is due to a bleed in the brain, it could be caused by problems with the platelets due to the lupus, in which case the person is treated with platelet transfusions and steroids; it could be due to blood-thinning medicines such as aspirin, Plavix or warfarin (Coumadin), in which case the causative medication would need to be stopped.

## Demyelinating Syndrome

Many nerves of the body are covered with a very thin layer of tissue called a myelin sheath. The purpose of this sheath is to increase the speed of electrical impulses up and down the nerve. If there is a loss of the myelin sheath, this is called demyelination. Multiple sclerosis (MS) is the most common disease that causes demyelination of the nerves in the central nervous system. MS is an autoimmune disease. People who have SLE can develop CNS demyelination that looks exactly like MS. It is impossible to tell whether this represents the lupus attacking the myelin and looks like MS, or whether the person has both SLE and MS. The demyelinating syndrome is often referred to as "lupoid sclerosis."

Common symptoms of lupoid sclerosis include weakness and numbness in an arm or leg, weakness or numbness in the face, blurred vision, double vision, tremors, balance difficulties, and problems with coordination of the arms or legs. Difficulty with memory and moodiness are other common problems. A particular complication called optic neuritis may occur with inflammation of the main nerve of the eye, causing blurred vision. These problems will often come and go over time, worsening and improving for no apparent reason.

An MRI of the brain is usually done. Lupoid sclerosis may show findings similar to those of classic MS, with abnormalities called plaque by the radiologist (a doctor that reads x-rays) or neurologist (a doctor who specializes in nerve disorders). A lumbar puncture (spinal tap) can also be very helpful. The procedure is explained in the section on meningitis. The cerebrospinal fluid may show an elevation of a particular type of protein of the immune system called IgG immunoglobulins, as well as an abnormal protein called myelin basic protein and other immune proteins called oligoclonal bands. These immunoglobulins, myelin basic protein, and oligoclonal bands are substances formed by the immune system in greater quantities in people who have multiple sclerosis and lupoid sclerosis.

The treatment of lupoid sclerosis is usually with high doses of steroids, as well as immunosuppressants such as azathioprine or mycophenolate. Some people have high levels of antiphospholipid antibodies. It is believed that tiny blood clots caused by the antiphospholipid syndrome may also be responsible for lupoid sclerosis and blood thinners such as warfarin may be needed (see the discussion of antiphospholipid antibody syndrome in chapter 9).

1. The demyelinating syndrome due to SLE appears similar to MS, causing fluctuating symptoms of numbness, weakness, and balance problems, as well as difficulties with speech, thinking, and walking.

2. "Plaques" are visible on MRI, and spinal fluid contains proteins often seen in MS.

3. Another term commonly used for this syndrome is "lupoid sclerosis."

4. Lupoid sclerosis is treated with high doses of steroids and immunosuppressant medicines.

## Headache (including Migraine and Pseudotumor Cerebri)

People who have SLE have an increased chance of having headaches compared to people who do not have SLE (they occur in up to 72% of SLE patients). In fact, the most common types of headaches seen in lupus patients are migraine headaches and tension headaches. Another not uncommon cause of headaches in people who have lupus is a condition called fibromyalgia (see the self-survey test in the first section of chapter 27). Therefore, in the vast majority of patients, headaches are not considered to be due to lupus at all. It is important for doctors to figure out if the headaches are tension headaches, migraine headaches, or due to fibromyalgia, and treat them the same way that they are treated in people who do not have SLE. Occasionally, headaches can occur during a severe flare of lupus as a part of the flare. These lupus-related headaches respond to treatment of the flare itself (e.g., they go away or get much better with the other lupus problems when treated with steroids).

One cause of headache in lupus deserves special mention: pseudotumor cerebri (also called benign intracranial hypertension). Pseudotumor cerebri occurs in 1% of people who have SLE. It is due to an increase in the pressure of fluid around the brain and spinal cord, causing headaches that are often severe, as well as blurred and double vision. On physical exam, the doctor will note swelling around the optic nerve in the back of the eye. This type of swelling in the eye (called papilledema) can also be caused by a tumor in the brain, so an MRI or CT scan is performed to make sure there is no tumor. If there is no tumor or cancer causing the problem, it is called pseudotumor cerebri. "Pseudo-" means "false" and "cerebri" means "of the brain." So "pseudotumor cerebri" means "a false tumor of the brain." In other words, it is a condition that causes some symptoms that are similar to those of a brain tumor, but there is no tumor. A lumbar puncture (spinal tap) is usually required as well (see the section on meningitis for a discussion of a lumbar puncture). The lumbar puncture will show an elevated pressure. In fact, it is this increased pressure of the cerebrospinal fluid (CSF) that causes the symptoms. Draining some of the CSF from the spinal canal (which also decreases the amount around the brain) during the lumbar puncture is a way to treat it and lessen the symptoms. This elevated pressure is also the source of the other name for the disorder—"benign intracranial hypertension" where "benign" means "nonmalignant" or not related to cancer. "Intracranial" means "inside the brain" and "hypertension" means that the pressure is increased.

In addition to draining extra CSF during a lumbar puncture, other therapies include treating lupus with steroids and other immunomodulating therapies. In addition, a diuretic called acetazolamide can be helpful in decreasing the fluid pressure. In more resistant cases, surgery on the eyes can relieve the amount of increased pressure around the brain, usually providing a more permanent treatment.

Some people who have SLE develop pseudotumor cerebri caused by a blood clot in the brain (called a dural venous sinus thrombosis) due to antiphospholipid antibodies. This is treated with blood thinners such as warfarin. See the section on antiphospholipid antibody syndrome in chapter 9 for more information.

---

### KEY POINTS TO REMEMBER

1. Most headaches in people who have lupus are most likely not due to SLE, but more commonly are tension headaches or migraine headaches.

2. Fibromyalgia is also a common cause of headaches in people who have SLE. You can take the home self-survey at the beginning of chapter 27 to see if you have fibromyalgia as a possible cause of headaches.

3. If headaches occur due to a lupus flare, they improve when the flare is treated.

4. Pseudotumor cerebri (also called benign intracranial hypertension) can occur in SLE patients as a cause of headache and is treated with acetazolamide. Surgery may be needed in severe cases.

5. It is important to rule out a blood clot in the veins of the brain due to antiphospholipid syndrome if pseudotumor cerebri occurs.

---

## Movement Disorders

There are several types of movement disorders in SLE. The most common is tremors, where the hands or head shake back and forth either when at rest or when moving. Tremors can occur for many possible reasons. Medications, such as steroids and some antidepressants, as well as caffeine intake are some of the most common causes of tremors.

The most common type of movement disorder seen in SLE due to the lupus itself is called chorea (which comes from the Greek word for "dance"). This occurs in 1% to 4% of people who have SLE. It causes sudden, uncontrollable, brief movements of the arms, legs, or head. These episodes may last several weeks at a time and often resolve on their own with no treatment. However, sometimes steroids and neurologic medicines are required. There are rarer types of movement disorders that have been described in SLE patients, but they are so rare I omit them from this discussion.

Some movement disorders (including chorea) are seen in people who are positive for antiphospholipid antibodies, and it is felt that they may be due to the antiphospholipid antibody syndrome. In these people, blood thinners like warfarin are the treatment of choice. For more information, see the section on antiphospholipid antibody syndrome in chapter 9.

1. Tremors in people who have SLE are most commonly due to other causes, such as medications or caffeine.

2. The most common movement disorder is chorea, which causes uncontrollable, sudden movements of the arms, legs, or head, and is treated with steroids. However, it is not uncommon for it to resolve without treatment.

3. Antiphospholipid antibodies are a potential cause of movement disorders in SLE.

## Myelopathy

"Myelo-" comes from the Greek word for both "spinal cord" and "bone marrow." In fact, the ancient Greeks considered the spinal cord to be the "bone marrow" within the vertebral bones of the spine. "Myelopathy" refers to abnormalities of the spinal cord itself. Other terms for lupus myelopathy include "lupus myelitis" and "transverse myelitis." Myelopathy is a rare but dangerous complication of lupus. It is due to inflammation and loss of blood flow to a section of the spinal cord. When it occurs, it does not allow communication between the brain and the section of the body below the level of spinal involvement. This causes paralysis and loss of sensation below this level (e.g., total loss of sensation from the waist down) and loss of bowel and bladder control. Unfortunately, most people have permanent paralysis and numbness below this level, leaving them paraplegic (paralyzed in the legs) or quadriplegic (paralyzed in the legs and arms), even with aggressive, rapid therapy. Myelopathy is treated with high doses of steroids given intravenously, as well as very strong immunosuppressants, especially cyclophosphamide. Many patients are positive for antiphospholipid antibodies, suggesting blood clots as a possible cause, and are treated with blood thinners such as warfarin. Transverse myelitis is included as one of the American College of Rheumatology's classification criteria used in helping to diagnose SLE.

1. Lupus myelitis is also called transverse myelitis and is one of the classification criteria used to help diagnose SLE.

2. Myelopathy can be a devastating and fortunately rare complication of SLE.

3. Myelopathy causes complete loss of sensation in the lower part of the body on both sides, as well as paralysis of both legs (paraplegia) or all four limbs (quadriplegia).

4. Myelopathy is treated with high doses of steroids, cyclophosphamide, and blood thinners. Unfortunately, it has a poor prognosis, with most patients not recovering their baseline neurologic status.

### Seizure Disorders

Seizures (also known as epilepsy) are due to repeated episodes of abnormal electrical activity occurring in the brain. The symptoms depend on which part of the brain is affected. It is one of most common neuropsychiatric problems in people who have SLE, occurring in anywhere from 10% to 20% of them. Seizures are included as one of the American College of Rheumatology's classification criteria used in helping to diagnose SLE.

When most people think of seizures (or epilepsy), they probably think of the person whose body is shaking uncontrollably, who is biting her or his tongue, and who is unconscious during the episode. This certainly can happen and is called a generalized tonic-clonic seizure. However, numerous other types of seizures can also occur, and not all of them cause a loss of consciousness. Sometimes only one part of the body will shake uncontrollably. Some seizures do not cause abnormal movements at all, but instead may cause the person to experience hallucinations. The affected person may see, hear, or even smell things that are not real.

Conditions other than lupus, such as infections, stroke, drugs, cancer, and metabolic problems, can also cause seizures. For that reason, a thorough blood workup, lumbar puncture, and brain MRI are required in the person who has recent-onset seizures to make sure there is no other explanation for the seizures. An EEG (electroencephalogram) is also done. This is a special test, usually done by a neurologist (a doctor specializing in nerve disorders), where electrodes are taped to various parts of the head and the electrical activity of the brain is observed to see if there is any abnormal seizure activity.

Lupus can cause seizures in several different ways. First, seizures can be due to immune-mediated inflammation, in which case it is treated with high doses of steroids and possibly other immunosuppressant medicines. If the person has antiphospholipid antibodies, then the seizures may be due to blood clots in the brain due to the antiphospholipid antibody syndrome. In this case blood thinners such as warfarin would be used. Sometimes there can be a tiny area of permanently damaged area of the brain left by scarring from previous inflammation of the brain from SLE or from a previous CVA (stroke). This tiny area of scar is called an "epileptic nidus" ("nidus" comes from the Latin word for "nest" and refers to a place where something originates) and can lead to recurrent bouts of irritation of the nerves. This problem usually cannot be identified on MRI or other imaging studies but is presumed to be the reason for seizures when other causes are ruled out. In this case, steroids and immunosuppressants will not be helpful. The treatment of choice is to use drugs that treat seizures called antiepileptic medicines. Examples include phenytoin (Dilantin), carbamazepine (Tegretol), clonazepam (Klonopin), gabapentin (Neurontin), and pregabalin (Lyrica).

### KEY POINTS TO REMEMBER

1. Seizures are caused by uncontrollable, repetitive electrical activity occurring along the nerves of the brain and can result in numerous possible symptoms, such as loss of consciousness, jerking movements, twitching, and hallucinations.

2. Another term for seizures is "epilepsy."

3. Seizures are one of the criteria used to help diagnose SLE.

4. If seizures due to SLE are due to active inflammation of the brain, they are treated with high doses of steroids.

5. If the seizures are due to blood clots, they are treated with blood thinners such as heparin and warfarin (Coumadin).

6. If the seizures are due to an area of permanent scarring in the brain (from previous inflammation, blood clot, or stroke), they are treated with anti-seizure medicines.

## Acute Confusional State

Acute confusional state is also called delirium. It usually occurs suddenly, with the person having difficulty staying fully alert. There may be mild drowsiness on one end of the spectrum to complete coma (unable to be awakened) on the other. If awake, the person has difficulty focusing and has problems answering questions appropriately. She or he may show inappropriate behavior and act in a bizarre way, not responding or reacting appropriately to the environment and other people. This can be a very scary situation for the person's loved ones. It is included as one of the American College of Rheumatology's classification criteria used to help diagnose SLE. It is usually seen in the person who has a severe lupus flare with significant inflammation throughout the brain. Other brain problems (such as infections, medicines, and metabolic problems) can cause similar symptoms. Hence, thorough testing, including MRI of the brain, blood tests, and a lumbar puncture, is usually done in the person who has acute confusional state or delirium.

If acute confusional state is found to be due to lupus, then it is treated with high doses of steroids and other immunosuppressant medicines, such as azathioprine, mycophenolate, cyclophosphamide, or rituximab (Rituxan). IVIG (see chapter 35) or plasmapheresis (see chapter 35) may be needed for severe cases.

### KEY POINTS TO REMEMBER

1. Acute confusional state (or delirium) is a severe complication of SLE, causing difficulty with thinking and responding to the environment correctly. Coma is the most severe form of an acute confusional state.

2. It is important to rule out other causes, such as brain infection.

3. Acute confusional state is one of the classification criteria used to help diagnose SLE.

4. Acute confusional state is treated with high doses of steroids and other immunosuppressants, such as azathioprine, mycophenolate, cyclophosphamide, or rituximab (Rituxan). IVIG or plasmapheresis are used for severe cases.

## Anxiety Disorder

Anxiety is a problem where excessive worrying is the predominant symptom and the individual focuses on bad things that may occur in the future. It is often accompanied by other symptoms, such as feeling nervous or "on edge," decreased appetite, difficulty relaxing or sitting still, and being easily annoyed, irritable, or moody. About 25% of people who have SLE will have problems with anxiety. When diagnosed with any chronic disease it is normal to exhibit some anxiety. However, if the symptoms are moderate or severe, affect the person's quality of life, impact relationships, or cause other significant problems—such as difficulty sleeping, fatigue, memory problems, and body pains—then it is considered to be a health problem. In addition, SLE can be worsened by stress, and people who have anxiety disorder can become more easily stressed, which theoretically could in turn worsen their SLE. At the extreme end of the disorder, panic attacks may even occur, manifested by sudden bouts of chest pain, shortness of breath, heart palpitations, sweating, dizziness, and having a general sense of doom. Some people may also develop phobias, such as a fear of being around other people in social situations.

Most lupus experts do not believe that anxiety is actually caused by lupus itself. In other words, there is doubt that it is due to the immune system attacking the brain. However, it was included in the neuropsychiatric syndromes of SLE to make it easier to study anxiety problems in patients who have lupus in a research setting.

Anxiety disorder is thought to be due to chemical imbalances that occur in the brain (such as a lack of neurochemicals like serotonin). These chemicals are very important for normal functioning of the brain and help in dealing with stress and life situations more appropriately. In addition, steroids used in many people who have lupus can actually cause or exacerbate anxiety. In fact, if anxiety is due to steroids, it can be treated by trying to decrease the dose of steroids. Many people who suffer from anxiety may blame all of their problems on stress or may be quick to blame others for their problems, not realizing that they have a chemical imbalance. It can be helpful to take a self-survey such as the GAD-7 (Generalized Anxiety Disorder-7) questionnaire (table 13.2) to see whether you have anxiety disorder. If you score 5 or higher, then you may have an anxiety disorder and you should show the results to your doctor for proper evaluation.

As far as treating anxiety, it is important for people to accept that they have the condition. Many people are resistant to accepting a diagnosis of anxiety. This interferes with their obtaining the proper treatment and prevents them from getting better. It is common for people suffering from anxiety to feel that their symptoms are all due to stress. They may think that how they feel and act is their own fault; they may have feelings of guilt and believe they should be able to control it themselves. Once people accept the diagnosis of anxiety disorder and realize that it is due to chemical imbalances in the brain instead of their own fault, this problem can become easier to treat.

Psychological counseling can be helpful. Counselors can be sociologists, psychologists, or psychiatrists. A counselor can help people learn new coping skills for dealing with the disease and how to interact more appropriately with others and handle life stressors. It has been shown that people with good disease coping strategies do better in the long term with their ability to control mood disorders such as depression and anxiety compared to people who do not have good coping strategies.

Table 13.2  GAD-7 (Screening Test for Anxiety)

| Over the last two weeks, how often have you been bothered by the following problems? | Not at all | Several days | More than half the days | Nearly every day |
|---|---|---|---|---|
| Feeling nervous, anxious, or on edge | 0 | 1 | 2 | 3 |
| Not being able to stop or control worrying | 0 | 1 | 2 | 3 |
| Worrying too much about different things | 0 | 1 | 2 | 3 |
| Having trouble relaxing | 0 | 1 | 2 | 3 |
| Being so restless that it is hard to sit still | 0 | 1 | 2 | 3 |
| Becoming easily annoyed or irritable | 0 | 1 | 2 | 3 |
| Feeling afraid as if something awful might happen | 0 | 1 | 2 | 3 |
| Column totals | ____ | +____ | +____ | +____ |
| Total score = ____ | | | | |

Circle the appropriate number to the right of each list of problems.

Add up each column of numbers; then add the column totals to get your total score.

If you score 5 points or higher, you may have anxiety disorder.

Many people improve significantly using medications that try to adjust the brain chemical imbalances. Most of these medications are listed as antidepressants, but many of them are used to treat other disorders such as anxiety and panic attacks as well. It has also been shown that regular aerobic exercise may be as helpful as medications in some cases, so it is important to try to exercise regularly. Some examples of aerobic exercise include stationary bicycling, walking on a treadmill, brisk walking, jogging, exercising on an elliptical machine, and participating in aerobics or dance classes.

**KEY POINTS TO REMEMBER**

1. Anxiety disorder causes excessive worrying about potential future bad events, and is often accompanied by feeling "on edge," moodiness, difficulty sleeping, and fatigue.

2. Anxiety disorder can sometimes be accompanied by panic attacks, characterized by shortness of breath, chest pain, heart palpitations, excessive sweating, and a general sense of doom.

3. Take the GAD-7 self-survey (table 13.2). If you score 5 points or higher, you may have an anxiety disorder, and you should show the results to your doctor for proper evaluation.

4. Treatment options include counseling, regular aerobic exercise, and medications to try to normalize the chemical imbalances in the brain.

## Cognitive Dysfunction

Cognitive dysfunction means having problems with long-term and/or short-term memory. It can also be accompanied by problems with concentration, judgment, abstract thinking, and personality changes. Up to 90% of people who have SLE have been found to have some problems with memory on formal testing (called neuropsychiatric testing). In most people it is not noticeable, but many people note significant, bothersome problems. On the extreme side, it can even cause overt, severe memory problems called dementia, and the person has difficulty even caring for himself or herself. The memory and concentration problems of SLE are sometimes referred to as "lupus fog." Unfortunately, in some people, the memory problems can be quite devastating, causing great difficulties in their jobs, social interactions, and family life, and can significantly affect their quality of life.

Many possible, different problems can cause the cognitive dysfunction in people who have SLE. These include depression, anxiety disorder, fibromyalgia, medications such as steroids, sleep disorders such as sleep apnea, and many others. The doctor attempts to determine if there are any potentially treatable causes of the cognitive dysfunction, such as depression. Two 2012 studies from the University of California, San Francisco, found that 15% of their patients with SLE had cognitive dysfunction. Being obese, having high blood pressure or a history of stroke, not exercising, and being positive for antiphospholipid antibodies were found more commonly in these patients with memory problems. This suggests that hardening of the arteries (accelerated arteriosclerosis as discussed in chapter 21) may play an important role in this occurring. Therefore, it is important for people who have SLE to do the measures discussed in chapter 21 (dieting, exercising, lowering cholesterol, maintaining normal body weight, not smoking, etc.) in trying to prevent memory problems.

Another study showed that close to one-third of patients with recently diagnosed SLE and cognitive dysfunction also had depression, a well-known cause of memory difficulties. If you have significant problems with memory and your doctor has determined that your lupus is not particularly active, and other problems such as abnormal thyroid levels have been ruled out, then depression, anxiety, and fibromyalgia are some of the most common causes of cognitive dysfunction in people who have SLE. You can take the self-surveys at the beginning of chapter 27 and in tables 13.2 and 13.4 in this chapter to see if you may have fibromyalgia, anxiety, or depression. If depression, anxiety, or fibromyalgia is found to be the cause of the memory problems, it needs to be treated. However, treatment may not be 100% successful. It is important to try other means to improve memory as well (see table 13.3).

Antiphospholipid antibodies may be responsible for memory problems in some people and a trial of blood thinners such as warfarin may be considered. In people who have had definite CNS neuropsychiatric lupus (such as stroke, meningitis, or acute confusional state), residual cognitive dysfunction from previous brain injury may be more common. Organic brain syndrome occurs when a person is left with severe, permanent brain damage due to previous inflammation from CNS lupus. People who have lupus can also develop unrelated causes of dementia such as Alzheimer's disease that may not be due to their lupus at all. In others, the exact cause of the memory problems is never established. Most chronic diseases have been associated with cognitive dysfunction. In fact, a study in 2011 showed no difference in the amount of cognitive dysfunction seen in patients who had lupus compared to that in patients who had rheumatoid arthritis. Therefore, it appears that memory problems are not unique to lupus. They could be related to the problems of dealing a chronic disease; they could share a common cause such as damage to the blood vessels supplying blood to various parts of the brain; or they could be due to the effects on the brain from the inflammation of the autoimmune disorder. Nonetheless, cognitive dysfunction can be a significant problem in many people who have lupus and deserves to be addressed.

Treatment of cognitive dysfunction is aimed at the cause if it can be determined— for example, treating sleep disorders or depression, or using blood thinners if there are high levels of antiphospholipid antibodies. Moderate doses of steroids may be helpful in some people if there is evidence of active lupus in other areas (blood and urine tests will show evidence of this). Unfortunately, treatment can be very frustrating because very few modalities have been shown to be helpful. It can be helpful to learn how to deal with the memory problems by seeing a memory specialist to learn how to cope with forgetfulness using special techniques. Help can be found in clinics dealing with dementia, Alzheimer's disease, and closed head injury. Seeing a neurologist or psychiatrist (the experts who most commonly treat people with cognitive dysfunction) can be helpful. There are also things you can do on your own to try to improve your memory (table 13.3). It usually requires a strong effort on the affected person's part to work on improving memory, but the rewards can also be significant in terms of quality of life.

One key recommendation is regular exercise. More studies are consistently showing the importance of exercise and its role in cognitive dysfunction, especially in diseases such as Alzheimer's disease. Studies show that people who exercise regularly are less likely to develop these problems compared to people who do not exercise. A 2012 study further validated the importance of exercise to help with the memory problems of lupus. The study evaluated 138 women who had SLE and found that only 5% of physically active women had cognitive dysfunction, while 23% of those who were not physically active had memory problems. The women who had cognitive dysfunction in this study were also much more likely to be obese as well. Lupus experts do not know why exercise is so important for retaining good memory and thinking abilities. It may very well play a role in the maintenance of good blood supply to the brain, but more research is needed. If you have lupus, it is very important to exercise regularly. Make sure to read and put into practice the measures recommended in chapters 7 and 38 regarding exercise and SLE.

### KEY POINTS TO REMEMBER

1. "Cognitive dysfunction" is the term used when there is difficulty with memory.

2. Cognitive dysfunction is a very common problem in people who have SLE.

**Table 13.3** Ways to Cope with Cognitive Dysfunction

- Decrease distractions in your environment to make it easier to focus (such as turning off the TV and music).
- Do not multitask; learn to concentrate on one activity at a time.
- Eliminate clutter in your life; learn to throw away or give away excessive objects and papers. Take a class on how to de-clutter.
- Keep organized.
- Carry around a small notepad to take notes and do so frequently. Review your notes later that day.
- Use sticky notes at home and work and put them in appropriate places to help you remember things.
- Keep a calendar and list of addresses and phone numbers with you at all times. Cell phones and smart phones easily serve this purpose.
- Ask that only one person speak at a time during conversations.
- During a conversation, concentrate on listening to the other person. Do not do anything else such as looking at your cell phone or newspaper or eating.
- Do not be afraid to ask people to repeat themselves when they speak if you miss something.
- Get into the habit of repeating things over and over out loud or in your head. For example, when you first meet someone, make a concentrated effort to say the person's name in your mind several times, and then repeat her or his name in the conversation as well.
- "Train the brain": do mental exercises such as crossword puzzles, Scrabble, or Sudoku daily.
- Use books to learn how to improve your memory such as *The Memory Book* by Harry Lorayne and Jerry Lucas or *The Memory Bible: An Innovative Strategy for Keeping Your Brain Young* by Gary Small.
- Keep your mind active: volunteer, continue working if possible.
- Challenge your brain by learning new skills, hobbies.
- Increase interactions with others to stimulate your mind: establish new friendships and relationships.
- Get treatment for disorders that can cause cognitive dysfunction. Take the self-surveys for anxiety disorder (table 13.2), depression (table 13.4), and obstructive sleep apnea (table 6.3).
- Exercise regularly.
- Decrease stress in your life; simplify your life; learn to say "no" when asked to do favors if you are a "yes" person.
- Be open about your memory problems with friends and family so they can understand and help.
- Get plenty of sleep, and practice all the good sleep hygiene techniques listed in table 6.2 regularly.

3. Cognitive dysfunction can be caused by depression, fibromyalgia, medications, sleep disorders, or thyroid disorders, which may occur along with lupus.

4. Take the self-surveys for fibromyalgia (beginning of chapter 27), anxiety (table 13.2), and depression (table 13.4) if you have cognitive dysfunction to determine if these may be the cause of your memory and concentration problems.

5. Treatment is aimed at the cause of the memory problem (such as treating depression).

6. Steroids or blood thinners may be tried in some situations to see if they help.

7. Seeing a neurologist, psychiatrist, or someone experienced in helping people with memory problems can be helpful. Attending clinics specializing in dementia, Alzheimer's disease, and closed brain injuries can be beneficial.

8. Do everything listed in table 13.3 to learn to cope with memory problems.

## Mood Disorder

Mood disorders include depression and bipolar disorder. There is a disturbance of mood causing either a depressed mood (depression) or an elevated mood (called mania or hypomania depending on severity). Mood disorders are one of the most common neuropsychiatric problems occurring in people who have SLE, affecting up to 57% of them. Lupus experts do not feel that depression is due to the immune system abnormalities of lupus itself, but rather is due to the complex problems of dealing with a chronic disease, taking multiple medications, and having difficulty coping. It is due to chemical imbalances in the brain. Depression is the most common psychological problem in people who have lupus. People who are depressed may feel "down in the dumps" or "have the blues." They often have difficulty sleeping, have increased or decreased appetite resulting in a gain or loss of weight, and may withdraw from social situations because of the way they feel. People who have depression may have difficulty with memory and forget things to the point that they are afraid they have developed dementia or Alzheimer's disease. Many depressed people will stop doing activities that they used to find enjoyable (called anhedonia) and often lose interest in sex (loss of libido). Some people who have depression also have feelings of guilt above and beyond what is rational. Depression can also cause problems that the person may not even realize are due to depression, such as body pain, severe fatigue, and stomach upset. Extremely depressed people may feel like it is not worth living and feel like they cannot go on. They may even consider committing suicide. Unfortunately, some people who have depression will carry this through. Depressed people are more apt to be noncompliant with their lupus treatment. They are less likely to take their medications as directed and to follow through with treatment recommendations. This leads to a higher rate of severe complications from their lupus.

Identifying depression and treating it in people who have SLE is very important as it does not always correlate with how severe the lupus is and can be more disabling than the lupus itself. It can be a major cause of memory problems, insomnia, body pain, and poor life quality. It is not uncommon for people who suffer from depression to be resistant to the diagnosis and treatment. It is easier to blame their lupus, stress, or pain as the cause of their depression than to acknowledge that it may be the depression itself that is causing problems with coping with stress and causing pain, fatigue, and insomnia. A 2011 study in the journal *Lupus* showed that among 125 patients who had SLE, patients were more apt to have a poor quality of life due to depression instead of having severe lupus disease activity. This means that getting lupus under better control would not necessarily help them feel better at all, but treating the depression would be more important in terms of helping them feel better. This is why I strongly encourage you to take the depression screening test if you suffer from fatigue, insomnia, uncontrolled pain, and difficulties with memory; if you are depressed, it is very important that it be treated to help you deal with these particular problems.

Just as with anxiety disorder, it is important for the person who has depression to first accept the diagnosis to get proper treatment. There are numerous self-surveys that can determine whether you are depressed or not. Since depression occurs so commonly in people who have SLE and responds well to treatment, I would encourage you to take one of these tests. One of them is called the PHQ-9 (Patient Health Questionnaire-9) depression questionnaire (table 13.4). A score of 5 or higher suggests that you may have depression, while a score of 10 or above means that you most likely have major depression. If you score 5 or higher, then you should show the results to your doctor for a proper evaluation. In particular, if you have any thoughts at all of hurting yourself or others, please contact your doctor immediately. Suicide and injuring others are two of the most dangerous complications of severe depression and are avoidable with proper treatment.

If you score high on these self-survey tests, you may want to consider exercising first as a form of treatment. Quite a few studies have shown that regular aerobic exercise can be just as effective as antidepressant medications in the treatment of depression. Therefore, consider doing activities such as brisk walking, stationary bicycling, swimming, using an elliptical machine, and doing aerobics five days a week. Of course, you should get approval from your doctor first about what is safe for you to do in terms of exercise. Another nonmedical way to treat depression is to see a psychotherapist or cognitive behavioral therapist. These are most commonly psychologists and sociologists and may be found in lists of counselors, psychologists, and sociologists with a special interest in treating depression. They can help by talking to you, usually over multiple sessions, to learn if there are particular reasons why you are depressed. They can help you focus on stressors and behavioral issues that you may have control over to try to lessen the severity of your depression. If depression significantly affects the quality of life, there are numerous antidepressants available to treat depression. The number of available treatments and their proper use are beyond the scope of this book. If you are affected significantly by depression, make sure to consult your rheumatologist or primary care provider for assistance. The expertise of a psychiatrist is sometimes needed for severe cases.

It is very common for people who have depression to feel like it is their fault, or that it is just a normal reaction to their illness. Certainly, it is normal to have some reactive depression when faced with a chronic disease, but when it interferes with your quality of life and how you react to those around you and your environment, it becomes a significant health problem. Just as with anxiety disorder, it is treated with psychologi-

Table 13.4 PHQ-9 Depression Questionnaire

| Over the last two weeks, how often have you been bothered by any of the following problems? | Not at all | Several days | More than half the days | Nearly every day |
|---|---|---|---|---|
| Little interest or pleasure in doing things | 0 | 1 | 2 | 3 |
| Feeling down, depressed, or hopeless | 0 | 1 | 2 | 3 |
| Trouble falling or staying asleep, or sleeping too much | 0 | 1 | 2 | 3 |
| Feeling tired or having little energy | 0 | 1 | 2 | 3 |
| Poor appetite or overeating | 0 | 1 | 2 | 3 |
| Feeling bad about yourself, or that you are a failure, or have let yourself or your family down | 0 | 1 | 2 | 3 |
| Trouble concentrating on things, such as reading the newspaper or watching television | 0 | 1 | 2 | 3 |
| Moving or speaking so slowly that other people could have noticed. Or the opposite, being so fidgety or restless that you have been moving around a lot more than usual | 0 | 1 | 2 | 3 |
| Thoughts that you would be better off dead or of hurting yourself in some way | 0 | 1 | 2 | 3 |
| Column totals Total score = _____ | ____ | + ___ | + ___ | + ___ |

Circle the corresponding number score to the right of each list of columns. Add up the circled numbers in each column, then total these results. Score of 5–9 suggests mild depression; score of ≥ 10 suggests major depression.

cal counseling, learning new coping skills, medications, and exercise. If the depression has been caused by or exacerbated by steroids such as prednisone, it also may be important to lower the dose of steroids. This should always be done under the direct supervision of your doctor to prevent a flare in your lupus and potential severe withdrawal problems that can occur when steroid doses are decreased too quickly.

The opposite mood disorder from depression are mania and hypomania where mood is elated, euphoric, and people feel like they are on top of the world, require little sleep and have lots of energy. It usually coexists with alternating bouts of depression or what is called bipolar disorder. Bipolar disorder is not nearly as common in people who have SLE as depression. It is essential for people who have bipolar disorder to take medications regularly to decrease the severity of their illness.

1. Mood disorders include depressed mood (depression) on one end of the spectrum and elevated mood (mania and hypomania as a part of bipolar disorder) on the other end of the spectrum.

2. Mood disorders are chemical imbalance disorders of the brain and are not considered to be directly due to inflammation of the brain from SLE.

3. Take a self-survey (table 13.4) to see if you may be depressed.

4. If you have suicidal thoughts or think about injuring others, see your doctor immediately.

5. Consider regular aerobic exercise, or seeing a counselor who specializes in depression. Antidepressant medications may be needed if these modalities do not work.

6. Many people who have depression or bipolar disorder do not realize it and often refuse treatment.

7. People who suffer from bipolar disorder need to take medications regularly to lessen the effects of their mood swings.

## Psychosis

Psychosis is characterized by disordered and bizarre thinking, including delusions and hallucinations. A delusion refers to a person believing that something is occurring when the facts show otherwise. Some classic examples would be thinking that people, such as the CIA, are out to get you, or that you are actually someone else, such as Napoleon. Hallucinations mean that a person senses things are present that are not really there. These can occur with all the senses, such as hearing voices that are not there, seeing things that are not there, smelling unusual smells that are not present, and feeling things such as ants crawling on the body. Psychosis can present along with an acute confusional state (discussed earlier in this chapter). Psychosis can occur in up to 10% of people who have SLE, typically within the first year. It has been included as one of the American College of Rheumatology's classification criteria used in helping to diagnose SLE. Most people who have SLE who have psychosis do so because of the effects of the lupus on the brain and require high doses of steroids for treatment. Occasionally, psychiatric medications that are used to treat psychotic conditions such as schizophrenia are prescribed to help control these bizarre processes.

It is also important for the doctor to make sure that there is not another reason for having psychotic episodes. For example, using illicit drugs such as cocaine and methamphetamines may cause psychosis. Just as with mood disorders, occasionally steroids such as prednisone can cause psychosis, especially when given in high doses. This can present quite a challenge to physicians because the way to treat lupus psychosis is to increase the steroids, but the way to treat steroid-induced psychosis is to reduce the steroids. It is not always possible to tell which is the cause, and various blood and brain tests may not be helpful.

234

1. Psychosis is characterized by disordered, bizarre thinking and includes problems with hallucinations and delusions.

2. Other important causes of psychosis must be ruled out, such as the effects of medications like steroids and the use of illicit drugs such as cocaine.

3. If psychosis is due to SLE, it can be due to inflammation of the brain and requires the use of high doses of steroids or other immunosuppressant medicines.

4. Therapies used to treat psychotic disorders such as schizophrenia may need to be used as well.

## Peripheral Nervous System

The peripheral nervous system involves all the nerves that travel to and from the brain and spinal cord to the rest of the body. Lupus can affect them in many ways. Just as with SLE affecting the CNS, many other factors can potentially affect the peripheral nervous system, such as diabetes, toxins, medications, metabolic problems, or infections such as Lyme disease. Therefore, multiple tests are necessary such as blood tests, EMG testing (as discussed in the myositis section of chapter 7), and sometimes a lumbar puncture (as discussed previously in the CNS section).

### Acute Inflammatory Demyelinating Polyradiculoneuropathy (Guillain-Barré Syndrome)

Acute inflammatory demyelinating polyradiculoneuropathy is a rare neurologic problem in SLE, with very few cases actually being reported. It occurs when SLE causes the loss of myelin sheaths around the nerves of the peripheral nervous system. The myelin sheath is the coating surrounding nerves that allows them to transmit electrical signals more quickly. This disorder causes the rapid onset of weakness and paralysis of the legs. The doctor will note the loss of reflexes on examination and a lumbar puncture and EMG testing confirm the diagnosis. As with many severe lupus nerve problems, it is treated with high doses of steroids. Sometimes a type of treatment called plasmapheresis can help as well. Plasmapheresis is a highly specialized treatment most commonly performed at large hospitals and major medical centers. It entails blood being taken from a person's body; antibodies are then filtered out. The treated blood (with the good parts remaining) is then transfused back into the person's body. The person usually recovers well as long as treatment is started soon enough. However, sometimes this syndrome can turn into a chronic neurologic problem (called chronic inflammatory demyelinating polyneuropathy, or CIDP for short) causing permanent problems with leg and/or arm weakness along with tingling sensations in the legs and/or arms.

1. Acute inflammatory demyelinating polyradiculoneuropathy is more commonly known as Guillain-Barré syndrome.

2. This disorder is a rare problem in SLE that causes abrupt onset of weakness in the legs and is suspected by finding the loss of normal reflexes on physical examination.

3. This syndrome is treated with high doses of steroids and sometimes with plasmapheresis.

## Autonomic Disorders

The autonomic nervous system is responsible for the electrical activity of all of the bodily functions over which we do not have conscious control. Autonomic nerves are the nerves that keep the heart beating correctly, constrict and dilate the pupils of the eyes, keep the muscles moving in the intestinal tract to transport digesting food in the right direction, and cause the sweat glands to secrete sweat when a person is hot or excited. Autonomic nerves are also responsible for some functions that you can sometimes control, such as breathing and blinking. SLE can affect these nerves, but usually not significantly in the vast majority of people. However, if these nerves are affected, it can lead to constipation, dizziness when standing up, and excessive sweating, among other difficulties. These problems can also be seen due to various medications as well as other medical problems, which makes a proper diagnosis challenging. If a problem is found to be due to SLE, the person is treated with steroids.

1. The autonomic nervous system refers to the peripheral nerves that cause our bodies to do things that we usually do not consciously control (such as blinking, beating of the heart, sweating, moving food through the intestinal tract, and regulating the blood pressure).

2. An autonomic disorder rarely causes any problems in people who have SLE.

3. When problems of the autonomic nerves occur, it is very important to make sure it is not due to medications.

4. If an autonomic disorder is felt to be due to SLE, a trial of steroids may be considered.

## Mononeuropathy and Mononeuritis Multiplex

When SLE attacks one large nerve of the peripheral nervous system it is called a mononeuropathy ("mono-" means "one"). If it attacks several large nerves that are not related to each other (i.e., occurring in different parts of the body), then it is called mononeuritis multiplex. These types of neuropathies usually cause a combination of weakness and numbness and/or tingling sensations in one part of the body. Developing "foot drop" in one foot (not being able to raise the foot upward) while the other muscles of the legs work fine would be an example of a mononeuropathy. If someone has a right foot drop, an inability to move the left wrist, and tingling in these two extremities, it would be considered mononeuritis multiplex. If one large nerve coming directly from the spinal cord is affected, then it is called a radiculopathy and is considered a type of mononeuropathy as well. These problems are felt to be most likely due to vasculitis (inflammation of the blood vessels) affecting the blood supply to these particular nerves and causing severe damage, resulting in weakness and numbness. Sometimes a nerve biopsy, especially of the sural nerve in the leg, may be done to confirm the diagnosis. It is treated with high doses of steroids and other immunosuppressants such as azathioprine, mycophenolate, or cyclophosphamide. It may take a person a long time to recover strength—up to a year until maximum improvement is reached. The severity of the damage to the nerve and the length of time prior to initiation of treatment tend to predict whether full recovery is possible or not. If a long time passes before it is treated, or if the involvement is particularly severe, there may be permanent weakness and numbness in the affected area.

**KEY POINTS TO REMEMBER**

1. If one large peripheral nerve is affected by SLE, it is called a mononeuropathy. One of the most common forms is foot drop where there is difficulty lifting the foot up, causing problems with walking.

2. If two or more large nerves are affected by SLE, it is called mononeuritis multiplex.

3. Vasculitis due to SLE is the most common cause of these problems and is usually treated with high doses of steroids, along with other immunosuppressant medicines.

## Cranial Neuropathy, Plexopathy, and Polyneuropathy

*Cranial Neuropathy.* The cranial nerves are the peripheral nerves that come out directly from the brain and are responsible for such functions as blinking, smiling, moving the tongue, moving the eyes, seeing, maintaining balance, and hearing. When lupus affects any of these nerves, the person may have double vision, drooping of the eyes or mouth, numbness of the face, loss of eyesight, vertigo (a type of dizziness), ringing in the ears, and hearing loss. One example of a cranial neuropathy is commonly called Bell's palsy (more appropriately called seventh cranial nerve palsy or facial nerve palsy). Involvement of this nerve causes the muscles on one side of the face to become weak causing difficulty with smiling and difficulty closing the eye. It especially can be seen in people who have secondary Sjögren's syndrome along with their SLE.

Cranial nerve palsies are most commonly due to inflammation of the nerves—either due to local meningitis or due to vasculitis of the nerve, which causes a decreased supply of blood to the nerve—and is treated with high doses of steroids. However, sometimes it can be due to antiphospholipid antibodies causing blood clots in the arteries, leading to nerve damage, in which case blood thinners such as warfarin (Coumadin) would be required (see the discussion of antiphospholipid antibody syndrome in chapter 9). In some people who have high levels of antiphospholipid antibodies in their blood, the exact cause may not be easy to establish. In this case, both high doses of steroids and blood thinners would be used.

*Plexopathy.* The peripheral nerves that directly connect to the spinal cord are called radicular nerves with one pair of nerves (one for the left side of the body and one for the right side) branching from each vertebral segment of the spine. For example, there are usually five lumbar vertebrae in the lower back, and each vertebra has its own pair of radicular nerves leaving the spinal cord, and they are numbered L1–L5. However, these radicular nerves actually intertwine together into what is called a plexus (which comes from the Latin word for a braid). This occurs throughout the spinal cord. If lupus causes damage or inflammation to this collection of nerves, then it is called a plexopathy. A plexopathy would typically cause both numbness and weakness in one arm or one leg. Usually there is significant pain in the arm or leg, described as a burning pain, often with tingling or numbness. Sometimes this pain can be excruciating. It is also treated with high doses of steroids and is diagnosed with an EMG test. This type of nerve problem is rare in people who have lupus.

*Polyneuropathy.* Polyneuropathy is more commonly called peripheral neuropathy by doctors. It typically affects the nerves that are responsible for sensation and feeling things more so than with muscle strength and motor activity. Typical symptoms are numbness and tingling of the feet more commonly than the hands. This can feel like a "pins and needles" sensation, and can sometimes be associated with burning pain or pain that feels like an electrical sensation that comes and goes. Often the pain is worse at night when the person is in bed, causing difficulty sleeping. It occurs in 10% to 20% of people who have SLE. If it occurs abruptly and severely it is treated with steroids. However, in most people it comes on very slowly and steroids may not be that helpful. It is also diagnosed using an EMG test. If the symptoms are mild, it may not need to be treated at all, but if the discomfort is severe enough, medications that can reduce nerve pain are prescribed. There are many different medications that can be used, including opioids such as tramadol, antidepressants such as nortriptyline and duloxetine (Cymbalta), and antiepileptic medicines such as pregabalin (Lyrica). The Patient Resources at the end of this book lists some useful books that can help lupus patients deal with the problems from peripheral neuropathy.

### KEY POINTS TO REMEMBER

1. Cranial neuropathy, plexopathy, and polyneuropathy occur due to inflammation or damage to peripheral nerves and cause weakness, numbness, or burning pain in the areas affected.

2. Cranial neuropathy generally affects the nerves of the face and can cause difficulty with speaking, hearing, balance, seeing, and facial movements.

3. These conditions may be treated with steroids and other immunosuppressant medicines.

4. Nerve pain medicines may also be needed if pain is particularly severe.

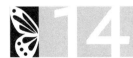

# The Exocrine Gland System

## The Most Common Overlap Syndrome with Lupus

In 1933, Dr. Henrik Sjögren (pronounced SHOW-grin), a Swedish ophthalmologist (eye doctor), published a paper describing nineteen patients who had dry eyes (keratoconjunctivitis sicca) and dry mouth entitled "On Knowledge of Keratoconjunctivitis Sicca. Keratitis Filiformis due to Lacrimal Gland Hypofunction." Loosely translated in layperson's terms, this means "What I have learned about dry eyes. Inflammation of the clear part of the eye due to the tear gland not producing enough tears." Most of his patients who had dry eyes had rheumatoid arthritis. It was eventually discovered that this was a common problem in systemic autoimmune diseases, and the autoimmune condition that could cause dry eyes and dry mouth became linked to his name. If Sjögren's syndrome occurs alone it is called primary Sjögren's syndrome. If it occurs in conjunction with another autoimmune disease, such as with SLE, it is called secondary Sjögren's syndrome.

As discussed in chapter 2, Sjögren's syndrome (SS) is an autoimmune disease that causes inflammation and damage to the glands of the body called the exocrine glands that produce moisture. Dry eyes and dry mouth are the two most common problems that it causes. Sjögren's syndrome occurs most commonly along with rheumatoid arthritis, but about 10% of SS patients have SLE. On the other hand, about one-third of people who have SLE have secondary Sjögren's syndrome. Therefore, Sjögren's syndrome occurs commonly in people who have lupus. This is a type of overlap syndrome and is in fact the most common overlap syndrome that doctors see in SLE patients. Recall from chapter 2 that an overlap syndrome occurs when a person has two or more systemic autoimmune diseases; in other words, he or she has two autoimmune diseases that overlap each other. People who have SLE who are positive for anti-SSA and/or anti-SSB antibodies are especially at increased risk of developing Sjögren's syndrome.

Just as in primary Sjögren's syndrome, dry eyes and dry mouth are the most common problems in secondary Sjögren's syndrome. However, the throat, nose, ears, skin, and vagina can also become excessively dry. Many people who develop Sjögren's syndrome do not even realize that it is related to their lupus. They often regard the dryness problems as not being important until they become severe enough to discuss with their doctor. The doctor may observe the dryness on physical examination and ask the patient about it. Another common route of being diagnosed with Sjögren's is when someone reads about it in a pamphlet, on a poster, or in a magazine, or hears about it on the news. This information can cause affected persons to realize that they may have an important medical condition causing dryness and bring it up to their physicians. With the announcement in 2011 of the famous tennis player Venus Williams having Sjögren's syndrome, it has become more public. On average, people who have Sjögren's syndrome have problems with dryness for an average of six to seven years before a person brings it to the attention of her doctors and a proper diagnosis is made. Although, initially, these dryness problems may be looked upon as being mild and annoying, over time they can become severe, interfering with many important aspects of a person's life and altering the quality of life. However, much can be done to decrease these problems. This chapter goes into more detail about this common complication of SLE.

· · · ·

The exocrine glands are glands that secrete fluids through tubes (called ducts) to the outside of the body—"exo-" means "outside" (table 14.1). They are different from endocrine glands (such as the thyroid gland), which secrete substances directly into the bloodstream of the body—"endo-" means "inside." The exocrine glands include lacrimal glands (see figure 16.1) that secrete tears in the eyes, salivary glands that secrete saliva, sebaceous and sweat glands that secrete oils and sweat on the skin, and mucosal glands that secrete lubricating fluids to lubricate areas such as inside the nose, ear canals, and vagina.

People who have primary Sjögren's syndrome may require a biopsy of the minor salivary glands in the lip to accurately diagnose the condition (discussed in chapter 2). However, in people who have SLE, this usually is not required. The finding of significant dryness in the eyes or mouth is usually sufficient to support the diagnosis (as long as other factors such as medications that cause dryness are not present). Being

Table 14.1 Exocrine Gland Involvement in Sjögren's Syndrome

- Lacrimal glands: secrete tears; Sjögren's syndrome can cause dry eyes, lacrimal gland swelling

- Meibomian glands: secrete oily film on eyes; Sjögren's syndrome can cause dry eyes and lid inflammation

- Salivary glands: secrete saliva; Sjögren's syndrome can cause dry mouth, dental cavities, gingivitis, thrush, sore mouth, mouth sores, trouble swallowing, hoarseness, and parotid gland enlargement

- Sebaceous glands, ear canal: secrete lubrication in ear canals; Sjögren's syndrome can cause dry, itchy ear canals

- Nasal mucosa glands: moistens inside of nose; Sjögren's syndrome can cause dry nose, bleeding from nose, sinus congestion

- Sebaceous and sweat glands: secrete oils and sweat; Sjögren's syndrome can cause dry, itchy skin

- Vaginal mucosal glands: secrete vaginal lubrication; Sjögren's syndrome can cause vaginal dryness, painful intercourse

positive for auto-antibodies commonly seen in Sjögren's syndrome (such as rheuma-toid factor, SSA antibodies, and SSB antibodies) are also supportive. In fact, being SSB antibody positive carries a very high risk for developing Sjögren's syndrome. It is very unusual to be positive for SSB antibody and not develop Sjögren's syndrome at some point.

### Dry Eyes (Lacrimal and Meibomian Glands)

When SS causes inflammation and damage to the glands that secrete tears (the lac-rimal glands—"lacrima" is Latin for "tear") it causes decreased tear production. The potential problems of dry eyes from SS are numerous and are listed in table 14.2. Tears are very important for coating the clear part of the eye (the cornea) and they allow the eyelids to blink comfortably over the cornea. If your eyes are healthy, tears should be in your eyes all day, every day, not just when you are crying. Tears keep the cornea hydrat-ed and protect it. The medical terms often given for dry eyes include "keratoconjuncti-vitis sicca" ("kerato-" refers to the cornea and "sicca" means dry, therefore it means in-flammation of the cornea and conjunctiva of the eye due to dryness), "xerophthalmia" ("xero-" meaning dry and "-ophthalmia" refers to the eyes), and "dysfunctional tear syndrome." These terms are interchangeable and refer to the same thing.

In addition to decreasing tear production from the tear gland, Sjögren's syndrome also causes the Meibomian glands of the eyes to malfunction. The Meibomian glands are located on the rims of the eyelids and secrete an oily film called meibum that coats the tear film on the eyes to decrease its evaporation. Meibum also lubricates, allowing the eyelids to move even more smoothly over the eyeballs. With less production of mei-bum, the tear film evaporates more quickly, which is especially problematic in the per-son who has SS where there is less tear film being produced already. In addition, there is less oily lubrication, which adds to the overall dryness of the eye. The combination of the less production of tears by the lacrimal glands, the faster evaporation of the tear film due to the decreased production of the oily layer of meibum, plus its lack of oily lubrication, all add up to cause significant problems with lubrication of the eyeballs and overlying eyelids.

**Table 14.2** Symptoms of Dry Eyes in Sjögren's Syndrome

- Dry, gritty eyes
- Sensation of a foreign object in the eye
- Redness of the white (sclera) of the eyes
- Blurred vision
- Photophobia (intolerance of light)
- Ropey, thick secretions in the eyes, especially when first awakening from sleep
- Difficulty opening eyes in the morning due to dryness
- Red, tender eyelids (blepharitis)

Common symptoms of dry eyes include a feeling of grittiness in the eyes; feeling like a foreign object is in the eyes; having thick, ropey secretions at the inner portion of the eyes, especially after first waking up from sleep; and having redness and a burning sensation in the eyes. Less tears are normally produced while sleeping, so the dryness is especially pronounced when first waking up. Eye dryness is an important problem to identify, diagnose, and treat. If left untreated, it can potentially cause permanent damage to the cornea, and this can cause permanent problems with vision. Usually the symptoms of dry eyes come on very slowly—over several to many years. If you have any of these symptoms, you should inform your doctor sooner rather than later.

Occasionally, but not very often, SS can also cause the lacrimal gland of the eye, located at the upper outer portion of the eye, to become swollen due to the inflammation. The upper outer eyelid will appear puffy if this occurs.

Since the eyelids of the person who has SS are moving over a drier, less lubricated surface, some of the skin of the eyelids can become irritated, causing a condition called blepharitis (which means inflammation of the eyelids). The eyelids may become sore and reddish in color, often accompanied by a gritty sensation in the eyes along with some crusting.

Diagnosing dry eyes can be done in several different ways. One test is called the Schirmer test (photograph 14.1). A small strip of sterile paper is placed under the lower eyelid, with part of it hanging down outside of the eye. The person closes her or his eyes for five minutes. Although there is some slight irritation during the test, it is a painless procedure. After five minutes, the paper is removed from the eyes and the amount of paper that is wetted with tears is measured in millimeters. If less than 5 mm of the paper is moistened with tears, it is considered abnormal, and the person is considered to have decreased tear production.

Another test is the Rose Bengal stain test. This is performed by an eye doctor (either an ophthalmologist or an optometrist). Some drops of Rose Bengal stain are applied to the eyes, and then the eyes are examined with a special instrument called a slit lamp. If there is any damage to the cornea due to dry eyes, the doctor will see it appear in color on the exam due to the Rose Bengal staining. This stain is temporary and goes away quickly.

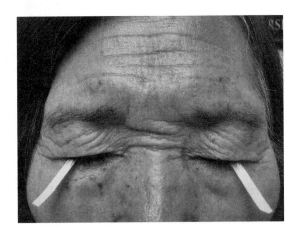

**Photo 14.1** Schirmer test to diagnose dry eyes in Sjögren's syndrome.

Another test that can measure dry eyes is the "tear break-up time" test, also performed by an ophthalmologist or an optometrist. A liquid containing fluorescein is added to the eyes. Fluorescein is a lime green–colored liquid that makes it easier to see the layer of tears on the surface of the eye. Then the person is asked not to blink while the eye doctor watches the coloration of the tear film. When the doctor starts to see dry spots appear on the surface of the eye, then that is the time entered as the tear break-up time. The more tears, and the better quality of tears that someone has, the longer this time is. Normally it should take more than ten seconds for the dry spots to start to appear on the eye.

People who have Sjögren's syndrome can do many things to help with the various dryness problems (table 14.3). Therapies specifically aimed at keeping the eyes moistened are listed in table 14.4. Some medical studies suggest that taking supplements that are high in omega-3 fatty acids may be beneficial, and there is at least one good medical study showing them to be effective. Omega-3 fatty acids can be found in fish oil and flaxseed oil supplements.

If dryness continues to be a problem even using these measures, doctors can try other measures to help. For example, using a prescription medication called cyclosporine (Restasis) can be very useful. Cyclosporine is an immunosuppressant medication. One drop is placed in each eye twice a day. Restasis decreases the amount of inflammation in the lacrimal and Meibomian glands, allowing them to produce more tears and meibum so that the eyes and eyelids are better lubricated. If this does not work, another intervention involves the ophthalmologist (eye doctor) inserting tiny plugs into the ducts of the eyes. The lacrimal ducts (tear ducts) are located at the inner lower portion of each eye. After the ophthalmologist plugs the ducts, tears will drain away from the eyes slower, allowing the tear film to increase and the eyes become moister.

### Dry Mouth (Salivary Glands)

When SS causes inflammation and damage to the glands that secrete saliva (the salivary glands), it causes decreased saliva production. Along with dry eyes, these are the two most common complaints in people who have SS (dry eyes and dry mouth), or at least they are often the two most bothersome problems. Just as with dry eyes, dryness

**Table 14.3** General Measures to Alleviate Dryness in Sjögren's Syndrome

- Drink plenty of fluids, especially water, throughout the day.

- Avoid dehydrating fluids such as alcohol and caffeine.

- Avoid smoking, which dries out the mouth, eyes, and nose.

- Use a humidifier in each room of your house where you spend significant time, especially the bedroom. Keep air humidity about 50%. Clean and dry out humidifiers daily to prevent mold and fungus. Another option is to have a centralized humidifier installed in the furnace but make sure to also have a central air UV light plus filter to decrease risk of spreading infections such as fungus and mold throughout the house.

**Table 14.4**  Keeping the Eyes Moist in Sjögren's Syndrome

- Do everything listed in table 14.3.
- Use artificial tears every several hours throughout the day. Make sure to use preservative-free preparations. Use regularly; do not wait for your eyes to dry out.
- Use artificial tears more often when flying (drier air), or when reading or doing computer work (you blink less during these activities).
- An alternative to artificial tears is to get a prescription for Lacrisert from your doctor (it is inserted in the lower eyelids to moisturize the eyes all day).
- If you have sore, irritated eyelids due to blepharitis, try cleaning them daily with baby shampoo. Use warm, moist cloths on the eyes intermittently to keep them comfortable.
- Carry a wet washcloth in a zip-lock bag when you travel to apply to your eyes when needed.
- Clean eyelids daily with warm water.
- If light bothers your eyes, wear sunglasses or have the lenses in your eyeglasses tinted with FL-41 (a rose-colored filter).
- Keep makeup and lotions away from your eyelids.
- Use a lubricating eye ointment or gel at night before you go to bed. At first, you can apply it just to your eyelids and lashes to see if it helps. If not, apply one-eighth inch under your lower eyelids.
- Consider wearing moisture chamber glasses, moisturizing goggles, or wrap-around sunglasses to keep your eyes moister (such as from Eye Eco brand).
- When reading, watching TV, watching a movie, or doing computer work, blink your eyes regularly on purpose to keep them moist. We naturally blink a lot less when doing these activities.
- Do not rub your eyes.
- Avoid wearing contacts unless under direct supervision of an ophthalmologist.
- Take fish oil, flaxseed oil, or omega-3 fatty acid supplements. (Natural sources such as fish, flaxseed, walnuts, and olive oil are even better.)
- Ask your doctor to prescribe Restasis eye drops.
- Systemic medicines such as pilocarpine (Salagen) and cevimeline (Evoxac) may be helpful.
- Ask your ophthalmologist to insert tear duct plugs, which decrease the drainage of fluids from the eye surface.

of the mouth can cause many different problems (table 14.5), including dryness of the passages that lead down to the esophagus (the tube that leads to the stomach), as well the trachea (windpipe), and vocal cords. Dryness in these areas can cause difficulty swallowing, coughing, and hoarseness.

The larger major salivary glands are the parotid, submandibular, and sublingual salivary glands (see figure 14.1). The parotid glands are located on both sides of the face just below the ears and covering the angle of the jaw. The submandibular glands ("sub-" means "under," and the mandible is the large lower jawbone) are located underneath the jaw in the soft tissue back toward the throat. The sublingual glands are located underneath the tongue ("lingua" means "tongue"). Although the parotid and sublingual glands are usually not noticeable in a healthy person, the submandibular glands can be felt as soft, rounded areas located above the Adam's apple toward the sides.

Inflammation of these glands from SS can cause the glands to enlarge, making them more noticeable, especially the parotid glands. This can sometimes cause a chipmunk-like appearance. If a lot of inflammation occurs in the salivary glands, they can become tender and painful in addition to being swollen. This is not uncommon with the parotid glands and is called parotitis.

**Table 14.5**  Symptoms of Dry Mouth in Sjögren's Syndrome

- Swelling of the parotid glands on the sides of the jaw
- Parotid gland pain due to parotitis
- Tongue sticking to the roof of the mouth
- Increased feeling of needing to drink fluids throughout the day
- Insomnia, waking up with dry mouth, and having daytime fatigue
- Difficulty swallowing crackers and other dry food without fluids
- Sore throat
- Dry, cracked, sore lips
- Difficulty tasting food
- Difficulty talking for very long
- Worsening of heartburn
- Hoarseness
- Dry cough
- Thrush (white patches in mouth, sore red tongue, or sore corners of the lips)
- Increased dental cavities
- Gingivitis (sore, bleeding gums)
- Loss of teeth
- Bad breath

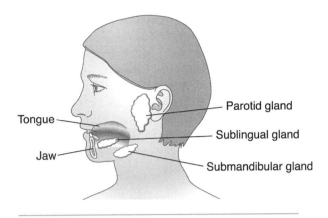

Figure 14.1 Major salivary glands

More commonly, people who have SS will notice dryness of the mouth. They may feel like they have to drink more water than other people do, and often will get into the habit of carrying a water bottle around with them. People who have Sjögren's syndrome will often note the locations of water fountains in their daily routine. This allows them locate and use them easily throughout the day. They may have difficulty swallowing dry food such as crackers without drinking fluids. The dryness especially can get worse while sleeping, sometimes awakening the person from sleep, which can cause insomnia and daytime fatigue. Dryness in the back of the mouth can cause a sore throat. The lips can also become dry, sore, swollen, and cracked due to the loss of moisture in the mouth, but also due to less production of oils from the sebaceous glands on the skin of the lips.

Saliva is also very important for the sense of taste. It helps dissolve molecules in food so that the taste buds can detect flavors properly. Therefore, it is not uncommon for the person with significant dry mouth from SS to notice a decreased ability to taste and enjoy food.

Since fluids from the mouth flow down the esophagus to keep acidic stomach contents from backing up, the dry mouth can also cause gastroesophageal reflux problems to be worse, causing heartburn and even chest pain. Moisture is also important for keeping the windpipe (trachea) moistened. Having a dry trachea (called xerotrachea) can cause a dry cough and even hoarseness. Sometimes the person who has SS will have difficulty when speaking for a prolonged length of time due to the xerotrachea resulting in hoarseness and coughing.

Saliva is very important as well for keeping bad bacteria and other organisms out of the mouth. Normally, the continuous production of saliva helps to wash away harmful bacteria, which are swallowed and destroyed by stomach acids. However, when the mouth becomes dry with less saliva, harmful organisms are allowed to multiply and cause damage in the mouth such as dental caries (cavities) and gingivitis (infection of the gums). The gums may become sore and bleed easily. These problems can unfortunately cause the early loss of teeth in people who have SS. The extra bacteria increase the chances of having halitosis (bad breath) as well.

One infection that is particularly problematic in people who have SS is thrush. Thrush is an infection in the mouth due to a fungus called *Candida albicans*. Doctors also call thrush oral candidiasis. Often this will show up as white patches of the fungal infection on the tongue, palate, and insides of the cheeks. However, if the mouth is particularly dry, the fungus will infect the tissues of the mouth, especially the tongue, causing the tongue to become tender and red. The *Candida* infection can also affect the corners of the mouth, causing them to become sore and tender. This is called angular cheilitis ("cheil-" comes from the Greek word for "lips"), angular stomatitis ("stoma-" comes from the Greek word for "mouth"), or perlèche. If you develop these problems from *Candida* infection, make sure you see your doctor for treatment. The treatments available for these infections are discussed in chapter 22.

Just as with dry eyes, there are many things that can be done to help with dry mouth (table 14.6). Most of these suggestions are self-explanatory. If all of these measures are taken and you still have difficulty with dry mouth, especially if it is causing dental problems or infections, then a doctor can prescribe either pilocarpine (Salagen) or cevimeline (Evoxac) to help the salivary glands to make more saliva. Pilocarpine is taken four times a day and cevimeline is taken three times a day. These medications cause the salivary glands to work harder at secreting saliva. They need to be taken regularly all the time, and it can take up to three months for them to work. Potential side effects of these two medications include heart palpitations, stomach upset, increased sweating, flushing, and increased urinary frequency. They can potentially worsen closed-angle glaucoma, asthma, COPD (e.g., emphysema), and some heart conditions, so they should be used with caution in people who have these conditions.

Rituximab (Rituxan) is a biologic medicine (discussed in detail in chapter 33) that has been studied in Sjögren's patients. It works by decreasing the number of B-cells in the immune system of the body. Several studies have shown that some patients who have Sjögren's syndrome may have significant improvements in mouth moisture and saliva flow when they are treated with rituximab. In fact, one study looked at salivary gland biopsies done before and after treatment. The salivary glands after rituximab treatment showed significantly decreased inflammation and improvement in how the glands looked under the microscope. Additional studies need to be done to see if this is truly a beneficial medication to treat Sjögren's syndrome. Another lupus medication used to decrease B-cells called belimumab (Benlysta; see chapter 34) is also being studied as a possible therapy in Sjögren's syndrome. I have one SLE patient whose dry mouth and swollen parotid glands improved significantly after he was treated with belimumab.

People who have a dry mouth should consider seeing their dentist more often than the commonly recommended twice a year schedule due to the increased chances for developing gingivitis, dental cavities, and tooth loss. Your dentist can identify problems at an early stage so that proper treatment can be given before things get out of hand, such as the permanent loss of teeth.

If you have signs of a *Candida* infection (white patches, sore red tongue, or sore corners of the mouth) make sure to see your doctor for antifungal medications. It is also important to realize that it is just as important to treat the mouth dryness as well. If someone develops these infections, they should take either pilocarpine or cevimeline to improve saliva production to try to keep the fungal infection from recurring.

**Table 14.6** Keeping the Mouth Moist in Sjögren's Syndrome

- Do everything listed in table 14.3.
- Use gum and mints that contain xylitol throughout the day. Other sugarless gums will not prevent tooth decay. Examples include sugarless Spry and Starbucks gum and mints.
- Drink water throughout the day; make sure each swallow moves through your teeth. Taking multiple small sips works better than larger drinks of water less often.
- Use lubricating sprays such as Biotene mouth spray or artificial saliva as needed to keep your mouth moist. Using these frequently in the evening can decrease the need for water and having to get up to urinate throughout the night. Keep some on your bedside stand.
- Apply vitamin E oil to sore, dry parts of your mouth. You can squirt out the gel from vitamin E gel capsules or get vitamin E oil.
- Eat soft, moist food if you have trouble swallowing.
- Eat smaller, more frequent meals to stimulate saliva flow more regularly.
- Avoid salty, spicy, acidic foods (including fruit juices) as well as carbonated beverages (the acid can irritate your dry mouth).
- Use lip balm or petroleum jelly (such as Vaseline) on your lips regularly throughout the day.
- Use moisturizing toothpastes and mouthwashes (such as Biotene or TheraBreath products) two to three times a day. Avoid any mouthwash containing alcohol or witch hazel, which dries out the mouth.
- Avoid whitening toothpastes—they may irritate teeth and gums.
- Floss daily (to decrease risk of gum infection).
- Avoid snacks between meals.
- Rinse your mouth with water or Biotene or TheraBreath mouthwash after eating anything.
- Brush or scrape your tongue at least once a day to remove bad bacteria and fungus (*Candida*).
- Remove and disinfect dentures, which can harbor bacteria and fungus, daily.
- See your dentist more often than twice a year.
- If you get cavities, ask your dentist for a fluoride tray or high-fluoride toothpaste.
- If you get cavities, consider crowns from your dentist instead of fillings.
- For thick mucus take guaifenesin (e.g., Mucinex).
- Ask your doctor to prescribe either pilocarpine (Salagen) or cevimeline (Evoxac) to stimulate saliva flow (see the text).
- The biologic medication rituximab (Rituxan) may be beneficial.

When a person has xerostomia (dry mouth) and thrush due to Sjögren's syndrome, deep furrows may develop in the tongue caused by the persistent dryness. Thrush (*Candida* infection) can appear either as a redder-than-normal color on the tongue or as a white coating on the tongue. The infection can cause the tongue to be very sore and make it difficult to taste food. The papillae (taste bud bumps) of the tongue may be much smaller (atrophied) than normal. *Candida* infection usually resolves with antifungal medication, and dryness improves with pilocarpine (discussed above). Lip balm helps keep dry lips more moist.

## Dry Nose (Nasal Mucosa Glands)

When dryness related to SS occurs inside the nose, the nose can become itchy and uncomfortable. Sometimes the blood vessels just beneath the mucosal surface can even bleed, causing a bloody nose. Since the sinus passages connect to the inside of the nose, dryness in this area can also cause other problems such as sinusitis (sinus infections) as well as increased problems from allergies (itching, sneezing, and nasal congestion). Measures to help with dry nose are listed in table 14.7.

## Dry Ear Canals (Ear Canal Sebaceous Glands)

When SS causes inflammation and damage to the glands that secrete moisturizing oils in the ear canals, the ears can feel itchy, uncomfortable, and even painful. Ringing in the ears (tinnitus) also occurs more often in people who have Sjögren's syndrome. Hearing may also decrease due to the buildup of wax that obstructs the ear canals.

**Table 14.7**  Keeping the Inner Nose Moist in Sjögren's Syndrome

- Do everything listed in table 14.3.
- Use a moisturizing spray or gel every several hours. Available brands include Ayr, Ponaris, Nasogel, Rhinaris, and Alkalol. The oil-based products usually work better and last longer than the saline-based products.
- Use Vaseline, Neosporin, or Polysporin every few hours if the outer nasal passages are particularly sore and dry.
- Use saline irrigation products (such as Sinus Rinse, Simply Saline, Ocean Spry, Nasal Comfort, or SinuPulse) regularly to keep the nasal passages moist.
- Avoid systemic antihistamines (Benadryl, Claritin, Alavert, and Zyrtec), which can dry out the nose more.
- Avoid systemic decongestants (Sudafed and antihistamines that end with a "-D" such as Claritin-D), which can dry out the nose more.
- A prescription for a nasal steroid may be more beneficial and less harmful to treat allergy symptoms compared to antihistamines and decongestants.
- Ask your doctor to prescribe pilocarpine (Salagen) or cevimeline (Evoxac).

**Table 14.8** Treating Itchy, Dry Ear Canals in Sjögren's Syndrome

- Do everything listed in table 14.3.

- Use a drop of mineral oil or ear wax removal oil once a day initially, then once weekly when you are feeling better, to lubricate the ear canals. Sweet Oil and other squalane oils work well because squalane is a natural component of earwax (sebum).

- For particularly itchy ears, use the cortisone drop DermOtic Oil (five drops in the ear twice a day for one to two weeks).

- Avoid systemic decongestants and antihistamines, which can worsen the dryness.

- For eustachian tube dysfunction, nasal saline and sinus irrigation (see table 14.7) can be helpful. Prescription nasal steroids may also help. Nasal decongestants (such as Afrin) may be used, but never for longer than three days to avoid significant side effects.

A condition called eustachian tube dysfunction may also occur. The eustachian tube connects the middle ear (behind the eardrum) to the very back of the nasal passages (called the nasopharynx). Its purpose is to keep air pressure normal behind the eardrum and allow fluids to drain from the middle ear down the back of the throat. The dryness from Sjögren's syndrome can cause the tube to get sticky and close up, causing abnormal pressure to build up behind the eardrum and even allowing fluid to collect behind the eardrum. This buildup of fluid or air pressure can cause ear pain, a feeling of fullness in the ear, decreased hearing, and tinnitus. Measures to help relieve these symptoms are listed in table 14.8. Never stick anything in your ears, such as cotton swabs, because this will only push the hard wax against the eardrums and can potentially cause irreversible damage.

## Dry Skin (Sebaceous and Sweat Glands)

Another common problem in people with SS is dry skin. When the skin becomes dry due to decreased sweat and oil production by the sweat and sebaceous glands of the skin, the skin often becomes itchy as well. This becomes especially apparent in the wintertime when the artificial indoor heat makes the dry winter air even drier. If fact, many of the dryness problems of Sjögren's syndrome are often exacerbated in winter. The itchiness can sometimes be quite intense, even causing difficulty sleeping at night. The scratching of the skin while trying to alleviate the itching can cause irritation and inflammation of the skin, as well as the development of red patches on the skin. It is not uncommon for people to complain of itchy skin, not realizing very dry skin is the cause. Suggestions for caring for dry skin are listed in table 14.9.

## Dry Vagina (Vaginal Mucosa Glands)

More than half of women who have Sjögren's syndrome have dryness of the vaginal area. It can cause a persistent feeling of itchiness and discomfort, pain during inter-

**Table 14.9** Treating Dry, Itchy Skin in Sjögren's Syndrome

- Do everything listed in table 14.3.
- Do not use soap on most body surfaces, except underarms and private areas, more than a couple of times per week. Soap removes natural, lubricating oils from your skin.
- Use an oil-based soap such as Eucerin Calming Body Wash Daily Shower Oil instead of other soaps (even those that claim to contain moisturizers).
- Shower or bathe in lukewarm water, not hot water. Hot water removes the natural, lubricating oils from your skin. Whatever your bath or shower temperature is currently, make it slightly cooler (the cooler the better).
- Take shorter baths and showers.
- After bathing or showering, pat the skin dry; do not rub (rubbing removes moisturizing oils).
- Apply a moisturizer to dry body areas immediately after bathing.
- Use a heavy-duty moisturizer that contains urea, glycerin, lactic, or alpha hydroxyl acids—for example, CVS Healing Skin Therapy Lotion, AmLactin Cream, or Carmol Cream.
- Consider moisturizers that contain ceramides, which can help repair the skin's protective barrier (such as Aveeno Eczema Care, CeraVe, TriCeram, or Remergent Barrier Repair Formula).
- For areas of very dry skin, consider using petrolatum (Vaseline) or bath oil (such as Neutrogena bath oil, RoBathol, or Aveeno Shower and Bath Oil) right after you bathe and while your skin is still moist to trap moisture in the skin.
- Reapply a moisturizer several times a day.
- Avoid using fabric softeners. They irritate dry skin.

**Table 14.10** Treating Vaginal Dryness in Sjögren's Syndrome

- Use Replens Long-Lasting Vaginal Moisturizer (available over the counter), one application every few days.
- Use the prebiotic moisturizer Luvena or the Yerba Santa containing Feminease as needed for increased moisture. These are available over the counter.
- Do not use hand or body lotions in the vaginal area because they will irritate the vagina.
- To decrease painful intercourse, use silicone-based lubricants each time.
- Sexual activities (including masturbation) help to keep vaginal tissues soft and flexible.
- See your gynecologist and ask about the use of an estrogen cream, ring, or suppository.

course, vaginal bleeding, and vaginal discharge. It also increases the risk of developing recurrent yeast infections due to *Candida albicans*. Another compounding issue is that estrogen hormones are very important to maintaining healthy vaginal tissue structure, as well as maintaining proper lubrication. Since a large number of women who have SS have gone through menopause (it is more common in women who are in their fifties and older), this lack of estrogen makes the situation worse. Some helpful recommendations on treating vaginal dryness are listed in table 14.10.

**KEY POINTS TO REMEMBER**

1. Sjögren's syndrome occurs when inflammation and damage occur to the exocrine glands of the body, which can cause varying degrees of dry mouth, dry eyes, dry itchy skin, dry nose, dry ears, and dry vagina.

2. Dry mouth can cause significant health problems, including gingivitis, dental cavities, and loss of teeth if not identified and treated.

3. White patches in the mouth or a red, sore tongue may indicate an infection due to *Candida albicans* (thrush) and needs to be treated with antifungal medications, as well as taking measures to increase mouth moisture.

4. Dry eyes can cause problems with vision if not addressed and treated.

5. If you have itchy skin, especially in the winter, consider dry skin from Sjögren's syndrome as a possible cause.

6. Numerous measures can be taken to help the dryness of Sjögren's syndrome. Refer to tables 14.2–14.10.

7. For mouth dryness, the medications pilocarpine (Salagen) or cevimeline (Evoxac) may be used to help the salivary glands produce more saliva.

8. For dry eyes, prescription cyclosporine (Restasis) eye drops can help the tear glands produce more tears.

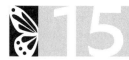

# The Digestive System

## From the Mouth to the Intestines

The digestive system (see figure opposite) handles what we eat and drink, breaking nutrients down into tiny molecules so they can be absorbed into the bloodstream and distributed throughout the body. The digestive system includes the gastrointestinal (GI) tract, which starts at the mouth, where food and fluids are taken into the body and ends at the anus, where the final waste products are eliminated in the feces. In between, there are the esophagus, the stomach, and the intestines. In addition to the GI tract, other organs in the digestive system also aid in digestion; these include the liver, gall bladder, and pancreas.

Many parts of the digestive system can be affected by inflammation in SLE. I discussed involvement of the salivary glands (which are part of the digestive system) from Sjögren's syndrome with SLE in chapter 14. The main problem in the mouth is oral ulcers, which I covered under cutaneous lupus in chapter 8. Not all parts of the digestive system are involved in SLE (e.g., the stomach, the gall bladder, and the small intestine). This chapter discusses the major areas of the digestive system that are affected by lupus.

## Pharynx

The pharynx is the area behind the mouth and nose. Anything that comes into this area from the mouth or nose is directed either to the gastrointestinal tract by way of the esophagus when you eat or drink, or to the respiratory system by way of the trachea (windpipe) when you breathe, cough, or sneeze. These tissues can become irritated either by direct inflammation from SLE itself, similar to how SLE can cause oral and nasal ulcers, or because of dryness due to Sjögren's syndrome. Either way, this can cause the person to have a sore throat. Therefore, a sore throat in a person with SLE can either be due to inflammation, which would be treated with steroids and other anti-inflammatory medications, or be due to dryness, which would be treated by treating the Sjögren's syndrome. However, sometimes there can be other causes of a sore throat, such as thrush (*Candida* infection), other infections such as strep throat or viral pharyngitis, or severe gastroesophageal reflux due to acidic contents backing up from the stomach. All of these possibilities need to be considered by the doctor when evaluating a sore throat in a person who has SLE.

**KEY POINTS TO REMEMBER**

1. Inflammation of the pharynx from lupus or dryness from associated Sjögren's syndrome can cause a sore throat in people who have SLE.

2. The doctor will consider other possibilities, such as strep throat, *Candida* thrush infection, or irritation from acidic stomach contents due to gastroesophageal reflux.

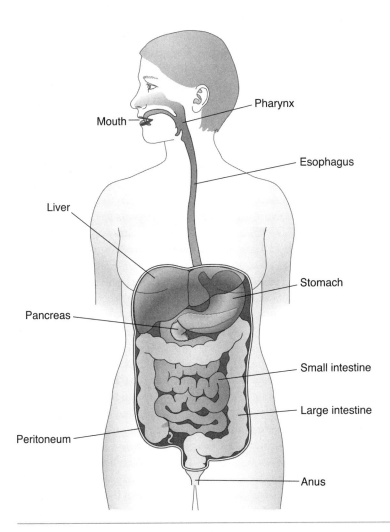

The digestive system

## Esophagus

The esophagus is a muscular tube that connects the pharynx to the stomach. Between the esophagus and the stomach, there is a ring of muscle called the lower esophageal sphincter (or LES for short). A sphincter is a muscle that squeezes a tube-shaped passageway closed. The role of the esophagus is to squeeze the food that you swallow downward into the stomach. The initial part of swallowing is performed consciously with squeezing of the muscles of the pharynx and upper part of the esophagus. Additional muscles lower in the esophagus subsequently continue this downward squeezing without conscious effort. The LES then automatically relaxes to allow the food to be propelled into the stomach by the muscles of the esophagus. After the food enters the stomach, the LES constricts and tightens up again to make sure that the swallowed food or liquid remains in the stomach and does not go back up into the esophagus.

Up to 25% of people who have SLE will develop a problem where the muscles of the esophagus do not work properly. This is termed "esophageal dysmotility" ("dys-" means "abnormal" and "-motility" means "motion or movement"). This means that the muscles do not work properly when moving swallowed food or fluids from the mouth down to the stomach and/or the LES may not function properly. This may be due to inflammation from SLE, scarring of the muscles of the esophagus, or a decrease in blood supply to these muscles. Esophageal dysmotility is more common in people who have SLE who are positive for RNP antibodies (discussed in chapter 4) and in those who have Raynaud's phenomenon. This can lead to difficulty swallowing, heartburn, and chest pain. The acidic contents coming up from the stomach into the esophagus are quite damaging because the esophagus does not have a protective barrier to this acid as the stomach does. With recurrent exposure to this acid, problems such as ulcers and scar tissue can form over time, causing permanent damage to the esophagus. In fact, over time, this irritation can even lead to a condition called Barrett's esophagitis, which is a pre-cancerous condition of the esophagus (pre-cancerous means that it currently is not cancer, but over time, it could turn into cancer) if not treated appropriately. Another harmful complication that can occur is that the gastric contents can potentially go back up the esophagus when a person is lying down. This acidic content and food might go down into the lungs, which can possibly cause lung damage or pneumonia.

Esophageal dysmotility can be diagnosed by having tests called an upper GI, esophagram, or barium swallow (the three tests are similar, but have some minor differences). During these tests, the person is asked to swallow a liquid (barium) that can be seen on x-rays. The barium coats the esophagus so that its shape shows up on the x-ray. Sometimes the person is asked to swallow a soft piece of food (such as bread or a marshmallow) coated with the barium. As it is swallowed, x-rays are performed to see how the esophagus is working. Another test, which is not as commonly done, is an esophageal manometry ("mano-" means "thin" and "-metry" means "measurement"). For this test, a thin, flexible tube is inserted into the nose, down the esophagus, and into the stomach. Then the person being tested takes sips of water, while the technician or doctor measures the pressures exerted by the muscles as the water goes down the esophagus.

If your doctor suspects that the esophageal dysmotility may be due to active inflammation, he or she may treat it with steroids to see if it improves. However, often the esophageal dysmotility is a permanent problem due to irreversible damage to the muscles. In this case, the person is instructed to change her or his eating and drinking habits to decrease problems from the esophageal dysmotility (table 15.1). These are the same measures recommended for people who suffer from gastroesophageal reflux disease (or GERD) and heartburn.

**KEY POINTS TO REMEMBER**

1. SLE can cause esophageal dysmotility, where the esophagus muscles do not move food down as well through the esophagus.

2. Esophageal dysmotility can cause difficulty swallowing, heartburn, and chest pain, and, if severe, it can cause stomach contents to go down into the lungs when a person is lying down.

3. Esophageal dysmotility is diagnosed by an upper GI, esophagram, barium swallow, or esophagus manometry.

4. Esophageal dysmotility is treated with medicines that decrease stomach acidity. However, the most important part of the treatment is to do everything listed in table 15.1.

5. If esophageal dysmotility is directly due to active inflammation from SLE, then steroids may be useful.

**Table 15.1** Measures to Help with Esophageal Dysmotility and GERD

- Eat smaller, more frequent meals.
- Take small instead of large bites of food and sips of liquids at a time.
- Promote saliva formation by using sugar-free candies and gum (sweetened with xylitol).
- Avoid caffeine, tobacco, chocolate, peppermint, high-fat food, and alcohol. These all relax the lower esophageal sphincter, which increases gastroesophageal reflux.
- Avoid highly acidic foods such as soda, citrus juices, tomatoes, and wine.
- Avoid tight clothing and belts (they increase pressure on the stomach).
- Maintain normal weight (fat on the abdomen puts pressure on the stomach).
- Do not lie down for at least two to three hours after eating or drinking.
- Avoid exercise and bending at the waist for one to two hours after eating.
- Maintain good posture; sit and stand upright.
- Elevate head of bed on six- to eight-inch blocks.

## Stomach and Intestines

Other than rarely being affected by mesenteric vasculitis (discussed later in this chapter), the stomach is not typically affected by SLE.

Inflammation of the intestines is called inflammatory bowel disease, which primarily includes Crohn's disease (also called regional ileitis) and ulcerative colitis. These disorders can cause many problems, including abdominal pain, anemia from blood loss, bloating, and diarrhea. They appear to be rarely seen in people who have SLE, with only twelve cases of Crohn's disease and twenty-three cases of ulcerative colitis in the medical literature as of the time of this writing. Therefore, inflammatory bowel disease most likely occurs as a coincidence of two different diseases occurring in the same person instead of SLE being a direct cause of inflammation of the intestines.

Another autoimmune disease called celiac disease (also called nontropical sprue and gluten-sensitive enteropathy) can affect the small intestine. This is an autoimmune disorder where the person develops difficulty with absorbing foods that contain gluten (which is especially common in wheat products). This can cause a multitude of problems, including diarrhea, stomach upset, weight loss, and anemia. A 2006 study found that 2.4% of celiac disease patients also had SLE, suggesting that they may occur together more than previously thought. This needs to be further studied to sort this out for sure. A larger 2012 study looked at 29,000 patients in Sweden and the United States and found that people who had celiac disease were three times more likely to also be diagnosed with SLE compared to the general population. Therefore, there does appear to be a link between these diseases.

The diagnosis of celiac disease begins with blood tests for the auto-antibodies against IgA gliadin, IgA endomysial, and IgA tissue transglutaminase (discussed in chapter 4). However, IgA gliadin antibodies are commonly found in people who have SLE (up to 25%) and therefore this particular blood test is not useful in diagnosing celiac disease in these individuals. If a person is positive for endomysial or tissue transglutaminase antibodies, or if the doctor suspects the person has celiac disease, the best test is a small bowel biopsy. During this procedure, the person undergoes an esophagogastroduodenoscopy (or EGD for short) where the doctor passes a thin fiber-optic scope through the person's mouth, then down the esophagus and stomach, until it goes into the small intestine. The doctor can then snip off a tiny piece of the small intestinal wall and send it to the laboratory for examination under a microscope to make the diagnosis. Celiac disease is treated by avoiding foods that contain gluten. Gluten-free foods are becoming easier to find in most grocery stores.

Another rare complication of SLE in the intestines is called protein-losing enteropathy. This is a problem where the intestines are not able to absorb proteins very well. Protein is important of course for normal nutrition, but it (especially albumin) is also essential for keeping fluids inside the blood vessels. People who have protein-losing enteropathy have very low albumin levels in the blood, and as a result develop profound edema, which means that fluid leaks from the blood and enters the soft tissues instead. This fluid builds up in areas closest to the ground due to the effects of gravity, so the feet, ankles, and legs can become very swollen. The condition worsens throughout the day as the person walks, sits, and stands, but improves after he or she lies down for a while. About 50% of people will also have diarrhea associated with protein-losing enteropathy. It is treated with high doses of steroids and sometimes stronger immunosuppressant medications such as cyclosporine or cyclophosphamide. Additional causes of edema are more common in people who have SLE other than this condition. Common causes of edema include medications, circulation problems, obesity, as well as having disorders of the heart, liver, and kidneys. The doctor evaluating edema would consider all of these possibilities. Protein-losing enteropathy from lupus is a very rare cause of edema, and I mention it only to be complete.

### KEY POINTS TO REMEMBER

1. Lupus does not generally involve the stomach.

2. Inflammatory bowel disease (such as Crohn's disease and ulcerative colitis) rarely occur in SLE.

3. Celiac disease (also called celiac sprue and nontropical sprue) is an autoimmune disorder related to sensitivity to gluten (found especially in wheat products and other grains).

4. Celiac disease causes malabsorption of nutrients, diarrhea, stomach upset, anemia, and potentially other problems as well.

5. Celiac disease may be suspected in people who are positive for IgA endomysial or tissue transglutaminase antibodies, but is best diagnosed with a duodenal mucosa biopsy performed by upper endoscopy.

6. A positive gliadin antibody is not useful in people who have lupus in diagnosing celiac disease.

7. Whether celiac disease occurs more commonly in people who have SLE is not known for sure at this time and more studies need to be done.

8. Celiac disease is treated by avoiding products containing gluten.

## Peritoneum

The abdominal contents are surrounded by a lubricating sac called the peritoneum (see figure on p. 255), just as the heart is covered by a pericardium and the lungs are surrounded by the pleura. These lubricating sacs are called serosae (the singular form is serosa). SLE commonly can cause inflammation of the serosae of the body to such an extent that it is considered one of the classification criteria for SLE, as discussed in chapter 1. Autopsy studies show that up to 70% of people who have SLE have had inflammation of the peritoneum (called peritonitis—"-itis" means "inflammation of") at some point in life. However, it is not identified by doctors very often due to its nonspecific symptoms (i.e., the symptoms caused by lupus peritonitis may be similar to symptoms caused by other conditions). Peritonitis typically causes abdominal discomfort and rarely can cause increased fluid in the abdomen (called ascites). Doctors treat it with steroids and other immunosuppressant medications. However, there are other important potential causes of ascites in people who have SLE, including kidney disease, heart disease, liver disease, and protein-losing enteropathy. Therefore, if a doctor notes ascites in someone who has SLE, he or she needs to consider all of these possible causes.

### KEY POINTS TO REMEMBER

1. The serosa surrounding the abdominal contents is called the peritoneum. It can become inflamed from SLE causing peritonitis.

2. Although autopsy studies show that 70% of SLE patients have evidence of having had peritonitis during their lives, it is rarely diagnosed by doctors, most likely because it causes nonspecific symptoms.

3. Peritonitis should be considered in any person who has SLE who has abdominal pain. It is treated with steroids.

## Mesenteric Vasculitis

As discussed in chapter 11, vasculitis occurs when there is inflammation of the blood vessels of the body. This causes narrowing of the blood vessels, which decreases blood supply to the particular organ or system that depends on those particular blood vessels for nourishment and oxygen, and leads to tissue damage, pain, and even death of those particular tissues. The mesenteric arteries ("mes-" means "middle" and "-enteric" means "related to intestines") supply blood to the stomach and intestines. If these become involved with vasculitis due to SLE, it can be one of the most dangerous complications of SLE, causing abdominal pain, fever, vomiting, bloody diarrhea, and even perforation (a hole) in the wall of the intestine. It usually occurs in people who have severe SLE. Fortunately, it does not occur very often, only affecting about 1% of people who have lupus. It is diagnosed by doing a study called an arteriogram, where x-ray contrast dye is injected into the arteries of the body, and x-rays are taken to look at the shapes of the arteries of the abdomen. Vasculitis can be seen as areas of abnormal dilations and constrictions of the arteries. It is treated by surgically removing any dead parts of the bowel, and using high doses of steroids and other immunosuppressants medications such as cyclophosphamide. Unfortunately, it has a high mortality rate even when treated quickly and appropriately.

Some people who have mesenteric artery blockages may also be positive for antiphospholipid antibodies (as discussed in chapters 4 and 9), causing blood clots in the arteries that can also cause severe intestinal problems and even death to part of the bowel. These people are treated with blood thinners such as warfarin (Coumadin).

1. Mesenteric vasculitis occurs when the blood vessels that supply blood to the stomach and intestines become involved with inflammation from SLE.

2. Mesenteric vasculitis causes abdominal pain, vomiting, diarrhea, and bloody feces.

3. Mesenteric vasculitis is diagnosed with an arteriogram x-ray.

4. Mesenteric vasculitis is treated with high doses of steroids and immunosuppressants such as cyclophosphamide.

5. Unfortunately, mesenteric vasculitis has a high mortality rate because it can cause bowel perforation (a hole in the bowel) and death of the bowel.

## Liver

The liver is the largest internal organ of the body (with the skin being the largest organ overall). The liver is located in the upper right side of the abdomen, just underneath the lower rib cage. It is a vital organ performing many different jobs, including producing energy for the body, important proteins, hormones, and bile (which aids in digestion). It is also important for removing many toxic products from the bloodstream. The liver can be affected by lupus in many different ways. The most common is an enlarged liver (called hepatomegaly—"hepato-" means "liver" and "-megaly" means "enlargement"). This occurs in about 25% of people who have SLE. It can sometimes be felt by the physician on physical examination or seen on x-ray studies, but it rarely is a significant problem.

Liver blood test abnormalities are very common in people who have SLE. The liver blood tests (also called liver enzymes and liver function tests) include AST, ALT, alkaline phosphatase, and bilirubin (all of which are explained in more detail in chapter 4). These blood tests are checked regularly in people who have SLE to ensure there is nothing wrong with their liver, either from SLE itself or from medication side effects. The most common reasons for elevated liver enzymes are medications (especially nonsteroidal anti-inflammatory drugs, or NSAIDs), alcohol use, and fatty liver. Fatty liver occurs when there is an increased amount of fat in the liver and it is usually due to obesity. However, there are other potential causes of elevated liver enzymes that doctors may need to rule out, such as infection from viral hepatitis B and C, as well as gall stones and other problems. Hepatitis simply means inflammation of the liver—"hepato-" means "liver" and "-itis" means "inflammation of"—and can be due to many different reasons, including medicines, viral hepatitis B and C, alcohol, or even genetic disorders. When someone has unexplained elevated liver tests (and therefore possibly hepatitis), the doctor will often stop any medicines that may possibly be the cause to see if they go back to normal. Other tests such as imaging studies of the liver (such as ultrasound or CT scan), as well as blood tests for viral hepatitis B and C may also be performed.

If the doctor rules these out, one possible cause is lupus hepatitis. Lupus can cause inflammation of the liver just as it can cause inflammation anywhere else in the body. The only way to know for sure if someone has hepatitis due to SLE is to get a liver biopsy. This is done by the doctor numbing up the skin and tissues overlying the liver, and then inserting a thin biopsy needle through the numbed-up area to remove a small amount of liver tissue. It is then examined under a microscope to try to figure out what is causing the liver problem.

Lupus hepatitis occurs in up to 5% of people who have SLE. It may be more common in children compared to adults, and appears to be seen more often in people who are positive for ribosomal-P and anti-SSA antibodies (discussed in chapter 4). The vast majority of the time the inflammation is mild, causing no significant problems other than the elevated liver enzymes on blood testing. These liver enzymes appear to become higher when SLE is more active in other parts of the body, and decrease toward normal when lupus is better controlled. However, rarely there can be enough inflammation to cause serious problems, including hepatomegaly, upper right abdominal discomfort, ascites (excessive fluid in the abdomen), jaundice (yellowish discoloration of the eyes and skin due to excessive bilirubin in the blood), and cirrhosis. Cirrhosis is the most severe consequence of hepatitis, where irreversible scarring and damage occur in the liver. Fortunately, this complication is rare in lupus hepatitis. A 2011 study found no progression to cirrhosis in fourteen patients followed over ten years. Lupus hepatitis is treated with steroids as well as other immunosuppressant medicines such as azathioprine. If cirrhosis develops, then a liver transplant can be done.

Hepatic vasculitis occurs when vasculitis (inflammation of the blood vessels) occurs in the arteries of the liver. It is a rare problem in SLE and can cause abdominal pain and elevated liver enzymes. It is treated with steroids and other immunosuppressant medicines.

Antiphospholipid antibody syndrome (see chapter 9) can also affect the liver, but liver involvement from them is rare. Antiphospholipid antibodies can cause blood clotting in the arteries or veins of the liver, leading to various problems. The most common complication occurs when they cause clotting of blood in the large veins that drain blood from the liver. Doctors call this problem Budd-Chiari syndrome and it causes blood to back up into the liver, which becomes enlarged (hepatomegaly). The blood pressure in the blood vessels of the liver increases (called portal hypertension), and the liver stops functioning normally. This can cause fluid to build up in the abdomen (ascites). It is treated with blood thinners such as heparin and warfarin (Coumadin).

## KEY POINTS TO REMEMBER

1. Hepatitis refers to any inflammation of the liver.

2. Although 5% of people who have SLE will develop hepatitis due to their lupus, most lupus patients who develop hepatitis do so because of other causes such as drugs, hepatitis B or C infection, alcohol, or fatty liver.

3. Hepatitis is suggested by elevated liver enzyme blood tests (especially ALT).

4. Usually drugs that may irritate the liver (such as NSAIDs and methotrexate) may be stopped, but additional blood studies, liver ultrasound, CT scan, and sometimes even a liver biopsy may be needed to figure out the cause of hepatitis in people who have lupus.

5. Lupus hepatitis is usually mild and rarely progresses to cirrhosis.

6. Vasculitis of the blood vessels of the liver is very rare, but it is dangerous when it occurs.

7. Antiphospholipid antibody syndrome may cause blood clots in the blood vessels of the liver, requiring blood thinners for treatment.

## Pancreas

The pancreas is an endocrine gland organ that lies in the upper abdominal area. An endocrine gland secretes hormones directly into the bloodstream (see chapter 17 for more information). I discuss the pancreas here because it also makes many enzymes that are important in digesting food. It secretes these substances directly into the bile, which is then excreted into the small intestine to aid in digestion. Inflammation of the pancreas is called pancreatitis and occurs in 2% to 7% of people who have SLE; it more commonly occurs in children. Adults who have SLE who are at increased risk of developing pancreatitis include those who have elevated triglyceride levels (part of the lipid and cholesterol blood tests), those who have had pleurisy (see chapter 10), those who have psychosis (see chapter 13), those who have secondary Sjögren's syndrome (see chapter 14), and those who are positive for anti-SSA (La) antibodies. Pancreatitis is most apt to occur during the first few years of having lupus.

The typical symptoms of pancreatitis include severe abdominal pain, which often radiates (spreads) to the back, nausea, and vomiting. Although SLE itself can cause pancreatitis, numerous other things can also cause pancreatitis and must be considered by doctors. These include gall bladder stones, alcohol, trauma, high triglyceride levels, high calcium levels, and even some congenital disorders. Some of the medications used to treat SLE can also cause pancreatitis, including azathioprine, steroids, diuretics, and NSAIDs. If any of these is found to be the cause, then it is very important to treat these causes and to stop the medications. If steroids are possibly the cause, then they may need to be decreased in dosage very slowly. However, if the pancreatitis is due to SLE itself, the treatment is to use medicines such as steroids and azathioprine. Therefore, the presence of pancreatitis in someone who has lupus and who is taking steroids or azathioprine presents some difficult management decisions for doctors.

Treatment includes hospitalization. The person is not allowed to eat or drink anything to allow the pancreas to rest. Intravenous (IV) fluids must be given since the person cannot eat or drink. Usually a tube is inserted through the nose down into the stomach so that stomach contents can constantly be suctioned out, which also allows the pancreas to rest.

Lupus pancreatitis is usually due to vasculitis involving the blood vessels of the pancreas; therefore, steroids are usually needed once other possible causes are ruled out. Azathioprine is also commonly used. If the person has high levels of antiphospholipid antibodies, then blood clots in the pancreas blood vessels may be another cause of the pancreatitis, and blood thinners such as heparin and warfarin may be needed as well.

Pancreatitis is a potentially severe problem with a high mortality rate. Overall, studies show that anywhere from 3% to 60% of people die from their pancreatitis attack. Severe pancreatitis occurs more commonly and more severely in children who have SLE (compared to adults who have SLE) with a death rate approaching 60%. Recent studies in adults show a lower death rate varying from 3% to 20%.

### KEY POINTS TO REMEMBER

1. Pancreatitis in people who have SLE is rare.

2. Pancreatitis causes severe abdominal pain, often radiating (spreading) to the back, nausea, and vomiting.

3. Pancreatitis is treated with hospitalization, not eating or drinking, having the stomach drained with a nasogastric tube, and using IV fluids to rest the pancreas.

4. Some medicines used to treat SLE (such as steroids and azathioprine) can actually cause pancreatitis and may need to be stopped.

5. Other more common causes of pancreatitis are alcohol and gall bladder stones.

6. If the pancreatitis is due to SLE, it is treated with high doses of steroids and sometimes azathioprine.

7. Pancreatitis due to SLE can have a high mortality rate, especially in children.

# Eyes

## See Your Ophthalmologist Once a Year

The vast majority of people who have SLE develop a close relationship with their eye doctors (ophthalmologists) on the direction of their rheumatologists. This is usually because the eyes need to be monitored and examined once a year while a person takes hydroxychloroquine (Plaquenil) to make sure that no side effects occur from the medication. Up to half of people who have SLE may develop dry eyes due to Sjögren's syndrome. Some people may develop other complications from their lupus affecting the eyes, but these problems are not common. This chapter discusses some of the ways that lupus may affect the eyes.

· · · ·

By far the most common condition involving the eyes in people who have SLE is Sjögren's syndrome (see chapter 14), which can cause dry eyes, swelling of the lacrimal (tear) gland, keratoconjunctivitis sicca (inflammation of the cornea and conjunctiva of the eye due to dryness), and blepharitis (swelling or inflammation of the eyelids). However, other parts of the eye can be involved as well (figure 16.1).

Iritis occurs due to inflammation of the colored portion, or iris, of the eye that surrounds the black pupil. The iris is part of a section of the eye called the uvea, so sometimes doctors use the term "anterior uveitis" instead of "iritis." The purpose of the iris is to increase or decrease the size of the pupil to allow the proper amount of light to enter the eye. The iris also helps to adjust focusing, depending on whether you are focusing on something near (the pupil gets smaller due to the iris constricting) or far away (the pupil becomes larger due to the iris relaxing). When iritis occurs, it causes discomfort in the eyes and blurred vision with light exposure due to the difficulty the inflamed iris has while constricting and relaxing. Often there is redness of the eye as well. It is important to treat iritis quickly. Over time, uncontrolled inflammation can cause scar tissue to develop, leading to permanent vision problems. Doctors usually treat iritis with steroid eye drops, which can be very effective in calming down the inflammation in the eye. These steroid drops have little to no side effects in areas of the body away from the eye. If used repeatedly, however, steroid eye drops can cause eye problems such as elevated pressures in the eye (called glaucoma) or clouding of the lens (called cataracts). Therefore, if the steroid eye drops do not control the iritis very well, or if the eye doctor has difficulty decreasing the use of the steroids, he or she

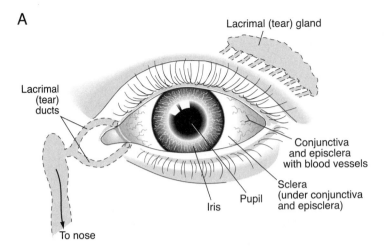

A

Lacrimal (tear) gland

Lacrimal (tear) ducts

Conjunctiva and episclera with blood vessels

Sclera (under conjunctiva and episclera)

Iris   Pupil

To nose

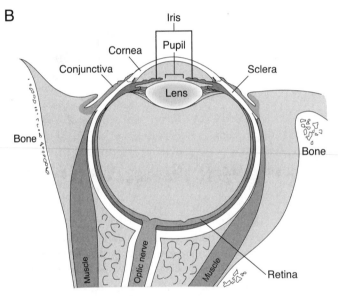

B

Iris

Pupil

Cornea

Conjunctiva

Sclera

Lens

Bone

Bone

Muscle

Optic nerve

Muscle

Retina

**Figure 16.1** The eye

may ask the rheumatologist to use systemic immunosuppressant medications such as those described in chapters 30–34. Fortunately, iritis does not occur very often in SLE.

Scleritis is inflammation of the sclera (white part of the eye), while episcleritis is inflammation of the thin layer of tissue that covers the sclera. Scleritis is rare in SLE, but occasionally episcleritis can occur, causing an intense redness of the white part of the eye. It is usually a mild problem and often will resolve on its own. Steroid eye drops and non-steroidal anti-inflammatory drugs (NSAIDs) are also useful in treating episcleritis.

The retina is located in the back of the eye. Light contacts the eye in the retina and forms an image. This is what makes us able to visualize what we see. The most common abnormality seen within the eyes of people who have lupus is retinal vasculopathy. This is a catchall term that includes all abnormalities of the blood vessels of the retina. The vast majority of the time these are mild problems picked up by the ophthalmologist when he or she examines the back of the eye. The doctor often will see something called "cotton-wool spots" as a sign of mild retinal vasculopathy. Most of the time, retinal vasculopathy is a sign of permanent damage to the blood vessels from previous lupus problems and requires no additional treatment. However, rarely, the retinopathy may be severe due to active inflammation (retinal vasculitis) or due to blood clots in the retinal arteries caused by antiphospholipid antibodies. Retinal vasculitis is a dangerous situation, causing blurred vision and often eye pain as well. Treatment for retinal vasculitis includes high doses of steroids and other systemic immunosuppressants such as azathioprine, mycophenolate, or cyclosporine. Retinal vasculitis only occurs in people who have severe SLE. If the retinopathy is due to blood clotting from antiphospholipid antibodies, then the treatment is the use of blood thinners like warfarin (Coumadin).

The optic nerve is located in the back of the eye and is responsible for transmitting information from the light contacting the retina to the brain so that it can be interpreted into vision. One percent of people who have SLE may develop inflammation of the optic nerve (called optic neuritis or optic neuropathy). The person affected by optic neuritis usually develops blurred vision or even blindness. This is actually a form of CNS lupus, as discussed in chapter 13, and it is sometimes seen in a multiple-sclerosis-like involvement from SLE (called lupoid sclerosis). It can be due to direct inflammation of the nerve, or of the covering around the nerve, or due to vasculitis (inflammation of the blood vessels). High-dose steroids and other immunosuppressants such as azathioprine, mycophenolate, or cyclophosphamide are useful for treatment. There have also been cases reported that were related to antiphospholipid antibodies that can cause blood clots in the blood vessels that feed the optic nerve. In these cases, blood thinners such as warfarin (Coumadin) need to be used and usually end up being a lifelong treatment. Approximately 50% of people who have optic neuropathy due to lupus fully recover their eyesight; unfortunately, about 50% have permanent visual impairment.

Another condition called orbital myositis (also known as orbital pseudotumor and orbital inflammatory syndrome) occurs when there is inflammation of the muscles or other tissues that surround the eye. This is a rare complication of lupus and can cause blurred vision, eye pain, or a bulging eye when it occurs. It typically responds to treatment with steroids.

An increasing popular eye surgery deserves special attention. People who have SLE should not get laser refractive surgery (commonly known as LASIK surgery, which stands for laser-assisted in situ keratomileusis). Systemic autoimmune diseases such as SLE can cause difficulties with healing of the cornea after surgery. In addition, a common complication after LASIK surgery is dry eyes. This problem would be worsened in the one-third of SLE patients who are bound to develop Sjögren's syndrome.

1. By far the most common problem in the eyes from SLE is dry eyes due to Sjögren's syndrome (see chapter 14).

2. Iritis, also called anterior uveitis, can cause blurred vision, red eyes, and difficulty tolerating light. Steroid eye drops treat iritis; fortunately, it occurs rarely in SLE.

3. Episcleritis is more common than scleritis, but both occur rarely in SLE. These problems cause red eyes, sometimes with eye discomfort. Doctors treat it with steroid eye drops.

4. Retinal vasculopathy is an abnormality in which SLE affects the blood vessels in the back of the eye. It can be caused by active inflammation (vasculitis), which is treated with high doses of steroids and immunosuppressant medicines, or by blood clots (due to antiphospholipid antibodies), which are treated with blood thinners. Most often, the vasculopathy is old damage that requires no treatment.

5. Optic neuritis is a type of CNS lupus (see chapter 13) that causes blurred vision and even blindness. It may occur in people who have SLE in a condition often called lupoid sclerosis since it can mimic multiple sclerosis. Treatment includes high doses of steroids.

6. People who have SLE should not get LASIK surgery.

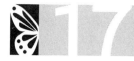

# The Endocrine System

## Internal Glandular Problems

The exocrine ("exo-" means "outside") system consists of glands that secrete fluids outside of the body (such as sweat and tears) and can be affected by Sjögren's syndrome in SLE (discussed in chapter 14). The endocrine ("endo-" means "within") glands secrete substances, called hormones, directly inside of the body. Many organs also act as endocrine organs by secreting hormones—these include the skin, kidneys, intestines, liver, pancreas, and heart. Sometimes lupus involvement of these organs can cause them to have difficulty in secreting the hormones they are supposed to secrete. For example, this is why people who have lupus nephritis often become anemic—their kidneys start making less erythropoietin, which is an important hormone that tells the bone marrow to make more red blood cells. Although numerous organs in the body have endocrine functions, the primary endocrine organ not mentioned so far that is commonly affected in people who have lupus is the thyroid gland. This chapter focuses on the thyroid gland involvement in lupus.

••••

The endocrine organ that most people have heard of is the thyroid gland (figure 17.1). This is a soft gland located underneath the Adam's apple in front of the cartilage of the windpipe (or trachea). It is responsible for secreting thyroid hormones that are very important for numerous metabolic processes in the body (the metabolism). In 1961, it was first noted that thyroid diseases occurred more frequently in people who had SLE compared to people who did not have SLE. It has been shown that people who have SLE can develop auto-antibodies directed at the thyroid gland, causing it to become either overactive (which is called hyperthyroidism—"hyper-" means "over") or underactive (which is called hypothyroidism—"hypo-" means "under"). About 24% of people who have SLE also have one of the autoimmune thyroid diseases. This is why rheumatologists typically check these thyroid function tests frequently in their SLE patients.

Hypothyroidism occurs in up to 15% of people who have SLE at some point in life. It is most commonly caused by a condition called Hashimoto's thyroiditis (also called chronic lymphocytic thyroiditis), which is an autoimmune disease of the thyroid gland associated with positive thyroglobulin and thyroid peroxidase antibodies (see chapter 4). Inflammation occurs in the thyroid gland (thyroiditis), occasionally initially caus-

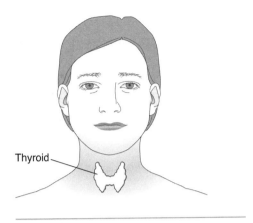

**Figure 17.1** The thyroid gland

ing an overactive thyroid (hyperthyroidism) followed by hypothyroidism. The hypo-thyroidism is caused by destruction of a large part of the thyroid gland due to the thy-roiditis to the extent that it is not able to make enough thyroid hormone anymore. The hypothyroidism of Hashimoto's thyroiditis is diagnosed by finding an elevated TSH level associated with thyroglobulin and thyroid peroxidase antibodies (see chapter 4) in the blood. Most people who have hypothyroidism do not have any symptoms at all. Most doctors test for TSH on a regular basis since hypothyroidism is such a common problem. Therefore, it is usually identified and treated before problems start. How-ever, if not identified quickly enough, some people will develop symptoms of hypo-thyroidism, which can include hair loss, cold and clammy skin, fatigue, mental slug-gishness, weight gain (even though the appetite is less than normal), and feeling cold while others feel warm. These symptoms are reversible with treatment. Treatment is a thyroid supplement that usually must be taken for the rest of the person's life.

Hyperthyroidism is just the opposite. It occurs due to an overactive thyroid gland releasing too many thyroid hormones into the body. It can be seen in the early stages of Hashimoto's thyroiditis, with overactive thyroid nodules (swollen areas in the thyroid gland), or in a condition called Grave's disease. Grave's disease is another autoimmune thyroid disorder that is associated with an auto-antibody found in the blood called thyrotropin (or TSH) receptor antibody. Grave's disease usually causes an enlarged thyroid gland (called a goiter) and hyperthyroidism. The symptoms of hyperthyroid-ism include anxiety, increased frequency of bowel movements, shortness of breath, weight loss, heart palpitations, heat intolerance, warm skin with increased sweating, and muscle weakness. It can be treated with medications such as methimazole or pro-pylthiouracil, which decrease thyroid activity. Some people who have Grave's disease are treated with nuclear iodine 131 treatments to destroy the thyroid gland to keep it from being overactive; then when the thyroid gland stops working, they take a thyroid supplement for the rest of their life. Others may require that the gland be surgically removed (called a thyroidectomy) for treatment.

Other endocrine organs include the pituitary gland in the brain, the parathyroid hormones that lie behind the thyroid gland, the reproductive glands such as the testes and ovaries, and the adrenal glands, which sit on top of the kidneys. These other endocrine glands are rarely affected by lupus directly.

## KEY POINTS TO REMEMBER

1. An endocrine gland secretes hormones directly into the body, as opposed to exocrine organs, which secrete substances outside of the body.

2. Many organs (such as the skin, liver, pancreas, and kidneys) also act as endocrine organs.

3. Lupus-induced inflammation of these organs can disrupt their ability to release important hormones. For example, lupus nephritis can decrease the kidneys' ability to release the hormone erythropoietin, resulting in anemia, which can be treated with erythropoietin medications.

4. Approximately one-fourth of everyone who has SLE will develop an autoimmune thyroid disease.

5. Hashimoto's thyroiditis is common and is diagnosed by finding an abnormal TSH level along with positive thyroglobulin or thyroid peroxidase antibodies.

6. Many people who have Hashimoto's thyroiditis have to take thyroid supplements for the rest of their life due to permanent hypothyroidism.

7. Another autoimmune thyroid problem is Grave's disease, which causes an enlarged thyroid gland, hyperthyroidism, and goiter.

8. Grave's disease is treated with either medications to calm down the thyroid gland or with nuclear iodine 131 treatments (which destroy the thyroid gland). Sometimes the thyroid gland is removed surgically.

9. People who have Grave's disease usually need to take a thyroid supplement the rest of their life after iodine 131 treatment or after surgical removal of the thyroid gland.

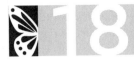

# The Reproductive System and Pregnancy

## Problems during Pregnancy

While SLE often affects other organ systems in the body, it does not typically cause inflammation and damage to the reproductive organs, such as the uterus (womb) and ovaries in women or the testes in men. It can, however, potentially cause problems with menstruation, pregnancy, and even problems after pregnancy. These particular problems will be discussed in detail in this chapter. Chapter 41 is devoted to measures that women who have SLE can take in dealing with these potential problems with pregnancy.

## Menstrual Cycles and Fertility

Other than difficulties during pregnancy, the other primary problem seen with the reproductive system is that it is not uncommon for women who have SLE to have irregular menstrual cycles. These irregularities primarily occur when their SLE is more active and is manifested by changes in how often they menstruate, how long the menstrual cycles last, and how much menstrual flow they have. The exact reason for these changes is not known, but it may be related to the stress the body is going through during lupus flares. When SLE is less active, the menstrual cycles generally tend to be more normal.

When lupus is highly active, it may be difficult to become pregnant as well. However, overall fertility rates in women who have lupus appear to be normal.

The most common cause of infertility in women who have lupus is the previous use of cyclophosphamide, which is a strong immunosuppressant used to treat severe SLE (especially lupus nephritis and CNS lupus). Unfortunately, some women who use cyclophosphamide will have damage to their ovaries due to the medication and end up becoming infertile. The ovaries are the reproductive organs in women that produce eggs. Cyclophosphamide can markedly decrease or even halt the production of eggs. Previous use of cyclophosphamide may also cause decreased sperm counts in men who have SLE. These infertility problems can be sometimes avoided by using a medication called Lupron (leuprolide) in women taking cyclophosphamide who wish to become pregnant later on. Leuprolide essentially causes the ovaries to temporarily stop making eggs—the hope is that the cyclophosphamide will not permanently injure the resting eggs since cyclophosphamide primarily damages cells that are actively multiplying in the body. Menstrual cycles will temporarily cease after leuprolide is started.

It is recommended that men who have SLE consider storing sperm at a sperm bank before cyclophosphamide is started. However, since cyclophosphamide is used for severe SLE, it is usually started in most people in an urgent manner during severe disease activity at a time when planning for sperm donation is not very practical.

### KEY POINTS TO REMEMBER

1. Menstrual cycles may be irregular and menstrual flow either lighter or heavier than normal when SLE is more active.

2. Although it may be difficult for a woman who has SLE to become pregnant during a severe flare, women who have SLE have normal fertility rates.

## During Pregnancy

### Lupus Flares

One common concern about women who have SLE who become pregnant is whether their SLE will become more active during pregnancy. This is an important concern for several reasons. First, it is not uncommon for lupus to become more active during pregnancy, presumably due to the hormonal changes that occur. Second, if SLE becomes more active during pregnancy, then there is an increased risk for having other complications (such as kidney problems, seizures, high blood pressure, or miscarriage).

Although most lupus flares that occur during pregnancy are mild, severe flares do occur in anywhere from 10% to 29% of pregnancies. Certain factors tend to predict which women are at highest risk for developing severe flares. These include women whose lupus has not been under good control during the six months before the start of pregnancy, those who have had severe disease in the past (especially lupus nephritis), elevation of anti-double-stranded DNA levels, and decreased complement (C3 and C4) levels during pregnancy. It also appears that African American women may have an increased chance of having lupus flares during pregnancy.

Women who have severe SLE have an increased chance of developing severe flares during pregnancy. This group especially includes those who have active lupus nephritis, myocarditis, or pulmonary hypertension. These women in particular need very close monitoring by their rheumatologist and a high-risk obstetrician. Although it is rare for a woman who has SLE to die during pregnancy, the chances are particularly increased in people who have these problems.

In women who have an increased risk of having lupus flares during pregnancy, it is recommended that they see their rheumatologist more regularly (at least monthly) during pregnancy to monitor for the possibility for lupus flares. In addition, all pregnancies in women who have SLE are considered to be high-risk due to the possibility of lupus flares during pregnancy and the increased risk for problems with the fetus. For that reason, seeing a high-risk obstetrician should be seriously considered as well.

If lupus flares during pregnancy, it causes problems not only for the mother but also for the fetus. Women who have SLE have increased chances for other complica-

273

tions during pregnancy—including preeclampsia, eclampsia, premature birth, intra-uterine growth restriction (IUGR), and even miscarriage. Preeclampsia is a condition where high blood pressure and protein in the urine occur during pregnancy. It is called eclampsia when seizures (epilepsy) also occur in a woman who has preeclampsia. Either of these conditions increases the risk for problems with the fetus from developmental delays to the worst-case scenario of miscarriage or death. IUGR means that the fetus's weight is in the lower 10% of normal as compared to that of other fetuses and babies of the same gestational age. Having IUGR increases the chances for premature birth and its associated complications. Increased lupus activity during pregnancy, having a history of lupus nephritis, having high blood pressure, and being positive for antiphospholipid antibodies (discussed in the following section in more detail) especially increase these risks. In addition, having an increased amount of protein in the urine, a low platelet count, anti-thyroid antibodies, autoimmune thyroid disease, low C3 and C4 complement levels, and high anti-double-stranded DNA levels, as well as being African American, appear to increase these risks as well (table 18.1).

Studies show that if a woman's lupus is under excellent control for six months before becoming pregnant, the chances of having a successful pregnancy is near normal. Therefore, it is essential to practice good birth control techniques, appropriately planning for pregnancy, and making the effort to not get pregnant until your rheumatologist says it is safe to do so. In addition, preventing lupus flares during pregnancy is one of the most important measures to take to try to have a successful pregnancy. A very important step in trying to ensure having no flares during pregnancy is to take the medication hydroxychloroquine (Plaquenil) throughout pregnancy. Hydroxychloroquine has been shown to be safe to take during pregnancy. Stopping hydroxychloro-

**Table 18.1** Factors That Increase the Risk for Complications during Pregnancy in SLE

- SLE not being in good control for six months prior to conception
- Active lupus during pregnancy
- Having a history of lupus nephritis
- Having severe lupus problems such as myocarditis, CNS lupus, or pulmonary hypertension
- Having protein in the urine, low C3, low C4, or low platelet counts
- Having positive anti-ds DNA, anti-thyroid antibodies, anti-SSA, or anti-SSB antibodies
- Having autoimmune thyroid disease
- Being positive for tests that identify antiphospholipid antibodies (false positive syphilis tests, anticardiolipin antibodies, lupus anticoagulant, beta-2 glycoprotein I antibodies, or antiphosphatidyl antibodies). Lupus anticoagulant may be the most important of these.
- Being African American
- Stopping hydroxychloroquine (Plaquenil)

quine during pregnancy increases the chances for the lupus to become active during pregnancy.

Many medications should not be taken during pregnancy, as most pregnant women know. This can be quite challenging for the woman who has SLE because it can be even worse if she stops her medicines and her lupus flares as this greatly increases the chances of her not having a successful pregnancy. It is vital that a woman who has SLE inform her rheumatologist immediately when she becomes pregnant so that the proper instructions can be given about what to do with her medications. A woman's obstetrician should not stop any of the lupus medications unless discussed with her rheumatologist as well. Hydroxychloroquine (Plaquenil) is generally continued throughout pregnancy because it is not associated with any problems with the fetus. Steroids, such as prednisone and methylprednisolone, are also usually continued as well. There is a small increased risk of the baby developing a cleft palate when steroids are used during the first fourteen weeks of pregnancy. The usual rate of cleft palate is about one out of a thousand births, but when steroids are used in pregnancy, the chances increase to one out of three hundred births. However, it is very important that steroids not be stopped abruptly during pregnancy because the problems of a severe lupus flare are worse than the potential problems of the fetus developing a cleft palate. Steroids should always be tapered down slowly under the direction of the rheumatologist to make sure that severe side effects do not occur due to going off or down on the dose of the steroids too quickly. Azathioprine is another commonly used medicine for SLE that can be continued during pregnancy. However, other medications such as methotrexate, leflunomide (Arava), or mycophenolate (CellCept and Myfortic) should not be taken during pregnancy because they can potentially cause a miscarriage or congenital deformities in the fetus. The very strong immunosuppressant cyclophosphamide should also not be taken during pregnancy because it is associated with congenital deformities. However, sometimes a woman who has severe SLE needs to be placed on a strong medicine such as cyclophosphamide. There have been cases reported of women using cyclophosphamide during the last three months of pregnancy (third trimester) with no problems since this is a time period when the vast majority of the fetus's organs have already reached a critical stage of development. When cyclophosphamide has to be used, it is usually because SLE is particularly severe and life threatening. In these cases, the chances of having a good outcome from the pregnancy (delivery of a healthy baby) are much lower whether cyclophosphamide is used or not.

Non-steroidal anti-inflammatory drugs (NSAIDS) are also usually safe to take during pregnancy during the first two trimesters. These include medications such as ibuprofen (Motrin) and naproxen (Naprosyn), which are often used for joint pain and headaches. However, it is important that they be stopped during the third trimester because they can cause a particular problem with the fetus's blood vessels called patent ductus arteriosus if they are continued. The ductus arteriosus is a blood vessel that connects the pulmonary artery directly to the large aorta. This blood vessel diverts blood directly from the right side of the fetus's heart to the large aorta, where it can go to the rest of the fetus's body. This way it bypasses the fetus's lungs, which at this time are not needed to oxygenate the blood since the mother's blood is providing all the necessary oxygen to the fetus, as well as disposing of carbon dioxide made by the fetus. Soon after birth, this blood vessel closes up, allowing the blood in the newborn baby to go from the right side of the heart directly into the lungs where it can be properly oxygenated. However, if NSAIDS are taken soon before birth, they can prevent this blood vessel from closing up, therefore causing the baby's blood to bypass the lungs and not get oxygenated. The blood vessel, ductus arteriosus, is still open or patent ("patent" comes from the Latin word for "to be open"). That is why the condition is called patent ductus arteriosus. All normal births and the vast majority of premature births occur during the third trimester, which is why NSAIDs should not be taken during this time to prevent this from happening.

A fairly recent study also showed that women who take NSAIDS during the first trimester may have an increased chance for their baby developing a type of heart problem called a cardiac septal defect. It had previously been accepted that it was permissible for a pregnant woman to take NSAIDs during the first trimester. However, this may change if additional studies confirm this finding.

One interesting phenomenon that can occur during pregnancy is that some women will actually have decreased lupus activity during pregnancy. This may be related to the fact that the fetus and placenta actually produce steroids such as cortisone and progesterone during pregnancy. These steroids can enter the mother's bloodstream and help to decrease lupus activity, especially during the second and third trimesters.

## KEY POINTS TO REMEMBER

1. While most flares of lupus during pregnancy are mild, between 10% and 29% of women will have a severe flare.

2. SLE flares during pregnancy increase the risk for pregnancy complications such as preeclampsia, eclampsia, and miscarriages.

3. Risk factors for either having a flare of lupus during pregnancy or complications such as preeclampsia, eclampsia, premature birth, or miscarriage include not having been in remission for six months prior to becoming pregnant, being African American, having had a history of lupus nephritis and high blood pressure, having myocarditis or pulmonary hypertension, having severe SLE, being positive for antiphospholipid antibodies, having low C3 or C4 levels, having low platelet counts, and having a high anti-ds DNA level.

4. All women who have any of these risk factors should consider seeing their rheumatologist monthly during pregnancy.

5. All pregnancies in women who have SLE are considered to be high-risk. Pregnant women who have SLE should consider being followed by an obstetrician who specializes in high-risk pregnancies.

6. Women who take hydroxychloroquine (Plaquenil) during pregnancy have a better chance of doing well.

7. Steroids and azathioprine (Imuran) can generally also be taken during pregnancy to help control SLE activity.

8. Methotrexate, leflunomide (Arava), and mycophenolate (CellCept and Myfortic) should not be taken during pregnancy. Cyclophosphamide can be considered for se-

vere SLE during the third trimester, but there is a high risk for miscarriage, probably related to the severity of the woman's lupus.

9. NSAIDs can be generally taken during the first two trimesters, but should be stopped in the third trimester to prevent the fetus from developing patent ductus arteriosus.

## Antiphospholipid Antibody Syndrome and Pregnancy

As discussed in chapter 9 in the section on the antiphospholipid antibody syndrome (APLS), women who are positive for antiphospholipid antibodies (such as anticardiolipin auto-antibody, lupus anticoagulant, and beta-2 glycoprotein I) have an increased chance of having a miscarriage during pregnancy. This occurs due to these antibodies causing blood clots in the placenta, which is the organ that connects the fetus's umbilical cord to the blood supply of the mother. These blood clots can then interrupt the blood flow between the mother and fetus, causing death and miscarriage of the fetus. Women who are positive for these antibodies are also at increased risk for preeclampsia and eclampsia during pregnancy. As discussed previously, preeclampsia and eclampsia increase the chances for having a premature birth, miscarriage, or stillbirth.

The majority of women who have lupus and who are positive for these antibodies do not develop miscarriages. However, in those in whom it does happen, these problems have an increased chance of repeating themselves during subsequent pregnancies. If a woman who has lupus is positive for these antibodies but has not had a problem with miscarriages, the doctor may recommend that she take a small dose of aspirin (such as 81 mg a day), which can thin the blood and hopefully prevent these problems from happening.

Miscarriages before the tenth week of pregnancy are common even in healthy women. Most of the time, this is due to genetic abnormalities of the embryo (which is what an unborn baby before the eleventh week of pregnancy is called). Therefore, one or two early miscarriages during the first ten weeks of pregnancy would not be considered to be due to the presence of these antibodies since early miscarriages are so common. However, if a woman who has these antibodies has three or more early miscarriages (and if there were no genetic abnormalities when the embryo was examined), then that person is diagnosed as having antiphospholipid antibody syndrome (APLS). Women are also diagnosed with APLS if there is the death of any fetus for otherwise unknown reasons (such as no genetic abnormalities) after ten weeks, or if there is a premature birth due to eclampsia, preeclampsia, or placenta problems.

Stronger blood thinners can be used in women who have pregnancy problems due to the APLS. Usually this includes heparin-like medications, either alone or in combination with low-dose aspirin. Keeping the blood thin with these medicines can greatly increase the chances of having a normal pregnancy and birth.

Of course, if a woman has APLS and a history of blood clots and has been taking blood thinners prior to pregnancy, then she should take blood thinners as well during pregnancy to prevent blood clots. However, warfarin (Coumadin) is changed to a heparin-like medicine because warfarin can cause fetal abnormalities.

1. Thirty to 50% of women who have SLE are positive for antiphospholipid antibodies.

2. Tests that can identify antiphospholipid antibodies include false positive tests for syphilis, anticardiolipin antibodies, lupus anticoagulant, beta-2 glycoprotein I antibodies, and phosphatidyl serine antibodies (see chapter 4).

3. If a woman is positive for any of these antibodies and has three or more miscarriages before the tenth week or a stillbirth after ten weeks (in the absence of genetic abnormalities of the embryo or fetus), or has had eclampsia or preeclampsia, then she is said to have antiphospholipid syndrome (APLS).

4. Women who have APLS causing pregnancy problems are more apt to have a successful pregnancy if they take heparin either with or without low-dose aspirin during pregnancy.

5. Women who are positive for these antibodies but do not have APLS may decrease their chances for miscarriage by taking low-dose aspirin during pregnancy. They should discuss this with their rheumatologist or OB/GYN doctor.

## Fetal Heart Block due to SSA and SSB Antibodies

When a woman is positive for anti-SSA (also called Ro antibody) or anti-SSB (also called La antibody), these antibodies can go through the placenta and enter the baby's bloodstream and cause neonatal lupus—either in the form of fetal heart block (discussed here) or in the form of a lupus rash after birth (discussed later in this chapter). Fortunately, neonatal lupus only occurs 2% to 3% of the time in women who are positive for anti-SSA or anti-SSB antibodies. Although anti-SSA and anti-SSB antibodies are the most common reasons for neonatal lupus, it can more rarely occur in mothers who are positive for anti-RNP antibodies as well.

Rarely, these antibodies can cause problems with the fetus's heart, especially the electrical conduction system. The electrical conduction system of the heart is a very important system of nerves that keep the heart beating correctly—making sure that it beats quickly enough and that the four chambers constrict and beat in the proper sequence to ensure that blood is properly circulated through the body and lungs. If these antibodies damage this electrical system at an important point in the fetus's development, then permanent damage may occur, causing what is called fetal heart block. This can result in persistent heart block, often requiring the permanent need for a pacemaker, inserted into the baby immediately after birth, to ensure that the heart beats normally. In addition, babies born with complete heart block due to neonatal lupus can potentially develop a severe heart condition called endocardial fibroelastosis, where severe scar tissue forms on the inside of the heart. These babies usually require a heart transplant.

It is essential that fetal heart block be diagnosed as early as possible because there is the possibility that treatment with steroids can make it less severe. Although steroids may not help most babies, especially those with more severe heart block, their use may prevent worsening of the condition in fetuses in which it is caught early enough. There-fore, it is recommended that women who are positive for anti-SSA or anti-SSB antibod-ies have their fetus's heart monitored using special tests, such as echocardiograms, beginning the sixteenth to eighteenth week of pregnancy. Monitoring is usually con-tinued weekly until around the twenty-sixth week, when it is decreased to every other week. If heart block is detected in the fetus, then steroids such as dexamethasone or betamethasone may be given to the mother to try to improve the heart block. A 2012 report from Italy suggested that the addition of IVIG (intravenous immunoglobulin) therapy (see chapter 35) and plasmapheresis (see chapter 35) may also be beneficial.

Therefore, it is very important that a woman who has lupus know whether she is positive for SSA or SSB antibodies before pregnancy and to let her obstetrician know. Women with these antibodies should be followed by a high-risk obstetrician and set up for fetal heart monitoring beginning at the sixteenth to eighteenth week of pregnancy.

Unfortunately, women who have had one child with neonatal lupus causing fetal heart block are at increased risk of having another baby with heart block. This risk is approximately 18%, and therefore they should be watched very closely with fetal heart monitoring during later pregnancies.

### KEY POINTS TO REMEMBER

1. Two percent to 3% of women positive for SSA and SSB antibodies will have their babies develop neonatal lupus.

2. One form of neonatal lupus is congenital heart block, which can be potentially treated if it is caught early during pregnancy.

3. Women positive for these antibodies should have fetal heart monitoring per-formed weekly from the sixteenth to eighteenth week up to the twenty-sixth week of pregnancy after which the frequency can be decreased to every other week.

4. If heart block is detected in the fetus, the mother can take steroids to try to treat it. IVIG and plasmapheresis may also be beneficial.

5. If a woman has a baby with neonatal lupus fetal heart block, there is an 18% chance of it recurring with a subsequent pregnancy.

## Problems after Pregnancy

### Lupus Flares

The fetus's part of the placenta actually makes steroids (such as cortisol and proges-terone) during pregnancy, and these steroids enter the mother's body. These steroids can actually decrease lupus activity in some mothers who have SLE during pregnancy. After delivery, this source of extra steroids is abruptly withdrawn. This causes a flare of lupus in up to 20% of women who have lupus after the baby is born. Some lupus experts advocate that their patients who have SLE take extra steroids or get a steroid shot after pregnancy to prevent a flare of their lupus.

1. Up to 20% of women who have SLE may flare during the first few weeks after giving birth due to the abrupt withdrawal of steroids secreted by the fetal part of the placenta.

2. Post-pregnancy lupus flares may potentially be prevented by taking extra steroids after delivery.

## Blood Clots due to Antiphospholipid Antibodies

There is an increased risk for blood clots in women who are positive for antiphospholipid antibodies after delivery. After delivering a baby, it is common to not walk very much and to be more sedentary. This decrease in activity is a prime setup for blood clots to occur in the veins of the legs when antiphospholipid antibodies are present. The blood clots that are of primary concern include deep venous thrombosis (DVT), which are blood clots that form in the veins of the legs, and pulmonary emboli (PE), which are blood clots that dislodge and travel to the lungs, creating a potentially deadly situation. Many experts recommend that women who required blood thinners during pregnancy for antiphospholipid antibody syndrome should continue taking blood thinners for at least six weeks after delivery to prevent these from occurring. Not all experts are in agreement on this issue, so it is best to let your rheumatologist and obstetrician make the decision as to whether blood thinners (such as warfarin or heparin) should be used after pregnancy or not.

1. Women who have APLS, which previously caused a miscarriage during pregnancy, may be at increased risk of developing DVT or PE in the weeks following delivery of the baby.

2. Continuing heparin or warfarin should be considered during this time period (approximately the first six weeks after pregnancy). However, not all doctors are in agreement with this.

## Neonatal Lupus

As mentioned in the section on fetal heart block, women who are positive for anti-SSA or anti-SSB antibodies have a 2% to 3% chance of having a baby with neonatal lupus, either in the form of fetal heart block or a lupus rash (cutaneous neonatal lupus erythematosus). Cutaneous neonatal lupus occurs due to the reaction of the anti-SSA and anti-SSB antibodies with the baby's skin. The rash is rarely evident at the time of birth; in most babies it requires exposure to ultraviolet light before it occurs. This may occur soon after birth or weeks or months later (on average first becoming apparent six weeks after birth). The rash is similar to subacute cutaneous lupus (discussed in chapter 8) in appearance and on biopsy. It causes circular-shaped red areas, especially on the face (particularly around the eyes) and scalp. The most important part of treatment is protecting the baby from light and using sunscreen. The anti-SSA and anti-SSB antibodies disappear from the baby's system within six to eight months. Therefore, the cutaneous neonatal lupus does go away by 8 months of age. It usually does not scar the skin significantly, but it may leave some mild discoloration.

Women who have a baby with neonatal cutaneous lupus have a high chance for a subsequent baby having neonatal lupus. Close to 50% of later pregnancies have a chance of being associated with some form of neonatal lupus. Fetal heart block has been shown to occur in 18% of these pregnancies and 30% have a recurrence of cutaneous neonatal lupus. Therefore, the mother who has had a baby born with cutaneous neonatal lupus needs to be extra vigilant during later pregnancies because there is a high risk for it recurring—not only the skin involvement, but also the heart involvement.

Fetal heart block due to neonatal lupus was discussed in detail in the preceding section. A baby born with heart block due to neonatal lupus may require a pacemaker implanted to keep the heart beating normally. This is required in more than 65% of babies born with congenital heart block, especially if complete (third-degree) heart block is present. Rarely, a heart transplant may be needed, especially if there is endocardial fibroelastosis or heart failure due to myocarditis. Overall, most babies born with fetal heart block do well. However, approximately 20% will die. This is usually seen in those who have complete heart block, or in those who have endocardial fibroelastosis or cardiomyopathy due to myocarditis.

A 2010 study suggested that if the mother is taking hydroxychloroquine (Plaquenil) during pregnancy, it may decrease the risk of neonatal lupus. The study looked at a group of fetuses with fetal heart block due to neonatal lupus. Only 14% of the mothers were taking hydroxychloroquine during their pregnancy. This is the first study to look at this particular question and needs to be followed up by additional studies. However, it is one additional study showing the importance of women who have lupus staying on their hydroxychloroquine throughout pregnancy.

There are some less common neonatal lupus complications that deserve mention. Occasionally, inflammation of the liver (hepatitis) may occur, causing elevated liver enzymes on blood tests and occasionally an enlarged liver or even jaundice (yellowish discoloration of the skin and whites of the eyes) may occur. Decreased platelet counts (thrombocytopenia) and white blood cell counts (leukopenia) may also occur. All these problems tend to resolve without any long-lasting effects.

### KEY POINTS TO REMEMBER

1. Two to 3% of women positive for SSA and SSB antibodies will have a baby born with neonatal lupus.

2. Neonatal cutaneous lupus erythematosus causes a red rash especially on the face and scalp and is made more prominent after exposure to ultraviolet light.

3. Neonatal cutaneous lupus erythematosus is treated with avoidance of light and the use of sunscreen.

4. Neonatal cutaneous lupus erythematosus goes away by the sixth to eighth month due to the elimination of the mother's anti-SSA and anti-SSB antibodies from the baby's body.

5. If the baby is born with neonatal lupus fetal heart block, a pacemaker will be needed more than 65% of the time (generally for third-degree complete heart block).

6. A heart transplant may be needed in more severe cases of heart block, especially if myocarditis or endocardial fibroelastosis occurs.

7. Neonatal lupus can rarely cause hepatitis or low blood cell counts. These also resolve by the eighth month.

8. If a mother has a child born with cutaneous neonatal lupus, she has close to a 50% chance of having another baby with neonatal lupus (either fetal heart block or cutaneous neonatal lupus).

9. Taking hydroxychloroquine (Plaquenil) during pregnancy may decrease the risk of having a baby born with fetal heart block due to neonatal lupus.

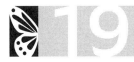

# Special Populations and Surgery

## Young and Old, Man and Woman, Rich and Poor

When I first started studying to specialize in rheumatology, I was a rheumatology fellow at Walter Reed Army Medical Center in Washington, DC. The pediatric department of the hospital consulted on me to see a young girl who was very ill. I will never forget how sick she was. She was about 8 years old. I reviewed her chart, which showed that she was running very high fevers of 101°F to 102°F. Her blood counts were very low, she had evidence of hepatitis with very high liver enzymes, and she was in kidney failure. When I saw her, my heart could not help but be touched by this sweet-looking girl who was so ill. She had the classic red butterfly rash on her cheeks and nose, but her lips were also inflamed and swollen. The inside of her mouth and tongue was covered with open sores and was very dry. She had difficulty concentrating and thinking, and her joints were swollen and very tender as well. It was not very difficult to diagnose systemic lupus erythematosus in this young girl. A kidney biopsy was done, showing that she had the most severe type of lupus nephritis, class IV diffuse proliferative glomerulonephritis. We treated her with high doses of steroids, strong chemotherapy, and the universal lupus drug Plaquenil.

She quickly improved, changing into a beautiful, healthy-appearing girl. She really surprised me at how good she was about using her sunscreen every day and taking her medications regularly. Her father was in the military, which probably had something to do with her excellent compliance. When I left the military to enter private practice, her disease was quiet, her liver and kidneys were no longer affected, and you could not tell that she had ever had a rash on her skin. I can still remember her sweet smile and how intelligent she was. I have often wondered how she ended up doing. Maybe she will read this someday and contact me to let me know.

This was my introduction to how SLE affects different groups of people. This was a classic example of how lupus can affect children. They often have much more severe disease than adults who have SLE and are more likely to have severe kidney disease. The age, sex, ethnicity, and even the socioeconomic status (income level) of a person can have a significant influence on how SLE affects the person. These issues are discussed in more detail in this chapter.

## Age

SLE most commonly appears in women who are of childbearing age. However, occasionally it can occur before puberty or after menopause. SLE tends to have some differences in these age groups compared to the lupus that affects women of childbearing age.

### Children

Development of SLE in children younger than 5 years old is rare. The youngest child ever reported on in the medical literature was only 6 weeks old (excluding those with neonatal lupus, as discussed in chapters 1 and 18). In fact, only fourteen cases of SLE have been reported in children younger than 1 year old (again, excluding children who have neonatal lupus). SLE, however, is not that rare in children from 5 years of age to the onset of puberty. In fact, approximately 20% of people who have SLE develop it while they are children. Among children, there is a relatively higher number of boys compared to girls—with there being one boy for every three girls who have SLE (compared to only one man to every ten women during childbearing years). Therefore, in this age group, factors other than hormones must be playing a more important role in the development of SLE. Genetic factors probably play a larger role. Children who have SLE are more apt to have mothers who are positive for anti-SSA antibodies and to have family members who are positive for antiphospholipid antibodies. Children who have SLE also tend to have a higher chance of having their SLE associated with a genetic immune problem, especially with having deficiencies in complements (especially C2 and C4 complements, which are molecules important for a properly functioning immune system). They are also more likely to be deficient in a particular protein of the immune system called IgA immunoglobulin.

Children who have SLE unfortunately tend to have more severe major organ disease compared to adults who have SLE. Their lupus is more likely to affect the blood cells, heart, lungs, nerves (seizures and psychiatric problems), and kidneys. They also appear to be more prone to developing low blood counts, mouth sores, fevers, and swollen lymph nodes, and are more apt to develop the classic butterfly rash of lupus. On the other hand, children tend to have fewer problems with discoid lupus and Raynaud's phenomenon than adults who have lupus do, and Sjögren's syndrome in children is rare.

Children especially tend to have an increased risk of developing lupus nephritis, which is usually more aggressive, often requiring the use of strong immunosuppressants such as cyclophosphamide, compared to lupus nephritis affecting adults who have SLE. Approximately 65% to 70% of children who have SLE have lupus nephritis compared to 40% to 50% of adults.

About half of children who have SLE have psychiatric manifestations from their lupus. Three-quarters of these children even have hallucinations (seeing or hearing things that are not truly there). Much of the time, they do not let their parents or doctors know they are having these hallucinations because they do not want to be seen as crazy.

Since 80% of children who have SLE develop major organ disease involvement (while less than half of adults who have SLE do), they usually require more aggressive treatment. High doses of steroids and immunosuppressant medications such as cyclophosphamide, azathioprine, or mycophenolate are often needed.

The treatment of SLE in children certainly presents some unique problems. For example, the use of high doses of steroids may interrupt the growth of the bones and can cause shortened stature as the child gets older. The need to use cyclophosphamide in adolescent girls who have severe SLE causes an increased risk of their becoming sterile and not being able to have children when they get older.

The use of steroids can cause weight gain, body shape changes, and acne. Cutaneous lupus can cause rashes, skin color changes, and loss of hair. These problems can set up difficulties with self-esteem at a pivotal point in the child's physical, mental, and social development. Unfortunately, other children may ridicule a child with these physical changes.

The child who has SLE often faces other problems such as fatigue and difficulty thinking and concentrating that may interfere with schoolwork, learning, socializing with other children, playing, and participating in school and extracurricular activities. One recent study even showed that all the children who had SLE they studied had significant cognitive dysfunction causing difficulties in memory leading to poor grades. Fortunately, these problems tend to improve with treatment of their lupus. These difficulties, such as the social aspects, can be especially problematic for the adolescent. Adolescence is a time of development when learning to belong and to be accepted by one's peers can be so important. This unfortunately often leads to noncompliance with treatment. When people who have lupus stop taking their medications properly, it usually causes worse lupus disease activity. The problems facing the parents of children who have SLE as well as the children themselves can be daunting.

Since false blood tests for syphilis (a sexually transmitted disease) can occur in people who have SLE, it is important for parents to know if their child is positive for this test or not. If a blood test for syphilis is done for any reason during the school years (especially high school and college) and it turns up positive, this is usually reported to the local health department. This may be followed by measures aimed at diagnosing and treating syphilis, as well as investigation into potential sex partners of the student. If parents arm themselves with the knowledge of their child having a false positive test for syphilis, it can mitigate potential embarrassment, unneeded testing, and unnecessary administrative interventions.

## Late-Onset Lupus

Late-onset lupus refers to the onset of SLE after the usual age of menopause (50 to 60 years old). Late-onset lupus tends to be overall milder compared to that occurring in younger people.

Approximately 10% to 15% of people who have SLE develop it after the age of 50. There tends to be relatively more males diagnosed during this age range—roughly a one-to-one ratio (male to female)—compared to the onset of SLE during childbearing years. Again, this most likely represents the decreased influence of female hormones compared to the role they play during childbearing years. In addition, late-onset SLE tends to involve major organs less often, occurring in less than 20% of people (compared to 50% of women of childbearing years and 80% of children who have SLE). Because of this, older people who have lupus are overall less likely to require as much treatment with steroids and immunosuppressant medications compared to younger people who have SLE. Sjögren's syndrome, pleurisy, and arthritis tend to occur more often, while cutaneous lupus, fevers, lymphadenopathy, low blood cell counts, Raynaud's phenomenon, nephritis, and neuropsychiatric lupus are less common.

While the severity of SLE is overall milder compared to that in younger people, the toll it takes on older individuals is greater. Older people who have SLE actually develop more damage in the affected organs and have an increased mortality overall compared to younger people who have lupus (and when compared to their own age peer groups who do not have SLE as well). Although they may have less aggressive inflammation from lupus, it tends to damage the internal organs of older individuals more easily.

## Lupus in Men

Although the majority of people who have SLE are female, about 10% of all patients are male. Men are as likely to develop SLE at a young age as they are at an older age. This is in contrast to women who are more likely to develop SLE when they are in their child-bearing years compared to when they are children or when they are past menopause.

There have been multiple studies looking at men who have SLE and what their characteristics are compared to women who have lupus. Men may have a higher chance of having fevers, weight loss, serositis (such as pleurisy), low blood counts, and neurological problems (such as seizures and psychosis as described in chapter 13) compared to women. Studies suggest that men may have more severe disease activity, more permanent damage to organs, and a higher mortality rate compared to women. These findings were confirmed by a 2012 report from Johns Hopkins University Hospital in Baltimore, Maryland.

However, these findings are not universal. A 2012 study looked at the differences in men and women who had SLE seen at the University College of London Hospital from 1976 to 2005 and they found that women had higher rates of oral ulcers, kidney failure, and death (just the opposite of the Johns Hopkins group). In fact, Dr. David Isenberg, MD (one of the authors of this study), said in his 1994 editorial on this subject, "a set of distinguishing features for the male lupus patient suggests that like the Loch Ness monster, real proof of its existence is still lacking despite many claims that it has been sighted!" In other words, people report seeing the Loch Ness monster in his home island of Great Britain every few years; however, the existence of the monster has never been proven. The same goes with male versus female lupus. Every couple of years a large study comes out suggesting major differences between the genders who have SLE only to be countered by another study showing no significant differences.

Another study looking at men who had SLE in Brazil suggested that men who have SLE may have increased chances for erectile dysfunction, fertility problems, and gonadal dysfunction (i.e., problems with male hormones causing problems with proper function of the testicles) compared to men who do not have SLE. It is not known for sure whether these differences may be related to SLE itself, to genetic-related hormonal problems, or to the medications used to treat SLE. However, these possibilities need to be investigated further.

## The Role of Ethnicity

With SLE being primarily a genetic-driven disease, and because different ethnic groups carry different groupings of genes, some ethnic groups stand out when it comes to the frequency of developing SLE and how severe it is. For example, SLE is more common in blacks than it is in Caucasians. One study showed that it occurs approximately three times more often among black Americans compared to Caucasians. Black people who have SLE also tend to more commonly have certain manifestations such as discoid lupus, neuropsychiatric lupus, and serositis while also having higher rates of anti-Smith and anti-RNP antibodies compared to Caucasians who have SLE.

Studies comparing the use of two different medicines, azathioprine (Imuran) and mycophenolate (CellCept and Myfortic), show that African Americans and Hispanics do better with mycophenolate compared to azathioprine. Why some medications would work better in some ethnicities compared to others is not understood at this time. It will hopefully become more apparent in the future so doctors can use genetic testing to make decisions in medical treatments. African Americans also tend to require higher doses of the medication mycophenolate compared to Caucasians. This need for a higher dose may be due to African Americans having a higher metabolism of mycophenolate compared to that in Caucasians.

Mexican Americans, along with blacks, tend to have a worse outcome when they have lupus nephritis. Blacks tend to have more severe kidney disease overall, which seems to be more difficult to control with the medication cyclophosphamide, compared to their Caucasian counterparts. However, it can be difficult to figure out from the medical studies whether these differences are truly related to ethnicity (genetic tendencies) or whether they are due to socioeconomic factors. In lower socioeconomic groups, the lack of money, insurance coverage, and education certainly plays a large role in reduced access to better healthcare.

An ongoing, important study aimed at evaluating the differences of SLE in different ethnic populations (primarily Hispanic, African American, and Caucasian), called the LUMINA study, was initiated in 1994 by Dr. Graciela Alarcón at the University of Alabama at Birmingham. LUMINA, stands for LUpus in MInorities: NAture versus Nurture. The LUMINA study includes a large number of SLE patients—mainly from Alabama, Texas, and Puerto Rico—and should prove valuable in learning more about ethnic differences. So far it has suggested that lupus nephritis is much more common in Hispanics and African Americans (about 60%), compared to only 25% in Caucasians and Puerto Ricans. SLE also appears to be more severe with a higher mortality rate in non-Puerto Rican Hispanics and African Americans. The authors of this study suggest that socioeconomic factors may play a more important role for these differences than do genetic ethnicity. In fact, poverty was found to account for increased mortality rates instead of ethnicity. In other words, being poor (and therefore not having as good access to healthcare) probably plays a larger role in having more severe disease instead of what ethnic background a person has. In fact, this same finding emerged from a large recent Canadian study that was also designed to look at different ethnic groups.

## Allergies in People with SLE

Allergies to pollen, animals, foods, medicines, and other things in the environment are very common in the general population. Many people who have SLE also have allergies and often wonder if this is due to their altered immune systems from their lupus. Although some earlier studies suggested the possibility of more allergies in lupus patients, studies that are more recent have failed to show this association. However, people who have SLE do have an increased reaction to sulfa antibiotics, as discussed previously, but this is a different type of reaction than what doctors classify as a true allergic reaction. One popular therapy for allergies is to get allergy shots or what doctors call allergy immunotherapy. Due to the increased formation of auto-antibodies after immunotherapy, in 1989 the World Health Organization (WHO) recommended that people who have autoimmune diseases (such as SLE) not receive immunotherapy. Therefore, it is most likely better to try other therapies to control allergies instead of immunotherapy. This is not to say that allergy shots absolutely cannot be given to people who have SLE. However, if immunotherapy ends up being the only way a person who has lupus can get relief from allergies, then it is important to realize that there is always the possibility of her or his SLE flaring after immunotherapy.

### KEY POINTS TO REMEMBER

1. Major organ involvement (e.g., kidneys, brain, heart, etc.) requiring the use of stronger immunosuppressant medicines and steroids tends to occur more frequently in younger people who have lupus (e.g., 80% of children) compared to older people who have lupus (e.g., 20% of people older than 50 years old).

2. Taking care of adolescents who have SLE presents numerous unique problems for the teenagers and their parents—including problems with school, socialization, and subsequent compliance with taking medications—compared to older people who have SLE.

3. Although older people who have SLE may have a lower risk for severe major organ involvement from SLE, they do tend to get a larger amount of permanent damage to organs. The increased susceptibility of aging organs to damage from inflammation most likely explains this problem.

4. Men may have more severe disease than women who have SLE; however, this has not been proven.

5. African American and non-Puerto Rican Hispanic patients tend to have more severe disease compared to their Caucasian counterparts. However, this may be related more to an increased incidence of poverty in these ethnic groups.

6. African Americans may have more difficulty responding to some therapies such as cyclophosphamide and azathioprine for lupus nephritis, and often require higher doses of mycophenolate compared to their Caucasian counterparts.

7. Most true allergies probably do not occur more often in people who have SLE.

8. Most people who have SLE should probably avoid allergy shots (immunotherapy).

## How to Have a Successful Surgery

Most of us will require surgery at some point in our lives, but for a person who has lupus, preparing for and having a successful surgery presents some unique challenges. Many of the medications taken by people who have lupus must be stopped around the time of surgery to prevent problems such as bleeding and infections, while some medications, such as steroids, may need to be increased. The cold operating room may cause problems with poor blood flow in a person who has Raynaud's phenomenon, while the dryness of the surgical suite can cause significant problems for those who are already dealing with the dryness of Sjögren's syndrome. The person who has lupus will need to prepare thoroughly and let the surgical team members know what special needs he or she has.

This section provides general information for people who have lupus who are preparing for surgery, but it will not provide all the information they need. All surgeries are different and have different requirements in terms of preparation and recuperation. You must consult with your surgeon and the surgical team for specific advice.

Most surgical procedures are routine, not emergencies, which means that you will have adequate time to prepare for the surgery. However, sometimes surgery needs to be done on an urgent or emergency basis. In those situations, you may not have time to do everything discussed in this section; much of this information can still be helpful, however, even if you do not have much time to prepare. Your surgical team will provide you with general instructions in how to prepare for your surgery; this section of the book is to help people who have lupus prepare in a way that addresses their needs specifically in terms of lupus. Table 19.1 lists the major steps for you to take in preparing for surgery; these steps are discussed in more detail in this section.

Table 19.1  Surgical Preparation Checklist Specifically for People Who Have SLE

- Gather together your records as listed in table 19.2.
- See your rheumatologist and fill out medicine start and stop dates as listed in table 19.3.
- See any other specialists for major organ involvement from lupus to prepare for surgery.
- Prepare information to deal with Raynaud's phenomenon during surgery.
- Prepare information to deal with Sjögren's syndrome during surgery.
- Write this information down so it can be given to all nurses and doctors who care for you before and after surgery.
- Take all medicines with you to the hospital in case the hospital does not carry them.

Preparation for surgery begins with your first appointment with a surgeon. The surgeon and his or her team need to know your complete medical history. Table 19.2 is a checklist of items you should take with you when you see your surgeon and your anesthesiologist. Do not forget to include all over-the-counter medicines and supplements that you take. For example, some over-the-counter items, such as vitamin E, Advil, and Aleve, can thin out the blood. You will need to stop these before the surgery. Do not forget to include eye drops, skin lotions, and any other special therapies that you require for your lupus; this includes all moisturizing products used for the dryness of Sjögren's syndrome.

Ask your surgeon if you need to obtain special surgical recommendations from any of your other doctors. Usually, you should obtain a surgical evaluation or advice from at least your primary care physician and rheumatologist. Some people who have systemic lupus have significant involvement of internal organs such as the kidneys, lungs, heart, and liver. If you have these types of problems, you may also need recommendations from other specialists such as your cardiologist (heart), pulmonologist (lungs), nephrologist (kidneys), or gastroenterologist (liver). Ask your surgeon, your rheumatologist, and your primary care physician which of your doctors, or additional doctors, you should see before surgery.

It is best to plan doing all of this well in advance of your surgery. If you wait until too close to the surgical date, you may find that your surgery has to be postponed if any of these specialists require any special medical studies to be done before the surgery.

You should be prepared to tell your surgeon about your medical history and all the ways that your lupus affects you. For example, if you have significant dryness from Sjögren's syndrome or if your fingers and toes lose blood supply easily from Raynaud's phenomenon, you need to bring these problems up.

## Your Medications

Many medicines that people with lupus take require special attention around the time of surgery. Of course, it is important to ask all of your doctors what you should do with

Table 19.2 Checklist of What to Bring to Your Surgeon and Anesthesiologist

- List of all prescription medications with dosages, how often taken, and what they are used for
- List of all over-the-counter medicines (including vitamin and herbal supplements)
- List of all of your medical problems (including what your lupus manifestations are)
- List of all surgical procedures done in the past
- List of all drug allergies and intolerances
- List of the names and phone numbers of all of your doctors
- List of names and phone numbers of people you consider your emergency contacts
- Special instructions from your rheumatologist on how to prepare for surgery
- Surgery recommendations from your primary care provider and any other doctors you see

your medications before and after surgery. It is usually best to ask each doctor specifically about the medicines that he or she has prescribed. For example, your surgeon may tell you to "stop all aspirin-like medicines." However, some medicines related to aspirin (such as celecoxib, meloxicam, or salsalate) may not need to be stopped. This section goes into detail about some of the common medicines used by people who have lupus to help you understand what you should do with your own medicines. All medical situations are different, so your rheumatologist may provide recommendations different from those outlined here, depending on your individual needs. If you obtain any conflicting recommendations from your surgeon regarding these medicines, make sure to ask the prescribing physician (such as your rheumatologist) to discuss these issues with the surgeon. Communication, either written or verbal, between them is very important.

If you take a lot of medicines, it can be difficult to remember when to stop and start each medicine. I would recommend using a chart similar to table 19.3 to keep track of medication stop and restart times. Ask the doctor who prescribes each medicine when that particular medicine should be stopped and then restarted before and after surgery. Then you can write these stop and start dates on a calendar that includes your surgical date to simplify and organize this information better. Events may occur requiring some dates to be changed. For example, if your surgical wound does not heal well after surgery, or if an infection occurs, you may have to delay restarting any medicines that suppress the immune system.

Hospitals only carry a certain number of medications. It would be too difficult to carry every medicine available. It is best to bring your own medicines with you to the hospital. *Ask your surgeon to write an order stating that you can take your own medicines for any that are not carried by the hospital.*

This section specifically discusses several groups of drugs commonly used to treat lupus: steroids, non-steroidal anti-inflammatory drugs (NSAIDs, or "aspirin-like drugs"), blood thinners, immunosuppressants, pain medicines, Sjögren's syndrome systemic medicines, and herbal preparations.

*Steroids.* Never stop your steroids for surgery. As discussed in chapter 26, the adrenal glands in the body produce larger amounts of steroids during stressful events such as surgery. This surge of steroids is very important to ensure that bodily functions react appropriately to the surgery. Unfortunately, the adrenal glands stop working properly

**Table 19.3** Medication Stop and Restart Dates for Surgery

Date of Surgery: _____

| Medication Name | Prescribing Doctor | Stop Date | Restart Date |
|---|---|---|---|
|  |  |  |  |
|  |  |  |  |
|  |  |  |  |

if you take steroids for an extended period or at high doses. Refer to table 26.2 to find out if you will need extra steroids around the time of your surgery. Doctors often refer to this as providing "stress doses of steroids." For example, if you have gained weight from steroids (called Cushing's syndrome), then you most likely have adrenal insufficiency and should receive extra steroids. Even people who have received smaller doses of steroids than those listed in this table for long periods may need extra steroids at the time of surgery. If you have taken steroids for less than three weeks, you most likely do not require extra steroids (unless you took them more than once a day). You should ask your rheumatologist if you require extra amounts of steroids at the time of surgery. If you do, then let your surgeon and anesthesiologist know so that they make the appropriate arrangements.

Another problem with steroids is that they can cause difficulty with wound healing. Higher doses of steroids are associated with increased problems with surgical site healing, and they increase the risk for infections. Therefore, your doctors will also want you to be on the lowest doses of steroids possible. Your doctors will decide how much steroids you require to control your lupus. Your rheumatologist is usually best in deciding how much steroids you should be taking before and after surgery.

*"Stop Aspirin-like Medicines."* Medical professionals call medications related to aspirin non-steroidal anti-inflammatory drugs (NSAIDs), discussed in chapter 36. Most of these medicines prevent platelet cells in the blood from clotting the blood properly. Therefore, if you take them around the time of surgery, you could bleed excessively. Once the dangers for bleeding have decreased sufficiently, you can restart them, often as soon as twenty-four hours after surgery. Many people who have lupus take NSAIDs to control pain and inflammation; it is important to find out when you can start your medicine up after surgery so that you do not suffer more than you need to from pain.

Some surgeries have such a low risk for bleeding that none of the NSAIDs, including aspirin, need to be stopped prior to the surgery. These include cataract surgery as well as minor dental and skin surgeries. Check with your surgeon before surgery to find out if you need to stop aspirin-like medications.

Other surgeries have such a high risk for bleeding complications that NSAIDs are usually stopped for the surgery. These include operations on the brain, around the spinal cord, inside of the middle ear, and in the back of the eye.

The effects of the NSAIDs on clotting differ between the different medicines. The effects of aspirin on clotting last longer than those of the other NSAIDs and therefore aspirin needs to be stopped sooner than the others are. In general, you should stop aspirin seven to ten days before most major surgeries. However, stopping aspirin before surgery does not apply to everyone or to all surgeries. Some people take aspirin to prevent heart attacks and strokes. Some of them have such a high risk for these problems that they should actually not stop taking aspirin because the chances of their getting a heart attack or stroke is higher than the chances of developing a bleeding problem from the aspirin. This may include people who have stents inside of the arteries of their heart, arms, or legs. Stents are tiny tubes that keep the blood flowing in blood vessels affected by hardening of the arteries. Stopping aspirin may cause a stent to become blocked with a blood clot and can potentially cause a heart attack or similar problem due to the loss of blood flow. Therefore, if you have significant heart, blood vessel, or brain problems, make sure to ask your cardiologist (heart doctor), vascular surgeon, or neurologist (brain doctor) if you should stop your aspirin before surgery or not. If you are instructed to do so, make sure to ask how many days before surgery you should stop taking it.

A group of NSAIDs called the non-acetylated salicylates often does not need to be stopped before surgery since they do not cause bleeding problems. Table 36.1 lists these NSAIDs, which include choline magnesium trisalicylate, salsalate, and diflunisal. Another special group of NSAIDs is the COX-2 inhibitors and includes celecoxib and meloxicam (see table 36.1). These NSAIDs also do not thin out the blood and can often be continued up to the day before surgery. However, as with other NSAIDs, the COX-2 inhibitors and non-acetylated salicylates may increase blood pressure or decrease blood flow to the kidneys in certain situations. Therefore, it is best for some people to stop them prior to some surgeries. Your rheumatologist and surgeon should make this decision.

All of the other NSAIDs can cause bleeding problems and generally should be stopped prior to major surgery. Many doctors recommend stopping them at least three to four days before your surgical date. However, the effects of ibuprofen (Motrin) do not last very long, and it can usually be stopped twenty-four hours before surgery. Again, check with your rheumatologist for recommendations for your particular situation.

*Other Blood Thinners.* Some people who have SLE need to take blood thinners such as warfarin (Coumadin), clopidogrel (Plavix), enoxaparin (Lovenox), fondaparinux (Arixtra), dabigatran (Pradaxa), rivaroxaban (Xarelto), apixaban (Eliquis), and dalteparin (Fragmin). The decision on when and if to stop these medicines is complex and depends on why they are being used. The doctor who prescribes and monitors the particular blood thinner is the one who should give instructions on what to do with the medicine before surgery.

*Immunosuppressant Medicines.* Many people who have lupus need to take strong medicines that suppress the immune system. Taking these medicines can increase the risk for getting infections and therefore may need to be stopped before surgery and then restarted when all infection risk is gone after surgery (usually after the surgical wounds have healed sufficiently). Different medicines may require stopping before surgery and restarting after surgery at different times. Although methotrexate is an immunosuppressant, it appears to not increase the risk of infections from surgery; therefore, you may not need to stop methotrexate for surgery if your kidney function is normal. It is important to get this information from your rheumatologist, and then relay it to your surgical team. Hydroxychloroquine (Plaquenil) is not an immunosuppressant and does not cause any problems with surgery. You can take your hydroxychloroquine up to the day before surgery. The recommendations on which medicines to stop and when to stop them is complex. It is always important to get written recommendations from your rheumatologist regarding what you should do with your medicines.

*Pain Medicines.* Most pain medications need to be continued throughout your surgical period. In fact, stopping some of them, especially the opioids, can cause withdrawal symptoms and severe pain if stopped abruptly. Let your surgeon know all of your pain medicines so that they are not stopped accidentally.

*Sjögren's Syndrome Systemic Medicines.* Some people who have lupus who have Sjögren's syndrome take the medications cevimeline (Evoxac) and pilocarpine (Salagen) to increase saliva in the mouth. These two medications can potentially cause the airway passages to constrict, lower the blood pressure and heart rate, as well as cause urination problems. Therefore, some experts recommend that these not be taken around the time of surgery. Both of these medicines are out of the system quickly after stopping them. It is sufficient to not take them the day before your surgery and then restart them at a time after surgery when you are recovering well and able to take your pill medications again.

*Herbal Medicines and Supplements.* No herbal products are proven to improve the results of surgery. Some, including vitamin E, garlic, gingko, and ginseng, can actually cause problems such as increased bleeding. Others (including kava, valerian, and St. John's wort) can have dangerous interactions with the medicines used for anesthesia. Ephedra can cause cardiac instability, while ginseng can cause the blood glucose levels to drop causing hypoglycemia. Some of these effects in the body can take a long time to get out of your system (e.g., garlic supplements should be stopped at least a week before surgery). Therefore, it is best to stop all herbal products and supplements at least one week before surgery.

## Raynaud's Phenomenon

If your fingers, toes, and ears become cold and turn colors with stress or cold temperatures, you may have Raynaud's phenomenon (see chapter 11). Hospitals, especially the operating room, tend to be a bit colder than normal. This is required to meet standards in keeping things as sterile as possible to prevent transmission of infections as well as preserving medications optimally. These conditions can potentially cause a loss of blood flow to the fingers and toes and can become painful and even dangerous in some people.

It is most important to let the anesthesiologist and nurses know about your Raynaud's phenomenon. In fact, the anesthesiologist may be able to increase the temperature inside of the operating room ahead of time. You should ask for additional blankets, socks, a hat, and covers for the hands and feet to decrease the severity of Raynaud's attacks in the operating room and the recovery room.

## Sjögren's Syndrome

Another important consideration that is often overlooked in preparing for surgery is how to protect you from the complications of Sjögren's syndrome. Surgery can worsen the dryness of Sjögren's syndrome because humidity levels in operating rooms and hospitals tend to be very low. Medications used for pain, anesthesia, and cleaning the skin can be very drying. In addition, tubes inserted in the nose and throat during surgical procedures can be very irritating if those areas are dry.

Before your surgery you will be told not to eat or drink anything (called being NPO) for a certain amount of time. This usually does not include using artificial saliva. Therefore, if you require the use of artificial saliva, it is usually fine to keep using it, and it is recommended that you continue doing so.

Make sure to communicate to your surgeon, anesthesiologist, and nurses before and after surgery about your Sjögren's syndrome and about how important it is to make sure that you maintain proper moisture. Ask the anesthesiologist to humidify your oxygen supply if oxygen is required. Request a humidifier in your room, if possible. Make sure to bring all eye, mouth, ear, nose, and skin moisturizers to the hospital with you. Use them immediately prior to your surgery (if allowed), and ask the nurses in the recovery room to use them immediately afterward. Ask the anesthesiologist to take extra care in using a moisturizing gel in your eyes when they are closed during surgery to prevent any damage to the corneas. Remind the surgical team that they may need to use extra lubrication on any tubes inserted into the nose or throat during surgery. Even if you do not typically use anything for your nose, make sure to bring a moisturizing nose spray or gel (see table 14.7), as the nose commonly will dry out during and after surgery. This can be very uncomfortable if you do not take proper precautions to keep it from occurring. Also, do not forget to bring some Vaseline or other lip moisturizer, as you will need it.

During and after surgery, you may be treated with antibiotics. One problem with antibiotics is that they can increase the risk of *Candida* (yeast) infections. People who have Sjögren's syndrome are at even higher risk for developing these infections. If you develop a sore and red tongue, a sore throat, a white coating inside of the mouth, red and sore angles of the mouth, or a vaginal discharge, then you may very well have a *Candida* infection. You should bring any of these developments up to your doctor's attention for evaluation and possible treatment.

## KEY POINTS TO REMEMBER

1. Be prepared when you see your surgeon and anesthesiologist by taking a list of items (table 19.2) to your appointment.

2. List all your medications—prescription, over the counter, and supplements (table 19.3). Ask each prescribing doctor when to stop and restart each of these medicines.

3. Take all of your medicines with you to the hospital just in case some of them are not available from the hospital pharmacy.

4. If you have Raynaud's phenomenon or Sjögren's syndrome, let your surgeon, anesthesiologist, and surgery nurses know.

5. Request that extra measures be taken to keep you warm during and after surgery if you have Raynaud's.

6. Ask the anesthesiologist to increase the operating room temperature as high as is practical if you have Raynaud's phenomenon.

7. Take all moisturizing products with you if you have Sjögren's syndrome and use all of them before and immediately after surgery. Use lip and nose moisturizers even if you do not normally use them.

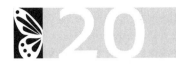

# Prognosis

## "How long do I have to live?"

> The wolf, I'm afraid, is inside tearing up the place. I've been in the hospital 50 days already this year. At present I'm just home from the hospital and have to stay in bed. I have an electric typewriter and I write a little every day but I'm not allowed to do much.
> —Flannery O'Connor, July 5, 1964

Flannery O'Connor was one of America's great writers. She was stricken with SLE in 1950 at the age of 25. She inherited the disease from her father, who passed away at a young age due to his lupus at a time when there were no treatments for SLE. The doctors told her mother, Regina, that Flannery was dying when she first became ill due to the "wolf." (Recall from chapter 1 that the word "lupus" comes from the Latin word for wolf.) At the time her doctor diagnosed Flannery with lupus, doctors considered SLE a terminal illness with no effective treatments. Fortunately, Flannery O'Connor developed her SLE right at the time that steroids first became available. Her physician prescribed adrenocorticotropin hormone (a type of steroid) followed by cortisone and then by prednisone. These medications enabled her to live another fourteen years (much longer than expected without the steroids). She would go on to write some of America's most critically acclaimed stories during periods when she felt well. However, she suffered the side effects of cortisone, including avascular necrosis or osteoporosis of the hips (discussed in chapters 24 and 25), which required her to walk with crutches, and she had periods when her lupus caused significant illness. She realized the double-edged sword of her treatment with steroids, writing, "So far as I can see, the medicine and the disease run neck & neck to kill you." Later, after being on steroids for ten years she went on to write to a friend, "What they found out at the hospital is that my bone disintegration is being caused by the steroid drugs . . . to keep the lupus under control . . . it is better to be alive with joint trouble than dead without it. Amen." Systemic lupus caused her to suffer from severe arthritis (or as she spelled it, "AWTHRITUS," giving us a hint of her southern accent from her home of Milledgeville, Georgia). It also caused severe anemia, requiring multiple blood transfusions, and lupus nephritis (kidney inflammation). After writing the introductory letter above about "the wolf . . . tearing up the place," she died less than a month later at the young age of 39 from the very "wolf" that she called her lupus.

Times have changed a lot since the 1950s and 1960s. Most people who have lupus today live long, normal lives. Significant research on lupus includes great discoveries that make the reality of living a long life with SLE even brighter for more people. However, there are certainly people who have severe disease who die at much too young of an age. There are also those who appear to have very mild disease but unexpectedly end up experiencing serious complications.

"Prognosis" is the medical term describing how a disorder affects a person and whether it may shorten a person's lifespan or not. This chapter discusses this topic in detail. If people who have SLE learn as much as they can about it, and about its potential complications, then they can take action to live better and longer lives. At times when SLE can appear overbearing, this can be a powerful and important message for the person who lives with lupus. The person who has SLE who arms herself or himself with knowledge empowers herself or himself with a degree of control over a disease that can at times seem uncontrollable. For example, did you know that the most common cause of death in people who have lupus is not the lupus at all? It is actually cardiovascular diseases such as strokes and heart attacks. Infections round out the top three causes of death (along with cardiovascular disease and SLE itself) in people who have lupus. Therefore, if people who have SLE recognize this and learn how to prevent heart attacks, strokes, and infections as well as treating their lupus, they will go a long way in taking control of their lives and destiny. Other factors also increase the risk of doing poorly from SLE, such as how old you are, whether you are married or single, how much money you make, what gender you are, and even what region of the United States you live in. This chapter on prognosis discusses these issues in more detail.

· · · ·

"Prognosis" comes from the Greek word for "to know beforehand" or "foresee." Almost everyone diagnosed with any illness wants to know what is in store for them in the future. How will it affect their lives? How long do they have to live? These are all very important questions. This chapter answers some of them. Since SLE affects every person differently and can affect any part of the body, prognosis is an especially difficult issue for the person diagnosed with SLE.

There are numerous aspects to the prognosis of a disorder such as SLE. Chapters 5–19 discuss the numerous ways that lupus can affect the body of someone who has the disease and what can happen with and without proper treatment. However, factors other than lupus itself can also affect the person who has lupus and these impact prognosis as well. For example, some medications can potentially cause significant side effects in someone who has lupus. Other problems not directly due to the inflammation of lupus itself can also potentially cause harm to someone who has lupus. Chapters 21–28 go into detail about all these aspects. Then, finally, there is the question of mortality. Will the disease cause the person who has it to die earlier than expected? This chapter covers life expectancy and mortality in people diagnosed with SLE. If people diagnosed with SLE know which problems can potentially kill them, then they can also learn how to prevent those things from occurring in the first place.

Unfortunately, some people are afraid of taking medicines due to their fear of potential side effects from these medications. In fact, in the patients whom I have seen die from their systemic lupus, the vast majority were either those who refused to take medications or those who did not have adequate insurance and were unable to get the best medical help until after it was already too late. The people who refused to take medicines wanted to take herbal supplements instead, or they were afraid of the potential side effects of the medicines used to treat lupus. If people understand what SLE does if not treated properly, they could be more motivated to trust their doctors and accept the recommended treatments.

Before modern medicine, people who had systemic lupus had a very poor outcome. SLE was a fatal disease. The first real treatment for systemic lupus was steroids, which became widely available around 1950. Before 1950, only 40% of people diagnosed with severe SLE survived the first year, and up to 83% of all people who had SLE died within the first two years. A study by Dr. Paul Klemperer from 1941 showed that while many patients who had SLE died from the disease itself, 55% actually died from infection. These patients had SLE before both steroids and antibiotics were available. This underscores the importance of preventing and treating infections in people who have SLE because infection continues to be one of the top three causes of death in people who have SLE.

After steroids became widely available in the 1950s, a remarkable improvement in survival rates began in people who had SLE (as illustrated in the case of Flannery O'Connor), especially in those who had severe brain and kidney involvement. About two-thirds survived two years and about 50% lived at least five years. In the early 1960s, the next big changes in lupus treatments occurred with the ability to treat kidney dis-

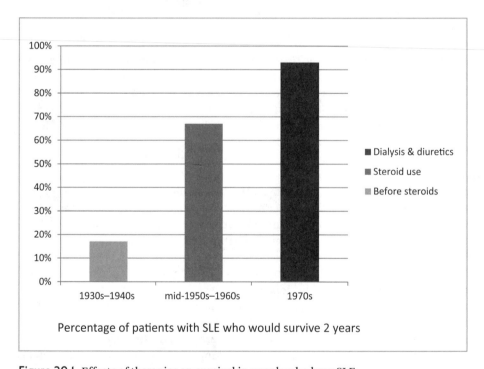

Figure 20.I  Effects of therapies on survival in people who have SLE

ease with fluid pills (diuretics) and dialysis machines. Survival increased to more than 90% living at least two years and about 75% living to at least five years (figure 20.1).

Recent studies of SLE patients show that 91% to 98% of patients diagnosed with SLE will live ten years or longer, the highest rates occurring in those who have private medical insurance. This underscores the importance of having good medical care and taking the prescribed medications to combat this disease. This greatly added lifespan over the past twenty to thirty years is due to the use of medicines that calm down the immune system to treat lupus directly, as well as to treatments for high blood pressure, diabetes, heart disease, strokes, infections, and cancer.

Another important reason for longer lifespans in people who have SLE is doctors' ability to diagnose lupus at an earlier stage. For example, before the current blood tests became widely available, doctors usually could not diagnose SLE until its more severe stages (and in most cases not until after the person had already died). Today doctors are able to diagnose many people when they have very mild problems. Some people are diagnosed with SLE even when they feel perfectly fine (e.g., people who only have mildly low blood counts). Therefore, doctors are able to make a diagnosis of SLE during periods of milder disease when prompt treatment can help prevent it from progressing to more severe disease.

Unfortunately, 2% to 8% of people diagnosed with SLE will still die within ten years of their diagnosis. They have two to five times the risk of dying compared to people who do not have SLE. The vast majority of the deaths in people who have lupus are due to their lupus, cardiovascular disease, infections, and cancer. If people who have SLE learn how to minimize and prevent problems from each of these conditions, then they can greatly improve their chances for survival. The rest of this chapter and later chapters go into more detail about these issues. Since they are quite complex, I have also included a chapter at the end of the book (chapter 44) which I call the "The Lupus Secrets Checklist" that lists these recommendations in an easy-to-read, comprehensive version.

## The Four Most Common Causes of Death in People Who Have SLE

### Lupus

One of the major reasons for people who have lupus living longer over time is that therapies are gradually getting better. However, the disease can still kill people. Lupus nephritis is the most common cause, but major organ system involvement affecting the brain, heart, and lungs or severely low blood counts can also be the culprits. More commonly, it is a combination of factors. Death due to lupus itself more often occurs during the first five years after the diagnosis is made. Then the risk gradually decreases over time after that. Doctors divide the major causes of death in people who have SLE into two large periods. They call this a bimodal pattern ( "bi-" refers to two, and "-modal" refers to time periods). In other words, a bimodal pattern means that there appears to be two periods of increased risk of death in people who have SLE. During the first five years death tends to occur due to the disease itself or from infection, while during the years after that death is more often due to cardiovascular disease or infection. However, death from lupus itself can occur at any time in the lifespan of a person who has lupus. Therefore, people who have SLE should stay vigilant with taking their medications and make sure to see their doctor regularly as recommended throughout their lives.

## Cardiovascular Disease

Cardiovascular (CV) refers to the heart and blood vessels of the body. When doctors talk about cardiovascular disease, they generally are referring to heart attacks, strokes, and blood clots in the blood vessels. The number of people who have SLE who die from CV disease unfortunately is not improving very much. Cardiovascular disease is the number one cause of death after the first five years of having SLE in the United States. Although the treatments for CV disease risk factors such as high blood pressure, diabetes, and high cholesterol have continued to improve over time, other risk factors such as obesity are worsening while problems such as cigarette smoking continue to play a big role. It is vital that everyone who has SLE work diligently with their primary care providers to decrease their CV risk factors to lower the chances of developing heart attacks, strokes, and blood clots. Chapter 21 discusses CV disease and its prevention in more detail.

## Infections

Although CV disease mainly occurs after the first five years of disease, infections can occur at any time and are included with SLE and CV disease as the top three causes of death in people who have lupus. In some parts of the world, infection is the number one cause of death. Two separate 2011 studies (one from Korea and one from China) showed this result. One reason for the increased risk for infections is that people who have moderate to severe lupus require medications that suppress the immune system, and the immune system is very important for fighting infections. In addition, the altered immune systems of people who have lupus make it more difficult for them to fight off infections adequately. To illustrate this point, in the 1930s and 1940s before either antibiotics or steroids became available, 60% of people who had SLE had a severe infection at the time they died. Therefore, it is imperative that the person who has SLE take every step possible to prevent infections (such as getting proper vaccinations) and see a physician immediately at the first signs of any infection. Chapter 22 discusses these measures in detail.

## Cancer

After lupus, CV disease, and infection, cancer is the fourth most common cause of death in people who have SLE. People who have SLE have an increased chance of getting certain cancers and of dying from those cancers compared to people who do not have SLE. The reasons for this may be partly due to their abnormal immune systems. Other potential causes include smoking cigarettes or using certain medications. People who have SLE must have proper screenings for cancer and maintain good lifestyle habits to help prevent cancer. Chapter 23 goes into detail about cancer and lupus.

## Factors Causing Increased Mortality in SLE

Some people who have lupus have certain characteristics (table 20.1) that increase their risk of not doing well with their lupus. Some of these are modifiable (such as being compliant with taking medicines) while others are not (such as age and gender).

### Potentially Modifiable Risk Factors

*Compliance with Treatment.* "Compliance" is a term that medical professionals use to describe how well patients stick to the recommended management of their disorders by their healthcare providers. It includes taking medications as prescribed, keeping doctor appointments, improving lifestyle habits (such as not smoking, eating right, and exercising), and getting medical studies (such as x-rays and labs) done as directed. Certainly, it can be confusing to try to do everything the doctor asks a person to do, especially if she or he has a complicated medical situation. Being compliant with these various parts of treatment can have a profound effect on outcome—that is, improving the chances for being healthier with a good quality of life versus becoming very sick and even possibly dying from lupus complications. People with SLE who are not compliant with their therapy are especially at higher risk of having worse lupus disease activity, requiring hospitalization for severe disease, requiring more trips to the emergency room, having a higher chance for developing significant kidney damage, and unfortunately dying from lupus complications. One study in patients who had SLE showed that 51% of them were not taking their most important medication, hydroxychloroquine (Plaquenil). This shows that noncompliance is a common problem. In my own practice, I have noticed that people who do everything as directed do much better over the long run compared to those who do not.

Factors predicting noncompliance include being younger, being single, having a lower income, having a lower educational level, being unemployed, having a history of missed appointments, having had lupus for a longer period, and having psychologi-

**Table 20.1**  Factors Associated with Increased Mortality in SLE

Modifiable risk factors:
   Noncompliance with treatment

Non-modifiable risk factors (you do not have control over these):
   Ethnicity (actually lower socioeconomic status)
   Gender (men)
   Age at onset
      - children have more severe lupus inflammatory disease
      - older people have more severe organ damage due to aging

   Poverty/insurance coverage
   Geography
   Disease activity

cal problems. Of course, some of these factors cause significant hardships that make it very difficult for the person to be compliant. For example, the person who has little money or does not have good insurance may not be able to afford transportation to get to doctors' appointments, or be unable to afford the medications and tests required for optimal healthcare. People who have a lower educational level may have more difficulty understanding what lupus is and how it may affect them if they do not treat it properly. Psychological issues and psychiatric disorders cause complex difficulties in following through with the numerous requirements for proper healthcare. Younger people are more apt to have a sense of denial about their disease, feel invulnerable, and not take it as seriously as they should. They often say they are too busy (work, family, life) to keep up on their healthcare, and are more apt to stop taking medicines especially when they are feeling well. Single people lack the support structure provided by partners or spouses (who could encourage their partners or spouses to keep taking their medicines and to see their doctors regularly). So if you identify yourself as being in one of these groups who have an increased chance of being noncompliant, it may take extra effort on your part to stay compliant.

Compliance is important in doing well. The person who has lupus has some control over this particular aspect of health. Overall, noncompliance is the number one cause of lupus flares and with doing poorly from lupus, including developing severe kidney disease and even dying. Compliance not only refers to taking medicines—it includes using sunscreen every day, not smoking, seeing doctors regularly, and so on. The vast majority of people who have SLE who are fully compliant with therapy will do very well. Refer to the "Lupus Secrets" in chapter 44 to ensure that you are doing everything you can to be compliant.

Although some people cannot stay compliant due to economic and psychological reasons, most people are able to control compliance. If people who have SLE go to all of their doctors' appointments, take their medications regularly, get all of their tests, and keep up good lifestyle habits (such as using sunscreen daily, not smoking, maintaining a good weight, eating well, getting plenty of sleep, and exercising regularly), they will go a long way in doing well with their SLE. However, people should not take medicines blindly. They should make sure that they understand what the medicines are for and what potential side effects can occur. Compliance is the one thing that the person who has SLE has control of, so it is very important to do everything possible to be a compliant patient.

## Non-Modifiable Risk Factors

*Ethnicity.* Studies in general show that Caucasians have better outcomes and lower death rates compared to other ethnic groups such as African Americans. Recent studies, however, show that socioeconomic status is more important than ethnicity. In other words, having a lower income is a better predictor of not doing well with lupus instead of what ancestral background a person is. Since some ethnic groups (such as African Americans and Hispanics) have higher poverty rates compared to others (such as Caucasians), this may explain why previous studies showed these differences among ethnic groups.

Another compounding issue is the effect of cultural beliefs among ethnic groups. For example, members of some ethnic groups (such as some Asian and Hispanic groups) may place a higher trust in home remedies or non-Western medicine practices and may be less likely to take the medications prescribed to them (i.e., the compliance issue discussed previously).

*Gender.* Males make up close to 10% of people who have SLE. Most studies suggest that men as a group have more severe disease and may have a higher death rate than women who have SLE. However, a few studies do not show a marked difference between the sexes. Although one study from the 1980s showed Asian American women to have more severe disease than Asian American men, there are more studies showing that men may overall have more severe disease and a higher mortality rate compared to women.

*Age at Onset.* As discussed in chapter 19, children tend to have more severe disease overall compared to older people. Infants who have SLE have the highest mortality rates. Unfortunately, the death rate approaches 50% in infants less than 1 year of age (this only refers to infants who have SLE, not to those who have neonatal lupus, as discussed in chapters 1 and 18). Older children generally do well with treatment, but they have a higher mortality rate compared to that of adults who develop SLE. In fact, a 2008 study showed that when deaths in adult SLE patients are assessed, those adult SLE patients who had developed SLE while they were children had an overall higher death rate compared to adults who had developed their disease while they were adults.

At the other end of the spectrum are people who develop late-onset SLE. Late-onset lupus occurs after the ages of 50 to 60 (after the childbearing years). Although this group tends to have overall less severe disease activity from their lupus (as discussed in chapter 19), they tend to develop more actual damage to their organs. This most likely occurs because their aging organs are more susceptible to damage from the inflammation of their lupus compared to the organs of their younger counterparts. Because of this, they have a higher mortality rate overall compared to younger people who have SLE. This is not unexpected; "healthy" people over the age of 50 also have higher death rates compared to those who are less than 50 years old.

*Poverty/Insurance Coverage.* Numerous studies have shown that having a lower socioeconomic status (in other words, having a low income) plays a major role in disease activity and mortality. People with low incomes are less likely to have good insurance, are less likely to have the money required to pay for medications and medical tests, and are more likely to have difficulty in obtaining transportation to see their doctors. It is not surprising that this would translate into having more severe disease and having a higher chance of dying. I have included this in the section on non-modifiable risk factors for having severe lupus. You may think that this factor is modifiable since we live in America, and everyone in America has the chances of advancing to a higher socioeconomic status or making more money simply by studying hard, making good grades, and working hard. However, the fact is that if someone develops severe SLE and she or he is already in a lower socioeconomic group, it becomes a vicious cycle of poverty and continued poor healthcare. When a person who has a low income becomes severely ill with lupus, it is harder to get well because of the problems with having poor to no insurance at all and not being able to afford the proper medical care. When a person is sick, it becomes very hard, if not sometimes impossible, to work or study. I have seen with my own eyes patients who were working or studying very hard while they were healthy only to have their dreams crushed because of the devastation of their illness, and it had nothing to do with their motivation. Certainly, America's health-care system needs vast improvements to provide all Americans with good healthcare; however, I will not turn this section into a political statement. I hope that things will change for the better in the future.

*Geographical Location.* Certain sections of the United States have higher mortality rates from SLE compared to other areas. The three most important factors found to explain these differences are poverty, increased Hispanic populations, and increased ultraviolet B (UVB) light exposure in the areas of higher death rates. Areas of highest death rates are the southwestern United States (especially around Southern California to southeastern New Mexico), while the lowest rates are clustered around the north-eastern United States (particularly the New Hampshire area). However, the states of Washington, Minnesota, Illinois, and Ohio have lower death rates as well compared to other parts of the country. The higher death rates seen in some areas of larger Hispanic populations may be reflective of the higher poverty rates in those particular areas. It certainly makes sense that areas of high UVB exposure would have higher rates of severe SLE activity and deaths—chapter 3 explained how important a role ultraviolet light plays in making SLE active.

I have placed geographical location in the "non-modifiable" factors section. How-ever, you could argue that it is "modifiable" because if you live in southeastern New Mexico in Chaves County (the area of highest death rates from SLE), you could move to areas in the study that had the lowest death rates (Strafford County, New Hampshire; Roseau County, Minnesota; or Lewis County, Washington). However, moving is a very difficult thing to do and is contingent upon being able to find a good job in the area that you move to, not to mention the difficulties of moving to a place where you have no support structure (friends and family). In addition, if you are able to just pick yourself up and move at a whim like that, you are more apt to have the money to do so, which is a good prognostic factor (i.e., you have a lower chance of dying from SLE due to not having a low income). In addition, there are no studies to show that if people move from a place of high death rates for SLE to an area of low death rates that their chances of dying decrease. However, this is an interesting question and not to be discounted as a possible choice to increase your chances of doing well.

*Disease Activity.* It makes sense that having increased lupus disease activity would place someone at greater risk of having worse disease and an increased chance of dy-ing from SLE. A recent study showed that 83% of patients who had lupus nephritis sur-vived ten years or longer, which is lower than the overall survival of 92% to 98% of all people who have SLE at ten years, as mentioned previously.

When a person who has SLE is doing well and has no evidence of active disease, doctors label him or her as being "clinically quiescent." This means that the disease is "quiet" ("quiescent" comes from the Latin word for "to rest" or "to become quiet") in a clinical sense as far as the history and physical exam are concerned, and that blood and urine tests demonstrate that organs such as the kidneys and liver as well as blood counts are doing well. A recent study showed that patients labeled as being clinically quiescent were much less likely to have flares of their lupus or to develop severe disease (such as lupus nephritis) compared to patients who had active disease. In addition, they were even less likely to develop heart attacks (one of the most common causes of death in people who have SLE) compared to those with active disease. However, it also showed that people who have SLE who are clinically quiescent can develop more active lupus over time. Sixty percent of clinically quiescent patients ended up having a flare of their SLE over time. Therefore, this study also shows that it is still very important that even people who are labeled as being "clinically quiescent" be diligent about being compliant (one of the modifiable risk factors) with their therapy, keeping their doctors' appointments, and keeping up on their lab tests.

Another term often used with "clinically quiescent" is the term "serologically active." These terms deserve explanation because people who have SLE may read these in their doctor's notes and should know what they mean. "Serologically" pertains to the blood test results that assess the activity of the immune system. In SLE, this specifically refers to the level of anti-ds DNA and C3 and C4 complement levels. Recall from chapter 4 that a high anti-ds DNA or low levels of C3 and C4 complement can occur when SLE is more active. When the ds DNA is high, or either of these complement levels are lower than normal, a person is "serologically active." This means that there is evidence of the immune system being active with inflammation due to SLE. If someone is "clinically quiescent but serologically active," this means that her or his lupus is not causing any active or major problems, and it appears to be under control. However, there is some background evidence of lupus activity in the immune system. The person who is "clinically quiescent but serologically active" is at higher risk for lupus flares compared to someone who has normal ds DNA and normal complement levels. This person is especially at increased risk for developing inflammation of the kidneys (lupus nephritis). Therefore, the person's rheumatologist will want to continue watching this person very closely to make sure that nothing does flare in the near future.

However, things in lupus are never clear-cut. Although I watch my patients who are serologically active very closely, I have had some patients who are "clinically quiescent but serologically active" who stayed this way for many years, never developing any lupus flares and never developing any lupus nephritis while taking their treatments (such as Plaquenil and using their sunscreen). Yet, there have also certainly been those patients who did unfortunately develop flares of their lupus, and worse, developed lupus nephritis. With watching them more closely (because of being serologically active), though, these problems were identified quickly and at early stages to prevent a bad outcome.

### KEY POINTS TO REMEMBER

1. Currently, about 91% to 98% of patients diagnosed with SLE survive ten years or longer after the diagnosis.

2. This increased life expectancy is primarily due to diagnosing SLE at earlier stages of disease, improved therapies to treat SLE, and the use of antibiotics to treat infections.

3. The most common causes of death in people with SLE are lupus disease activity, infections, and cardiovascular disease (such as heart attacks and strokes).

4. Cancer is the fourth most common cause of death in people who have lupus; however, it is much less common than the top three causes.

5. To decrease the risk of developing severe disease and dying, it is extremely important to stay compliant with taking medications, see doctors as directed, and obtain the recommended medical tests.

6. People who have SLE should be diligent about preventing and treating infections and heart attacks, and they should keep up with their cancer screenings.

7. Read "The Lupus Secrets Checklist" in chapter 44 for a simplified list of things to do to improve compliance on these issues.

# PART III

# Other Complications of Lupus and Their Treatments

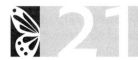

# Heart Attacks and Strokes

## Work at Preventing Heart Attacks and Strokes!

In our clinic, we ask that all of our lupus patients have a primary care doctor and that they see him or her regularly. In fact, this is as important as seeing a rheumatologist regularly for treatment of lupus even if the person is young and feels perfectly fine. The reasons?

- Cardiovascular problems (heart attacks, strokes, and blood clots) are the number one cause of death in people who have SLE after the first few years of their diagnosis.

- These problems occur at a much younger age than in their peers (I have SLE patients in their twenties who have had heart attacks and strokes).

- Primary care doctors are the experts at preventing these problems from occurring by monitoring and treating the cardiovascular risk factors of high blood pressure, high cholesterol, diabetes, obesity, lack of exercise, poor diet, and smoking.

If you are serious about living a long, normal lifespan with your SLE, then you have to make it a priority to prevent these complications from occurring. Read this chapter, and make that appointment with your primary care doctor (preferably an internal medicine doctor or a family practice doctor) right away and see him or her at least every six months to monitor you closely. Remember that preventative medicine is the best medicine.

••••

"Cardiovascular events" (or "CV events" for short) is a medical term that includes problems with the heart and blood vessels of the body. "Cardio-" refers to the heart, and "-vascular" refers to the blood vessels of the body. Cardiovascular events are the number one cause of death in people who have SLE in the United States. As mentioned in chapter 20, causes of death in people who have lupus occur in a bimodal distribution (in other words, in two different periods—"bi-" means two) that are associated with different patterns of death. In the first five years, if a person who has SLE dies, it is more likely to be from lupus or infection. After the first five years, death is more commonly due to cardiovascular events, followed by lupus activity and infections. Dr. Murray Urowitz in Toronto, Ontario, Canada, first described this bimodal pattern in SLE. He found that after having lupus for five years or more, people who had SLE were more likely to have either heart attacks or sudden cardiac death (discussed later), and this does not even count other cardiovascular problems such as strokes and blood clots. Since CV events are the most common cause of death, it is incredibly important that people who have SLE do everything that they can to decrease their chances of developing these complications. Although heart attacks and strokes are two of the most common CV events, other possibilities include angina, heart rhythm problems, congestive heart failure, peripheral vascular disease, and blood clots.

Chapter 11 discussed how SLE could attack the heart and blood vessels, causing inflammation and damage; this chapter focuses on how people who have lupus can develop problems with the heart and blood vessels for other reasons. These same cardiovascular problems occur in people who do not have lupus. In fact, cardiovascular disease is the most common cause of death in people in the United States overall and becomes more common as we get older.

This is a good point to define some medical terms associated with hardening of the arteries. Doctors describe hardening of the arteries using both "arteriosclerosis" and "atherosclerosis." "Arterio-" refers to the blood vessels called arteries, and "-sclerosis" means "scarring" or "hardening of"—therefore, "arteriosclerosis" is literally "hardening of the arteries." The Greek word "athero" means "paste." "Atherosclerosis" refers to the buildup of a paste-like substance called plaque within the hardening blood vessels. Plaque is composed of cholesterol and clotted blood. As plaque builds up (figure 21.1), it decreases blood flow in the artery. The tissues and organs of the body that have these clogged arteries end up getting less blood flow, and this lack of blood results in inadequate amounts of nutrition and oxygen. If the blood vessel gets completely clogged with plaque, then the person can get a heart attack if it occurs in the blood vessels that feed the heart muscle; a stroke if it occurs in the brain; bowel ischemia if it occurs in the intestines; as well as problems in other parts of the body. Doctors call arteriosclerosis in the arteries of the heart (also called the coronary arteries) coronary artery disease. When it occurs in the blood vessels of the brain they call it cerebrovascular disease (see chapter 13), and when it occurs in other blood vessels it is called peripheral vascular disease.

People who have SLE develop arteriosclerosis (or atherosclerosis), causing cardiovascular disease, cerebrovascular disease, and peripheral vascular disease, at a younger age than other people. The faster than usual onset of these problems has been termed "accelerated arteriosclerosis" or "accelerated atherosclerosis." Some of the causes of arteriosclerosis are similar in people who have lupus and the rest of the population (such as high blood pressure, diabetes, obesity, high cholesterol, and cigarette smoking). However, direct inflammation from lupus itself also plays an important role. This chapter discusses these various causes and gives recommendations to decrease the possibility of developing CV events.

## Types of Cardiovascular Events

### Coronary Artery Disease (Angina and Heart Attacks)

When atherosclerosis occurs in the blood vessels of the heart (the coronary arteries), it is called coronary artery disease (CAD for short). This occurs when the insides of the arteries narrow due to plaque. Eventually, the blood flow to a section of the heart mus-

A

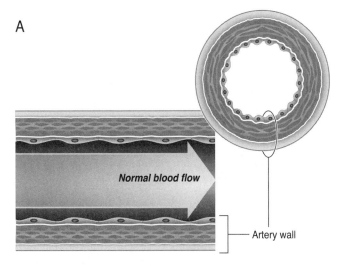

**Normal blood flow**

Artery wall

**Cross-sections of Normal Coronary Artery**

B

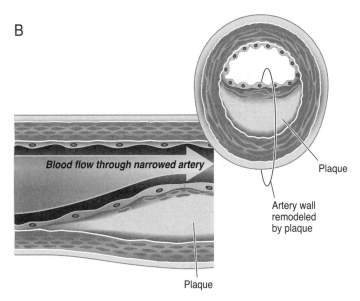

**Blood flow through narrowed artery**

Plaque

Artery wall
remodeled
by plaque

Plaque

**Cross-sections of Atherosclerotic Coronary Artery**

**Figure 21.1** Views of a normal artery and an artery with plaque (due to arteriosclerosis) decreasing blood flow

cle decreases to the point where it cannot get enough oxygen from the bloodstream. When the heart muscle has to work harder (such as during exercise, walking, or even during stress), it requires more blood flow to supply the necessary increased amounts of oxygen and nutrition. However, if there is narrowing of the arteries due to CAD, there is decreased blood coming through the narrowed blood vessels, so the muscle does not get enough oxygen to function properly. This can cause a type of pain in the chest area called angina. The person often feels this pain underneath the breastbone as a pressure-like discomfort. Sometimes it will travel (or "radiate") to the arm (often the left one) or the jaw. Angina typically occurs during periods of exertion and stress, then gradually resolves once the person rests or after the person takes something such as nitroglycerin (which opens the coronary arteries up wider to allow more blood flow to the heart muscle). Some people will also get shortness of breath or nausea along with the angina. Some people will get these other symptoms of angina without the chest pain—that is, they will only get jaw discomfort, arm discomfort, nausea, or shortness of breath. In fact, it has become increasingly clear that women especially can get shortness of breath or nausea without the classic chest pain of angina. This can cause difficulties in making a correct diagnosis of heart disease in women.

If a blockage completely obstructs one of the coronary arteries, then that particular part of the heart muscle loses its supply of blood. This causes a complete lack of vital oxygen and nutrients. That section of heart muscle quickly begins to die and causes symptoms similar to those of angina, but they are usually more intense and prolonged. Physicians call this complete loss of blood flow to a section of heart muscle a myocardial infarction (or "heart attack" in layperson's terms). "Myocardial" refers to the muscle ("myo-") of the heart ("-cardio"), and "infarction" is the medical term describing death of tissue due to the lack of oxygen because of a blocked artery.

The problem of CAD causing heart attacks in people who have SLE cannot be over-emphasized. By the age of 45, one out of every three people who have SLE has evidence of coronary artery disease. Studies show that women who have SLE are fifty times more likely to have a heart attack and to die from a heart attack compared to women their same age who do not have SLE. This problem seems to be especially prevalent in African American women—a 2010 study showed that they develop coronary artery disease and get heart attacks about twenty years younger than African American women who do not have lupus. However, this same study showed that men and women who have SLE of all ethnicities developed coronary artery disease at younger ages than people who do not have SLE. Overall, the average age for SLE patients admitted to the hospital with a heart attack was about ten years younger than patients who did not have lupus. Another 2013 study supported these findings by showing that people who had SLE had the same amount of coronary artery disease on cardiac catheterization studies compared to non-lupus patients who were 20 years older.

These problems can be diagnosed using various types of heart tests, including an ECG (electrocardiogram, also called an EKG), stress test (where an ECG is monitored while a person exercises), and an echocardiogram (see chapter 11). If a myocardial infarction (heart attack) is suspected, then the person should be admitted to the hospital to have these tests done and be treated immediately. In addition, doctors will obtain blood tests to look at cardiac muscle enzymes that become elevated after a myocardial infarction due to the damage done to the heart muscle. It is very important that a person experiencing unexplained chest pain go to an emergency room (ER) immediately for evaluation. If the person is evaluated quickly enough, doctors are able to use medications that can open up the clogged arteries and prevent permanent damage to the heart. It can be a potentially fatal mistake to experience chest pain, and then wait to see if it goes away instead of immediately going to the hospital.

## Heart Rhythm Problems (Arrhythmias)

The way that the heart normally beats is due to electrical impulses that travel along the nervous system of the heart—called the electrical conduction system. This system normally makes sure that the two atria of the heart squeeze blood at the same time, followed by the two ventricles. It also makes sure that the heart does this at a particular rate or frequency (which we can measure as the heartbeat, or how many times the heart beats in a minute). The correct regulation of the heartbeat and the sequence of when the atria and the ventricles beat are very important to ensure that the proper amount of blood is sent through the lungs to absorb enough oxygen, and then throughout the body to feed and oxygenate all the cells of the body. If there is an abnormality of the electrical conduction system and the electrical activity of the heart becomes abnormal, then the heart can beat too fast or too slow, or the order of when the atria and the ventricles beat in relationship to each other can be abnormal. If any of these abnormal events occur, then the heart pumps blood improperly, causing decreased blood flow through the lungs and the rest of the body. Doctors call this group of problems, where the electrical conduction system of the heart works incorrectly, arrhythmias; "-rhythmia" refers to the rhythm of the beating of the heart, and the prefix "a-" is the Greek term indicating "a lack of" or "absence of." Therefore, an arrhythmia is the lack or absence of a normal rhythm of the beating of the heart muscle. There are numerous types of arrhythmias. Some of the common names for arrhythmias include atrial fibrillation, atrial flutter, supraventricular tachycardia, sick sinus syndrome, bradycardia (slow heartbeat), and tachycardia (fast heartbeat).

One study at the Heart Rhythm Society 2011 meeting showed that SLE patients had a 60% higher risk of having atrial fibrillation compared to people who did not have lupus. These problems can certainly occur because of damage due to inflammation from lupus, as described in chapter 11. However, they more commonly occur due to a lack of oxygen and nutrients to the electrical conduction system because of coronary artery disease. These problems may also occur when the electrical conduction system stretches abnormally. This can happen when the heart muscle becomes thicker or larger than normal due to coronary artery disease, high blood pressure, or valvular heart disease (see chapter 11).

The person who has an arrhythmia can have various symptoms. These include having heart "palpitations" where the person can actually feel the beating of the heart in the chest. It can feel faster or more prominent than normal. These palpitations are due to the abnormal heartbeat. Other symptoms have to do with the problems associated with not enough oxygenated blood flowing to the lungs and rest of the body. This can include having chest pain, being lightheaded or dizzy, and having shortness of breath. If severe enough, the person can even pass out when a severe arrhythmia occurs.

An ECG is usually required to diagnose an arrhythmia. Sometimes the doctor will ask the person to wear an ECG device called a Holter monitor. This can be worn for twenty-four hours or longer to pick up recurrent arrhythmias. Many arrhythmias are minor and require no treatment at all, while medications are required to treat arrhythmias that are more significant. In severe cases, the person may require a pacemaker or defibrillator implanted under the skin of the chest to make sure that the heart beats properly. Some people can benefit from electrical cardioversion, where paddles placed on the chest send an electric shock to the heart to cause it to beat properly. The person is typically sedated with medication during cardioversion so that she or he is as comfortable as possible and does not feel the electrical shock. Some people can even have a surgical procedure called ablation therapy where a part of the electrical conduction system is blocked (ablated) to prevent excessive, unwanted electrical impulses from occurring.

## Congestive Heart Failure

Congestive heart failure (CHF) occurs when the heart muscle is not able to pump blood adequately to the lungs and the rest of the body. When this occurs, the entire body lacks the appropriate amount of nutrients and oxygen. Blood backs up into the blood vessels of the lung, causing a leakage of fluid into the lungs, and in the veins of the body since there is difficulty with blood passing through the heart properly. This fluid backup can cause swelling of the legs (called edema). People who have CHF usually have shortness of breath that gets worse with exertion, and they feel fatigued. When they lie down, more fluid collects in the lungs, causing worsening of their shortness of breath. Therefore, they often find that they breathe better if they sleep on extra pillows or even while sitting up.

CHF is a severe heart problem, and is one of the most common causes of death in older people. However, it can occur in anyone of any age who has a severe enough heart condition. It can be due to any problem of the heart that keeps it from working properly, including high blood pressure, coronary artery disease, myocarditis (see chapter 11), arrhythmias, and valvular heart disease (see chapter 11). Doctors treat it by initially identifying the heart condition that is causing the CHF and then treating that particular heart problem (such as controlling the blood pressure in the person who has high blood pressure). The physician may prescribe "water pills" (called diuretics) to get rid of excessive fluid from the body. The person who has severe CHF may also require oxygen to help her or him breathe properly.

## Sudden Cardiac Death

Sudden cardiac death occurs when someone dies abruptly without warning due to the heart stopping. This is most commonly due to a massive heart attack (from CAD) or a severe arrhythmia.

## Peripheral Vascular Disease

When arteriosclerosis or atherosclerosis occurs in the arteries other than the blood vessels of the heart (which is called CAD), it is called peripheral vascular disease (PVD) or peripheral artery disease (PAD), which both mean the same thing. "Peripheral" refers to the arteries that are "away from" the heart. Blockage of the peripheral arteries can cause problems with whatever organ the blocked arteries supply. Arteriosclerosis of the arteries in the legs can cause muscle cramping or leg muscle pain with walking (called claudication in medical terms). It can also cause the feet to be cooler than normal. The feet and toes may have a bluish discoloration due to the lack of oxygen getting to the tissues of the feet. PVD of the legs is treated by treating the causes of arteriosclerosis (discussed later in this chapter), but surgery and medicines can also be helpful to open up the arteries of the legs.

If PVD occurs in the arteries of the kidneys, then there may be decreased kidney function. A low eGFR on blood tests (see chapter 4) signifies a decrease in kidney function. Blood pressure can even become elevated due to the decreased blood supply to the kidneys. If the arteries of the intestines are blocked, then abdominal pain can occur along with bleeding from the rectum due to the damage occurring in the intestines from the lack of oxygen and nutrients (called bowel ischemia).

The carotid arteries are the large arteries in the neck that supply blood to the brain. If plaque from atherosclerosis clogs these arteries, doctors call it carotid artery disease (which is a type of peripheral vascular disease). This can potentially cause decreased blood flow to parts of the brain and can be the cause of a stroke (called a cerebrovascular accident, or CVA for short). Sometimes, if there is plaque buildup in the carotid arteries due to arteriosclerosis, a small piece of plaque can become loose (at which time it is called an embolus) and travel to the brain to cause a stroke. If an embolus travels to the arteries that go to the eyes, it can cause temporary (or even permanent) blindness in one eye. Physicians call this temporary loss of sight amaurosis fugax ("amaurosis" comes from the Greek word for "darkening of" and "fugax" from the Greek term for "fleeting"). In other words, there is a fleeting (or temporary) moment of darkening of vision in one of the eyes. This can be a very important clue to the possibility of carotid artery disease due to atherosclerosis. An ultrasound of the carotid arteries can find the plaque buildup in the carotid arteries to make a diagnosis of carotid artery disease. This is very important to figure out because the person who has amaurosis fugax due to carotid artery disease is at high risk of developing a stroke if it is not treated. In addition to treating the causes of arteriosclerosis (which will be discussed below), it can also be treated with surgery to open the artery up. Doctors call peripheral vascular disease in the arteries located within the brain itself cerebrovascular disease (see chapter 13).

In addition to causing decreased blood to areas of the body, peripheral vascular disease can also cause the walls of the arteries to become dilated and thinner than normal. Doctors call this dilatation of an artery an aneurysm. An aneurysm can occur in most arteries of the body, but most commonly in the largest artery of the body (called the aorta) and in the blood vessels of the brain. The danger of aneurysms is that they can potentially burst due to the thinned out and weakened arterial wall. This can become a potentially deadly situation. A person who has an aneurysm may need surgery to decrease the chances of it rupturing. Physicians can also prescribe medicines to try to prevent an aneurysm rupture.

## Cerebrovascular Disease

Chapter 13 discusses cerebrovascular disease in more detail. Cerebrovascular disease can be due to the direct influence of inflammation from lupus in the brain, but it also can be due to other causes, including arteriosclerosis in the arteries of the brain. Doctors call arteriosclerosis of the brain cerebrovascular disease—where "cerebro-" refers to the brain.

## Blood Clots (Thrombi and Emboli)

Chapter 9 discusses the problem of blood clots due to the antiphospholipid antibody syndrome in people who have SLE. However, blood clots can also occur in people who do not have antiphospholipid antibodies, and are due to many of the problems that can cause arteriosclerosis (obesity, smoking, diabetes, high blood pressure, etc.). Therefore, people who have SLE can also get blood clots due to these risk factors even in the absence of having antiphospholipid antibodies.

## Some Causes of Accelerated Arteriosclerosis in SLE

### Diabetes

Diabetes is a disease where the level of glucose (a type of sugar) is elevated in the body due to problems with the body handling it correctly. Diabetes is a well-known cause of atherosclerosis due to its causing damage to the blood vessels of the body and causing arteriosclerotic plaques to occur in the blood vessels of the body. People who have SLE are at increased risk of developing diabetes due to their increased risk of obesity. In addition, steroids used to treat SLE can cause diabetes or make diabetes worse in people who already have it.

There are several ways that doctors diagnose diabetes (table 21.1). One way is by measuring hemoglobin A1C. Hemoglobin A1C is a blood test that can estimate the amount of glucose in the body over approximately a three-month period. An A1C level $\geq$ 6.5% is sufficient to make a diagnosis of diabetes when reproduced on more than one occasion. Another way is to measure a fasting glucose level. The chemistry blood test that your rheumatologist orders at each visit usually also measures the glucose level. However, if you are not fasting for the test, it is not an accurate way to measure the glucose level because eating anything with sugar in it can artificially raise the glucose level. If you fast for eight hours before your blood work (not taking anything by mouth except for water and your medicines), then your glucose level can be relied upon to determine your risk of having diabetes. Your doctor may diagnose you with diabetes if the fasting glucose is greater than or equal to 126 mg/dL. A glucose level $\geq$ 200 mg/dL can also indicate diabetes even if the person was not fasting for the blood test. Another way to diagnose diabetes is by doing a two-hour fasting plasma glucose test. This involves measuring the glucose level first after fasting, then drinking some glucose in water, and then repeating the plasma glucose test two hours later. You have diabetes if your two-hour glucose test is $\geq$ 200 mg/dL.

**Table 21.1**  How Diabetes Is Diagnosed

| |
|---|
| Hemoglobin A1C $\geq$ 6.5% |
| Fasting glucose $\geq$ 126 mg/dL |
| Blood glucose (either non-fasting or fasting) $\geq$ 200 mg/dL |
| Two-hour plasma glucose $\geq$ 200 mg/dL |

## Obesity

Overweight people are at increased risk of developing arteriosclerosis. Obese people also are more prone to having other related problems such as diabetes, high blood pressure, and high cholesterol. People who have SLE are at increased risk of being obese due to the use of steroids, which can cause weight gain. In addition, the fatigue and pain that can occur with SLE can cause the person who has SLE to move around and exercise less, therefore causing weight gain.

Studies show that 50% or more of people who have SLE are obese. Obesity is a medical condition where there is excessive body fat accumulation to the point where it has adverse effects on health. Various measurements can diagnose obesity—most commonly, the body mass index (or BMI for short), the waist circumference (WC), and the weight:hip ratio (WHR).

BMI is measured by the formula BMI = (weight in pounds X 703) ÷ (height in inches X height in inches). A BMI chart (table 21.2) or an online BMI calculator can determine your BMI. However, you can also figure it out by using this formula yourself. For example, a person who is 4 feet 8 inches (or 56 inches) and weighs 150 pounds is not included on the BMI chart below. This person can calculate her or his own BMI: (150 X 703) ÷ (56 X 56) = (105,450) ÷ (3,136) = 33.6. So what does this number mean? In general, a person who has a BMI of 25 or higher is considered overweight. A person who has a BMI of 30 or higher is considered obese. A BMI of 40 or higher is labeled extremely obese (also called morbidly obese), while a BMI of 50 or higher is considered super morbidly obese.

Most people who are 10% to 20% heavier than their ideal body weight are considered overweight if that extra weight is not due to additional muscle (as seen in athletes). Overweight people are at increased risk for developing cardiovascular disease compared to those whose weight is normal. Obese people are at a higher risk for health problems, including cardiovascular disease. People who are morbidly obese and super morbidly obese are at the highest risk for health problems such as cardiovascular disease and numerous other obesity-related medical problems that cause great disability and early death. I hope that everyone who is reading this section will calculate his or her own BMI. Many people become more motivated to lose weight if they realize exactly how overweight they are.

BMI, however, does have some limitations. People who are athletic or muscular can have a higher BMI due to their having increased weight because of more muscle mass. Using BMI alone could incorrectly classify them as being obese or overweight, while in reality they are very healthy with low amounts of body fat. On the opposite end of the spectrum are people who have lower than normal amounts of muscle mass, such as the elderly and people who are ill or who do not exercise. They can potentially have a normal BMI (defined as a BMI between 18.5 and 29.9), yet in reality be overweight or even obese since they may have very little actual muscle and instead have too much fat in their bodies. Many people who have SLE fall into this latter category. The use of steroids such as prednisone causes the breakdown of muscle in the body and the increased accumulation of fat. Many people treated with steroids are actually obese or overweight even though they may have a normal BMI. Other people who have SLE do not move around or exercise due to the pain and fatigue caused by their disease. This

**Table 21.2  BMI**

| BMI, kg/m² | Good Weight | | | | | | Overweight | | | | | Obese | | Morbidly Obese |
|---|---|---|---|---|---|---|---|---|---|---|---|---|---|---|
| | 19 | 20 | 21 | 22 | 23 | 24 | 25 | 26 | 27 | 28 | 29 | 30 | 39 | 40 |
| Height, inches | Weight, pounds | | | | | | | | | | | | | |
| 58 | 91 | 96 | 100 | 105 | 110 | 115 | 119 | 124 | 129 | 134 | 138 | 143 | 186 | 191 |
| 59 | 94 | 99 | 104 | 109 | 114 | 119 | 124 | 128 | 133 | 138 | 143 | 148 | 193 | 198 |
| 60 | 97 | 102 | 107 | 112 | 118 | 123 | 128 | 133 | 138 | 143 | 148 | 153 | 199 | 204 |
| 61 | 100 | 106 | 111 | 116 | 122 | 127 | 132 | 137 | 143 | 148 | 153 | 158 | 206 | 211 |
| 62 | 104 | 109 | 115 | 120 | 126 | 131 | 136 | 142 | 147 | 153 | 158 | 164 | 213 | 218 |
| 63 | 107 | 113 | 118 | 124 | 130 | 135 | 141 | 146 | 152 | 158 | 163 | 169 | 220 | 225 |
| 64 | 110 | 116 | 122 | 128 | 134 | 140 | 145 | 151 | 157 | 163 | 168 | 174 | 227 | 232 |
| 65 | 114 | 120 | 126 | 132 | 138 | 144 | 150 | 156 | 162 | 168 | 174 | 180 | 234 | 240 |
| 66 | 118 | 124 | 130 | 136 | 142 | 148 | 155 | 161 | 167 | 173 | 179 | 186 | 241 | 247 |
| 67 | 121 | 127 | 134 | 140 | 146 | 153 | 159 | 166 | 172 | 178 | 185 | 191 | 249 | 255 |
| 68 | 125 | 131 | 138 | 144 | 151 | 158 | 164 | 171 | 177 | 184 | 190 | 197 | 256 | 262 |
| 69 | 128 | 135 | 142 | 149 | 155 | 162 | 169 | 176 | 182 | 189 | 196 | 203 | 263 | 270 |
| 70 | 132 | 139 | 146 | 153 | 160 | 167 | 174 | 181 | 188 | 195 | 202 | 209 | 271 | 278 |
| 71 | 136 | 143 | 150 | 157 | 165 | 172 | 179 | 186 | 193 | 200 | 208 | 215 | 279 | 286 |
| 72 | 140 | 147 | 154 | 162 | 169 | 177 | 184 | 191 | 199 | 206 | 213 | 221 | 287 | 294 |
| 73 | 144 | 151 | 159 | 166 | 174 | 182 | 189 | 197 | 204 | 212 | 219 | 227 | 295 | 302 |
| 74 | 148 | 155 | 163 | 171 | 179 | 186 | 194 | 202 | 210 | 218 | 225 | 233 | 303 | 311 |
| 75 | 152 | 160 | 168 | 176 | 184 | 192 | 200 | 208 | 216 | 224 | 232 | 240 | 311 | 319 |
| 76 | 156 | 164 | 172 | 180 | 189 | 197 | 205 | 213 | 221 | 230 | 238 | 246 | 320 | 328 |

can cause them to lose muscle mass and gain fat instead. A 2011 study suggested that a BMI of 26.8 or higher more accurately predicts obesity in women who have SLE instead of the commonly used BMI of 30. Women who have lupus who have been on steroids and/or have not exercised very much are more likely to be obese if the BMI is 26.8 or higher.

Another easy way to diagnose obesity is by measuring the waist circumference (WC). To measure the WC, stand up relaxed without wearing a shirt or top. With your fingers, find your waist, which is the soft portion above your hipbones. Exhale slightly, then, at approximately the level of or just above the belly button, wrap a tape measure around this area. Make sure it is snug but not compressing the skin and that it is parallel to the floor. Place one finger on the tape at the point where the zero end of the tape hits your waist measurement and read the measurement (figure 21.2). Repeat this two more times. Use an average of the two numbers that are closest to each other. A WC of greater than 35 inches in women and of greater than 40 inches in men is associated with an increased risk of developing cardiovascular disease. However, the same study mentioned above looking at obesity in women who have SLE suggests that a WC of more than 33.4 inches (instead of 35 inches) more accurately diagnoses obesity. It should be noted that this study did not include any men who have lupus. Therefore, if you have SLE and have been on steroids or do not exercise regularly, it is most likely more accurate to use the 33.4 inches cutoff for obesity.

Measuring the waist to hip ratio (WHR) is another way to diagnose obesity. To calculate your WHR, measure your waist circumference in inches using the method in the above paragraph. Then measure your hip circumference at the widest part of your buttocks in inches (see figure 21.2). Then divide the number for your waist size by the hip size. The normal WHR in women is 0.8 or less and in men is 0.95 or less. Women are considered to be obese if the WHR is 0.85 or higher, and in men if it is 1.0 or higher.

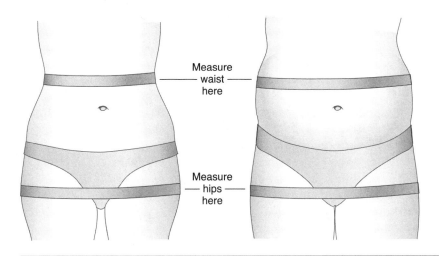

Measure waist here

Measure hips here

**Figure 21.2** Measuring waist and hip circumferences

However, the study mentioned above in women who have SLE suggests that a WHR of greater than 0.8 more accurately diagnoses obesity. Table 21.3 summarizes the definitions of obesity using these different measurements.

I need to offer my opinion here on men who have SLE and diagnosing obesity. Just as in women, I suspect that men who have SLE who have been on steroids or who do not exercise regularly should probably use lower numbers than those listed in the table. There has not been a study in men who have lupus, to my knowledge, to answer this question. This most likely is due to the lower numbers of men who have SLE, which makes it difficult to do this kind of study.

However, it is becoming clearer that these measurements underestimate the number of people who are obese. A more accurate measurement for detecting the percentage of the body that is muscle versus fat is by the use of an x-ray technique called a dual-emission x-ray absorptiometry (DXA scan for short, pronounced "DECKS'uh"). This scan also diagnoses osteoporosis by measuring the strength of bone in the body, but it is also helpful for measuring the amount of body fat. Many rheumatologists, endocrinologists, and radiology offices have DXA machines. In 2010, Dr. Eric Braverman showed that out of 1,234 people, only 20% of them were considered to be obese by using BMI, while 56% of them were considered obese by using the more accurate DXA scan. At this time, most insurance companies do not cover the use of DXA scans to diagnose obesity by measuring body fat. However, if you are interested in obtaining a more accurate reading of your body composition (i.e., body fat measurement), then you may want to consider asking your doctor to order a body fat measurement on a DXA machine, realizing that you will most likely have to pay for it yourself. In 2013, DXA scans to measure body fat cost anywhere from $75 to $150 nationwide. There is no one accepted definition of obesity by percentage of body fat. One commonly used definition for obesity (by www.emedicine.medscape.com) is having a body fat of more than 33% in women and more than 25% in men.

**Table 21.3** Definitions of Obesity

Women who have SLE who have been on steroids or who do not exercise regularly
    BMI $\geq$ 26.8 kg/m$^2$
    WC > 33.4 inches
    WHR > 0.80

Women who have SLE who have not been on steroids and who exercise regularly
    BMI $\geq$ 30.0 kg/m$^2$
    WC > 35 inches
    WHR $\geq$ 0.85

Men who have SLE
    BMI $\geq$ 30.0 kg/m$^2$
    WC > 40 inches
    WHR $\geq$ 1.0

BMI, body mass index; WC, waist circumference; WHR, waist to hip ratio

## Hypertension (High Blood Pressure)

"Hypertension" is the medical term for high blood pressure. Hypertension causes repetitive damage to the arteries of the body over time, predisposing them to arteriosclerosis. It is one of the primary risk factors for developing strokes, heart attacks, and kidney disease. People who have SLE are at increased risk of developing hypertension due to the use of steroids, becoming obese, and the development of lupus nephritis (which can also increase blood pressure).

Your blood pressure is determined by your doctor using an inflatable cuff filled with air (called a sphygmomanometer), which is placed on your upper arm—it compresses the blood in the arteries of your arm while a stethoscope is used to listen to the blood flowing in the arteries below the cuff. The person taking your blood pressure slowly deflates the cuff; the pressure at the point when blood first starts to flow back through the arteries is the "systolic" blood pressure, which is the top number of your blood pressure reading. The point at which the blood flow stops making noise in the stethoscope is the "diastolic" blood pressure, which is the bottom number of your blood pressure reading. You have hypertension if your systolic blood pressure is $\geq 140$ mm Hg (abbreviation for millimeters of mercury) or if the diastolic blood pressure is $\geq 90$ mm Hg.

## High Cholesterol

Cholesterol is a normal and necessary part of the body. Millions of individual cells make up the body, and a very thin cellular membrane surrounds each of these cells, keeping them intact. Cholesterol is a very important component of these cellular membranes and is vital to the body's normal function, helping to protect these inner portions of the cells from the outside world. Cholesterol also has other very important functions. Cholesterol is required to produce sex hormones such as estrogen and testosterone. In addition, some types of cholesterol are vital in the absorption of excess fat from the body and bloodstream. However, too much of anything can be bad, and that includes cholesterol. Too much cholesterol can accumulate inside your body if you either eat too much of it in your food, or if your body produces too much cholesterol (which is usually determined by genetics). This excess cholesterol can then cause problems in the blood vessels of the body. Cholesterol is a primary component of the plaque that clogs up the arteries in people who have atherosclerosis. People who have SLE can develop high levels of cholesterol due to treatment with steroids or from becoming obese.

There are many different types of cholesterol in the body, and your doctor can measure several of these in your blood. Low-density lipoprotein (LDL) cholesterol is a "bad" type of cholesterol that plays a major role in plaque formation in the arteries. High-density lipoprotein (HDL) cholesterol is "good" cholesterol. The purpose of HDL is actually to remove excess cholesterol from the cells that produce plaque buildup and take that cholesterol to the liver where it can be disposed of. Therefore, you want a low amount of the "bad cholesterol" LDL and high levels of the "good cholesterol" HDL. A complete cholesterol test (also called a lipid panel, lipid profile, or cholesterol panel) is a blood test that measures the amount of cholesterol and triglycerides (a type of fat) in your blood. It is very important to fast for eight hours for this blood test to obtain an accurate reading—just as you do to get an accurate glucose result. The normal values for the different cholesterol tests vary by age, gender, and race and therefore are determined by the laboratory based on these factors. Doctors must be very careful when evaluating the results of these cholesterol tests. As mentioned in a subsequent section, HDL cholesterol is not always "good cholesterol" in people who have SLE.

## Smoking Cigarettes

Smoking cigarettes is a major cause of atherosclerosis. Smoking causes plaque build-up in the arteries along with its associated problems of heart attacks and strokes. This can occur from cigarettes even in the absence of other risk factors such as high cholesterol and high blood pressure. Cigarettes contain many harmful substances. These dangerous chemicals have profound adverse effects on the body. Cigarette smoking causes cholesterol levels to become abnormal, and this leads to arteriosclerotic plaque. It also directly damages the blood vessels of the body, making it easier for plaque to form. Cigarette smoking increases homocysteine levels (discussed below) in the blood, which also has been associated with atherosclerosis. Cigarettes also contain the chemical nicotine that causes the blood vessels of the body to constrict. These areas of arterial constriction from the nicotine further decrease blood supply to important parts of the body (such as the brain, heart, and kidneys). Nicotine also increases the heart rate. The muscle cells of the faster-beating heart require more oxygen and nutrients than the blocked arteries can provide to them. This can potentially cause angina or a heart attack.

## Immune-Related Effects of SLE

All of the above risk factors are the typical risk factors for atherosclerosis seen in people who do not have SLE. However, they do not fully explain why people who have SLE get arteriosclerosis at a younger age than other people do. It appears that many diseases that cause systemic inflammation (including rheumatoid arthritis, psoriatic arthritis, and gout) also cause arteriosclerosis more often and at a younger age in affected individuals compared to the rest of the population. This is an area of intense investigation. Understanding why these diseases cause atherosclerosis can help doctors figure out how to keep it from happening in the first place.

Diseases that cause a lot of inflammation (such as SLE) are often associated with an elevated C-reactive protein (CRP) level. Doctors have identified high CRP levels as a risk factor for developing arteriosclerosis. In other words, people who have heart attacks and strokes due to arteriosclerosis are more likely to have high levels of CRP compared to the general population. People who have arteriosclerosis who do not have a systemic inflammatory disease (like SLE) often have elevated CRP levels. Physicians do not know why this occurs, but inflammation occurring in the blood vessels is a possible explanation. Systemic inflammatory diseases, such as SLE, appear to cause inflammation directly in the blood vessels of the body, increasing the chances of developing atherosclerosis.

In particular, people who have SLE who have had lupus nephritis seem to have an increased chance of developing accelerated arteriosclerosis. This may be due to the increased amounts of lupus-related inflammation occurring in the blood vessels, the elevated levels of blood pressure that occur in people who have lupus nephritis, or the use of high doses of prednisone (discussed below). Kidney disease also raises homocysteine levels in the blood, which increases the chances of developing atherosclerosis (discussed below). Another lupus complication that has been associated with arteriosclerosis is vasculitis. This is not too surprising because vasculitis is due to lupus directly attacking and causing inflammation and damage to the blood vessels.

On the opposite end of the spectrum, people who have SLE who have less disease activity appear to have a lower chance of developing coronary artery disease compared to people who have high disease activity. A 2010 study showed that people who had SLE who had active disease developed coronary artery disease more than four times more often than those SLE patients who had no disease activity (known as clinically quiescent) over a ten-year period.

Research looking at accelerated arteriosclerosis in patients who have SLE is also finding other interesting possible causes. The altered immune system in people who have SLE can cause antibodies directed at cholesterol itself, and there is evidence of the immune system directly causing damage to the blood vessel walls as well. These findings parallel the evidence that patients who have more severe SLE appear to be at higher risk of developing accelerated arteriosclerosis compared to patients who have milder SLE.

Having antiphospholipid antibodies also increases the risk for developing heart attacks and strokes. This most likely is due to the tendency for these antibodies to cause blood clots in the arteries. Doctors prescribe blood thinners such as Coumadin (warfarin) to treat heart attacks or strokes due to antiphospholipid antibody syndrome (see chapters 9, 11, and 13).

### When Is HDL "Good Cholesterol" Not So Good?

As previously discussed, having a large amount of HDL is usually considered an important lab finding by doctors. HDL cholesterol helps to remove bad fats and cholesterol from the blood vessels, decreasing the risks for heart attacks, strokes, and blocked arteries. However, as many people who have SLE can attest, lupus does not necessarily play by the rules; this is one of those situations where lupus likes to cause confusion. Lupus experts have found that this is the case when it comes to HDL levels in SLE. Dr. Bevra Hahn and associates from the David Geffen School of Medicine at the University of California, Los Angeles showed that abnormal HDL called proinflammatory HDL is present in SLE patients, and that this unusual HDL contributes to early-onset atherosclerosis. The inflammation of lupus actually converts "good cholesterol" HDL to an abnormal proinflammatory HDL. Instead of decreasing atherosclerotic plaque and inflammation, this type of cholesterol actually increases plaque formation and increases inflammation. In their 2006 study, they showed that while only 4% of "normal" people had proinflammatory HDL, 45% of people who had SLE had this abnormal HDL and was directly associated with having atherosclerosis.

Unfortunately, doctors are currently unable to tell the difference between good HDL and proinflammatory HDL as this blood test is new and only available in research studies. If someone who has SLE has this bad HDL present, it is included along with the good HDL in the total HDL reading. People who have SLE may be told that their cholesterol is fantastic because the HDL is high. In reality, they may have a significant amount of proinflammatory HDL as a part of that reading and be at high risk for heart attacks and strokes while having the false impression that they are at low risk based on this lab test result. One word of caution: I doubt that most doctors (especially non-rheumatologists) know about this possibility, as it is such a recent finding. In addition, having this bad HDL does not necessarily cause a high HDL level; it is even more likely to be present if the HDL is low or normal in people who have SLE.

Dr. Hahn's group subsequently showed in 2010 that SLE patients who exercised regularly had significantly lower amounts of this proinflammatory HDL and less hardening of the arteries. This finding carries a very strong message that people who have SLE need to emphasize regular exercise as a part of their lifestyle to try to prevent this number one cause of death in people who have SLE (cardiovascular disease).

## Steroids

For a long time, it has been noted that people who have SLE and have received high doses of steroids or who have taken steroids for a long time have a higher chance of developing complications of arteriosclerosis than people who have SLE who have not taken steroids. Whether the steroid drugs themselves generate the blocked arteries, or whether the use of steroids simply reflects the higher severity of lupus inflammation in those patients is not clear. In a related matter, a 2009 study showed that another medicine used in SLE, azathioprine (Imuran), was also associated with higher rates of arteriosclerosis. The authors of that study suggested that this was most likely due to patients who had more severe SLE developing arteriosclerosis instead of the medicines themselves causing the arteriosclerosis.

However, the use of steroids also increases problems known to cause arteriosclerosis. These include weight gain, diabetes, high blood pressure, and elevated levels of cholesterol—all of which increase the chances of developing arteriosclerosis.

## Hyperhomocysteinemia

Homocysteine is a protein (specifically, an amino acid) normally found in the body. When it is present in excessive amounts, doctors call the condition hyperhomocysteinemia. High levels of homocysteine have been associated with atherosclerosis in people who have SLE. Some potential causes of elevated homocysteine levels in people who have lupus include vitamin deficiencies (specifically folic acid, vitamin B-12, or vitamin B-6), cigarette smoking, and kidney disease. Homocysteine appears to damage blood vessels when present in higher than normal amounts, increasing the risk of developing arteriosclerosis. Taking additional folic acid, vitamin B-12, and vitamin B-6 supplements can decrease homocysteine levels. However, studies using these supplements do not show any decreases in the numbers of heart attacks and strokes even when these supplements are able to correct the high levels of homocysteine. Therefore, many experts do not currently recommend these vitamin supplements in patients who have hyperhomocysteinemia. This is controversial, though. Some doctors do prefer to treat their patients with these vitamins in the hopes that they will decrease their risk of developing cardiovascular disease.

## Genetics

People who have family members who have had heart attacks and strokes at younger ages (e.g., men younger than 50 years old and women younger than 60 years old) are at increased risk of developing arteriosclerosis due to the genes they inherit. The genetics of arteriosclerosis is quite complex and extends beyond just elevated cholesterol levels, high blood pressure, and diabetes. The bottom line is that if you have family members who have had problems from arteriosclerosis or who have elevated cholesterol levels or high blood pressure and diabetes, then you are at increased risk of developing arteriosclerosis as well. Unfortunately, you have no control over this particular risk factor, as you cannot control what genes you were born with.

## Preventing Cardiovascular Disease

The actual treatment of cardiovascular disease events such as strokes and heart attacks once they do occur is beyond the scope of this book. For more information on this topic, consider reading *Living with Coronary Heart Disease* by Jerome E. Granato, MD, FACC. There are some important measures you can take to decrease the risk of developing these problems. Everyone should practice these interventions because the damage to blood vessels occurs over time and at all ages. Early prevention is important. While you are not able to do anything about the genes you were born with causing cardiovascular disease, you do have control over many other things.

I recommend that my patients who have SLE follow up regularly with a primary care provider, such as a good family practice or internal medicine doctor. Primary care doctors are the experts who assess and manage these risk factors for cardiovascular disease. Your doctor should check you regularly for high cholesterol, high blood pressure, and diabetes. If any of these occur, it is very important that you get treatment. Doctors should treat SLE patients more aggressively for these problems than people who do not have SLE. For example, the proper treatment of a 30-year-old female who has elevated cholesterol, who is overweight, but who has no other risk factors for cardiovascular disease may be with diet, exercise, and weight loss without prescribing medications. The 30-year-old woman who has SLE who is overweight and has high cholesterol should also diet, exercise, and lose weight. However, there should be strong consideration given to using a medication to lower her cholesterol level as well. In fact, a group of cholesterol-lowering medications called statins also has anti-inflammatory properties. While it has not been shown (or adequately studied yet) that statins improve the inflammatory state of lupus, they have been shown to decrease the chances of developing heart attacks and strokes in people who do not have lupus who have high cholesterol. People who have SLE should take the following measures to try to prevent accelerated arteriosclerosis.

## Diet

Eating a proper diet is essential for many reasons for people who have SLE (see chapter 38). Preventing atherosclerosis is one of those reasons. It is very important to eat a diet that is low in fat and cholesterol, while high in omega-3 fatty acids, fiber, fruits, and vegetables. Most Americans do not eat a proper diet due to numerous adverse cultural influences and the increasingly easy access to "fast food," which is generally unhealthy. In addition, the use of unhealthy components in food, such as high fructose corn syrup, enhances the taste of food but decreases its nutritional value. In fact, the explosion in the use of high fructose corn syrup in food may be one of the primary reasons for the obesity epidemic in America. It also may be one of the main reasons for the increase in numerous health problems such as cardiovascular disease, diabetes, high blood pressure, cancer, and gout. The proper diet that people should be on varies from person to person, depending on their need to lose weight and if they have other problems such as diabetes, hypertension, high cholesterol, or kidney disease. You should consider asking your doctor to refer you to a dietician or nutritionist to teach you how to eat properly based on your own situation. Eating properly does not equate to eating foods that do not taste good. Many people are surprised at how good tasting a proper diet can be once they learn how to eat right. If you can motivate yourself enough to learn lifelong proper eating habits, it can really go a long way in ensuring you a long, healthy life, including decreasing your risk of developing the dreaded accelerated arteriosclerosis of SLE. Chapter 38 goes into more detail about dietary recommendations in people who have SLE.

## Alcohol Intake

Many studies have shown that drinking alcohol has numerous potential health benefits when done in moderation; this includes the prevention of cardiovascular disease. Alcohol can increase the amounts of HDL "good cholesterol" and is associated with decreased complications from cardiovascular disease such as strokes and heart attacks. Two servings of alcohol a day or less in men and no more than one serving a day in women are the recommended amounts of alcohol in a healthy lifestyle. One serving is approximately 12 ounces of beer, 8 ounces of malt liquor, 5 ounces of wine, 3–4 ounces of fortified wine (such as sherry and port), 2.5 ounces of 24% alcohol liqueur, or 1.5 ounces of 80-proof liquor. However, drinking too much alcohol certainly has negative effects, including the dangers of drunk driving and the numerous health and social consequences of alcoholism. Therefore, people predisposed to alcoholism should avoid any form or quantity of alcohol. In addition, people who have had previous problems with substance abuse, those with a family history of alcohol and substance abuse, and those who have psychological problems, such as depression or bipolar disorder, should not drink. In addition, people on certain medicines and those who have liver disease should also not drink. There does appear to be an increased risk of breast cancer in women who drink alcohol regularly, but taking a folic acid vitamin supplement may decrease this risk. Since alcohol consumption can have potential benefits and risks, it is best to discuss this topic with your physicians to get adequate guidance based on your particular medical situation.

## Exercise

The lack of exercise is another risk factor for developing atherosclerosis and the complications of cardiovascular disease. Regular exercise has many health benefits beyond preventing cardiovascular disease. All people who have SLE should exercise regularly to improve their overall health and increase their chances of living a long, normal life. Aerobic exercise, in particular, appears to decrease weight, decrease blood pressure, help with glucose control, and elevate HDL "good cholesterol." However, strengthening exercises most likely help with these issues as well. As previously mentioned, regular exercise is probably very important in eliminating proinflammatory HDL from the body to decrease the risk of getting heart attacks and strokes.

The added muscle mass from strengthening exercises helps the body to use more calories on a regular basis, which helps to maintain proper weight. Strength training also helps to keep the bones strong to prevent broken bones from osteoporosis. A balanced, regular exercise regimen should include aerobic exercises, strengthening exercises, and proper stretching. You should see your doctor and ask what type of exercise program you should do and what is safe for you to do based on your medical condition.

## Not Smoking

For numerous reasons, it is important that people who have SLE not smoke cigarettes. Of course, this is "easier said than done" because the nicotine in cigarettes is a highly addictive substance. People addicted to smoking face problems of withdrawal from nicotine when they stop, as well as the loss of the behavioral motions and activities associated with the act of smoking itself. However, the cigarette smoker needs to realize how important it is to stop smoking. For example, a study has shown that when cigarette smokers stop smoking cigarettes after their first heart attack, it decreases the chances of getting another heart attack by 50% in the first year. Two years after they stop smoking, their chance of having a heart attack is the same as someone who has never smoked. Therefore, stopping smoking can make a huge difference in the health of people who are at high risk of cardiovascular diseases, such as people who have SLE.

There are many different methods available to stop smoking. Combining behavioral modification therapy with using medications to decrease the urge to smoke has the highest success rates for stopping smoking. Behavior modification programs are usually available through most hospitals, and there are increasing numbers of programs available on the internet as well. Medications used to decrease the desire to smoke include varenicline (Chantix), bupropion (Zyban and Wellbutrin), and nicotine replacements (in the forms of patches, gum, lozenges, and even inhalers). You should talk to your physician to see which medications may be best for you to use to stop smoking.

## Taking Plaquenil

Hydroxychloroquine (Plaquenil) is the most common medication used to treat people who have SLE. Plaquenil decreases the severity of lupus, increases how long people who have SLE live, and decreases the chances of getting blood clots. Several studies have demonstrated that hydroxychloroquine decreases cholesterol levels, including a 2012 study that showed that its use decreases total cholesterol by 7.6% and LDL "bad" cholesterol by 13.7% within three months of using the medication.

## Taking Low-Dose Aspirin

Platelets are fragments of blood cells that cause the blood to clot. They play an important role in helping to form the plaque and the blood clots that cause strokes and heart attacks. Aspirin interferes with the ability of platelets to clump together and therefore decreases the possibility that plaque and blood clots will form. In addition, aspirin has anti-inflammatory properties that may help to decrease the inflammation involved in causing arteriosclerotic plaque. Therefore, taking aspirin in small doses, such as 81 mg a day, may be beneficial in preventing cardiovascular events such as heart attacks and strokes. However, aspirin also increases the risk of bleeding. People who may have problems with bleeding already, people who have low platelet counts, people who are on other blood thinners, and people who are at increased risk for bleeding into the gastrointestinal tract (such as people who have problems with gastric ulcers) may be especially at increased risk of bleeding from taking aspirin. Although many people who have SLE should take aspirin daily to decrease their chances of having cardiovascular events, your doctor should help you figure out if the potential benefits outweigh the potential risks of taking the aspirin.

### Diabetes

The actual treatment of diabetes is quite complex and involves proper diet, exercise, and the use of medications. People who have SLE who have diabetes should work closely with their primary care doctor or with a diabetic specialist (called an endocrinologist) to get their diabetes under excellent control.

### Obesity

Just as stopping smoking can be very difficult for the person who smokes, losing weight can be very challenging to a person who is overweight. The weight loss industry makes billions of dollars yearly through multiple diets, medications, supplements, exercise programs, and weight loss programs—all fueled by the fact that many people want to lose weight. Even with this exploding weight loss industry, more people are becoming overweight and obese every year. Successful long-term weight loss generally comes from adopting good lifestyle habits of proper diet and exercise along with realizing that these lifestyle changes need to continue for the rest of one's life. Working with one's primary care provider to design a proper weight loss program can be helpful. In addition, legitimate programs such as Weight Watchers are available to give excellent guidance. In those people who are not able to lose weight on their own and who have medical problems related to being obese, weight loss surgery (such as gastric bypass, sleeve gastrectomy, or gastric banding) is also an option. In fact, studies show that people who have BMIs of 35 and above have a much higher long-term success rate of losing weight through weight loss surgery compared to people who try exercise and diet alone.

### Hypertension

Regular exercise combined with proper diet can help lower blood pressure in people who have hypertension (high blood pressure). For example, people who have hypertension should generally decrease their intake of sodium (salt) and avoid caffeine. Working with a dietician can be helpful in designing a proper diet. However, people who have SLE who have hypertension should take blood pressure lowering medicines if diet and exercise do not control their blood pressure enough to prevent cardiovascular complications. The blood pressure goal recommended by most experts is to keep the systolic blood pressure (the top number) below 140 mm Hg and the diastolic blood pressure (the bottom number) below 90 mm Hg. However, in people who have kidney disease, and in those who have already had cardiovascular events such as a stroke or heart attack, many experts recommend keeping the systolic blood pressure below 130 mm Hg and the diastolic blood pressure below 80 mm Hg. Again, it is very important that you work closely with your primary care provider to keep your blood pressure un-

**Table 21.4** Statins Used to Control Cholesterol Levels

atorvastatin (Lipitor)

fluvastatin (Lescol)

lovastatin (Mevacor)

pitavastatin (Livalo)

pravastatin (Pravachol)

rosuvastatin (Crestor)

simvastatin (Zocor)

der good control. Other doctors who can also do this include heart experts (called cardiologists) and kidney experts (called nephrologists).

## High Cholesterol

A diet low in fat and cholesterol helps to decrease levels of total cholesterol and LDL "bad cholesterol." Regular aerobic exercise helps to increase levels of HDL "good cholesterol" and most likely decreases the chances of having the bad proinflammatory HDL (mentioned previously). People who have SLE who have abnormal cholesterol levels should employ these healthy lifestyle habits. In addition, as mentioned above, moderate intake of alcohol can also help to increase HDL levels while taking hydroxychloroquine (Plaquenil) decreases both total and LDL "bad" cholesterol levels. Many people who have SLE should consider taking medications, especially the statins (see table 21.4), to control their cholesterol levels. Some lupus experts go so far as to recommend that everyone who has SLE should take a statin. It probably is a good idea for anyone who has SLE who has had any of the previous mentioned risk factors and who is therefore at increased risk for atherosclerosis to take a statin.

The statins are generally safe medications. Headaches and upset stomach are the most common side effects. These are generally mild and resolve when people stop the medicine. Your doctor will want to check blood tests for the liver regularly if you take these medications to make sure that you do not develop any irritation of the liver from them. A few people can get inflammation of the muscles while taking statins. If you develop muscle pain or muscle weakness while taking a statin, it is very important to see your doctor right away to see if it is due to the statin or due to some other reason. People who have severe liver disease and pregnant women should not take statin medications.

### KEY POINTS TO REMEMBER

1. After the first five years of having SLE, cardiovascular events such as heart attacks, strokes, and blood clots are the most common causes of death in people who have SLE. Therefore, it is very important that all people who have SLE do everything they can to avoid these problems from occurring.

2. Accelerated arteriosclerosis (also called accelerated atherosclerosis) occurs in people who have SLE. For example, African American women develop heart attacks about twenty years younger than their peers who do not have SLE.

3. The reasons that people who have SLE develop accelerated arteriosclerosis include diabetes, obesity, hypertension, abnormal cholesterol levels, inflammation of the blood vessels due to lupus, lupus nephritis, antiphospholipid antibodies, elevated levels of homocysteine, lack of exercise, a family history of cardiovascular disease, using steroids, and smoking cigarettes.

4. It is very important that all people who have SLE follow up regularly with a primary care provider (internal medicine or family practice doctor) to monitor and treat cardiovascular risk factors—such as diabetes, high cholesterol, obesity, and hypertension.

5. A high HDL "good cholesterol" reading in SLE is not necessarily "good." The inflammation of SLE can create proinflammatory HDL that can actually cause heart attacks and strokes. This is especially a concern in people who have SLE who do not exercise on a regular basis.

6. Practicing healthy lifestyle changes such as eating properly, exercising regularly, not smoking cigarettes, and maintaining proper weight can decrease cardiovascular problems.

7. Consider taking 81 mg of aspirin a day, if approved by your doctor, to decrease your chances of having a heart attack, stroke, or blood clot.

8. Taking hydroxychloroquine (Plaquenil) decreases the chances of getting blood clots.

9. Try to keep your blood pressure below 140/90. If you have kidney disease, or have had a heart attack or stroke, try to keep your blood pressure below 130/80.

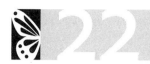

# Infections

## Avoiding Being One of the 30,000 Americans Who Die Each Year from the Flu

My patients are used to my recommending that they get a flu shot every fall, and some of them unfortunately become "victims" as a consequence of not doing so. One of my patients always refused to get a flu shot in spite of my yearly lecture. I do not remember exactly what her reason was, but like most patients, it probably was something like "I never get the flu," "my aunt got the flu after her flu shot," or "I'm afraid of the side effects." One year she came in distraught. Her husband who was in his fifties had gotten the flu while at a business conference. Shortly afterward, he died from its complications. Prior to that, her husband was a very healthy man; he had never had the flu before. I was very saddened by this news, as I could see how devastated she was from this loss and how the rest of her life would be changed forever. However, at that appointment, she asked for a flu shot and has gotten one every year since. It is easy to ignore prevention as one of the most important aspects of medical care, and sometimes it takes something to hit "close to home" to learn its importance.

Infections are among the top three (and possibly top two) causes of death in people who have SLE—the other top causes being cardiac conditions and lupus itself. However, lupus experts feel that most of these infectious deaths are preventable with vaccinations, immediate treatment with antibiotics, and people doing everything they can to control their lupus through measures that do not require suppression of the immune system. Because infection is one of the most common causes of death in people who have lupus and is preventable in most of them, this chapter is one of the most important ones in this book. A large percentage of this prevention is in your control.

Complications from influenza (or "the flu" for short) kill on average 30,000 Americans every year, most commonly during the months of October through April. People who have altered immune systems (such as the elderly, infants, and people who have SLE) as well as people who have chronic medical illnesses (such as lung disease, heart disease, and diabetes) comprise the majority of the people who do not fare well with influenza. However, it is a preventable infection. Although the flu shot may not 100% prevent someone from getting the flu, it can significantly decrease the severity of the infection. Getting a yearly flu shot is an easy way to avoid becoming a statistic when it comes to influenza.

Infections are one of the top three causes of death in people who have SLE due to their already abnormal immune system, but also because of the need for immunosuppressant medications (discussed in chapters 31, 32, 33, 34, and 37). It is possible to decrease infections significantly in lupus by following some simple precautions. People who take the necessary steps to prevent infection in the first place go a long way in living longer and healthier with their SLE. This chapter explains how to prevent and treat infections.

. . . .

Treatments for systemic lupus erythematosus (SLE) have improved substantially over the past few decades. Before antibiotics and steroids became available, the vast majority of people who had SLE died within the first two years of the disease. Now, more than 90% can expect to live past ten years. The majority of those who have mild disease and who have no major internal organ involvement can plan on living normal lifespans as long as they keep up with their healthcare to keep their lupus and its potential complications under control. Knowing what those potential complications can be is the first step in knowing what to do. Infections are a major potential complication in people who have SLE.

Deaths of people who have SLE occur in two time-periods marked by different causes of death. The first period is the first five years after the diagnosis. The vast majority of people who die during this period do so from a combination of the lupus itself and major infections. These infections are due to the abnormal immune systems these people have due to their lupus, as well as their immune systems being suppressed from the medications that are needed to treat their lupus. Generally, these people have severe lupus. They usually have major organ involvement such as kidney, lung, heart, or brain involvement.

After the first five years, cardiovascular disease (including strokes, heart attacks, and blood clots) is the major cause of death, followed closely by infections. Infections appear to play a larger role in some parts of the world than in others. For example, a 2011 study from Hong Kong showed that infection was the cause of death in 60% of patients who had SLE. Another 2011 study from China showed that infection was the number one cause of death in patients who had lupus. Chapter 21 dealt with how to prevent the cardiovascular events. This chapter covers how to prevent infection complications.

Infections are an important potential cause of death at any time during the life of a person who has lupus. Doctors estimate that 20% to 50% of all people who have lupus will have an infection as a contributing cause of death. This is why it is so important for you to know how to prevent, identify, and treat infections.

## What Is an Infection?

Infections occur when disease-causing organisms, commonly called germs, get into the body, use the body for nourishment, reproduce, and cause damage to the body. The immune system, most importantly white blood cells, detects these invaders and attacks them to protect the body. This battle between the germs and the immune system can end up causing inflammation. The signs of inflammation are pain, heat, redness, and swelling. For example, strep throat (due to infection from streptococcus bacteria in the back of the throat) causes a painful, sore throat. The sick person may have a fever due to the inflammation, and when the doctor looks at the back of the throat, he or she will see redness, swelling, and sometimes pus (the collection of white blood cells fighting against the invading bacteria). Often, these infections are mild and readily treatable. However, if an infection is severe and spreads throughout the entire body, or severely injures a major organ (such as the lungs from pneumonia), it can potentially be deadly.

## Why People Who Have SLE Get Infections

People who have SLE are more prone to getting infections than people who do not have SLE. This is due to several reasons. First, the person who has SLE has an abnormal immune system that may not be able to fight off infections as well as the immune system of a healthy individual. Before medications were available to treat lupus, and before antibiotics were available to treat bacterial infections, approximately 55% of people who had SLE died from complications of severe infection. Therefore, even in the absence of medicines that suppress the immune system, people who had SLE had an increased risk of developing uncontrolled infection.

Today there are medications that suppress the immune system. People who have moderate to severe SLE may require the use of medications such as methotrexate, azathioprine, cyclophosphamide, mycophenolate, biologic medications, or high doses of steroids. All of these medications can work miracles in controlling the disease of lupus, but they can also lower the immune system's ability to fight off infection. Although most people who take these medications do not develop more infections or severe infections, they are at increased risk of doing so and need to be constantly vigilant in preventing infections.

The final reason for increased infections is that lupus can damage parts of the body that are important for protecting against infections. For example, the skin plays a very important role in keeping invading organisms from getting into the body, but if a person has an open sore from cutaneous lupus, that person has lost part of this natural protection. Similarly, if lupus has damaged the lungs, the affected person has lost some of her or his natural protection against infection. That person is at increased risk of developing pneumonia from infection. The person who has decreased saliva production due to secondary Sjögren's syndrome (see chapter 14) has lost an important protective element because saliva is important in maintaining healthy bacteria in the mouth. When there is a decrease in saliva in the mouth, harmful organisms (such as the fungus *Candida albicans*) can become abundant, causing an infection in the mouth (thrush in the case of *Candida*). Bad bacteria can also grow out of control causing problems with gum infection (gingivitis) and dental cavities as well.

## Preventing Infections

If you have lupus, the most important thing you can do is to prevent infections in the first place. Preventative medicine is always better than waiting until bad things happen and then treating them after the fact. That is why doctors insist that people try as hard as they can to exercise, eat well, maintain normal weight, get enough sleep, and not smoke cigarettes because these preventative measures can go a long way in preventing the damage from diseases such as diabetes, high blood pressure, heart attacks, and strokes. Unfortunately, preventative medicine is often the most difficult to get people to accept because it requires extra effort and work on their part to prevent something that has not even happened to them.

You can do many things to prevent infections (table 22.1). One of the most important is to take care of your lupus, using all the therapies available that can keep it under control without suppressing the immune system. All people who have SLE should be taking Plaquenil (hydroxychloroquine) daily as long as they are not allergic to it. This medicine is by far the safest medicine to treat SLE. It does not suppress the immune system, and it can help decrease the need for stronger medicines that do. While some people develop severe lupus requiring strong immunosuppressant medications, many people have milder disease and have the power to prevent more severe lupus from developing. Unfortunately, it can be easy to become complacent when you have mild lupus and feel well. People who have mild SLE are particularly at increased risk of becoming noncompliant with taking their hydroxychloroquine and even stopping visits to their rheumatologist. Doing so can cause their disease to flare and become severe, requiring the use of strong immunosuppressant medicines. Studies show that if patients who have mild SLE take their hydroxychloroquine regularly and stay compliant with their doctor visits and labs, their disease is much less likely to evolve into a more severe form of SLE.

People who have lupus should not smoke cigarettes. At first mention, this is apt to bring a questioning look. What does not smoking cigarettes have to do with keeping lupus under control? There are several reasons for this recommendation. Cigarettes contain chemical substances that cause the immune system to become more active and this will lead to a lupus flare. One such chemical found in cigarettes is hydrazine. Hydrazine can actually cause a lupus-like autoimmune reaction. In addition, cigarette smoke contains other substances that cause damage to cells, abnormalities in the DNA of cells, and increased activity of the immune system. These substances include carbon monoxide, cyanide, and hydroquinone. In fact, studies show that cigarette smoking increases the chances of developing numerous autoimmune diseases, such as lupus, rheumatoid arthritis, and autoimmune thyroid disease due to these abnormal influences on the immune system.

Another way that smoking may increase lupus disease activity is that it may prevent hydroxychloroquine from working properly. Doctors do not understand how this occurs, but a couple of studies have shown that people who have lupus who smoke cigarettes do not respond to anti-malarial therapies (such as hydroxychloroquine) as well as those who do not smoke. One study showed that only 40% of patients who had cutaneous (skin) lupus and smoked responded to anti-malarial medications. Yet, more than twice as many (90%) of the people who did not smoke responded.

In addition, smoking causes repetitive damage to the lungs and to the passageways that lead to them. People who smoke cigarettes are more likely to get lung infections such as bronchitis and pneumonia than people who do not smoke. They are also more likely to get more severe infections that last longer, and they are more likely to die from these infections as well. Therefore, it is essential that people who have SLE not smoke cigarettes for numerous reasons.

Table 22.I  How to Prevent Infections in SLE

Control SLE activity using therapies that do not suppress the immune system.

> Take hydroxychloroquine (Plaquenil) regularly.
>
> Do not smoke cigarettes.
>
> Protect yourself from UV light (table 38.3).

Vaccinations

> Get an influenza ("flu") shot every fall.
>
> Get a pneumonia vaccine (Pneumovax). Those who are on immunosuppressant medicines or who have had their spleen removed should get revaccinated five years later, then again after age 65.
>
> Get a PCV-13 pneumonia vaccine if you take immunosuppressant medications, have had your spleen removed, or if you are 50 years old or older.
>
> Get a shingles vaccine (Zostavax) if not on certain immunosuppressants; it is FDA-approved for people over 50 years old.
>
> Get the human papillomavirus vaccine (Gardasil) if 26 years old or younger. Consider getting it if older than 26 and not in a permanent, monogamous relationship.
>
> Get a hepatitis B vaccine if you are at increased risk for hepatitis B.
>
> Get a meningococcal vaccine if you have had your spleen removed, if you have a complement deficiency, if you are a freshman in college living in a residence hall, or if you are a military recruit.
>
> Get a vaccine for tetanus-diphtheria every ten years.
>
> Receive vaccines before Rituxan and Benlysta treatments instead of after the treatments.

General measures

> Wash your hands frequently during the flu and cold season.
>
> Avoid contact with people who are sick.
>
> Urinate right after having sexual intercourse if you are female (UTI prevention).
>
> Wipe front to back after bowel movements if you are female (UTI prevention).

Avoidance of ultraviolet (UV) light exposure should be as important as taking medications in treating lupus. The reason for this is that UV light contacts the skin and causes reactions that cause the immune system to become more active, making systemic lupus more active inside of the body (see chapters 3 and 38). All people who have lupus should be using sunscreen on all exposed body areas every day, even if they do not go outside because indoor lighting has UV activity. On sunny days, people who have lupus should reapply sunscreen several times throughout the day. Other measures to decrease UV light exposure include wearing a wide-brimmed hat when exposed to the sun, avoiding the sun in the middle of the day, and wearing clothing with additional sun protection (such as Rit Sun Guard). Chapter 38 goes into more detail about UV protection.

People who have lupus should also get eight hours of sleep each night, try to decrease their daily stress levels, eat a well-balanced diet that includes omega-3 fatty acids, and exercise regularly. All of these things will improve their health and their immune function.

Vaccinations can prevent certain infections from occurring. Currently, doctors in the United States are able to decrease problems from seventeen different infections using vaccinations. Unfortunately, many people do not take advantage of these miracles of modern medicine. The Centers for Disease Control estimates that approximately 45,000 adult Americans die every year from vaccine-preventable infections; the majority of these deaths are from influenza (commonly called the flu). This is a sad statistic since these are preventable deaths.

Everyone who has SLE and takes an immunosuppressant medication should get a Pneumovax. This vaccine is for *Pneumococcus*, which are the most common bacteria causing pneumonia. In fact, pneumonia is the most common cause of death due to infection in people who have SLE. The Centers for Disease Control estimates that the Pneumovax prevented 211,000 serious infections and 13,000 deaths from pneumococcal pneumonia between 2000 and 2008. Therefore, this is a very important recommendation to follow through. People who have lupus who are at the highest risk for developing a serious infection and those who are at an increased risk for the vaccine wearing off over time should get a second vaccination in their lifetime. This should be done five years after the initial vaccination. This group includes those who are receiving immunosuppressant medicines (see the subsequent discussion on live vaccines for a list) and long-term steroid treatments. People who are 65 years old or older should receive an additional Pneumovax if it has been five years or longer since the previous Pneumovax. Therefore, many people who have SLE should receive up to three Pneumovax shots during their lifetime.

There are actually ninety different types of pneumococcal bacteria. The Pneumovax vaccine helps to protect against twenty-three of the most common ones. Currently, the Centers for Disease Control (CDC) recommends that people who take immunosuppressant medications also get another type of pneumococcal vaccination called the pneumococcal conjugate vaccine 13 (PCV13). Getting both types of vaccine gives additional immunity against pneumococcal infection. The PCV13 should be taken at least one year after receiving the Pneumovax and is a once-in-a-lifetime vaccine. If you have not received a Pneumovax yet, the CDC recommends getting the PCV13 first followed by the Pneumovax at least eight weeks later. The PCV13 is also FDA indicated for all people 50 years old and older. Therefore, people who have SLE but who are not on immunosuppressant medications should get a PCV13 once they reach 50.

People who have SLE should also get the influenza vaccine, commonly called the flu shot, every fall before the flu season occurs. As mentioned in the first section of this chapter, influenza kills on average 30,000 Americans every year. This number can range from as low as 3,000 to as high as 49,000. The vast majority of those who die are the elderly, the very young, and the immunosuppressed (including people who have SLE), as well as people with chronic diseases such as lung disease, heart disease, and diabetes. The "flu shot" never gives anyone the flu. This is unfortunately a common, incorrect belief that keeps many people from getting one. A couple of reasons explain why this misperception exists. First, medical professionals give flu shots during the time of year when respiratory conditions such as allergies, colds, the flu, bronchitis, and sinusitis commonly occur. Therefore, if someone develops one of these problems any time after getting the flu shot, it is very easy to blame the flu shot. However, in reality, this is simply a coincidence. Another reason is that one possible side effect of the flu shot is having a "flu-like syndrome." This is not actually the flu, but it can feel like the flu. People who develop a "flu-like syndrome" from any vaccine can get muscle and joint achiness with low-grade fever, which can last for a few days after the vaccination. Doctors consider this a mild and uncommon reaction. Taking acetaminophen (Tylenol) can help to alleviate these symptoms if they occur.

In the past, it was recommended that people who were allergic to eggs not receive the flu vaccination. Seventeen studies on 2,600 egg-allergic patients showed no association between egg allergy and having an allergic reaction to the flu shot. The Advisory Committee on Immunization Practices recommends that people who have only experienced hives due to eggs should still receive a flu shot, but they should be observed for thirty minutes in the medical facility after the shot is given. In addition, it should only be done in facilities that are able to treat severe allergic reactions (just in case a reaction occurs).

Human papillomavirus (HPV) infection occurs through sexual contact and can cause certain types of cancer. These HPV-associated cancers are even more common among people who have SLE (see chapter 23). The HPV vaccine decreases the chances for getting some of these cancers, including cervical, vulvar, vaginal, and anal cancer, all of which occur more commonly in people who have SLE. HPV is also a cause of genital warts, and getting the vaccination (specifically Gardasil) can help protect from those as well. There are two types of vaccines available. The human papillomavirus quadrivalent vaccine (Gardasil; "quadri-" means "four") protects against four strains of HPV, and the human papillomavirus bivalent vaccine (Cervarix; "bi-" means "two") only protects against two strains. Cervarix only protects against cervical cancer, but not the other complications of HPV. Therefore, "at-risk" people who have SLE should get the Gardasil vaccine. The CDC recommends that lupus patients get this series of vaccinations between 11 and 27 years of age. Doctors prescribe the vaccine as a series of three shots with the second shot given two months after the first and the third given six months later.

Although the FDA approval is for adults younger than 27 years old, people older than 26 who are sexually active and who are not in permanent, monogamous relationships are still at risk of HPV infection. Therefore, consideration should be given to being vaccinated if you are in this situation. However, this is an "off label" use of the vaccine. This primarily means that insurance companies are much less likely to cover the cost of the vaccination. Since it is best to get vaccinated prior to the age of sexual activity, the Centers for Disease Control recommends that boys and girls who are 11 years old or older receive the vaccination. This provides better protection for them. Since there are several different strains of HPV, the Centers for Disease Control also recommends that people receive the vaccine even if they know that they have been infected before (such as in someone who already has genital warts, for example). The Gardasil vaccine can potentially prevent further infections with the other strains of HPV.

People should also get a tetanus-diphtheria toxoid vaccine (Td vaccine) every ten years. The diphtheria bacterium predominantly affects the respiratory tract, causing sore throat and hoarseness, but it can also cause pneumonia, nerve and heart damage, and sores on the skin. Prior to introduction of the vaccine in the 1930s, infections from diphtheria were common and they carried a high mortality rate of 5% to 10%. Although it has a high mortality rate, diphtheria infection has become rare in the United States due to regular immunizations of the general population.

Tetanus is a bacterial infection that attacks the nervous and muscle systems of the body, causing paralysis and a high death rate. It is now rare in the United States due to regular immunizations of children and adults, in addition to the use of tetanus toxin shots for "dirty" puncture and trauma wounds to prevent infection.

People who have SLE should also receive other vaccines under certain circumstances. People who have SLE who have a household member who has chronic hepatitis B infection should get the hepatitis B vaccine. This vaccine is given as a series of three shots. People who have had their spleen removed (sometimes done for severe low blood count problems in people with lupus) should receive the meningococcal vaccine. Other people with SLE who should receive the meningococcal vaccine include those who have a complement component deficiency, those who live in a college dormitory or residence hall, and those who join the military.

One question that sometimes comes up concerns how many vaccines are safe to get in one day. It is actually OK to get any number of the above-mentioned vaccines on the same day with no differences in safety or response rates to the vaccines. In fact, the Centers for Disease Control recommends getting both the Pneumovax and the influenza vaccine at the same time if the person needs both. This improves compliance rates with getting these vaccinations by decreasing the possibility of forgetting to get one or the other.

People who take immunosuppressant medicines (making it more difficult to fight off infections) should not receive vaccines that have live organisms as part of the vaccine. Some of the medications that can suppress the immune system include prednisone (at 20 mg a day or more), methotrexate, Arava, Imuran (azathioprine), CellCept (mycophenolate), cyclophosphamide, Humira, Enbrel, Remicade, Benlysta, Rituxan, Actemra, and Orencia (see chapters 31, 32, 33, 34, and 37 for all of them). The live-virus vaccines include MMR (measles, mumps, and rubella), OPV (polio), BCG (tuberculosis), vaccinia (small pox), varicella (chicken pox), rotavirus, typhoid, yellow fever, and Flu-Mist (nasal flu vaccine) (table 22.2). The previously mentioned vaccines (Pneumovax, flu shot, tetanus-diphtheria, hepatitis B, and meningococcal vaccine) are not live vaccines and can be used safely in people who are on immunosuppressants.

People who are 50 years old and older should strongly consider getting the Zostavax. This helps to prevent shingles, which is a very painful rash that is due to the chicken pox virus. About one-third of all people will suffer from shingles at some point in life, and it occurs more commonly in people who have SLE, especially if they require immunosuppressant medicines. Although it is a live vaccine, an official statement from the Centers for Disease Control has stated that it is safe to give to individuals who are on lower doses of immunosuppressant medications. People who take less than 20 mg of prednisone a day, methotrexate at a dose of 0.4 mg/kg a day, and azathioprine at a dose of 3.0 mg/kg a day or less may safely get the Zostavax. The American College of Rheumatology has added leflunomide (Arava) to the list of immunosuppressants that Zostavax can be taken with safely. People who use other immunosuppressant medications should not get the Zostavax. However, they can get it if they have been off the immunosuppressant medication for at least three months. In addition, it is recom-

## Table 22.2 Vaccines Containing Live, Attenuated Organisms

Adenovirus type 4, 7 (oral)

BCG (Bacille Calmette-Guérin, tuberculosis)

FluMist (nasal flu vaccine)

MMR (measles, mumps, rubella)

OPV (polio)

RV (rotavirus)

Typhoid (oral vaccine)

Vaccinia (smallpox)

VZV (varicella zoster virus, varicella, chicken pox)

Yellow fever

Zostavax (varicella zoster virus, herpes zoster, shingles). Read further information in the text.

*Note:* These vaccines should be avoided by people who are taking immunosuppressant medications.

mended that the vaccine be given at least two weeks before an immunosuppressant medication is started if the person wants to get the vaccine.

If someone receives a live vaccine, he or she can potentially infect someone else with it for a short period after the vaccination. This is usually only a potential problem for immunosuppressed people. If a close friend or family member receives the OPV for polio, the immunosuppressed person should avoid contact for four weeks. A better vaccine alternative than the OPV for the close contact person would be the eIPV. The eIPV does not contain any live poliovirus. If a close friend or family member receives the vaccinia vaccine, contact should be avoided for two weeks. If a close contact develops a rash after getting the varicella (chicken pox) or the Zostavax (herpes zoster) vaccine, he or she can spread the virus to other people and contact should be avoided until the rash has resolved. An infant who gets the rotavirus vaccine can excrete rotavirus in his or her feces for up to a week after the vaccination; immunosuppressed people need to avoid any contact with potential fecal soiled items for at least a week. In addition, all members of the household should practice strict hand-washing with soap and water after any possible exposure to the child's feces.

None of these vaccines is 100% effective. In other words, you can still get the infection after you get the vaccine. However, if you get the infection after getting the vaccination, the infection is usually less severe compared to what could have happened without the vaccine. It is easy for people to say that the flu shot or Pneumovax did not work because they still developed the flu or pneumonia. However, what they do not realize is that the infection would probably have been more severe if they had not received the vaccine beforehand.

Do not get any vaccination while your lupus is very active because vaccines can sometimes cause lupus to become even more active. You should also probably not get a vaccine while on 40 mg of prednisone a day or more, because you are less likely to respond to the vaccine. You should always ask your rheumatologist whether it is safe to get any vaccine before you do so.

Some immunosuppressant medications may prevent the immune system from responding adequately to a vaccine. For a vaccine to work, the immune system needs to recognize the components of the vaccine. Then the B-cells (a type of white blood cell) of the immune system respond by making antibodies directed toward the particular organism for which the vaccination is intended. For example, after a person gets the Pneumovax vaccine, the B-cells of the immune system are primed to remember to make antibodies directed toward the pneumococcal bacteria. If the person vaccinated with Pneumovax becomes infected with the pneumococcal bacteria, these B-cells recognize the bacteria because of the vaccine, and they produce a lot of that antibody to fight against the infection. The medication rituximab (Rituxan) has been shown to decrease the response to vaccinations. Rituximab works by decreasing the number of B-cells, and these are the cells of the immune system required to make the necessary antibodies in response to vaccinations. Therefore, it is recommended that people who have SLE and are immunosuppressed be given immunizations such as the flu shot and the Pneumovax before their rituximab treatment. This may also potentially become an issue with belimumab (Benlysta). Belimumab also decreases the number of B-cells in the body, but its effects on immunizations have not been studied yet. It would probably be best for people who have SLE to get all of their necessary vaccines before they start on belimumab therapy as well.

This is a good point to talk about the prevention of endocarditis. Endocarditis is an infection of the heart valves that can cause severe heart valve damage, leading to congestive heart failure and even death. People who are at high risk for developing this should receive antibiotics around the times of dental procedures, such as teeth cleaning, to prevent this type of infection from happening. In fact, many rheumatologists had previously recommended that most (and, in some cases, all) SLE patients take antibiotics during dental procedures to prevent endocarditis. However, more recently, the American Heart Association has relaxed these recommendations. It has determined that many patients are actually at low risk of developing endocarditis and are at higher risk of developing side effects from the antibiotics. Therefore, they now recommend antibiotics only for people who have the most severe heart valve problems, who have had heart valve or congenital heart surgeries, or who have had endocarditis before. It is no longer recommended that people who have milder forms of heart valve problems (such as mitral valve prolapse) take antibiotics at the time of dental procedures.

An undervalued yet very important form of infection prevention is to avoid hand contact with infected persons who are sneezing and coughing. Avoiding those who are sick along with practicing frequent hand washing is important, especially during cold and flu season.

It is also important to learn to avoid urinary tract infections. Urinary tract infections (UTIs) are common in women because the urethra (the tube through which urine passes to exit the body) is very short, allowing easier access for bacteria to enter the urinary bladder from the vaginal area. Contamination with bacteria from the rectal area and infection related to sexual intercourse are two of the most common ways women can develop UTIs. Methods to prevent UTIs include urinating right after having sexual intercourse to flush out any bacteria and wiping from front to back after having a bowel movement. In addition, using spermicidal gels and an intrauterine device (IUD) may also increase the risk of getting UTIs; therefore, other forms of birth control may be more optimal. Eating or drinking cranberry-containing products (juices, food, supplements) on a regular basis also appears to decrease the risk of getting UTIs.

## Treating Infections

All people who have SLE should see their physician immediately if they have an infection. Fevers and chills especially should make a person think about the possibility of having an infection. Although fever can happen due to lupus itself, this should never be assumed. Infection can do the same thing, and the treatment of an infection is vastly different from what doctors use to treat a lupus fever. Other symptoms of an infection depend on the area in which it occurs—for example, coughing up sputum in pneumonia, painful and frequent urination with a urinary tract infection, and warm, tender skin with a skin infection (cellulitis). Infections should be assessed and treated by your primary care physician. If it is after hours, a weekend, or your doctor is not available, you may be directed to go to the local emergency room or urgent care center. Although an ER visit can end up being a long waiting affair, it is very important to do this because a potential infection could be very dangerous if not diagnosed and treated promptly. Your primary care physician may also ask you to see your rheumatologist if there is the possibility that your lupus may be the cause of your symptoms. Sometimes, it can be difficult to figure out if the symptoms are due to lupus or infection, and you may be treated for both.

Some common infections deserve special mention. Thrush is a yeast infection from *Candida albicans*. Classic thrush causes patches of white to occur inside of the mouth. However, sometimes there may just be redness and soreness of the mouth and tongue. Thrush occurs most commonly in people who have SLE who have dry mouth (which can occur due to Sjögren's syndrome, medications, or cigarette smoking), who have diabetes, and who take immunosuppressant medications (especially steroids). If you notice white patches in your mouth or develop a red sore tongue, it is important to see your doctor to determine if you have this infection.

Thrush is treated with several different anti-fungal antibiotics. Clotrimazole troches (Mycelex) can be very useful. It comes as a lozenge that you allow to dissolve in your mouth. However, it should be used five times a day, which can be very difficult to do. Fluconazole (Diflucan) is much easier to take as it is taken by tablet just once a day. Miconazole tablets (Oravig) can also be used. The tablet is placed between the gum and lip once daily and allowed to slowly dissolve. However, it is expensive because there is not a generic version, and it may not be very effective in people who have dry mouth if there is difficulty with the tablet dissolving. Nystatin "swish and swallow" is also commonly prescribed. It comes in liquid form and is taken by swishing it throughout the mouth for several minutes then swallowing it four times daily. Nystatin should not be used by people who have dry mouth (such as from Sjögren's syndrome) nor by people with recurrent dental problems such as dental cavities and gingivitis. Nystatin contains the sugar sucrose that can cause bad bacteria to grow in the mouth, increasing the risks for dental problems from bacterial infections.

If you develop a band of burning, painful red rash on one side of the body, often associated with small blisters, this could be due to shingles. Shingles (also called herpes zoster) is due to the virus that causes chicken pox. When a person is infected with the chicken pox virus (usually as a child), the virus continues to live in the nerves next to the spinal cord. When the immune system becomes less effective at keeping the virus under control (such as in elderly people or in people who have abnormal immune systems such as in SLE), the virus can multiply and attack one of these nerves, causing pain and the rash. The rash occurs in the area of skin to which the nerve gives sensation. Shingles should be treated as soon as possible with antiviral medicines to try to prevent permanent damage to the nerve, which can cause long-lasting, severe pain in some people when not treated quickly.

Another type of herpes virus infection is due to *Herpes simplex* virus. This virus also lives inside of our bodies for our entire lives after we are infected, but it is contracted from someone else by direct contact. It causes painful open sores most commonly on the lips (called herpes labialis, coming from the Latin word for "lips") or on the genitals (herpes genitalis). When it occurs on the lips, it often begins as a burning sensation followed by the appearance of itchy bumps that then open up into painful sores. In addition to being painful, it can be cosmetically unappealing and embarrassing to the person who has the infection. Nonmedical people often call them "cold sores" or "fever blisters." Stress, illness, and dry chapped lips can cause them to occur repeatedly throughout the person's lifetime. When they occur on the genitals, it can be quite distressing as it is possible to spread the infection to someone else through sexual contact (it is a sexually transmitted disease). An important thing to remember is that if someone with recurrent *Herpes simplex* infection has to take an immunosuppressant medication for SLE (discussed in chapters 31, 32, 33, 34, and 37), he or she may develop these outbreaks more often, and they can become more severe. It is important to contact your doctor right away if you have an outbreak while you are taking an immunosuppressant medication to get treatment. The quicker an anti-herpes medication is used, the easier it is to treat. If the outbreaks occur more often, then a daily prophylactic anti-herpes antibiotic may be needed to prevent these more frequent outbreaks. Anti-herpes antibiotics include acyclovir (Zovirax), famciclovir (Famvir), and valacyclovir (Valtrex). These are the same antibiotics that are also used to treat herpes zoster (shingles).

Not all infections are treatable. For example, infections due to some viruses, such as sinus infections, bronchitis, and colds, do not respond to antibiotics. Your doctor may not recommend any treatment except over-the-counter medicines to help you feel better. Too many people are inappropriately given antibiotics. This unnecessary overuse of antibiotics leads to organisms becoming resistant to antibiotics, making them much more difficult to treat over time. Taking vitamin C and Echinacea (an herb from the purple coneflower) have not been shown to be effective for the common cold. People who have SLE should not take Echinacea because it can potentially make lupus worse. One possible treatment for the common cold is to use over-the-counter zinc lozenges (such as Cold-EEZE) that have been shown to possibly decrease the duration of symptoms of the infection. Zinc lozenges appear to work best if used immediately at the first appearance of cold symptoms and must be used regularly (such as every few hours).

People who have SLE need to remember that they should always list sulfa antibiotics as one of their allergies, even if they have never taken them before. Sulfa antibiotics—such as Septra, Bactrim, trimethoprim-sulfamethoxizole, Gantrisin, and sulfadiazine—can cause lupus to flare, and people who have lupus have a high chance of being allergic to them as well.

## KEY POINTS TO REMEMBER

1. Infections are among the top two or three causes of death in people who have SLE.

2. People who have SLE are prone to infections due to their altered immune systems, as well as due to medications they may take to control their lupus.

3. You can improve your chances of not needing to take stronger immunosuppressant medications by taking Plaquenil, not smoking cigarettes, and doing everything you can to decrease your exposure to UV light.

4. Everyone who has SLE should get a flu shot every fall.

5. SLE patients who are on immunosuppressant medicines should get two Pneumovax vaccines five years apart from each other. If you are 65 years old or older, you should get a third vaccination if it has been at least five years since your previous Pneumovax.

6. SLE patients who are not on immunosuppressant medications should get a Pneumovax when they are 65 years old.

7. All SLE patients should get a PCV13 vaccine when they reach 50 years old or older.

8. SLE patients who take immunosuppressant medications should get a PCV13 as soon as possible before the age of 50, but it needs to be coordinated with the Pneumovax (one year after the Pneumovax, or at least eight weeks before the Pneumovax if the Pneumovax has never been received).

9. Consider getting a Zostavax (against shingles) if you are 50 years old or older and not on strong immunosuppressant medicines. If you are on hydroxychloroquine, methotrexate, leflunomide, azathioprine, or prednisone less than 20 mg a day, it is safe to get the Zostavax.

10. Get the tetanus-diphtheria vaccine every ten years.

11. Avoid live vaccines (table 22.2) if you are on immunosuppressant medicines.

12. Do not get vaccinated if your SLE is very active or if you are on 40 mg or more of prednisone a day.

13. If you are prescribed rituximab (Rituxan) or belimumab (Benlysta), try to get any vaccinations before your treatments.

14. If you develop a fever or any symptoms of an infection, call and see your primary care physician, or go to an emergency room or urgent care center for assessment and treatment as soon as possible. Do not wait!

15. Always list sulfa antibiotics (such as Bactrim and Septra) as an allergy because they can cause flares of lupus.

16. Most cases of infections in people who have lupus are preventable by following the above recommendations.

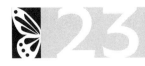

# Cancer and SLE

## A Vaccine to Prevent Cancer?

People who have SLE have a slightly increased risk of getting cancer compared to people who do not have SLE. This is not surprising since lupus is an abnormality of the immune system and a properly working immune system is important for constantly policing the body and getting rid of cancerous cells as they form. A large 2011 study from Europe showed that there were an increased number of cancers in SLE patients due to human papilloma virus (HPV). HPV is transmitted sexually and can live inside the body for many years. Infections with HPV have been associated with malignancies such as cervical cancer, anal cancer, throat cancer, and even skin cancer. Why people who have lupus get HPV-associated cancer more often than other people is not entirely known. It may be due to their immune systems not being very good at fighting against HPV, or it may be due to the immunosuppressant medicines that they take. Fortunately, there is now a vaccine available called Gardasil that can actually prevent infection from some strains of HPV. Therefore, this vaccination could potentially decrease the risk for getting HPV, and therefore certain cancers in people who have lupus.

Many other cancers can be prevented as well. Read this chapter to learn about important strategies to prevent cancer or to detect it at early, curable stages.

. . . .

Cancer is the second most common cause of death in Americans (after heart disease). In people who have SLE, cancer is the fourth most common cause of death (after lupus itself, cardiovascular events, and infections). Cancer is not emphasized very much in the lay literature about lupus. However, it is a very important topic because people who have SLE are at higher risk of developing cancer (15% more likely) than people who do not have SLE. Some cancers occur more commonly in people who have SLE (table 23.1), and some of these are potentially preventable. Screening tests can detect some of these cancers at very early stages, allowing possible cures with appropriate treatment. Interestingly, some cancers may occur less commonly in people who have SLE.

The increased risk of getting cancer is greatest during the first year or two after the diagnosis of SLE. However, the higher cancer risks persist throughout the affected person's lifespan. In addition, people who have SLE tend to get cancer at a younger age than their peers who do not have SLE.

This increased risk for cancer is probably partly due to the abnormal immune system of the person who has SLE. The immune system not only protects the body from infections, but also from cancer. The human body regularly produces abnormal cells that are potentially cancerous. However, the immune system is responsible for recognizing these abnormal cells and removing them. This is one reason why cancer becomes more prevalent as people age. The aging immune system becomes less able to recognize and remove cancerous cells from the body. The same thing may occur in SLE. The immune system in people who have SLE may not be as efficient at policing the body and removing these cancerous cells compared to the immune systems of people who do not have lupus. The risk of developing cancer is also highest in people who have more severe lupus disease, which certainly would support this theory.

Another potential reason for people who have lupus having an increased risk for developing cancer may be the use of some medications. For example, studies show that the use of cyclophosphamide in particular may be associated with an increased risk of developing cancer. Cyclophosphamide increases the risk of developing lymphoma (a cancer of the lymph glands) and cervical cancer. Cyclophosphamide given in pill form can also cause bladder cancer, but people who have lupus rarely take oral cyclophosphamide. Doctors usually prescribe the IV form instead. Cyclophosphamide is main-

**Table 23.1** Cancers in SLE

Cancers that occur more often in people who have SLE

    Lymphoma (especially non-Hodgkin's lymphoma): More common in those who have more active SLE, in those who have secondary Sjögren's syndrome, and in those treated with cyclophosphamide

    Lung cancer: Especially in those who smoke cigarettes

    Liver cancer

Cancers due to human papilloma virus infection

    Cervical cancer

    Vulvovaginal cancer

    Anal cancer

    Non-melanoma skin cancer (basal cell carcinoma and squamous cell carcinoma)

Cancers that may possibly occur more often in people who have SLE (increased numbers seen in one or just a few studies)

    Kidney cancer (also called nephroma)

    Thyroid cancer

Cancers that may occur less often in people who have SLE (possibly due to sex hormone differences)

    Breast cancer

    Ovarian cancer

    Uterine (endometrial) cancer

    Prostate cancer

ly used in people who have the most dangerous forms of SLE, such as severe kidney, brain, or lung disease. Other immunosuppressant medications used in lupus have not been proven to cause cancer.

Another possible reason for increased cancer in people who have lupus is the possible decreased ability of their immune systems to fight against cancer-causing viruses. For example, human papillomavirus (HPV) causes several types of cancer. Several studies have shown that lupus patients are more likely to develop cancers due to HPV. One study in particular followed 576 Danish SLE patients over an extended period (up to thirty-eight years) and found a marked increase in the number of HPV-related cancers compared to the number of cancers in people who did not have SLE. For example, the lupus patients were twenty-seven times more likely to develop cancer of the anus, nine times more likely to develop vulvovaginal cancer, and twice as likely to develop non-melanoma skin cancer and mouth cancer. All of these can be caused by HPV.

One group of medications may actually decrease the risk for certain cancers. Studies suggest that non-steroidal anti-inflammatory drugs—called NSAIDs for short (such as ibuprofen and naproxen)—may actually decrease the chances of developing some cancers such as colon cancer, breast cancer, and prostate cancer. People who have SLE are more likely to take NSAIDs to treat aches and pains compared to people who do not have SLE. Although we do not know if people who have lupus develop colon cancer more or less often, recent studies suggest that women who have SLE may have a lower chance of developing breast cancer compared to other women. In addition, men who have SLE may actually develop prostate cancer less often than other men do.

## Specific Cancers and SLE

### Lymphoma

Lymphoma is a group of cancers affecting cells of the immune system called lymphocytes. People who have systemic autoimmune diseases as a group, including SLE, have an increased chance of developing lymphoma, especially non-Hodgkin's lymphoma (NHL for short). The risk for NHL is highest for people who have primary Sjögren's syndrome, who have about a forty-four times increased risk of developing NHL compared to the general population. People who have severe rheumatoid arthritis (RA) have about a twenty-five times increased chance of developing it. This risk appears to be substantially less in people who have SLE compared to those who have primary Sjögren's syndrome and severe RA. However, people who have SLE still are three times more likely to develop lymphoma than the general population. This increased risk for lymphoma is probably due to the B-cells of the immune system being overactive in SLE. Recall from chapter 1 that it is the B-cells (also called B-lymphocytes) of the immune system that produce the many auto-antibodies in SLE. Therefore, this increased activity of B-lymphocytes (which carries an increased risk of some of them becoming cancerous), in combination with an abnormal immune system that is less efficient at removing cancerous cells, increases the chances of some of these cancerous cells surviving to evolve into lymphoma.

Rheumatologists had suspected that cyclophosphamide caused a slight risk of developing lymphoma. A large 2013 study addressed this question directly (whether lupus medications can cause lymphoma or not). This study involved numerous lupus experts, led by Dr. Sasha Bernatsky from McGill University in Canada, and their patients from multiple lupus centers. They did find that the use of cyclophosphamide was associated with increased risks for developing lymphoma (but still less than 0.1% of patients per year). However, other medications used in lupus did not show any increased risk. This is comforting because for years rheumatologists had wondered if any other medications, especially azathioprine (Imuran) caused lymphoma or not. Another study suggested that patients who have low blood counts due to their SLE, secondary Sjögren's syndrome, or lung involvement due to their lupus may be at increased risk for developing lymphoma compared to other SLE patients.

Lymphoma is a rare cancer overall, and even though it may appear more often in people who have SLE, it is still a rare cancer in them as well. However, it is important to understand what the symptoms are so that you know what to look out for. Lymphoma usually causes enlargement of the lymph glands. Therefore, it is not uncommon for a person who has lymphoma to have lymph gland swelling in areas that have a lot of lymph nodes—such as the arm pits, anywhere in the neck, just above the elbow on the inside of the arm (epitrochlear lymph nodes), and in the groin. Other symptoms include weight loss, fever, and night sweats.

A compounding issue is that SLE itself can also cause lymph node swelling (called lymphadenopathy), weight loss, and fever. Flares of lupus are much more common than lymphoma. Therefore, if a person who has SLE develops these symptoms, the doctor treats the person for a possible lupus flare, usually using steroids. If the lymph node swelling, fever, and weight loss resolve with treatment, then the symptoms were most likely due to lupus instead of lymphoma.

Another possible cause of lymph node swelling is infection. Therefore, the doctor may treat a person with antibiotics to see if this resolves the lymph node swelling. If the swollen lymph nodes persist after treatment with steroids and antibiotics, then the only way to make sure it is not due to lymphoma is to obtain a biopsy. A surgeon uses local anesthesia to numb up the area around the lymph node and then removes the lymph node for examination. Even in this situation, it is more likely for the biopsy to show that the lymph node swelling is due to lupus instead of lymphoma, but it is a very important distinction to make since lymphoma usually needs treatment with chemotherapy and possible radiation therapy.

The most common NHL that occurs in people who have SLE is a type called diffuse large B-cell lymphoma. This is a particularly aggressive form of NHL, meaning that it typically can kill the affected person within a few months if not treated. However, with proper treatment (usually chemotherapy and radiation therapy), it is a potentially curable form of cancer. One study showed that people who have SLE are as likely to respond to treatments for NHL as patients who do not have SLE. Therefore, it is important to let your doctor know if you develop any persistent lymph node swelling, especially if it occurs with fevers, weight loss, and night sweats.

## Lung Cancer

Lung cancer is the most common cause of death among all cancer-related deaths in the United States. Many studies have shown that people with SLE have an increased risk of developing lung cancer (about 1.4 times more often) compared to the general population. While 70% to 85% of these lung cancers are in lupus patients who smoke, they also can occur in lupus patients who do not smoke. Some rare types of lung cancers appear to occur more commonly among people who have lupus for unknown reasons. However, smoking cigarettes remains the primary reason for people who have SLE developing lung cancer. This is another very important reason why people who have lupus should not smoke cigarettes.

## Cervical Cancer

The cervix is in the back of the vagina at the entranceway to the uterus (or womb). It is through the cervix that sperm must travel to fertilize an egg. Cancer of the cervix is almost always due to infection from human papillomavirus, which is transmitted by sexual contact. The Pap smear (short for Papanicolaou, the last name of the doctor who developed it) and testing for HPV are the screening tests done to look for early cervical cancer. Since the Pap smear was introduced in 1941, the incidence of and death rates from cervical cancer have decreased substantially. Cervical cancer is potentially curable when caught at an early stage. Recently, this has been improved upon even more by testing directly for HPV infection. The Pap smear and HPV testing are performed by taking a specimen of cells and fluid from the cervix during a pelvic exam for evaluation in the laboratory.

Women who have SLE have higher rates of cervical cancer and precancerous lesions of the cervix compared to women who do not have SLE. This is due to a higher number of women with SLE being infected with HPV. The immune systems in people who have SLE may have more difficulty guarding against an infection from HPV compared to those of people who do not have SLE. In addition, immunosuppressant medicines increase the risk of developing cervical cancer, and studies in lupus patients show that the use of cyclophosphamide in particular has been associated with an increased risk of developing cervical cancer.

Women should begin having screening tests for cervical cancer with Pap smears and HPV testing three years after they begin sexual activity, or beginning by the age of 21, whichever comes first. It is recommended that most women have these tests every three years until the age of 30, then every two years after that. However, women who are at increased risk (such as those who take immunosuppressant medicines and women infected with HPV) should be screened for cervical cancer yearly. Therefore, it would be prudent for women who have SLE to consider having a pelvic exam, including Pap smear and HPV testing, on an annual basis.

A recent advance in the prevention of cervical cancer has been the availability of a vaccination against some types of HPV called Gardasil (see also chapter 22). Gardasil protects against infection from four types of HPV (strains 16 and 18, which cause 70% of all cervical cancers, and strains 6 and 11, which cause 90% of genital warts). Doctors give it as a series of three vaccines over a six-month period. The Centers for Disease Control recommends that all boys and girls receive Gardasil beginning at 11 years old. It would be advisable for people who have SLE to get vaccinated with Gardasil to try to prevent these potentially preventable cancers. Gardasil decreases the chances of getting genital warts from HPV as well as cervical, anal, vulvar, and vaginal cancers. Even if you have been found to be infected with HPV, it is still recommended that you get the Gardasil vaccine because it is possible to get infected with an additional strain of HPV, which can increase the risk of developing cervical cancer or genital warts.

## Breast, Ovarian, and Uterine Cancer

There is evidence that estrogen-sensitive cancers (breast, ovarian, and uterine [or endometrial] cancer) may actually occur less often in women who have SLE. This is interesting since SLE is a female hormone-driven disease, and people who have SLE may have different levels of sex hormones in their bodies than normal. Another possible reason for a decrease in these cancers in women who have lupus could be that they often do not take estrogen hormones (which can increase the risk of developing these cancers). Doctors are less likely to prescribe them to women who have lupus for birth control and for treatment of menopausal symptoms (such as hot flashes) in the fear that the hormones may increase their lupus activity. Therefore, these statistics could simply reflect a decreased rate of getting these cancers since there are fewer women who have lupus taking hormone supplements. In addition, some women who have SLE stop producing eggs (stop ovulating) prematurely due to using medications such as cyclophosphamide to treat their SLE, and this causes a decrease of estrogen in the body. In addition, taking NSAIDs (such as ibuprofen and naproxen) for pain may decrease the risk of getting breast cancer. Nonetheless, these cancers still occur in women who have lupus and so it is still very important that they undergo mammograms and pelvic exams regularly.

## Other Cancers

Other cancers shown to be more common in people who have lupus include liver cancer and cancer of the vagina and vulva (often grouped together under the term "vulvovaginal cancer"). As mentioned above, the Gardasil vaccine can decrease the risk of developing vaginal and vulvar cancers, which are related to HPV infections.

Liver cancer may cause pain in the right upper area of the abdomen just under the ribs, or it may cause jaundice (where the eyes and skin turn yellow). However, more commonly it is discovered by the doctor finding an elevation of liver function tests on the blood tests, followed by imaging studies of the liver such as an ultrasound or CT scan. Although cancers of the vagina and vulva (the skin flaps that surround the vagina) appear to be increased in people who have SLE compared people who do not have SLE, they are rare. Regular visits to your gynecologist and an annual pelvic exam are very important in finding these types of cancer at an early stage.

A study from Iceland showed an increased occurrence of a type of skin cancer called squamous cell carcinoma in patients who had SLE. Another study from California showed an increased number of kidney and thyroid cancers, in addition to lung cancer, liver cancer, and lymphoma. Kidney cancer can cause pain on the side of the lower chest and upper abdominal area as well as blood in the urine. Usually the blood is in very small quantities and is identified when a urine sample is examined in the lab. People who have SLE are at increased risk for autoimmune thyroid disease, and therefore should have their thyroid examined regularly on physical examination, in addition to having blood tests for thyroid function. Thyroid cancer is most commonly discovered when the doctor feels a swollen area in the thyroid at the front of the neck.

Interestingly, the study from California found a lower number of prostate cancers in its male lupus patients. It would not be surprising if this lower risk of prostate cancer is reproduced in future studies since prostate cancer is a male sex hormone–driven disease, and there is evidence that there is an offset in the normal balance of estrogen and testosterone in men who have SLE. In addition, NSAIDs taken by many people who have SLE for pain may decrease the chance of developing prostate cancer.

## Screening for and Prevention of Cancer in SLE

Unfortunately, studies show that people who have SLE have lower rates of cancer screenings, such as mammograms and PAP smears, compared to people who do not have SLE. It is not known why this would occur since patients who have SLE typically see doctors much more frequently than other people do. However, maybe this is exactly the reason why. I see in my own patient population that many patients who have SLE become tired of seeing doctors frequently, and they may possibly forgo certain important health maintenance visits such as recommended cancer screenings.

People who have SLE are at increased risk for developing cancer overall and in particular lymphoma, lung, liver, vulvovaginal, cervical, kidney, and thyroid cancers and possibly squamous cell carcinoma of the skin. Therefore, it is important that they undergo the necessary cancer screenings because many of these cancers are curable when caught early. Good primary care physicians and/or gynecologists should ensure that people who have SLE get their mammograms, pelvic exams, PAP smears, colonoscopies (done to look for colon cancer), PSA blood tests (for prostate cancer), and prostate exams (table 23.2) regularly.

Of course, cancer prevention also includes not smoking cigarettes because cigarettes clearly have a driving effect in causing lung cancer in people who have SLE. Obesity is also a risk factor for many cancers, such as colon cancer, so maintaining normal body weight may be beneficial as well. Diets rich in omega-3 fatty acids, fruits, vegetables, and fiber may also decrease the risk of some cancers. Doctors ask all people who have lupus to use sunscreen every day. Regular use of sunscreen helps to decrease the risk of developing squamous cell carcinoma as well as the more potentially deadly skin cancer malignant melanoma.

Table 23.2  Recommended Cancer Screenings

Women

    Pelvic exam, Pap smear, HPV screening yearly starting at 21 years old

    Mammograms yearly between 50 and 75 years old (some recommend starting screening at 40)

Men

    PSA blood test and prostate exam yearly 50–74 years old (start at 40 years old if positive family history or if African American)

Everyone

    Colonoscopy regularly starting at 50 years old (40 years old if there is a family history of colon cancer)

## Cancer Treatments in People Who Have SLE

If chemotherapy for cancer is needed by someone who has SLE, it may actually be beneficial for that person's lupus since many types of chemotherapy suppress the immune system. However, since many of the immunosuppressant medications used to treat lupus can potentially increase the risk for infections and cause low blood counts (which may also occur with cancer chemotherapy), some lupus medications may need to be stopped during chemotherapy. The cancer doctor (called an oncologist) and the rheumatologist should discuss this issue. However, it is very important to still take anti-malarial medications such as hydroxychloroquine (Plaquenil) while taking chemotherapy.

The safety of radiation therapy in people who have SLE is less clear. A couple of studies have demonstrated more long-term side effects from the radiation therapy in people who have SLE. However, if the radiation therapy is recommended as a potential lifesaving therapy, it usually should be done. This is a decision that should be made through discussions between the radiation oncologist and the rheumatologist.

### KEY POINTS TO REMEMBER

1. People who have SLE have a higher risk of developing various cancers than people who do not have SLE.

2. People who have SLE tend to get cancer at a younger age, and this risk is increased especially during the first couple of years of being diagnosed with SLE.

3. People who have SLE are three times more likely to develop non-Hodgkin's lymphoma, which usually causes lymph node swelling, fevers, weight loss, and night sweats.

4. Do not smoke. Smoking greatly increases your risk for lung cancer.

5. Cervical cancer occurs more often in women who have SLE due to human papilloma virus, which is a sexually transmitted infection.

6. Vulvovaginal, liver, kidney, and thyroid cancer also occur more often in people who have SLE.

7. Get the Gardasil HPV vaccine series if you are not in a monogamous relationship and are sexually active.

8. Women who have SLE should get a pelvic exam, a Pap smear, and HPV testing yearly, beginning at 21 years old.

9. Women should get yearly mammograms starting at 40 to 50 years old.

10. Get a colonoscopy regularly starting at 40 to 50 years old.

11. Men should have a blood PSA and prostate exam yearly beginning at 40 to 50 years old.

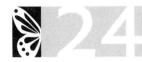

# Osteoporosis

## A Silent Killer

M. was one of my favorite patients, but then I must admit that most of my patients are "my favorite patients." She was in her early seventies, but she was a very young 70-year-old woman who was very friendly, always had a smile, was very active and independent, and insisted that I call her by her first name. She also had a wonderful husband whom I still see as a patient who was very devoted and loving toward her. Unfortunately, her SLE caused her to have a particularly severe form of skin disease that caused blistering and required the use of steroids to keep it under control. Even before this, M. had been diagnosed with a bone disorder called osteoporosis. Osteoporosis occurs when the bones are fragile and can fracture more easily than normal. Doctors call it a "silent disease" because people who have osteoporosis feel no discomfort nor do they have any symptoms at all until they actually break their bones.

I repeatedly advised M. that it would be best if she would take a medication, such as alendronate (Fosamax), to make her bones stronger to prevent her from getting a broken bone. However, M. insisted numerous times that she had seen "bad things" on the news and in magazine articles about the dangers of side effects from alendronate and other osteoporosis medicines. She constantly said that she was afraid to take any medicines for osteoporosis because of these side effects and would add, "Why should I take a medicine for something that I don't feel bad from?" I would repeatedly remind her that the dangers of broken bones from osteoporosis were much worse than the potential side effects of alendronate. I would tell her that if side effects do occur from alendronate, they are generally mild and resolve after the patient stops taking it. I would also tell her how bad osteoporosis was, including facts such as 20% of people dying if they fracture their hip. This went on for several years, with my advising her to take an osteoporosis medicine (along with the reasons why) and her telling me why she did not want to take them.

One day, her husband made an urgent appointment for M. to see me. When I walked into the examination room, I was shocked. M. was in a wheelchair, slumped forward. It was the fear in her eyes, though, that really got me. She told me how a few days before she had felt severe pain in her back when she stood up from a chair. Immediately she had difficulty walking and urinating. Her lumbar (lower) spine was very tender, and it had an angle in it, forcing her to be bent forward. Her abdomen was bloated and tender due to a very full bladder. I knew immediately what was most likely wrong: a fractured spine from her osteoporosis pushing on the nerves of the spine causing leg weakness and inability to urinate. I sent M. and her husband immediately to the emergency room. M. passed away within a few weeks.

One of my patients asked me not to put any stories of patients doing poorly with their SLE in this book. I agree with her in that respect because unfortunately many people hear about people doing poorly and even dying from lupus, not realizing that the vast majority of people who have lupus actually do well and live long, normal lives. However, I feel it is important to stress how severe of a disease osteoporosis is since it is a silent disease that has potentially grave consequences if ignored. So many people are similar to M. in that they refuse treatment because "I don't want the side effects of the medicine," or "I don't want to take a medicine for something that I don't feel badly from," or "I don't want to take another pill." Every year I have a patient like M. get a severe fracture in the hip or spine due to not accepting treatment for osteoporosis. Every several years, a patient of mine dies from the consequences of not taking a medicine for osteoporosis. If people realize how horrible the disease can be, they can make a better-educated decision to do something about it. I also remind my patients that although I have seen severe problems from osteoporosis (as illustrated here), I have never had a patient get a severe reaction from the osteoporosis medicines, and I have treated a large number of osteoporosis patients.

Therefore, I invite you to read this chapter about the silent disease called osteoporosis. I miss M. very much, and I like to think of her smiling, friendly face I saw every time she came in to see me instead of the scared, frail person she became toward the end. If her story can convince even one person to take osteoporosis seriously and treat it to prevent the complications from a bone fracture, then her story and her life have served a wonderful purpose.

· · · ·

Osteoporosis is a disease of the bones where the bones become more fragile due to the loss of hard minerals such as calcium and phosphorus from the bone. "Osteo-" comes from the Greek word for "bone," while "-porosis" comes from the Greek word for "pore" or "passageway." Normal bones have pores and passageways between the layers of hard mineral to allow blood vessels to flow through them to provide nutrients and oxygen to the cells that maintain the bones. There is a fine balance in normal bone: there is a lot of hard mineral structure with just enough pores or passages for the blood vessels. In the person who has osteoporosis, however, there is a decrease in the amount of hard, bony, mineral-rich architecture and an overabundance of pores or passages (figure 24.1). This ends up causing less strength in the bones; they become brittle and are at increased risk of breaking.

The most common cause of osteoporosis is menopause. Female hormones such as estrogen are very important for keeping bones strong and keeping the correct amount of hard, calcium-rich supports intact. After women go through menopause, their estrogen levels decrease substantially. This causes the bones to lose calcium and women can develop osteoporosis, which can lead to broken bones, most commonly occurring in the spine, hips, and wrists.

This can be devastating, as these fractures can cause numerous problems with the quality of life of the person, and they can be deadly as well. For example, when people who have osteoporosis develop broken bones in the vertebra, the spine typically

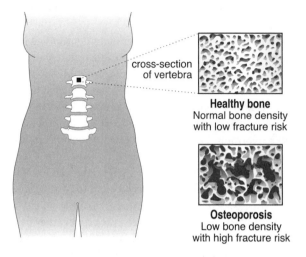

cross-section
of vertebra

**Healthy bone**
Normal bone density
with low fracture risk

**Osteoporosis**
Low bone density
with high fracture risk

**Figure 24.1** A section of normal bone compared to bone with osteoporosis. The sample of normal bone on the top has many white, calcium-rich supports while the osteoporotic bone on the bottom has very little calcium-rich supports and more passageways or pores (hence the term "osteoporosis"). The osteoporotic bone on the bottom is more fragile, and the person is at high risk of developing broken bones.

begins to arch forward (figure 24.2). The arched spine compresses the lungs, making it more difficult to breathe normally. Women with multiple vertebral fractures are at increased risk of early death due to lung infections because they have difficulty taking in complete, full breaths. The lower rib cage is thrust down and forward toward the bones of the pelvis. This causes the abdominal wall to become rounded forward, and the intestinal contents become compressed, causing problems with digestion. Women who have osteoporosis are also plagued by recurrent problems with digestion causing gastroesophageal reflux (heartburn), stomach upset, and constipation. The person who has an arched back from osteoporosis also cannot stand up straight. This often causes the person to have poor self-esteem due to the dramatic changes in body appearance. So not only can these vertebral fractures cause early death, but they also decrease the quality of someone's life through problems with breathing, digestion, and self-esteem.

Fractures of the hips are even worse. If someone gets a fracture of the hip due to osteoporosis, she or he has about a 20% chance of dying from the hip fracture. This is because of the numerous medical problems that can occur due to the immobility of people who have hip fractures. They are at high risk of developing blood clots and other complications such as pneumonia due to the forced inactivity. If they are fortunate enough to survive the hip fracture, a significant proportion of people end up greatly debilitated from the hip fracture, with difficulties in walking and standing for the rest of their lives. Many end up in nursing care centers due to their family's inability to care for them.

As discussed in the first section of this chapter, osteoporosis is considered a silent disease. Silent diseases are disorders that occur in people, who have no idea the disorders are occurring until significant damage has already happened. One of the most common silent diseases is hypertension (high blood pressure). People who have hypertension have no idea they have it until it actually begins to cause significant damage with heart attacks, strokes, and kidney failure. Since hypertension has been treated aggressively by doctors with blood pressure medicines in the last half century, the lifespans of Americans have increased significantly.

Doctors now are dealing with a similar situation with osteoporosis. When I was a medical student and an internal medicine resident, osteoporosis was an accepted part of the aging process. There was very little doctors could do about it. It was just a fact of life that most women would get broken bones as they got older, causing hip fractures as well as curved spines; doctors had no effective treatments to prevent these things from happening. The FDA approval of alendronate (Fosamax) in 1995 completely changed the scene. Doctors finally had a safe medication that was proven to significantly decrease the number of broken bones in people who have osteoporosis. No more could osteoporosis be considered a fact of aging. Doctors finally could stop people from fracturing their bones. Keeping people who have osteoporosis from getting vertebral fractures (and therefore not becoming hunched over as they age) and hip fractures (which can cause significant problems in walking) have provided people with a much better quality of life as they age compared to previous generations.

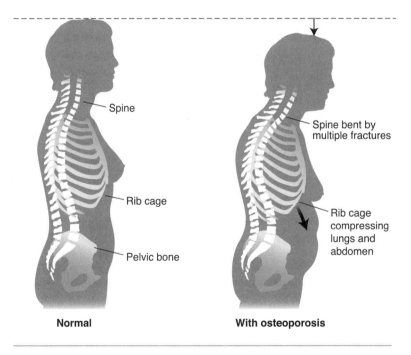

Spine

Rib cage

Pelvic bone

**Normal**

Spine bent by multiple fractures

Rib cage compressing lungs and abdomen

**With osteoporosis**

Figure 24.2  Effects of vertebral fractures due to osteoporosis

## How Osteoporosis Occurs

Bones are constantly remodeled. Some bone is removed while new bone is laid down by the cells of the bones. This process can be compared to a brick or stone wall where some workers are responsible for removing parts of the wall that are aging and crumbling, while other workers are responsible for putting in fresh, strong brick or stone replacements. The cells responsible for making new calcium-rich bone are called osteoblasts, while the cells that dissolve the bone are called osteoclasts. You can think of them as diligent construction workers who are constantly trying to improve the architecture of the bones to help them support the weight of the body better all the time. The driving force for where they make stronger bone occurs in areas where the bones feel more stress and weight. In areas of bone where there is more stress, the osteoblasts will lay down extra mineral-enriched bony supports. This explains the reason astronauts develop decreased bone density when they travel to outer space. Their bones feel very little stress while in outer space since there is no gravitational pull on the bones. The osteoclasts dissolve bone in those areas of bone feeling very little weight, and the osteoblasts do not have any incentive to build up the bone since they do not feel weight or stress on the bones. It is also one of the reasons why obese and muscular people have stronger bones than people who do not exercise or who are very thin.

Anything that disrupts this orchestrated cycle of bone dissolving by the osteoclasts and bone-building activity by the osteoblasts can end up causing abnormal bone formation. If the osteoclasts dissolve too much bone and/or the osteoblasts stop making more bone, then less mineral-rich bone structure is formed, more passageways or pores develop, and weak bone due to osteoporosis occurs. As mentioned above, menopause with its lack of estrogen is the most common cause of osteoporosis. Yet there

**Table 24.1** Risk Factors for Having Osteoporosis

- Menopause
- A family history of osteoporosis (especially if a parent had a broken hip)
- Drugs (table 24.2)
- Weight $\leq$ 126 pounds
- Cigarette smoking currently or in the past
- Drinking more than two servings of alcohol per day
- Some medical diseases (table 24.3)
- Vitamin D deficiency
- Lifelong low calcium intake (such as in people who are lactose intolerant)
- History of broken bones as an adult
- Advanced age (the older you are, the higher the risk)
- Increased risk of falling (frail, nerve or muscle problems, dementia, poor balance, arthritis, weak)

are many other factors involved that can also cause this to occur. Table 24.1 lists risk factors (or causes) of osteoporosis. When going through these risk factors for osteoporosis, it can be very helpful to circle the ones that apply to you. The more risk factors people have for developing osteoporosis or getting broken bones, the more aggressive they and their doctors should be at trying to reverse the potentially reversible risk factors and use medicines to make the bones stronger.

## Genetics

Certainly, genetics play a role in the development of osteoporosis. People from certain ethnicities, such as northern European and Asian ancestry, are at higher risk of developing osteoporosis compared to other ethnicities such as African Americans. However, all ethnic groups have problems with osteoporosis (although the percentage of people who get osteoporosis may vary substantially within each ethnic group). Even though African Americans may have a lower risk of osteoporosis compared to some other ethnic groups, it certainly occurs.

One of the biggest risk factors found to be particularly predictive of someone being at high risk for developing osteoporosis and broken bones is if the person has a parent who had a hip fracture. For example, if a woman has a parent who has had a hip fracture, this increases her risk of getting broken bones from osteoporosis by a factor of 2.

## Drugs

Certain drugs cause osteoporosis by causing the cells of the bones not to work properly or interfering with the proper metabolism of calcium and vitamin D by the body. Drugs that can cause osteoporosis include steroids (such as prednisone and methylprednisolone), anti-seizure medicines, and medicines that decrease acidity of the stomach (which causes less calcium to be absorbed). A list of drugs that can adversely affect bone strength is provided in table 24.2. Medications are one of the biggest reasons people who have lupus are at increased risk for developing osteoporosis. Many people who have SLE are treated with osteoporosis-causing medications such as steroids, anti-seizure medicines, blood thinners, and anti-acid medications.

## Low Body Weight

Weighing less than 127 pounds is a risk factor for osteoporosis most likely due to having smaller and therefore weaker bones.

## Cigarette Smoking

The chemicals in tobacco keep the cells of the bones from forming strong bone and increase the chances of getting broken bones from osteoporosis.

## Excessive Alcohol Use

As with cigarettes, excessive alcohol also prevents the cells of bones from forming strong bone. Excessive alcohol is defined as having more than two servings of alcohol a day. One serving is approximately 12 ounces of beer, 8 ounces of malt liquor, 5 ounces of wine, 3–4 ounces of fortified wine (such as sherry and port), 2.5 ounces of 24% alcohol liqueur, or 1.5 ounces of 80-proof liquor. Interestingly, the effects of alcohol on bone formation appear to be related to how much alcohol is consumed. The largest

**Table 24.2** Drugs That Can Cause Decreased Bone Strength

**Drugs That Cause Bone Loss**

  Steroids
    prednisone
    methylprednisolone (Medrol)

  Anti-seizure medicines (cause decreased vitamin D levels)
    phenobarbital
    phenytoin (Dilantin)
    carbamazepine (Tegretol)

  Blood thinners
    heparin

  Hormones
    medroxyprogesterone (Depo-Provera) (when used in "high doses")

  Loop diuretics (fluid pills) (increase the excretion of calcium from the kidneys)
    furosemide (Lasix)
    bumetanide

  Chemotherapy
    methotrexate (high doses for cancer; not the low doses used in lupus)
    ifosfamide (Ifex)
    imatinib (Gleevec)

  Aromatase inhibitors (used to treat breast cancer)
    anastrozole (Arimidex)
    letrozole (Femara)
    exemestane (Aromasin)

  Proton pump inhibitors (decrease stomach acid; decrease absorption of calcium)
    esomeprazole (Nexium)
    lansoprazole (Prevacid)
    omeprazole (Prilosec)
    pantoprazole (Protonix)
    rabeprazole (AcipHex)

  Thiazolidinediones (used to treat diabetes)
    rosiglitazone (Avandia)
    pioglitazone (Actos)

  HIV antiviral medications
    tenofovir (Viread)

  Anti-androgen therapies (for prostate cancer)
    bicalutamide (Casodex)
    cyproterone

  Thyroid hormone (when taken in excessive amounts)
    levothyroxine (Synthroid)

**Drugs That Possibly Cause Bone Loss***

  warfarin (Coumadin) (a blood thinner)
  cyclosporine (an immunosuppressant)
  vitamin A (when taken in high doses)
  antidepressants (could be related to increased risk for falling due to dizziness)

* Studies are conflicting.

study ever to look at risk factors for developing osteoporosis showed that women who drank no alcohol at all as well as those who drink too much both had a higher chance of developing broken bones from osteoporosis compared to women who drank alcohol in small to moderate amounts.

## Medical Diseases

Many medical diseases can cause osteoporosis in numerous ways, ranging from directly affecting the health of bones, to causing decreased absorption of calcium and vitamin D, to effects of the medicines used to treat the diseases (table 24.3).

## Vitamin D Deficiency

Vitamin D is very important for the proper handling of calcium in the body. Inadequate amounts of vitamin D cause decreased absorption of calcium from the intestines, increased excretion of calcium from the kidneys, and subsequent decreased amounts of calcium in the bones. We naturally get vitamin D through sun exposure. Ultraviolet light from the sun contacts the skin and actually causes the skin to produce vitamin D. Since people who have lupus are asked to avoid the sun and to use sunscreen daily, most of them have vitamin D deficiency and should take a vitamin D supplement regularly.

There are several other reasons most people who have lupus are deficient in vitamin D (table 24.4). Melanin, the dark pigmentation of the skin, prevents ultraviolet light from penetrating the skin, and subsequently less vitamin D is produced. Therefore, darker-colored people such as African Americans and Hispanics have higher rates of vitamin D deficiency than lighter-colored individuals do. Since lupus occurs more commonly in African Americans and Hispanics, this is another reason people who have lupus have vitamin D deficiency. Vitamin D is also fat absorbable. Overweight people have lower amounts of vitamin D circulating in their bodies since a lot of it dissolves into the fat cells of their bodies instead of being used effectively by the bones,

**Table 24.3** Medical Diseases That Can Cause Osteoporosis

HIV infection

Rheumatoid arthritis

Systemic lupus erythematosus

Diabetes (both type I and type II)

Inflammatory bowel disease (Crohn's disease and ulcerative colitis)

Celiac disease (gluten hypersensitivity, non-tropical sprue)

Cystic fibrosis

Hyperthyroidism (overactive thyroid such as Graves' disease)

Kidney disease

Liver disease

Hyperparathyroidism

**Table 24.4**  Reasons Most People Who Have Lupus Are Deficient in Vitamin D

- Avoidance of the sun as part of their treatment
- Darker skin color in African American and Hispanic people
- Obesity
- Use of steroids

intestines, and kidneys where it is needed. Fat acts as a "sink hole" for vitamin D. Obesity occurs more commonly in people who have SLE due to the use of steroids and due to more inactivity because of their aches and pains. Lastly, steroids themselves cause the active form of vitamin D (25-OH vitamin D, pronounced 25-hydroxy vitamin D) to be metabolized more quickly in the body, causing decreased levels as well. Therefore, there are multiple reasons vitamin D deficiency is so common in people who have lupus.

Low vitamin D levels have been associated with other problems besides osteoporosis and broken bones. One large study showed that people who have vitamin D levels less than 15 ng/mL have an increased risk of having cardiovascular events such as strokes and heart attacks. Increasing vitamin D levels may decrease this risk. This is a very important matter since people who have SLE develop heart attacks and strokes at an earlier age than other people (see chapter 21). Vitamin D levels lower than 20 ng/mL have been associated with an increased risk of dying from breast, colon, ovarian, and prostate cancer. A couple of studies have shown that taking vitamin D supplements may actually decrease the chances of dying from cancer. Since people who have SLE have a higher chance than normal of getting cancer, this is another important reason for taking a vitamin D supplement if you have lupus.

Adequate amounts of vitamin D are required for the immune system to function properly. Some cells of the immune system (such as B-cells, T-cells, and macrophages) actually have receptors on their cell walls to which vitamin D attaches to help keep them working correctly. People who have more severe lupus disease activity have lower levels of vitamin D compared to those who have less severe disease. This vitamin D deficiency is seen even when they are first diagnosed with SLE (before they have been instructed to avoid the sun). It has been theorized that supplementing vitamin D levels may potentially help the immune systems of people who have SLE, but this has not been studied adequately yet nor proven. Since a higher number of African Americans and Hispanics are vitamin D deficient (due to increased skin pigmentation), and low vitamin D levels may be a cause for the immune system to work improperly, vitamin D deficiency has even been postulated as a potential contributor for developing lupus in the first place, but this also has not yet been proven.

Low vitamin D levels have also been shown to be associated with increased fatigue in people who have SLE. Fatigue is one of the most common and most difficult problems to improve in many people who have SLE. Several studies have shown that vitamin D supplementation may potentially decrease the severity of fatigue in some patients.

## Inadequate Calcium Ingestion

A big factor in bone density has to do with how much calcium people ingest throughout their lives. This is especially important when people are in their teens and twenties when they are building bone density up the most. People reach their maximum bone density at about 30 years old; after that, bone density slowly begins to decline over time. People who have an inadequate intake of calcium during their teens and twenties are particularly at increased risk of starting with a lower bone density when they reach 30 compared to other people. They are therefore at higher risk of developing osteoporosis as they age. Dairy products are the major dietary sources of calcium; therefore, those who do not eat or drink many dairy products are at increased risk of having decreased bone density. Sometimes this is due to reasons beyond the person's control. For example, people who are lactose intolerant have great difficulty tolerating dairy products and therefore learn to stay away from them. This automatically causes them to have a deficiency in calcium intake, and they are at increased risk for osteoporosis as they get older.

## Additional Risk Factors for Getting Osteoporotic Fractures

*History of Broken Bone as an Adult.* Having had a broken bone as an adult from minimal trauma increases the risk of developing broken bones from osteoporosis as it can signal that there is something wrong with the bones.

*Advanced Age.* Age definitely plays a large role in the chances of having broken bones from osteoporosis for numerous reasons. Aging people are at increased risk of falling and their bone architecture (i.e., how well the bone is actually constructed) is not as strong as that of people of younger ages. For example, if a 50-year-old and an 80-year-old each have similar bone density measured by x-ray (DXA scan discussed later), the 80-year-old would be at higher risk of getting broken bones compared to the 50-year-old since his or her bone structure is not as strong architecturally as the bones of the 50-year-old. Although they may have the same amount of mineral in them, the quality, and therefore the actual strength, of the 50-year-old person's bones is better than that of the 80-year-old person's bones. This increased risk for broken bones with advancing age is very important to take into account when deciding if someone should go on a medication for osteoporosis or not.

*Recurrent Falls, Use of Walking Aids, Dementia, Poor Health, and Frailty.* These problems can be lumped together as factors that increase the risk for getting broken bones from osteoporosis. People may have just a mild decrease in bone density and yet be at high risk of getting broken bones simply because they are at increased risk of falling and injuring their bones more often.

## How Osteoporosis Is Diagnosed

The most accurate way to diagnose osteoporosis is by getting a bone biopsy. However, this is rarely ever done, as it is a painful, invasive procedure. Yet it is the best way to know that someone has osteoporosis. If doctors tried to do this painful procedure on everyone who is at risk of having osteoporosis, though, they would have many unhappy patients.

Therefore, doctors have to rely on less invasive ways to make the diagnosis. Currently, the best method of making a diagnosis of osteoporosis (other than the bone biopsy) is by using an x-ray technique called dual-energy x-ray absorptiometry (DXA scan for short). This type of x-ray is done on an outpatient basis in the offices of rheumatologists, endocrinologists, primary care doctors, gynecologists, and radiologists. The most accurate measurements are taken at the hip, spine, and forearm. Most of the time the hip and spine are the preferred areas to be measured. The forearm is used if there is some reason that either the hip or spine measurements cannot be used, or for some diseases (such as hyperparathyroidism) where the forearm is the more accurate place to measure the bone density. The machine sends a small amount of radiation through the body to measure the density (and therefore the presumed strength) of the bones. A complete DXA scan uses approximately the same amount of radiation that you would encounter if you were to take a round-trip airplane flight from New York City to Los Angeles and back.

The DXA scan measures the density of the bones in several different areas and then compares it to the density expected of someone with the same height and weight at the age of 30 years old (when people typically have the greatest bone density). A statistical analysis is performed on this comparison to come up with a number called the standard deviation (a calculated statistical number) from this expected number for a 30-year-old. This standard deviation number is called the T-score. If your T-score is zero, that means that your bone density is similar to a 30-year-old with your same height and weight. A negative T-score means that your bone density is less, and a positive T-score would mean that your bone density is stronger than the bones of a 30-year-old person. The World Health Organization (WHO) has come up with a system using the T-score to diagnose osteoporosis (table 24.5).

This brings up a new medical term: "osteopenia." "Osteo-" means "bone," and "-penia" comes from the Greek word for "deficiency." Therefore, osteopenia means a deficiency of bone or decreased bone density. You can think of osteoporosis and osteopenia as being parts of a continuum of bone density where osteoporosis represents a more severe loss of bone density along with its associated higher risk for broken bones compared to osteopenia where there is an increased risk of broken bones but not as much as with osteoporosis.

There are important caveats to consider when using the T-score result when diagnosing osteoporosis and the potential for someone getting broken bones. For exam-

**Table 24.5** Using the T-score from a DXA Scan to Diagnose Osteoporosis

| T-score | Diagnosis |
| --- | --- |
| -1.0 or more positive | Normal |
| -1.1 to -2.4 | Osteopenia (also called low bone density) |
| -2.5 or more negative | Osteoporosis |

ple, the test can be inaccurate. Since the DXA scan measures only the density of bone, not the type of bone, it can overestimate density if a person has additional bone matter such as bone spurs. Almost everyone will develop a type of arthritis of the spine and hips as they get older called osteoarthritis (or degenerative joint disease). It causes bony growths called bone spurs to form around the joints. The DXA machine does not make a distinction between bone spurs and the bones of the spine and hip and will add up this bony density along with the bone density within the bones themselves, calculating a higher (and inaccurate) amount of bone density than there actually is. Therefore, people who have many bone spurs from osteoarthritis may look like they have very strong bone strength on their DXA scans, but may in fact have weak bones due to osteoporosis. Because of this, there are some people who have osteoporosis and get broken bones even though their T-scores are completely normal. To clarify this point, studies show that one out of every three women who have SLE who have a vertebral fracture due to osteoporosis actually have "normal" bone density when measured with DXA scans at the spine and hip. Unfortunately, the DXA scan is not a perfect test for osteoporosis, but it is currently the best doctors have without doing a bone biopsy.

Not all T-scores mean the same thing. Any particular T-score can represent a different risk for getting broken bones in different people. For example, a very healthy, active 50-year-old woman who went through menopause a year ago has a T-score of –1.5, giving her a diagnosis of osteopenia. Her risk of getting broken bones due to her osteopenia would be very different from that of a 100 pound, frail 80-year-old woman with a T-score of –1.5 who has to use a walker because she is very unsteady on her feet and is at high risk for falling. Although their T-scores are the same, the 80-year-old most likely has overall weaker bones due to her bone health (the actual structure of the bones) being worse. Her bones are not nearly as strong as those of the 50-year-old woman. In addition, the 80-year-old is at high risk for falling, and this greatly increases her risk for getting a broken hip or spine compared to the 50-year-old. Therefore, most osteoporosis experts would treat the 80-year-old more aggressively with medications to get her bones stronger. The 50-year-old is at much lower risk for getting broken bones and therefore can be treated with calcium, vitamin D, and exercise instead of medications. This is where the use of the risk factors for developing osteoporosis and getting broken bones comes in handy. For any given T-score, the more risk factors someone has, the higher are her or his chances of getting broken bones due to osteoporosis.

Relying only on the T-score is not a very accurate way to try to determine someone's risk for getting broken bones. Doctors now have a way to more accurately determine the risk for someone getting broken bones by using the WHO's calculation method called the Fracture Risk Assessment Tool (or FRAX for short). FRAX takes into account the bone density (T-score) at the femoral neck (hip) of the person as well as other risk factors for getting broken bones such as smoking, excessive alcohol use, family history of broken bones, medical diseases associated with osteoporosis, use of steroids, and a personal history of broken bones. These known risk factors are used to come up with an estimate of getting broken bones over a ten-year period by plugging them into a formula. These FRAX estimates may be done by the DXA machine itself, or by your doctor plugging the numbers into a calculation formula to determine the results. This formula calculates the ten-year risk for developing any major broken bone from osteoporosis as well as the risk for getting a broken hip. Currently, the National Osteoporosis Foundation (NOF) recommends that medications, such as bisphosphonates like alendronate (Fosamax), be used if the ten-year risk for getting any major fracture is 20% or higher or if the ten-year risk for getting a hip fracture is 3% or higher.

However, the FRAX formula is not foolproof. For example, if someone has many bone spurs around the hip joint due to osteoarthritis, the DXA scan can give a falsely high T-score result (and therefore be interpreted incorrectly as being strong bone). The FRAX calculation in this example would underestimate the risk for getting broken bones (FRAX uses the bone density of the hip but not of the spine in its calculations). In addition, the FRAX formula does not use all known risk factors for osteoporotic fractures. For example, a very important one that it does not use is if the person is at risk for falling or not. If someone has a high risk for falling (such as the 80-year-old woman in the preceding example), yet her FRAX calculation shows a ten-year risk for broken bones of 18% instead of the 20% cut off for treatment recommended by the NOF, most osteoporosis experts would recommend treating her. Her risk for getting broken bones would be much higher than this calculated 18% since falling was not used in the FRAX calculation.

Another problem with the FRAX is that it does not take into account the quantity of steroids the person has taken or if the person is currently taking steroids versus has taken them in the past. It uses an "all or none" factor as far as steroids are concerned. If the person has ever been on steroids, then that is plugged into the formula no matter what dose was used or when it was used. The problem with this is that there is a higher risk for getting broken bones from osteoporosis in those who are currently on steroids, and the risk is higher for those who take higher doses. All other things being equal, if there is one person who was on prednisone 5 mg a day for a few months a few years ago, and another person who currently takes 60 mg a day for the past month, their FRAX calculations would be the same. However, in reality the person on the 60 mg a day currently is at much higher risk for broken bones. Therefore, even the FRAX cannot be used in isolation to determine whether someone should take medicines for osteoporosis or not. It takes a doctor experienced at treating osteoporosis to put all the variables together to reach the proper treatment regimen for any particular person.

Another way (besides bone biopsy and DXA scan T-score) to diagnose osteoporosis is if someone has developed what is called a fragility fracture. A fragility fracture occurs when a fracture occurs because of minimal trauma in a bone that would not normally be expected to break. One definition of a fragility fracture is if someone breaks a bone by falling from standing height—for example, if a woman falls down by tripping over something, sticks out her hand to catch her fall, and then breaks her wrist. That would be considered a fragility fracture and would be enough to make a diagnosis of osteoporosis even if the person has a normal T-score. Another example would be if someone were found to have a vertebra fracture on x-ray and does not remember ever breaking his or her spine, never had any trauma to explain it, and does not remember having any back pain. A large percentage of vertebral fractures never cause pain and are picked up accidently when x-rays are done for other reasons. This would also be enough to say the person has osteoporosis (once other reasons for having a broken vertebra are ruled out by the doctor) and to start her or him on treatment.

Most people who have lupus who have had vertebral fractures actually are not aware of the fact. This is not completely understood, but a large number of vertebral fractures cause no pain. This has been shown in multiple studies. A 2010 study showed that 29% of patients who had SLE had at least one vertebral fracture on x-ray. The vast majority of these patients did not know that they had them, nor did their doctors. Another surprise is that 40% of these patients who had vertebral fractures actually had normal bone density on DXA scans (which are not foolproof in diagnosing osteoporosis). Therefore, a large number of these SLE patients had osteoporosis complicated by a vertebral fracture yet had no idea they had it. Once someone has had a vertebral fracture, that person is at higher risk of developing other fractures of the spine and hips than similar people (as far as age, gender, build, and T-score). The use of steroids is a major contributing factor in these vertebral fractures.

Due to the inaccuracy of DXA scans and the high incidence of undiagnosed vertebral fractures, it is recommended that people who have SLE who have been treated with steroids for any significant time or amount in the past have a special type of x-ray called a vertebral fracture assessment. This is a very simple x-ray of the entire spine that can be done by a DXA machine. It uses much less radiation compared to normal x-rays of the spine and can be ordered by your doctor at the same time that he or she orders your DXA scan.

## Why Lupus Patients Are at Increased Risk for Getting Osteoporosis

Women who have SLE are five times more likely to develop broken bones due to osteoporosis compared to other women. Several studies have shown that between 20% and 29% of women who have SLE have at least one vertebral fracture, and the surprising thing is that most of them did not even know they had a broken vertebra in their spine. Once someone has had a vertebral fracture, she or he is at high risk of developing other broken bones, of which hip fractures are the most dreaded complications. These facts further point out why this is such an important concern in people who have SLE.

People who have SLE are at increased risk of developing osteoporosis due to multiple reasons, as mentioned above. Steroids are often used to treat lupus, and they are a major cause of osteoporosis. Other medications that can cause osteoporosis are also commonly used in treating SLE, including PPI inhibitors to decrease stomach acidity, anti-seizure medications for epilepsy, and blood thinners if the person has had blood clots due to SLE. In addition, most people who have lupus are deficient in vitamin D. This occurs partly because they are asked to use sunscreen daily and to avoid the sun, which is the major natural source of vitamin D production. As discussed earlier, vitamin D is essential for the absorption and proper metabolism of calcium and bone. Many people who have SLE move around less and do not exercise very much due to being ill or having fatigue or pains. Exercise and activity are essential for the bones staying strong and healthy. Therefore, osteoporosis is a major concern in people who have SLE.

## How Osteoporosis Is Prevented and Treated in People Who Have SLE

### Measures to Prevent Osteoporosis

Many of the risk factors for osteoporosis can be dealt with and fixed. Of course, there are some which you have no control over such as your genetics, but others, such as smoking, you do have control over (table 24.6).

There are a number of things you can do to decrease your risk for osteoporosis and certainly things you should do if you are diagnosed with osteoporosis.

*Do not smoke.*

*Do not drink more than two servings of alcohol a day.* One serving of alcohol is approximately 12 ounces of beer, 8 ounces of malt liquor, 5 ounces of wine, 3–4 ounces of fortified wine (such as sherry and port), 2.5 ounces of 24% alcohol liqueur, or 1.5 ounces of 80-proof liquor. However, the metabolism, and therefore the tolerance to alcohol, varies depending on body weight and fat content of the body. People (especially women) who are of smaller build and who weigh less should most likely not drink more than one serving a day. An exact body weight has not been determined for this recommendation. In addition, daily alcohol use may increase the risk of breast cancer in women. Taking 1 mg of folic acid (a B vitamin) daily may decrease this risk. Of course, women who have liver disease or who take medications that can potentially affect the liver (such as methotrexate) should discuss alcohol use with their doctor as it may be better for them not to drink any alcohol or to drink it in more limited quantities.

*Perform weight-bearing exercise five days a week, thirty minutes at a time.* This can include activities such as brisk walking, low-impact aerobics, and weight-training/toning exercises. Swimming does not help with osteoporosis as the water removes the stress from the bones necessary to stimulate bone growth.

*Get adequate calcium from dietary means or through supplements.* It was recommended by the Institute of Medicine in 2010 that women 50 years old or older and men 71 years and older get 1,200 mg or more a day while others should get 1,000 mg a day or more of calcium. However, the American College of Rheumatology recommends that anyone taking steroids (such as prednisone and methylprednisolone) should get 1,200 mg to 1,500 mg of calcium a day regardless of age and gender. The reasons are discussed in more detail in the following section on steroids. Some calcium-rich foods are listed in table 24.7. If you cannot get enough calcium intake daily through these

Table 24.6  Non-Medicine Ways to Treat and Prevent Osteoporosis

- Do not smoke.
- Do not drink excessive amounts of alcohol.
- Exercise (which stresses the bones) five days a week, thirty minutes at a time.
- Get adequate calcium.
- Get adequate vitamin D.
- Prevent falling.

**Table 24.7** Calcium-Rich Foods

| Food Item | Serving Size | Estimated Calcium Content (in mg) |
|---|---|---|
| American cheese | 1 ounce | 175 |
| Bok choy (Chinese cabbage), raw | 8 ounces (1 cup) | 75 |
| Broccoli, cooked and drained | 8 ounces (1 cup) | 60 |
| Cereal with added calcium, without milk | 8 ounces (1 cup) | 100–1,000 |
| Cheddar cheese, shredded | 1 ounce | 205 |
| Cottage cheese, 1% milk fat | 1 cup | 140 |
| Dried figs | 2 figs | 55 |
| Frozen yogurt, vanilla (soft serve) | 1 cup (8 ounces) | 205 |
| Fruit juice with added calcium | 6 ounces | 200–345 |
| Ice-cream, low-fat or high-fat | 1 cup (8 ounces) | 140–210 |
| Kale, cooked | 8 ounces (1 cup) | 95 |
| Milk, low-fat or fat-free | 1 cup (8 ounces) | 300 |
| Mozzarella cheese, part-skim | 1 ounce | 205 |
| Oranges | 1 whole | 50 |
| Parmesan cheese, grated | 1 tablespoon | 70 |
| Ricotta cheese, part-skim | 4 ounces (½ cup) | 335 |
| Salmon, pink, canned with bones | 3 ounces | 180 |
| Sardines, canned in oil with bones | 3 ounces | 325 |
| Shrimp, canned | 3 ounces | 125 |
| Soy milk with added calcium | 8 ounces (1 cup) | 80–500 |
| Soybeans, mature, cooked and drained | 8 ounces (1 cup) | 175 |
| Swiss cheese | 1 ounce | 220–270 |
| Tofu prepared with calcium | 4 ounces (½ cup) | 205 |
| Turnip greens, fresh, cooked and drained | 8 ounces (1 cup) | 200 |
| Yogurt, low-fat or fat-free (plain) | 8 ounces (1 cup) | 415 |

*Source*: National Osteoporosis Foundation.

foods (especially if you are lactose intolerant and cannot tolerate dairy products), it is important to take additional calcium supplements.

If you are on a proton pump inhibitor (or PPI for short; see table 28.3 for a list of PPIs), which are medications that decrease the acidity of the stomach, then you will not absorb much calcium from food or from many supplements. Calcium carbonate (the calcium found in supplements such as OsCal and Caltrate) as well as calcium phosphate (one of the main calcium sources found in food) require acid for optimal intestinal absorption. Therefore, people who take PPIs daily for problems such as gastroesophageal reflux disease, ulcers, gastritis, esophagitis, and hiatal hernia do not absorb adequate amounts of calcium and are at increased risk for broken bones from osteoporosis. Calcium citrate is much better absorbed as it does not require acid to be absorbed and should be taken regularly if you are on a PPI. You should assume that if you are taking a PPI medication that you are not absorbing much calcium, even if you have a diet high in dairy products (which primarily contain calcium that requires acid for absorption). You should take 1,000 mg to 1,500 mg of calcium citrate a day. Calcium citrate is a very large molecule, so calcium citrate usually comes in 250 mg tablets or chews, and therefore, you should take two at a time twice a day (in other words, four a day total) to equal 1,000 mg of calcium a day. There is also a slow-release brand of calcium citrate called Citracal Slow Release 1200. This latter formulation is convenient since it only needs to be taken once a day instead of twice a day. Two tablets taken once a day of this form of calcium citrate provides 1,200 mg of calcium citrate and 1,000 international units (IU) of vitamin D.

While I advocate taking calcium citrate if a patient needs to take a PPI, many osteoporosis experts feel that calcium carbonate may be adequate as long as they are taken along with food. The reasoning is that eating food causes the stomach to produce more acid, allowing the calcium carbonate to be absorbed. However, taking a PPI decreases this amount of acid production. No rigorous comparison studies have been performed comparing taking calcium carbonate supplements with food versus taking calcium citrate by people needing PPIs for stomach acid. I prefer that my patients take calcium citrate, as I know these supplements do not rely on the production of acid in the stomach.

*Consume an adequate amount of vitamin D.* The Institute of Medicine also updated guidelines for vitamin D intake in 2010. It recommends that women over 70 years old get 800 IU a day or more of vitamin D; 600 IU a day or more is recommended for everyone else over 1 year of age. It is very difficult for most people to get enough vitamin D through food sources alone (see table 24.8 for vitamin D content in food). Unless you are willing to swallow a half tablespoon of cod liver oil each day or you get regular sun exposure (which is not recommended in people who have lupus), you are likely to have low levels of vitamin D. Studies show that most people who have SLE are deficient in vitamin D. Your vitamin D level can be easily measured by your doctor through a blood test. Your vitamin D level (measured as 25-OH vitamin D; also called 25-hydroxy vitamin D) should normally be 20 ng/mL or higher. However, the American College of Rheumatology recommends that anyone taking steroids (such as prednisone or methylprednisolone) should have a vitamin D level greater than 30 ng/mL. The reasons are discussed in more detail in the following section on steroids. If your level is lower than that, then you should take a vitamin D supplement. This can be done by

Table 24.8  Vitamin D Content of Food

| Food | IUs per Serving |
|---|---|
| Cod liver oil, 1 tablespoon | 1,360 |
| Salmon (sockeye), cooked, 3 ounces | 447 |
| Mackerel, cooked, 3 ounces | 388 |
| Tuna fish, canned in water, drained, 3 ounces | 154 |
| Milk, nonfat, reduced fat, and whole, vitamin D–fortified, 1 cup | 115–124 |
| Orange juice fortified with vitamin D, 1 cup (varies) | 100 |
| Yogurt, fortified with 20% of the DV for vitamin D, 6 ounces | 80 |
| Margarine, fortified, 1 tablespoon | 60 |
| Liver, beef, cooked, 3.5 ounces | 49 |
| Sardines, canned in oil, drained, 2 sardines | 46 |
| Egg, 1 large (vitamin D is found in yolk) | 41 |
| Ready-to-eat cereal, 0.75 to 1 cup (varies by brand) | 40 |
| Cheese, Swiss, 1 ounce | 6 |

taking an over-the-counter form of vitamin D3. Your doctor may recommend that you take anywhere from 1,000 IU to 50,000 IU a day. Another approach would be to take a prescription form of vitamin D2 called ergocalciferol, which is commonly prescribed as 50,000 IU (or 1.25 mg) taken weekly. After starting a vitamin D supplement when you are vitamin D deficient, it typically takes about three months to restore your body's supply of vitamin D; therefore, it is best to wait about three months before having your vitamin D levels checked again to make sure you are taking enough vitamin D.

*Prevent falling.* This is one of the most important yet often overlooked measures to prevent broken bones in osteoporosis. It especially needs to be followed by people who are frail and who are at increased risk of falling, such as those who have balance problems, difficulty walking, weakness, or arthritis in the legs and back. Table 24.9 lists ways to reduce your risk of falling.

*If you are on steroids such as prednisone or methylprednisolone, you should be concerned about preventing osteoporosis.* Taking steroids greatly increases the risk of getting osteoporosis. They do this several different ways. They cause the intestines to absorb less calcium. (Fortunately, taking a vitamin D supplement helps to reverse this calcium absorption problem from steroids.) Steroids also cause the kidneys to excrete more calcium than they should. Therefore, there is less calcium in the body in the person taking steroids due to less absorption coupled with more kidney excretion. In addition, steroids prevent the cells of the bones from producing bone properly. They actually decrease the activity of osteoblasts (which are the cells important for producing new bone) and increase the activity of osteoclasts (which are the cells that destroy

**Table 24.9**  Preventing Falls

- Always use a cane or walker when walking.
- Remove throw rugs and any loose or frayed rugs.
- Remove electrical cords from walk areas.
- Remove all items from floors that could cause tripping.
- Ensure adequate lighting throughout the house, at all entranceways, and in all pathways outside the house.
- Avoid walking on any icy surfaces, wet floors, polished floors, and any slippery surfaces. Always get someone to help you do so if you must walk on these surfaces.
- Avoid walking in any unfamiliar places outside.

bone). So not only do people taking steroids have less calcium in their bodies to make good strong bones, but the bones themselves are breaking down bone (due to more osteoclasts) and producing less of it (due to lower amounts of osteoblasts).

The chances of losing bone density, developing osteopenia/osteoporosis, and breaking bones are also dependent on the dose of steroids taken. The risks for losing bone increase with the daily dose of steroids used and how long they are taken. Bone loss can begin within a few weeks of starting on steroids and increases after that, especially during the first six months of taking the medication. The other problem with steroid-induced osteopenia is that the bones are not as strong due to abnormal bone architecture. For example, if someone has been on prednisone 10 mg a day for six months and has a T-score of –1.5 on a DXA scan that person's bones are not going to be as strong as those of someone else of the same age who has a similar T-score of –1.5 but who is not on steroids. The steroids cause the cells of the bones to make bone that is structurally less strong compared to bones not affected by steroids. The steroids cause the formation of less structural supports in the bone and more gaps and holes in the bones, making them weaker.

Anyone who is on steroids for lupus should be doing all of the recommendations for preventing osteoporosis (see table 24.6). The American College of Rheumatology (ACR) in 2010 recommended that patients on steroids take in more calcium and vitamin D than people who do not take steroids. People who take steroids should take 1,200 mg to 1,500 mg of calcium a day, regardless of age and gender. This increased recommendation is because of the fact that steroids cause the body to absorb and retain less calcium overall compared to normal. The ACR also recommends that the vitamin 25-OH vitamin D level in the blood be kept above 30 ng/dL (instead of the 20 ng/dL recommended by the Institute of Medicine). This higher vitamin D level will help the intestines absorb more calcium as well as help with keeping the bones stronger. If you are one of those few people who have lupus who have a normal vitamin D level, then the ACR recommends that you take 800 to 1,000 IU of vitamin D3 a day through food (table 24.8) or supplements if you are on steroids.

As far as whether you should also take a medication to keep or make your bones strong is quite a complex and difficult question to answer. The ACR did give updated recommendations on the use of medications in patients on steroids in 2010. However, these recommendations are difficult to reproduce here in an easy to understand manner. The bottom line is that every person's case must be considered individually because the risks for getting osteoporosis and broken bones depends on numerous factors, such as age, gender, body weight, how much steroids are taken, and other risk factors for broken bones. Using the FRAX formula for risk for broken bones can be helpful because if there is an increased risk based on these calculations, the decision for taking a medication for osteoporosis is easy. However, even the FRAX formula is not fully accurate in people who take steroids. One reason for this is that steroids typically cause bone loss to occur primarily in the bones of the spine more than the hips. The FRAX equation only uses the bone density measurement at the hip. Therefore, FRAX can underestimate the risk for getting broken bones in people who are on steroids. However, I will go out on a limb and say that in my own experience, most people who are on more than 7.5 mg of prednisone (or 6 mg of methylprednisolone) per day should probably be on a medication for osteoporosis. People who are particularly at increased risk for broken bones and osteoporosis should be on medications even if they are on much lower doses of steroids. It is very important for you to discuss this issue with your rheumatologist.

## Medications Used to Treat and Prevent Osteoporosis

Whether someone should take a medication for osteoporosis is a complex question and depends on what that person's risk for getting broken bones is. Sometimes a medication may be used in someone who has known osteopenia or osteoporosis to prevent broken bones. They may be used in someone who has normal bones to prevent that person from developing osteoporosis in the first place (called preventative or prophylactic therapy). Your physician is the best person to decide whether you should take a medication for osteoporosis or not. In this section, I go over the medications currently used to treat and prevent osteoporosis and then discuss some complementary or "alternative" therapies as well.

### Bisphosphonates

The bisphosphonates (table 24.10) are the workhorse group of medications used to treat osteoporosis. These medications are the most commonly prescribed due to their proven effects of increasing bone density and decreasing the risk for getting broken bones combined with their ease of usage and relative safety. They have also been used longer than most of the other medications, starting with the FDA approval of alendronate (Fosamax) in 1995. Therefore, there are numerous long-term studies looking at the effectiveness of these medicines and the potential side effects that they may cause.

*Generics available*: Yes, but only for Fosamax (alendronate) and Boniva (ibandronate). A generic for Actonel may be available as soon as 2013.

*How bisphosphonates work*: Bisphosphonates treat osteoporosis by keeping osteoclasts from working correctly. The osteoclasts are the cells in the bones that absorb or break down bone. The bisphosphonate medication actually attaches directly to the bone itself. When an osteoclast tries to absorb that particular part of the bone, the

371

**Table 24.10**  Bisphosphonates Used to Treat Osteoporosis

| Name | Medication Form and How Often Taken |
| --- | --- |
| alendronate (Fosamax, Binosto) | Pill form, 5–10 mg a day, or 35 mg to 70 mg a week; strawberry-flavored effervescent tablet 70 mg dissolves in water (Binosto) |
| ibandronate (Boniva) | Pill 2.5 mg a day or 150 mg a month, or 3 mg IV infusion every 3 months |
| risedronate (Actonel, Atelvia) | Pill 5 mg a day, 35 mg a week, or 150 mg a month also comes in a delayed-release form (Atelvia) that can be taken with food |
| zolendronic acid (Reclast) | 5 mg IV infusion once a year |

bisphosphonate causes the osteoclast to stop absorbing bone. This allows the cells that produce bone (the osteoblasts) to keep working, while slowing down how quickly the osteoclasts are breaking down bone. This offsets the balance of bone formation toward the direction of more bone production compared to bone resorption, and therefore more bone is produced overall.

*What benefits to expect from bisphosphonates*: The goal of taking bisphosphonates is to decrease the risk of getting broken bones from osteoporosis. They are slow to work, generally taking six to twelve months before significant bone density is increased. They will not work, however, unless you are also taking adequate amounts of calcium and vitamin D (see previous discussions). Your doctor can repeat your DXA scan, usually after one to two years, to see if there is improvement in your bone density or not. Most osteoporosis experts agree that even if your bone density has remained stable (in other words, not worsened nor gotten stronger) your risk of getting broken bones is still decreased due to the bisphosphonates improving the actual architecture of the bones themselves, causing them to be stronger. Studies show that increasing the bone density by a mere 3% decreases the risk of getting broken bones by 50%.

If your bone density actually gets worse while taking a bisphosphonate, it could be because you are taking the medicine incorrectly. For example, bisphosphonate pills (except Atelvia) should be taken on an empty stomach first thing in the morning, and it is important to not eat or drink anything or take any other medicines for at least thirty minutes after taking the medicine. It is also important to ensure that you are not missing any doses, not smoking, and not drinking too much alcohol. It is also important to get an adequate amount of vitamin D and calcium and to exercise regularly. If you are following these guidelines and your bone density worsens, then your doctor may recommend that you switch from a pill form to one of the IV forms (Boniva and Reclast), or that you switch to a stronger medicine (such as Forteo or Prolia).

*How bisphosphonates are taken*: The bisphosphonates can be administered by pill form or intravenously (IV) directly into a vein. The pill forms (table 24.10) can be taken either daily, weekly, or monthly. The pill forms are not absorbed very well from the stomach and intestines if there is any other food, medicines, or liquid (other than water) present. Therefore, they need to be taken first thing in the morning on an empty stomach, and it is important not to eat or drink anything (other than water) or take any other medications for at least thirty to sixty minutes after taking the medication. Even one sip of coffee can prevent the stomach from absorbing these medicines. There is now one exception. Risedronate comes in a delayed-release form called Atelvia, which can be taken along with breakfast (instead of waiting thirty minutes to eat). This makes Atelvia less complicated to take compared to the other pill forms of bisphosphonates.

The bisphosphonates can be potentially irritating to the lining of the esophagus and stomach. If the pill or the dissolving particles of the pill contact the lining of the esophagus for very long, it can be irritating, causing stomach upset, heartburn, and even potentially an ulcer. Therefore, it is very important to take the bisphosphonate with 8 ounces of water and not lie down for at least thirty minutes after taking it. Due to this irritating effect, the pill forms should be avoided in people who have severe esophagus and stomach problems such as hiatal hernia, severe gastroesophageal reflux, or esophageal dysmotility (as discussed in chapters 15 and 28).

The IV forms have the advantage of not causing the stomach and esophagus problems of the pill forms, so they are often preferred in people with these difficulties. Two IV forms are FDA-approved for osteoporosis. Ibandronate (Boniva) is infused every three months, and zolendronic acid (Reclast) is only given once a year. Therefore, they also have the advantage of not having to be taken as often as the pill forms.

So which bisphosphonate is the best one to take? There are numerous reasons for choosing one over another. One important factor is cost. At the time of this writing, alendronate (Fosamax) and ibandronate (Boniva) were the only bisphosphonates that come in a generic form. These are usually much cheaper compared to the other forms that do not (such as Actonel). Certainly, this is an important factor if you are paying out of pocket for the medications, or if you do not have a good prescription plan. However, even if you have good insurance, most prescription plans ask you to pay more for a brand name medication (such as Actonel, or Atelvia) compared to taking a generic (such as alendronate or ibandronate).

If you absolutely do not want to put up with the complicated regimen of taking an oral form of bisphosphonate thirty to sixty minutes before eating anything or before taking your other medications, then you may want to consider the delayed-release form of risedronate (Atelvia). If you can afford the higher cost of the medication, and you are on a complicated medicine regimen where you do not want to be bothered by the added complexity of taking the other bisphosphonate pills, then Atelvia may be a better choice for you.

For people who have difficulty swallowing pills and who prefer liquid medications, Binosto is another option. Binosto is a strawberry-flavored form of alendronate, which is dissolved in 4 ounces of room-temperature water. After the bubbles (effervescence) have dissipated, it is stirred and then consumed. This must still be taken on an empty stomach first thing in the morning with no other food or medications being taken for at least thirty minutes afterward. Although the pill form of Fosamax (alendronate) has a cheaper generic equivalent, this form of alendronate does not and is therefore more expensive.

People who have esophagus and stomach problems may have difficulty tolerating the bisphosphonate pills or may want to avoid their potential digestive side effects altogether. These people should consider taking either ibandronate (Boniva) by IV every three months or zolendronic acid (Reclast) by IV once a year.

There may be differences in how effectively these medications prevent broken bones, as some studies indicate. Therefore, your physician may suggest a particular bisphosphonate over the others if he or she feels that one may be better at preventing broken bones.

*Alcohol/food/herbal interactions of bisphosphonates*: Drinking alcohol can exacerbate inflammation of the esophagus and stomach, increasing the risks for stomach problems with bisphosphonates. Drinking more than two servings daily may prevent your bones from getting stronger.

Always take the pills on an empty stomach first thing in the morning with a full glass of water. Do not eat or drink anything except water for at least thirty to sixty minutes after taking the pills (except for Atelvia). If there is anything else present in the stomach (medicines or food), these will prevent proper absorption of the oral bisphosphonate. Atelvia can be taken with food.

No specific interactions with herbal products are known.

*Potential side effects of bisphosphonates*: As far as the potential for side effects, generally most people tolerate the bisphosphonates with little to no problems (table 24.11). A general word about side effects is in order here. Whenever you decide to take a medication or not, it is important to learn what the potential side effects of the medication are. However, it is also very important to understand how often they occur. Out of all the medications doctors use in lupus patients, the bisphosphonates are some of the most misunderstood. There are many patients (like M. in the first section of this chapter) who refuse to take them. This is unfortunately fueled by the popular media (news, magazines, etc.) reporting on the side effects of medicines. It is important that people realize that news agencies, magazines, and other lay publications often report on items based on sensationalism. Their job is to make money and the more sensational a story is, the more likely people will watch, listen to, or read their news. The bisphosphonates in particular have been a favorite subject with agencies reporting on medical subjects. However, they often do this in an unbalanced fashion. People not trained in how to interpret the medical studies accurately are often the ones who report on them.

Whenever you take a medication, you always want to weigh the risks versus the benefits of taking the medication. For example, if a medication has significant benefits that far outweigh the potential for severe side effects, then it generally is a good idea to take the medication. For example, penicillin kills approximately four hundred Americans each year due to severe allergic reactions. Yet, it would be unusual for someone to refuse to take penicillin prescribed by her physician. Maybe this is because she does not consciously take into account the potential for side effects from penicillin, not realizing that it can cause potentially severe reactions. However, subconsciously, the person is weighing the risks and benefits of the medicine. She realizes that the potential benefits of penicillin in successfully treating an infection far outweigh the possibility of getting a severe side effect from the penicillin (such as being one of the four hundred Americans who will die from penicillin that year). Therefore, she will take the penicillin.

**Table 24.11** Potential Side Effects of Bisphosphonates

|  | *Incidence* | *Side Effect Therapy* |
|---|---|---|
| **Nuisance side effects** | | |
| Low calcium and phosphate levels | Common | No intervention usually needed. |
| Stomach upset, heartburn, nausea, gas, diarrhea | Common | Usually do not occur when the medicine is taken correctly. Stop the medicine if these side effects occur. |
| Chest pain due to esophagus irritation | Uncommon | Stop the medicine. |
| Body aches and pains | Uncommon | Take pain relievers or do nothing if mild. Stop medicine if problematic. |
| Flu-like symptoms with IV Reclast (achiness, low-grade fever) | Common | Taking acetaminophen (Tylenol) for a few days after the infusion can decrease the severity of the symptoms or prevent them from occurring. Usually does not recur with subsequent infusions. |
| **Serious side effects** | | |
| Ulcers | Uncommon | Stop the medicine. Take ulcer medicines. |
| Atypical femur fractures, subtrochanteric fractures | Very rare | Stop the medicine. Rest. Sometimes surgery. May avoid by taking a "drug holiday" off of medicine after taking it for five to ten years. |
| Osteonecrosis of the jaw | Very rare | Avoid by stopping medicine three months before invasive dental procedures and by maintaining good dental health. Very difficult to treat once it occurs. |

Side effect incidence key (these are approximations as they can vary widely study to study): rare < 1% occurrence; uncommon 1%–5% occurrence; common > 5% occurrence

You should use this same logic when considering taking a bisphosphonate for your osteoporosis. If you have osteopenia, your FRAX calculation can give you a very rough estimate of what your risk of getting broken bones is. If you were to break a bone in your spine, then you could potentially suffer the ravages of spinal fracture, as discussed previously. If your hip fractures, then you have a 20% chance of dying from the fracture. If you are lucky enough to survive it, you have up to a 50% chance of needing to be in a long-term nursing facility (nursing home) due to you and your family not being able to adequately care for you. These realistic, big problems often occur due to inadequately treated osteoporosis. Certainly, you may never get a broken bone, but you do not have a crystal ball to be able to predict this. If there is a medication (such as a bisphosphonate) which has a much lower chance of causing significant side effects (which is true) compared to your chances of having to deal with the broken bones of osteoporosis, then the wiser choice would be to take the medication.

Many medication side effects are mild, are transient, and go away when the medicine is stopped. Some people do not want to take medicines because they do not want any stomach upset. The vast majority of medications, including simple vitamins, can potentially cause stomach upset. However, this is usually considered a mild side effect with most medications. If stomach upset occurs, it usually goes away soon after the medicine is stopped. So why not try the medicine anyway? If it upsets your stomach, just stop taking it and let your doctor know so he or she can prescribe something to take its place.

By the way, I am not at all trying to belittle the importance of severe side effects from medications. Anyone who has had a severe side effect from a medicine or knows of someone who has had one can attest that severe side effects do exist with almost all prescription medications. This possibility should not be taken lightly. I am just trying to point out that it is a healthier approach to put them into perspective in the larger scheme of things by assessing the benefits of taking the medicine versus how often these side effects occur. It is better to educate yourself about potential side effects so that you know what to look for and let your doctor know right away if you develop any.

One rare, potential side effect of bisphosphonates is an unusual fracture of the hip. Medically doctors specifically are referring to atypical femoral shaft fractures (also called subtrochanteric fractures). "Atypical" refers to these fractures (broken bones) as being different from the typical fractures (called intertrochanteric fractures) that occur in the neck of the femur bone. The femur is the large bone of the leg that connects to the hip. If someone breaks his or her hip, it occurs in the femoral neck, which is right next to the hip joint high up in the leg. However, the rare type of atypical hip fractures occurs farther down the bone in the main part of the femur called the shaft. This causes pain in the thigh and difficulty with walking when it occurs. These fractures have primarily been seen in relatively younger, active women. These types of fractures have been reported rarely in people who have taken bisphosphonates. These types of hip fractures also occur in people who have osteoporosis (and who are often given bisphosphonates to treat it in the first place). One problem is that it is not even known whether this is truly a side effect of bisphosphonates or not since these fractures also occur in people who have osteoporosis. The largest study so far to address this question was from Denmark; it looked at a population of 160,505 patients, 5,187 of whom took alendronate. This study showed no difference in how often patients who had osteoporosis who did not take a bisphosphonate developed these fractures versus those who took the bisphosphonate alendronate.

Between 1996 (soon after Fosamax first came into use) and 2006, the number of admissions to hospitals for broken hips decreased from 600 per 100,000 admissions to 400 per 100,000 admissions (reflecting the marked decrease in hip fractures due to treatments for osteoporosis). During this same time period, the numbers of these atypical subtrochanteric hip fractures remained the same. If the bisphosphonates were causing these types of fractures, there should have been an increase during this period. However, a 2012 study suggested that atypical fractures had increased between the years 1999 and 2010, but this was a small study looking at only 477 people who were admitted to hospitals with broken hips.

Therefore, it is not known if these fractures occur more often or not due to bisphosphonates, and it certainly has not been proven yet. If they do occur, they are very rare and are most likely to occur after people have taken the medication for many years. There is some theoretical concern, though, that the long-term use of bisphosphonates may potentially increase this risk. This is only a theory, but it is possible that some people could develop unusual areas of weak bone with the long-term use of bisphosphonates. However, this is just theory and has not been borne out in studies. For example, there have been research studies on alendronate for up to ten years of treatment that show that it is safe and effective when used for ten years as far as causing a low number of side effects and decreasing broken bones.

At this time, the osteoporosis experts recommend that a "drug holiday" be given to some people who have osteoporosis, just in case there is a chance for weaker bones after prolonged use. There is no one agreed-upon method, but stopping bisphosphonates after five years of use in people who have mild osteoporosis and after seven to ten years in those who have moderate to severe osteoporosis has been suggested. Then the medication can be restarted after one to five years, depending on the person's particular circumstances.

Another potential rare side effect of bisphosphonates is osteonecrosis of the jaw. "Osteo-" means bone while "-necrosis" refers to death. Therefore, "osteonecrosis" means "death of a piece of bone." This has primarily been seen with large doses of IV bisphosphonates that have been infused on a more frequent basis in people who have cancer of the bone. It has only rarely been reported in people treated with bisphosphonates for osteoporosis. To put it into perspective, it is estimated that it only occurs in one out of every 100,000 to 160,000 people who take a bisphosphonate to treat their osteoporosis. Therefore, it truly is a very rare side effect, especially compared to how often untreated osteoporosis causes significant problems. In fact, osteonecrosis of the jaw occurs so rarely in people who take bisphosphonates for osteoporosis (excluding those who use high doses to treat bone cancer) that it has not even been proven to be a definite side effect at all. The FDA had a special meeting about this in September 2011 to go over the data of potential side effects of the bisphosphonates and they found "no clear evidence of clear risk" for the development of osteonecrosis of the jaw from these medicines.

In osteonecrosis of the bone, a small part of the bone of the jaw dies (becomes necrotic in medical terms). A person who has osteonecrosis develops discomfort in the jaw and an open sore in the gums. It has most commonly been seen in people who have undergone dental procedures such as teeth removal and other types of dental surgeries. Even though it is very rare in people treated for osteoporosis, it is recommended that good oral hygiene be maintained such as seeing the dentist as well as brushing and flossing the teeth regularly. In addition, if any major dental procedures are being planned, it is recommended that they be done prior to starting these medications if feasible. If someone has been on a bisphosphonate for three years or more and then requires a major dental procedure, some doctors recommend that the bisphosphonate be stopped three months prior to the procedure and then restarted after the mouth has healed. However, this is a controversial recommendation.

Another potential side effect of bisphosphonates is muscle, joint, and bone pain. Although this is reportedly a rare side effect, and some experts question whether it truly occurs, I do think that it can occur, although not very commonly. I have had a few patients who were convinced that their bisphosphonate caused bone pain. Fortunately, this resolved after they stopped taking it. In addition, zolendronic acid (Reclast) can cause a flu-like reaction twenty-four to seventy-two hours after getting the medication infused. It is called flu-like because it can cause muscle and joint pain as well as low-grade fevers similar to how the flu can act. Taking acetaminophen (Tylenol) after the infusion can decrease the chances of this occurring or make it tolerable. It appears to be very unusual to have this recur with the second infusion of the medicine if it occurred with the first infusion.

By far the most common side effects of the bisphosphonates are the gastrointestinal side effects that occur when taken in pill form. The symptoms can include heartburn, stomach upset, nausea, chest pain, difficulty swallowing, and bloating. Fortunately, the vast majority of the time these are mild and resolve by stopping the medicine. They are also much less likely to occur if the medicine is taken with a full glass of water on an empty stomach and the person taking it does not lie down immediately afterward. However, occasionally, these medicines can cause ulcers causing abdominal pain and may require a special procedure called an esophagoduodenoscopy (EGD for short) as discussed in chapter 15 to diagnose. People who have pre-existing esophagus and stomach problems such as esophageal dysmotility, hiatal hernia, or severe gastroesophageal reflux disease should not take the pill forms of the bisphosphonates.

*What needs to be monitored while taking bisphosphonates*: Your doctor will most likely want to check blood tests for calcium, vitamin D, and kidney function before and while you are on the medicine. A DXA scan can be repeated after one to two years to see if the medicine is working.

*Reasons not to take bisphosphonates (contraindications or precautions)*:

• If you have esophagus problems such as esophageal dysmotility, esophageal strictures, achalasia, or severe hiatal hernia you should probably not take the pill forms.

• If you cannot sit or stand upright for at least thirty minutes after you take the pill forms.

• If you have persistently low calcium levels (such as if you have hypoparathyroidism).

• If your kidney function (measured as eGFR or CrCl) is < 30 ml/min to 35 ml/min. There are some studies suggesting that lower doses may be safe to use, but this is a decision that only your doctor should make.

*While taking bisphosphonates*: Tell your doctor:

• If you get stomach upset, nausea, vomiting, chest pain, or body pain.

• If you develop an open sore on your gums, especially if bone is exposed (it could be a sign of osteonecrosis of the jaw), but keep in mind that other causes not related to bisphosphonates (such as gingivitis) are much more common.

• If you develop thigh or hip pain (your doctor will need to rule out atypical hip fracture).

*Pregnancy and breast-feeding while taking bisphosphonates*: Should not be taken during pregnancy. Adequate studies have not been done in pregnant women. If taken during pregnancy, bisphosphonates may cause the baby's blood calcium levels to be abnormal. It is recommended that women of childbearing age who want to become pregnant generally not take bisphosphonates unless their risk for broken bones due to osteoporosis is increased. If you are taking a bisphosphonate and want to become pregnant, it is recommended that you wait six months after stopping it before becoming pregnant.

It is not recommended to take bisphosphonates while breast-feeding.

*Geriatric use of bisphosphonates*: No change in dosage required.

*What to do with bisphosphonates at the time of surgery*: It is always best to double-check with your rheumatologist and surgeon regarding specific instructions. However, bisphosphonates are generally safe to take up to the time you are told to stop taking medications by mouth before surgery.

*Patient assistance program for bisphosphonates*: For Reclast call 1-800-245-5356. Also see chapter 42.

*Drug helpline for bisphosphonates*: Unaware of any.

*Website to learn more about bisphosphonates*: For Actonel go to www.actonel.com. For Binosto go to www.binosto.com. For Reclast to go www.reclast.com.

## Teriparatide (Forteo)

*Generic available*: No.

*How teriparatide works*: Teriparatide is a form of parathyroid hormone (PTH for short). PTH is a natural hormone made by the parathyroid glands. These glands are located behind the thyroid gland that sits in the front of the neck just below the Adam's apple. PTH is very important in causing the cells of the body to process calcium and vitamin D correctly. It increases the production of the cells that form new bone (called osteoblasts), causing increased bone formation. This is very different from all other currently available osteoporosis medicines, which work by causing decreased bone resorption by the osteoclasts (which allows the osteoblasts to "catch up"). Teriparatide actually stimulates the bones to make additional, stronger bone faster. It appears to be the quickest and most effective medication currently available to treat osteoporosis, causing significant increases in bone density within the first few months of use. In addition to rapidly building bone strength and decreasing the risk of broken bones, it also appears that teriparatide may decrease pain from vertebral fractures as well. The reason for this effect is not known.

*What benefits to expect from teriparatide:* Teriparatide is currently the fastest-acting medication available to cause the bones to increase in strength. Bone density begins to increase within a few months of starting the medicine and by eight months, evidence for decreased broken bones appears.

*How teriparatide is taken*: Teriparatide is given by subcutaneous injection, similar to how insulin shots are given. It comes in a "pen" that contains four weeks' worth of medication. Each day a fresh, new small needle is attached to the "pen," and the patient inserts the needle into the skin of either the stomach or thigh, and then pushes a button on top of the "pen" to inject it.

*Alcohol/food/herbal interactions with teriparatide*: Drinking more than two servings of alcohol a day will decrease the chances of your bones getting stronger with teriparatide.

You should make sure you are getting enough calcium and vitamin D; see previous discussions.

No herbal interactions are known.

*Potential side effects of teriparatide*: The most commonly reported side effects from teriparatide are headaches, nausea, and dizziness (table 24.12). If dizziness occurs, it appears to occur most commonly with the first few doses and then resolves over time. One of the most important side effects to monitor is that it can potentially increase calcium levels, so your doctor will want to check blood work for calcium after you start it to make sure this does not happen.

Animal studies with teriparatide showed an increased risk for a particular cancer of the bone called osteosarcoma, which occurred in rats given teriparatide. However, it should be pointed out that rat bones and human bones differ in that bones in rats continue to grow throughout their lives (as opposed to human bones, which stop growing after puberty). The effects of teriparatide may be much different on the active growth plates of rat bones compared to adult human bones that lack these growing sections of bone. In addition, much higher doses of teriparatide were used in the rat studies than are used in humans. Thus far, no increases in osteosarcomas have occurred in humans taking teriparatide. To decrease the potential risk of this occurring,

**Table 24.12**  Potential Side Effects of Teriparatide (Forteo)

|  | *Incidence* | *Side Effect Therapy* |
|---|---|---|
| **Nuisance side effects** | | |
| Elevated blood calcium | Common | Decrease calcium intake or stop Forteo. May be temporary and of no clinical significance. |
| Light-headed, dizzy | Common | Usually goes away with regular use. Stand up slowly if you get dizzy. If it does not get better, you may need to stop it to prevent falls. |
| Gout attacks if you have gout | Uncommon | Increase gout medicines. |
| Nausea, upset stomach | Common | Usually goes away with regular use. May need to stop teriparatide if it does not go away or if it is particularly bothersome. |
| **Serious side effects** | | |
| Passing out due to dizziness | Uncommon | Call ambulance or have someone take you immediately to hospital. Stop teriparatide. |

Side effect incidence key (approximations, as side effects can vary widely study to study): rare < 1% occurrence; uncommon 1%–5% occurrence; common > 5% occurrence

the FDA recommends using teriparatide for only two years. Therefore, most osteoporosis experts prescribe teriparatide for two years followed by a bisphosphonate.

*What needs to be monitored while taking teriparatide*:

- Calcium and phosphate levels.

- Uric acid levels in people who have gout.

- Blood pressure if you are prone to having low blood pressure.

- DXA scan after two years to see how bone strength is doing.

*Reasons not to take teriparatide (contraindications or precautions)*:

- If you have elevated calcium levels (such as in hyperparathyroidism).

- Use with caution if you are prone to getting calcium kidney stones.

*While taking teriparatide*:

- Tell your doctor if you get dizzy or light-headed.

- Tell your doctor if you get gout attacks (very painful, red, hot swollen joints).

- Tell your doctor if you get kidney stones.

*Pregnancy and breast-feeding while taking teriparatide*: Should not be used during pregnancy.

Breast milk excretion is not known. Not recommended for use if breast-feeding.

*Geriatric use of teriparatide*: No dosage adjustments needed.

*What to do with teriparatide at the time of surgery*: It is always best to double-check with your rheumatologist and surgeon regarding specific instructions. To prevent any problems with calcium levels around the time of surgery, it may be best not to use Forteo for a few days before surgery.

*Patient assistance program for teriparatide*: 1-866-568-8942. Also see chapter 42.

*Drug helpline for teriparatide*: 1-866-436-7836.

*Website to learn more about teriparatide*: www.Forteo.com.

## Denosumab (Prolia)

*Generic available*: No.

*How denosumab works*: Denosumab is the new kid on the block when it comes to osteoporosis medications. The FDA approved it on June 1, 2010. It is the only osteoporosis medication that is considered a biologic medicine (biologics are discussed in chapter 33). It works by connecting to a molecule called RANKL and keeping it from doing its job. RANKL stands for Receptor Activator of Nuclear factor KappaB Ligand. That is why it is preferable to say RANKL (pronounce RAIN-kel), which is much simpler to say. RANKL is a molecule that attaches to osteoclasts to cause them to break down and reabsorb bone. Therefore, when denosumab is given, it connects to these RANKL molecules, keeping them from attaching to the osteoclasts. The osteoclasts work less hard and do not reabsorb as much bone. This allows the osteoblasts to make more bone and make the bones stronger.

*What benefits to expect from denosumab:* Denosumab increases bone density and decreases the risk for broken bones from osteoporosis. Your doctor can do a DXA scan after one to two years while you are on the medicine to see if it is working or not.

*How denosumab is taken*: Denosumab is very easy to take. It is given just twice a year (six months apart) by an injection under the skin in the doctor's office.

*Alcohol/food/herbal interactions*: Drinking more than two servings of alcohol daily can decrease the chances of denosumab increasing your bone density.

Ensure you are taking enough calcium and vitamin D (see previous discussions). No herbal interactions are known.

*Potential side effects of denosumab*: There may be an increased risk for infections in people taking denosumab. However, in the studies, this chance was very small. If there is an increased chance of an infection, skin infection (cellulitis) appears to be the most common. Therefore, it is very important to let your doctor know if any symptoms of infection occur such as red, hot, painful skin or fevers. Potential side effects are listed in table 24.13.

*What needs to be monitored while taking denosumab*:

- Calcium level before treatment and ten days after injection (if you have chronic kidney disease stage 3 or worse).

- Kidney function blood test before treatment (eGFR).

*Reasons not to take denosumab (contraindications or precautions)*:

- Caution in people who have chronic kidney disease.

- Vitamin D deficiency should be normalized before starting therapy.

- Latex allergy. Packaging and needle cover may contain latex.

*While taking denosumab*:

- Call and see your doctor right away if you develop an area of red, warm, tender skin. This could be a sign of cellulitis (skin infection).

**Table 24.13**  Potential Side Effects of Denosumab (Prolia)

|  | *Incidence* | *Side Effect Therapy* |
| --- | --- | --- |
| **Nuisance side effects** | | |
| Eczema (rash) | Uncommon | Seek your doctor's advice. |
| Low calcium levels | Uncommon unless there is kidney disease | Make sure you are taking enough calcium and vitamin D. |
| **Serious side effects** | | |
| Cellulitis (skin infection) red, hot painful skin | Rare | Call and see your doctor right away for antibiotics. |

Side effect incidence key (approximations, as side effects can vary widely study to study):  rare < 1% occurrence; uncommon 1%–5% occurrence;  common > 5% occurrence

*Pregnancy and breast-feeding while taking denosumab*: Not recommended during pregnancy. No human studies done. Studies in pregnant monkeys showed no adverse events on the fetus.

Breast milk excretion unknown. Use during breast-feeding is not recommended.

*Geriatric use of denosumab*: No changes in dosing needed.

*What to do with denosumab at the time of surgery*: It is always best to double-check with your rheumatologist and surgeon regarding specific instructions. It may be best not to use Prolia for several weeks before surgery to decrease the risk of infection.

*Patient assistance program for denosumab*: 1-877-776-5421. Also see chapter 42.

*Drug helpline for denosumab*: www.Prolia.com.

*Website to learn more about denosumab*: www.Prolia.com.

## Raloxifene (Evista)

*Generic available*: Not at the time of this writing. A generic may become available as soon as 2014.

*How raloxifene works*: Raloxifene is a type of medication called a selective estrogen receptor modulator. This means that it works the same as estrogen in some tissues of the body (such as the bone), but not in others (such as in the breasts and uterus). Therefore, it has some estrogen (female hormone) effects in some parts of the body but not in others. Recall that the most common cause of osteoporosis is the loss of estrogen after menopause. Taking raloxifene helps to provide estrogen-like bone-building effects back in the bone. It works similar to estrogen in this respect, but it is a little weaker than estrogen overall in building bone density. It has been shown to decrease the risk of getting broken bones in the spine, but not in the hips. Therefore, it is considered one of the weaker medicines to use for treating and preventing osteoporosis.

One potential major advantage of raloxifene is that it decreases the risk for getting breast cancer. Since one out of nine women will develop breast cancer at some point in life, this may be an excellent choice for women who want to decrease this risk, especially if they have a strong family history of breast cancer. It is a good choice for women who want this additional breast cancer prevention and who have mild osteoporosis or who want to take a medicine to prevent osteoporosis from occurring in the first place.

*What benefits to expect from raloxifene*: Raloxifene should help to increase your bone density and decrease your risk of getting broken bones. However, it is not as strong as the bisphosphonates, teriparatide, or denosumab. It is not known whether it is very good at decreasing the risk of getting hip fractures or not. If you do not have osteoporosis yet, it can be used prophylactically to keep you from getting it. Your doctor can perform a DXA scan one to two years after starting it to see if it is working or not.

If you have a family history of breast cancer or if you have had lobular breast cancer *in situ*, then taking raloxifene regularly can decrease the chances of your developing breast cancer. It has not been studied adequately in women who are not at high risk for breast cancer to see if it decreases their risk or not.

*How raloxifene is taken*: Raloxifene comes in a 60 mg tablet and is taken once a day with or without food.

*Alcohol/food/herbal interactions*: Drinking two or more servings of alcohol a day can prevent raloxifene from helping to strengthen the bone density.

Raloxifene can be taken with or without food. You need to make sure you are getting enough calcium and vitamin D (see previous sections).

No interactions with herbal products are known.

*Potential side effects of raloxifene*: Raloxifene is one of the easiest to tolerate osteoporosis medicines. Very few women stop it due to side effects (which are listed in table 24.14). Although most medicines can cause allergic reactions (such as rash) and stomach upset, I have rarely had patients report these problems with raloxifene. The most common problems appear to be hot flashes and muscle cramps. Anywhere from 10% to 25% of women who take raloxifene can have hot flashes (similar to what can occur with menopause). Usually these are mild and tolerable. However, if you already have hot flashes, this medication may not be a good choice for you. Ten percent of women can develop muscle cramps while on raloxifene. These also tend to be mild and tolerable in most women, but occasionally can be uncomfortable enough to cause the person to stop taking it.

One very important potential side effect of raloxifene is that it can increase the risk for blood clots. Therefore, women who are at increased risk for blood clots should not take it. This includes people who are positive for antiphospholipid antibodies (see chapters 4 and 9), those who smoke cigarettes (smoking increases the risk for blood clots), and anyone who has had a blood clot before.

*What needs to be monitored while taking raloxifene*:

- DXA scan after one to two years to see how it is doing.

*Reasons not to take raloxifene (contraindications or precautions)*:

- If you are positive for antiphospholipid antibodies (increased risk of blood clots).
- If you smoke (increased risk of blood clots).

**Table 24.14** Potential Side Effects of Raloxifene (Evista)

|  | Incidence | Side Effect Therapy |
|---|---|---|
| **Nuisance side effects** | | |
| Hot flashes | Common | None if mild. Stop if bothersome. |
| Leg cramps | Common | None if mild. Stop if bothersome. |
| Leg swelling (edema) | Common | None if mild. Stop if bothersome. Or wear vascular support stockings. |
| **Serious side effects** | | |
| Blood clots (strokes, pulmonary embolism, deep venous thrombosis) | Rare | Go to emergency room immediately or call doctor immediately |

Side effect incidence key (approximations, as side effects can vary widely study to study): rare < 1% occurrence; uncommon 1%–5% occurrence; common > 5% occurrence

- If you have had blood clots or a stroke before.

- If you already have bothersome postmenopausal hot flashes.

- If you have had a heart attack before.

- If you are still having periods or have not gone through menopause yet.

- It is not known how safe it is if the kidneys or liver do not work properly.

*While taking raloxifene*:

- Contact your doctor if you develop possible symptoms of a blood clot or stroke such as a painful swollen calf, shortness of breath and chest pain, numbness or weakness, or slurred speech.

- Stop taking it seventy-two hours before any prolonged immobilization (surgery, long car or plane trips) to prevent blood clots.

*Pregnancy and breast-feeding while taking raloxifene*: Do not take if you are pregnant. Do not take if you are breast-feeding.
*Geriatric use of raloxifene*: No adjustment in dosage needed.
*What to do with raloxifene at the time of surgery*: It is always best to double-check with your rheumatologist and surgeon regarding specific instructions. You should not take Evista for two to four weeks before surgery to decrease the risk of getting blood clots.
*Patient assistance program for raloxifene*: Call 1-855-559-8783. Also see chapter 42.
*Drug helpline for raloxifene*: None.
*Website to learn more about raloxifene*: www.Evista.com.

## Calcitonin (Miacalcin, Fortical):

*Generic available*: Yes.
*How calcitonin works*: Calcitonin is a hormone produced by the thyroid gland. It attaches to the osteoclasts and prevents them from breaking down bone; therefore, the osteoblasts can make more bone. It is considered one of the weakest medicines used to treat osteoporosis and is not used very often. However, calcitonin can help to decrease the amount of pain that can occur when a broken bone happens from osteoporosis. It is not known how this pain-reducing effect occurs. Therefore, it is most commonly prescribed to people who have osteoporosis who have pain due to a broken bone to try to decrease the pain as well as to help the bones get stronger.
*What benefits to expect from calcitonin*: Calcitonin is considered the weakest FDA-approved medicine to use for osteoporosis. It increases bone density but has not been proven to decrease the risk of getting a broken hip. It can help to decrease the pain from broken bones due to osteoporosis, and this is one of the more common reasons for using it. A DXA scan can be done after one to two years to see if it is helping to increase bone density.
*How calcitonin is taken*: Although it can be prescribed as an injection, it is most commonly prescribed as a nasal spray. One spray in one nostril is done daily, alternating nostrils every other day.
*Alcohol/food/herbal interactions*: Drinking two or more servings of alcohol a day can prevent it from making the bones stronger.

**Table 24.15** Potential Side Effects of Calcitonin Nasal Spray (Miacalcin, Fortical)

|  | Incidence | Side Effect Therapy |
|---|---|---|
| **Nuisance side effects** |  |  |
| Nose irritation and runny nose | Common | Stop using it if bothersome enough. |
| Nasal ulceration | Uncommon | Stop using it. |
| Headache | Uncommon | Stop using it if bothersome enough. |
| **Serious side effects** | None |  |

Side effect incidence key (approximations, as side effects can vary widely study to study): rare < 1% occurrence; uncommon 1%–5% occurrence; common > 5% occurrence

Ensure you are getting enough calcium and vitamin D (see previous sections).

No interactions with herbal products are known.

*Potential side effects of calcitonin*: The most common side effects of the nasal spray forms of calcitonin are nausea, irritation in the nose, and headaches (table 24.15). These quickly resolve when the medication is stopped.

*What needs to be monitored while taking calcitonin*: No blood work needed.

*Reasons not to take calcitonin (contraindications or precautions)*: Do not take if you have sores in your nose.

*While taking calcitonin nasal spray*:

• Let your doctor know if you get any ulcerations inside your nose.

*Pregnancy and breast-feeding while taking calcitonin*: Calcitonin does not cross the placenta. Low birth weights were seen in animal studies. It has not been studied in human pregnancies. Doctors may prescribe it during pregnancy if the benefits of the medicine outweigh the potential risks.

Calcitonin has been shown to decrease breast milk production in animals. It has not been studied in humans. Use during breast-feeding is not recommended.

*Geriatric use of calcitonin*: No dosage adjustments needed.

*What to do with calcitonin at the time of surgery*: It is always best to double-check with your rheumatologist and surgeon regarding specific instructions. You can use calcitonin nasal spray up to the day before surgery.

*Patient assistance program for calcitonin*: See chapter 42.

*Drug helpline for calcitonin*: None.

*Website to learn more about calcitonin*: www.fortical.com.

## Estrogen

As discussed, the loss of estrogen after menopause is the most common cause of osteoporosis. However, due to increased risks for breast cancer, strokes, blood clots, and possibly heart attacks, estrogen is not prescribed very often to treat or prevent osteoporosis. In women who have significant menopausal problems (such as hot flashes, vaginal dryness, and aches and pain), estrogen can decrease these menopausal symptoms while treating osteoporosis at the same time. Gynecologists appear to prescribe estrogen more commonly than primary care doctors and rheumatologists.

## Other Potential, but Not Proven, Therapies for Osteoporosis

### Vitamin K

Vitamin K is necessary for the formation of a hormone called osteocalcin. Osteocalcin is secreted by osteoblasts (the cells that make bone) and is important for making bones stronger. Green, leafy vegetables as well as some fruits such as grapes and avocado are primary sources of vitamin K. Studies show that vitamin K increases bone density in Japanese women. However, studies on men and women in the United States and Scotland showed no improvements in bone density. This may possibly be due to an increased problem with vitamin K deficiency in Japanese women compared to people in other countries. Vitamin K deficiency can also occur in older people, especially those who do not eat very many leafy, green vegetables. Therefore, taking a vitamin K supplement may be beneficial for people who are at increased risk of vitamin K deficiency, but most people who have osteoporosis would probably not benefit from taking a vitamin K supplement. Anyone taking warfarin (Coumadin), a medicine used to prevent blood clots, should not take vitamin K supplements. Vitamin K prevents warfarin from working properly.

### Vitamin B-12

Vitamin B-12 deficiency may increase the chances for developing osteoporosis since vitamin B-12 appears important for the proper functioning of osteoblasts to build bone. While it is not a major cause of osteoporosis or broken bones, it is important that anyone diagnosed with vitamin B-12 deficiency take a vitamin B-12 supplement regularly to keep the levels normal. A common regimen is to take 1,000 mcg to 2,000 mcg of vitamin B-12 a day in the form of an over-the-counter oral supplement. Vitamin B-12 can also be administered through a prescription-strength nasal spray (Nascobal) used once a week, or vitamin B-12 injections can be administered by your doctor.

### Isoflavones

Isoflavones are estrogen-like substances classified as phytoestrogens. They occur naturally in soybeans, lentils, and chickpeas as genistein and daidzein. A synthetic form called ipriflavone is also available as a supplement. Isoflavones have been promoted as possibly useful for the treatment of osteoporosis. In one study subjects who took 54 mg of genistein a day increased their bone density. However, a couple of studies looking at ipriflavone, and another study where 200 mg of isoflavone was taken daily, showed no improvements in bone density. There have been no medical studies proving that any of these substances decrease broken bones due to osteoporosis. This may sound a little confusing, but when doctors evaluate research studies on osteoporosis, they are more interested in their proving that substances decrease broken bones from occurring and not just increase bone density by itself (as seen in the study on genistein). The reason for this is that therapies used in the past that increased bone density (examples include fluoride and a medicine called etidronate) in medical studies actually caused the bone to become weaker, causing an actual increase in fractures. This is because these substances (fluoride and etidronate) increased the density of bone but in an abnormal way that actually did not strengthen the bone at all. The bottom line is that it may be helpful to eat more soybeans, lentils, and chickpeas or to take a genistein supplement if you have osteoporosis. However, be careful. There is not enough evidence to recommend doing this alone without taking proven medications for osteoporosis; no studies with these supplements have shown an actual decrease in broken bones.

Since these substances have weak estrogen effects, they should probably be avoided by women who have estrogen-sensitive tumors such as breast cancer, and by women who are at increased risk for getting blood clots (such as those who are positive for antiphospholipid antibodies). They should also not be taken by women who take a type of antidepressant called MAOIs (monoamine oxidase inhibitors) as they increase the risk for side effects from this class of medications. These supplements may also potentially interact with multiple other medications such as non-steroidal anti-inflammatory drugs (NSAIDs), blood thinners, antibiotics, cholesterol-lowering medicines, blood pressure medicines, diuretics, diabetes medicines, iron, and thyroid medicines. Therefore, you should check with your doctor prior to taking these supplements.

### KEY POINTS TO REMEMBER

1. Osteoporosis is a disease of the bones where they are fragile and it can cause broken bones.

2. People who have SLE are at increased risk for osteoporosis due to medications (steroids, anti-seizure medicines, blood thinners, and proton pump inhibitors) as well as being less active.

3. Osteoporosis is a silent disease, causing no symptoms at all until the bones start to break.

4. Osteoporosis is treatable and preventable.

5. Osteoporosis is often diagnosed by DXA scan.

6. If you have risk factors for having osteoporosis (table 24.1) ask your doctor to order a DXA scan and a vertebral fracture assessment, both of which can be done on a DXA scan machine.

7. Do the things listed in table 24.6 to prevent and treat osteoporosis.

8. Most people who have lupus should be taking a vitamin D supplement. Make sure you have your vitamin D level measured regularly.

9. If you take a proton pump inhibitor to lower stomach acidity, take calcium citrate supplements daily to ensure that you absorb calcium adequately.

10. If you take steroids regularly you need more calcium and vitamin D than other people, and you may need to be on a medicine for osteoporosis.

11. The most effective medicines for osteoporosis are the bisphosphonates, teriparatide, and possibly denosumab.

12. Raloxifene (Evista) can help treat osteoporosis and prevent breast cancer.

13. Do not take raloxifene (Evista) if you are positive for antiphospholipid antibodies.

14. Calcitonin can help decrease pain from osteoporotic fractures, but is a weak osteoporosis medicine for making the bones stronger.

15. Natural supplements such as vitamin K, vitamin B-12, genistein, soybeans, soy milk, lentils, and chickpeas may be beneficial to help strengthen bones with osteoporosis but are not good enough to use by themselves in place of osteoporosis medicines to prevent broken bones. None of these have been shown to prevent fractures due to osteoporosis.

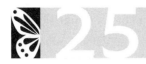

# Avascular Necrosis of Bone

## How Bone Can Die in Lupus

Dr. Edmund L. Dubois (pronounced doo-BOYZ') is credited with organizing the very first and largest clinic in the world dedicated to the treatment of SLE patients. His clinic, called the Collagen Disease Clinic, was located at the Los Angeles County General Hospital. In 1966, he published the first edition of his groundbreaking textbook *Lupus Erythematosus*, which was based on his experience with 520 SLE patients whom he had cared for. He discussed his findings in detail and presented an extensive review of the medical literature about SLE. His textbook is now in its seventh edition and has grown from an initial 479 pages to its current 1,414 pages. It is an invaluable resource for any rheumatologist with a special interest in treating patients who have SLE.

In 1960, Dr. Dubois and his associate Dr. Lewis Cozen reported the cases in the medical literature of eleven patients who had SLE who developed a problem where the bone of their joints developed "necrosis" ("necrosis" is the medical term for "death"). Most of these patients had progressive pain in their hips, two patients had pain in their knees, and one patient had developed signs of necrosis on x-ray but had no pain at all. Prior to this report, there had been no reports of patients who had SLE developing this condition. The only difference between these eleven cases and previous reports on patients who had SLE was the use of steroids in these patients. Steroids began to be used to treat SLE regularly in the 1950s. Ten of Dr. Dubois's eleven patients who had necrosis of the bone were treated with steroids at some point for their SLE. It was becoming apparent that although steroids were a miracle drug in extending the longevity of life and the quality of life for people who had lupus, treatment with steroids was also a "double-edged sword" due to its potential side effects. When Dr. Dubois later reported on his experience in 520 SLE patients, the number of patients affected by necrosis of the bone had jumped up to 26 patients. All but one had been treated with steroids.

Necrosis of the bone is most commonly called avascular necrosis of the bone where "avascular" means "a lack of blood supply." Doctors often abbreviate avascular necrosis as AVN. Another commonly used term is "osteonecrosis," which literally means "death of bone." It is an important potential complication of steroid use in people who have SLE. Anywhere from 5% to 10% of people who have SLE will develop AVN over their lifetimes, and it is most commonly related to taking high-dose steroids. This chapter goes into detail about AVN, what problems it causes, how it is diagnosed, and how it is treated. Although many people end up requiring surgery, such as total joint replacement, the disease process can potentially be slowed down if caught early enough. This chapter gives you information on how to identify this condition and what you can do to slow it down if you do develop it.

．．．．

Avascular necrosis (AVN) happens when the supply of blood in an area of bone is disrupted, causing a piece of the bone to die. It most commonly occurs in the large bone of the leg (femur) connecting to the hip joint, but it also may occur in the knees and shoulders as well. Although it may affect just one joint, many people will develop AVN in the same joint on each side of the body.

The hip joint is a ball and socket joint; the ball of the femur bone (called the femoral head) fits like a ball into the acetabulum of the pelvic bone (acting as the socket of the joint). This ball and socket joint allows the hips to move widely in many different directions. AVN typically occurs in the femoral head of the hip. This section of dead bone softens over time and can no longer bear the weight placed on it. It eventually collapses, causing the normal ball-shaped configuration of the femoral head to flatten out. This loss of the smooth ball shape of the femoral head makes it much more difficult for it to move within the acetabulum socket of the pelvic bone. This causes loss of range of motion and pain. The hip joint eventually develops arthritis (joint damage) because of the AVN.

The hip joint is located in the groin area; therefore, people most commonly feel discomfort in the groin when they develop AVN of the hip. Many people find this surprising, thinking that hip arthritis would cause pain on the side of the hip, but this is incorrect. (The most common cause of pain on the side of the hip is actually hip bursitis.) As the AVN worsens, people usually will lose range of motion and will experience groin pain from the arthritis. They may have difficulty bending the hip to put on their shoes, and they may have difficulty bearing weight on the hip, causing them to limp when they walk.

The primary reason people develop AVN is the use of steroids. The vast majority of people who have SLE who develop AVN have taken steroids, often in high doses (more than 20 mg a day). However, there are people who have developed AVN even with taking smaller doses. There have even been very small numbers of people who have taken no steroids at all, suggesting that there may be other reasons people who have SLE develop AVN. These additional reasons are not fully known. Numerous studies have been done trying to answer this question, but so far they have had conflicting results. Some studies have suggested that lupus inflammation, having high cholesterol, having Raynaud's phenomenon (where the fingers turn pale and blue with exposure to cold), antiphospholipid antibodies, or vasculitis (inflammation of the blood vessels) may increase the chances of people who have SLE developing AVN. However, there are other very good studies showing that these problems do not increase the risk of AVN. The one common denominator in all the studies is that the patients who have SLE who develop AVN have overwhelmingly been treated with steroids. In fact, there are no reported cases of SLE patients having AVN until after steroids came into use in the 1950s. This certainly illustrates the "double-edged sword" problem involving steroids and lupus. Although steroids are lifesaving medicines in many people who have lupus, they can potentially cause significant problems as well.

Most people who develop AVN do not have SLE at all, as it can be caused by problems other than using steroids to treat SLE (listed in table 25.1). Since people who have SLE can potentially have these other problems in addition to having SLE, it is important to consider these other possible causes of AVN as well.

Exactly how the use of steroids to treat lupus causes AVN in the first place is not known. It appears that somehow steroids cause the blood vessels of the bone to develop a decreased blood supply, which ends up causing the bone to die. Since steroids can cause increased cholesterol and fat to form in the blood, it has been suggested that maybe the steroids cause tiny globs (called emboli) of cholesterol and fat to form in the blood vessels and that maybe these end up clogging the blood vessels. Steroids can also cause osteoporosis, as discussed in chapter 24. There is a theory that people on steroids may first develop osteoporosis in the femoral head and then develop tiny microscopic breaks or fractures in these areas of weakened bone. The steroids may not allow the blood vessels to supply enough blood flow to allow the body to fix these tiny fractures. The fractures may worsen and eventually cause the bone to die.

Since doctors do not fully understand why people who have SLE who take steroids develop AVN, they do not completely know how to prevent it from happening in the first place. One study showed that taking a blood thinner called warfarin (Coumadin) was able to decrease, but not eliminate AVN from happening in SLE patients who took steroids. This study would need to be repeated before doctors would consider putting patients who take steroids on warfarin, because warfarin can potentially cause significant bleeding problems. Studies would have to prove that warfarin prevents more cases of AVN than produces side effects before doctors would consider using it as standard therapy. In addition, since the vast majority of people who have lupus who take steroids never develop AVN, it would be a tough call to put such a high number of people on warfarin if it only prevents a few of them from getting AVN in the first place.

Doctors most commonly diagnose AVN by looking at an x-ray of the hip. However, early in the disease process, x-rays can be normal. If there is significant joint pain (or groin pain with the hip joint) and the x-ray is normal, an MRI is the next best way to

**Table 25.1**  Causes of AVN Other Than High-Dose Steroids

- Excessive alcohol drinking
- Sickle cell disease
- Trauma
- Gaucher disease (a rare genetic disorder)
- Decompression disease (when underwater divers ascend too quickly from deep water)
- Kidney transplantation
- HIV infection
- Radiation therapy for cancer
- Legg-Calvé-Perthes disease or slipped capital epiphysis (developmental disorders occurring in children)

diagnose AVN. An MRI can identify AVN at a very early stage. It is a good idea to get an x-ray or MRI of the opposite joint as well since it is common for AVN to occur on both sides of the body.

Once AVN is diagnosed, doctors can grade its severity on a scale of 0 to 4 where 0 is the mildest and 4 is the most severe. It is helpful to know how severe your AVN is if you have been diagnosed with it. Occasionally, a person with the least severe stages, stage 0 or 1, may stay the same and not worsen. AVN is usually picked up on x-ray or MRI done for other reasons, and the person may have no symptoms associated with it at all or the symptoms (discomfort) may be minimal or mild. Sometimes AVN can actually get better over time, or at least not worsen. One study looked at people who had SLE who had AVN on MRI, but no hip pain. Over a three-year period, 75% of these patients did not worsen, while 25% did get worse. Therefore, if a person has AVN, and it is causing very few problems, there is the potential for it not to necessarily get worse.

People who have stage 3 or 4 AVN are on the opposite side of the spectrum. They already have significant damage to the femoral head and may already have significant arthritis of the hip joint. These people more commonly require a total hip replacement for adequate treatment. Surgery may not be needed right away, but usually it is required at some point to decrease the pain and to improve their ability to walk and stand. People who have stage 2 AVN have a better chance of doing well. This group already has damage to the femoral head but do not have arthritis of the hip joint yet. Most people who have stage 2 AVN appear to worsen over time, or at least do not improve; however, they are not destined to absolutely need a hip replacement as much as people who have stage 3 or 4 AVN.

## Treatment of AVN

There are three ways to treat AVN: joint protection, conservative management (non-surgical therapy), and surgical therapy.

### Joint Protection

Joint protection is extremely important no matter what stage of AVN you have. If you have stage 0 or 1, it could potentially make a big difference in preventing your AVN from becoming worse because the goal of joint protection is to decrease stress on the bone and cartilage of the joint. All people who have AVN should review the joint protection advice given in tables 7.2 and 7.3 for the particular joint involved. If you have involvement of the knee or hip, it is extremely important to use a cane whenever you walk. A cane can greatly decrease the amount of pressure and weight placed on the affected joint as you walk and stand. It is important to use the cane in the hand opposite of the joint involved as this is most effective in decreasing weight on the affected joint. In addition, weight loss is very important in achieving this goal if you are overweight.

Too many people do not abide by the principles of joint protection. Instead, they rely too much on pain medications that do nothing to prevent the progression of AVN. In addition, many people are uncomfortable with the thought of being seen in public using a cane. It is very important to learn to put your health first at some point and realize that it is more important than worrying about what other people think of you.

Exercise is important to maintain muscle strength and flexibility, and to help with weight loss. However, you want to use low-impact exercises such as swimming or stationary bicycling instead of jogging or doing aerobics. You really should consider asking your doctor to refer you to a physical therapist to get the best exercise advice.

### Conservative Management (Nonsurgical Therapy)

Nonsurgical, conservative treatments include using medications for pain such as acetaminophen (Tylenol), non-steroidal anti-inflammatory drugs (NSAIDs), and opioid medications. You can try to use over-the-counter medications as described in chapter 7 to decrease your discomfort, but if these are ineffective, you should see your doctor for prescription pain relievers. These therapies do nothing to prevent the AVN from getting worse, but they can potentially decrease your pain, improve your ability to use the affected joint, and improve the quality of your life.

Another potential therapy for AVN is the use of alendronate (Fosamax). Alendronate is a bisphosphonate used to treat osteoporosis (see chapter 24). There have been a couple of studies that suggest that taking alendronate may decrease the progression of AVN if taken in very early stages, before flattening of the surface of the femoral head occurs. Currently, it really is not known if it truly makes a difference in the end or not. One study showed that by the eighth year of taking alendronate, it delayed the amount of time before surgery was needed, but it did not completely prevent the need for surgery. Since the vast majority of people who take alendronate tolerate it, it may be a good option for those who have early AVN. It certainly is worth asking your doctor to consider prescribing it in the hopes that it may slow down the progression of AVN.

### Surgical Therapy

Unfortunately, most people who have stage 2, 3, or 4 AVN eventually require total joint replacement surgery. The decision for getting a total joint replacement is usually up to the patient. Doctors usually recommend surgery if medicines do not control the pain adequately, and if the person's quality of life is greatly affected. An older person who is not very active could potentially have severe stage 4 AVN with only mild discomfort. If this is the case, she should probably not undergo a joint replacement. The potential for adverse consequences from surgery are probably higher than the benefits she would receive from the joint replacement (since she does not have much discomfort nor is it affecting the quality of her life very much). In comparison, a very active 30-year-old who enjoys hiking, exercising, and dancing could have a milder case of stage 2 AVN but be severely impacted. If she has severe pain and is unable to do the activities that she enjoys, then her quality of life could be greatly affected. This person should consider getting a total joint replacement as it could potentially make a huge impact in decreasing or even totally getting rid of her pain and allowing her to return to many of her previously enjoyed activities. The decision to get a joint replacement is complex, involving a detailed discussion of the potential risks and benefits with an orthopedic surgeon.

Doctors recommend having surgery, such as total joint replacement, if significant life-altering pain continues after taking pain medications, performing regular exercise, and abiding by joint protection advice. A joint replacement is a complex procedure performed under anesthesia and involves removing the bone of the joint that contains the necrotic (dead) bone and replacing it with a new replacement part called a prosthesis. The other part of the joint may also need to be replaced as well. There are many types of joint replacements that are performed using numerous different materials (e.g., cement, metal, etc.). It takes a detailed evaluation by a good orthopedist to determine which is the best procedure for you to undergo. The different potential options are certainly beyond the scope of this chapter.

People who feel they may need a joint replacement for AVN should find an orthopedic surgeon in the area who has done numerous joint replacements. Studies show that one of the best predictors for how well you do from surgery is the number of surgeries that the surgeon has done. Getting advice from your rheumatologist and primary care provider is essential when making this decision. Ask them which surgeon they would personally go to in your area if they needed to get the same surgery done (or whom they would send a family member to). Another way to help make this decision is to ask friends and family. Talk to people who have had joint replacements and ask them how their experience was, whom they saw, and how happy they were with the outcome.

Check out patients' reviews on the internet. As of the time of this writing, some potentially useful internet sites include www.angieslist.com, www.vitals.com, www.ratemds.com, www.healthgrades.com, and www.wellness.com. However, you should use caution when reviewing online ratings of doctors. There is quite a bit of controversy in the medical community over the accuracy of these sites because reviewers typically can leave comments anonymously without enforced accountability. Patients who have had negative experiences are more apt to leave comments on these sites compared to the numbers of patients who have had positive experiences. However, it can be helpful to check these sites for a recurrent pattern. For example, if there is a doctor who has had numerous reviews on multiple sites and the vast majority of ratings have been positive, then he or she is probably a doctor who is overall liked as a good physician. Even the best physicians can have bad outcomes since medical therapies are not 100% effective. If you find that a physician has had numerous reviews on multiple sites and the vast majority are negative, then that would be a physician that you should have some reservations about seeing.

After you have chosen an orthopedic surgeon, go to the initial consultation fully prepared. Bring all x-ray and MRI films with you and any notes on your recent visits to your rheumatologist and primary care physician (doctors call these "progress notes"); a list of all of your medical problems, surgeries, and medications; and any recent lab study results. (In fact, it is a good idea to bring this type of information to any new doctor you see.) Prepare a brief list of questions to ask the surgeon about the surgery:

- Do you recommend that I have surgery? If so, what type and why?

- Approximately how many of these surgeries have you done?

- If I undergo this surgery what are my chances of having a good outcome (decreased pain and increased ability to be more active in my life)?

- If I undergo surgery what are my chances of having complications from the surgery, how often do they occur, and how bad are they?

- If I undergo this surgery what is the rehabilitation process afterward? How long can I expect to be out of work?

Another surgery performed for AVN, which is somewhat controversial, is a type of surgery called core decompression. This involves the surgeon drilling a hole into the area of bone affected by the AVN to release built up pressure inside of the bone. By decreasing this pressure in the bone, the surgeon hopes to slow down the progressive worsening of the AVN. Studies suggest that it may slow down or stop the progression of the AVN in 50% to 77% of patients who have early (stage 0, 1, or 2) AVN. However, it is a surgery, and is therefore not an easy decision to make. When contemplating this type of surgery you want to see a surgeon who has expertise in this area. Other surgeries can be done as well, including bone-grafting and a procedure called osteotomy. All of these options can be discussed with an experienced orthopedic surgeon.

### KEY POINTS TO REMEMBER

1. AVN (also called osteonecrosis) is a disorder where part of the bone dies, usually in a bone next to a joint.

2. AVN occurs in 5% to 10% of people who have SLE most commonly due to steroid therapy.

3. AVN most commonly occurs in the hip, causing groin pain and difficulty walking, and putting shoes and socks on. The shoulders and knees can also be affected.

4. AVN is diagnosed by x-ray or MRI.

5. Doctors grade the severity of AVN on a scale ranging from 0 to 4.

6. If picked up very early (stage 0 or 1) and you have no symptoms, you have a 75% chance of not getting worse.

7. Core decompression surgery may decrease the chances of progressing in early AVN (such as stages 0–2).

8. Taking the medication alendronate may potentially decrease progression in very early AVN, but this has not been proven.

9. All people who have AVN should abide by strict joint protection measures to try to slow down or prevent their AVN from progressing (tables 7.2 and 7.3).

10. Most patients with stage 2, 3, or 4 AVN will eventually need a total joint replacement.

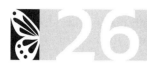

# Adrenal Insufficiency

## Why You Must Decrease Steroid Doses Slowly

In 1855, Dr. Thomas Addison of England described a group of patients who had an unusual set of problems that included loss of energy, weakness, stomach upset, nausea, diarrhea, weight loss, and a peculiar increased coloration of the skin. Autopsies showed that the adrenal glands (which sit on top of the kidneys) had shrunk or had been replaced by fat in these patients. This led him to theorize that this gland was very important for bodily functions and that the destruction of these glands caused their problems. Doctors eventually called this disease involving destruction of the adrenal glands Addison's disease in honor of Dr. Addison. In 1855, the most common cause of Addison's disease was tuberculosis. Today the most common cause of Addison's disease (albeit a rare one) is autoimmune in nature, where the immune system destroys the adrenal glands. Another reason for the adrenal glands to stop working normally ("adrenal insufficiency") is due to the use of steroids. However, this form of adrenal insufficiency is not called Addison's disease since the steroids do not actually destroy the adrenal glands. However, the use of steroids causes many of the same problems as first described by Dr. Addison.

It was determined over time that the adrenal glands were responsible for making numerous hormones in the body, including steroids and epinephrine (also known as adrenalin). These hormones were determined to have essential life-sustaining properties in the body, including the production of sex hormones, maintenance of blood pressure, proper handling of salts, and other vital functions. One of these steroids produced by the adrenal gland is cortisol, which is related to cortisone and prednisone. Soon after cortisone and prednisone came under widespread use in the 1950s for diseases such as SLE, it was noted that if people's steroid doses were decreased too quickly or stopped abruptly, they could become ill with profound fatigue and body aches. Most people had symptoms that improved when their steroid doses were increased again. Then in 1953, the case of someone dying after surgery due to adrenal insufficiency from prolonged cortisone treatment was reported. In 1954, the case of a patient treated with steroids for asthma who went into a coma after the steroids were abruptly stopped was reported. It soon became apparent that adrenal insufficiency due to steroid treatment was a significant problem.

Adrenal insufficiency is an important concept for anyone who takes steroids (such as prednisone and methylprednisolone) to understand. It is the very reason that doctors tell their patients not to lower the doses of their steroids too quickly or to stop taking steroids abruptly. People who take steroids can potentially develop this problem, yet it is completely avoidable in the vast majority of cases and is discussed in detail in this chapter.

· · · ·

The adrenal glands (also called suprarenal glands) sit on top of the kidneys. In fact, this is where they get their name since "renal" is another name for "kidney"; "ad-" means "near" and "supra-" means "on top of." Although they are small, they have incredibly important functions as endocrine glands. Endocrine glands (see chapter 17) are organs that produce and secrete hormones within the body. The adrenal glands produce about fifty different steroids that have numerous functions in the body, including maintenance of blood pressure; the proper handling of salts by the kidneys; metabolism of nutrients such as glucose (sugar), fats, and proteins; and helping with how the body responds to stress. They also produce other very important hormones such as the sex hormone DHEA (dehydroepiandrosterone) and epinephrine (called adrenaline), which is very important for keeping blood pressure up, keeping the heart beating, and keeping the lung passages open. All of these hormones are very important for normal, daily living.

"Adrenal insufficiency" is the term for when the adrenal glands stop making enough of some of these hormones, especially the steroids. To understand how this can occur in people who take steroids, it is helpful to know some basics on how the adrenal glands produce steroids.

The adrenal glands do not work independently. Instead, they work with the help of two other organs that are in the brain, the hypothalamus, and the pituitary gland (figure 26.1). These three areas of the body work in conjunction with each other in a finely orchestrated way to ensure that each of them is working properly. The medical term for this interaction between these three organs is the "hypothalamic-pituitary-adrenal axis."

The hypothalamus is the primary organ in charge of this whole operation. The hypothalamus continuously secretes a hormone called corticotropin-releasing hormone (CRH for short). CRH travels in the blood to the pituitary gland to cause it to secrete another hormone called adrenocorticotropic hormone (ACTH for short). In turn, ACTH travels to the adrenal glands to tell them to secrete a certain amount of steroids (such as cortisol, which is related to cortisone, prednisone, and methylprednisolone). In fact, the body normally makes about the equivalent of 5 mg to 7 mg of prednisone (or 4 mg to 6 mg of methylprednisolone) every day.

Increased amounts of steroids are needed for more intense activity or in times of stress. When the hypothalamus senses less cortisol in the bloodstream than there should be, or soon after people first wake up and become active, or during periods of stress (such as during infections or surgery), it secretes higher amounts of CRH. This in turn causes the pituitary gland to secrete more ACTH, and subsequently the adrenal glands dutifully make more cortisol as initially demanded by the hypothalamus. After this, when the hypothalamus senses the increased amounts of cortisol being produced in the blood by the adrenal glands, it backs off again and produces less CRH. This system of each organ talking to each other with these chemical messages in the blood helps to maintain a proper amount of cortisol in the blood for the body to func-

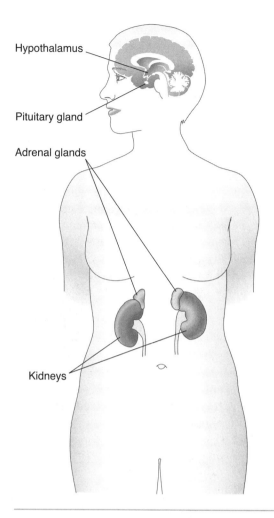

**Figure 26.1** Locations of the hypothalamus, the pituitary gland, and the adrenal glands

tion normally under various conditions. This ensures that there is more cortisol in the body during periods when it is needed most (stress and increased periods of activity), and less cortisol during other periods (periods of rest).

When someone takes steroid medications, such as prednisone and methylprednisolone, on a regular basis, the hypothalamus senses this increased amount of cortisol-like steroids in the blood. When taken on a regular basis, especially at higher doses (such as more than 7 mg of prednisone a day), the hypothalamus produces a smaller amount of CRH because it thinks the adrenal glands are making too much cortisol. In turn, the pituitary gland makes less ACTH, which tells the adrenal glands to stop making steroids. The adrenal glands respond just as a muscle responds to the lack of exercise. Since they think they are not needed anymore to make steroids, the adrenal glands atrophy (shrink in size). The adrenal glands become even smaller if higher doses of steroids are taken and if they are taken over prolonged periods. Therefore, by taking steroids, such as prednisone and methylprednisolone, at higher doses and for extended periods, a person develops adrenal insufficiency.

As long as someone stays on large doses of steroids, she will not realize that she has a problem from adrenal insufficiency. The steroid medicine that she is taking will replace the steroids usually produced by her adrenal glands. The problem is not realized until one of two things happen. One situation occurs if is she becomes stressed while taking relatively small doses of steroids, and the second is if the steroids are decreased too quickly to small doses or are stopped abruptly.

During stressful situations such as infections, trauma, and surgery, the adrenal glands normally secrete higher amounts of cortisol (as ordered by the hypothalamus and the pituitary gland). In fact, the adrenal glands can produce the equivalent of about 20 mg of prednisone a day during periods of stress, and this amount is essential to help bodily functions during stress. During periods of severe stress, the adrenal glands may produce up to the equivalent of 100 mg of prednisone a day.

Here is an illustrative example. Let us say that someone has lupus pleurisy (inflammation of the lining of the lungs) and requires 40 mg of prednisone a day for a few weeks. The rheumatologist may then start to decrease the prednisone dosage gradually. After a few more weeks, the patient is down to 8 mg a day of prednisone at which point she gets the flu (because she forgot to get her flu shot that year). The hypothalamus senses the infection, which is causing a high fever, coughing, nausea, and severe fatigue, and realizes the body needs more cortisol-like steroids during the infection. It sends an increased amount of CRH to the pituitary gland, which in turn produces an increased amount of ACTH. The smaller than normal adrenal glands sense this high ACTH level. Although they know they are supposed to make more cortisol in response to this elevated ACTH, they cannot do so. It is like asking a 90-pound weakling to lift 200-pound dumb bells. Since the adrenal glands are unable to produce the proper amount of cortisol steroids in the body, this person becomes much sicker than a person who does not have adrenal insufficiency. Her fatigue becomes incapacitating; her aches and pains are unbearable; and she is so light-headed and dizzy that she can hardly get up out of bed.

A few different scenarios could play out from this point. In one scenario, the person may try to tough it out at home. By doing so without extra steroids or cortisol, she will be more miserable and will probably take a lot longer to recuperate from the flu than a person who does not have adrenal insufficiency. In another scenario, she may stay home in bed but eventually get sick enough where she has to go to the hospital. Chapter 22 mentioned how 30,000 Americans die yearly from the flu, and immunosuppressed people (such as people who have lupus) are at high risk of being in that group. Hopefully, she will be seen quickly enough so that antiviral antibiotics can be given to help her, and she can be treated with extra doses of steroids to help save her life.

The best scenario occurs when the well-educated person (like you, since you are putting in the effort and time to read this information) calls her primary care physician to be seen immediately in the office (as she knows she is supposed to see her doctor ASAP with any type of infection) to get prompt antiviral therapy. In addition, she realizes that she may have adrenal insufficiency and calls up her rheumatologist to see if she needs an extra dose of steroids. Her rheumatologist tells her to increase her prednisone to 20 mg a day for a few days, then to taper the dose down slowly over the next week or two. Her internist puts her on an antiviral antibiotic medicine. Within a day or two, she is feeling markedly better. This temporary increase in steroid dose is called a stress dose of steroids. The dosage of steroids used for stress varies, depending on how much stress the person is in and how long the stressful event is expected to last. If she had not taken this additional stress dose of steroids, she would have felt much sicker for a longer time.

This last scenario is extremely important to remember. Whenever you have been on steroids for more than a few weeks, you should consider the possibility that you may have adrenal insufficiency. If you ever go through a period of stress such as an infection, if you have significant trauma, or if you are preparing for surgery, always call your rheumatologist to see if you should increase your steroid dose.

The second situation where adrenal insufficiency typically rears its ugly head is in the person who has lupus who has been taking steroids for a prolonged period and is decreasing the steroid dose or completely stopping it. Normally, after a person has been on significant doses of steroids for more than a few weeks, it is important to decrease the dosage slowly over time. Doctors call this a steroid taper. This is where the "art of medicine" plays a more critical role than the science of medicine. All people are different as far as how their bodies (and adrenal glands) react to steroids and a steroid taper. A steroid taper relies a lot on the doctor's experience to determine how quickly and safely to taper the steroids. After the steroid dose is decreased to 7 mg a day and lower, the taper needs to be done slowly enough to allow the adrenal glands to learn to become more active, stronger, and larger. They must learn to start making their own cortisol-like steroids again. If the taper is done properly, the patient will hopefully never have any symptoms of adrenal insufficiency. However, if it is done too quickly, symptoms of adrenal insufficiency will set in causing fatigue, weakness, loss of appetite, weight loss, body aches and pains, light-headedness, and depression (table 26.1).

These symptoms can occur gradually, making it more difficult to pinpoint them to the steroid taper itself. This reminds me of one of my patients who had been on steroids for several years due to a flare of lupus nephritis (inflammation of the kidneys). With proper treatment, her nephritis went into remission and she started a slow ste-

Table 26.1 Symptoms Suggesting Adrenal Insufficiency Due to Steroid Withdrawal

- Fatigue
- Weakness
- Loss of appetite
- Weight loss
- Body aches and pains
- Light-headedness
- Depression
- Longer recovery from mild infections such as colds

roid taper. After she got down to about 3 mg of prednisone a day she came in for her regular office visit. She had lost all of her prednisone weight (she previously had gained a lot of weight on prednisone), which she was very happy about, but she had absolutely no energy, had very little appetite, was light-headed, and had headaches. Simply by increasing her prednisone by 1 mg (up to 4 mg daily), she felt markedly better, like a new person. Even this tiny increase in prednisone made a huge difference in resolving her symptoms of adrenal insufficiency due to steroid withdrawal, but it was not a high enough dose to give her any steroid side effects. Initially, she was very discouraged at my suggestion that she increase her steroids. However, when she felt like a new person again on the extra milligram a day of prednisone, she changed her mind quickly.

A person who has been on prednisone for a couple of months may be able to safely taper off of the steroid within a couple of weeks, while a person who has been on prednisone for a year or two may take a couple of years to taper off slowly. It often takes a lot of trial and error on the part of the patient and the physician to know how quickly to taper the steroids. While you are going down on your dose of steroids, if you feel symptoms of adrenal insufficiency (see table 26.1), it is important to communicate this to your rheumatologist so that the steroid can be tapered a little bit more slowly. Most of my patients who have been on steroids for a while know that if they taper their steroids and they develop these symptoms, then they should increase the prednisone back to the previous dose at which they felt fine.

It can sometimes be challenging to know how quickly to taper steroids, and it can be frustrating for the patient (who usually wants to get off them as soon as possible). The good news is that the adrenal glands do start to work again in everyone, although it can occasionally take quite a while if a person has been on steroids for a long time.

As far as how much steroids it takes to develop adrenal insufficiency varies a lot from one person to another. Doctors do use some "rules of thumb" that help them decide which patients are at highest risk of having adrenal insufficiency (table 26.2). However, these rules are not set in stone. For example, many people who take 10 mg to 20 mg of prednisone a day for a few weeks will develop adrenal insufficiency, and there are even people who will develop it while taking doses lower than 10 mg a day. It also varies by how long the steroid is taken. For example, a person who has been on just 9 mg of prednisone a day for three months most likely will develop adrenal insufficiency.

**Table 26.2** People Who Probably Have Adrenal Insufficiency Due to Steroids

- Anyone who has taken 20 mg a day of prednisone (or 16 mg a day of methylprednisolone) for three weeks or longer

- Anyone who has taken any dose of prednisone (excluding Rayos brand) in the evening for three weeks or longer (evening doses of steroids suppress the adrenal glands more than morning doses)

- Anyone who has gained weight or become puffy from steroids (called a Cushingoid appearance, discussed in chapter 31)

It is important to take steroids first thing in the morning instead of at nighttime. When steroids are taken in the morning, they are much less likely to cause adrenal insufficiency than when they are taken in the evening. This is why your doctor usually prescribes the steroid to be taken each morning. The sooner you take it in the morning when you get up, the better it will work, and the fewer side effects you will get from taking it. However, if you miss your dose of steroids in the morning, take it later in the day (even if it is at nighttime). This is far better than not taking it at all when you miss a dose. Missing the daily dose of steroids could possibly cause problems with your lupus becoming more active or could cause you to develop symptoms of adrenal insufficiency that day or the following day.

The other time you should take a nighttime dose of steroids is if your doctor asks you to do so. There are several instances where your doctor may ask you to do this. If you are having a particularly severe attack of your SLE, taking steroids two to three times a day is more effective compared to taking them all in the morning. For example, taking 20 mg of prednisone twice a day (a total of 40 mg a day) is stronger than taking all 40 mg a day in the morning. It works a lot faster dosing it this way; however, it also has more side effects. One reason that 20 mg taken twice a day is stronger lies in the fact that prednisone does not last very long in the body. When 40 mg is taken in the morning, there is minimal to no prednisone in the body for about seven to eight hours each night. This allows the adrenal glands to have some time to function properly (not be suppressed by the prednisone), yet there is no more prednisone left to decrease inflammation. However, 20 mg taken twice a day produces a significant amount of prednisone within the body twenty-four hours a day. This is excellent at decreasing inflammation better, but at the cost of more side effects. Therefore, doctors usually only do this for a short period.

Another common reason for asking patients to take an evening dose of steroids is if they have severe morning stiffness and pain with their lupus arthritis. In this instance, doctors may ask patients to take a small dose of steroids (such as 1 mg to 3 mg of prednisone) at nighttime as it can help the severe morning stiffness and pain from arthritis. However, even this small dose at night will increase the chances of developing adrenal insufficiency.

A new and safer alternative to this approach is to take the delayed-release form of prednisone called Rayos. When taken at night before bed, it provides significant relief of pain and stiffness from inflammatory arthritis in the morning when the person first wakes up.

A final aspect of adrenal insufficiency and steroids is the concept of wearing a medical alert bracelet that states you take steroids. People can order medical alert bracelets from most pharmacies and drug stores. Anyone who has been on steroids for a few months or longer and who may have to continue using them should wear a bracelet regularly. If you end up in an emergency room for any type of illness, trauma, or emergency surgery, the medical personnel will immediately know that you require extra doses of steroids to help you survive the stressful event. This could potentially be lifesaving.

The bottom line is that anyone who has been on steroids for more than a few weeks is at risk for having adrenal insufficiency. If you know it is a possibility, you should not decrease your steroids too quickly, not stop them abruptly, and take extra steroids during periods of stress. If you follow these rules, you should do very well with minimal to no problems. Wearing a medical alert bracelet is also an important thing to do as well.

1. Adrenal insufficiency occurs when someone has been on steroids for a prolonged period. The adrenal glands atrophy and are unable to produce enough of the body's life-sustaining steroids on their own.

2. Adrenal insufficiency is most likely to occur in those who have been on steroids for more than a few weeks, those who have taken steroids in the evening, those who have taken higher doses, and those who have gained weight while they took steroids.

3. You should always take your steroid medicine as soon as you wake up in the morning (instead of at nighttime) to decrease the chances of developing adrenal insufficiency. Take steroids in the evening only if your doctor tells you to, or if you missed your morning dose of steroids that day.

4. People who have possible adrenal insufficiency must taper their steroid dose slowly, especially after they get down to 7 mg of prednisone a day and lower. People should never abruptly stop steroids on their own. Always follow your doctor's instructions carefully.

5. People who have possible adrenal insufficiency must take higher doses of steroids during stressful events (called stress doses of steroids) such as during infections, after trauma, or before and after surgery.

6. If you develop any symptoms of adrenal insufficiency (table 26.1) as you are decreasing your steroids, let your doctor know right away because your taper probably needs to be slowed down a bit.

7. Wear a medical alert bracelet if you have been on steroids for a significant amount of time and may have to continue taking them. Ask your rheumatologist if you should wear one.

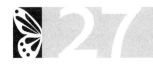

# Fibromyalgia

## Self-Survey for Fibromyalgia

Are you fatigued and tender? Do you ache all over? Are you having difficulty with memory and headaches? Take this survey if you have had any of these symptoms for three months or longer.

I. **Pain Score**: Circle each **body part** where you have had pain in the past week:

o Left shoulder region

o Left upper arm

o Left lower arm

o Left buttock or side of hip

o Left upper leg

o Left lower leg

o Left jaw

o Chest

o Upper back

o Neck

o Right shoulder region

o Right upper arm

o Right lower arm

o Right buttock or side of hip

o Right upper leg

o Right lower leg

o Right jaw

o Abdomen

o Lower back

Each area circled is 1 point. Add up each circled area for your Pain Score.

**Total points for part I Pain Score** = _____

II. **Symptom Score**: For each of the following three **symptoms** (a, b, and c), circle the number corresponding to how much it bothers you.

### Scoring method for Symptom Score

For a, b, and c, use this scale:

0 = You have not had this problem at all.

1 = The problem is very mild and comes and goes.

2 = It causes considerable problems, or is often present at a moderate severity.

3 = The problem is severe, constant, or life-disturbing.

a. How fatigued and tired are you?                                                           0 1 2 3
b. Do you feel like you did not get a good night's sleep when you wake up?   0 1 2 3
c. Do you have difficulty remembering things or concentrating?                 0 1 2 3

For d, use this scale:

    0 = no problems

    1 = few problems

    2 = a moderate number of problems

    3 = a large number of problems

d. How many problems (like pain, fatigue, weakness, drowsiness, difficulty thinking, insomnia, headaches, stomach upset, diarrhea, constipation, numbness, feeling too hot or cold, etc.) do you have?   0 1 2 3

Add up each number for a, b, c, and d for Symptom Score total points

**Total points for Symptom Score** = _____

You may have fibromyalgia if:

- Your pain score is $\geq 7$ and your symptom score is $\geq 5$
- or your pain score is 3–6 and your symptom score is $\geq 9$

If you scored positive for fibromyalgia, show these results to your doctor.

Fibromyalgia can be one of the most difficult and bothersome problems in people who have SLE. It is not due to the autoimmune or inflammatory aspect of SLE, but rather is due to a problem with the pain nerves of the body. It can cause pain, fatigue, insomnia, headaches, and difficulty with memory and concentration; in some people it can be quite life altering.

If your scores on this survey are high, then you have a very good chance of having fibromyalgia. In fact, you actually meet the diagnostic criteria to diagnose fibromyalgia. However, some people can have the features of fibromyalgia, not meet the diagnostic criteria, and yet still have fibromyalgia (as this set of criteria is not 100% foolproof). If you have any of the symptoms, take this survey. If you score high on the test, show the results to your primary care doctor and rheumatologist and see what they think about this possibility.

Fibromyalgia is important to identify because it is not treated with steroids or immunosuppressant medicines; instead, there are other treatments that can be helpful. If you may have fibromyalgia, read this chapter as it goes into detail about this problem and how it is treated.

••••

Any serious book about lupus must include a discussion of the disorder called fibromyalgia (pronounced fi-bro-my-AL-juh) because fibromyalgia affects about 20% of people who have systemic lupus erythematosus. Fibromyalgia causes many problems, including aches and pains, fatigue, and interrupted or inadequate sleep. Many people who have fibromyalgia have seen many doctors over time and may have received numerous individual diagnoses such as tendonitis, bursitis, tennis elbow, back arthritis, or nerve damage. Although anyone can have pain from any one of these diagnoses, sometimes what the person has is not numerous individual problems (like tennis elbow) but rather fibromyalgia as the cause of all of them. Fibromyalgia can cause pain or discomfort in one area of the body at a time initially, and then cause pain in multiple areas as it worsens over time. In other words, fibromyalgia can sometimes masquerade as tendonitis, bursitis, or nerve problems.

Although they may have received many different diagnoses and treatments, most people who have fibromyalgia do not get adequate relief from these therapies because fibromyalgia does not usually respond well to the usual treatments. In fact, some people who have fibromyalgia will even undergo unnecessary surgeries on the spine when their back and neck pain from the fibromyalgia is diagnosed as bulging discs (seen on x-ray or MRI) instead of fibromyalgia. It is also not that uncommon for people who have fibromyalgia to show up at a rheumatologist's office taking high doses of narcotics prescribed by well-meaning physicians to try to help with their pain—and yet they still have severe pain. The narcotics typically help with the pain initially, but they do nothing for the disorder itself and the body soon becomes tolerant of the narcotic. Many people in this situation become addicted to narcotics yet do not get long-term relief from their pain.

Fibromyalgia is a common problem, affecting approximately 4% of women and 1% of men. It is much more common in people who have had other stressful, painful disorders (such as SLE). The hallmark symptom of fibromyalgia is multiple areas of pain and tenderness. In some people, it will begin with pain all over, while in others it may start in just one body part. It is not uncommon for people to be diagnosed with, for example, plantar fasciitis as a cause of their foot pain, then tennis elbow as a cause of their elbow pain, and then costochondritis (inflammation of the cartilage that connects a rib to the breastbone) for severe chest pain. However, over time, it typically adds pain to more and more areas of the body, eventually making the diagnosis of fibromyalgia clear as the cause of all of these pains instead of the individual diagnoses by themselves. People who have fibromyalgia often will state, "I hurt all over" or "I feel like I have the flu," as it can cause pain in joints, muscles, bones, back, and neck, and commonly will cause recurrent headaches as well.

Another problem some people will have is a sensation of numbness and tingling, especially in the arms and legs. In fact, many people will undergo an uncomfortable nerve test (called an EMG test; see chapter 7) for these symptoms only to find out that it is not a nerve damage problem at all. Fibromyalgia can also cause stiffness in the joints and muscles. Often this occurs after a person has been sitting or has been still for a while or when getting out of bed. However, some people will have stiffness that can last all day long. Another common pain problem in fibromyalgia is muscle spasms, commonly called myofascial pain by doctors. This will cause areas of painful or tender "knots" in the muscles, especially in the shoulders, neck, and back.

The aches and pains of fibromyalgia can vary a lot from person to person. Some people can have mild discomfort not requiring any treatment at all, while others can have severe, incapacitating pain. The pain can also fluctuate in severity, with mild discomfort on some days and severe, diffuse body pain on others. Sometimes there is no rhyme or reason to these fluctuations. At other times, the pain may worsen due to weather changes, periods of increased stress, or during periods of inadequate sleep.

Besides pain, fibromyalgia can cause numerous other symptoms as well (table 27.1). A large number people will have fatigue and difficulty sleeping. Some may have noticeable insomnia, while others may feel like they sleep all night yet wake up in the morning feeling like they did not get a good night's sleep at all (called non-restorative sleep). Although some people do not feel fatigued, the vast majority do, and it is not uncommon to receive a diagnosis of chronic fatigue syndrome at some point from a doctor because of the profound tiredness. The fatigue seems to be intimately tied in with the sleep problem. Some people who have fibromyalgia say, "No matter how much sleep I get, in the morning it feels like a truck ran over me."

Some people's memory and concentration may be affected. This is often called "fi-bro fog," where the person can have problems with staying focused, concentrating, and remembering things. "Fibro fog" can greatly affect the quality of life at home and at work. Some people also get ringing in the ears (called tinnitus) and dizziness. Each person who has fibromyalgia has different symptoms and different severity of symptoms. Some have just mild achiness in their muscles and joints and do not have the memory, sleep, fatigue, or other problems. Others have most or all of these symptoms to a severe, disabling degree.

Because pain from fibromyalgia is perplexing and can affect any part of the body, many people seek assistance from many different types of specialists (table 27.2). Women may see a gynecologist to treat chronic pelvic pain, or a urologist to treat a condition called interstitial cystitis, which can feel exactly like a recurrent urinary tract infection with pain and burning while urinating. Some people end up seeing a stomach doctor (gastroenterologist) for a condition called irritable bowel syndrome that can cause recurrent abdominal pain often associated with diarrhea and/or con-

Table 27.1 Common Symptoms of Fibromyalgia

- Multiple areas of pain (joints, muscles, bones, head, abdomen, pelvis)
- Skin and body tenderness
- Tingling or numbness of the face, arms, hands, legs, and feet
- Headaches
- Stomach upset
- Pain while urinating
- Fatigue
- Difficulty sleeping
- Non-restorative sleep (feeling very sleepy after waking; feels like you had inadequate sleep)
- Memory and concentration problems ("fibro fog")
- Ringing in the ears
- Dizziness

**Table 27.2** Other Common Pain Problems in People Who Have Fibromyalgia

- Chronic pelvic pain
- Interstitial cystitis (also called painful bladder syndrome)
- Irritable bowel syndrome
- Migraine headaches
- Restless legs syndrome
- Temporomandibular joint disorder (TMJ)

stipation. Some people may see a headache specialist (usually a neurologist) for recurrent migraine headaches from their fibromyalgia. A person can have achiness in the legs, causing difficulty getting them into a comfortable position especially while in bed. Doctors call this restless legs syndrome, which is often treated by neurologists. Some people can have severe jaw pain with great difficulty opening their mouths and eating, causing them to need treatment for temporomandibular joint disorder (TMJ for short). For many people, it is only after they have seen many different specialists that a doctor finally realizes that all of their problems are due to the same disorder: fibromyalgia.

To make things even more complex, fibromyalgia can also cause problems that are commonly seen in systemic autoimmune diseases such as SLE. Of course, pain and fatigue can be seen in all these disorders, but, in addition, fibromyalgia can cause Raynaud's phenomenon (where the fingers turn pale and blue with exposure to cold) and dry mouth and eyes (just like in Sjögren's syndrome; see chapter 14). One of the most common reasons for a patient to be sent to a rheumatologist is if he or she has a positive antinuclear antibody (ANA) discovered while working the patient up for problems such as aches and pains. Although the ANA is the most important initial screening test to help diagnose SLE, it is also common in people who do not have SLE. The most common reason to be ANA positive and have a lot of pain is to have fibromyalgia. This can be quite confusing for patients as well as for their doctors since both fibromyalgia and lupus can cause many of the same problems (pain, fatigue, tingling of the hands and feet, Raynaud's phenomenon, dry mouth and eyes). This sharing of symptoms becomes even more problematic in that unfortunate 20% of SLE patients who have fibromyalgia in addition to their lupus. These are the patients who can be the most difficult to help and treat due to this overlap of problems.

If you have SLE, have some of the symptoms of fibromyalgia, and do not know whether you have fibromyalgia or not, you should take the self-test at the beginning of this chapter. Another clue that you may have fibromyalgia includes if you "hurt all over." People who have lupus arthritis typically will have pain, stiffness, and swelling in just the joints of the body, especially in the elbows, wrists, knuckles, middle joints of the finger, and knees. People who have SLE who have true inflammatory arthritis due to their lupus typically do not say that they "hurt all over" (unless they also have fibromyalgia), although there are certainly exceptions. Another important clue is the location of the pain. Lupus arthritis does not affect the neck, muscles of the neck and upper back, lower back, buttock areas, or the sides of the hips. If these areas are hurting, then fibromyalgia is more likely the cause than lupus. This is a very important distinction to make because the aches and pains of fibromyalgia require different therapies than the arthritis of lupus. In fact, too many people who have lupus receive improper prescriptions of steroids for aches and pains that are actually due to fibromyalgia. There are much safer and more effective medicines to use for the pain of fibromyalgia than steroids.

## What Causes Fibromyalgia?

It is unclear why some people get fibromyalgia and others do not. It is more common in people who have disorders such as arthritis and lupus. This is important for doctors to recognize because the problems of fibromyalgia rarely respond well to the typical treatments for arthritis and lupus.

Fibromyalgia occurs more commonly in people who have experienced traumatic events. It is not uncommon to develop it after having been in a motor vehicle accident or after having had surgery. Some people will develop it after having a severe infection such as the flu, mononucleosis, or Lyme disease.

Unfortunately, studies show that many people who have fibromyalgia have a history of a profound psychological stress, especially abuse. This may have taken the form of emotional, physical, or sexual abuse, and occurs more frequently in people who have fibromyalgia than in people who do not have fibromyalgia. Other major psychological stresses such as the loss of a parent while young have also been noted more frequently in people who have fibromyalgia. Why people who have gone through these traumatic events are more prone to develop fibromyalgia is unknown. Most people do not volunteer this information to their doctors, as most patients do not realize its importance; nor do they realize that it may be associated with having the pain in the first place. Many people will also refuse to accept the fact that they may be related when a doctor raises this possibility. Another problem is that admitting to abuse can be emotionally stressful and embarrassing. However, experts agree that people who have had these sorts of events have a much better chance of improving when they get psychological and psychiatric assistance in dealing with these very deep, scarring issues. For these people, pain rarely improves until they get adequate psychological help as well as medical treatment for their pain.

Doctors have conducted an amazing amount of research addressing what is going on in people who have fibromyalgia. Although they may feel severe pain in the muscles, joints, and bones of the body, there is not anything wrong going on in these areas (except of course in people who may have arthritis along with fibromyalgia). This can be very difficult for the person who has fibromyalgia to learn to accept. Normally our bodies are programmed to tell us there is pain somewhere only when damage or injury is taking place in that body part. For example, you burn your finger on the stove. Your body (via the nervous system) alerts your brain of the burn injury by way of severe pain so that it can tell the arm and hand to pull away from the stove. This is the normal function of pain.

How do people normally feel pain? Most areas of the body have special sensory nerves that sense injury or damage to the body. Their role is to let the brain know that damage is happening, which in turn causes the body to make an appropriate response (such as pulling back a burned finger) to protect itself. There is a complex network of interacting pain nerves throughout the body. The sensory nerves that initially sense the injury will release chemical messages (called neurotransmitters) to adjacent nerves. These will do the same thing to other nerves in a sequence from the body part that is affected to nerves in the spinal cord, which then alert the brain about where the damage or injury is noted. The brain will "feel" the injury or damage in the form of conscious pain. In tiny fractions of a second, it will in turn send neurotransmitter messages along additional nerves back down the spinal cord. These nerves then alert the appropriate muscles so that they can withdraw the injured body part from the injuring source.

If the injured body part (such as the burned finger) continues to be damaged even after it is pulled away, the sensory nerves continue to note this injury and to send painful neurotransmitter messages up to the brain. If this were to continue until the body part completely healed, then we would be in misery with constant, severe pain for a long time. However, the body protects us from sensing continuous pain by releasing other neurotransmitters in the brain and spinal cord (such as serotonin and norepinephrine) that work by calming down these pain messages coming up from the sensory nerves of the body. This allows the painful messages to decrease so that we are not in constant, severe pain for a long time. However, we still notice that there is an injury or damage going on which allows us to be conscious of this and to take care of the injured area (such as running cold water over the burned finger or applying some soothing lotions on it until it heals).

These neurotransmitters are essential in feeling pain. The pain nerves can sometimes send these chemicals to each other even if there is no injury going on. Unfortunately, this is what happens in fibromyalgia. Numerous very good medical studies (table 27.3) have demonstrated this occurrence. For example, people who have fibromyalgia have an increased amount of a pain neurotransmitter called substance P in the spine. Levels are about two to three times higher in people who have fibromyalgia compared to people who do not have fibromyalgia. Substance P is one of the neurotransmitters that are sent from one nerve to another to tell the brain that there is pain going on in the body.

In addition to these overactive pain nerves in the person who has fibromyalgia, there is also a lack of inhibition of these pain messages as well. Normally, levels of neurotransmitters such as serotonin and norepinephrine in the brain are sufficient to calm these pain pathways down. However, the person who has fibromyalgia has a decreased amount of these inhibitory chemicals. These deficiencies allow the pain nerves to stay overactive and not calm down. This combination of the pain nerves being overactive along with a lack of the inhibitory neurotransmitters calming down the pain nerves has been called central pain amplification. It appears that some stressful events (e.g., SLE, arthritis, accidents, surgery, infections, abuse, etc.) probably initiate this problem of central pain amplification and cause it to continue. In turn, this subsequently causes the numerous problems in fibromyalgia, especially the multiple areas of aches and pains.

This problem with an abnormality of neurotransmitters also illustrates why people who have fibromyalgia often also have depression and anxiety. Depression and anxiety are disorders caused by chemical (neurotransmitter) imbalances in the brain leading to problems with mood, worrying, sleep problems, and fatigue. They typically have a lack of proper amounts of serotonin and norepinephrine in the brain, just as people who have fibromyalgia do. In fact, between 30% and 50% of people who have fibromyalgia also have depression and/or anxiety. It is important for doctors to treat depression and anxiety. If you do have fibromyalgia, it is a good idea to take the screening tests for depression (table 13.4) and anxiety disorder (table 13.2) to see if you may have either of these problems in addition to fibromyalgia.

Fibromyalgia disrupts the sleep cycle, causing fatigue that can sometimes be quite severe. Very interesting studies have shown that many people who have fibromyalgia do not go into the deepest parts of sleep. The brain emits different electrical signals and energy during different activities and these can be measured by a test called an electroencephalogram (EEG for short). During normal wakefulness and conscious activities, the brain exhibits a lot of electrical activity on the EEG called alpha waves. As a person falls asleep, these alpha waves become different electrical waves that show she or he is going into deep sleep. However, in the person who has fibromyalgia, there are periods of alpha waves occurring during times when the person who does not have fibromyalgia would be in deep sleep. This signifies that people who have fibromyalgia are not sleeping deeply at all. This helps explain why they wake up feeling as if they did not have a good night's sleep.

Other sleep problems can also be associated with fibromyalgia. For example, the condition called obstructive sleep apnea occurs more often in people who have fibromyalgia, especially in men. In fact, many fibromyalgia experts recommend that all men who have fibromyalgia undergo a sleep study to make sure they do not have sleep apnea as the cause of their fibromyalgia. However, sleep apnea occurs in women as well. It is a good idea if you have fibromyalgia to take the STOP questionnaire for sleep apnea (table 6.3). If you score 2 or more points on the questionnaire, then you should get a sleep study done to make sure you do not have sleep apnea as a potential cause of your fibromyalgia.

Restless legs syndrome is another sleep problem that occurs more commonly in people who have fibromyalgia. People with restless legs syndrome feel an achiness or pain in the muscles, joints, or bones of the legs when they are resting. It causes them to feel like they cannot get their legs into a comfortable position. When it occurs while they are trying to sleep, it can cause great difficulty with sleeping. This condition is associated with improper amounts of another neurochemical in the brain called dopamine. This is why restless legs syndrome is often treated with medicines designed to treat Parkinson's disease, another disorder due to improper amounts of dopamine in a different part of the brain.

Fibromyalgia can run in families, but doctors do not know whether this is because of environment or genetics. Genetic studies demonstrate that there may be some abnormal genes passed down from parents to children that may cause these neurochemical imbalances to occur. If additional studies confirm these findings, they may represent the best chances of finding better treatments in the future.

## "It is all in your head"

Even with all the sound medical evidence showing that fibromyalgia is a definite medical disorder, some physicians still do not believe fibromyalgia is an actual condition. However, there are volumes of research studies that show numerous abnormalities going on in the bodies of people who have fibromyalgia that explains their increased pain, fatigue, and other symptoms (table 27.3). These tests can only be done in a research setting (instead of in a clinical setting such as the doctor's office) due to their complexity and expense. Going over each of these abnormalities is beyond the scope of this book, but I have listed some of them here to help the person who has fibromyalgia realize that his or her suffering is real.

Why do some doctors still not believe that fibromyalgia is a disorder? Partly it is because of the lack of physical exam, lab, and x-ray abnormalities in fibromyalgia. Since the problem is due to neurochemical imbalances of the nervous system of the body, doctors do not have any special tests to diagnose it. These chemical imbalances are certainly occurring, as proven in research studies, but these types of tests are too complex, expensive, and impractical to do in a doctor's office outside of a research situation. There are no simple blood tests or x-rays to diagnose fibromyalgia.

**Table 27.3** Abnormal Findings in Research Studies of People Who Have Fibromyalgia

- Elevated substance P (a pain neurotransmitter) in the spine (this causes increased pain)
- Alpha waves (wakefulness brain waves) increased during sleep on EEG testing interfering with non-REM sleep (this causes fatigue and probably contributes to difficulty thinking)
- Low cortisol (a steroid released during increased stress) levels
- Decreased growth hormone (which can cause low energy, muscle weakness, difficulty thinking, cold intolerance)
- Low blood testosterone and DHEA levels (male hormones that help with muscle strength and energy)
- Lower estrogen levels (this may increase pain)
- Lower levels of serotonin (this can cause increased pain and depression symptoms)
- Genetic abnormalities that cause low serotonin levels, increased pain, and increased depression
- Increased inositol and glutamate levels in the amygdala of the brain (as shown in MRIs)
- Increased blood flow in areas of the brain responsible for pain perception (as demonstrated in brain imaging)
- Increased activation of pain perception areas of the brain (as shown in MRIs)

If you have fibromyalgia, it absolutely is a medical condition proven through very good medical studies. It is "in your head" in that there are significant problems with the way the pain nerves of the brain are functioning, but you are not imagining it or making it up. My best advice to the person who has had a bad experience with a doctor, who has told her that she is making it up or that it is all in her head, is to find a doctor who is familiar with the medical studies of fibromyalgia and knows how to diagnose and treat it.

## How Doctors Diagnose Fibromyalgia

The doctor's first clue that a patient may have fibromyalgia is from her or his history. Often the person who has fibromyalgia will have pain in multiple areas of the body, have difficulty with fatigue, have non-restorative sleep, or have difficulty with memory and concentration. However, people who have severe arthritis in many different areas, uncontrolled thyroid problems, infections, metabolic disorders, and other conditions can have similar symptoms. Therefore, additional testing is usually needed in the person who has these problems. The doctor's first order of business is to do a physical examination. If the person who has a lot of pain has arthritis as the cause, then the physical exam will show evidence of the arthritis affecting the joints; the affected joints are tender and swollen. However, in the person who has fibromyalgia, there will also be tenderness in places away from the joints. In fact, this is one of the most helpful clues to the doctor in figuring out whether someone just has arthritis or whether he or she has arthritis plus fibromyalgia. The person who has just arthritis will have tender joints on examination, while the person who has arthritis plus fibromyalgia will have tenderness not only in and around the joints but also in the muscles, on the skin, and on top of bones, ligaments, and tendons that are away from the joints. People who have fibromyalgia and no arthritis can have tenderness in the joints as well as these other places as well.

In 1990, the American College of Rheumatology came out with classification criteria for fibromyalgia. These criteria were established to ensure that doctors in different medical centers and in different parts of the world were including similar types of patients in fibromyalgia research studies and were diagnosing fibromyalgia patients in the same way. To have a diagnosis of fibromyalgia with these criteria, the person has to have had pain on both sides of the body, above and below the waist, for at least three months. In addition, eighteen tender points on the body were defined (figure 27.1). If a person also has eleven tender points in addition to having the chronic, widespread pain, then she or he has fibromyalgia.

This set of classification criteria has been very useful for doctors to use in diagnosing fibromyalgia because most people with fibromyalgia do satisfy the criteria. However, these criteria are not foolproof. In fact, about 15% of patients who have fibromyalgia do not fulfill the criteria. For example, the tender points can fluctuate from day to day. Some days a person may have a lot of pain with tender points in multiple areas of the body and therefore easily have eleven tender points or more, while on good days she or he may have hardly any tender points. Not everyone who has fibromyalgia will have pain all over the body; some will have pain mainly on the right side of the body or

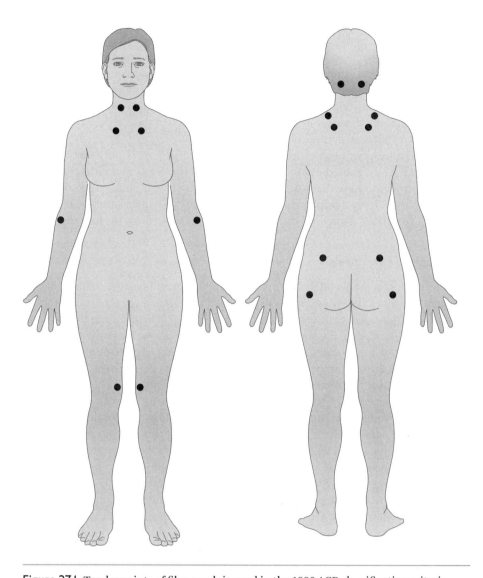

**Figure 27.1** Tender points of fibromyalgia used in the 1990 ACR classification criteria

the left side, or in the back, neck, and arms instead of in the legs. Although they have fibromyalgia, they would not meet these particular criteria.

Nonetheless, testing for these areas of tenderness on exam is very important in diagnosing fibromyalgia, and most doctors experienced in treating fibromyalgia will look for their presence. It is important to realize, though, that a person can have fibromyalgia and have less than eleven of these tender points.

Since not everyone with fibromyalgia will have eleven or more tender points on examination, fibromyalgia experts have established an additional set of diagnostic crite-

415

ria for fibromyalgia. This new set of criteria is the self-test presented at the beginning of this chapter. Currently, doctors use both the older classification criteria of 1990 as well as the newer diagnostic criteria to help them diagnose fibromyalgia.

After a physical examination, a doctor will next most likely do some blood tests and possibly some x-rays to look for other causes of diffuse body pain. Some medical conditions can act exactly like fibromyalgia. An example is a disease called polymyalgia rheumatica, which causes severe pain in older people. When these types of conditions are identified and treated, then the pain should resolve.

Then there are other people where another disorder (such as SLE or other causes of arthritis) may be diagnosed. However, if this disorder is treated appropriately and the person continues to have the widespread pain and the tender points, then he or she most likely has fibromyalgia plus this other disorder. In these situations, it is important that the doctors treat all medical conditions in addition to treating the fibromyalgia.

## Treatment of Fibromyalgia

Many therapies can be useful in treating the symptoms of fibromyalgia (table 27.4). The first area of business when a person is diagnosed with fibromyalgia is education about the disorder. Your reading this chapter will do a great deal in helping your understanding fibromyalgia, its diagnosis, and its treatment. Studies show that patients who have fibromyalgia and are educated about the disorder are more likely to follow their doctors' recommendations for therapy and have better improvements in their symptoms. Unfortunately, fibromyalgia tends to be a chronic disease, meaning that it lasts for years if not the rest of the person's life, and there is no cure for fibromyalgia. The person who has fibromyalgia usually has to deal with discomfort, fatigue, and insomnia in one degree or another for a long time. Simply realizing this fact can go a long way. It is important that people who have fibromyalgia direct their efforts toward learning how to change their lifestyle and expectations in dealing with chronic pain instead of constantly seeking a cure. Since no cure for fibromyalgia exists, the constant search for one by an afflicted individual can just cause increased disappointment, anxiety, and even more pain. There are fibromyalgia educational groups that can help people who have fibromyalgia learn how to deal with the many problems fibromyalgia can cause as well as keep them up on the latest in research and treatments. One of these groups is the National Fibromyalgia Association (www.fmaware.org).

Numerous studies show that exercise is important in decreasing the symptoms of fibromyalgia. Exercise most likely helps in many different ways, including reconditioning the muscles of the body, helping to relieve stress and depression, helping with relaxation, and even reversing some of the neurotransmitter imbalances seen in fibromyalgia. It is a huge mistake to think that simply taking medicines for fibromyalgia or taking a pain pill is going to do the trick. If you truly want to get better from your fibromyalgia, then you absolutely must force yourself to exercise.

The resistance to exercising is understandable. When you are in such severe pain, have muscle spasms, and have severe fatigue, how can you possibly exercise? That is the last thing on someone's mind when she has severe fibromyalgia symptoms. She typically will say, "I can't exercise" or "I feel worse when I exercise." I really do not know the best way for people to get over this barrier to exercising. However, I can say from

**Table 27.4** Treatments Used for Fibromyalgia

Education

Exercise

    Regular low-impact aerobic exercise

    Stretching exercises

    Tai chi

    Yoga

Measures to improve energy levels (table 6.1)

Improvement of sleep hygiene (table 6.2)

Treatment for conditions that make fibromyalgia worse

    Take the self-survey for depression (table 13.4).

    Take the self-survey for anxiety disorder (table 13.2).

    Take the self-survey for sleep apnea (table 6.3).

Improvement of memory skills (table 13.3)

Psychological therapies

    Cognitive behavioral therapy

    Psychotherapy and counseling aimed at areas of previous abuse

Acupuncture?

Medications

personal experience with my own patients that when people finally force themselves to exercise on a regular basis, they typically improve. Many people will in fact have an "ah, hah" moment when they realize that they do feel better overall when they exercise regularly compared to times in their life when they do not exercise.

You usually are not harming or injuring your joints and muscles when you exercise. When they first start to exercise, most people will typically ache. It is easy to conclude that you are injuring yourself, give in to the pain, and stop exercising when you feel this. If you are fearful that you may be hurting or injuring yourself, it can be helpful to work with your doctor, a physical therapist, or a personal trainer in a gym to ensure you are using proper exercise techniques. As long as you are exercising properly, you need to force yourself to do the exercises.

Ease yourself into an exercise program slowly. Make sure to do proper warm up and cool down exercises. Start with exercising just a little bit at a time and gradually increase the duration and exertion over time. For example, do not jump right in and try to do a thirty-minute aerobics class or the stair climber machine for thirty minutes. Instead, you should consider participating in a low-impact aerobics class or water exercise class designed for people who have arthritis initially, or do the stair climber machine for just five minutes at a time initially. Do this on a regular basis, then every few weeks you can increase the amount of time and exertion you put into the exercise.

A good exercise regimen for someone who has fibromyalgia should consist of some sort of aerobics exercise five days a week for about thirty minutes at a time. As mentioned above, you should first start with just a few minutes at a time and very slowly work your way up to the thirty minutes. Examples of appropriate aerobics activities include water exercises, low-impact aerobics classes, aerobics classes designed for people with arthritis, elliptical climber machines, stationary bicycle (especially a recumbent bike if you have back problems), treadmill, and brisk walking.

Incorporate gentle stretching exercises into your routine as well. Fibromyalgia typically will cause tightness and spasm of the muscles; therefore, it is very important to gently stretch them and improve flexibility and range of motion. This can help to lessen the spasms and pain. Proper stretching techniques can be learned from a physical therapist (ask your doctor for a referral), a personal trainer, or an exercise instructor at a gym.

Tai chi (also known as tai chi chuan) can also benefit people who have fibromyalgia. Studies looking at fibromyalgia patients who do tai chi twice a week have shown that it can decrease pain and improve sleep and energy. Tai chi is a Chinese low-stress form of martial arts that combines gentle movements of the body with using the mind to control body movements and help with relaxation. It is becoming popular for health reasons and it is becoming easier to find classes at exercise centers, hospitals, martial arts clinics, and seniors' centers. Tai chi is best performed in a group setting, although videos for doing tai chi at home are also available.

Yoga is another popular form of activity, originally from India, which incorporates combinations of various body movements and poses in conjunction with breathing and relaxation techniques. It is helpful in decreasing the severity of pain, fatigue, and moodiness of fibromyalgia as well as aiding the person in learning to accept and live with daily discomfort. Just as with tai chi, yoga classes are becoming popular and easier to find even in rural areas.

Most people who have fibromyalgia have a sleep quality problem where their brains do not go into the deepest parts of sleep while sleeping. This problem accentuates the severity of their fatigue and pain. Therefore, it is essential that all people who have fibromyalgia abide by proper sleep hygiene (table 6.2) even if they feel they are sleeping OK. You should also take the surveys to see if you may have sleep apnea (table 6.3), depression (table 13.4), or anxiety disorder (table 13.2) since people who have fibromyalgia have an increased chance of having these problems. It is very difficult to treat the pain, fatigue, and other problems of fibromyalgia if these problems are not addressed and treated as well. If you score high on these tests, make sure to show the results to your doctor to see if you have these problems and make sure you get proper treatment for them. Memory and concentration problems ("fibro fog") are also very difficult in many people who have fibromyalgia. Using measures to help with memory (table 13.3) can be beneficial in dealing with these problems.

Numerous psychological therapies can also be helpful when dealing with the problems of fibromyalgia. Do not let the term "psychological" turn you off to these recommendations. "Psychological" does not refer to being crazy or anything like that. Rather, it refers to techniques often employed by psychology experts in helping people learn how to decrease pain by using the power of their minds. It is amazing how strong the mind is when it comes to dealing with pain. I see this every day in my clinic. Rheumatologists frequently give cortisone injections into the joints of patients. There are patients who naturally prepare themselves mentally to relax and who subsequently say that they feel little to no discomfort during the procedure. Then there are patients who work themselves up mentally before they are even touched with a needle. They are visibly tense, already saying that it is going to hurt and miserable even before anything is done. In their defense, this latter group of patients may have had some sort of bad experience in the past, or may be naturally anxious and tense. Patients in this latter group can learn to calm down, relax, and use mental imagery (taking themselves somewhere pleasant in their minds) to make the injection a more comfortable experience. Those who force themselves to use these psychological relaxation techniques are usually very surprised at how little discomfort they feel, while those who cannot (or will not) do them usually have a very unpleasant, painful experience.

These are simple examples of psychological techniques that can be used to help with pain. They belong to a large group of psychological techniques called cognitive behavioral therapy. Cognitive behavioral therapy consists of a number of different psychological practices people can learn to do to lessen pain. They include learning to use mental imagery, relaxation, self-hypnosis, and stress reduction techniques. Biofeedback is another example of a type of cognitive behavioral therapy. A biofeedback specialist (often a psychologist) attaches instruments that measure brain electrical activity, heart rate, muscle tension, and body temperature to different parts of a person's body. He then helps the person learn to have her or his own mind decrease stress and pain perception in the body. Unfortunately, insurance does not often pay for these types of treatments, although they can have a long-lasting, beneficial effect on dealing with the problems of fibromyalgia. It can be well worth the price to consider seeing someone who specializes in cognitive behavioral therapy techniques for chronic pain.

Other forms of psychological therapy can be helpful and are very important for the person who has had significant abuse in the past. Sexual, mental, and physical abuse can all cause significant problems in some people with fibromyalgia. It is amazing what the mind can do to try to suppress and deal with a history of abuse. The mind cannot function without neurotransmitters signaling the nerves of the brain to think the way they do. Abnormalities of these neurotransmitters in people who have a history of abuse can result in the problems seen in fibromyalgia. In this scenario, it is extremely important to get help from someone who is an expert in the field of abuse. Experts who can provide psychological counseling and psychotherapy to deal with suppressed abuse include psychiatrists, psychologists, and some sociologists. If someone who has a history of abuse and fibromyalgia does not undertake this form of therapy, but instead tries to rely on pain medicines for fibromyalgia, he or she rarely gets significantly better.

I put a question mark next to "acupuncture" in the table about therapies for fibromyalgia (table 27.4) because it really has not been proven beneficial yet. There have been studies addressing this form of therapy, however, the best-run studies failed to show any significant improvement. Acupuncture is safe to undergo and will not make lupus or fibromyalgia worse. It can be expensive, however, and usually has to be done several times a week over a prolonged period. There is also insufficient evidence (research studies) to support biofeedback (as discussed above), hypnosis, massage therapy, salt/mineral baths, and therapeutic ultrasound. However, this lack of evidence may be because large, adequate studies have not been done yet to see if they work for fibromyalgia.

## Medicines Used to Treat Fibromyalgia

Numerous medications can be used in the treatment of fibromyalgia. The most effective ones work by changing the abnormal chemical imbalances occurring in the disorder. Since these are similar to the chemical imbalances that occur in depression, many of these medications are also antidepressants. This is an important point for people who have fibromyalgia to realize. Some people become upset when their doctor prescribes an antidepressant, concluding that he or she thinks it is all in their head or that they are depressed. It is true that 30% to 50% of people with fibromyalgia also have depression, but that is not why these medications are prescribed for most people who have fibromyalgia.

Another group of medicines that can be helpful is anti-seizure medications. Seizures are a problem where the nerves of the brain are overactive and can cause uncontrolled body movements. These anti-seizure medicines work by calming down the activity of the nerves. This is also how they can help with fibromyalgia by calming down the activity of the pain nerves of the brain. Therefore, you will more likely than not be treated with an antidepressant or an anti-seizure medicine for your fibromyalgia; your doctor is not making a mistake by giving you this prescription.

None of these medications has been proven better than the others, so choosing the correct medication for a patient can sometimes be difficult. Doctors do not know the best choice for any particular person. However, some medications have certain beneficial effects that may work in some patients and may be better choices (table 27.5). There have not been enough comparison studies to help physicians decide which medicine is best to use in which patients overall.

Three medications are FDA-approved to treat fibromyalgia: pregabalin (Lyrica), duloxetine (Cymbalta), and milnacipran (Savella). Although these are the only three medicines specifically approved by the FDA, this does not mean that they are any better than the others are. Seeking FDA approval is a very lengthy and expensive process that usually can only be afforded by pharmaceutical companies that are producing new medications. These companies have to recuperate the expensive research costs put into developing these medications. The medications that are not FDA-approved have cheaper generic equivalents. It is too expensive for makers of generic medications to do research studies to try to obtain FDA approval. Generic drug companies would never regain the money they would have to put into the FDA approval process.

When a medication is prescribed for a disease (like fibromyalgia) although that medicine is not FDA approved for that disorder, doctors say it is being prescribed "off label." This does not mean that off label medicines do not work as well as the more expensive FDA-approved medicines. It all comes down to the business side of developing medications. Prescribing medications off label is a very common practice in treating rheumatologic diseases. The vast majority of medicines that rheumatologists prescribe to treat diseases (especially SLE) are used off label. Although they are prescribed off label, they have been shown to be effective in treating fibromyalgia by research studies that were done after the drug's initial FDA approval process. For example, amitriptyline is FDA-approved as an antidepressant. However, numerous studies have shown that it can be effective in treating the pain and insomnia of fibromyal-

**Table 27.5** Possible Benefits of Some Fibromyalgia Medicines over Others

| Drug | Pros | Cons |
|------|------|------|
| amitriptyline (Elavil) | May be the most helpful for insomnia, improving energy, and decreasing pain, and is inexpensive. Usually taken one time a day (usually night time). | Numerous potential side effects (table 27.6). Not tolerated well by older individuals. |
| pregabalin (Lyrica) and gabapentin (Neurontin) | Possibly a good second choice when insomnia is a big problem if amitriptyline does not work. Gabapentin has a generic, less expensive form. | Weight gain and difficulty thinking occur more often. May not be as good for pain as amitriptyline. Pregabalin is expensive. Most often prescribed two to three times a day. |
| duloxetine (Cymbalta) | May be better for pain than milnacipran. May be a good second choice to help with energy levels if amitriptyline does not work. Usually taken once a day. | May not be as good for pain as amitriptyline. More commonly causes headaches, nausea, and diarrhea. Cymbalta is expensive. |
| milnacipran (Savella) | May be a good second choice to help with energy levels if amitriptyline does not work. | May not be as good for pain as amitriptyline, pregabalin, or duloxetine. More commonly causes headaches, nausea, and diarrhea. Savella is expensive. |

gia as well. Now many fibromyalgia experts consider it as one of the initial therapies of choice for people who have fibromyalgia. It is markedly cheaper, works just as well (some feel it works better), and is just as safe as the three FDA-approved medications for fibromyalgia.

Most arthritis pain medications, other than tramadol (Ultracet, Ultram), have not been shown to be effective in treating the pain of fibromyalgia. In addition, most fibromyalgia experts recommend not using scheduled opioid medications, commonly called narcotics, as they only cause addiction without providing significant long-term benefits. In this section on medications for fibromyalgia, I only discuss medications that have shown significant benefit in research studies.

Often, fibromyalgia can be very hard to treat. Many people have less pain, insomnia, and fatigue when taking these medications (along with doing the recommendations in table 27.4). However, there are people who do not get much benefit from the medicines. In addition, one medication may work fantastic in one person but do nothing at all or cause side effects in another person. Therefore, doctors may need to try various medicines until the best medication is found. Sometimes a combination of medicines helps since they work through different mechanisms. For example, taking an antidepressant at night and an anti-seizure medicine in the morning may work great in one person, while using two different antidepressants that work in two different ways may be better in another person.

To try to improve the chemical imbalances responsible for causing the symptoms of fibromyalgia, the medications must be taken on a regular basis all the time exactly as prescribed (the only exception to this is tramadol, which works quickly, but even it works best when taken regularly). To improve the chemical imbalances, it can take anywhere from three to eight weeks to get the benefit of the medicine. These medications do not work when taken on an as needed basis. In addition, most of these medicines are started out at low doses then increased in dosage gradually. It is not uncommon for a person who has fibromyalgia to stop taking a medication soon after starting it because it "didn't work." Usually doctors want patients to keep taking their medications because if they are not any better after one or two months (the length of time it usually takes these medicines to work), they usually plan on increasing the dose. The only time you should stop the prescribed medicine is if you develop side effects. If you develop side effects, you should contact your doctor. Some of these medicines need to be decreased gradually to prevent withdrawal symptoms. Withdrawal symptoms occur when the body is used to taking a medicine, then develops unpleasant side effects (such as nausea, insomnia, sweating, moodiness, stomach upset, aches and pains) if it is stopped too quickly.

Unfortunately, studies have shown that a large number of patients are noncompliant with taking their medication either on purpose or by accident. A 2004 study showed that this occurred in 47% of women who had fibromyalgia. This is one of the biggest reasons for not getting better with fibromyalgia. Another big mistake people who have fibromyalgia make is to have high expectations for the medicine to help yet not put any effort into exercise, proper sleep habits, and other advice. People who are most successful with managing their fibromyalgia not only take their medications regularly and consistently, but also exercise regularly, work on sleep hygiene, and practice relaxation techniques as well as the other principles discussed earlier in this chapter. This absolutely requires a lot of work, but with due diligence, most people are able get some improvement in their symptoms.

There are, of course, people who have severe symptoms who have tried everything and still are greatly affected by debilitating pain, profound fatigue, memory problems, and insomnia from this disorder. This fact, along with the fact that most patients must deal with pain from fibromyalgia for a long time, illustrates the great unmet need for better therapies to treat it. There is a lot of research currently being done in this field, and I certainly hope that it results in better therapies that work in more people. Although many medications have been used to treat fibromyalgia, including some experimental therapies, I discuss the most widely recommended medicines in this chapter.

## Tricyclic Antidepressants

The tricyclic antidepressants (table 27.6) have been around for a long time and are some of the most common medicines used to treat fibromyalgia. Amitriptyline has been the most studied and is probably the most prescribed of this group of medicines for fibromyalgia. They are generally given in much lower doses than those used to treat depression, and are usually best taken two to three hours before bed each night.

*Generic available*: Yes.

*How TCAs work*: TCAs increase levels of the neurotransmitters serotonin and nor-

Table 27.6  Tricyclic Antidepressants (TCAs)

| Generic Name | Brand Name | Usual Doses Used | Maximum Recommended in Geriatric Individuals | Special Situation When Used for Fibromyalgia |
|---|---|---|---|---|
| amitriptyline | Available only as generic | 10–150 mg | 150 mg | Most-studied TCA |
| nortriptyline | Pamelor | 10–150 mg | 150 mg | Often better tolerated by older people |
| desipramine | Norpramin | 10–150 mg | 100 mg | Do not take if you have a family history of heart disease |
| amoxapine | Only available in generic | 25–200 mg | 150 mg | Used more for depression than fibromyalgia |
| clomipramine | Anafranil | 25–100 mg | 100 mg | Can be used for chronic pain |
| doxepin | Silenor | 3–150 mg | 75 mg | Can be used for chronic pain |
| protriptyline | Vivactil | 5–60 mg | 20 mg | Used more often for depression than fibromyalgia |
| trimipramine | Surmontil | 25–200 mg | 100 mg | Used more often for depression than fibromyalgia |

epinephrine. This can help decrease pain nerve pathway activity in the brain. They also help with sleep.

*What benefits to expect from TCAs*: TCAs are slow working medications usually taking three to six weeks for the full benefit at any particular dose. They can help decrease pain, fatigue, and insomnia from fibromyalgia.

*How TCAs are taken*: TCAs are best taken starting at a low dose two to three hours before bedtime each night. If taken too soon before bedtime, they often will cause a hung over, groggy sensation in the morning.

*If you miss a dose of your medicine*: If you miss a dose of your TCA, it is usually best not to take it and wait until the next evening to take your next dose at the usual scheduled time if you typically get very drowsy from taking it. However, if you tolerate your TCA well, and it does not tend to cause you side effects such as drowsiness or dizziness, you could take one-half to a full amount of your dose right before you go to bed (instead of two hours before bed). However, you have an increased chance of feeling groggy or hung over if you take it right before bedtime. Consult with your prescribing doctor to double-check these instructions, but these guidelines will suffice for most people.

*Alcohol/food/herbal interactions with TCAs*: Do not drink alcohol, which will increase side effects of drowsiness, dizziness, and difficulty thinking while on these medicines.

Do not eat grapefruit or drink grapefruit juice, which can increase blood levels of TCAs, causing increased side effects.

Avoid valerian, St. John's wort, kava kava, and gotu kola, which can increase drowsiness when taken with TCAs.

*Potential side effects of TCAs*: The side effects that occur with the TCAs have to do with how they change the levels of neurotransmitters (table 27.7). Norepinephrine and serotonin not only occur in pain and brain nerves, but also are found in numerous other nerves throughout the body. This includes those used to maintain blood pressure, heart function, vision, sweating, urination, sexual function, and numerous others. The vast majority of these side effects occur at high doses and less commonly at lower doses. Since usually the lowest dosages of TCAs are used in people who have fibromyalgia (as opposed to the high doses that are used more to treat depression), most people who have fibromyalgia do not get the majority of these side effects.

The most common side effects are dizziness, grogginess, and dry mouth. These are particularly more common among older people. If any of these side effects occur, let your doctor know right away as the dose can be decreased or the medicine can be stopped completely if needed. It is usually best to take the medication two or three hours before going to bed. This decreases the likelihood of having grogginess and a "hung over" feeling when you wake up. Make sure that you are getting about eight hours of sleep when you take these medicines. For example, do not take the medicine at 10:00 PM to go to bed at midnight expecting to get up at 5:00 AM for work (only five hours of sleep). You must become serious in changing lifestyle habits to fit in that full eight hours of sleep. If you take a TCA too close to bedtime, or if you only get five hours of sleep or so, you most likely will not tolerate the medicine.

*What needs to be monitored while taking TCAs*: If you are over 40 years old, make sure that you have had an ECG to make sure your heart is OK before taking a TCA.

*Reasons not to take TCAs (contraindications or precautions)*:

• If you have any form of heart disease.

• Desipramine (Norpramin), in particular, should not be taken if you have a family history of any type of heart disease.

• If you have a history of seizures.

• Inform your doctor if you have closed-angle glaucoma (also called angle-closure and narrow-angle glaucoma) before taking the medicine. Note that most people with glaucoma have open-angle glaucoma. It is safe to take this medicine if you have open-angle glaucoma. It is also usually safe to take this medicine if your closed-angle glaucoma has already been surgically treated (ask your eye doctor).

• Inform your doctor if you take an MAOI antidepressant. The combination could cause deadly side effects.

• Do not plan to start taking TCAs if you are going to drive, climb, or use machinery until you know how you react to the medicine to make sure it does not make you too drowsy or cause you to have difficulty thinking.

**Table 27.7**  Potential Side Effects of TCAs

|  | *Incidence* | *Side Effect Therapy* |
|---|---|---|
| **Nuisance side effects** | | |
| Dry mouth | Common | Decrease dose or stop medicine. |
| Grogginess | Common | Decrease dose or stop medicine. |
| Difficulty thinking, confusion | Common | Decrease dose or stop medicine. |
| Dizziness (can be mild to severe) | Common | Decrease dose or stop medicine. |
| Fluid retention | Common | Decrease dose or stop medicine. |
| Weight gain | Common | Decrease dose or stop medicine. |
| Blurred vision | Common | Decrease dose or stop medicine. |
| Sexual dysfunction, de-creased libido and arousal, difficulty achieving orgasm | Common | Decrease dose or stop medicine. |
| Sweating | Common | Decrease dose or stop medicine. |
| Heart palpitations, fast heart rate | Uncommon | Decrease dose or stop medicine. |
| Tremor, shaking | Uncommon | Decrease dose or stop medicine. |
| Difficulty urinating | Uncommon | Decrease dose or stop medicine. |
| **Serious side effects** | | |
| Severe dizziness | Uncommon | Decrease dose or stop medicine. |
| Heart rhythm problems at high doses | Uncommon (usually small doses are used for fibromyalgia) | Stop medicine. |
| Hepatitis | Rare | Stop medicine. |
| Seizures at high doses | Uncommon | Seek medical attention immediately. |
| Closed-angle glaucoma worsening | Uncommon | Seek medical attention immediately. |
| Death | Very rare with fibromyalgia where low doses are used. | |

Side effect incidence key (approximations, as side effects can vary widely study to study):  rare < 1% occurrence; uncommon 1%–5% occurrence;  common > 5% occurrence

*While taking TCAs*:

- If you develop heart palpitations, fast heart rate, chest pain, or shortness of breath, call your doctor immediately.

*Pregnancy and breast-feeding while taking TCAs*: TCAs have not been linked to birth defects. However, they may potentially cause withdrawal symptoms in the newborn baby while the drug levels in the baby decrease after birth. The preferred TCAs to use during pregnancy are nortriptyline and desipramine as they are less likely to cause any adverse effects on the newborn baby. However, for insomnia, low doses of amitriptyline and imipramine are recommended. Amitriptyline is often the most effective TCA for fibromyalgia. Higher doses of TCAs may be required during pregnancy due to increased metabolism during pregnancy.

Small doses of TCAs do enter the breast milk. The American Academy of Pediatrics Committee on Drugs notes that all of these drugs' "effects are unknown" and that they may be "of concern" in breast-feeding. Doxepin should not be taken as there has been a report of side effects in a nursing infant. Studies on amitriptyline, nortriptyline, imipramine, desipramine, and clomipramine have shown no side effects in nursing infants

*Geriatric use of TCAs*: Older people are more sensitive to the side effects of TCAs and usually lower doses should be used, as shown in table 27.6. Nortriptyline is usually the best tolerated and is considered the drug of choice for older people if a TCA is prescribed.

*What to do with TCAs at the time of surgery*: It is important to get specific instructions from your surgeon and anesthesiologist. Some experts recommend stopping tricyclic antidepressants seven to fourteen days before surgery to decrease the risk of heart problems during surgery.

*Patient assistance program for TCAs*: See chapter 42.

*Drug helpline for TCAs*: Unaware of any.

*Website to learn more about TCAs*: Unaware of any.

## Selective Serotonin Reuptake Inhibitors

Selective serotonin reuptake inhibitors (SSRIs for short) are some of the most widely prescribed medications to treat depression (table 27.8). Of the currently available SSRIs in the United States, fluoxetine (Prozac) was the first one to be FDA-approved in December 1987.

*Generic available*: Yes.

*How SSRIs works*: Serotonin is an important neurotransmitter (a chemical released by a nerve to send a message to another nerve). It has many duties to do in the nervous system, one of which is to decrease the amount of pain that the brain is sensing from pain nerves of the body. People who have fibromyalgia have a decreased amount of serotonin in their brains. This lack of serotonin allows pain nerves to tell the brain that there is pain going on in multiple areas of the body even if there is no damage going on at all. This also allows the pain signals that are being sent to the brain appropriately (such as those due to pain from arthritis) to be magnified and not calm down as quickly as they normally would. The chemical serotonin is typically released by a nerve so that it can send a signal or message to another nerve. The nerve that originally

Table 27.8 Selective Serotonin Reuptake Inhibitors (SSRIs) Studied in Fibromyalgia

| Generic Name | Brand Name | Usual Doses Used | Special Situation When Used for Fibromyalgia |
|---|---|---|---|
| Fluoxetine | Prozac | 20–80 mg | Usually doses higher than 20 mg a day are needed for fibromyalgia. |
| Paroxetine | Paxil | 12.5–62.5 mg | Most effective at higher doses. |
| Fluvoxamine | Luvox | 50–100 mg | One study showed it to be as effective as amitriptyline for pain and with less side effects. |
| Citalopram | Celexa | 20–40 mg | Studies are inconsistent on how helpful it is for fibromyalgia. |

produces the serotonin is also reabsorbing (or reuptaking, as the "reuptake" in the name of this group of medications implies) serotonin to recycle it. SSRIs decrease the ability of the nerves to reabsorb (or reuptake) serotonin. This allows more serotonin to build up in the nervous system, which helps to calm down the pain nerve signals to the brain.

*What benefits to expect from SSRIs*: Decreased severity of pain, improved sleep, and better energy level. It usually takes four to eight weeks to achieve these effects at any particular dose.

*How SSRIs are taken*: Varies depending on which one is prescribed. People will often respond differently to different SSRIs. If an SSRI causes drowsiness, it is best to take it at night. If an SSRI causes insomnia, it is best to take it in the morning.

*If you miss a dose of your medicine*: If you miss a dose of your SSRI, it depends on how you react to it and how often you take it that determines what you should do. For example, if you take it every morning and you know that it can cause you to have trouble sleeping if you take it too late in the day, you may want to skip that day's dose if you remember too late in the day. If you usually take it at nighttime because it makes you drowsy when you take it earlier in the day, you may want to skip the dose you missed if you do not realize you missed your nighttime dose until the next morning. If it does not make you drowsy or cause problems with sleeping, you can take it as soon as you realize you missed it on the day you were supposed to take it and then resume your normal dosing schedule the next day. If you take it twice a day and it has been just a few hours since you missed your dose, then take the dose you missed as soon as you realize it and take your next dose at the regularly appointed time. For example, if you take your SSRI at 7:00 AM and 7:00 PM every day and you forget to take your 7:00 AM dose but do not realize it until 10:00 AM, go ahead and take it at 10:00 AM. Then take your 7:00 PM dose at the usual time. However, if you do not realize you missed your morning dose until 2:00 PM, just skip the dose and resume taking your medicine at 7:00 PM. Consult with your prescribing doctor to double-check these instructions, but these guidelines will suffice for most people.

*Alcohol/food/herbal interactions with SSRIs*: Avoid alcohol as it can increase the side effects of SSRIs.

Can be taken with or without food.

Avoid valerian, St. John's wort, SAMe, and kava kava (may increase risk of drowsiness). Avoid alfalfa, anise, bilberry, bladderwrack, bromelain, cat's claw, celery, chamomile, coleus, cordyceps, dong quai, evening primrose, fenugreek, feverfew, garlic, ginger, ginkgo biloba, ginseng (American), ginseng (Panax), ginseng (Siberian), grape seed, green tea, guggul, horse chestnuts, horseradish, licorice, prickly ash, red clover, reishi, SAMe (S-adenosylmethionine), sweet clover, turmeric, and white willow (may cause increased bleeding).

*Potential side effects of SSRIs*: The most common side effects of SSRIs are listed in table 27.9. There are numerous potential side effects to look out for and it is best to get a list of these from your pharmacist. However, it is not uncommon to get a side effect from one SSRI, but not from another. Therefore, if you do not tolerate one SSRI, your doctor may switch to a different one to see if it is tolerable. The side effects are also usually dose dependent, meaning that they are less likely to occur at lower doses. Therefore, lowering the dose of the medicine if a side effect occurs is also a common practice. In addition, it is not uncommon for side effects to be mild and tolerable when the medicine is first started. They then go away the longer the person takes the medication as the body gets used to it. Withdrawal symptoms can occur if the medicine is stopped abruptly; therefore, it is a good idea to decrease the dose slowly if the decision is made to stop it.

A rare side effect called serotonin syndrome can potentially occur when SSRIs are taken along with other medications that are also known to cause this same problem. These include other antidepressants, pain relievers, migraine medicines, illicit drugs such as cocaine and Ecstasy, and the herbal supplement St. John's wort. The symptoms of serotonin syndrome include anxiety, agitation, difficulty thinking, increased sweating, feeling hot, increased heart rate, stomach upset, and muscle spasms. If these symptoms occur, let your doctor know right away. In severe cases, this problem can be potentially deadly.

*What needs to be monitored while taking SSRIs*: Blood tests for kidney function and liver function should be checked before starting SSRIs as sometimes a lower dose of the SSRI may be needed in people who have decreased kidney or liver function. Whether the dose needs to be decreased varies with each medicine. Blood tests are not required after starting these medicines.

*Reasons not to take SSRIs (contraindications or precautions)*:

- Some SSRIs may need to be avoided in people who have severe liver or kidney disease.

- Inform your doctor if you are taking an MAO inhibitor antidepressant, as life-threatening side effects may occur with this combination.

- Inform your doctor if you have closed-angle glaucoma (also called angle-closure and narrow-angle glaucoma) before taking the medicine. Note that most people with glaucoma have open-angle glaucoma. It is safe to take this medicine if you have open-angle glaucoma. It is also usually safe to take this medicine if your closed-angle glaucoma has already been surgically treated (ask your eye doctor).

**Table 27.9**  Potential Side Effects of SSRIs

|  | *Incidence* | *Side Effect Therapy* |
|---|---|---|
| **Nuisance side effects** | | |
| Sexual dysfunction, loss of libido, difficulty with orgasm | Common | Decrease dosage, stop medicine (taper off gradually), or change to a different SSRI. |
| Drowsiness | Common | Take it at bedtime. |
| Weight gain, anxiety, or dizziness | Common | Decrease dosage, stop medicine (taper off gradually), or change to a different SSRI. |
| Insomnia | Common | Take it in the morning. |
| Headaches | Common | Decrease dosage, stop medicine (taper off gradually), or change to a different SSRI. |
| Dry mouth | Common | Decrease dosage, stop medicine (taper off gradually), or change to a different SSRI. |
| Blurred vision, nausea, or rash | Common | Decrease dosage, stop medicine (taper off gradually), or change to a different SSRI. |
| Tremor | Common | Decrease dosage, stop medicine (taper off gradually), or change to a different SSRI. |
| Stomach upset or constipation | Common | Decrease dosage, stop medicine (taper off gradually), or change to a different SSRI. For constipation, try taking Miralax or senna (Senekot) daily. |
| Easy bruising and bleeding | Rare | Decrease dosage, stop medicine (taper off gradually), or change to a different SSRI. |
| **Serious side effects** | | |
| Serotonin syndrome (see the text) | Rare | Seek immediate medical attention. |
| Seizures | Rare | Seek immediate medical attention. |

Side effect incidence key (approximations, as side effects can vary widely study to study): rare < 1% occurrence; uncommon 1%–5% occurrence; common > 5% occurrence

- Inform your doctor if you have bipolar disorder. SSRIs may exacerbate bipolar mania symptoms.

- Do not start using while planning on driving, climbing, or using machinery until you make sure you do not get too drowsy or have difficulty with thinking from the medicine first.

*While taking SSRIs*:

- Inform your doctor if any side effects occur.

- If you are taken off the medicine, it is usually better to taper off it slowly to prevent withdrawal side effects.

*Pregnancy and breast-feeding while taking SSRIs*: SSRIs cross the placenta and enter the baby's body. There are some studies suggesting that paroxetine may increase the risk of heart problems in the fetus (however, this is controversial). Fluoxetine, sertraline, and paroxetine have been associated with possibly increasing the risk of pulmonary hypertension in newborns. Whether SSRIs truly cause birth defects or not is controversial. Many experts regard sertraline as the antidepressant of choice in pregnant women.

They are known to cause potential transient problems in the baby after birth either due to the effect of the medicine itself or due to withdrawal as the drug levels decrease. This may be most evident with fluoxetine, which lasts longer in the body than the others. The benefits of the medicine should be weighed against this potential side effect. SSRIs (especially sertraline) can be taken during pregnancy if there is significant benefit. Discuss this with your doctor.

Enters breast milk (fluoxetine has the highest transmission rate). Use with caution or not at all during breast-feeding.

*Geriatric use of SSRIs*: Usually lower doses are used due to increased risk of side effects in older individuals.

*What to do with SSRIs at the time of surgery*: It is important to get specific instructions from your surgeon and anesthesiologist. SSRIs can potentially cause increased bleeding during surgery and may need to be stopped several weeks before surgery.

*Patient assistance program for SSRIs*: See chapter 42.

*Drug helpline for SSRIs*: Unaware of any.

*Website to learn more about SSRIs*: Unaware of any.

## Dual Uptake Inhibitors

Dual uptake inhibitors are also called serotonin norepinephrine reuptake inhibitors (SNRIs for short) and are classified as antidepressants. Duloxetine (Cymbalta) and milnacipran (Savella) are two of the FDA-approved drugs for the treatment of fibromyalgia. Venlafaxine (Effexor XR) is not formally FDA-approved for fibromyalgia, but there are studies suggesting that it is effective in some people who have fibromyalgia.

*Generic available*: Yes.

*How SNRIs works*: Like SSRIs, SNRIs prevent the reuptake or reabsorption of both serotonin and norepinephrine by nerves in the pain nerve pathways of the body. Serotonin and norepinephrine are important neurotransmitters (chemicals released by nerves to send messages to other nerves). They have many duties to do in the nervous system, one of which is to decrease the amount of pain that the brain is sensing from pain nerves of the body. People who have fibromyalgia have a decreased amount of serotonin and norepinephrine in their brains. The lack of these chemicals allows pain nerves to tell the brain that there is pain going on in multiple areas of the body even if there is no damage going on at all. This lack of serotonin and norepinephrine also allows the pain signals that are being sent to the brain appropriately (such as from the pain of arthritis) to be magnified and not calmed down as quickly as they normally would.

The chemicals serotonin and norepinephrine are typically released by nerves so that they can send signals or messages to other nerves. The nerves that originally produce the serotonin and norepinephrine also reabsorb (or reuptake, as the "reuptake" in the name of this group of medications implies) these neurotransmitters to recycle them. SNRIs decrease the ability of the nerves to reabsorb (or reuptake) both serotonin and norepinephrine. This allows more of these chemicals to build up in the nervous system, which helps to calm down the pain nerve signals to the brain.

*What benefits to expect from SNRIs*: Decreased severity of pain, improved sleep, and better energy level. It usually takes four to eight weeks to achieve these effects at any particular dose.

*How SNRIs are taken*: Varies depending on which one is prescribed. Everyone responds differently to them. Cymbalta is usually best taken right after the evening dinner; however, if it causes difficulty sleeping, it should be taken after breakfast.

*If you miss a dose of your medicine*: If you miss a dose of your SNRI, it depends on how you react to it and how often you take it that determines what you should do. For example, if you take it every morning and you know that it can cause you to have trouble sleeping if you take it too late in the day, you may want to skip that day's dose if you remember too late in the day. If you usually take it at nighttime because it makes you drowsy when you take it earlier in the day, you may want to skip the dose you missed if you do not realize you missed your nighttime dose until the next morning after you wake up. If it does not make you drowsy or cause problems with sleeping, you can take it as soon as you realize you missed it on the day you were supposed to take it and then resume your normal dosing schedule the next day. If you take it twice a day and it has been just a few hours since you missed your dose, then take the dose you missed as soon as you realize it and take your next dose at the regularly appointed time. For example, if you take your SNRI at 7:00 AM and 7:00 PM every day and you forget to take your 7:00 AM dose but do not realize it until 10:00 AM, go ahead and take it at 10:00 AM. Then take your 7:00 PM dose at the usual time. However, if you do not realize you missed your morning dose until 2:00 PM, just skip the dose and resume taking your medicine at 7:00 PM. Consult with your prescribing doctor to double-check these instructions, but these guidelines will suffice for most people.

*Alcohol/food/herbal interactions with SNRIs*: Avoid alcohol as it can increase the side effects of SNRIs.

Can be taken with or without food.

Avoid valerian, St. John's wort, SAMe, kava kava, tryptophan, and gotu kola, which can increase side effects from these medicines.

*Potential side effects of SNRIs*: The most common side effects of SNRIs are listed in table 27.10. There are numerous potential side effects to look out for and it is best to get a list of these from your pharmacist. However, it is not uncommon to get a side effect from one of the SNRIs, but not from another. Therefore, if you do not tolerate one SNRI, it is not unreasonable for your doctor to switch to a different one to see if it is tolerable. The side effects are also usually dose dependent, meaning that they are less likely to occur at lower doses. Therefore, lowering the dose of the medicine if a side effect occurs is a common practice. In addition, it is not uncommon for side effects to be mild and tolerable when the medicine is first started. They then go away the longer the person takes the medication as the body gets used to it. Withdrawal symptoms can occur if the medicine is stopped abruptly; therefore, it is a good idea to decrease the dose slowly if the decision is made to stop it.

A rare side effect called serotonin syndrome can potentially occur when SNRIs are taken along with other medications that are also known to cause this same problem. These include other antidepressants, pain relievers, migraine medicines, illicit drugs such as cocaine and Ecstasy, and the herbal supplement St. John's wort. The symptoms of serotonin syndrome include anxiety, agitation, difficulty thinking, increased sweating, feeling hot, increased heart rate, stomach upset, and muscle spasms. If these symptoms occur, let your doctor know right away. In severe cases, this problem can be potentially deadly.

*What needs to be monitored while taking SNRIs*:

• Blood tests for kidney function and liver function should be checked before starting SNRIs as sometimes a lower dose of the SNRI might be needed in people who have decreased kidney or liver function. Whether the dose has to be decreased varies with each medicine.

• Blood pressure, blood glucose, and cholesterol levels should be monitored.

• Inform your physician if you have ever had a seizure.

*Reasons not to take SNRIs (contraindications or precautions)*:

• Some SNRIs may need to be avoided in people who have severe liver or kidney disease.

• Inform your doctor if you are taking an MAO inhibitor antidepressant as life-threatening side effects may occur with this combination.

• Inform your doctor if you have closed-angle glaucoma (also called angle-closure and narrow-angle glaucoma) before taking the medicine. Note that most people with glaucoma have open-angle glaucoma. It is safe to take this medicine if you have open-angle glaucoma. It is also usually safe to take this medicine if your closed-angle glaucoma has already been surgically treated (ask your eye doctor).

• Inform your doctor if you have bipolar disorder. SNRIs may exacerbate bipolar mania symptoms.

• Do not start using while planning on driving, climbing, or using machinery until you make sure you do not get too drowsy or have difficulty with thinking from the medicine first.

**Table 27.10** Potential Side Effects of SNRIs

|  | Incidence | Side Effect Therapy |
|---|---|---|
| **Nuisance side effects** | | |
| Nausea | Common | Decrease dosage, stop medicine (taper off gradually), or change to a different SNRI. |
| Dry mouth | Common | Decrease dosage, stop medicine (taper off gradually), or change to a different SNRI. |
| Constipation or diarrhea | Common | Decrease dosage, stop medicine (taper off gradually), or change to a different SNRI. Over-the-counter Miralax or senna (Senekot) can be taken daily to combat constipation. |
| Upset stomach | Common | Decrease dosage, stop medicine (taper off gradually), or change to a different SNRI. |
| Headaches | Common | Decrease dosage, stop medicine (taper off gradually), or change to a different SNRI. |
| Nervousness and tremors | Common | Decrease dosage, stop medicine (taper off gradually), or change to a different SNRI. |
| Insomnia or drowsiness | Common | First try taking the medicine in the morning if it causes insomnia, or taking it at night if it causes drowsiness. Also can decrease dosage, stop medicine (taper off gradually), or change to a different SNRI. |
| Dizziness | Common | Decrease dosage, stop medicine (taper off gradually), or change to a different SNRI. |
| Sweating | Common | Decrease dosage, stop medicine (taper off gradually), or change to a different SNRI. |
| Increased bleeding or bruising | Uncommon | Decrease dosage, stop medicine (taper off gradually), or stop any unnecessary blood thinners. |
| Elevated liver enzyme blood tests | Uncommon | Decrease dosage or stop medicine (taper off gradually). |
| Elevated blood pressure, sugar levels, and cholesterol | Uncommon | Decrease dosage or stop medicine (taper off gradually). |
| Withdrawal symptoms when stopped | Uncommon | Taper off dose slowly when discontinuing it. |
| **Serious side effects** | | |
| Serotonin syndrome (see the text) | Rare | Seek immediate medical attention. |

433

**Table 27.10** (*Continued*)

|  | Incidence | Side Effect Therapy |
|---|---|---|
| Passing out (syncope) | Rare | Seek immediate medical attention. |
| Worsening of narrow-angle glaucoma | Common in people who have untreated narrow-angle glaucoma | Should not be taken if you have narrow-angle glaucoma that has not been treated. |
| Seizures | Rare | Seek immediate medical attention. |

Side effect incidence key (approximations, as side effects can vary widely study to study): rare < 1% occurrence; uncommon 1%–5% occurrence; common > 5% occurrence

*While taking SNRIs*:

• Inform your doctor if any side effects occur.

*Pregnancy and breast-feeding while taking SNRIs*: SNRIs cross the placenta to enter the baby's body and are known to cause problems in the baby after birth either due to the effect of the medicine itself or due to withdrawal as the drug levels decrease. As of the time of this writing, there have been no reports of birth defects from SNRI use during pregnancy. Discuss with your doctor whether the benefit of taking the drug during pregnancy outweighs this possible problem.

Enters breast milk. It is recommended not to use SNRIs during breast-feeding.

*Geriatric use of SNRIs*: Usually lower doses are used due to increased risk of side effects in older individuals.

*What to do with SNRIs at the time of surgery*: It is important to get specific instructions from your surgeon and anesthesiologist. SNRIs can usually be continued up to the day before surgery.

*Patient assistance program for SNRIs*: For Savella call 1-800-851-0758. For Cymbalta call 1-855-559-8783. Also see chapter 42.

*Drug helpline for SNRIs*: Unaware of any.

*Website to learn more about SNRIs*: For Savella go to www.savella.com. For Cymbalta go to www.cymbalta.com.

### Anti-Seizure (Antiepileptic) Medicines

One of the three FDA-approved medicines for use in fibromyalgia is an anti-seizure medicine called pregabalin (Lyrica). Another closely related medicine to pregabalin called gabapentin (Neurontin) has also been shown in studies to be effective in some patients who have fibromyalgia.

*Generic available*: Neurontin is available in its generic form, gabapentin.

*How pregabalin and gabapentin work*: These medications are believed to decrease the over-activity of pain nerves that are sending too many pain messages to the brain.

*What benefits to expect from pregabalin and gabapentin*: Decreased pain, improved sleep, and improved quality of life. They usually take four to eight weeks to achieve the full effect at any one dose.

*How pregabalin and gabapentin are taken*: Taken one to three times a day. Both are often started at a low dose and increased slowly. Pregabalin usually requires 300 mg to 600 mg a day in divided doses, but some people (especially older individuals) can respond to doses as low as 50 mg a day. Gabapentin usually requires 1,200 mg to 3,600 mg a day in divided doses. It takes four to eight weeks to achieve the effect of these medicines. Gabapentin now comes in a once-daily, slow-release form, Gralise, which is taken with the evening meal. This can provide a convenient alternative to the generic and Neurontin formulations that often need to be taken up to three times a day. However, Gralise is expensive, and it may be difficult to get prescription insurance plans to cover its cost.

*If you miss a dose of your medicine*: If you miss a dose of your medicine, it depends on how you react to it and how often you take it that determines what you should do. For example, if you take it every morning and you know that it can cause you to have trouble sleeping if you take it too late in the day, you may want to skip that day's dose if you remember too late in the day. If you usually take it at nighttime because it makes you drowsy when you take it earlier in the day, you may want to skip the dose you missed if you do not realize you missed your nighttime dose until the next morning after you wake up. If it does not make you drowsy or cause problems with sleeping, you can take it as soon as you realize you missed it on the day you were supposed to take it and then resume your normal dosing schedule the next day. If you take it twice a day and it has been just a few hours since you missed your dose, then take the dose you missed as soon as you realize it and take your next dose at the regularly appointed time. For example, if you take your medicine at 7:00 AM and 7:00 PM every day and you forget to take your 7:00 AM dose but do not realize it until 10:00 AM, go ahead and take it at 10:00 AM. Then take your 7:00 PM dose at the usual time. However, if you do not realize you missed your morning dose until 2:00 PM, just skip the dose and resume taking your medicine at 7:00 PM. Consult with your prescribing doctor to double-check these instructions, but these guidelines will suffice for most people.

*Alcohol/food/herbal interactions with pregabalin and gabapentin*: Avoid alcohol, which can increase the side effects of these medicines.

Pregabalin should be taken with food. Generic gabapentin and Neurontin can be taken with or without food. The once-daily formulation of gabapentin, Gralise, should be taken with food since it is not absorbed as well on an empty stomach. The manufacturer recommends that it be taken with the evening meal.

Avoid valerian, St. John's wort, SAMe, kava kava, and tryptophan.

*Potential side effects of pregabalin and gabapentin*: Potential side effects are listed in table 27.11.

*What needs to be monitored while taking pregabalin and gabapentin*: No blood tests have to be monitored.

*Reasons not to take pregabalin and gabapentin (contraindications or precautions)*:

**Table 27.11** Potential Side Effects of Pregabalin and Gabapentin

|  | Incidence | Side Effect Therapy |
|---|---|---|
| **Nuisance side effects** | | |
| Edema (ankle swelling) | Common | Decrease dosage or stop medicine. |
| Dizziness | Common | Decrease dosage or stop medicine. |
| Sleepiness, drowsiness | Common | Try taking the medicine only at night. Also can decrease dosage or stop medicine. |
| Dry mouth | Common | Decrease dosage or stop medicine. |
| Difficulty with concentration | Common | Decrease dosage or stop medicine. |
| Increased appetite, weight gain | Common | Decrease dosage or stop medicine. |
| Blurred vision | Common | Decrease dosage or stop medicine. |
| Increased feelings of well-being, addiction, and dependency with pregabalin (in those with a history of drug or alcohol abuse) | Rare | Taper off medicine slowly to prevent withdrawal symptoms. |
| **Serious side effects** | None | |

Side effect incidence key (approximations, as side effects can vary widely study to study): rare < 1% occurrence; uncommon 1%–5% occurrence; common > 5% occurrence

- Caution should be used in people with a history of drug or alcohol abuse as there is an increased risk of drug dependency using pregabalin.
- Decreased doses are used if there is decreased kidney function.

*While taking pregabalin and gabapentin*:

- Initially, do not take if you are driving, climbing, or operating machinery. You want to make sure it does not make you drowsy first.
- Alert your doctor if any side effects occur.
- Do not abruptly stop the medicine. It is best to decrease the dose gradually.

*Pregnancy and breast-feeding while taking pregabalin and gabapentin*: Cause birth defects in animals. Have not been studied in humans. It is probably best to avoid using these drugs during pregnancy.

Secreted in breast milk. Effects in infants is unknown. Probably best to avoid while breast-feeding.

*Geriatric use of pregabalin and gabapentin*: Lower doses are usually used due to increased risk of side effects.

*What to do with pregabalin and gabapentin at the time of surgery*: It is important to get specific instructions from your surgeon and anesthesiologist. These can usually be continued up to the day before surgery.

*Patient assistance program for pregabalin and gabapentin*: For Lyrica go to www
.phahelps.com or call 1-866-706-2400. Also see chapter 42.

*Drug helpline for pregabalin and gabapentin*: Unaware of any.

*Website to learn more about pregabalin and gabapentin*: For Lyrica go to www.Lyrica
.com.

## Cyclobenzaprine (Flexeril, Amrix, Fexmid)

Cyclobenzaprine is a muscle relaxant that works like tricyclic antidepressants. Therefore, it is not a surprise that it can be effective in treating fibromyalgia. Much of the
information in this section is similar to that of the section on TCAs.

*Generic available*: Yes.

*How cyclobenzaprine works*: Similar to TCAs. See section on TCAs.

*What benefits to expect from cyclobenzaprine*: Decreased pain and improved sleep.
Studies show that approximately 20% of people who have fibromyalgia have significantly decreased pain. It takes about four weeks to work.

*How cyclobenzaprine is taken*: The immediate-release forms (generic cyclobenzaprine, Flexeril, and Fexmid), are usually taken two to three hours before bedtime to
prevent morning hangover feeling; sometimes a low dose can be taken in the morning
as well if it does not cause drowsiness. Extended-release Amrix is taken two to three
hours before bedtime. Never crush or bite on Amrix as it would be absorbed too quickly and could potentially cause significant side effects.

*If you miss a dose of your medicine*: If you miss a dose of your cyclobenzaprine and
typically get drowsy from taking it, it is usually best not to take it and wait until the
next evening to take your next dose at the usual scheduled time. However, if you tolerate your cyclobenzaprine well, and it does not tend to cause you side effects such as
drowsiness or dizziness, you could take one-half to a full amount of your dose right
before you go to bed. However, it is important to realize that you have an increased
chance of feeling groggy or hung over if you take it right before bedtime. Consult with
your prescribing doctor to double-check these instructions, but these guidelines will
suffice for most people.

*Alcohol/food/herbal interactions with cyclobenzaprine*: Alcohol should be avoided to
prevent increased side effects.

The extended-release form (Amrix) has increased absorption when taken with food.
The immediate-release forms (generic cyclobenzaprine, Flexeril, and Fexmid) can be
taken with or without food.

Avoid valerian, kava kava, and gotu kola.

*Potential side effects of cyclobenzaprine*: The side effects of cyclobenzaprine are
similar to those of TCAs (table 27.12). See the section on TCAs.

*What needs to be monitored while taking cyclobenzaprine*: No blood work needs to be
monitored.

*Reasons not to take cyclobenzaprine (contraindications or precautions)*:

- Should be avoided in people who have heart disease and those who have
difficulty urinating (such as benign prostatic hypertrophy).

- Inform your doctor if you have closed-angle glaucoma (also called angle-closure
and narrow-angle glaucoma) before taking the medicine. Note that most people

**Table 27.12** Potential Side Effects of Cyclobenzaprine

| | Incidence | Side Effect Therapy |
|---|---|---|
| **Nuisance side effects** | | |
| Drowsiness, hung over feeling when waking up | Common | Make sure to take it two to three hours before going to bed. Otherwise, decrease dose or stop it. |
| Dizziness | Common | Decrease dose or stop it. |
| Dry mouth | Common | Decrease dose or stop it. |
| Constipation | Common | Decrease dose or stop it. Can also take over-the-counter Miralax or senna (Senekot) daily to combat constipation. |
| Difficulty urinating | Uncommon | Seek immediate medical attention. |
| **Serious side effects** | | |
| Heart problems (shortness of breath, chest pain, palpitations) | Rare | Seek immediate medical attention. |
| Worsening of narrow-angle glaucoma | Common in people who have untreated narrow-angle glaucoma | Should not be taken if you have untreated narrow-angle glaucoma. |

Side effect incidence key (approximations, as side effects can vary widely study to study): rare < 1% occurrence; uncommon 1%–5% occurrence; common > 5% occurrence

with glaucoma have open-angle glaucoma. It is safe to take this medicine if you have open-angle glaucoma. It is also usually safe to take this medicine if your closed-angle glaucoma has already been surgically treated (ask your eye doctor).

• Inform your doctor if you are taking an MAO inhibitor antidepressant as life-threatening side effects may occur with this combination.

• Inform your doctor if you have an overactive thyroid (hyperthyroidism).

• Do not begin taking if you plan on driving, climbing, or using machinery until you make sure it does not make you groggy or cause difficulty with thinking.

*While taking cyclobenzaprine*:

• Contact your doctor if any side effects occur.

*Pregnancy and breast-feeding while taking cyclobenzaprine*: No adverse effects are known; however, this drug has not been studied in humans. Use with caution during pregnancy. Check with your doctor.

Excretion in breast milk is unknown. Use only with caution. Check with your doctor.

*Geriatric use of cyclobenzaprine*: Increased risk of side effects. Generally avoided in older people or used in smaller doses.

*What to do with cyclobenzaprine at the time of surgery*: It is important to get specific instructions from your surgeon and anesthesiologist. Cyclobenzaprine can usually be continued up to the day before surgery.

*Patient assistance program for cyclobenzaprine*: See chapter 42.

*Drug helpline for cyclobenzaprine*: Unaware of any.

*Website to learn more about cyclobenzaprine*: Unaware of any.

## Tramadol (Ultracet, Ultram, Ultram ER, Ryzolt, Rybix, ConZip)

*Generic available*: Yes.

*How tramadol works*: Tramadol is an opioid pain reliever. Opioids work by attaching to opioid receptors on pain nerves, decreasing the pain messages to the brain. "Opioid" may sound familiar as it comes from the word for opium produced from poppies. Opioids include narcotics such as heroin, morphine, hydrocodone, and oxycodone. However, tramadol is rarely ever addictive. There have been rare cases of addiction in people who had previous addiction problems but this is not common. Tramadol also blocks the reuptake of both serotonin and norepinephrine, which helps to decrease pain (see the section on dual uptake inhibitors).

*What benefits to expect from tramadol*: Most people can get a 50% or more reduction in pain.

*How tramadol is taken*: The immediate-release forms (generic tramadol, Ultracet, Ultram, and Rybix) are generally taken three to four times a day. The extended-release forms (tramadol ER, Ultram ER, ConZip, and Ryzolt) are generally taken once a day. Rybix is an orally disintegrating form; therefore, it may be more desirable in people who have difficulty swallowing pills. Do not crush or bite tramadol ER or Ultram ER as these are extended-release forms. They would be absorbed too quickly and could potentially cause significant side effects.

*If you miss a dose of your medicine*: If you miss a dose of your immediate-release tramadol, take the dose you missed as soon as you realize you missed taking it. Usually immediate-release tramadol is taken a similar number of hours apart from each other while you are awake; for example, you may take one or two tablets every six hours while you are awake (e.g., 8:00 AM, 2:00 PM, and 8:00 PM). If you realize at 10:00 AM that you missed your morning dose, go ahead and take the morning dose, then take your next dose six hours later at 4:00 PM and then the last dose of the day six hours later at 10:00 PM. If it is too late in the day and past your bedtime to take the last dose, just skip the last dose and resume your regular dosing schedule the next day.

If you take the extended-release form tramadol ER or Ultram ER, take your dose as soon as you remember you missed it that day, then resume your usual dosing schedule the next day. If you do not realize you missed your dose until the next morning, do not try to make up for it by taking an extra dose. Just resume your usual dosing schedule. Check with your prescribing physician as well to make sure these instructions apply to you, but these guidelines suffice for most people taking tramadol.

*Alcohol/food/herbal interactions with tramadol*: Avoid alcohol, which can increase the side effects of tramadol.

The extended-release forms (tramadol ER, Ryzolt, and Ultram ER) are absorbed faster if taken with fatty foods. Therefore, it is usually best to take them on an empty stomach to prevent unwanted side effects. The immediate-release forms are not affected by food.

Avoid chamomile, valerian, St. John's wort, kava kava, and gotu kola.

*Potential side effects of tramadol*: If you are taking the extended release forms (tramadol extended release, Ultram XR, or Ryzolt), it is best to take the medicine on an empty stomach and avoid fatty foods after taking it to decrease the risk of side effects. Table 27.13 lists the potential side effects.

*What needs to be monitored while taking tramadol*: No labs need to be monitored.

*Reasons not to take tramadol (contraindications or precautions)*:

- If you have a history of drug or alcohol abuse let your doctor know as you may have an increased risk for addiction.

- Should generally be avoided if you have ever had seizures.

- Usually lower doses are taken by people who have decreased kidney or liver function.

- Inform your doctor if you have been diagnosed with increased intracranial pressure (such as pseudotumor cerebri) or have had a brain injury.

*While taking tramadol*:

- Let your doctor know if you develop any side effects.

- Do not stop the medicine abruptly to avoid withdrawal symptoms.

*Pregnancy and breast-feeding while taking tramadol*: Crosses the placenta during labor and can cause seizures, withdrawal, and even death in the baby. Do not take during pregnancy.

Enters breast milk. Do not use while breast-feeding.

*Geriatric use of tramadol*: Causes increased side effects in older people; therefore, usually lower doses are used.

*What to do with tramadol at the time of surgery*: It is important to get specific instructions from your surgeon and anesthesiologist. When tramadol is stopped, there is the risk for developing withdrawal symptoms. Your surgical team may need to give you an alternative around the time of surgery to prevent withdrawal symptoms and pain.

*Patient assistance program for tramadol*: www.access2wellness.com for Ultram and Ultracet. Also see chapter 42.

*Drug helpline for tramadol*: Unaware of any.

*Website to learn more about tramadol*: Unaware of any.

**Table 27.13** Potential Side Effects of Tramadol

|  | Incidence | Side Effect Therapy |
|---|---|---|
| **Nuisance side effects** | | |
| Drowsiness | Common | Decrease dose or stop it (taper off the medicine gradually). |
| Nausea | Common | Decrease dose or stop it (taper off the medicine gradually). |
| Itchiness | Common | Decrease dose or stop it (taper off the medicine gradually). |
| Constipation | Common | Consider taking something for constipation every day such as over-the-counter Miralax or senna (Senekot). Decrease dose or stop it (taper off the medicine gradually). |
| Dizziness | Common | Decrease dose or stop it (taper off the medicine gradually). |
| Headaches | Common | Decrease dose or stop it (taper off the medicine gradually). |
| Withdrawal symptoms if stopped abruptly (anxiety, stomach upset, pain, sweating, insomnia) | Common | First try not to miss any doses. Taper off tramadol slowly if you plan to stop taking it. |
| **Serious side effects** | | |
| Seizures | Rare | Seek immediate medical attention. |
| Serotonin syndrome (anxiety, agitation, difficulty thinking, increased sweating, feeling hot, increased heart rate, stomach upset, and muscle spasms) | Rare | Seek immediate medical attention. |

1. Fibromyalgia is a problem with the pain nerves of the body being overactive, causing numerous problems, including body pain, fatigue, difficulty sleeping, numbness, headaches, stomach upset, and difficulty thinking.

2. Fibromyalgia occurs in about 20% of people who have SLE.

3. You can take the self-survey at the beginning of this chapter to see if you may have fibromyalgia. If you score high on the test, show your results to your doctor.

4. The pain of fibromyalgia is not treated with immunosuppressant medicines such as steroids.

5. Fibromyalgia is treated with medications that improve the chemical imbalances that are occurring in the pain pathways of the body.

6. Treatment should include a combination of therapies as outlined in table 27.4. Medications alone usually are not effective.

7. Antidepressants and anti-seizure medicines are the most common and most effective medicines used in treating fibromyalgia.

8. Although there are three FDA-approved medicines to treat fibromyalgia (Cymbalta, Savella, and Lyrica), there is no evidence that they work any better than the other medicines discussed in this chapter.

9. Medications for fibromyalgia need to be taken on a regular schedule. Most take three to eight weeks to work at any particular dose. Often a low dose is started and gradually increased every four to eight weeks.

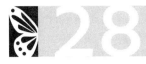

# Gastroesophageal Reflux and Stomach Ulcers

## Using Antibiotics to Treat Ulcers?

The chief of gastroenterology (gastroenterologists are stomach doctors) from one of the large hospitals where I have worked used to recall the story of how he went to visit China in the 1970s to learn more about Chinese medicine. At the time, they were using antibiotics to treat ulcers of the stomach. He just laughed to himself about how "backward" they were in some of their therapies.

The interest in using antibiotics to treat ulcers is not new. It was first suggested in 1875 that an infection might be the cause of ulcers, and during the 1880s, it was shown that bacteria seemed to be found in the stomachs of humans and animals. However, it was assumed that there was no way bacteria could possibly survive the harsh, acidic environment of the stomach. Respected experts in the field of gastroenterology for decades considered any signs of bacteria in stomach samples in people who had ulcers to be contaminants (in other words, the bacteria infected the stomach specimens after they were removed from the patients instead of the bacteria actually living in the patients' stomachs). Beginning in 1951, there were physicians who dared to recommend using antibiotics to treat ulcers. In fact, one particular doctor in Greece, Dr. John Lykoudis, treated his own ulcers with antibiotics successfully in 1958 and became a big proponent of their usage for ulcers. He built up quite a practice using antibiotics for treatment of ulcers and had many very grateful patients. The Disciplinary Committee of the Athens Medical Association considered his practice to be a form of quackery and fined him 4,000 drachmas.

A 1972 study from China demonstrated the successful use of antibiotics to treat ulcers. This led to their increased use in China. The Western world, however, did not acknowledge the potential importance of this finding.

In the early 1980s, Dr. J. Robin Warren, an Australian pathologist, noted that about half of the stomach samples from ulcer patients that he examined in his laboratory had bacteria in them. He was convinced that they probably played a role in causing the ulcers. He enlisted the help of an internal medicine doctor, Dr. James B. Marshall. Together they tried to grow the bacteria to identify it but without success. One Easter holiday, they accidentally left a stomach sample in a warm incubator. When they returned to the lab, they found an abundance of bacteria in the sample. However, finding bacteria, or any type of potential infectious agent, in the body is not enough to say that it is the cause of any disease. This is because the body is full of many beneficial organisms. In addition, tissues can become contaminated accidentally after they are taken out of the body. It is important to demonstrate that when humans are actually infected with a suspected organism (such as a virus or bacteria) that that particular organism then actually causes the disease in question.

Dr. Marshall then did a very daring experiment. He and a volunteer each swallowed a collection of the bacteria. Both of them subsequently developed inflammation of the stomach called gastritis (which can potentially lead to ulcers). This finally proved that this infection caused gastritis. This discovery opened up the way for further studies that quickly demonstrated that antibiotic therapy could cure people of ulcers if it were due to these bacteria. Doctors named the ulcer causing bacteria *Helicobacter pylori* (or *H. pylori* for short). Subsequently, studies have shown that infection from *H. pylori* is the most common cause of ulcers in the stomach, and that antibiotics are best in treating it. Dr. Barry Marshall and Dr. J. Robin Warren subsequently received the Nobel Prize in Physiology or Medicine in 2005 for proving this association after a previous century of major disagreements among doctors over this question. The chief of gastroenterology at the large hospital I attended became humbled as the antibiotic therapies (previously demonstrated by his Chinese counterparts) became the standard of medical care worldwide for people who have ulcers due to *H. pylori* infection.

This story has many lessons:

• Many medical discoveries are made by accident; the bacteria did not grow until a specimen was left in the incubator over the Easter holiday. This gave it the longer amount of time it needed to reproduce (compared to the shorter amounts of time needed by other bacteria).

• The "absence of proof" is not the same as a "proof of absence." In other words, just because a medical study has not been done to prove something in medicine does not mean that it is not the correct thing to do or that it does not exist.

• Some people take extraordinary risks in search of the truth to help humankind (such as Dr. Marshall and a volunteer ingesting the bacteria in the hopes of it causing them to get ulcers and proving the bacteria was the cause of ulcers).

• "Modern medicine" does not have all the right answers, and doctors will constantly be learning newer and better things to help their patients. Doctors must always keep an open mind.

• However, doctors still must rely on the proof of causes of disease and their treatments to take care of their patients safely. There can be a fine line between practicing good medicine and quackery. Yet, sometimes the "quacks" of yesterday (like Dr. Lykoudis) end up being the brilliant ones in history.

Although lupus does not directly cause ulcers, ulcers and related problems (such as acid reflux) are very common problems that must be dealt with by many people who have lupus. Read on in this chapter about how to deal with these issues, including the possibility of this infection causing ulcers in people who have lupus.

. . . .

Gastroesophageal reflux disease (commonly called GERD) and peptic ulcer disease (which includes ulcers of the stomach and intestines) are usually not caused by lupus directly (except in the case of esophageal dysmotility causing GERD). Nonetheless, they are common problems in people who have SLE mainly related to the medications that are commonly used to treat SLE. Therefore, it is fitting to discuss these two diseases in detail.

## Gastroesophageal Reflux Disease

Gastroesophageal reflux disease, often shortened to GERD, is also commonly called acid reflux. It is a very common problem not only in people who have lupus, but also in the general population. GERD occurs when acidic contents of the stomach back up (also called reflux) from the stomach into the esophagus. There is a tight, circular muscle (called a sphincter) between the esophagus and the stomach. This sphincter normally prevents acidic contents from the stomach going backward up into the esophagus (figure 28.1). It normally relaxes when swallowed food travels from the esophagus down into the stomach, then it tightens up again after the food enters the stomach.

There are numerous reasons GERD can develop (table 28.1). It can occur if the sphincter is too relaxed. This may happen with some medicines commonly used to treat lupus, such as when taking calcium channel blockers that are used to treat Raynaud's phenomenon to prevent the fingers from losing blood flow with exposure to the cold. These medicines relax the muscles of the arteries to the hands and feet to allow more blood flow, but they also can relax the muscles of the lower esophageal sphincter. Other substances that also relax this muscle (causing reflux) include tobacco, caffeine, chocolate, peppermint, alcohol, and fatty foods. That is why typical instructions for treating GERD include avoiding these substances.

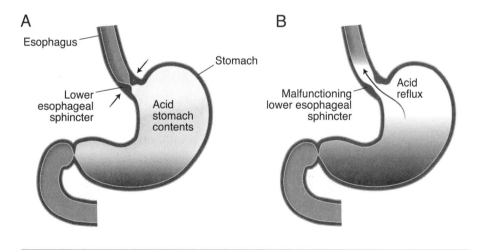

Figure 28.1  How the lower esophageal sphincter works to prevent GERD

**Table 28.1**  Causes of Gastroesophageal Reflux Disease (GERD)

Medications that relax the lower esophageal sphincter

    **calcium channel blockers** (such as nifedipine, amlodipine, etc.) used for blood pressure and Raynaud's phenomenon

    beta blockers used to treat high blood pressure

    antihistamines used for allergies

    antidepressants and anti-anxiety medicines

    sedatives (sleeping aids)

    **pain relievers** (such as tramadol and opioids)

    Parkinson's disease medicines

    theophylline and other asthma medicines

    medicines used for urinary incontinence

    some glaucoma medicines

    progestin female hormones (used for birth control, menopause, and to decrease uterine blood flow)

Other substances that relax the lower esophageal sphincter

    tobacco, cigarettes

    alcohol

    caffeine

    chocolate

    peppermint

    fatty foods

Drugs that exacerbate GERD by other means

    **non-steroidal anti-inflammatory drugs** (table 36.1)

    **steroids** (such as prednisone)

    **bisphosphonates** for osteoporosis (table 24.10)

    tetracycline antibiotics (such as doxycycline and minocycline)

    potassium and iron supplements

Conditions that exacerbate GERD

    hiatal hernia

    obesity

    wearing tight clothes and belts

    pregnancy

    **esophageal dysmotility**

    **decreased saliva flow** (Sjögren's syndrome and some medicines that cause dry mouth)

Terms in **bold** can be causes of GERD in people with lupus.

Having a hiatal hernia can also cause this sphincter muscle to work improperly and not keep acidic contents in the stomach. A hernia is a hole or gap in a body cavity that allows an organ to protrude through that gap. A hiatal hernia specifically refers to when part of the stomach protrudes through a gap in the diaphragm muscle (figure 28.2). Normally the entire stomach is below the diaphragm. With a hiatal hernia, part of the stomach extends above the diaphragm through the weakened muscle up into the chest cavity where the lungs are located. This can cause the lower esophageal sphincter to be ineffective and allow acidic stomach contents to reflux up into the esophagus. This typically worsens when there is increased pressure on the abdominal contents such as when coughing, bending over, wearing a tight belt, or when the person is overweight (the abdominal fat pushes up against the stomach).

Being overweight is a common cause of GERD and, unfortunately, studies show that the majority of patients who have SLE are obese due to numerous reasons, including the use of steroids, inactivity, and eating a bad diet coupled with lack of exercise. Obesity can cause an excessive amount of fat to accumulate in the abdomen. This exerts increased pressure on the stomach at the top of the abdomen, causing it to push its acidic contents up through the lower esophageal sphincter and into the esophagus.

Pregnancy can also cause GERD for a couple of reasons. First, the increase in female hormones causes the lower esophageal sphincter to become relaxed, allowing reflux of stomach acid contents. In addition, the enlarging uterus and fetus increase pressure on the stomach, which causes the contents to back up into the esophagus.

Some people who have SLE can have esophageal dysmotility (see chapter 15). This causes problems with moving food down from the esophagus into the stomach and can cause the esophageal sphincter to be weaker than normal. Thirty to 50% of people

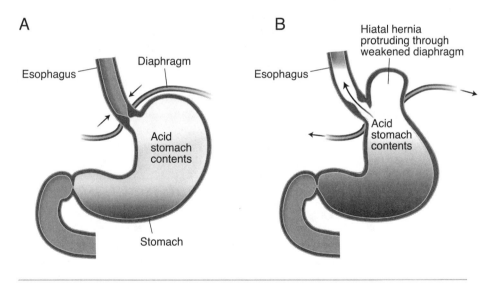

**Figure 28.2** Hiatal hernia

who have SLE can also have decreased saliva formation due to secondary Sjögren's syndrome (see chapter 14). The normal, constant flow of saliva down from the mouth and through the esophagus helps to keep fluids moving down into the stomach. However, when there is decreased saliva formation, this forward flow of saliva from the esophagus into the stomach is not present. Hence, a backup of stomach contents occurs more easily. This also can occur with some medications that can cause dry mouth such as antidepressants, blood pressure medicines, and pain relievers.

The symptoms of GERD are due to the irritation that the acidic contents exert when they go up into the esophagus. These include heartburn, difficulty swallowing, a feeling of having a lump in the throat, increased salivation, nausea, and even stomach contents coming up into the mouth. Sometimes heartburn can cause chest pain that can feel just like a heart attack or angina. It is not uncommon for someone to develop a sensation of severe chest pressure radiating into the arm, go to the emergency room, and find out it was due to GERD and not a heart attack. (However, never assume this on your own because heart attacks and strokes are the number one cause of death in people who have SLE, and a doctor should always evaluate these symptoms.) Some unusual symptoms of GERD can include hoarseness of the voice (if the acid drips on the vocal cords, called laryngopharyngeal reflux) and cough (from the acid contents going down the windpipe into the lungs). In fact, some people will only have a cough or hoarseness and no other symptoms of GERD at all.

Not only can GERD be uncomfortable, but also if left untreated, it can potentially cause significant complications (table 28.2). The complications occur due to sensitive tissues of the esophagus, vocal cords, and lungs being exposed repeatedly to the acid. While the stomach normally has a protective lining that prevents damage from acid, these other tissues do not. The esophagus can develop inflammation (called esophagitis). If the inflammation becomes severe, it can even cause an actual hole in the lining of the esophagus, called an esophageal ulcer, which will often cause pain and trouble swallowing. Scar tissue can also end up forming in the esophagus, causing an esophageal stricture (a "stricture" is a medical term meaning a narrowing of a passageway) which can cause trouble swallowing food. The cells of the esophagus can actually become cancerous from repeated exposure to acid contents. Initially this can occur as Barrett's esophagitis, which is a precancerous condition. However, this can transform into esophageal cancer if not treated appropriately.

If the acid contents drip down the trachea (windpipe), it can cause inflammation of the larynx (voice box) causing laryngitis that will produce hoarseness while talking. Scar tissue can also form in the trachea causing a stricture (narrowing) and even cancer if it occurs repeatedly over a long period. If the acid contents drip farther down into the lungs, then a persistent cough or even asthma may occur. The treatment of GERD is important not just to help the person feel better, but also to prevent these potentially serious complications from occurring.

Doctors can usually diagnose GERD from the symptoms alone. Someone who has classic symptoms of GERD such as heartburn, which may get worse with eating or when lying down, can be diagnosed and treated for GERD without further testing. Of course, this is not 100% accurate because there is no way to know if any of these complications of GERD have occurred without further testing. Sometimes other conditions, such as stomach ulcers, can cause similar symptoms. However, stomach ulcers

**Table 28.2**  Potential Complications of Gastroesophageal Reflux Disease

- Esophagitis (inflammation of the esophagus)
- Esophageal ulcer
- Esophageal stricture (narrowing of the esophagus due to scar tissue)
- Barrett's esophagitis (a precancerous condition)
- Esophageal cancer
- Laryngitis and hoarseness
- Stricture of the trachea (narrowing of the windpipe)
- Throat cancer
- Asthma
- Cough

and many of these GERD problems are treated the same way, and therefore it is easier, less invasive, faster, and less expensive in most cases to treat GERD without further testing.

If the symptoms thought to be due to GERD do not improve with proper treatment, or if the person has some worrisome symptoms that could potentially indicate a significant GERD complication (such as trouble swallowing, which occurs with esophageal strictures, esophageal ulcers, or even esophageal cancer), then it is appropriate to proceed with additional testing. One of the most commonly performed tests is an upper endoscopy, also called an esophagogastroduodenoscopy (or EGD for short), where a doctor inserts a thin, fiberoptic tube down the esophagus so that the esophagus ("esophago-"), stomach ("-gastro-"), and duodenal portion of the small intestine ("-duodeno-") can be visualized directly by the doctor. This procedure is usually done while the patient is sedated, so most patients have very little if any memory of the procedure at all. The advantage of this procedure is that these structures can be viewed directly. The doctor can see any inflammation, ulcers, cancers, or other problems. In addition, biopsies can be performed on anything that appears abnormal, and these can be sent to the laboratory to look for any signs of infection, inflammation, or cancer.

The doctor can also order a barium swallow. This is performed by having the patient swallow a substance that coats the esophagus and stomach and shows up on x-ray. It can show if stomach contents are refluxing up into the stomach, and it can visualize problems such as a hiatal hernia, strictures, tumors, or ulcers as well (if they are large enough to be seen on x-ray). However, the problem with a barium swallow is that it can miss up to 25% of cases of mild GERD as well as small ulcers and tumors. Therefore, a "normal" barium swallow does not mean that nothing is wrong, and an EGD usually needs to be done anyway. There are other studies used to diagnose GERD (such as manometry and pH monitoring) but they are not done very often; therefore, I will not discuss them.

The first step in treating GERD is to change lifestyle habits that make GERD worse (see table 15.1). This addresses many of the causes of GERD listed in table 28.1 such as obesity, wearing tight clothing, smoking, and drinking alcohol. Avoiding many of these habits may be enough to control GERD without even using medications in some people. People who have GERD must follow these rules religiously. Many people continue to have bad problems from GERD by trying to rely too much on medications alone, and often are very surprised at how much better they do when abiding by these important lifestyle changes. In addition, the medicines used to treat acid reflux only decrease the acidity of the stomach contents that are refluxed, but they do not decrease the amount of fluid refluxed. Therefore, the same amount of fluid continues to reflux up the esophagus regularly while taking anti-GERD medications. The fluid can continue to irritate the esophagus, trachea, vocal cords, and even the lungs if lifestyle changes are not made to prevent this from happening. In addition, if there are any medicines making the GERD worse, and they are not needed or can be changed to medicines that do not cause GERD, then this is an appropriate step to take as well.

If changing lifestyle habits or changing offending medications does not relieve the problems of GERD, then the use of medications may be important. If symptoms are mild and intermittent, then over-the-counter preparations such as Tums, Alka-Seltzer, Pepto Bismol, Mylanta, Rolaids, Prilosec OTC, Pepcid Complete, Pepcid AC, Tagamet HB, or Zantac 75 can be taken. However, before taking any of these, check with your doctor first as some of these can have potential interactions with other medicines or should not be used if you have certain medical problems.

If these measures are ineffective, then your doctor will put you on a prescription medicine. This not only will help you feel better, but it also can help prevent the complications of GERD. The main medications used to treat GERD are medications that lower the acidity of the stomach contents. Prescription-strength medications used to lower stomach acidity are divided into two main groups: proton pump inhibitors (PPIs) (table 28.3) and H2 blockers. H2 blockers include ranitidine (Zantac), cimetidine (Tagamet), famotidine (Pepcid), and nizatidine (Axid). PPIs usually work better compared to H2 blockers. However, H2 blockers tend to be less expensive than PPIs. Therefore, some insurance companies require people to take an H2 blocker before they can take a PPI. Most PPIs work as well as another. However, in any one person, one PPI may work better than another; therefore, trials of different medicines at different doses sometimes need to be done to figure out the best PPI for any particular person. Some people also do better if they take a combination of a PPI and an H2 blocker because they work in two different ways that can complement each other when used together. These medicines are not a cure for GERD. They can help decrease symptoms of GERD and prevent some of the complications (such as ulcers, strictures, or cancer), but they do not prevent the stomach contents from backing up into the esophagus and lungs where it can still potentially cause damage.

Long-term use of PPIs is generally safe, and it is unusual to develop any severe side effects from them. However, they can decrease the absorption of vitamin B-12, calcium, and magnesium. Studies show that people who take a PPI regularly are at increased risk of getting broken bones from osteoporosis. This most likely occurs due to their preventing the proper absorption of most types of calcium. Calcium carbonate and calcium phosphate are the primary types of calcium found in most foods and supplements, and they require acid in the stomach for proper absorption. Calcium citrate, on the other hand, does not require acid for absorption. Anyone who is taking a PPI

**Table 28.3**  Proton Pump Inhibitors

dexlansoprazole (Dexilant)

esomeprazole (Nexium)

omeprazole (Prilosec)

lansoprazole (Prevacid)

pantoprazole (Protonix)

rabeprazole (AcipHex)

regularly should consider taking calcium citrate supplements to prevent osteoporosis, as discussed in chapter 24. In addition, it is a good idea to have your vitamin B-12 and magnesium levels checked regularly while taking a PPI.

For severe cases of hiatal hernia, surgery can be performed such as a Nissen fundoplication, which gets rid of the hiatal hernia. However, this is usually reserved for severe cases that do not respond to the lifestyle change and medication therapies listed above.

**KEY POINTS TO REMEMBER**

1. GERD is common in people who have SLE due to multiple reasons, including obesity, esophageal dysmotility, secondary Sjögren's syndrome, and taking medications such as steroids, non-steroidal anti-inflammatory drugs (NSAIDs), medicines for Raynaud's (such as calcium channel blockers like nifedipine), bisphosphonates for osteoporosis (like alendronate), antidepressants, and pain relievers.

2. The most common symptoms seen with GERD include heartburn, chest pain (which can even feel like a heart attack), and difficulty swallowing.

3. If chest pain occurs, do not assume it is GERD. Heart attacks and strokes are the number one cause of death in people who have lupus; therefore, chest pain requires a doctor's evaluation.

4. Surprising symptoms that can occur from GERD include hoarseness (from laryngopharyngeal reflux), cough, and asthma symptoms. These can even occur without any heartburn.

5. You must abide by all lifestyle habit changes listed in table 15.1 because medicines for GERD only cover up the symptoms but do nothing to decrease the amount of fluid that refluxes up from the stomach.

6. For mild or intermittent GERD, you can try over-the-counter heartburn preparations.

7. If over-the-counter medicines do not work, then your doctor may prescribe a prescription-strength PPI and/or H2 blocker.

8. If you take a PPI, consider taking calcium citrate supplements regularly to prevent osteoporosis and broken bones. You should also have your vitamin B-12 and magnesium levels checked regularly.

## Peptic Ulcer Disease

"Ulcer" is a medical term describing a condition where a hole occurs on the surface of a part of the body. "Peptic" refers to the digestive juices of the stomach. Therefore, "peptic ulcer disease" is the term doctors use when they talk about ulcers that occur in the gastrointestinal system, specifically those that occur in the esophagus, the stomach, and the small intestine due to irritation from the highly acidic stomach contents (figure 28.3). SLE itself does not generally cause peptic ulcer disease, but it can occur due to medications, specifically the non-steroidal anti-inflammatory drugs (NSAIDs).

Peptic ulcers occur when the acidic stomach contents erode through the lining of the esophagus, the stomach, or the first part of the small intestine (duodenum). Stomach contents normally should not be in the esophagus at all, and therefore it is not normally equipped to protect itself from acid. The main cause of esophageal ulcers is recurrent GERD.

Ulcers occurring in the stomach are called gastric ulcers, where "gastric" refers to the stomach. The lining of the stomach is normally coated with a protective layer of mucus (think of a slimy layer) that is continuously produced by the cells lining the inside of the stomach. This mucus protects the inner lining of the stomach from the acidic stomach contents. The acidity of gastric contents is primarily due to the production of hydrochloric acid by the stomach, giving it a pH of about 2 (which is similar to that of strong lemon juice or vinegar). This high acidity is important in helping to start digestion of food. If anything causes a problem with proper formation of the

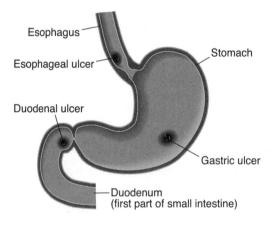

**Figure 28.3** Possible locations of peptic ulcers

mucous layer, the acid contents of the stomach will damage and eat away at the lining of the stomach. In the early, mildest stages, there may just be some inflammation of the stomach lining, which is called gastritis. If a very shallow layer of the lining of the stomach erodes away, it is called a gastric erosion. If a larger hole erodes into the stomach wall, it is called a gastric ulcer. These terms are used to represent severity where gastritis is the mildest form of peptic ulcer disease and an ulcer is the worst (an erosion is in between). Stomach acid contents can also cause similar problems in the first part of the small intestine (the duodenum) causing duodenitis, duodenal erosions, or even duodenal ulcers.

Ulcers can produce a multitude of possible symptoms. The classic stomach ulcer pain is a discomfort in the upper part of the abdomen that has a burning, gnawing, or "hunger-like" quality to it. Eating food or taking an antacid often relieves this discomfort. However, sometimes the discomfort can be more vague or described as "crampy," or it may be more on the right side or the left side of the abdomen. Ulcers do not always follow this classic description. Some people will have stomach upset that actually gets worse with eating food, or may get stomach bloating, nausea, or an early feeling of fullness when they eat (just the opposite of the previously described "classic" symptoms). Others will just get heartburn or a feeling of acid reflux related to their stomach ulcers.

Duodenal ulcers usually behave differently. They typically are worse a few hours after eating. After eating food, the digested food in the stomach tends to decrease the acidity of the stomach contents so that when this goes into the duodenum (the first part of the small intestine); it does not bother the duodenal ulcer. However, three to five hours after eating, the food is gone from the stomach, and instead, acidic stomach contents are being leaked into the small intestine, where they irritate the ulcer and cause pain. It is not unusual to experience abdominal pain from a duodenal ulcer at 11:00 PM to 2:00 AM for this reason.

Unfortunately, some people can have severe complications from their ulcers. Sometimes they can bleed. If a stomach ulcer bleeds and the person throws up, usually it looks like there are "coffee grounds" in the vomit due to the coagulated blood. If the blood instead goes through the intestines and is excreted in the feces, they usually appear very black and tarry (i.e., sticky and thick) and have a very strong, foul, hard-to-forget smell (called melena). A bleeding ulcer can be a potentially deadly situation. If you ever vomit up "coffee grounds" or notice black, tarry, foul-smelling feces, you should seek medical attention (such as have someone take you to your nearest emergency room) immediately.

Occasionally a bleeding ulcer can cause severe bleeding abruptly with no warning at all. In this case, the person may feel faint and light-headed all at once or may even pass out without ever noticing any blood in the feces (melena) at all. On the opposite end of the spectrum, some people will have such a slow, small amount of bleeding over time that their ulcer is not picked up until they are noted to be anemic (have a low red blood cell count or low hemoglobin level, as explained in chapter 9) by their doctor. This is why your doctor sometimes wants a fecal specimen from you if you are anemic. The laboratory can check the feces to see if there is any blood present.

Another potential complication of an ulcer is a perforation. This occurs when a hole has eroded completely through one side of the stomach or small intestinal wall and out the other side. The stomach and intestinal fluid then leak into the abdominal cavity. This can be catastrophic and potentially deadly. The person who has an ulcer perforation typically will have severe abdominal pain that will lead her or him to seek immediate medical attention. The other most dreaded complication of an ulcer is an obstruction. If the ulcer occurs close to where the stomach empties into the small intestine, sometimes it can narrow this opening and make it very difficult for any food to get through. This causes difficulty with eating, and the person typically vomits up food repeatedly. This too will cause the person to seek immediate medical attention. Surgery is required to treat perforations and obstructions from ulcers.

The two most useful tests to diagnose an ulcer are a barium swallow x-ray and an esophagogastroduodenoscopy (both discussed in the previous section on GERD). However, getting an EGD (esophagogastroduodenoscopy) is usually the best test as it can visualize smaller ulcers. In addition, if biopsies are needed (to look for the possibility of infection or cancer), an EGD would be required.

As far as what causes peptic ulcers to occur, there are some well-known ones such as stress and cigarette smoking. Ulcers have been diagnosed more commonly in populations affected by great stressors, such as the Great Kobe Earthquake of Japan in 1995 and the German bombing of London in World War II. Problems from ulcers increased dramatically in these populations because of the stress from these disasters. They also appear to occur more commonly in people who have depression and anxiety as well as those exposed to increased stressors in the family and at work. Smokers also get ulcers more often than nonsmokers do. On the other hand, alcohol does not seem to increase the risk of getting ulcers. However, alcohol abuse appears to hinder the ability of people to be compliant with the treatment of ulcers, making it more difficult to eradicate an ulcer after diagnosis. Although there is a lot of talk about certain foods being associated with ulcers, this does not pan out in medical studies. Certainly, some foods can cause increased stomach upset and heartburn, but none has been proven to increase the risk of getting ulcers.

By far, the two most common causes of peptic ulcer disease are infection from *Helicobacter pylori* (*H. pylori* for short) or taking non-steroidal anti-inflammatory drugs (NSAIDs for short).

*H. pylori* is a bacterium that loves to live in the harsh, acidic environment of the stomach. It is the most common bacterial infection in humans. It is spread from person to person, and most adults are infected with it. Factors that increase *H. pylori* include poor sanitation and close human contact. It is most common to be infected with it as a child and it is most prevalent in families that have a large number of siblings. People who came from a family of lower income, shared a bed as a child, or who had a lack of running water have a higher chance of infection. *H. pylori* infections are becoming less common as sanitation practices have generally improved. Adults born in recent decades, such as the 1960s and later, compared to those born in the 1940s and earlier have lower rates of infection. While it is gradually becoming less common in developed countries (such as the United States) with recent generations, it is still a large problem in the rest of the world. Doctors estimate that *H. pylori* has infected at least 50% of the world's population. Once infected by the bacteria, people will have the bacteria in their stomachs for the rest of their lives unless they take special antibiotics to get rid of it.

*H. pylori* bacteria attach to the cells that line the wall of the stomach and secrete substances that cause the protective mucous layer to become thinner than normal.

The infection also causes the cells of the stomach to make less mucus as well. The immune system notes the presence of these bad bacteria, so it also fights against them via inflammation (as discussed in chapter 1). This inflammation formed by the body trying to protect itself also plays an important role in perpetuating the formation of the erosions and ulcers. Ulcers are not the only problem it can cause. *H. pylori* is also capable of causing cancer of the stomach. Most people infected with *H. pylori* do not get ulcers. Why some do and some do not is not known. Although people who have systemic lupus are at increased risk of having infections, there is no evidence that they get *H. pylori* infection more than people who do not have lupus. Remember, *H. pylori* infection is most commonly acquired when people are children, usually far in advance of when their lupus occurs.

The other leading cause of peptic ulcer disease is the use of NSAIDs prescribed to treat arthritis pains and serositis (such as pleurisy) in people who have lupus. NSAIDs help decrease pain and inflammation in numerous ways. One of the best studied and well known effects is how these medications decrease the production of a group of substances in the body called prostaglandins. Prostaglandins are essential for many different body functions. One of these is sensing pain. Prostaglandins are important for how the spinal nerves transmit pain messages up to the brain. When a person takes an NSAID, there is less production of these prostaglandins; therefore, the spinal nerves transmit less pain signals up to the brain. Prostaglandins are also important for inflammation production in the body, so when an NSAID is taken, there is less inflammation. Due to these properties, the severe pain produced by the inflammation of lupus arthritis and serositis (like pleurisy) can be decreased in intensity.

Prostaglandins have many other uses in the body as well. For example, they are essential in how the stomach produces its protective mucous layer (protecting itself from those harsh acid contents). When NSAIDs are used, there are less prostaglandins produced by the cells of the stomach, causing the lining to become thinner and less protective. This can allow the acidic stomach fluids to damage the stomach lining, eventually causing inflammation (gastritis), erosions, or ulcers.

Of course, most people do not get ulcers when they take NSAIDs. Sometimes there is no rhyme or reason why one person will get an ulcer and someone else will not get one. It is possible to predict, however, which people are at highest risk of developing ulcers from NSAIDs. The American College of Gastroenterology (ACG) has come up with guidelines suggesting which people are at highest risk of getting ulcers when they take an NSAID (table 28.4). People at moderate to high risk for developing ulcers should consider taking extra steps to decrease the risk of getting an ulcer while they take an NSAID.

Most of the time, ulcers caused by NSAIDs do not cause any abdominal pain. This may be due to the NSAID decreasing any discomfort, which makes sense since NSAIDs decrease pain in the body. Most people who get an ulcer while taking an NSAID do not realize they have the ulcer until they actually develop a significant complication. These complications include anemia due to slow bleeding from the ulcer, or they may have a large bleed causing them to vomit up "coffee grounds" or develop melena (black, tarry, foul-smelling feces). Unfortunately, some will not have any warning signs at all until they pass out from massive blood loss, or develop severe abdominal pain or vomiting due to a perforation of the ulcer through the wall of the gastrointestinal tract or due to

**Table 28.4** Risk Level for Getting Ulcers When Taking NSAIDs

High risk (either of the following)

- A history of a previously complicated ulcer (such as one that caused bleeding)
- Having three or more of the moderate risk factors below

Moderate risk (one to two of these risk factors)

- Age > 65 years old
- Taking a high dose of a prescription NSAID (dose varies from NSAID to NSAID)
- A history of an uncomplicated ulcer (such as one that did not bleed)
- Concurrent use of aspirin (even in low doses), steroids, or blood thinners

Low risk

- None of the risk factors listed

intestinal blockage. The reason I bring this up is that people are often reluctant to take an additional medication (such as a PPI or misoprostol as mentioned in table 28.5) to prevent ulcers while they are on NSAID therapy. They commonly say, "The medicine never bothers me; I never get belly pain, so I don't need a medicine to prevent ulcers." It is important that you realize that most people who take NSAIDs do not get any warning at all, so do not let this be an excuse for your not taking a PPI or misoprostol if your doctor recommends it.

If you need an NSAID and you fall into the medium- or high-risk category for developing stomach ulcers, then you should consider taking extra precautions to prevent an ulcer from occurring. Preventative medicine is always better than waiting for something bad (like an ulcer) to happen. There are several tactics useful in decreasing the chances of getting an ulcer while taking an NSAID (table 28.5).

One option is to take the medication called misoprostol. Misoprostol acts as a prostaglandin in the body. Remember, the reason people who take NSAIDs get ulcers is due to the NSAID decreasing the production of prostaglandins in the lining of the stomach. Misoprostol replenishes the stomach prostaglandins and therefore increases the production of the protective mucous lining. This is one of the most effective methods (possibly even the most effective method) for preventing ulcers. However, it has a couple of drawbacks. To begin with, for it to work most effectively, it needs to be taken four times a day. Anyone who takes medications regularly can vouch that it is hard enough to take any medicine two to three times a day and not miss any doses. It is almost impossible for most people to do that with a four-times-a-day medicine. The other problem is that many people get side effects from misoprostol, making it difficult to take. In particular, a significant proportion of people develop diarrhea and/or abdominal pain. Approximately 20% of people stop taking the medicine within a month of starting it because of diarrhea or stomach upset. Starting at the lowest-dose tablet (100 micrograms) three times a day and slowly increasing the dose to the 200 micrograms tablet four times a day can help prevent these side effects from occurring. This does not get rid of the problem of remembering to take it four times a day, though.

Another option is to take Arthrotec. Arthrotec is a pill that combines misoprostol with the NSAID diclofenac in three separate layers. The outer layer contains the misoprostol, which dissolves as soon as the tablet reaches the stomach where it can help the stomach keep its protective mucous lining. The middle layer is a protective layer that keeps the inner layer of diclofenac from dissolving until it reaches the small intestine. This delay tactic helps prevent the diclofenac from irritating the stomach directly and allows it to be absorbed in the small intestine instead of in the stomach. Arthrotec is taken two to three times a day. Studies show that fewer ulcers occur in people who take Arthrotec compared to those who only take the NSAID diclofenac.

There are a few downsides to taking Arthrotec. First, it does not yet have a generic equivalent. Consequently, it is relatively more expensive than taking generic medications. A generic equivalent to Arthrotec may possibly become available in 2014. Second, since the misoprostol portion is only being taken two to three times a day instead of the usual four times a day, it most likely does not work as well compared to taking the generic diclofenac by itself two to three times a day along with the generic form of misoprostol four times a day (as two separate medications). Lastly, there is an increased risk of diarrhea and stomach upset with Arthrotec compared to taking generic diclofenac without the misoprostol portion.

Taking a proton pump inhibitor (table 28.3) is another option. Proton pump inhibitors (PPIs) are very effective at decreasing the acidity of the stomach and decreasing the chances of ulcers forming due to taking an NSAID. They have two big advantages over misoprostol. First, they are only taken once a day (occasionally twice daily), which is more convenient than a four-times-a-day medicine. Second, they are tolerated more easily by most people causing much less problems overall with stomach upset or diar-

**Table 28.5** Strategies to Prevent Ulcers While Taking NSAIDs

Cytotec (misoprostol)

    Taken as an additional medication 200 micrograms four times a day

Arthrotec (the NSAID diclofenac plus misoprostol)

Proton pump inhibitors

    Taken as an additional medication (table 28.3)

    Vimovo (naproxen plus esomeprazole)

Non-acetylated salicylates (less likely to cause ulcers but also weaker pain medicines)

    diflunisal

    choline magnesium trisalicylate

    salsalate

COX-2 inhibitor (only when aspirin is not taken as well)

    celecoxib (Celebrex)

    meloxicam (Mobic) at the lowest dosage of 7.5 mg a day

Duexis (combination of the NSAID ibuprofen plus the H2 blocker famotidine)

rhea compared to taking misoprostol. However, as mentioned before, it is important to take a calcium citrate supplement regularly when you take a proton pump inhibitor, and you may need to have your vitamin B-12 and magnesium levels checked by your doctor while you take it.

Just as with misoprostol, there is a medication that combines a proton pump inhibitor (esomeprazole) with an NSAID (naproxen) in the same tablet called Vimovo. It is usually taken twice a day. The advantage of this formulation is that it negates the need to take naproxen separately from the esomeprazole. However, one downside of Vimovo is that it is more expensive since there is no generic equivalent. It all depends on what your pharmacy prescription plan costs you to pay for a brand-only medication versus paying for two generic medications. In some plans, there may not be a big difference, and Vimovo may be a good option. However, in other plans, it may be markedly less expensive to pay for the two generic medications separately compared to paying for one brand name (Vimovo) medication. Another downside is that people are more likely to miss doses on twice-a-day medications. It is easier to take a once-a-day generic PPI along with a once-a-day NSAID (such as meloxicam, piroxicam, nabumetone, or extended-release etodolac) to get a similar effect as taking Vimovo twice a day.

Duexis is another new combination medication. It contains the NSAID ibuprofen plus the H2 blocker famotidine to protect the stomach. As with Vimovo above, it is more expensive than taking generic equivalents by themselves and Duexis is a three-times-a-day medication that can be very difficult to take. However, for someone who already takes ibuprofen three times a day who is looking for a simpler alternative compared to adding an anti-acid medicine to their regimen, Duexis can be a suitable consideration if they can afford it with their drug prescription plan.

Another option is to take a COX-2 inhibitor. COX stands for cyclooxygenase, which is a very important enzyme produced by cells of the body. Enzymes are chemicals that cause some substances to be turned into other substances. Cyclooxygenases are the enzymes of the body that are essential in the production of prostaglandins. There are three different types of cyclooxygenases in the body named COX-1, COX-2, and COX-3. COX-1 is the one used to produce the prostaglandins in the stomach that maintain the protective mucous layer, while COX-2 is the one used to produce the prostaglandins that cause pain and inflammation. All NSAIDs work by stopping both COX-1 and COX-2 from working (or inhibiting these enzymes). However, a couple of NSAIDs inhibit COX-2 much more than COX-1. Therefore, they inhibit COX-2 a lot, and consequently decrease pain and inflammation. At the same time, they inhibit COX-1 much less, therefore allowing COX-1 to keep working in the stomach, permitting the protective mucous lining of the stomach to prevent ulcers from forming. Currently, there are two COX-2 inhibitors available. There is celecoxib (Celebrex), which is taken 100 mg to 200 mg once or twice a day. There is also meloxicam (Mobic). However, meloxicam works primarily as a COX-2 inhibitor when taken at its lower dose of 7.5 mg once a day. When taken at the higher dose of 15 mg once a day, it inhibits COX-1 a lot more and increases the risk of getting ulcers similar to that of other NSAIDs. When celecoxib (Celebrex) is taken at any dose, or when meloxicam (Mobic) is taken at 7.5 mg a day, they cause less ulcers compared to other NSAIDs.

If aspirin is taken along with COX-2 inhibitors, they lose this stomach protection ability. This is because aspirin is also an NSAID and inhibits both COX-1 and COX-2 even when taken in very small doses. Many people who have lupus need to take a small dose of aspirin daily to prevent heart attacks, strokes, and blood clots. In people who take aspirin, it is better to take either a PPI or misoprostol to prevent ulcers from their NSAID instead of relying on taking a COX-2 inhibitor.

Of course, trying to prevent ulcers from occurring in the first place, using the methods explained above is the best thing to do. However, prevention is not always 100% effective. If an EGD or barium swallow shows evidence of an ulcer, it needs to be treated. The doctor will usually test for *H. pylori* infection. This infection is diagnosed by taking a biopsy of the ulcer at the time of the EGD and sending it to the laboratory for testing. A breath test can also be done for *H. pylori*. This complex testing method usually has to be done at a doctor's office. Most often it is done by a gastroenterologist (the same type of doctor who most commonly does EGDs). *H. pylori* can also be detected through a blood test. However, the problem with the simple blood test is that it can miss a significant number of people who have the infection. In addition, a larger number of people who are positive for the test do not actually have the infection. In other words, it is much less accurate than either the biopsy by EGD method or the breath test method. The final option is a fecal test for *H. pylori*, which is better than the blood test, but probably not as good as the EGD biopsy or the breath tests. Your doctor will choose which option is best for your particular situation. Since EGD identifies most ulcers, a biopsy accurately diagnoses most *H. pylori* infections.

If there is an *H. pylori* infection, then there are several available treatment regimens. They combine a PPI plus two different antibiotics taken for one to two weeks. There are other medicine regimens that also add bismuth (which is found in Pepto Bismol) or even a third antibiotic. The doctor will choose which regimen is best for any particular situation.

The other important action, of course, is that NSAID medications need to be stopped during an active ulcer. A big question often arises as to whether the NSAID can be added after the ulcer heals or not. If the ulcer occurred in the course of an *H. pylori* infection, or if the person was not taking misoprostol or a PPI to prevent the ulcer in the first place, then it may be possible to add the NSAID back into the person's medical regimen. However, it is prudent to take a PPI or misoprostol along with the NSAID. This is especially important if the person has significant arthritis pains and quality of life issues become problematic. The person may require an NSAID to decrease the severity of arthritis pain. Another option would be to take either celecoxib (Celebrex) or a low dose of meloxicam (Mobic) as long as the person is not also taking aspirin (which increases the risk of developing ulcers if taken with celecoxib or meloxicam unless a PPI is taken as well).

Everyone who gets an ulcer needs to be treated with medications that lower stomach acid. PPIs are the most common medicines used to do this. However, a group of medicines called H2 blockers are also commonly used. Examples of H2 blockers include cimetidine (Tagamet), ranitidine (Zantac), and famotidine (Pepcid). They are used for various amounts of time depending on how large the ulcer is and whether there is *H. pylori* infection or not. It is also important to stop smoking cigarettes and to decrease how much alcohol you drink if you drink excessively to help the ulcer heal properly. Avoiding certain foods does not speed up the healing process, but it can cause less problems with heartburn or stomach upset if you identify any foods (such as acidic foods) that bother you. Although stress, depression, and anxiety appear to increase the risk of getting ulcers, there is no medical evidence that resolving these issues causes ulcers to heal any quicker. However, having these problems does increase the risk of an ulcer recurring after it is healed. Therefore, it is important to take measures to try to decrease stress, or to have depression and anxiety disorders treated appropriately.

### KEY POINTS TO REMEMBER

1. Peptic ulcers occur due to acid contents of the stomach eroding through the inner lining of the esophagus, the stomach, or the first part of the small intestine (duodenum).

2. Peptic ulcers occur more commonly in people who have lupus because they take NSAIDs for arthritis and serositis, but *H. pylori* infection is the other most common cause.

3. If you are at increased risk of developing ulcers from NSAIDs (table 28.4), then consider asking your doctor if you can take a PPI or misoprostol along with the NSAID.

4. Another option would be to take a COX-2 inhibitor like celecoxib (Celebrex) or low-dose meloxicam (Mobic). However, this strategy only works if you do not take aspirin.

5. Peptic ulcers can produce many different patterns of stomach upset and nausea. However, most people who get an ulcer while taking an NSAID have no warning signs (like abdominal pain) until they get a complication such as bleeding from the ulcer.

6. Vomiting up "coffee grounds" or having black, tarry, foul-smelling feces (called melena) can mean bleeding due to peptic ulcer disease. Seek immediate medical attention if either of these occurs.

7. Peptic ulcers are most commonly diagnosed by EGD (a type of endoscopy); however, large ones can be seen using a barium swallow x-ray. An EGD often is required to obtain a biopsy to rule out *H. pylori* infection, cancer, or other problems.

8. If *H. pylori* infection is identified (by EGD biopsy, breath test, blood test, or fecal test), then one to two weeks of a PPI plus two to three antibiotics are prescribed. Sometimes bismuth (like Pepto Bismol) is added to the regimen.

9. Doctors prescribe either a PPI or an H2 blocker to decrease stomach acidity to treat ulcers.

10. If you take a PPI or an H2 blocker, you should consider taking a calcium citrate supplement to ensure you are absorbing enough calcium into your body.

11. If you are on an NSAID when you develop an ulcer, it needs to be stopped.

12. To help ulcers heal properly, it is also helpful to stop smoking cigarettes and to decrease the amount of alcohol intake if you drink excessively.

# PART IV

# Treating Lupus

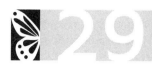

# General Treatment of Lupus

## Treatment of Lupus: That Was Then, This Is Now

As previously presented in the opening section of chapter 1 (photo on page 4), the very first case of lupus was described in the Middle Ages. Hildricus, the bishop of Liège (Liège was a city in Belgium), suffered from a disease called lupus that caused horrible, open sores on his skin but also affected the inside of his body. Although he was an upright, moral man, he developed lupus "by a secret judgment of God." He suffered greatly from the disease, not unlike people who have lupus today. His treatment was as follows. His physicians would have two young chickens freshly killed, plucked, and disemboweled. They would then place the raw chicken on the open sores of his body first thing in the morning. They would repeat this with two newly killed chickens later in the day. Supposedly, this was the only treatment that helped him feel better. This was an expensive form of therapy. Only a wealthy person in the Middle Ages could have afforded to use four chickens a day in this manner.

However, the use of chickens was not enough to cure Hildricus's lupus. He was about to die and realized that his physicians were not going to be able to cure him. Therefore, he traveled with a group of attendants to the tomb of Saint Martin in Tours, France. Like many devotees to Saint Martin, he was hoping that Saint Martin could cure him of his horrible disease. He and his attendants stayed and slept at the tomb for seven days and nights. It is written that Saint Martin, along with Saint Brice, who was buried close by, appeared to the bishop and cured him of his disease. The bishop was so thankful for his recovery that he gave a gift of silk tapestries and vessels made of gold and silver to the church of Saint Martin.

In the early 1800s, medical textbooks, in which doctors shared their experiences and recommendations for treatments, became more commonplace. Dr. Jonathan Green noted in his textbook published in 1835 that a healthy lifestyle, including nutritious food and exposure to open air such as at a seaside resort, were important in treating lupus. Of course, today doctors would not recommend a seaside resort due to our knowledge of how bad sun exposure is for people who have lupus. However, before the turn of the twentieth century, the disease lupus most likely comprised three totally separate diseases (lupus erythematosus [the subject of this book]; lupus pernio, which is due to a disease called sarcoidosis; and lupus vulgaris, which is due to tuberculosis). The latter two are not sun sensitive. In addition, Dr. Green was from England, where the beaches are not nearly as sunny as many others in the world.

Dr. Green also mentioned that it was common for doctors to use cauterization in the treatment of lupus sores. While cauterizing, physicians would apply heated metal instruments or fire to burn the sores of the skin. He was personally not an advocate of this form of therapy, but it continued to be used commonly for lupus throughout the 1800s. In fact, Dr. Alexander Squire wrote in 1868 that using cauterization was one of the quickest and most effective ways to treat lupus skin rashes, although it did leave significant scarring to the skin.

Dr. Green also recommended the use of arsenic as the first drug of choice for most patients (arsenic is a well-known poison). When applied to the skin, it appeared to decrease the severity and spread of the rashes of lupus. He also noted that mercury, sulfur, iodine, and silver compounds could be applied to the sores. These would cause significant inflammation with redness, pain, and heat after application. These were desired effects because it signified that the lupus-affected skin was being destroyed. He also recommended that blood-sucking leeches be applied around the edges of the sores followed by the use of narcotic-based salves to lessen the pain.

Dr. Thomas Hunt was a British dermatologist who wrote extensively on treatments of skin diseases from 1846 to 1864. For the treatment of lupus, he advised that patients should take lukewarm baths. Various therapies were recommended for the person who had lupus who had a fever, including going on a diet with decreased calories, taking the anti-inflammatory colchicum (now called colchicine, which is commonly used to treat gout), and medications that would cause the person to vomit. Bleeding (draining blood from the patient) was also recommended for fever. The practice of bleeding was done for many diseases back then to remove toxic substances from the body. Of course, now doctors know it probably contributed to the deaths of many more patients than it actually helped. Just like Dr. Green, Dr. Hunt also advocated using arsenic; however, he recommended that it be taken internally. He presented quite a few cases of lupus that were "cured" in this manner. He was also an advocate for people drinking cod liver oil for their lupus, and he presented cases where it was "curative" as well. The use of cod liver oil continued to have its advocates. In fact Dr. Tilbury Fox wrote in 1864 that cod liver oil was "the sheet-anchor in lupus," meaning that it was the best treatment of choice to treat people who had lupus. Doctors now know that cod liver oil is rich in anti-inflammatory omega-3 fatty acids and certainly may be helpful in lupus patients (chapters 38 and 39).

It is interesting that one of the people whom Dr. Hunt wrote about was treated with both arsenic and quinine. Quinine is an anti-malarial medication, and now doctors use the anti-malarial called hydroxychloroquine (Plaquenil) as the first drug of choice for most patients who have lupus. This is one of the first mentions of using an anti-malarial in someone with lupus.

In the mid-1800s, Dr. Moritz Kaposi first described the systemic problems from lupus. He advocated applying very irritating substances such as pure ammonia, acetic acid, arsenic, and hydrochloric acid to the lupus rash. He recommended that these substances should be rubbed into the borders of the rash with a hard brush to cause the skin to become raw. Severe pain at the treated area was thought necessary for the treatment to be successful. He also advocated using a sharp medical instrument called Volkmann's spoon to scrape away lupus-affected tissue. Supposedly, normal skin was resistant to the damage from the spoon while the lupus-affected tissue could be removed. Dr. Kaposi felt that treatments like these were effective for lupus involvement of the skin, but he did not recommend that anything be taken internally.

In 1868, Dr. Alexander Squire continued to recommend the use of arsenic internally for lupus along with quinine and cod liver oil, but he also added the use of walnut tree leaves and seawater as well. He went into quite a bit of detail about the proper diet for lupus, which needed to include well-seasoned, roasted or broiled mutton, beef, or game; coffee; and vegetables such as radishes. He also recommended that a glass or two of wine should be drunk at dinner each day as well.

Textbooks in the 1880s added that a treatment called linear scarification could be effective for treating lupus. This is a surgical procedure where numerous crisscrossed lines were cut into the lupus-affected areas of skin to cut off the blood supply so that the area of skin would essentially die and be easier to remove. Wine was even used to remove the crusts of cutaneous lupus.

Dr. J. F. Payne made the earliest mention of any modern forms of therapy in 1894. He went into detail about his success in using the anti-malarial quinine to treat people who had lupus. He would have them take 10 g to 30 g of quinine a day and noted that many of his patients had significant improvements in their lupus rashes. After that, anti-malarials would continue to play an important role in the treatment of lupus up until today, in the form of hydroxychloroquine (Plaquenil).

Throughout the first half of the twentieth century, it was strongly felt that lupus was due to an infection somewhere in the body. Many doctors felt that the best way to treat it was to remove any possible sources of infection. It became commonplace to remove tonsils or other infected parts of the body to try to "cure" lupus.

The next big "fad" for treating lupus was the use of gold. In 1890, the famous bacteriologist Dr. Robert Koch noted that the bacteria causing tuberculosis would die when exposed to gold while in a test tube. At that time, diseases such as rheumatoid arthritis and lupus were felt to be due to infections such as tuberculosis. Therefore, doctors and pharmacists began to make medications out of gold. Doctors prescribed gold for patients to take internally to see if it would help treat these diseases. It was actually quite successful in treating many people who had rheumatoid arthritis and was one of the most common therapies into the early 1990s. It was used a lot to treat people who had lupus in the 1920s to 1930s, but fell out of favor in the 1950s as medical studies showed that most patients who had lupus only had slight improvements from gold, or that its good effects wore off too quickly. In addition, cortisone arrived in 1949 and showed amazing effects in the treatment of lupus. Cortisone outshined gold and other worthless treatments for lupus at the time and truly ushered in the modern era of medicine.

Fortunately, doctors no longer use freshly killed, eviscerated chickens on their patients. Nor do they apply hot irons, hard brushes, or sharp spoons to scrape lupus sores. Doctors also do not use poisons such as arsenic or medications that cause patients to vomit (on purpose). Doctors do not treat patients with bad-tasting cod liver oil, nor do they remove the tonsils from every lupus patient they see. The treatment of lupus has come a long way. With today's methods, doctors are able to help the vast majority of people who have lupus to live a long, normal life. In others who have severe disease, doctors are able to extend their lives significantly and at least help ease their suffering to give them a better quality of life than what could be offered in the past. Part IV of this book (chapters 29–39) goes into detail about not only the medications your doctor can prescribe to help your lupus, but also things that you can do on your own to help your lupus out that can actually decrease the need for stronger medications (chapter 38). Many people are also interested in the use of complementary or alternative therapies, so chapter 39 discusses these treatments. This chapter explains how lupus is treated in general. It gives you some tools on how to assess the possibility of side effects of medicines, and offers advice on how to take medications appropriately to maximize your health to the fullest.

····

The treatment of lupus is complex. Since lupus is an autoimmune disease, where the immune system is overactive and attacks the body of the person, the primary treatment is to use medications that calm down the immune system. This chapter goes into detail about the thought processes that your doctor will go through when giving you treatments and medications while also giving you some insight into how best to take the medications. Subsequent chapters in part IV go into more detail about the medications and therapies themselves.

## How Your Doctor Chooses Medicines to Treat Lupus

There are many different ways to treat lupus, and it is possible to treat the exact same person in different ways successfully. Doctors choose therapies based on their own personal training and experience. Not all therapies work the same in everyone, so sometimes a trial-and-error approach to different medications may be needed before the best combination is found. For example, one person who has lupus arthritis may respond completely to taking only hydroxychloroquine, while another may fail numerous trials of medicines before the best therapy is found. Unfortunately, some people respond very poorly to most or all medicines, but this is uncommon.

Generally, when doctors evaluate people who have systemic lupus erythematosus (SLE), they note the different problems it is causing; identify which is the most severe problem; determine if any of the individual problems may require different therapies; and decide if the lupus is mild, moderate, or severe. Since every person who has lupus is different, every treatment decision is also different.

Most lupus experts treat all people who have lupus with hydroxychloroquine (Plaquenil), as discussed in chapter 30. It is by far the safest medicine that doctors have to calm down the immune system. It is very good for mild problems such as arthritis and rashes, it decreases the chances of developing severe internal organ involvement (such as lupus nephritis), it decreases the risk of getting blood clots, and it increases the chances of living a long, normal lifespan. The evidence is so strong in using Plaquenil that one group of doctors made this statement in their study from 2011: "Our analyses show that antimalarials [like hydroxychloroquine] are the only class of drugs that exerted a clear protective effect on survival [in people who have lupus]." One problem with hydroxychloroquine, though, is that it can take a long time to work in some people. The fastest it can work is about a month, while it can take up to a year to get the full effect in some people. If a person has mild lupus problems that do not bother her or him very much, then just taking hydroxychloroquine may be the only medicine required to treat her or his lupus successfully. However, if there are problems that are quite bothersome, such as joint pain, chest pain, disfiguring rash, profound fatigue, or other symptoms that cannot wait a month or so, then it is important to use something other than just hydroxychloroquine alone.

The only group of medications that works immediately for lupus is the corticosteroids (steroids for short) such as prednisone and methylprednisolone (see chapter 31). Anyone who does not feel very well, and definitely anyone who has any major internal organ involvement (such as the kidneys, lungs, brain, or heart), will need steroids initially along with the other medications (like hydroxychloroquine) that take longer to work. Some doctors call this bridge therapy, where they are using the steroid as a "bridge" to control the lupus quickly while they are waiting for better, but slower-working medicines to work. Some people can be resistant to using steroids for treatment, but in many situations it is very important to do so. While inflammation from lupus is occurring in the body, it can cause permanent damage to the organs it is attacking. The faster doctors can stop this inflammation, the better chances there are of preventing permanent organ damage. Therefore, for many problems in lupus, it is worth dealing with some of the side effects of the steroids compared to dealing with the permanent damage that could be caused by undertreating the lupus (such as not using steroids and allowing permanent, irreversible damage to occur). Doctors usually will use the steroids to calm down disease activity, then begin to lower the dose (called tapering the dose) once better control is obtained.

As far as how lupus is labeled as mild, moderate, or severe, there are no formal definitions of these terms for SLE. Doctors also usually do not write down "mild," "moderate," or "severe" in patients' charts or records; it is more or less an idea that doctors keep in their minds about how bad a given case of lupus is to help guide what the treatment should consist of. However, there are some disease characteristics or manifestations that the vast majority of rheumatologists would most likely agree on for these definitions. For example, if a person has mildly decreased blood cell counts, cutaneous lupus that is not very noticeable, or mild Raynaud's phenomenon (where the fingers turn pale or blue with exposure to cold), then she or he would most likely be felt to have mild lupus and hydroxychloroquine alone may be the treatment of choice.

On the other hand, if someone has major internal organ involvement, such as significant inflammation of the nerves, brain, heart, lungs, liver, or kidneys, then the person would be considered to have severe lupus especially if there was a chance for organ failure or death if not treated aggressively. People who have severe lupus are typically treated with high doses of steroids plus a strong medicine that suppresses the immune system such as cyclophosphamide, mycophenolate (CellCept and Myfortic), or azathioprine (Imuran).

Everything else would fall in between these two extremes, with many cases of lupus falling into the moderate category. People who have moderate lupus involvement usually also need another medicine in addition to hydroxychloroquine. It depends greatly on the exact circumstances to decide which medicines need to be used.

## Why So Many Medicines?

It is a normal reaction to be concerned about taking so many medications, and it is often difficult to convince someone to take so many especially when a person is young and may have never been on any medications at all previously. Sometimes different individual problems caused by lupus must be treated using different medications. In addition, sometimes doctors must also use medications to prevent or treat side effects of the medications that need to be used in people who have lupus. If you understand the reasoning for having to take so many medications, it can make it easier to accept the treatment plan and to stay compliant with taking the medicines.

The different, individual problems caused by lupus may require different types of therapies. Medicines that calm down the immune system are called immunomodulating medicines (table 29.1). These include hydroxychloroquine (Plaquenil), steroids, the numerous immunosuppressive medicines, and biologics (all discussed in the following chapters). The immunomodulating medicines are important to use for anything that is due to actual inflammation. This would include cutaneous lupus, arthritis, serositis (like pleurisy), and nephritis (kidney inflammation). However, some problems are not actually due to active inflammation and are not helped with these immunomodulating medications. These problems require other forms of therapies (table 29.2) in addition to taking the immunomodulating medicines to treat the active inflammation component of SLE.

One example of a non-inflammatory complication of lupus is Raynaud's phenomenon. This occurs when lupus causes the arteries that lead to the hands and feet to become smaller than normal, and the blood supply decreases during periods of stress and in cold temperatures. Sometimes the pale or blue fingers and toes can be accompanied by discomfort, or in severe examples, open sores can form on the fingertips. In these situations, medicines may be needed to open the blood vessels up and increase blood flow. The immunomodulating medicines and anti-inflammatory medicines (such as Plaquenil and prednisone) usually do not help decrease the Raynaud's attacks by very much.

Some people who have lupus have had blood clots due to antiphospholipid antibodies. These antibodies cause the blood to be thicker than normal. The drugs of choice for treating this problem are blood thinners such as warfarin (Coumadin). If someone is positive for the antibodies, but has never had a blood clot, then she or he may need to take an aspirin every day to try to prevent the blood clots from forming in the future.

Anywhere from 30% to 50% of people who have lupus will have Sjögren's syndrome, which causes dryness in numerous parts of the body, especially the mouth and eyes. Sometimes medications to increase fluid production may be needed such as Restasis eye drops for the eyes or pilocarpine (Salagen) and Evoxac for the dry mouth. Again, most of the immunomodulating medicines do not usually help very much with the dryness of Sjögren's syndrome (although Rituxan and Benlysta may have a role in the future).

Some people will need medications to decrease pain. One of the most common medicines used for this purpose, especially for arthritis and serositis, are the nonsteroidal anti-inflammatory drugs (NSAIDs) such as ibuprofen (Motrin) and naproxen (Naprosyn).

**Table 29.1** Immunomodulating Medicines Used to Treat SLE

Anti-malarial medicines (chapter 30)
    hydroxychloroquine (Plaquenil)
    chloroquine (Aralen)
    quinacrine
Corticosteroids ("steroids") (chapter 31)
    prednisone (Rayos)
    methylprednisolone (Medrol, Solu-Medrol)
    prednisolone
Immunosuppressant medicines (chapter 32)
    methotrexate (Rheumatrex, Trexall)
    azathioprine (Imuran)
    mycophenolic acid (CellCept, Myfortic)
    leflunomide (Arava)
    cyclosporine A (Neoral, Sandimmune, Gengraf)
    cyclophosphamide
Biologic agents
    TNF inhibitors (chapter 33)
        adalimumab (Humira)
        certolizumab pegol (Cimzia)
        etanercept (Enbrel)
        golimumab (Simponi)
        infliximab (Remicade)
    rituximab (Rituxan) (chapter 33)
    belimumab (Benlysta) (chapter 34)
Intravenous immunoglobulin (IVIG) (chapter 35)

**Table 29.2** Medications Other Than Immunomodulatory Medicines Used to Treat Problems from SLE

- Medications to dilate the arteries in Raynaud's phenomenon (chapter 11)
- Blood thinners for antiphospholipid antibodies (chapter 11)
- Medicines for the dry eyes and mouth of Sjögren's syndrome (chapter 14)
- NSAIDs and pain relievers for pain (chapters 7 and 36)

In addition to treating the problems of lupus itself, often other medications are needed to treat or prevent side effects from these medications (table 29.3). This is a very important part in the treatment of lupus. Although it adds a burden of having to take more medications and having to pay additional money for them, it can make a big difference in making sure that the medicines are used in the safest ways possible. For example, it is important to take a vitamin called folic acid or folinic acid (Leucovorin) to prevent side effects like low blood counts while taking the medicine called methotrexate. NSAIDs and steroids can sometimes cause significant stomach upset, heartburn, or even ulcers, so sometimes your doctor may want you to take a medicine to calm down the acidity of the stomach if these problems occur. If you have had an ulcer before, or if you are at increased risk of developing an ulcer, then your doctor may want to you to take an acid-lowering medicine such as a proton pump inhibitor like omeprazole (Prilosec) even if you feel perfectly fine. This is really a very important thing to do because most severe ulcers (such as a bleeding ulcer) occur without any warning at all (no abdominal pain), and it is best to prevent it from happening in the first place.

One of the worst side effects that can occur from taking steroids is a condition called osteoporosis where the bones become brittle and break. However, if you take calcium supplements, vitamin D, and medicines to keep the bones strong (especially the medicines called bisphosphonates), the chances for getting these broken bones are greatly reduced.

Some of the strong immunosuppressant medicines can increase the risk for infections, so sometimes it is important to take an antibiotic regularly along with the medicine (especially with the medicine called cyclophosphamide) to prevent infections from occurring in the first place. The biologic immunosuppressant medicines (such as the TNF [tumor necrosis factor] inhibitors) can potentially cause tuberculosis to become active in someone who has been exposed to the infection in their past. Therefore, if someone is positive for the TB (tuberculosis) skin test (called the PPD [purified protein derivative] test) or one of the blood tests for TB (QuantiFERON and the T-SPOT. TB), then she or he may need to take an antibiotic called isoniazid along with vitamin B-6 (to prevent side effects from the isoniazid) for nine months. As you can see these possibilities can be daunting; however, in the end, it is well worth taking these extra medicines compared to developing the potential bad complications that could occur without taking them.

For example, Lucy is a 25-year-old woman who has inflammatory arthritis and Raynaud's phenomenon from her SLE and is positive for anticardiolipin antibodies (a type of antiphospholipid antibody, as discussed in chapters 4 and 9). She is placed on hydroxychloroquine (Plaquenil) as almost all lupus patients are, but her pain from the arthritis is too uncomfortable to wait a few months for the hydroxychloroquine to work. Meloxicam (a type of NSAID) is added for the arthritis pain and it helps somewhat but not enough. Therefore, her rheumatologist ends up needing to put her on prednisone as well, which helps her feel much better. She is unable to tolerate her Raynaud's attacks (where her fingers turn pale and uncomfortable with cold temperatures); therefore, she is placed on nifedipine (Procardia), which is a blood pressure medicine used to dilate the arteries of the fingers and makes her Raynaud's much less uncomfortable. Since she has an increased chance of developing blood clots in the future due to her antiphospholipid antibodies, she takes 81 mg of aspirin a day to pre-

**Table 29.3** Medicines Used to Prevent or Treat Side Effects of Medicines
Used in SLE

- Vitamins folic acid or folinic acid (Leucovorin) used with the medicine methotrexate

- Anti-acid medicines (such as proton pump inhibitors; chapter 28)
    used for stomach upset caused by many medicines
    used to treat gastroesophageal reflux that may become worse with medicines
    used to prevent ulcers in people at increased risk of getting ulcers

- Used to prevent and treat osteoporosis in people on steroids
    bisphosphonate medicines (such as alendronate or Fosamax)
    calcium supplement with vitamin D

- Antibiotics used to prevent infections in people on immunosuppressant medicines
    dapsone or Septra for people on cyclophosphamide
    isoniazid for biologic agents in people exposed to tuberculosis

vent these blood clots from forming. She feels markedly better on this regimen, but unfortunately develops a lot of heartburn due to the steroid and the meloxicam. She changes her eating habits to try to control the heartburn, but this does not resolve the issue. Therefore, omeprazole (Prilosec) is added, which gets rid of her heartburn problems. In addition, since she is at increased risk of developing fragile bones (osteoporosis) on the steroid; she is asked to take a calcium supplement (calcium citrate, which is the best form to take while taking an acid-lowering medicine) twice a day plus alendronate (Fosamax) once a week to keep her bones strong.

Lucy feels markedly better, and therefore her rheumatologist begins to taper down the dose of her prednisone. As Lucy's prednisone dose is decreased to 7 mg a day, her arthritis flares. Although she is on a lower dose of prednisone, her rheumatologist realizes that he needs to put her on a medication that can help lower her need for steroids more or possibly get her off them eventually. Therefore, he places her on methotrexate once a week, plus one tablet of folic acid a day (to prevent any side effects from the methotrexate). She feels markedly better at this point and is able to decrease her prednisone dose down farther. However, to get to this point (resolving the arthritis pain plus tapering down her steroids significantly), it has required the use of many different pills to control the lupus and to prevent and treat complications (such as blood clots from the antiphospholipid antibodies and side effects from the medicines) (table 29.4).

This is a typical example of a person with moderate SLE who goes from being a person who has never taken any medicines in her life, to where she now must take nine different medicines on a regular basis for her lupus. Each medicine and vitamin has a specific purpose and is very important to take. In this example, you may ask why the meloxicam was not stopped when it did not control her arthritis pains well enough and the steroid had to be added to her medication regimen. The reason is that doctors generally try to do everything they can to keep people on the lowest doses of steroids (like prednisone) as possible. Taking the meloxicam regularly will most likely help to keep Lucy on lower doses of prednisone compared to if she did not take the

**Table 29.4** Example of Multiple Medications Used in a Patient Who Has SLE

- Hydroxychloroquine (Plaquenil) treatment for SLE taken by almost everyone who has SLE
- Meloxicam (Mobic), an NSAID for arthritis pain
- Aspirin (81 mg/day) to prevent blood clots resulting from antiphospholipid antibodies
- Prednisone (steroid) for arthritis not controlled well enough by the above
- Omeprazole (Prilosec) for heartburn from the above medicines
- Alendronate (Fosamax) to prevent broken bones from steroid-induced osteoporosis
- Calcium citrate to prevent broken bones from steroid-induced osteoporosis
- Methotrexate in place of steroids for arthritis
- Folic acid to prevent side effects from methotrexate

meloxicam. Although the prednisone can be an incredibly important medicine to give rapid pain relief from arthritis, when taken for a long time and at higher doses, eventually everyone will get side effects from it, as opposed to medicines such as meloxicam where most people do not get any significant side effects. After Lucy gets under good control from adding the methotrexate, the next step would be to begin tapering her prednisone again slowly to try to get her off it eventually. If her rheumatologist is able to get her off prednisone, then alendronate and the calcium could be stopped as well, possibly followed by stopping the meloxicam and omeprazole. If that is not possible, then, unfortunately, another lupus medicine may need to be added to try to get her off the prednisone.

## How to Approach Medicine Side Effects Like a Doctor

Anything taken internally into the body can potentially cause problems. When a substance is taken for a medical purpose and then causes an unwanted problem, doctors call it either a side effect or an adverse event. Even water, if drunk in excessive quantities, can cause problems in the body. Something as harmless appearing as a multiple vitamin can potentially cause the side effect of stomach upset. Taking vitamins in sufficient quantities, even in normal amounts recommended on bottles over the counter from a drugstore, can potentially cause side effects. For example, taking vitamin B-6 tablets as directed from an over-the-counter preparation can potentially cause nerve damage if levels of the vitamin build up high enough in the blood. Even food causes side effects. If people eat too much, or if they eat the wrong kinds of foods, then they can become overweight, or they can get heart attacks and strokes. People who have certain medical conditions can get side effects from certain foods. For example, people who have high blood pressure can possibly develop dangerously high blood pressures if they eat too much salt, or people who have gout can get a gout attack if they eat too much seafood. All of these examples are potential side effects. If people learn how to limit their intake of these things to levels that are safe, then they can greatly decrease the possibility of their causing side effects yet still reap the benefits of taking these particular substances. The same goes for medications.

Many people are afraid to take medicines because of their potential side effects. They seem to think that if a medication lists something as a side effect that they are going to get that particular side effect. Sometimes this turns out to be a self-fulfilling prophecy. Then there are others who seem to think that everyone who takes the medicine is bound to get the side effects that are listed.

It is very important for you to understand the potential for side effects from medications as it will greatly enhance your medical care if you learn how to address them in a rational manner. Side effects absolutely can be potentially very dangerous and even life threatening. Many people have probably known someone who has had a dangerous side effect from a medication or perhaps they have had a bad side effect from a medicine themselves. However, the reality is that most people never develop a severe reaction or side effect to medications.

When taking a medication, it is always important to weigh the risk of potential side effects against the benefit that the medicine can provide. For example, if you develop pneumonia (infection of the lungs) and your doctor prescribes penicillin for your infection, you may read on the side effects list provided to you by your pharmacist that one of the potential side effects from the medicine is severe allergic reaction and even death. It is true that close to four hundred Americans die every year from just taking penicillin. However, the number of lives saved from taking penicillin is markedly higher than that because it is rare to have that severe of a reaction to penicillin. Many people certainly are allergic to penicillin and learn over their lifetime to never take it if they have had an allergic reaction, but the vast majority of those allergic reactions are not life threatening. All antibiotics, in fact, can potentially cause dangerous, life-threatening side effects. Yet, the chance of dying or developing permanent body damage from an infection such as pneumonia is far greater than the chances of developing these severe side effects. In other words, the benefit of taking the antibiotic outweighs the potential side effects. This is an example of how doctors weigh the risks and benefits of a medication (figure 29.1). A medicine should always have a much greater chance of providing beneficial effects against a disease compared to the potential harm that they can cause.

Today new medications approved in the United States are studied far more extensively than at any other time in history. Due to public demand and the U.S. legal system, there is far greater scrutiny in the approval of new medications. When a drug first comes on the market today, you can be assured that it has been studied in more people and more intensely by doctors and scientists than older medications were.

The agency that is responsible for ensuring that medications are safe in America is the United States Food and Drug Administration (FDA for short). After a potential medication has undergone rigorous research in numerous trials on human subjects, panels of experts at the FDA review the results of the research studies to decide whether the medicine does what it is supposed to do for a disorder, and whether it is safe enough for people to take for that disorder. This determination, of course, will depend on the disease being treated. For example, a medicine used to treat a mild skin rash should have hardly any potential side effects at all and certainly no dangerous side effects. On the other hand, it may be more acceptable to have some potentially very

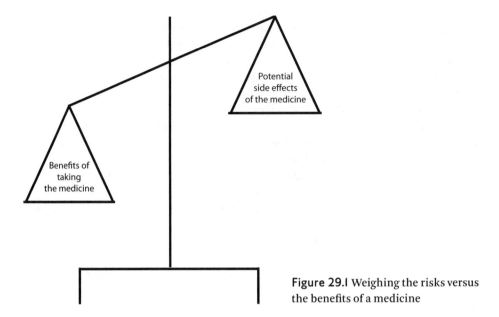

**Figure 29.1** Weighing the risks versus the benefits of a medicine

dangerous side effects in a medicine used to treat a rapidly deadly disease (such as some forms of cancer), especially if there are no other therapies available.

Even after a medicine is approved for use, though, it does not always mean that the medicine will be entirely "safe enough" for use. The reason for this is that research studies are incredibly difficult to do, are very expensive, and can realistically be done only on a finite number of people. There is no way to know every single potential side effect even with today's high standards established by the FDA. It is not until the medicine has been used more widely after its approval that doctors truly get a better idea of how safe the medicine is. Monitoring side effects of medications after they are approved by the FDA and become widely used by doctors and patients is called post-marketing surveillance. It is important for both patients and doctors to report any significant side effects that medications may cause after they come onto the market, especially if they are serious side effects. Patients and doctors can report medicine side effects by contacting the Adverse Event Reporting System of the FDA by sending an email to druginfo@fda.hhs.gov, calling (888) 463-6332, or by filling out a form on the internet at www.accessdata.fda.gov/scripts/email/cder/comment.cfm. Sometimes enough significant side effects are seen post-marketing on a drug that the medication is deemed unsafe and is taken off the market.

A practical way to evaluate the side effects of a medication is to think like a doctor. Physicians are much more apt to take medications than are many laypeople. Doctors prescribe so many medications on a daily basis that they have a better feel about how often the side effects actually occur and how severe they are. Doctors realize that the vast majority of side effects seen with most medications are more or less nuisance side effects that are mild and tolerable, or that easily resolve after the medicine is stopped.

In addition, doctors know how to assess the medical studies on medications to get a better sense of how often side effects occur. On the other hand, laypeople who are prescribed medicines deal with the unknown and are left with sheets of paper given to them by their pharmacists that simply list what side effects can potentially occur from the prescribed medicines. Therefore, it can be more helpful to think like a doctor when you are looking at the potential side effects from medicines.

Here is an example of how to do this. Table 29.5 is based on an FDA-approved drug insert on a commonly prescribed arthritis medicine. It includes the side effects that were seen and how often they occurred. On the left side of the table is the list of side effects and on the right is how frequently they occurred.

So look over the list. Most people's gut reaction would be that there is no way they would want to take this medicine that causes a headache in 20% of people who take it, or causes them to hurt themselves (accidental injury), or causes all of these infections. Therefore, what do you think of this therapy?

Actually, this is a list of the "side effects" seen in people who took the placebo (commonly called a sugar pill) in the studies for the anti-inflammatory pain reliever called

**Table 29.5** Frequency of Side Effects Seen in a Research Study on a Common Arthritis Medication

| Side Effect | People Who Had the Side Effect (%) |
| --- | --- |
| Abdominal pain | 2.8 |
| Diarrhea | 3.8 |
| Dyspepsia (stomach upset, heartburn) | 6.2 |
| Flatulence (gas) | 1.0 |
| Nausea | 4.2 |
| Back pain | 3.6 |
| Peripheral edema (swelling of the ankles) | 1.1 |
| Accidental injury | 2.3 |
| Dizziness | 1.7 |
| Headache | 20.2 |
| Insomnia | 2.3 |
| Pharyngitis (sore throat) | 1.1 |
| Rhinitis (runny nose) | 1.3 |
| Sinusitis (sinus infection) | 4.3 |
| Upper respiratory infection | 6.7 |
| Rash | 2.1 |

celecoxib (Celebrex). In the best medical studies, a large group of patients enters the study, but some of them take a placebo while others will take the actual study medicine. In the research, the placebo medicine and the actual medicine look the same. For example, if it is a pill, all of the pills are the same color, shape, and size, and have the same types of markings on them. Neither the patients taking the medicines nor the doctors conducting the study know who are taking the actual medicine and who are taking a placebo. However, it is monitored very closely by a secret code that is only known by the pharmacists who distribute the pills to the people participating in the research study. Only after the study is completely finished do the pharmacists reveal the results. Then mathematical calculations can be performed to figure out what percentage of people responded to the medicine and what percentage "responded" to the placebo and also what percentage had side effects.

So how can 20% of people get a headache due to taking a placebo? Of course, they did not get a headache from taking the "sugar pill." It is important to understand how these "side effects" are counted in research. In a medical study, patients who are taking the medicines (or placebos) see the doctors doing the research on a regular basis during the study. Each time they are seen, they fill out a long questionnaire asking them if they have had any problems at all during the previous period. They mark down "yes" to anything that they have experienced, including things such as headaches, colds, back pain, joint pain, upset stomach, and injuries. The bottom line is that many people get headaches, back pain, colds, and injuries in their daily lives on a normal basis not related to taking pills. When any of these occur in those who take the placebo, they are considered a "placebo effect" for side effects. The placebo is not causing any of these side effects; this is just background noise of things that happen in daily life normally. To show that a medicine actually causes side effects, it has to be demonstrated that the medicine causes more of that particular problem than what is seen in the people who take the placebo.

In addition, there has to be a statistically significant difference between the groups. Just because there are more people who report a problem (side effect) in a research study, it does not necessarily mean that the medicine actually causes more of that side effect because this difference could possibly be due to chance alone. For example, let us say that you want to do a research study to show how often a quarter comes up heads or tails when you flip it. Of course, we know intuitively that it is very close to 50:50; one-half the time it should come up heads and one-half the time it should come up tails. So, let us say that you decide you only want to flip the quarter four times for your study. You flip it four times. Three times, it actually comes up tails and one time it comes up heads. Therefore, you calculate from your "study" that when you flip a quarter, three out of four times (75% of the time) it will come up tails, and only one out of four times (25% of the time) it will come up heads. Of course, the results of this study are completely incorrect since we all know it should be closer to 50% for both. It is easy to see that this study should be done with a lot more flips of the coin. By intuition alone, we can realize that by only flipping the coin four times and it lands tails-up 75% of the time: this occurred simply due to chance. You should have flipped the coin a lot more times than four times to have a good-quality study that would give you a reliable result.

This is where the mathematical experts who specialize in statistics (called statisticians) come into play. They can actually figure out how many times the coin should be flipped to have a meaningful study result before the study is actually done. Then, after the study is finished, the statisticians can figure out whether the results are statistically correct (or statistically significant) and can be trusted. Even we as non-statisticians can easily tell that in this particular study there is not statistical difference between the 75% tails and the 25% heads and it is all because the quarter was not flipped enough times. In much larger studies, looking at a significant number of patients and many potential side effects with many possible response rates to a medicine, it becomes markedly more difficult. To tell whether there is a statistically significant difference in the percentage of people who developed a particular side effect to a medicine or not compared to placebo requires complicated mathematical calculations. It is the statistician's job to figure out whether a difference in numbers was simply due to chance or not. If the numbers are not statistically and significantly different than they would be just due to chance, then it cannot be concluded that the medicine causes that particular side effect. If there is a statistically significant difference by these calculations, therefore not occurring just by chance alone, then the side effect probably is actually due to the medicine.

So now let us look at the same numbers in the Celebrex study (table 29.6), but this time we will insert the amount of times that these side effects also occurred in patients who took Celebrex. By the way, it is very easy for you as a patient to obtain these kinds of results yourself. If your doctor has samples of medicines, these samples will contain the FDA prescribing information, and it will include a chart similar to this with the percentage of times that a potential side effect occurs with the medicine and the percentage of times it occurs in the people who took the placebo. It is also very easy to get this kind of information on the internet. Most medications have their own websites that use their name in the website. For example, to find this information for Celebrex, just go to www.celebrex.com (type in the name of whatever drug it is followed by .com). Then on the main page of the website, it should have a place that says "prescribing information" that you can click on to access this information. Alternatively, it may say something to the effect of "for healthcare professionals" where you can click on that section and it will take you to the prescribing information. If you cannot find the website of the medicine by using the name of the medicine followed by .com, another way to find it is to go to www.google.com (or any other search engine) and do an internet search using the keywords "prescribing information" and the name of the medicine.

So now, let us take a closer look at these numbers. Jump right to the headache side effect row. Note that only 15.8% of the people who took Celebrex got headaches. Compare that to the 20.2% of people who got headaches on the placebo. Quite a few more people got headaches on the placebo than from taking Celebrex. Of course, this does not mean that taking a placebo causes headaches. In the actual research studies, the statisticians would have done their calculations and figured out that there is actually no statistically significant difference between these two numbers. Although it appears that more people got headaches from taking the placebo, this increased number occurred simply due to chance alone.

However, the FDA does not include these statistically significant determinations in the prescribing information. This information is provided in the actual research studies that are available to doctors to review (usually in medical journals or in more in-depth study results that doctors can get from drug companies). Still, you can look

**Table 29.6** Frequency of Side Effects Seen in a Research Study on Celebrex

| Side Effect | Placebo Group % | Celebrex Group % |
|---|---|---|
| Abdominal pain | 2.8 | 4.1 |
| Diarrhea | 3.8 | 5.6 |
| Dyspepsia (stomach upset) | 6.2 | 8.8 |
| Flatulence (gas) | 1.0 | 2.2 |
| Nausea | 4.2 | 4.2 |
| Back pain | 3.6 | 2.8 |
| Peripheral edema (swelling of the ankles) | 1.1 | 2.1 |
| Accidental injury | 2.3 | 2.9 |
| Dizziness | 1.7 | 2.0 |
| Headache | 20.2 | 15.8 |
| Insomnia (difficulty sleeping) | 2.3 | 2.3 |
| Pharyngitis (sore throat) | 1.1 | 2.3 |
| Rhinitis (runny nose) | 1.3 | 2.0 |
| Sinusitis (sinus infection) | 4.3 | 5.0 |
| Upper respiratory infection (colds) | 6.7 | 8.1 |
| Rash | 2.1 | 2.2 |

at the numbers yourself and get a sense as to whether there is a big difference in the numbers or not.

For example, many of these side effect numbers are not very different when you compare them (such as accidental injury, dizziness, headaches, insomnia, sinusitis, upper respiratory tract infection, and rash). Therefore, there is a very good chance that Celebrex does not cause these side effects (at least when based on this particular study's results). It is more helpful to compare how much larger one percentage is than another to get a better feel for whether there is an important difference or not. For example, look at the numbers for flatulence (gas). An increased amount of flatulence (compared to their normal amount) occurred in 1% of people who took the placebo and in 2.2% of those who took Celebrex. While the difference between these two numbers is only 1.2% (2.2 − 1.0 = 1.2), it is more helpful to figure out their ratio difference by dividing the numbers. The 2.2% of the Celebrex group is more than double the 1.0% of the placebo group. While this particular example is easy to figure out intuitively (2.2% is more than twice as large as 1%), this can be figured out mathematically by dividing the two numbers: 2.2 divided by 1 is 2.2. Therefore, flatulence occurred 2.2 times more often in the people taking Celebrex than in those who took the placebo. It would be easy to figure out that this much of a difference is an important one.

Then you can ask yourself, "So what percent of people who take Celebrex probably get flatulence due to the Celebrex?" A rough way of estimating this is by subtracting the numbers. Subtract 1% (the placebo rate) from the 2.2% and you can suspect that about 1.2% of people who take Celebrex can expect to get an increased amount of flatulence due to the Celebrex.

Using this method does not tell you if there is truly a statistically significant difference between all the numbers or not. It is easy enough to figure out if the placebo numbers are bigger than the numbers for the drug itself. For example, since more headaches occurred in the placebo group than in the Celebrex group, it can be safe to assume that Celebrex probably does not cause headaches. Or if the ratio difference is large enough, such as flatulence occurring in more than twice as many people who take Celebrex, it is also easy to figure out if there is truly a difference or not. These simple mathematical determinations can give you a sense about whether there is truly a difference or not. Other side effects on this list that probably occur more commonly with Celebrex more often than just by chance include abdominal pain, diarrhea, dyspepsia (indigestion), edema (swelling caused by a collection of fluid in tissues), pharyngitis (inflammation of the throat), and rhinitis (inflammation of the nasal mucous membrane).

The FDA is not in the business of determining whether medicines definitely cause certain side effects or not. Its job is to determine whether medicines do what they are supposed to do for certain diseases and to make sure that they are safe enough to treat those diseases. As far as reporting the potential side effects, the FDA just states the numbers themselves and leaves it up to doctors to interpret these numbers. For example, in the prescription information on Celebrex, the FDA has decided to report which "side effects" occurred more than 2% of the time and it lists all the "side effects" that occurred that often.

Since headaches occurred in about 15% of people who took Celebrex (more than their 2% cutoff), headaches must be reported in this table of side effects. As we now see, this does not necessarily mean that Celebrex causes headaches. It is up to physicians (and patients) to question these numbers and look at them more closely. In the example analysis above, although 15% of people who took Celebrex got headaches, more people who took placebo got headaches so it probably is not a significant side effect due to Celebrex. In fact, doctors often prescribe Celebrex to treat headaches (as it works on all kinds of pain). Therefore, that is probably why there were fewer headaches in the Celebrex group. However, it is still listed as a potential side effect by the FDA simply because it was above that 2% mark. In fact, headaches will also be included in the list of side effects provided to you by your pharmacist when you pick up your prescription of Celebrex. This is just one of numerous examples of how you must be critical of medical information provided to you, and that it is always better to ask your doctor's opinion on any question you may have about medical information instead of relying on everything you read in print.

This same problem of FDA reporting of side effects also occurs with advertisements of drugs to patients, or what is termed "direct to patient advertising" in the medical field. The FDA requires that certain potential side effects be presented in a "direct to patient advertisement" without actually giving an indication of whether it is truly an actual side effect or not, or how often it realistically happens. This is one reason many doctors do not like advertisements on the television or in magazines that are directed toward patients. Often, they over-exaggerate potential side effects that may not be side effects at all or occur so rarely that they scare patients unnecessarily. Therefore, whenever you see an advertisement for a medicine, it is always a good idea to ask your doctor's opinion about what the advertisement says.

So let us put all this together and try to simplify how to look at potential side effects of a medicine. Let us say that your doctor has prescribed Celebrex. You get a list of side effects from your pharmacist (which by the way includes a list as recommended by the FDA) which includes things such as stomach pain, nausea, headaches, and back pain. There is an irrational way to think about these side effects and there is a rational way to think about them. The irrational way is to decide that you are not going to take that medicine because you do not want any of those side effects, and you are deathly afraid of getting headaches (which as you now know you would actually get more often with a placebo than from Celebrex). This is the wrong way to approach the issue.

The rational way to approach side effects is to do one of several different things. One method is to ask your pharmacist while you are at the pharmacy, "How often has Celebrex been shown to actually cause headaches compared to the placebo?" Then ask if she or he can show it to you in the package insert. Then you can ask what her or his opinion is of that particular side effect. That is one of the quickest ways to get better information about side effects. The second method would be to simply ask your doctor (but this may take longer if your next appointment is not scheduled for a while) and get his or her opinion.

The final way to investigate the potential side effects is to do a simple analysis on your own as outlined above using the following three steps (table 29.7).

For example, let us say that you are worried about the possibility of getting diarrhea from the drug. You would use the following method:

1. 5.6% (Celebrex) – 3.8% (placebo) = 1.8%.

2. 5.6% (Celebrex) ÷ 3.8% (placebo) = 1.47.

3. Since the ratio difference in step 2 is more than 1.25, diarrhea most likely does occur more often with Celebrex than placebo. Probably about 1.8% of people (the answer in part 1) could develop diarrhea due to the drug. This also means that 98.2% of people (the vast majority) who take Celebrex would not develop diarrhea due to Celebrex.

This calculation on your part provides a more realistic perspective on how often Celebrex may cause diarrhea and whether it is truly a potential side effect or not. Although diarrhea probably does occur as a true side effect from Celebrex, it occurs in only a tiny fraction of people who take it.

Let us do another example. Let us say that you are prone to getting colds (upper respiratory infections) so when you read that these infections occurred in 8.1% of people who took Celebrex, it really worries you. Again, the irrational approach would be to avoid taking Celebrex because you are afraid it will cause you to get sick with a cold. So you would be refusing to take a medicine that could potentially get rid of joint pain from your lupus arthritis and give you a better quality of life without thinking this through more clearly. The better way to approach this issue is to follow the previous steps on evaluating this potential side effect of colds:

**Table 29.7** Evaluation of Potential Side Effects of Drugs Compared to Placebo

1. What is the difference between how often this side effect occurred in those who took the drug itself and those who took the placebo? (Subtract the placebo percentage from that occurring from the drug.)

2. Is there a very big difference in the ratio of these two numbers to give an idea as to whether it is truly a statistically significant difference or not? (Divide the percentage number occurring with the drug by that occurring with the placebo group.)

3. If the ratio in the second part seems large (use a ratio of 1.25 or bigger), then it may actually be a true side effect from the medicine, and you can use the difference number obtained in question 1 to figure out approximately what percentage of people probably get that particular side effect.

1. 8.1% (Celebrex) – 6.7% (placebo) = 1.4%.

2. 8.1% (Celebrex) ÷ 6.7% = 1.21.

3. Since the answer in step 2 is less than 1.25 (see explanation below), it probably is not a definite side effect of Celebrex. In fact, Celebrex does not cause upper respiratory infections (colds) at all (even though it is in the list of potential side effects in the package insert). If you did not take the medicine because you were afraid of getting a cold from Celebrex, you would have been doing the wrong thing because Celebrex does not cause colds. It is better to do the calculation yourself, as we did here, or ask your doctor or pharmacist about it.

The above method can help you think more rationally about how to approach potential side effects of medicines. However, not everything is as easy as it looks. The second step, where I recommended a ratio of 1.25 and higher as the cutoff on considering a side effect as being real, is arbitrary and not completely accurate (remember, only the statisticians with their very complex formulas can truly determine this possibility). However, this does give you a close enough number to work with that will be correct much of the time. It is always a good idea to ask your doctor for her or his opinion if you are still worried about a particular side effect, especially if this ratio difference is below 1.25. The higher this number, by the way, the more likely it is truly a side effect, especially if it is close to 1.5 or higher.

Some side effects occur so infrequently that they do not show up very well in these studies. For example, a very small number of people can develop an allergic rash to Celebrex. This occurs in approximately 50% of people who have a sulfa allergy. The number of people who got a rash while on Celebrex is similar those who got it from the placebo. The reason for this is that people who had a known allergy to sulfa antibiotics were not allowed to be in the research study in the first place since it was known to be a possible side effect. This is a well-known side effect that your pharmacist and doctor would be aware of. Your doctor would warn you to stop the medicine if you get a rash or warn you about the possibility ahead of time if you get rashes when you take sulfa antibiotics.

It is also helpful to divide side effects into those that are considered mild and those that are potentially dangerous. Many side effects are considered mild or nuisance-type side effects. Many people are willing to put up with mild side effects and continue to take the medicine safely (especially if the medicine is helping a lot). Other acceptable responses to mild side effects include decreasing the medicine dosage, or your doctor may stop it and switch you to a different medication. If you ever get a side effect to a medicine, it is important to let your doctor know so that he or she can give you instructions on whether it is safe to continue taking the medicine or not. The severity of side effects can vary a lot from medicine to medicine as well. For example, mild stomach upset on an antibiotic may be considered very mild, not dangerous, and worth putting up with to get rid of an infection. However, the same amount of stomach upset on an anti-inflammatory medicine (e.g., Motrin) is more serious because sometimes it can be the warning sign of an ulcer in the stomach. Your doctor may want you to either stop the medicine completely or take an anti-ulcer medicine along with the Motrin.

It is best not to determine how mild a side effect of a medicine is on your own. It is always better to contact your doctor's office for advice instead. In this book, medications used to treat lupus are accompanied by charts containing a list of potential side effects to the medicine. I only list those that are definitely known to occur with the drug (taking the guesswork out on your part) and indicate whether they are considered mild or severe as well as how often they occur and what you should do if you get the side effect. Even with these charts, though, it is still a good idea to contact your doctor if you get a side effect on a medicine to get her or his advice.

Be careful about what you hear on the news. The news is a good source to learn about things for the first time, but when it comes to medical information, the media often get it wrong. The purpose of the news is to evoke interest and get people to watch or read reports. Therefore, it can be advantageous to the media to take the results of a medical study and report them as soon as possible, and even to sensationalize them. Unfortunately, this can sometimes lead to people worrying too much about something that may not be true at all or may be blown out of proportion. This is especially the case when it comes to news reports on studies showing possible side effects of medications. When doctors are watching television and see a news report on a medical study showing that a medicine does not work or causes certain side effects, most of them cringe. This is because they realize the report is oversimplifying the results of the study and is most likely not giving all of the facts, or fails to compare this particular study to other studies appropriately. In addition, doctors dread the barrage of phone calls from worried patients they expect to receive the day after the news report.

One recent example of this news-reporting phenomenon was when the media began reporting that the bisphosphonates (medicines, such as Fosamax, taken to treat osteoporosis) were causing a complication called osteonecrosis of the jaw. Osteonecrosis of the jaw occurs when a small piece of bone in the jaw dies, the overlying gum thins out to expose the dead bone, and there is great difficulty with its healing. This news caused many people to stop taking their osteoporosis medicines. In actuality, this particular potential side effect has mainly been seen in people who have bone cancer and took very high doses of these medicines in the intravenous (IV) form. However, in the typical patient with osteoporosis, this side effect is extremely rare, only reported in one out of 150,000 patients who take it. In fact, it is so rare that it still is not known whether it is truly a side effect of the medicine or not since osteonecrosis of the jaw can occur for many other reasons other than from taking a medicine (remember: it must be proven that a medicine causes a side effect more often than by chance alone). One out of every two women will develop a major bone fracture due to osteoporosis if it is not treated. It is much better to take the bisphosphonate instead of worry about osteonecrosis of the bone (figure 29.2). The bottom line is that if you hear something that worries you about your medical condition or a medication which you are taking, instead of becoming too excited and worried, make an appointment with your doctor to find out his or her opinion on the matter. Your physician can put things into better perspective for you.

## Cancer from Lupus Medicines

A large number of the medications that are used in treating lupus and that suppress the immune system carry warnings about their possibly causing cancer. This is primarily done from a theoretical standpoint in many cases. The immune system is very important in policing our bodies to get rid of any cancerous cells that form throughout our lives, so it makes sense that if a medication suppresses the immune system, that there could be an increased risk for developing cancer. So far, the TNF inhibitors (see chapter 33) have been studied the most regarding this question. Although there have been a few controversial results, overall, there appears to be no significant risk

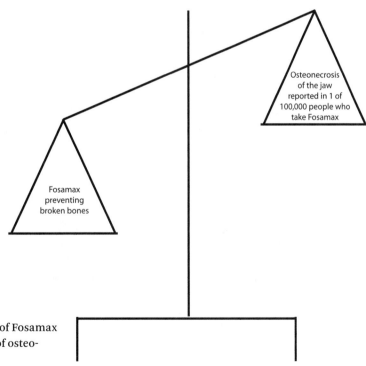

Osteonecrosis of the jaw reported in 1 of 100,000 people who take Fosamax

Fosamax preventing broken bones

**Figure 29.2** The benefits of Fosamax versus the potential risk of osteonecrosis of the jaw

for developing cancer from these medications according to the latest studies. Read the section on TNF inhibitors to learn more specifics. (Also see "Lymphoma," pp. 346–47).

## General Advice on Managing Your Medical Treatment

### Compliance

As discussed in chapter 20, compliance is one of the most, if not the most, important factor in doing well with lupus. One part of compliance is ensuring that you take your medications as directed by your doctor, plus seeing your doctor to get the necessary tests to ensure that the medicine is not causing any side effects. It is extremely important to take most medicines used to treat lupus on a regular basis because many of them must build up in the body and stay at steady levels in the blood to exert their beneficial effects. If you forget your medicine on a regular basis, then it is not going to work. When your doctor sees you and notes that your lupus is not doing well, but you keep forgetting to take your medicine, it is very important that you let him or her know this fact. Otherwise, your doctor will assume that the medicine is not working and either add something to your medicine regimen or switch to another medication. It is better to admit to not taking a medicine regularly, identify why that is happening, and then come up with a plan to help you take it regularly.

The most common reason for a medicine not working is due to not taking the medicine or not taking it properly. In fact, Dr. C. Everett Koop, former surgeon general of the United States, said, "Drugs don't work if people don't take them." Studies often show that drugs for chronic diseases (like lupus) are taken properly only about 50% of the time overall. A study focusing on this question in patients who had SLE supported these results, with only 49% of them taking their hydroxychloroquine (Plaquenil) on a regular basis. This is worrisome because rheumatologists know that Plaquenil is by far the safest medicine to treat lupus. People who take it regularly are much less likely to get severe internal organ involvement or even to die from their lupus. Therefore, this large number of patients who are not taking their hydroxychloroquine regularly are playing with fire and inviting their lupus to become more active. If this does occur, then they are facing the possibility of needing high doses of steroids and strong immunosuppressant medicines that have many more potential side effects compared to hydroxychloroquine.

It can be difficult to remember to take medications regularly, especially if they need to be taken at different times of the day or on different days of the week. There are some strategies that can help a lot in remembering to take your medications as instructed (table 29.8). The most important initial strategy is to convince yourself about how important it is to take your medications regularly. If you can convince yourself about what a serious disease SLE is, that you truly have the disorder, and that you must take your mediations regularly to do well, then you will be more motivated to take your medications. Some people (especially younger people who were previously very healthy) can go into denial about their illness, which then contributes to their not taking their medications as prescribed.

Depressed people are less likely to stick to a treatment regimen and take their medications regularly as prescribed. If you have depression, it needs to be treated. If you are being treated for depression, but still feel significantly depressed, then you need

**Table 29.8** Strategies to Ensure That You Take Your Medications Regularly

- Convince yourself about the importance of taking your medicines regularly.
- If you are depressed (table 13.4) make sure to see your doctor for proper treatment.
- Educate yourself about how the medicine works, how long it takes to work, and what lupus can do to you if you do not take the medicine regularly.
- Ask your doctor if there is an alternative medicine that is easier to take, such as a once-a-day medicine.
- If a medicine is too expensive for you, immediately ask if there is a cheaper alternative.
- Keep your medicines in places that will remind you to take them (such as on your desk at work or in your purse).
- Fill up a large pill organizer once a month to ensure you do not miss any medicines.
- Set alarms on your cell phone or smart phone to remind you to take your medicines.
- Ask a family member to help remind you to take your medicines.
- Stick to a particular regimen that will get you into the habit of taking your medicine (e.g., always taking it after breakfast or after you brush your teeth).
- If you miss doses of a medicine due to side effects, ask your doctor for an alternative.
- If you do not understand your medicine regimen, ask your doctor or a nurse to write it down in easy-to-understand language.
- Plan ahead for prescription refills to make sure you do not run out.
- If you can get a ninety-day supply of medicines with your prescription plan, this can save you time and money.

to see your doctor about it to try to get it under better control. If you have any symptoms of depression at all (such as feeling blue, not being motivated to do things, feeling tired, or having difficulty sleeping), take the self-test on depression in table 13.4 to see if you may be depressed. If you score high on this test, then make sure to see your doctor about evaluating you for possible depression.

Educating yourself about how the medicine works can also be very helpful with compliance. For example, if you realize that a medicine must be taken every day regularly plus that it takes three weeks to work, you will be more apt to take it regularly. A common mistake is to not realize this, take a pain reliever for just a few doses, and then stop it if it does not work, not realizing that it does not work unless taken for at least three weeks and on a regular basis (not just "as needed"). Education also helps if you realize what happens if you do not take your medicines. Your simple act of reading this book actually increases the chances that you will be compliant with taking your medicines regularly since you are learning what lupus can do if you do not get it under control with your therapies.

Another well-known fact is that it is much easier to take a medicine once a day compared to taking a medicine two or three times a day. Medicines taken three to four times a day are very hard to take regularly without missing doses. So another strategy, if you find yourself missing the second or third dose of a medicine every day, is to ask your doctor if there are simpler alternatives (such as a once-a-day medicine). While for some medicines, there may not be an alternative medicine with a simpler schedule, other medicines may very well have easier alternatives. However, sometimes this may come with a price. For example, a medicine may exist as a cheap generic in a two- or three-times-a-day tablet yet also exist in a once-a-day, slow-release version that does not come in a cheaper generic form. The once-a-day, slow-release form may cost quite a bit more than the two- to three-times-a-day alternative. Some people may find this price difference prohibitive and decide that it is better for them to be compliant taking their medicine more regularly two to three times a day. Other people may decide that it is worth it to spend more money to have the convenience of taking the once-a-day medicine.

Affordability of medications is an important issue. Doctors usually prescribe what they feel is best for their patients' medical conditions, which are going to be safest, and which medicine is more apt to be taken regularly. Therefore, doctors are more apt to prescribe a new medicine if it is taken once a day for a particular condition compared to a cheaper, generic medicine that is taken four times a day because they know the four-times-a-day medicine is rarely ever going to be taken properly. Doctors may have samples of a new medicine available and they may want to give patients some samples first to make sure that a particular medicine works and is tolerable before committing them to a full prescription of the medicine. However, medicines that doctors have samples for are the newer and more expensive medicines; they do not have cheaper generic alternatives. People have numerous different types of insurance prescription plans and different economic backgrounds. There is no way that physicians can keep track of all the insurance plans and what medicines they will cover for the patients who have each plan. If you are ever prescribed a medicine that ends up being one that you cannot afford, you are most likely not going to take the medicine at all, or you are going to take it only some of the time. Either way, that particular prescription is not going to work for you. It is very important that you let your doctor know that you cannot afford it and ask for an alternative. Most of the time (but not all the time) more affordable medicines are available. Many times, the cheaper generic medicines are just as good as the more expensive ones as long as they are taken regularly and properly. Your doctor would rather have you be upfront about the prohibitive cost of a medicine so that he or she can prescribe a more affordable version that you will be able to take correctly.

Make sure that you keep your medicines in locations that will remind you to take them. For example, keeping some in your purse and at your workplace can help keep you from missing medicines when you are not at home. There are also many types of pill organizers available to use as well. One of the most helpful is one that contains an entire month's worth of medicine containing sections for four separate weeks divided by individual days of the week. If you spend some time once a month filling it up, it can help make a big difference in ensuring that you do not miss any doses of medicine during the month.

Cell phones and smart phones that have software programs and applications (apps) placed on them also can make taking medications easier. There are actually apps available that can be downloaded from the internet or directly onto the phone wirelessly specifically for medication timers that you can set to go off throughout the day to remind you about what medicines to take at what times. Of course, there is also the old-fashioned way of being reminded of when to take your medicine. Ask for help from a family member. This can be especially important if you have difficulties with memory. If you do this, it is very important to remind yourself that you are giving that person permission to prompt you. Some people can get upset when a loved one is constantly reminding them to do something (such as taking their medicines), and it can become easy to get angry when they feel they are being nagged. However, if you remind yourself that you are giving this person permission to do so for your own good, and remind yourself not to get upset, it can go a long way in keeping a good, loving relationship with that caring family member.

Make taking your medicines habit forming. Pick a particular time of day or regularly performed activity that will remind you to always take your medicine and stick to it. For example, if you choose to take your medicine every time you brush your teeth in the morning or after you eat your breakfast, you will be more likely to stick to your regimen.

Sometimes people do not take their medicines regularly because they do not make them feel good. For example, if you take a medicine that gives you a little bit of stomach upset, you and your doctor may decide that it is OK for you to keep taking it (if this is considered a mild side effect). However, if this stomach upset ends up making you start to miss doses of it, then it is not a good idea to continue it. Let your doctor know to see if there may be a better alternative. This same line of thinking also goes with difficulty taking the medicine for other reasons. For example, if a pill is large and you have trouble swallowing it, ask your doctor if it comes in a different size, in an easier to swallow alternative, or in liquid or topical patch form.

Unfortunately, the medication regimens taken by people who have lupus can be complex and difficult. If your doctor changes your treatment regimen and you are not 100% clear on how to take your medicine, make sure to ask him or her to write down the instructions in easy-to-use terms before you leave the office. Never be afraid to tell your doctor that you do not understand something. Sometimes, what sounds simple to the doctor may not at all be simple to understand by a layperson, and sometimes doctors forget that. Doctors would rather have patients understand how to take their medicines instead of leave the office with unanswered questions.

An often easily missed part of being compliant with taking medicines is to ensure that you do not run out of your medicine. It is important to plan ahead of time in keeping up on your refills. When you pick up your medicine, make sure to note how many refills remain on the bottle. If it says, "0 refills," then it is important that you know when and how to get it refilled so that you do not run out. Some doctors want you to ask your pharmacist to fax them a request or send a request by computer for refills (called electronic prescribing or e-prescribing). Some doctors will want to see you personally for an appointment to give you the refill, while another doctor may want you to call her or his office to get your refill. Make sure you learn what your doctor's refill procedure is. In addition, you do not want to wait until the last minute. Make sure that you request your refills a week or so before they are needed. If your pills will be gone by Saturday morning, and you think you can call your doctor late on a Friday afternoon to get your prescription filled, that is asking too much of your doctor.

Also, find out if your prescription plan allows ninety days' worth of medicine at a time or not. If you only get thirty days at a time, that means you have to go to the drug store every thirty days to pick up your prescription. If you have multiple prescriptions that have different fill dates, this can become quite a daunting task. Many prescription plans now allow ninety days' worth of medicine to be filled at a time. This can make it much easier as you do not have to get your prescriptions filled as often. In addition, this is often done through mail-order pharmacies; this can save you even more time. Just make sure to let your doctor know to prepare your prescription for ninety days' worth at a time. In addition, this is often cheaper in the end compared to getting thirty days at a time. Many prescription plans have made cost-saving deals with certain pharmacies where they can save their members additional money by doing it this way.

## How to Take Medications

An important part of taking medications is knowing how to take them correctly. For example, some medications are best taken without food; some are better taken with food for better absorption. Some medicines should not be taken at the same time as other medicines. These instructions will often be on your pill bottle or on a printout given to you by your pharmacist. I go into detail about the most commonly used medicines in lupus in this book and supply much of this advice in the following chapters.

If you forget to take a dose of your medicine, find out from your pharmacist or your doctor what you should do. Sometimes it is best to wait until the next scheduled time to take the next dose of medicine, while at other times it may be better to take your next dose of medicine early. Another possibility may be to go ahead and take the missed dose of medicine right away; then take the next dose on time. This varies a lot from medicine to medicine. Specific instructions on how to deal with missed doses of medicines used to treat lupus are also included in the following chapters.

Sometimes crushing or cutting tablets can make it easier to take them (such as crushing up a pill and putting it in applesauce to help get a large tablet down easier). However, some medicines should never be chewed, crushed, or split in two. This especially should not be done with medicines that are designed for slow release. These medicines will often have the letters CR (controlled release), DR (delayed release), XR (extended release), SR (slow release), or XL (extended life) in their names. If these are cut or crushed, the medicine could be absorbed all at once instead of slowly and can cause dangerous side effects.

Other medicines have a protective coating on them to make them easier on the stomach or to allow them to be absorbed later in the intestines instead of in the stomach. These will often be followed by the letters EC (enteric coated). Then there are other medicines that may contain two different medicines or substances that are designed to be released at different times in the intestinal system (e.g., Arthrotec) or that may counteract each other on purpose if the pills are tampered with. It is always very important to ask your doctor or pharmacist first to see if it is safe to cut, crush, or chew any pills or capsules.

Make sure your medications are not expired before taking them. All prescription packages should have an expiration date on them. The medicine should always be stored in the original bottle with the appropriate identification information on it as well. Although it is very common for people to keep their medicines in the bathroom, the FDA recommends that medications not be stored there because heat and moisture can cause medicines to expire prematurely. Also, do not store them by any dangerous materials (such as cleaners) to avoid inadvertently opening up the wrong container.

## Medicine List

One of the most important things that I recommend patients do is keep an updated list of the medicines that they take and always carry it around with them. This can be extremely helpful for many reasons. Keeping an up-to-date medicine list can decrease the likelihood of medical mistakes occurring. A medication list similar to the one in table 29.9 is useful. Of course, it can be handwritten, but it is even better and more accurate to keep a copy on your computer. Every time there is a change in any medicine or prescription, you should immediately update your list and throw away the old one. Put a new copy in your pocketbook or wallet right away. The nice thing about keeping it on a computer is that it simplifies this process and a new one can be printed out each time a change is made. It is very easy to find medication list forms that you can download free off the internet.

At a minimum, you want the list to include the name of the medicine, what dose each tablet or capsule contains, how many you take at a time, and how often you take it. However, to be complete and if you have enough room, you should consider adding the other information as well. The dose section should have the dose per pill or tablet. This is usually labeled in milligrams (mg) on the bottle, but sometimes other units of measurement may be used such as micrograms (mcg) or international units (IU). If your medicine is a liquid, then make sure that you put the concentration of the liquid (e.g., 25 mg/mL for liquid methotrexate). You should also include all over-the-counter medicines, vitamins, and herbal supplements that you take because there can potentially be important interactions between any of these. Also, make sure you have written down exactly what you are taking. Your doctor wants to know exactly how you are taking your medicines and not how you should be taking your medicines. There is a big difference between them. For example, if your doctor wants you to be taking a medicine twice a day, but you have only been taking it once a day most of the time, be honest and indicate once a day on your list. When your doctor notes this discrepancy, it can lead to a discussion about why you are only taking it once a day, whether this may negatively impact your health, and if a better alternative may be available.

**Table 29.9** Medication List Form (Example)

| Drug Name | Dose | How Much Taken at a Time | How Often Taken | Why Taken (for what purpose) | Prescribing Doctor |
|---|---|---|---|---|---|
|  |  |  |  |  |  |
|  |  |  |  |  |  |
|  |  |  |  |  |  |
|  |  |  |  |  |  |

Keeping a list like this with you at all times can greatly enhance your medical care and prevent medical mistakes from happening. What a doctor prescribes and what the patient is actually taking are not always the same, and a list like this kept by the patient and double-checked by the doctor each visit can ensure that everyone is on the same page. It is not uncommon, for example, for the pharmacy to fill an older version of a medicine after the doctor has made a change in dosage. The patient may be taking exactly what is on the bottle, but this may be very different from what the doctor thinks she or he is taking. In addition, sometimes a prescription may be filled incorrectly. For example, some medicines can have very similar names, or an incorrect dose of a medicine may have been filled by mistake. If you always put down on your medicine list exactly what is on the pill bottle, it can help communicate to your doctor exactly what you are taking and these kinds of mistakes can be caught and corrected. It is also very important for doctors to know what other doctors are prescribing so they are aware of what other medical conditions you have and to make sure that they do not prescribe any medicines that may have important drug interactions. Lastly, if you have a list like this with you at all times and you end up in an emergency room, it will ensure that the medical personnel know what you are being treated for and medicines you are on so that you receive the best medical care possible.

Whenever you see a doctor, you will always (or should always) be asked what medicines you are taking. Usually a nurse or medical assistant does this. Instead of your answering "yes" and "no" to a list of questions about your medications, it is more accurate just to hand your current medicine list to the nurse or medical assistant. Then the list can be double-checked against what is written down in your chart. This will ensure that your medication list is accurate in your doctor's chart. Never assume that what is written in the chart is the same as what you have written down.

Some people do not want to keep a list of their medicines, or they find it too bothersome. An easy alternative is for them to bring all of their medicines and vitamins in a bag to every doctor's visit. Doctors would rather have their patients do this than possibly have an incorrect list of medicines in their charts.

## Pharmacy

Always go to the same pharmacy. One of the main reasons for this is that if you always go to the same pharmacy, the pharmacist will know all of your medications and can alert your prescribing doctor if a medicine has any important drug interactions with another medicine. If you go to several different pharmacies for different medications, you will miss having this very helpful safety net.

Another important reason to go to the same pharmacy is to help you build a good rapport with the pharmacist. Knowing your pharmacist can help a lot as far as you getting good, high-quality service and with having any questions answered. In addition, if you take a medicine that is difficult to get or requires special ordering, and if you always go to the same pharmacy, it is easier for you to contact your pharmacist a week or so before you need your refill so that you can remind him or her that it needs to be ordered for you. This can help prevent your running out of your medication.

When you pick up your medications at the pharmacy, always make sure to open the bottles before you leave and inspect them. If they are generic, they may come in different shapes, sizes, and colors each time. Pharmacies will often buy the least expensive generic medicine to help keep down healthcare costs. If your medicine looks different, you want to make sure that it is the correct medicine and that a mistake was not made in filling the prescription. You can simply ask the pharmacist to confirm that it is the correct medicine before you leave. If you are at home before you notice the difference, you can also find out on the internet whether it is the correct medicine or not. Internet sites, such as the American Association of Retired Persons (AARP for short), have "pill identifier" tools online. These make it easy to identify your pills (go to www.AARP .org).

Another reason for checking your pills before you leave the pharmacy is to make sure that you have the correct number of tablets. This is especially important with DEA (Drug Enforcement Administration) scheduled drugs (narcotics in nontechnical language). These particular drugs are potentially habit forming. Doctors have to go by strict laws regulating how many they can prescribe and how often. If you are short-changed (given too few pills), then you could run out of your medicine too soon and possibly develop withdrawal side effects. If you do not realize this until after you get home, then it is too late to do anything about it, and you will be stuck with taking less of the medicine or running out of it too early before you can get your next prescription. A potential reason for being shortchanged is simple human error in the prescribing process; however, you can never be 100% sure. Since these types of drugs are sometimes used for recreational purposes, abused, or sold on the street, someone in the pharmacy could potentially have an ulterior motive in taking some of the tablets out of your pill bottle. You want to figure this out while you are actually standing at the counter in full view of the pharmacy clerk and pharmacist.

## Disposing of Medicines

If for some reason you have to stop taking a medicine and have some left over, it is important to know how to dispose of the medicine correctly (table 29.10). If you have internet access, a good way to learn how to dispose of medications is to go to www .dea.gov. Under "Resource Center" click on "Drug Disposal" for complete information. Some drugs will have specific disposal instructions that are printed on the prescription package.

Most medications can be thrown out in the trash; however, you should take some precautions when doing this. To start with, make sure it is legal to do so in your location by contacting your local government agency or pharmacist. Make sure to mix the medicine in something unappealing such as coffee grounds or kitty litter. This will decrease the chances of children or pets eating it as well as the chances of a person using the medicine after rummaging through your garbage. Place it in a sealable bag, empty can, or other container and put it in the trash. Before throwing away your prescription packages, make sure to scratch out your identifying information to protect your identity and medical information, and to decrease the chances of someone else using this information to get refills of the medicine.

Never give your medicine to friends or relatives. You cannot be sure it is safe for them to take without a physician's prescription. Do not flush most medicines down the toilet; otherwise, it will end up in the drinking water at some point or in streams

**Table 29.10** Disposing of Medications

- Many medicines can be thrown out in the trash if not illegal in your community.
- Contact your local government and pharmacist for detailed information.
- Mix drugs in a substance such as kitty litter or coffee grounds and put into a container before throwing out in the trash.
- Scratch off all identifying information on prescription packages before discarding them.
- Most medicines *should not* be flushed down the toilet.
- Some medicines *should* be flushed down the toilet (e.g., Percocet, morphine, fentanyl patches, OxyCONTIN).
- Some communities have "Medication Take-Back" programs.

and lakes where significant harm may occur to wildlife and humans. However, the FDA recommends that some medicines should be flushed down the toilet. These instructions are often noted on the prescription bottle, and lists of these medicines can be found on the internet. Many opioid pain relievers (narcotics) are actually on this list (e.g., Percocet, morphine, fentanyl patches, and OxyCONTIN). The reasons for this recommendation are that these medicines are safe to flush into the sanitation system and that, by getting rid of them immediately by flushing, it is less likely that they will be accidently swallowed by children or pets or be stolen by other people for inappropriate usage.

Many localities also have special "Medicine Take-Back" programs. You can check with your pharmacist to see if your community has this option available. Your pharmacist can also be very helpful in answering any of your drug disposal questions.

## Handling of Sharps

Many of the newer medications must be given by injection instead of by pill form. These include the biologic medications discussed in chapters 33, 34, and 37. There are other medications, such as the osteoporosis medicine Forteo (see chapter 24), which also involve the use of needles as well. Learning how to properly handle sharp needles and other devices is very important to protect other people from getting cut, which would put them at risk for injury, getting exposed to your medicine, or even possibly contracting a blood-borne disease (such as viral hepatitis or HIV). Each state has its own laws on the proper handling and disposal of needles and other sharps. A good website to learn more about your particular state is at www.safeneedledisposal.org. The FDA also has additional information at www.acr.tw/y2zoyS. If you do not have access to the internet, contact your pharmacy or physician for additional guidance. In addition, many pharmaceutical companies provide assistance with proper disposal of needles. If you contact the company directly (usually the number is in the drug information that most patients receive), you can often ask for sharps containers to help in disposing of the needles and sharps (this is usually free of charge).

1. Sometimes it is necessary to take numerous medications to treat SLE. Some of these medicines are to calm down the immune system, some are used to treat symptoms (such as pain), while others are used to decrease the chances of side effects occurring.

2. Learn and understand the reason for taking each of your medicines. This can be helpful in ensuring that you stay compliant with taking that particular medicine.

3. When evaluating the potential side effects of any particular medicine make sure to do so rationally. Ask your pharmacist or your doctor, or use the steps outlined in table 29.7.

4. Always contact your doctor's office when you develop a possible side effect to a medicine to find out how you should respond to the side effect.

5. The most common reason for medicines not working is not taking them regularly or taking them incorrectly.

6. Use the strategies in table 29.8 to ensure you take your medications regularly.

7. Keep an updated medication list with you at all times (table 29.9).

8. Use one pharmacy to fill all of your medications.

9. Check your prescription for accuracy at the time you pick it up at the pharmacy.

10. Make sure to dispose of medications properly (table 29.10).

11. If you use injectable medicines, go to www.safeneedledisposal.org or www.acr.tw/y2zoyS on the internet for additional information on how to dispose of needles and syringes. Also, consider calling the drug company to see if it can provide you with sharps disposal equipment.

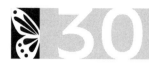

# Anti-Malarials

## How Antibiotics to Treat Malaria Became Important in Treating Lupus

Almost everyone who has systemic lupus reading this has most likely been treated with the anti-malarial medication called hydroxychloroquine (Plaquenil). It is classified as an anti-malarial because its initial purpose was to treat and prevent malaria. Malaria is a severe, sometimes deadly infection, which is transmitted to humans by mosquitoes in the tropics. So why do people who have lupus take a medicine that was intended to treat the tropical infection called malaria? This is a story that goes back several centuries (see table opposite).

The story begins with a beautiful woman. It was sometime between 1629 and 1633 in Lima, Peru. The Spaniards had been in control after invading Peru initially in 1527. Doña Francisca Henriquez de Ribera was described as a beautiful woman who was married to the Fourth Count of Chinchón (the Spanish viceroy of Peru), meaning that he ruled over Spanish-controlled South America. Legend says that she became very ill, almost dying, with a high fever (most likely malaria). The indigenous people (native Indians) south of Lima used the bark of a tree to treat fever. She took the remedy and was cured of the illness. The indigenous name for this bark was "quina-quina" (pronounced KEY-nuh KEY-nuh). She was so thankful that she procured large amounts of the bark and personally dispensed powder made from the bark to cure people stricken with fever (malaria). She reportedly took back some of the bark to Europe, where malaria was becoming problematic, and its medicinal qualities became renowned for curing people of the deadly disease. Due to this story, the powder of the bark was sometimes referred to as "The Countess's Powder."

A legend of a beautiful woman being saved by a simple tree bark that she then gives out to sick people and then brings to Europe to save millions makes for a wonderful story. As is true of many legends, however, this one turns out most likely to be fabricated. Nonetheless, it is still referenced in many lupus texts. According to the actual diary of the count himself, Doña Francisca was actually his second wife (his first wife, Countess Ana de Osorio, died before he even left Spain). Doña Francisca actually enjoyed excellent health and died while still in South America; she never even returned to Spain and therefore could not have taken the bark back to Europe. In fact, she had only been ill twice while in South America and neither time was a malaria-type illness described.

| | |
|---|---|
| Before 1527 | Indigenous South Americans used quina-quina bark to treat febrile illnesses. |
| 1632 | Jesuit priest Bernabé de Cobo took quina-quina bark from Peru to Spain. |
| 1629–1633 | Romantic legend of Countess of Chinchón cured with quina-quina bark. |
| 1600s–1700s | Use of Jesuit bark powder widespread throughout Europe and Asia for febrile illnesses. |
| 1742 | Quina-quina tree named Cinchona tree by the botanist Carolus Linnaeus after the legend of the Countess of Chinchón. |
| 1818 | Quinine isolated from cinchona tree bark; found to be useful for the treatment of malaria. |
| Mid-1800s | Quinine reported by dermatologists to treat lupus. |
| 1894 | Dr. J. F. Payne's in-depth report on the effectiveness of high doses of quinine to treat lupus. |
| 1930 | Quinacrine (Atabrine) developed as an alternative to quinine to treat malaria. |
| 1940 | Professor A. J. Prokoptchouk reported use of quinacrine for lupus in Russia. |
| World War II | British physicians noted soldiers who had inflammatory diseases improved on quinacrine. |
| 1946 | Chloroquine is FDA-approved to treat malaria. |
| 1951 | Dr. Francis Page reported remarkable effects of quinacrine in the treatment of lupus. |
| 1955 | Plaquenil is FDA-approved to treat malaria. |
| 1957 | Chloroquine is FDA-approved to treat lupus. |
| 1958 | Plaquenil is FDA-approved to treat lupus. |
| 1959 | Triquin (Plaquenil, chloroquine, and quinacrine) is FDA-approved to treat lupus. |
| 1972 | FDA approval for Triquin withdrawn and is pulled off the market. |
| 1992 | Winthrop Laboratories stops production of quinacrine due to loss of profits. |

The more likely true story is not as romantic. Bernabé Cobo, a Spanish Jesuit priest, probably brought the tree bark to Spain from Peru sometime between 1633 and 1643 to be used for its anti-fever effects. It was effective and became popularly known as Jesuit's bark, Jesuit's powder, and Peruvian bark. The medicinal qualities of this bark, which we need to truly credit to the native Indians of South America, changed medical history forever, leading to the production of medications for malaria (quinine) and heart rhythm problems (quinidine). In 1742, the tree from which the bark comes from was named the cinchona tree by the botanist Carolus Linnaeus in honor of the Fourth Countess of Chinchón from the legend. Jesuit's powder made from the bark quickly spread throughout Europe and even through the Far East. The powder became even more popular after curing such famous people as King Louis XIV of France and the Chinese emperor Kangxi, helping him to become the longest-reigning emperor in China's history.

Those who are reading this and are believers in homeopathic medicine should be interested to know that cinchona bark powder is also responsible for the birth of homeopathic medicine. The founder of homeopathy, Dr. Samuel Hahnemann, took large doses daily to test its effects in 1790. The high doses that he took caused him to develop numerous side effects, including light-headedness, weakness, and drowsiness. His cheeks turned red, "characteristic of intermittent fever." These symptoms were very similar to those of diseases that cause fever (such as malaria), the very symptoms that quinine was supposed to be treating in the first place. Dr. Hahnemann reported these effects, coming up with the idea of "like cures like," and homeopathy was born. The symptoms that Dr. Hahnemann developed from taking the medicine are now known to actually be a type of allergic reaction to the medicine.

Over the years, it was discovered that the bark actually contained many different chemicals, and eventually several different medications were developed from it. One of these was a medicine called quinine that was isolated from the bark in 1818. It eventually was useful in the treatment of malaria. However, several dermatologists also described its usefulness for lupus in the mid-1800s. However, none of these authors really seemed to recommend it very highly (instead, they recommended other therapies such as arsenic). A paper written by Dr. J. F. Payne in 1894 propelled quinine into the forefront as far as treating lupus. While he was a medical student, he learned to use large doses of quinine (produced from the cinchona tree bark) to treat patients who had typhoid fever. He noted that their severe fevers would resolve and that they would become very pale (white). He subsequently developed an interest in treating patients who had lupus. A hallmark of lupus was the erythema (medical term for redness) of the skin (hence the "erythematosus" in "systemic lupus erythematosus"). He theorized that since larger doses of quinine were needed to treat typhoid fever and would cause the skin of the treated patient to become very pale, that higher doses should also be used in the patients with lupus who had red skin.

Dr. Payne reported significant success with this approach in his report. He also noted that it was common for his lupus patients to develop side effects from the quinine (deafness and buzzing in the ears), but he felt this was an acceptable tradeoff at the time since there were no other effective treatments for lupus. Although Dr. Payne's article was important in pointing out the use of the anti-malarial medicine quinine in the treatment of lupus, other doctors seem to have ignored his findings. Although other doctors subsequently used quinine to treat lupus during the decades following the publication of his paper, it never was highly recommended. This raises some doubt as to whether it was truly very helpful, or maybe doctors thought that the side effects caused by these high doses (the deafness and buzzing of the ears) were too much to subject patients to.

During World War I, malaria re-emerged as an important infectious disease among soldiers. Supplies of quinine became unavailable when armies would prevent enemy troops from gaining access to places where cinchona tree bark was located. The leading industrial countries were on the hunt for better alternatives. Therefore, the race was on to synthesize better anti-malarials in laboratories so that governments would not be dependent on limited access to cinchona trees. In 1930, a German dye company developed quinacrine (also called Mepacrine and Atabrine) as an effective anti-malarial alternative.

In World War II, the Japanese occupied the Dutch East Indies (located in the South Pacific Ocean between China and Australia). The Dutch East Indies provided 90% of cinchona tree bark to the world, and therefore the war greatly interrupted access to the bark to make quinine. Without this access to quinine, malaria infected 60% to 85% of British and American forces in the Pacific, making them useless in the war effort. Therefore, quinacrine (Atabrine) was used as an alternative. About four million soldiers from the United States, Britain, Canada, and Australia used Atabrine regularly for three years, making it one of the most used and studied medicines ever. Quinacrine controlled the symptoms of malaria and is partially credited with being essential in helping the Allied forces win World War II.

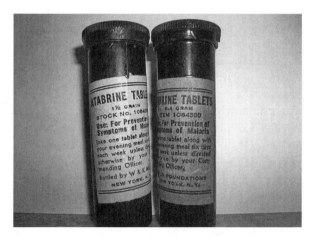

World War II Atabrine (quinacrine) bottles used by soldiers to prevent malaria. Military doctors like Dr. Page noted some soldiers who had inflammatory diseases (such as lupus and rheumatoid arthritis) got better when they took Atabrine.

During World War II, some astute British physicians noted that soldiers with cutaneous lupus and rheumatoid arthritis improved when they took quinacrine to prevent malaria. One of these physicians was Dr. Francis Page. While serving in the Royal Army Medical Corps in Burma and India, he had the chance to observe the effects of quinacrine in several thousand troops. He noted that military personnel affected by discoid lupus improved when they took quinacrine. After he got out of the military, he was a physician at Middlesex Hospital in London. In 1948, a 56-year-old man who had severe, scarring discoid lupus erythematosus came to the hospital seeking help for his severe lupus. Prior to that, he had been subjected to numerous unhelpful therapies, including various ointments, sulfonamide antibiotics, and even having his tonsils removed. The discoid lupus was causing severe scarring on his face and he was desperate for help. Several other treatments were then tried, including bismuth injections and local frozen carbon dioxide treatments, all of which failed.

Finally, based on his observations on the use of quinacrine during the war, Dr. Page started the man on 100 mg of quinacrine (called Mepacrine in Britain) a day. His lupus responded so dramatically to the treatment with almost complete resolution of the active rash that the patient remarked that it was the only therapy that had ever worked. From that point on, quinacrine was used on every lupus patient who presented to the dermatology department at Middlesex Hospital. In 1951, Dr. Page reported the results on the first eighteen lupus patients in the British medical journal *The Lancet*, noting that seventeen of the eighteen patients had remarkable responses to quinacrine. This was the first report in the English-language medical literature showing the effectiveness of quinacrine in treating lupus. Professor A. J. Prokoptchouk had also presented a study in 1940 in a Russian-language medical journal where he successfully treated thirty-five patients who had lupus using quinacrine. However, the English medical community had not noted this prior study. Other than the recent reports from America about the use of a new medicine called cortisone, never before had such a successful treatment been described in treating this disease. Thus began rheumatologists' love affair with anti-malarial drugs. After Dr. Page's initial landmark paper on the use of quinacrine in lupus, numerous other studies were soon published in the medical literature echoing his results, and anti-malarial medications became destined to be the first drugs of choice in treating lupus.

Soon after doctors began using quinacrine in lupus patients, they noted that around 25% of light-skinned patients developed a yellowish discoloration of the skin. Low blood counts occurred as well, although rarely. Therefore, the hunt was on for a safer anti-malarial medication. The anti-malarial chloroquine (Aralen) became popular since it did not cause the skin discoloration. In 1953, several reports were published in the medical journals on its successful use in lupus patients. Although chloroquine was originally approved to treat malaria in 1946, in October 1957 it became one of the first FDA-approved medicines for the treatment of lupus. Chloroquine is converted in the body to another chemical called hydroxychloroquine, and in 1950 there was success in synthesizing this substance as well. Doctors soon began to test it in patients who had lupus. Although hydroxychloroquine was weaker than both quinacrine and chloroquine in treating lupus, it was overall safer. Hydroxychloroquine (Plaquenil) was FDA-approved for the treatment of malaria in 1955 and then in 1958 for the treatment of lupus.

Additional studies showed that using these three anti-malarials (quinacrine, chloroquine, and hydroxychloroquine) was more effective when used in combination than when used individually. Therefore, in 1958, the FDA approved the medication Triquin made by Winthrop Laboratories to treat lupus. It contained all three anti-malarials. Although quinacrine was never FDA-approved to treat lupus by itself, it essentially became FDA-approved to treat lupus when used in this particular combination. However, the problem with this combination pill was that if someone developed a side effect (such as a rash or stomach upset) it was never certain which component was responsible. Therefore, doctors treating lupus prescribed it less often over time. The FDA eventually withdrew its approval for Triquin in 1972 after doctors campaigned against the use of combination drugs. Physicians also began to prescribe less quinacrine (Atabrine) for lupus and malaria over time (preferring to use hydroxychloroquine for lupus), and it ceased to be produced by any major pharmaceutical company in 1992 due to its not being profitable. However, the medicine was, and still is, available from compounding pharmacists (licensed pharmacists who mix medications ordered by physicians in a safe and controlled environment).

Most (if not all) people who have taken hydroxychloroquine (Plaquenil) know that they should get an eye exam regularly to ensure that they do not develop any problems from the medicine with their eyes. Although this problem does not occur very commonly with hydroxychloroquine, it does with chloroquine (Aralen). Even before its FDA approval in 1957, doctors reported eye problems from chloroquine. By 1959, this side effect became well established, and the FDA approval for the use of chloroquine for the treatment of lupus was eventually withdrawn.

Today, hydroxychloroquine (Plaquenil) is the only anti-malarial medication still FDA-approved to treat lupus. It is the first drug of choice in treating lupus by most lupus experts and most patients who have SLE have been treated with it. However, both chloroquine (Aralen) and quinacrine still have their place in the treatment of lupus under special circumstances when used in experienced hands.

We can still be thankful to the indigenous people of South America for their knowledge of their quina-quina bark curing fevers, which led to the current use of hydroxychloroquine (Plaquenil), quinacrine, and chloroquine (Aralen) as the drugs of first choice in treating lupus. In fact, each of these medicinal names still contains the original word for this miraculous bark, "quina-." This chapter goes into detail about the use of these three medications to treat lupus.

....

## "Why do medicines used to treat malaria also work for lupus?"

To answer this question, it is helpful to understand how the immune system works. One of the key things that occurs in the immune system is something called antigen presentation (figure 30.1A). Recall from chapter 1 that antigens are proteins that cause the immune system to make antibodies directed toward those specific antigens for protection. For example, let us say you are infected with parvovirus, which can cause a cold-like illness and sometimes even rash and joint pain. The immune system "sees" the proteins (which act as antigens) on this virus, recognizes that they do not belong to the body, and launches an all-out war against the virus. One way it does this is by making antibodies that can attach to the parvovirus antigens, which in turn identifies

499

A

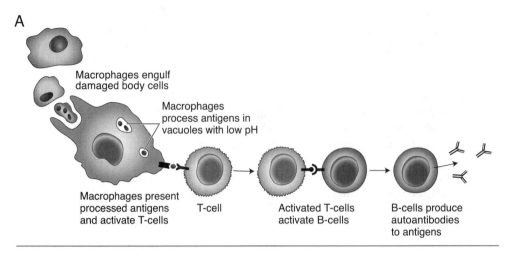

Macrophages engulf
damaged body cells

Macrophages
process antigens in
vacuoles with low pH

Macrophages present
processed antigens
and activate T-cells

T-cell

Activated T-cells
activate B-cells

B-cells produce
autoantibodies
to antigens

B

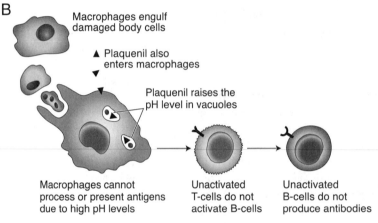

Macrophages engulf
damaged body cells

▲ Plaquenil also
▼  enters macrophages

Plaquenil raises the
pH level in vacuoles

Macrophages cannot
process or present antigens
due to high pH levels

Unactivated
T-cells do not
activate B-cells

Unactivated
B-cells do not
produce antibodies

**Figure 30.1**  (A) Skin antigen processing to T-cell causes lupus rash; (B) anti-malarial
Plaquenil interferes with skin antigen presentation to T-cell

the virus invaders as being the "bad guys." Subsequently, this alerts other white blood
cells of the immune system to attack the virus. These antibodies are then made for
the rest of your life. If you are infected by parvovirus ever again, you will hopefully be
immune to the virus and the white blood cells of your immune system can attack the
virus immediately so that you do not get sick from it ever again.

So now let us go a little deeper into how the body makes these antibodies in the
first place, focusing on a concept called antigen processing (figure 30.1A). This is a
very technical discussion that can be skipped by many people reading this book, but
it can be interesting for the person who wants to know more about how anti-malarial
medicines work. Macrophages are white blood cells that are responsible for identifying foreign antigens for the immune system. You can think of them as the frontline

soldiers that come into contact first with any unusual antigen proteins such as viruses and bacteria that may be invading the body.

Macrophages are often also called antigen-presenting cells in immunology. In lupus, where the immune system starts to attack parts of the body itself, the antigens it thinks are foreign are actually antigen proteins naturally occurring in the body. When the macrophages see these antigens (such as proteins found in the skin), they engulf them into little bubbles called vacuoles (follow along in figure 30.1A). The vacuoles then break down (or digest) these antigen proteins into numerous smaller components and reassemble them into structures that are then attached to the macrophage cell surface. The macrophages then show these antigens (antigen presentation) to other white blood cells of the immune system (especially T-cells) so that they can recognize them as being "bad" proteins. This in turn causes other white blood cells (called B-cells) to start making antibodies directed against these antigen proteins. However, in the case of lupus, these antigen proteins that end up being attacked belong to the person's own body. The antibodies produced to attack the body's own antigens are called "auto-antibodies." If the antigens belong to damaged cells of the skin (due to ultraviolet light, for example), the immune system attacks the skin, causing the rashes of lupus. If the antigens processed and presented in this way belong to the joints, then the immune system attacks the joints, causing the pain and swelling of lupus arthritis. If they belong to the kidneys, the person develops lupus nephritis.

For this antigen presentation to occur, the vacuoles within the macrophages must have a low pH level (in other words, must be acidic), otherwise, the enzymes of the vacuoles that are responsible in processing the antigens will not work. The anti-malarial medicines (such as Plaquenil) enter the macrophages and subsequently concentrate in large amounts inside of these vacuoles. The anti-malarials have a higher pH level and in turn cause these very important vacuoles to develop a higher pH level (figure 30.1B). Enzymes only work under precise pH conditions. This higher pH level in the vacuoles prevents the digesting enzymes of the macrophages from being able to break down the antigens for presentation to the T-cells. Therefore, the T-cells are unable to "see" these antigens and do not signal the B-cells to make antibodies against the skin, joints, or other parts of the body that may be targets for lupus. Therefore, the anti-malarial medicine calms down the immune system of the person who has lupus. Interestingly, though, it does not actually cause overt immunosuppression. In other words, the immune system is still able to function normally in other areas and still protects the person from infections and cancer.

A similar thing occurs in malaria. Malaria is an infection due to single-celled parasites called *Plasmodium* that get into humans from mosquito bites. The malaria organisms get into the red blood cells, where they ingest iron-rich hemoglobin. The malaria need to digest this hemoglobin inside vacuoles within their own bodies (similar to the macrophages of the immune system ingesting antigen proteins inside their vacuoles). The malaria organisms digest the proteins of the hemoglobin to use for food and for reproduction. Just as the macrophages of our bodies need an acidic environment to digest antigen proteins, the malaria organisms also require an acidic environment to digest the hemoglobin and dispose of the waste product (the iron-rich heme portion of the hemoglobin). The anti-malarial medicine dissolves into the vacuoles of the malaria organisms and raises the vacuole pH levels. The malaria organisms are unable to digest the hemoglobin and to get rid of the heme. The heme molecules actually combine with the anti-malarial medicine molecules and build up inside of the malaria organisms, trapped within their vacuoles. This is toxic to the malaria organisms, and they die (or at least stop reproducing inside of the human body).

The bottom line is that anti-malarials appear to work by increasing the pH of the vacuoles inside of malaria organisms and macrophages alike. These vacuoles usually ingest hemoglobin (in the case of malaria organisms) or antigen proteins (in the case of macrophages in people who have lupus). When the pH is increased, these vacuoles are unable to process these components. In the case of malaria, the malaria organisms die due to the buildup of toxic waste products. In the case of lupus, the macrophages cannot process antigens properly to present them to T-cells and therefore the immune system is calmed down so that it does not attack the body (such as the skin, joints, or kidneys) as much.

### "Plaquenil should be in the drinking water of lupus patients"

This is something I was told when I was first learning to become a rheumatologist many years ago, and it is still a common saying among rheumatologists. In fact, the book *A Clinician's Pearls and Myths in Rheumatology* has a section that is entitled "Hydroxychloroquine should be added in the water supply" where it even goes on to say that "Experienced lupus clinicians refer to this medication as 'lupus health insurance.'" In medicine, doctors are always trying to find therapies that do the best for patients while causing the least possible side effects and that is exactly a niche in which anti-malarials fall. They are immensely helpful in people who have lupus while causing very little in the way of significant side effects. This is especially true when you compare them to the potential side effects that steroids and immunosuppressant medicines can have. The anti-malarial medications have many benefits to people who have lupus (table 30.1).

In this discussion, I mainly talk about hydroxychloroquine (Plaquenil) since it is the best studied of the anti-malarial medications and is used in the vast majority of people who have lupus. However, chloroquine and quinacrine also have their places as well, and I discuss them separately toward the end of the chapter. Hydroxychloroquine is especially helpful for treating what are considered the milder problems from lupus; however, these "mild" problems can still be devastating to the person who has them. The medicine can especially be helpful for alleviating arthritis joint pain and stiffness, decreasing the severity of inflammation of the skin from cutaneous lupus, and calming down the inflammation of serositis (such as pleurisy). In people who have low blood counts (red blood cells, white blood cells, and platelets) it can also sometimes help in increasing these blood counts. Plaquenil also helps to resolve or decrease episodes of fever from lupus. In the person who has significant fatigue directly due to lupus, it can increase energy levels. However, you must be careful not to over-interpret this effect. As I discussed in chapter 6, fatigue is more commonly caused by other problems such as depression or fibromyalgia in many people who have lupus, and in these instances, hydroxychloroquine does not help with these causes of fatigue. Interestingly, the anti-malarial quinacrine especially appears to help increase energy levels in people who have lupus. In fact, quinacrine also stimulates the mind, which can

**Table 30.1** Benefits of Anti-Malarial Medicines in People Who Have Lupus

- Helps arthritis, rashes, serositis, fatigue, fevers, low blood counts
- Decreases lupus flares
- Prevents evolution to SLE (or delays its onset) in those who have undifferentiated connective tissue disease
- Decreases light sensitivity of the skin
- Makes stronger lupus medicines more effective
- Decreases the spread of lupus to the internal organs
- Decreases the need for higher doses of steroids
- Decreases the amount of permanent damage to organs
- Decreases blood clots from antiphospholipid antibodies
- Decreases total cholesterol and bad cholesterol (LDL) levels
- Decreases risk of developing diabetes
- Increases life expectancy of people who have lupus and take anti-malarial medicines
- Has very low chance of significant side effects compared to other medicines

increase energy levels as well as even improve memory and concentration abilities if these problems are directly due to SLE.

Anti-malarial medicines also decrease the number and severity of lupus flares. In a study by the Canadian Rheumatology Group, it was shown that 73% of patients who were not taking an anti-malarial medicine developed flares of their lupus during the study, while only 36% of those who took an anti-malarial had a flare, suggesting that anti-malarial medicines can decrease flares by half. Not only did they decrease the number of flares, but they also decreased the severity of these flares. Some of these lupus flares in the group that did not take an anti-malarial medicine involved major organs such as the kidneys. Those who took the anti-malarial medicines had much less kidney involvement from their lupus.

Although this book is mainly focused on people who have systemic lupus erythematosus (SLE), there are those who have symptoms suggestive of SLE but do not yet fully have full-blown lupus. This group of people is often diagnosed as having undifferentiated connective tissue disease (UCTD) or lupus-like disease (chapter 2). It has been shown that if people who have UCTD are treated with hydroxychloroquine that it can decrease the chances of them developing full-blown SLE, slow down how quickly they develop SLE if it does occur, and decrease the severity of their SLE compared to people who have UCTD who are not treated with hydroxychloroquine.

Ultraviolet light exposure to the skin causes lupus to become more active. One interesting effect of anti-malarials is that they decrease this light sensitivity. Although taking them does not negate the need to use sunscreen and avoid the sun, they do help.

While hydroxychloroquine helps with the milder problems from lupus, it unfortunately does not treat the severe problems such as brain or nerve involvement, kidney inflammation, or lupus involvement of other major organs such as the heart and lungs. In other words, if you have developed significant inflammation of any major organs, your rheumatologist needs to use stronger medicines such as steroids and/or immuno-suppressant medicines. However, hydroxychloroquine usually is used along with these stronger medicines. Studies have shown that lupus patients who have major organ in-volvement, such as the kidneys, do much better when they take hydroxychloroquine along with their stronger immunosuppressant medicines compared to if they did not take hydroxychloroquine. Unfortunately, this means that numerous medications should be taken to treat the lupus, but the good thing is that taking these combina-tions of medicines makes it much more likely that people will do well and get the lupus under better control. In addition, taking a very safe medicine, such as hydroxychloro-quine, can help decrease the doses needed of the other stronger medicines, which over-all decreases the chances of developing significant side effects from them.

Another important reason to take hydroxychloroquine is that it tends to decrease the chances of developing more severe involvement of major organs (like the kidneys). Some people who have mild lupus may not feel sick at all, and they are often resistant to taking any medicines. This is a natural human reaction, and many people will say, "Why should I take anything when I feel so good?" The reason is that over time, anyone who has SLE can develop more severe lupus. Anywhere between 40% and 50% of people who have SLE will develop lupus nephritis (inflammation of the kidneys). It can occur at any time in life and usually does so without any warning at all. If someone who has mild lupus takes hydroxychloroquine regularly, she or he is much less likely to develop lupus nephritis compared to someone who refuses to take it. That is why some lupus experts call hydroxychloroquine "lupus life insurance." It is important, however, to realize that you can still develop severe lupus while taking hydroxychloroquine, but it is less likely to occur compared to if you did not take it. In addition, if you do develop major organ involvement while taking hydroxychloroquine, you have a better chance of it not being as severe compared to if you were not taking the hydroxychloroquine.

Steroids can be lifesaving medications in people who have severe lupus. However, virtually 100% of people who take steroids for any significant amount of time will de-velop side effects. Therefore, any time doctors can use a medicine to decrease the need for steroids (called steroid sparing) is a good thing. Hydroxychloroquine decreases the need to use as much steroids since it decreases the severity of lupus and helps stronger immunosuppressants to work better. Therefore, people who have lupus who take hy-droxychloroquine regularly end up requiring fewer steroids compared to people who do not take hydroxychloroquine. Therefore, it is truly a steroid-sparing medication.

Studies show that anti-malarial medications also decrease the amount of perma-nent damage that occurs within organs affected by lupus inflammation. The damage from lupus occurs in two stages. The first is the inflammatory stage where the im-mune system of the person who has lupus attacks an area of the body (e.g., the kidneys from lupus nephritis). This is followed by a second, permanent damage stage as the in-flammation heals up, leaving behind permanent scar tissue. Unfortunately, this per-manent damage leaves behind sections and parts of an organ that no longer function properly. In the case of the kidneys, for example, there would be areas of the kidneys replaced by scar tissue. The kidneys' overall function decreases to where they cannot filter the blood adequately (which doctors call renal dysfunction, renal insufficiency, or chronic kidney disease). If enough permanent damage occurs, then the kidneys may stop filtering blood to the extent that the person may need to go on dialysis (end-stage renal disease). Therefore, when doctors treat people who have lupus, they think about treating them so they feel better right away (such as relieving them of their red rashes, pain, fever, fatigue, etc.). However, doctors also want to decrease the amount of inflammation as quickly as possible so that permanent damage does not occur in any organs of the body. Fortunately, regular usage of hydroxychloroquine decreases the accrual (adding up over time) of the amount of permanent damage that occurs in the body due to lupus inflammation.

As discussed in chapter 9, anywhere between 30% and 50% of people who have SLE will be positive for tests that identify antiphospholipid antibodies such as anticardio-lipin antibody, lupus anticoagulant, beta-2 glycoprotein I antibody, and false positive syphilis tests. Over time, approximately 50% of people positive with these antibodies can develop blood clots causing deep venous thrombosis in the legs, strokes in the brain, heart attacks, or pulmonary embolism in the lungs. Taking hydroxychloroquine regularly decreases the chances of these blood clots from forming. A 2010 Canadian study showed that lupus patients who took anti-malarial drugs had 68% less blood clot events compared to patients who did not take an anti-malarial medicine. One reason less blood clots form is that hydroxychloroquine decreases how much platelets in the blood stick together. Blood platelets are very important in forming blood clots due to their sticking together. In addition, a 2013 study showed that taking hydroxychloro-quine markedly decreases the levels of antiphospholipid antibodies. Eighty percent of the SLE patients in this study who initially had high levels of antiphospholipid anti-bodies developed normal levels while taking hydroxychloroquine.

In the United States, the most common cause of death in people who have SLE is heart attacks or strokes. Therefore, anything that decreases these from happening is very important. One of the risk factors for developing heart attacks and strokes is having high cholesterol. Interestingly, taking hydroxychloroquine regularly tends to decrease cholesterol levels (both total cholesterol and LDL "bad" cholesterol). There has even been a study that showed that people who had lupus who took hydroxychlo-roquine were less likely to develop diabetes (another risk factor for heart disease) com-pared to those who did not take it. While a study has not been done yet proving that hydroxychloroquine decreases the chances of people with lupus from getting heart attacks, these findings are certainly very encouraging.

Hydroxychloroquine also increases life expectancy in people who have lupus who take it regularly. Numerous studies have shown that hydroxychloroquine decreases death (mortality) by more than 50%. In other words, it decreases the risk of dying by more than half. Other studies have shown even better results. For example, a 2010 study from South America followed 1,480 patients who had lupus up to 9 years and found that 11.5% of the patients who did not take anti-malarial medicines died while only 4.4% of those who took anti-malarials died. That is a huge difference. The peo-ple who had lupus who did not take anti-malarial medicines were more than twice as likely to die during the study compared to those who did take an anti-malarial such as hydroxychloroquine. A 2011 study from China even went so far as to say, "Our analyses show that anti-malarials are the only class of drugs that exerted a clear protective ef-fect on survival." This study looked at about two thousand patients hospitalized with lupus. The researchers looked at all the medications that the patients were taking, and they found that those who were taking anti-malarial medicines at the time of admission were much less likely to die compared to those who were not taking an anti-malarial medication.

Much of the credit for anti-malarial medicines increasing life expectancy is due to their controlling lupus better. However, another important point is that when people take hydroxychloroquine regularly, they are less likely to need stronger immunosuppressant medicines and steroids, which increase the risk for infections. Recall from chapter 22 that infections are one of the leading causes of death in people who have lupus. Studies that look at the causes of death in people who have lupus frequently show that those who take hydroxychloroquine are less likely to die from infection compared to those who do not take hydroxychloroquine.

With hydroxychloroquine having so many good effects in lupus, as listed above, it is amazing that it rarely causes significant side effects. While 10% to 20% of people who take it may experience mild side effects such as stomach upset, difficulty sleeping, or headaches, these typically are either very mild and tolerable, or go away when the dose of the medicine is decreased. Severe side effects are rare.

Unfortunately, some people who have lupus refuse to take hydroxychloroquine due to their fear of it causing eye problems. This potential side effect deserves some in-depth discussion (see below) because the chances of getting an eye problem from hydroxychloroquine are very low and pale in comparison to the medicine's cumulative benefits.

One major down side of hydroxychloroquine is that it is slow to work. It takes about a month of taking it before any positive effects occur. Most people require three to six months of use to get the full benefit of the medicine, while others may take up to a year. Therefore, people who have lupus who do not feel well (such as those who have significant pain, fatigue, or severe rash) may require additional medicines such as steroids or pain relievers in addition to the hydroxychloroquine while waiting for it to take effect. In addition, hydroxychloroquine is not effective by itself for moderate to severe lupus where internal organs (such as the kidneys) are involved. It should always be used along with stronger medicines in these circumstances.

## Eye Problems and Anti-Malarial Medicines

Soon after the introduction of chloroquine to treat people who had lupus in the 1950s, there were reports of people who developed blurred vision. Eye doctors (ophthalmologists) noted that a problem was developing in the back of the eye involving the retina. The retina is that section of the eye that collects light to create an image of the visual world. Chloroquine was causing a loss of pigment in the central part of the retina along with an increased amount of pigment around it in the shape of a bull's eye (such as the bull's eye on a dartboard). Doctors called this abnormality of the retina chloroquine retinopathy. It also occurred in a particular part of the retina called the macula. The macula is that part of the retina where high definition and the central part of vision is located. Therefore, the condition was also called chloroquine maculopathy. Often, the term "bull's eye retinopathy" or "bull's eye maculopathy" was used because it looked a like a bull's eye (photograph 30.1). People who had this eye problem typically developed symptoms of blurred vision, difficulty reading, intolerance of bright light (photophobia), and sometimes episodes of flashes of light. Fortunately, most cases resolved after people stopped their chloroquine; however, some cases did become permanent. About 10% of people who took chloroquine regularly developed this eye problem over time. This is why the FDA retracted its approval for the use of chloroquine to treat lupus.

This problem occurs much less often with hydroxychloroquine (Plaquenil) than it does with chloroquine. Although chloroquine appears to be more effective in treating lupus problems, the higher chance of developing retinopathy with chloroquine has caused hydroxychloroquine to become the anti-malarial drug of choice. The chances of developing hydroxychloroquine-induced retinopathy in the past had been considered very rare. For example, by 2003, only nineteen cases of hydroxychloroquine retinopathy were in the world's medical literature, and this was out of millions of prescriptions written since the 1950s. In addition, these patients had decreased kidney function, or had taken the medicine for more than six years, or were on too high of doses of hydroxychloroquine.

Over the past decade, more cases of hydroxychloroquine retinopathy have been reported. However, it is still suggested that it probably occurs in only 1% to 3% of people when it is taken for more than 7 years. The risk for developing retinopathy coincides with the cumulative dose of hydroxychloroquine. Cumulative dose is calculated by adding up the dose taken daily. For example, 2 days' worth of hydroxychloroquine at 400 mg a day would be a cumulative dose of 800 mg. Retinopathy from hydroxychloroquine is very rare under a cumulative dose of 1,000,000 mg of hydroxychloroquine. Since most people who have lupus take 400 mg a day, that calculates out to be 7 years of hydroxychloroquine, meaning that it would be very rare to ever develop retinopathy after taking it for 7 years or less at this dose. If you take 300 mg a day (or take 200 mg

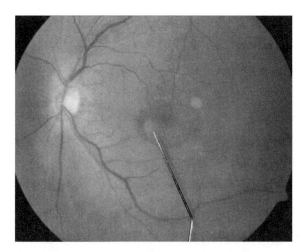

**Photo 30.1** Bull's eye maculopathy in a person taking hydroxychloroquine. The metal pin is pointing at the "bull's eye" (the dark ring surrounding a lighter-colored ring with a central red area). This woman was on hydroxychloroquine for treatment of lupus. She had no vision problems at all and this was picked up by her ophthalmologist during her routine Plaquenil exam. Photograph courtesy of retinologist Omar Ahmad, MD.

507

on one day and 400 mg the next day), then this would calculate out to be 9 years and 3 months. If you take 200 mg a day of hydroxychloroquine, then it would be rare to develop retinopathy after taking it for less than 14 years.

The chances of developing retinopathy from hydroxychloroquine also appear to be related to the dose of medicine taken per actual body weight (or ideal body weight if overweight). In people who are not overweight, it is recommended not to take more than 6.5 mg per kilogram of body weight. Going by this recommendation, you should take 200 mg a day if you weigh 101 pounds or less. If you weigh 102 to 135 pounds, you should not take more than 300 mg a day. If you weigh more than 135 pounds, then you can take 400 mg a day.

Dosing by ideal body weight is used when someone is overweight because hydroxychloroquine is not deposited in the excess fat of the body. A person's gender and height are used to calculate ideal body weight. The chance for developing this eye problem is much less as long as the dose of hydroxychloroquine is less than 6.5 mg of hydroxychloroquine per gram of ideal body weight. This can be simplified by referring to table 30.2. If you are a woman and are taller than 5 feet, 6½ inches, then it is very safe to take 400 mg a day of hydroxychloroquine. If you are between 5 feet, ½ inch, and 5 feet, 6½ inches, then you should take 300 mg a day or less of hydroxychloroquine to decrease this risk. These are new dosing recommendations, and most women who have SLE should have their dosage decreased downward from the most commonly prescribed dose of 400 mg a day. In my own practice, most of my patients require less than 400 mg a day based upon these new dosing guidelines. Everyone taking hydroxychloroquine should look at table 30.2. If you think you may be on too high of a dose of hydroxychloroquine, ask your doctor for his or her opinion and show him or her these recommendations.

Table 30.2  Recommended Dosing of Hydroxychloroquine Based on Height-Determined Ideal Body Weight

| | Height (feet, inches) | Recommended Average Daily Hydroxychloroquine Dose |
|---|---|---|
| Women | | |
| | ≥ 5' 7" | 400 mg |
| | 5' ½" to 5' 6 ½" | 300 mg |
| | < 5' ½" | 200 mg |
| Men | | |
| | < 5' 5" | 400 mg |
| | 4' 10 ½" to 5' 5" | 300 mg |
| | < 4' 10 ½" | 200 mg |

These recommendations are based upon a recommended hydroxychloroquine dose of < 6.5 mg/kg and an ideal body weight based upon height using the "method of Devine." If you are skinny or normal weight, use the dosing recommendations in table 30.3

If you are thinner than the average person, then you probably need to be on an even lower dose than what is recommended in table 30.2. If you weigh 101 pounds or less (whether you are a woman or a man), then you should take no more than 200 mg a day of hydroxychloroquine. If you weigh 102 pounds to 135 pounds then you should take no more than 300 mg a day.

Having decreased kidney function most likely plays a role in developing eye problems because many people who have been found to have hydroxychloroquine maculopathy have had decreased kidney function. This probably occurs because these medicines are metabolized (broken down) by the kidneys and liver. Therefore, if you have kidneys or a liver that do not function properly, then you may have higher amounts of these drugs circulating in your body where they can potentially cause side effects. However, it is not certain that people who have decreased kidney function necessarily need to be on lower doses than those listed in table 30.2 since those patients who had decreased kidney function in the medical reports who developed maculopathy were also on too high of doses.

In 2011, the American Academy of Ophthalmology (AAO) released new recommendations on how to prevent and screen for hydroxychloroquine retinopathy (listed in table 30.3). People starting treatment with hydroxychloroquine should have a thorough eye examination performed soon after starting treatment. This evaluation and subsequent ones need to include one of three different eye tests that are very sensitive for retina problems: a fundus autofluorescence (FAF), spectral-domain optical coherence tomography (SD-OCT), or a multifocal electroretinogram (mfERG). It is very important that you note (as a patient who is responsibly taking your healthcare into your own hands) that these three tests are not commonly performed by optometrists or some ophthalmologists. Optometrists have the letters OD (*Oculus Doctor*, or doctor of optometry) at the end of their names. Although good optometrists are highly capable in assessing vision and prescribing eyeglasses and contacts, most do not perform hydroxychloroquine evaluations using these new guidelines. It is OK if optometrists directly examine the eyes if they work with ophthalmologists who also have the expensive equipment to do these tests, however.

Ophthalmologists have either MD (medical doctor) or DO (doctor of osteopathic medicine) at the end of their names. Make sure that your primary eye doctor is an ophthalmologist. However, not even all ophthalmologists are able to do these three tests. Ophthalmologists who specialize in the retina are called retinologists, and they most certainly can do these tests. If you live in a large city, then you may have the luxury of having a retinologist who you can see to do your evaluations. In addition to having one of the three tests (FAF, SD-OCT, or mfERG), the AAO recommends that you also have a special visual field test performed called a 10-2 visual field examination. When you see the ophthalmologist or retinologist, she or he most likely will do a thorough examination of your eyes on one visit. The other tests, such as the 10-2 visual field exam, FAF, SD-OCT, and mfERG, may need to be done at a separate visit.

After your initial eye exam, it is then OK to wait five years before your next exam (since it is so rare to develop a problem before five to seven years); however, after that, you should have an exam performed every year. Some people who may be at increased risk for eye problems, such as older people, those who have other eye problems, or those who have kidney or liver problems, should have their exams done sooner than

**Table 30.3** How to Ensure That You Do Not Get Hydroxychloroquine Retinopathy

- Make sure your long-term dose of hydroxychloroquine is based on the criteria in table 30.2.
- If you are thinner than normal, you should take a lower long-term dose.
   If you are < 102 pounds do not take more than 200 mg a day.
   If you are 102 to 135 pounds do not take more than 300 mg a day.
- Have your first hydroxychloroquine screen exam done soon after starting hydroxychloroquine as a baseline.
- Make sure you have your exams done in the office of an ophthalmologist or retinologist (there should be an MD or DO after the doctor's name).
- Make sure that the doctor does a 10-2 visual field test as part of the exam (this may be scheduled at a separate visit in addition to the initial eye exam visit).
- Make sure that your ophthalmologist can do one of the following tests as part of your exam: SD-OCT, FAF, or mfERG.
- After the initial exam, start getting yearly exams performed beginning the fifth year after starting the hydroxychloroquine regimen.
- If you are at increased risk for eye problems (older age, kidney disease, liver disease, or other eye problems), your doctor may recommend eye exams more often and sooner.

five years. In addition, some people at higher risk for other eye problems may be asked to see their ophthalmologist more often than once a year. To simplify the recommendations of the AAO on how to prevent and screen for hydroxychloroquine retinopathy, refer to table 30.3.

If these recommendations are followed closely, then it should be rare for anyone to develop any significant eye problems from hydroxychloroquine. This will help keep its place as the safest medicine that doctors have to treat lupus. In fact, your ophthalmologist should detect any problems before you would ever notice any visual changes at all. When caught early, hydroxychloroquine retinopathy usually causes no symptoms whatsoever. However, if the proper screening tests are not done, as described above, and retinopathy is caught late, then there can be problems with vision. The good thing is that these problems usually improve or resolve over time. However, sometimes they can worsen, especially the first couple of years after the retinopathy first occurs. Keep in mind that this is still a very unusual problem. Ninety-seven percent of everyone who takes hydroxychloroquine for many years will never develop retinopathy. In addition, the 1% to 3% of patients who have been reported in the medical literature as having hydroxychloroquine retinopathy were not following the recommendations as listed in table 30.3. If all of these recommendations are followed closely, then these numbers would be even smaller.

If you are still nervous about taking hydroxychloroquine after reading this chapter, another thing you can do to add some "insurance" is to look at an Amsler grid regularly. An Amsler grid is a sensitive test to look for problems with vision that you can easily do at home. You can use the Amsler grid in figure 30.2.

- If you wear reading glasses, make sure to wear your glasses when looking at the grid.

- Hold the grid out at a comfortable reading distance where it is in good focus.

- Cover one eye and look directly at the dot in the center of the grid. You should be able to see all the lines on the grid clearly. They all should be straight, and they should all connect at 90-degree angles. You should also be able to see all four outer sides plus the corners. If any of the lines appear blurred, wavy, or distorted, or parts are missing, then there may be a problem with your vision, possibly involving the retina.

- Cover your other eye and repeat the above.

If the results of this test are abnormal, it can be due to other problems other than hydroxychloroquine retinopathy. For example, other problems with the retina such as from diabetes, high blood pressure, or macular degeneration can also cause the test to be abnormal. In fact, if your Amsler grid is abnormal, it is much more likely that it is due to one of these problems instead of being due to hydroxychloroquine. The bottom line is that if the test is abnormal, make an appointment with your ophthalmologist as soon as possible. The Amsler grid does not replace the need to have the 10-2 visual field or the FAF, SD-OCT, or mfERG tests done.

Chloroquine is used to treat some people who have lupus instead of hydroxychloroquine. It is actually a stronger medicine to treat lupus, but it is not used nearly as often since about 10% of people can develop retinopathy over long periods. It is also more likely to cause permanent eye damage, compared to hydroxychloroquine, which usu-

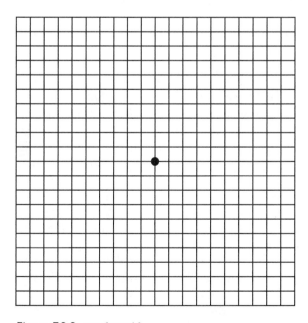

**Figure 30.2** Amsler grid

ally resolves after the medicine is stopped. People who take chloroquine should see a retinologist every 11 to 12 months and have the same studies performed as recommended above for hydroxychloroquine.

Quinacrine is the third anti-malarial sometimes used to treat lupus. One of its major advantages is the lack of retina problems. Out of millions of prescriptions of quinacrine used since the 1930s, there have only been two reported case of retinopathy in the medical literature. In one of those cases, the patient remained on quinacrine since her problem was not severe enough to stop it; after an additional four more years, her eye condition had not worsened. Another study reported on twenty-six patients who took quinacrine over thirty years and none of them developed retinopathy.

Of special note, retinopathy is not the only eye problem that can occur with anti-malarial medications. They can also be deposited in the clear, front part of the eye called the cornea. When this occurs, the affected person may see halos around lights and have difficulty tolerating light. Usually this is a very mild and transient problem; most people do not need to stop the medicine for this. However, if it is significant, it always goes away when the medicine dose is decreased or after it is stopped. Other eye problems can also cause these same symptoms. Therefore, it is very important to see your eye doctor for an evaluation to see if it is the anti-malarial medicine or some other reason instead of stopping the medicine on your own.

Very few medicines can rival the anti-malarials in terms of positive overall benefit and lower chances of side effects. Everyone who has SLE should be taking an anti-malarial medicine if they are not truly allergic to these medications. Please do not be one of those people who have SLE and refuse to take hydroxychloroquine (Plaquenil) due to your fear of developing eye problems. As long as the above recommendations are followed, it would be incredibly rare to have a problem from it. The numerous advantages of the medicine (better disease control, steroid-sparing effects, longer life expectancy, less chance for blood clots, etc.) far outweigh any risk for significant side effects from the medicine. The rest of this chapter discusses the three anti-malarial medicines currently used to treat lupus.

## Hydroxychloroquine (Plaquenil)

Hydroxychloroquine is considered the first drug of choice in treating SLE according to most lupus experts due to how safe it is and how many good things it does for people who have lupus. It may be the only medicine required by people who have mild lupus throughout their lifetime. In people who have more severe lupus, it can help to decrease the need for stronger medicines or to decrease the doses of steroids needed to treat their lupus. Whatever you do, do not refuse to take it if you have SLE because you are afraid of developing eye problems.

*Generic available*: Yes.

*How hydroxychloroquine works*: See "Why do medicines used to treat malaria also work for lupus?" earlier in this chapter.

*What benefits to expect from hydroxychloroquine*: Hydroxychloroquine is a slow working medication. It takes about a month before its effects are noted and it takes three to six months before its full effects are noted in most people. However, it can take up to a year in some people. It is most helpful for arthritis, rashes, mouth sores, serositis (such as pleurisy), fatigue, fevers, and low blood counts from SLE. It is not effective by itself to help with more severe lupus problems such as kidney, nerve, brain, heart, and lung involvement. However, it can help to decrease the doses of steroids and immunosuppressant medicines used to treat these disorders. It decreases the risk for blood clots in people who are positive for antiphospholipid antibodies and can help to decrease total and LDL "bad" cholesterol levels. For pregnant women who have SLE, hydroxychloroquine decreases the chances for miscarriage in those who are positive for antiphospholipid antibodies and may also decrease the chances of causing neonatal lupus in the baby.

*How hydroxychloroquine is taken*: The maintenance dose is based on ideal body weight determined by height and gender (table 30.2). It comes in 200 mg tablets. If you are on 400 mg a day, you can take both tablets at the same time once a day. If it bothers your stomach by taking both at the same time, you can split up the dose by taking one tablet twice a day instead (however, 2 tablets once a day helps improve compliance). If you take 300 mg a day (1 ½ tablets) based upon your height, an alternative is to take one tablet on one day (200 mg) alternating with 2 tablets (400 mg) the next day. Taking the one tablet on odd-numbered days of the month, and two tablets on even-numbered days is an easy way to remember how to take it. Some rheumatologists will prescribe more than 2 tablets a day initially as this can help hydroxychloroquine work faster compared to when it is started at lower doses.

*If you miss a dose of your medicine*: If you miss a dose of your hydroxychloroquine, take your next dose as soon as you remember that you forgot it on the same day. For example, if you usually take it at 11:00 AM every day and you realize at 8:00 PM that you forgot to take your medicine, go ahead and take your tablets for that day. Resume taking your next dose of hydroxychloroquine at 11:00 AM the next day. However, if you do not remember until the next morning that you forgot your previous day's dose, just wait until 11:00 AM, and take your usual dose for that day, totally missing the previous day's dose. Consult with your prescribing doctor to double-check these instructions, but these guidelines will suffice for most people.

*Alcohol/food/herbal interactions with hydroxychloroquine*: Avoid alcohol if you get stomach upset.

Hydroxychoroquine can be taken with or without food. Taking it with food can help decrease the chances for stomach upset.

Do not take Echinacea, which can increase immune system activity.

*Potential side effects of hydroxychloroquine*: The vast majority of people who take hydroxychloroquine do not get any side effects (listed in table 30.4). Stomach upset is by far the most common and easily goes away when taken at a lower dose. However, it is better to take it with food or to take Pepto Bismol with it to try to tolerate the full dose before decreasing your dose. It is rare to have any major side effects while taking hydroxychloroquine. Do not be afraid to take it because of the potential for eye problems. Read the section on retinopathy in this chapter for more information about retinopathy and how to prevent it (table 30.3).

*What needs to be monitored while taking hydroxychloroquine*: You must see an ophthalmologist (not an optometrist) when you first start the medicine, then every year after being on it for five years or longer. You need to have a 10-2 visual field test plus either an SD-OCT, FAF, or an mfERG yearly (see earlier in this chapter for more information). For extra "insurance," consider looking at an Amsler grid every month (figure 30.2).

**Table 30.4** Potential Side Effects of Hydroxychloroquine

|  | Incidence | Side Effect Therapy |
|---|---|---|
| **Nuisance side effects** | | |
| Stomach upset, nausea | Common | Try taking it with food or with Pepto Bismol. Or decrease the dose. |
| Blue-black or gray pigment changes of skin and gums | Common after many years | Decreases on lower doses. Resolves after medicine is stopped. |
| Insomnia, nervousness | Uncommon | Contact doctor. Usually resolves at lower doses. |
| Rash | Uncommon | Contact doctor. Resolves when medicine is stopped. May be able to start back at a lower dose. |
| Seeing halos around lights, light sensitivity due to corneal crystals | Uncommon | Usually mild and of minimal consequence not requiring intervention. Resolves if medicine stopped or dose is lowered. |
| Weight loss, loss of appetite | Rare | Resolves on lower doses or when stopped. |
| Low white blood count, anemia | Rare | Resolves when stopped. |
| **Serious side effects** | | |
| Retinopathy (maculopathy). No symptoms when picked up early. Can cause blurred vision if diagnosis is delayed. | Very rare < 7 years. Uncommon > 7 years | After medicine is stopped it can progress for a couple of years, but then usually resolves over time. It is rarely permanent. |

Side effect incidence key (approximations, as side effects can vary widely study to study): rare < 1% occurrence; uncommon 1%–5% occurrence; common > 5% occurrence

*Reasons not to take hydroxychloroquine (contraindications or precautions)*: If you are allergic to it. If you have a severe eye problem that makes it impossible to screen for retinopathy (the ophthalmologist would make this determination).

*While taking hydroxychloroquine*: If you experience any vision problems such as blurred vision, light sensitivity, or seeing halos around lights, see your ophthalmologist. These problems are usually due to something other than hydroxychloroquine, but you need to see the eye doctor to know for sure.

*Pregnancy and breast-feeding while taking hydroxychloroquine*: Never stop taking hydroxychloroquine during pregnancy if you have SLE unless your rheumatologist tells you to do so. Rarely should this be done. If your obstetrician (OB/GYN) tells you to stop taking it, discuss this with your rheumatologist first. Some women who have lupus are told to stop this along with their other medicines during pregnancy by physicians who are not familiar with the medicine. It would be much worse for you and your baby if your SLE flares during pregnancy due to stopping the hydroxychloroquine. Continuing hydroxychloroquine during pregnancy decreases the risk of lupus flaring during pregnancy as well as decreases the risk for miscarriage from antiphospholipid syndrome, and may decrease the chances of giving the baby neonatal lupus as well.

If you do get pregnant while taking hydroxychloroquine, consider contacting the Organization of Teratology Information Specialists (OTIS) Autoimmune Diseases in Pregnancy Project at www.otispregnancy.org or 877-311-8972 or email otisresearch@ucsd.edu so that more can be learned about what happens when women on medications used in treating lupus become pregnant.

Although a small amount of hydroxychloroquine enters breast milk, the American Academy of Pediatrics lists it as being "compatible" during breast feeding.

*Geriatric use of hydroxychloroquine*: Some older people may need to have their eye exams performed yearly as soon as they start the medicine or may need eye exams even more often than just once a year. This would mainly occur in people who have other eye problems or if they have significant liver or kidney disease. Otherwise, the doses used do not vary with age.

*What to do with hydroxychloroquine at the time of surgery*: It is always best to double-check with your rheumatologist and surgeon regarding specific instructions. However, hydroxychloroquine is generally safe to take up to the time you are told to stop taking medications by mouth before surgery.

*Patient assistance program for hydroxychloroquine*: Call 1-888-847-4877 or visit the Partnership for Prescription Assistance at www.pparx.org or call 1-888-477-2669.

*Drug helpline for hydroxychloroquine*: Unaware of any.

*Website to learn more about hydroxychloroquine*: www.rheumatology.org/practice/clinical/patients/medications/hydroxychloroquine.asp.

## Chloroquine (Aralen)

Chloroquine is sometimes used instead of hydroxychloroquine or is prescribed in addition to hydroxychloroquine in some people who have lupus because it works better and faster than hydroxychloroquine works. While hydroxychloroquine can take six to twelve months to achieve complete efficacy, the full effects of chloroquine are reached around two to three months. Therefore, sometimes it is used initially if someone has severe cutaneous lupus, especially discoid lupus, or if someone has severe mouth sores when a quicker response is desired to try to prevent permanent scarring of the skin or permanent hair loss. Another reason that chloroquine may be considered is if someone has an allergic reaction to hydroxychloroquine (such as rash); there is a chance that she or he may tolerate chloroquine without the same side effect.

*Generic available*: Yes.

*How chloroquine works*: See beginning of chapter "Why do medicines used to treat malaria also work for lupus?"

*What benefits to expect from chloroquine*: Chloroquine may set up its effects within a couple of weeks after starting it, and the full effect occurs around two to three months. It is most helpful for arthritis, rashes, mouth sores, serositis (such as pleurisy), fatigue, fevers, and low blood counts from SLE. It is not effective by itself to help with more severe lupus problems such as kidney, nerve, brain, heart, and lung involvement. However, it can help to decrease the doses of steroids and immunosuppressant medicines used to treat these disorders. It decreases the risk for blood clots in people who are positive for antiphospholipid antibodies and can help to decrease cholesterol levels.

*How chloroquine is taken*: Chloroquine comes in 250 mg and 500 mg tablets. The usual dose is 250 mg a day. If someone is kept on chloroquine for longer than a few months, often the dosage is decreased even farther to prevent side effects such as retinopathy.

*If you miss a dose of your medicine*: If you miss a dose of your chloroquine, take your next dose as soon as you remember that you forgot it on the same day. For example, if you usually take it at 11:00 AM every day and you realize at 8:00 PM that you forgot to take your medicine, go ahead and take your tablet for that day. Resume taking your next dose of chloroquine at 11:00 AM the next day. However, if you do not remember until the next morning that you forgot your previous day's dose, just wait until 11:00 AM, and take your usual dose for that day, totally missing the previous day's dose. Consult with your prescribing doctor to double-check these instructions, but these guidelines will suffice for most people.

*Alcohol/food/herbal interactions with chloroquine*: Alcohol should be avoided if stomach upset occurs.

Chloroquine can be taken with or without food. However, taking it with food can decrease stomach upset from chloroquine.

Do not take Echinacea, which makes the immune system more active.

*Potential side effects of chloroquine*: Potential side effects of chloroquine are listed in table 30.5. The most important thing to remember about chloroquine is that there is about a 10% risk for developing damage to the retina (retinopathy) with long-term use. Therefore, more frequent eye examinations from an eye expert (either an ophthalmologist or a retinologist) are needed. These should be done about every 11 to 12 months while taking chloroquine.

*What needs to be monitored while taking chloroquine*: You must see an ophthalmologist (not an optometrist) when you first start the medicine. Formal recommendations on follow-up are not available in the treatment of lupus since chloroquine is not used very often for long-term therapy. However, I would recommend that the eye exams be done every 11 to 12 months. You need to have a 10-2 visual field test plus either an SD-OCT, FAF, or an mfERG regularly (see earlier in this chapter for more information). For extra "insurance," consider looking at an Amsler grid every month (figure 30.2).

*Reasons not to take chloroquine (contraindications or precautions)*: If you are allergic to it. If you have a severe eye problem that makes it impossible to screen for retinopathy. In addition, it is important to make sure that you do not have a genetic enzyme deficiency called G6PD deficiency because you could develop severe anemia if you take chloroquine. This is easily tested by a simple blood test.

*While taking chloroquine*: If you get any vision problems such as blurred vision, light sensitivity, or seeing halos around lights, see your ophthalmologist.

*Pregnancy and breast-feeding while taking chloroquine*: The safety of taking chloroquine during pregnancy is unknown. It probably is safe during pregnancy, but it is recommended to switch to hydroxychloroquine during pregnancy, if possible. If you do get pregnant while taking chloroquine, consider contacting the Organization of

**Table 30.5** Potential Side Effects of Chloroquine

|  | Incidence | Side Effect Therapy |
|---|---|---|
| **Nuisance side effects** | | |
| Rash, itchy skin | Common | Contact doctor. Resolves when medicine is stopped. May be able to start back at a lower dose. |
| Stomach upset, nausea | Common | Try taking it with food or with Pepto Bismol. Usually resolves at lower doses. |
| Insomnia, nervousness | Common | Contact doctor. Usually resolves at lower doses. |
| Blue-black pigment changes of skin and gums | Common after many years | Decreases on lower doses. Resolves after medicine is stopped. |
| Weight loss, loss of appetite | Uncommon | Resolves on lower doses or when stopped. |
| Low white blood count, anemia | Uncommon | Resolves on lower doses or when stopped. |
| Seeing halos around lights, light sensitivity due to corneal crystals | Uncommon | Usually mild and of minimal consequence not requiring intervention. Resolves if medicine stopped. |
| **Serious side effects** | | |
| Retinopathy (maculopathy). No symptoms when picked up early. Can cause blurred vision if diagnosis is delayed. | Common | After medicine is stopped it can progress for a couple of years, but then usually resolves over time. It can occasionally be permanent. |

Side effect incidence key (approximations, as side effects can vary widely study to study): rare < 1% occurrence; uncommon 1%–5% occurrence; common > 5% occurrence

Teratology Information Specialists (OTIS) Autoimmune Diseases in Pregnancy Project at www.otispregnancy.org or 877-311-8972 or email otisresearch@ucsd.edu so that more can be learned about what happens when women on medications used in treating lupus become pregnant.

Although a small amount of chloroquine enters breast milk, the American Academy of Pediatrics lists it as being "compatible" during breast feeding.

*Geriatric use of chloroquine*: Since older people have a higher risk for some eye diseases such as macular degeneration, it is especially important that they be evaluated by a retinologist frequently while taking chloroquine.

*What to do with chloroquine at the time of surgery*: It is always best to double-check with your rheumatologist and surgeon regarding specific instructions. However, chloroquine is generally safe to take up to the time you are told to stop taking medications by mouth before surgery.

*Patient assistance program for chloroquine*: Call 1-888-847-4877 or visit the Partnership for Prescription Assistance at www.pparx.org or call 1-888-477-2669.

*Drug helpline for chloroquine*: Unaware of any.

*Website to learn more about chloroquine*: Unaware of any.

## Quinacrine

No major pharmaceutical companies have produced quinacrine since 1992 (since it is not profitable for them to manufacture). There are not enough lupus patients taking it to offset the costs of production. However, it can be made by compounding pharmacists. Since it is not made by any pharmaceutical companies, most insurance plans do not cover the cost (in my experience). In the Washington, DC, area my patients are currently able to obtain it for about $35 a month. Lupus experts use quinacrine in patients because it works much faster than hydroxychloroquine, and therefore it can be very useful to use along with hydroxychloroquine initially to try to get quicker control of lupus, especially for severe rashes, mouth sores, hair loss, and arthritis. Since it does not affect the retina, it can be used in people who have eye problems that prevent them from being able to use hydroxychloroquine. Lastly, if someone is on hydroxychloroquine and has persistent mild lupus problems (such as fatigue, memory problems, mild rash, or mild arthritis), but is not sick enough to warrant strong immunosuppressant medicines or steroids, then quinacrine can be a better and safer alternative. It especially may be helpful for energy and memory in some people if those problems are directly due to lupus (instead of being due to depression, fibromyalgia, or other disorders). It can have rapid, impressive results when treating severe discoid lupus, mouth sores, and hair loss in some patients. In addition, it can be helpful for swollen lymph nodes, fever, sun-sensitive rashes, and headaches as well.

*Generic available*: Yes; however, it is not inexpensive since the capsules must be individually manufactured by a compounding pharmacist.

*How quinacrine works*: How it exactly works in lupus is not fully known. It may work like other anti-malarials discussed in this chapter or by other mechanisms. For example, quinacrine has been shown to bind to DNA in the nuclei in cells and actually decrease the production of antinuclear antibodies (the hallmark lab finding in people who have SLE). Just like other anti-malarial medicines, it also decreases the effects of ultraviolet light activity in the skin. Ultraviolet light is one of the best-known activators of lupus activity.

*What benefits to expect from quinacrine*: Like hydroxychloroquine and chloroquine, quinacrine is most helpful for mild lupus problems such as rashes, arthritis, serositis (pleurisy), fever, fatigue, and low blood counts. One of its biggest advantages is that it appears to stimulate the brain better, so energy levels and memory often improve better with quinacrine compared to the other anti-malarial medications. It works a lot faster than hydroxychloroquine (which can take six to twelve months for its full effects). Quinacrine can start to work by a couple of months, and by three months its full effect is noticeable. In fact, it can rapidly improve severe discoid lupus, hair loss, and mouth ulcers within 4 to 12 weeks.

*How quinacrine is taken*: It is usually provided as a yellow powder in capsule form. The usual prescribing dose is 100 mg a day. The dose is then tapered down as needed when patients are doing well. However, most patients do best if they continue to take it for a long time even if only taking it once or twice a week. Although it can be taken by itself, it works even better if taken along with hydroxychloroquine and/or chloroquine.

*If you miss a dose of your medicine*: If you miss a dose of your quinacrine, take your next dose as soon as you remember that you forgot it on the same day. For example, if you usually take it at 11:00 AM every day and you realize at 8:00 PM that you forgot to take your medicine, go ahead and take your tablet for that day. Resume taking your next dose of quinacrine at 11:00 AM the next day. However, if you do not remember until the next morning that you forgot your previous day's dose, just wait until 11:00 AM, and take your usual dose for that day, totally missing the previous day's dose. Consult with your prescribing doctor to double-check these instructions, but these guidelines will suffice for most people.

*Alcohol/food/herbal interactions with quinacrine*: Alcohol should be avoided if you get stomach upset.

Quinacrine can be taken with or without food. However, taking it with food can decrease stomach upset.

Do not take Echinacea, which can increase immune system activity.

*Potential side effects of quinacrine*: The most significant potential side effect of quinacrine is that it can cause a severe blood problem called aplastic anemia (table 30.6). This is a condition where all the blood cell counts (red blood cells, white blood cells, and platelets) can become severely low, and unfortunately 50% of people who develop it can die from this complication. However, it is very rare, only occurring in one out of 50,000 people who take quinacrine. In patients who have lupus or rheumatoid arthritis, there have only been eleven patients ever reported who have developed this complication, and all but one were on much higher doses than the currently recommended dose. In addition, these patients were not having their blood work monitored carefully as is also currently recommended. Fifty percent of the patients who developed this severe complication developed an itchy skin rash called lichen planus before they developed the blood problem. Today because doctors monitor patients much more closely and use much lower doses of the medicine, as long as people stop the medicine if they get a rash, this side effect should be very rare, and potentially may not even occur at all. In fact, there are no reported cases of aplastic anemia in patients who take 100 mg a day and have their blood work monitored regularly. If anemia is noted while doing the blood work, it resolves when the medicine is stopped.

Another potential side effect to discuss is skin pigmentation. Quinacrine was initially developed as a yellow dye. Approximately 50% of people who take it will develop discoloration of the skin, eyes, or gums. Half of these people will have black and blue areas, and half will have a yellow tone to the skin. Interestingly, sometimes the skin can appear tan, and some patients actually like the esthetics of the tanned look. If the discoloration occurs, it goes away and the skin returns to its normal color when the dose is decreased or the medicine is stopped.

Other unusual rashes can occur with the use of quinacrine, including hair loss. Fortunately, these only occur in one out of two thousand people who take quinacrine. All skin changes should be pointed out to your prescribing doctor if they occur.

*What needs to be monitored while taking quinacrine*: Blood work for complete blood cell counts should be done monthly for the first few months, then every two to three months after that. No eye exams need to be done.

**Table 30.6** Potential Side Effects of Quinacrine

| | Incidence | Side Effect Therapy |
|---|---|---|
| **Nuisance side effects** | | |
| Headache or dizziness | Common | Contact your doctor. Resolves on lower doses or if medicine is stopped. |
| Stomach upset, nausea | Common | Try taking it with food or with Pepto Bismol. Usually resolves at lower doses. |
| Insomnia, nervousness | Common | Contact your doctor. Usually resolves at lower doses. |
| Blue-black or yellow pigment changes of skin and gums | Very common | Resolves on lower doses or if the medicine is stopped. |
| Weight loss, loss of appetite | Uncommon | Resolves on lower doses or when stopped. |
| Rash | Uncommon | Stop the medicine immediately and contact your doctor to get a blood test done for complete blood count (CBC). |
| **Serious side effects** | | |
| Difficulty thinking, bizarre thoughts or behavior | Very rare | Resolves after stopping the medicine. |
| Aplastic anemia; 50% of the time preceded by an itchy rash | Very rare (if ever) at current doses and with getting a CBC done regularly | Contact your doctor immediately. |

Side effect incidence key (approximations, as side effects can vary widely study to study):  rare < 1% occurrence; uncommon 1%–5% occurrence;  common > 5% occurrence

*Reasons not to take quinacrine (contraindications or precautions)*: Allergy to quinacrine.

*While taking quinacrine*: If you develop a rash, discontinue it immediately and contact your doctor to get a CBC blood test done.

*Pregnancy and breast-feeding while taking quinacrine*: Quinacrine crosses the placenta. No studies have been done on pregnant women. There have been reports of successful pregnancies in women who took quinacrine throughout pregnancy and no adverse effects. However, I would not personally be comfortable in recommending it to my patients during pregnancy without more information. If you do get pregnant while taking quinacrine, consider contacting the Organization of Teratology Information Specialists (OTIS) Autoimmune Diseases in Pregnancy Project at www.otispregnancy .org or 877-311-8972 or email otisresearch@ucsd.edu so that more can be learned about what happens when women on medications used in treating lupus become pregnant.

Adequate information is not available about breast-feeding while on this medication. I would not recommend its use.

*Geriatric use of quinacrine*: No changes from the above information.

*What to do with quinacrine at the time of surgery*: It is always best to double-check with your rheumatologist and surgeon regarding specific instructions. However, quinacrine is probably safe to take up to the time you are told to stop taking medications by mouth before surgery.

*Patient assistance program for quinacrine*: See chapter 42.

*Drug helpline for quinacrine*: Unaware of any.

*Website to learn more about quinacrine*: Unaware of any.

### KEY THINGS TO REMEMBER

1. Everyone who has SLE should be taking an anti-malarial medicine such as hydroxychloroquine unless there is a very good reason not to (a contraindication to taking it such as an allergy).

2. People who have SLE who take hydroxychloroquine regularly overall have less severe disease and live longer than people who refuse to take it.

3. Follow the recommendations in table 30.3 to ensure you are not one of those rare people who get retinopathy from hydroxychloroquine.

4. Use the Amsler grid (figure 30.2) as a way to screen for retina problems. See your ophthalmologist ASAP if it you do not see it properly. Usually it will be something other than hydroxychloroquine that will cause an abnormal test result.

5. If you are on chloroquine the risk for retinopathy is higher. You should see an ophthalmologist (or a retinologist is even better) every three months.

6. Quinacrine does not cause retinopathy.

7. If you ever get a rash while taking quinacrine, make sure to stop it immediately and contact your doctor to get a complete blood cell count.

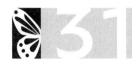

# Steroids

### Cortisone: The Miracle Drug

Before 1948, rheumatoid arthritis was uniformly a deadly and crippling disease. It caused severe deformities of the joints of the body to the point that most people afflicted with it were unable to work, to care for their families, and to care for themselves. Many had to rely on others to feed, wash, and clothe them. Many became bed bound and wheel chair bound. Not only was it a crippling disease, but it was a deadly disease, killing its victims ten to twenty years before their same-aged peers. There were no effective treatments at the time.

On July 26, 1948, a 29-year-old woman, Mrs. G, with severe rheumatoid arthritis for four and a half years was admitted to the Mayo Clinic in Minnesota for a research study using an experimental medicine. The medicine did not work. She had miserably failed the only effective treatment of the day, gold salts, but also had failed to respond to experimental antibiotics such as penicillin and streptomycin. She refused to leave the hospital, hoping for a cure. Her disease was so severe that she was mostly bed bound. She begged her rheumatologist, Dr. Philip Hench, to try anything; she was desperate for help. This was understandable because she went from being a very healthy young woman one day to someone crippled in bed the next.

Dr. Hench had been planning to try a substance called compound E at some point in patients who had rheumatoid arthritis. Compound E was one of several steroids recently discovered in the adrenal glands. There was only a tiny amount of it available from the drug company Merck and Company, but Dr. Hench was able to convince the company to allow him to use a small portion of it. On September 21, 1948, he gave the patient an injection of 100 mg of compound E in the muscle. Her arthritis at the time was so severe that she was barely able to roll over in bed on her own. Dr. Hench gave her one injection daily. By the third day, most of her painful stiffness was gone, and she could walk with a limp. One week after she began treatment, "she walked out of the hospital in a gay mood and went on a shopping trip." She reportedly shopped for three hours after being completely crippled with the disease just a week earlier. The results were no less than miraculous, so Dr. Hench and his associates began testing compound E on other people who had rheumatoid arthritis. They presented their findings at the usual staff meeting at the Mayo Clinic. He included a film showing one of the bed-bound patients walking out of the hospital effortlessly after its use and another man who danced a jig in joyous celebration. The results were so impressive that the doctors gave him a standing ovation. Doctors rarely ever give each other standing ovations, but this was truly a miracle. The scientific term for the adrenal hormone compound E was corticosterone. Not wanting compound E to be confused with vitamin E, Dr. Hench and his associate, Dr. Edward Kendall, renamed it "cortisone" as a shortened version of corticosterone in 1950. They both received the Nobel Prize for their discovery. Cortisone was destined to change the lives of arthritis patients forever.

Since lupus and rheumatoid arthritis are so closely related, doctors began to experiment with cortisone to treat people who had SLE the year after its first use by Dr. Hench. The early reports describe how quickly the rashes, fevers, and pain of SLE would resolve. Doctors wrote of miraculous cases of dying lupus patients becoming healthy. The same things doctors see today with steroid treatment were occurring back then with these initial treatments. I can only imagine the amount of jubilation on the parts of the doctors, their patients, and patients' family members. Doctors considered SLE a uniformly deadly diagnosis prior to cortisone, but now their patients had hope. The statistics would bear this fact out as well. As pointed out in chapter 20, before steroids, only about 15% of people who had SLE would survive two years, but after treatment with steroids became available, that number dramatically increased to more than 65% of patients living two years or longer.

People today like to complain about how expensive new medicines are, but this is not a new phenomenon at all. It took so much work, research, and production costs to make even small quantities of cortisone that initially it was very expensive. Cortisone was produced from cows, and it took 14,600 cows to produce a year's worth of cortisone for one patient. The total cost in producing cortisone was $4,800 a year, which was more than 100 times the cost of a similar amount of gold. The initial retail cost of cortisone was $20 a day for 100 mg of cortisone. When you factor in inflation, this comes to $182 a day in today's dollars. For one year's worth of treatment, cortisone initially cost about $66,000 for one person. Fortunately, as manufacturing improved, the price began to decrease. By November 1950, the price had dropped to $3.50 a day, which still comes out to close to $12,000 a year (in today's dollars). Most people at that time did not have insurance, and Medicare was not yet in existence.

As anyone who has taken steroids can guess, this jubilation was soon followed by judicial caution. Very quickly it was noted that many patients would gain significant weight, even becoming obese (or what doctors call Cushingoid) from the steroids. Other problems such as low potassium levels, elevated blood pressure, diabetes, avascular necrosis (see chapter 25), adrenal insufficiency (see chapter 26), and broken bones from osteoporosis (see chapter 24) were noted in many people who took the steroids. It appeared that cortisone would truly be a double-edged sword. On the one hand, it was a lifesaving medicine; on the other hand, it could cause numerous potential side effects.

Today steroids are still one of the most important medicines used to treat lupus when it is moderate to severe in nature. The effects of steroids are immediate, and they are truly lifesaving to many people who have lupus. This chapter goes into detail about steroids. It discusses how they work, what potential side effects they can cause, and how to minimize the chances of getting these side effects.

····

## When and Why Steroids Are Used to Treat Lupus

I use the word "steroids" throughout this chapter and book, but they are also commonly called glucocorticosteroids and corticosteroids. All three terms are used interchangeably. As noted in the first section to this chapter, this group of medicines is essential in the treatment of many people who have SLE so it is important to discuss them. Chapter 26 went into detail about how steroids are normally made by the body and are essential to normal, everyday functioning. It is a good idea to read that chapter before reading this one.

There are several reasons doctors use steroids to treat lupus (table 31.1). To begin with, it is essential to use them in people who have life-threatening lupus and in those who have major organ involvement (such as the kidneys, lungs, heart, or brain). They are the only medications that work immediately in lupus. The other immunosuppressant medications, such as cyclophosphamide, azathioprine (Imuran), or mycophenolate (CellCept), can take several months to get the full effects in treating severe lupus problems. When someone has life-threatening lupus or involvement of major organs several months' time is not an option; otherwise there would be irreversible damage to the organs. Not only can the steroids provide rapid improvement and save the life of the person, they can decrease the amount of permanent damage that occurs to the organs of the body.

When steroids are used to treat life-threatening lupus or lupus that is attacking major internal organs, high doses are needed. For example, prednisone is the most common steroid used, and when prednisone is used for severe lupus, the dosage is typically about 1 mg per kilogram of body weight per day. For a 130-pound person, this would amount to 60 mg per day. In the more severe cases, up to 2 mg per kilogram may be warranted. However, sometimes this is not enough. Sometimes, it is better to give even higher amounts intravenously (IV). When this is done, doctors often give 1,000 mg of methylprednisolone (Solu-Medrol) a day, often three days in a row. Rheumatologists call this method of giving high dose IV steroids "pulse steroids." This is especially helpful in calming down the severity of lupus more quickly compared to just using the pills.

Moderate lupus (such as serositis, severe arthritis, severe discoid lupus, and high fevers, for example) may require moderate doses of steroids. For example, prednisone

**Table 31.1** Reasons Steroids Are Used in Lupus

- To treat life-threatening lupus

- To treat lupus affecting major internal organs

- As "bridge therapy" for moderate lupus while waiting for other medicines (like hydroxychloroquine) to work

- As topical treatment for cutaneous lupus

- As intra-articular cortisone injections to treat arthritis

- As intramuscular cortisone injections to treat lupus flares may be prescribed anywhere between 10 mg and 40 mg per day for these problems. Again, this is needed because the other medicines used for these purposes (e.g., hydroxychloroquine, methotrexate, azathioprine, or mycophenolate) take too long to work by themselves. Doctors sometimes call this "bridge therapy." For example, a patient who has SLE who has severe joint pain from SLE is usually treated with hydroxychloroquine (Plaquenil), but it would take too long for it to work (one to six months). Therefore, prednisone can work as "bridge therapy" to calm down the inflammation and pain quickly to give the hydroxychloroquine time to start working. The goal of the doctor is to taper the prednisone down once the hydroxychloroquine starts to work.

Steroids are also used as topical therapies to treat the rashes of lupus. The medical term "topical" describes medicines applied to the skin surface. If cutaneous lupus is one of the primary problems and it does not cover a large area of the body, this can be a safer way to use steroids. Typically, a person who has cutaneous lupus may use a cream, lotion, or ointment containing steroids two to three times a day. It is often recommended to use it regularly for a couple of weeks at a time, then take a rest between each round of usage. One reason for taking a break is that if topical steroids are used continuously, the skin can become used to the medicine and actually stop responding to it (a condition called tachyphylaxis).

Steroids can also be injected into the muscles (intramuscular) or directly into the joints (intra-articular). A study from Johns Hopkins showed that an intramuscular injection of steroids in the buttock can be as helpful as increasing the dose of oral steroids. The muscle injection of steroids works faster than using oral steroids and is safe to use. This can especially be helpful for flares of lupus. If someone with lupus has a flare of arthritis causing swelling and pain of one or two joints more so than any other joints, it can be very helpful to give a steroid injection intra-articularly. This is much safer to do than giving steroids by mouth because the cortisone medicine is placed directly into the area of the body that needs it the most and there are far fewer side effects compared to taking steroids in pill form.

## Types of Steroids Used

There are many different steroids available for doctors to use. However, only a few of them are used regularly in people who have lupus, so I only mention those most commonly used (table 31.2). Prednisone is by far the most commonly used steroid to treat SLE. Some people have difficulty tolerating prednisone and may be prescribed prednisolone or methylprednisolone instead. When high doses of IV pulse steroids are needed, then Solu-Medrol is used. There are many types of steroids used for intra-articular injections, intramuscular injections, and topically for the skin. I do not go into detail about those forms. Your doctor will use his or her expertise to choose the one most appropriate depending on your situation.

## The Potential Side Effects of Steroids and How to Treat and Prevent Them

Although steroids are naturally produced by the body, when taken long enough and at high enough doses, most people do get side effects from them. Therefore, it is important to learn what the potential side effects are (table 31.3), how to try to prevent

**Table 31.2** Systemic Steroids Most Commonly Used to Treat Lupus

| Name of Steroid | Equivalent Dose to Prednisone | Usage |
|---|---|---|
| prednisone (Rayos) | 1 mg | Pill form usually. Rayos brand taken at night can work better for morning joint pain and stiffness. |
| prednisolone | 1 mg | Pill form usually. More tolerable in some people. May be a better choice if liver disease is present. |
| methylprednisolone (Medrol, Solu-Medrol) | 0.8 mg | Pill form and IV form. The IV form is often used for "pulse" IV steroids. |
| dexamethasone | 0.15 mg | Sometimes used to mature the fetus's lungs if a premature delivery is needed. Also used to prevent fetal heart block during pregnancy in women positive for SSA and SSB antibodies. |
| betamethasone | 0.12 mg | Sometimes used to mature the fetus's lungs if a premature delivery is needed. Also used to prevent fetal heart block during pregnancy in women positive for SSA and SSB antibodies. |

them (table 31.4), and how they are treated. Since most people want to know everything they can do to prevent all of the potential side effects from steroids instead of just a few of them, I list all of these preventative measures together in table 31.4 but also discuss them individually in the appropriate sections in the text below. The side effects of steroids are best dealt with by going through each organ system of the body. While other side effects for medications in this book are labeled as occurring "commonly," "uncommonly," or "rarely," I do not use this system when it comes to steroids. The potential side effects vary greatly, depending on the dose of the steroid, how long it is used, how often it is taken (daily, twice a day, or every other day, etc.), and how the individual person reacts to it. Some people are very sensitive to steroids, getting many side effects at relatively low doses, while other people can take high doses and have relatively few if any side effects.

It is very important to take steroid medications immediately when waking up in the morning (except for Rayos discussed later). This will actually minimize some of the side effects, especially the possibility of adrenal insufficiency (see chapter 26). Taking steroids more than once a day is much stronger in effect than taking them once a day. This is because when you take a tablet of a steroid, it actually stays in the blood system for only a few hours. Taking three 20 mg tablets of prednisone a day all at once in the morning (60 mg total) is not nearly as effective as taking each tablet by itself eight hours apart. The body ends up seeing a high dose of steroids for a much longer amount of time throughout the day when you divide the dose. The advantage of splitting up the dose is that it is much more effective for treating severe problems from lupus (such as brain and kidney disease), but it also causes a lot more side effects compared to taking it all at once in the morning. Doctors sometimes prescribe steroids divided up throughout the day for severe lupus, but then consolidate the dose to once each morning as soon as things stabilize. If you are prescribed more than one tablet of a steroid a day, make sure to ask if you are to spread out the dose or take it all in the morning. If you are told to spread out the dose, find out when you can consolidate the dose all in the morning to decrease your chances of getting side effects.

If you happen to miss a dose of your steroid, make sure to take it as soon as you remember that you forgot your dose. This is so that you do not develop any problems from adrenal insufficiency. Then take your next dose at the usual scheduled time.

## Bones

There are several potential problems relating to the bones that can occur from steroids. One is osteoporosis where the bones become fragile and become broken (see chapter 24). Another problem is avascular necrosis of the bone (see chapter 25). Those chapters also give recommendations on how to prevent those problems from occurring.

Children who have not completed their full growth may develop a stunting of their growth. Prolonged steroids, especially at high doses, can cause the growth plates of the bones to slow down growth and the limbs (arms and legs) can end up being shorter than normal.

## Muscles

Most everyone has heard about steroids used by athletes. They use a different type of steroid to make their muscles become large and strong, giving them an unfair advantage over their competitors. Those types of steroids are anabolic steroids. Anabolic steroids break down fat and produce more muscle. The types of steroids to treat lupus are just the opposite. They are classified as catabolic steroids, and they do just the opposite. They break down muscle and produce more fat.

When taken for long enough periods and at high enough doses, catabolic steroids will cause the muscles of the body to become smaller and weaker (called muscle atrophy). In severe cases, they can even cause myopathy ("myo-" comes from the Greek word for "muscle" and "-opathy" comes from the Greek word for "abnormality of"). Therefore, a myopathy is an abnormality of the muscle. In steroid myopathy, the individual muscle fibers themselves become smaller than normal. This especially occurs in the muscles of the shoulders, upper arms, thighs, buttocks, and upper legs. The person who develops steroid myopathy can have difficulty raising her arms up to brush her hair or teeth, and she can have problems standing up from a chair without using her hands to push herself up. It usually takes several weeks to months at higher doses of steroids for this to occur, and the treatment is to decrease the dose of the steroid. However, if the steroids are decreased in dosage, this can also potentially cause the lupus to become more active if the steroids were essential in keeping it under control.

This conundrum can potentially cause quite a bit of difficulty if it occurs in a person for whom the steroids are a critical treatment. It can also become a very difficult problem if the person has inflammation of the muscles (called myositis) due to lupus. Myositis (see chapter 7) also causes weakness in the upper arms and legs. It is treated with moderate to high doses of steroids. If someone with myositis develops more mus-

**Table 31.3**  Potential Side Effects of Systemic Steroids (Pill or IV Form)

Bones
    Osteoporosis (chapter 24)
    Avascular necrosis (chapter 25)
    Stunted growth in children
Muscles
    Muscle atrophy and overall body weakness
    Steroid myopathy
    Muscle spasms and pain
Joints
    Joint pain when tapered downward
Skin
    Thinning of the skin
    Stretch marks
    Bruising
    Acne
    Hair loss on the scalp
    Increased hair growth on the face
    Poor wound healing
    Increased blood vessels under the skin (telangiectasias)
    Worsening of psoriasis when the steroid dose is tapered down
Endocrine (hormone) and metabolic systems
    Increased hunger and craving for sweets, carbohydrates, and fats
    Weight gain
        Increased fat in central areas of the body
        Moon-shaped face
        "Buffalo hump" on upper back
    Salt (sodium) retention causing fluid retention and swelling
    Decreased potassium levels
    Elevated cholesterol and triglycerides
    Elevated glucose levels and diabetes
    Adrenal insufficiency (chapter 26)
    Irregular menstrual cycles
    Decreased fertility
Heart and blood vessels
    High blood pressure
    Hardening of the arteries, heart attacks, strokes, peripheral vascular disease
Brain and nerves
    Depression, anxiety, moodiness
    Restlessness, tremors, heart palpitations, increased energy
    Difficulty sleeping
    Psychotic, bizarre thinking and behavior
    Decreased memory
Eyes
    Cataracts
    Glaucoma
Gastrointestinal system
    Nausea
    Peptic ulcer disease when used with NSAIDs
    Bowel perforation from ulcers or diverticulitis
Immune system
    Increased infections

cle weakness as the steroid dose is decreased, the doctor has to figure out whether the weakness is coming from the myositis due to tapering the steroids, or if it is a steroid myopathy due to the steroids themselves. If it is due to myositis, the treatment is to increase the dose of steroids plus find another immunosuppressant medicine to use (such as methotrexate, azathioprine, mycophenolate, or IVIG [intravenous immuno-globulin]) to control the myositis better. If it is due to steroid myopathy, then the treatment is to continue tapering the steroid dose.

One clue that can help figure this out is that myositis usually causes the muscle enzyme (CPK, aldolase, LDH, AST, and ALT) levels to increase while they usually are normal in people who develop steroid myopathy. However, sometimes it may take a muscle biopsy to help figure this problem out.

The best way to prevent the possibilities of muscle atrophy or steroid myopathy is to perform strengthening exercises regularly. This is best done as soon as you start on the steroids to try maintaining or even building up muscle mass instead of waiting un-til you notice your muscles are getting weaker. Muscle-strengthening exercises should be done three days a week with a day of rest between each session to allow the muscles to heal. If you have never performed muscle-strengthening exercises before, you can join a gym and get assistance from a personal trainer to learn how. Another option, since this is a medical condition, is to ask your doctor to refer you to a physical thera-pist to learn how to do it on your own at home. Some inexpensive dumbbells may be all the equipment that you need to do proper exercising to keep your muscles strong.

Another common side effect of steroids are muscle spasms and muscle pain. This can occur at higher doses of steroids or when the steroid dose is being lowered. The muscle spasms may occur due to abnormalities of electrolytes such as potassium. Taking a potassium supplement from your doctor may be helpful to combat them. However, if you have kidney problems, or if you take a type of blood pressure pill called an ACE inhibitor or an angiotensin receptor blocker (ask your doctor), then you should not take potassium without consulting with your doctor as these can increase potassi-um levels on their own. Sometimes drinking tonic water can be helpful to treat muscle spasms. Exercising regularly, including a combination of stretching, strengthening, and aerobic exercises, can be helpful in decreasing the severity of muscle spasms and muscle pain. Again, using a personal trainer at a gym or seeing a physical therapist for assistance is a good way to learn how to do these types of exercises properly.

## Joints

As mentioned above, steroids can cause avascular necrosis of the bone (see chapter 25). This most commonly occurs in the shoulders, hips, or knees. When it does occur, some people will develop degenerative arthritis in the affected joints, which can cause pain, loss of range of motion, and difficulty using the particular joint. It is treated with pain relievers and exercise, but sometimes surgery is required.

Steroids can cause pain in the joints themselves without causing an actual arthri-tis. Doctors reserve the word "arthritis" to refer to actual damage or inflammation to the joints. Sometimes, especially when high doses of steroids are decreased, people can develop pain in the joints and muscles of the body due to a withdrawal type of reaction to this decreased steroid dose. Sometimes it can feel like lupus arthritis is flaring. Never increase the steroids on your own. This should only be done if the lupus itself is truly flaring with inflammatory arthritis. Your doctor should be the one to figure out what is causing the joint pain. If the pain is due to steroid withdrawal (instead of lupus arthritis), the pain will gradually decrease over several weeks as you stay on the current dose of steroids. The treatment is to take medications that help to decrease pain, exercise, and continue on the current dose of steroids (i.e., not increase the dose) until the pain goes away.

## Skin

When steroids are taken by mouth, especially at high doses or for long amounts of time, they can cause skin to become thinner than normal, so that it wrinkles and bruises easily; they can also cause stretch marks. The thin skin can become fragile and tear easily with minimal trauma as well in some people. Work with your doctor to find other medicines to try to allow your steroids to be tapered down to lower doses. Unfortunately, the stretch marks tend to be permanent. The skin thinning can improve once you are off steroids.

Acne can occur, especially on the face, upper back, and chest. Using acne medications can help decrease this effect, and the acne does resolve after the steroids are stopped.

High doses of steroids or long-term use of smaller doses can cause hair loss similar to what is seen in men (called male pattern baldness). Fortunately, this is reversible and hair growth resumes after the steroids are stopped. Increased hair growth may occur in areas of the face where it is unwanted, such as the eyebrows, side burns, chin, and upper lip. This usually improves when steroids are stopped.

Skin wounds, scratches, and cuts can take longer to heal when you have been on steroids a long time, especially at higher doses. This is one reason why surgeons like patients to be on the lowest possible doses of steroids before attempting surgery. However, never lower your steroid dose on your own without consulting your rheumatologist or other doctor who treats your lupus.

If you have psoriasis, you will most likely notice that it improves during steroid treatment. However, in people who have severe psoriasis, this can be potentially a very dangerous situation. As the dose of steroids is decreased, it is possible for the psoriasis to become much more severe than before to the point where it can actually be dangerous. Therefore, if you have significant psoriasis, it is essential that you see your dermatologist as soon as possible after being started on steroids and come up with a game plan as far as what to do if the psoriasis worsens as the steroid dose is decreased.

## Endocrine (Hormone) and Metabolic Systems

Most people who take steroids at moderate to high doses will experience increased hunger. Even people who have never considered themselves as having a sweet tooth may find themselves all at once driven to eat sweets, carbohydrates, and fatty foods that they previously would not have eaten. The sight and smell of cakes, cookies, donuts, bread, and pasta can cause an insatiable desire to eat them in large quantities. The only way to decrease this urge is to go on lower doses of steroids. Otherwise, it takes a very motivated, strong-willed person to try to overcome these intense cravings. Force yourself to eat a good diet that includes fresh fruits, vegetables, foods high in fiber, and low-fat (non-fried) meats to keep your hunger from getting out of control. If you are not sure how to eat a proper diet, you may want to ask your doctor to send you to a dietician or go to an organization such as Weight Watchers to learn how to do so. Learning to do this beforehand is better than waiting for the cravings to kick in.

One of the most dreaded problems from taking steroids (by mouth or by IV) is weight gain. As mentioned previously, the steroids used to treat lupus are catabolic steroids. They actually break down muscle tissue and cause the buildup of extra fat. This production of extra fat combined with the intense desire to eat too much of the wrong foods can spell disaster as far as weight gain. The fat typically forms in the central and middle parts of the body, including the face, the back, the chest, the shoulders, and the abdomen. The face can become rounded in shape and puffy. Medically doctors call this a moon facies, or moon face, as it can have the appearance of the moon. Fat can occur above the collarbones. When it happens on the upper part of the back, doctors call this a buffalo hump. This accumulation of fat and weight gain together are described as a Cushingoid appearance or having Cushing's syndrome due to the steroids.

Some people are fortunate and tend to have very little weight gain while on steroids, while there are others who develop significant weight gain even on smaller doses of steroids. By far the best way to minimize this side effect is to try to prevent it from happening in the first place. Make sure that you eat a proper diet or get some help from a dietician or Weight Watchers. Exercise regularly. Doing muscle-strengthening exercises several days a week to improve muscle strength and muscle bulk can help preserve as much muscle mass as you can, while aerobic exercises can help you burn up excess calories. Aerobic exercise includes exercises where you are moving large muscle groups continuously for a significant amount of time, such as stationary bicycling, treadmill, swimming, low-impact aerobic exercise, elliptical machines, and brisk walking. These should be done five days a week, and you should try to gradually increase how many minutes you do, striving to eventually do around thirty minutes at a time. A personal trainer at a gym or a physical therapist can be helpful. There are also many classes organized for senior citizens and people who have arthritis in most communities that can be very helpful. Breaking up the monotony by doing various types of exercise (instead of always doing the same things repetitively) can help keep up interest and motivation.

If you have gained weight and developed extra fat accumulation as stated above (Cushing's syndrome), then your adrenal glands are presumed to also not be functioning normally (adrenal insufficiency). It is very important for you to read the chapter on adrenal insufficiency (chapter 26) and follow its recommendations closely.

Steroids can cause the kidneys to retain extra amounts of sodium salt as well as lose potassium salt. When sodium salts accumulate in the body, the extra salt also retains additional water with it causing the person to swell with extra fluid that occurs especially in the legs and ankles but also in the hands and face. The swelling of the legs typically is worse after sitting or standing throughout the day and gets better after lying down for a while. Therefore, it usually is not noticeable when you first get up in the morning but becomes more evident toward the afternoon and evening hours. This swelling in the legs due to fluid and sodium accumulation is called edema. The best way to combat this is to decrease the amount of sodium salt in your diet. Of course, you should not add salt to your food; however, it is equally important to learn to avoid "hidden" sodium. Most pre-prepared foods are high in sodium. This includes anything in a can, fast food, any food that is prepared by most restaurants or convenience stores, pizza, many things in a bag (like chips, pretzels, etc.), and soda pop. These types of foods should be avoided. Instead, it is much better to cook your own food using fresh ingredients and spices (other than salt) to season your food. In addition, the largest single source of sodium in the American diet is bread. Therefore, it is important to limit the intake of bread as well. It can be very helpful to work with a dietician to learn what foods to avoid and which ones you can eat.

The sodium and fluid retention problem is especially problematic in people who have had congestive heart failure, severe kidney disease, or cirrhosis of the liver. This fluid retention can potentially make any of these problems worse and cause extra fluid to build up in the body, especially in the lungs, where it could cause significant breathing and heart problems. It is very important that you see your doctor more frequently if you have these problems and are taking steroids.

The loss of potassium can potentially cause muscle spasms and pain. You can use a salt substitute that contains potassium salts instead of sodium salts to help balance out this sodium and potassium problem. However, make sure to check with your doctor first because people who have kidney problems or who are on certain blood pressure medicines should not take too much potassium, or they should at least have potassium levels monitored regularly through a simple blood test.

Steroids can increase total cholesterol, bad cholesterol (LDL), and triglyceride levels. Since people who have SLE are at increased risk of having heart attacks and strokes, steroids can make this possibility even worse. See your primary care doctor regularly in addition to your rheumatologist to make sure that your cholesterol is checked regularly while you are on steroids. Exercising and eating right as described above can help to decrease this complication. However, if these levels are elevated, it is usually best to take a medication to lower the levels. It may be important for you to remind your primary care physician that people who have lupus get heart attacks and strokes younger than other people and that you would like to have your cholesterol problem treated more aggressively compared to the person who does not have lupus.

Glucose (sugar) levels can also become elevated. This especially can occur in people who have pre-existing diabetes or borderline diabetes, but also in people who have a family history of diabetes. People who are overweight, have high blood pressure, or have high cholesterol are also at increased risk of this complication. Proper diet and exercise as outlined above can help decrease this problem. However, if they do not, then diabetes medications, even insulin shots, may be needed to control it. Having high glucose levels increases the chances of developing heart attacks and strokes and it is very important to keep this in mind. If you have pre-existing diabetes, it is very important to follow up more often than usual with the doctor who treats your diabetes. You may need higher doses of your diabetic medicine while you are taking steroids.

A very serious complication of prolonged steroid usage is adrenal insufficiency. If you use steroids for a month or longer it is very important that you know about this side effect and how to deal with it. Read chapter 26 carefully and do as it recommends. At a minimum, if you are on steroids for a month or longer make sure to get a medical alert bracelet from your pharmacist that mentions that you are on steroids. Even better, medical history bracelets are now available that include a USB attachment that can be plugged into any computer. You can include your entire medical history (to include all of your medications) using your computer at home and keep it up to date. These are easily obtained at pharmacies and over the internet. If you are scheduled for surgery, you may need higher doses of steroids around the time of surgery. If you have a stressful event such as an infection or trauma, you may need to have extra doses of steroids and you should contact your rheumatologist to find out.

With high doses of steroids (greater than 10 mg a day usually) women can develop irregular menstrual cycles. High doses can also decrease fertility rates in both men and women. This is believed to be due to alterations in the production of sex hormones. These problems resolve on lower doses of steroids and are not permanent.

## Heart and Blood Vessels

Steroids can cause the blood pressure to become elevated. This more commonly occurs at higher doses of steroids. However, in people who have pre-existing hypertension, this can occur on lower doses as well. The sodium salt retention discussed above is one of the reasons this can occur. It is very important to exercise regularly and eat a diet low in sodium salt to prevent this from happening. If you have hypertension, you should see the doctor who treats your blood pressure more often as you may need higher doses of your blood pressure medicine while you are on steroids.

As I have said numerous times so far in the book, people who have SLE develop heart attacks, strokes and peripheral vascular disease at a younger age than other people. Especially African American women who have SLE tend to develop these complications twenty years younger than their peers do. Doctors call this condition "accelerated atherosclerosis" (see chapter 21). Unfortunately, people who have lupus who take steroids are particularly at risk for this possibility, especially those who have lupus nephritis. This may reflect the severity of the lupus itself because steroids are used in people who have more severe lupus and these people have been shown to develop significant inflammation in the blood vessels of the body, which can cause atherosclerosis (hardening of the arteries) to occur quickly. Having kidney disease (nephritis) itself is another risk factor for atherosclerosis. While helping to decrease the amount of inflammation occurring within the body and the blood vessels of people who have severe lupus, steroids can also increase cholesterol, glucose levels, and blood pressure, as discussed above. Each of these things contributes to the atherosclerosis and causes it to occur earlier than it would otherwise.

While eating a proper diet and exercising regularly are essential in helping to prevent this complication, it is also very important to have your cholesterol, glucose, and blood pressure checked regularly by your primary care physician and to have them treated aggressively with the proper medicines. It is also essential not to smoke cigarettes at all. Smoking cigarettes causes atherosclerosis to be more severe, and the nicotine in cigarettes causes the blood vessels to constrict. When the blood vessels constrict, this causes loss of blood flow to the heart or brain and can even precipitate a heart attack or stroke. Smoking if you have lupus is the equivalent of having an early death wish. It is essential if you smoke to concentrate on participating in a smoking cessation program and ask your primary care doctor for assistance as there are patches, gums, and medications that can help decrease the desire to smoke.

## Brain and Nerves

Steroids can cause significant moodiness in some people. Even people not predisposed to depression or anxiety may feel very nervous on the medicine, cry for no apparent reason, and get angry with others very easily. You need to inform your loved ones that you are taking steroids early on and that these are potential side effects. This is important because you may not notice this problem yourself at all. You may lash out at your loved ones without even realizing it. They need to understand that it is probably not their fault or your fault, but it is due to the steroids. They can point it out to you at an early stage so that you can discuss the problem sooner rather than later with your doctor. If your steroid dose can be decreased, this may help. However, sometimes a mood stabilizer or an antidepressant may help until your steroid dose can be decreased.

Learning how to minimize stress is also very important to decrease this impact from the steroids. Most people who develop lupus are women in their childbearing years and they often have more on their plate than they should. Learning how to say "no" when asked to do additional activities and responsibilities can be very helpful. It is important to learn how to prioritize the important things in life such as taking care of your own health. You need to learn how to ask for help and get assistance from your loved ones. Chapter 38 discusses coping strategies for stress in detail.

It is often difficult to sleep properly while on steroids. Steroids can make the mind race. While this can be helpful as far as you feel more energized, it is not helpful when you are trying to sleep. Do everything in the sleep hygiene section in table 6.2 to try to improve your sleep habits. However, sometimes it may be helpful to take a sleep aid prescribed by your doctor. Sleep aids with low abuse potential are available.

Steroids can also cause overactivity in general in the nervous system causing increased anxiety, tremors, restlessness, and heart palpitations (feeling the heart pounding in the chest). Avoid caffeine and tobacco if you develop any of these side effects at all because caffeine and tobacco will make these problems much more prominent.

A rare, but important potential side effect of steroids is a condition called steroid psychosis. Psychosis refers to a brain problem that causes bizarre thoughts and behavior and even hallucinations. The person may lose touch with reality and have delusions that are not real, or she or he can become irrationally paranoid. This typically occurs while using the higher doses of steroids at 20 mg a day or more. It occurs more commonly in people who have family members who have had problems with depression or alcoholism; therefore, there is probably a genetic basis for this reaction to the medicine. The treatment for steroid psychosis is to lower the steroid dose. However, sometimes this occurs in people who need the high doses of steroids due to the severity of their lupus. In this situation, the steroid dose cannot be decreased and antipsychotic medicines (the types used to treat conditions like schizophrenia and bipolar disorder) may be needed. Another complicating issue is that severe SLE can cause brain inflammation and psychosis. This of course has to be treated with high doses of steroids (just the opposite of what doctors do for steroid psychosis [i.e., decrease the steroids]). Therefore, it can sometimes become a very difficult situation for doctors to figure out if the psychosis is coming from the steroids themselves or from the lupus.

Memory problems can develop after using steroids. This typically occurs after using steroids at a prednisone dose of greater than 5 mg a day for three months or longer.

Most people require higher doses of steroids for a year or longer for this to occur. Older people are more prone to getting this problem than are young people.

## Eyes

Cataracts occur when the clear lens in the eye (the part of the eye that focuses light on the retina) becomes clouded. This can occur from the use of steroids. It is more common in people who take higher doses of steroids and in those who use them for a long time. It is one of the few side effects that can even occur on very low doses of steroids (less than 5 mg a day) or when used even every other day. The only way to try to prevent it is by working with your doctor to try to decrease your steroid dose as much as is possible and safe. Typical symptoms of cataracts include blurry vision and seeing halos around lights at night, as well as the loss of nighttime vision. You should be seeing an ophthalmologist regularly to follow the use of your anti-malarial medicine (such as hydroxychloroquine). During these visits, your eye doctor will also be checking to make sure that you are not developing cataracts. If they develop and become severe enough, cataract surgery, which replaces the damaged lens of the eye, is very successful in taking care of this complication. There have been no studies done to show a way of preventing steroid-induced cataracts from occurring. However, studies have suggested that eating a diet high in fruits and vegetables may decrease the onset of cataract formation due to aging.

Steroids can also potentially increase the pressure inside of the eye (called intraocular hypertension, or glaucoma). If you already have glaucoma or have been labeled as a "glaucoma suspect" by your ophthalmologist, it is important to see your eye doctor more regularly while taking steroids to keep track of your eye pressures. If you have a family history of glaucoma, it is also important to have your pressures checked and to let your eye doctor know that it runs in your family.

## Gastrointestinal System

Some problems with the gastrointestinal system can occur early on when using steroids. Nausea, heartburn, and upset stomach are the most common problems. You can try taking Tums or over-the-counter stomach acid reducers (e.g., Zantac, and Prilosec OTC) to see if they help. If they do not help, then make sure to contact your doctor for help. If you also take a non-steroidal anti-inflammatory drug (NSAID) (see chapter 36) such as ibuprofen, Motrin, naproxen, or Naprosyn, then you have an increased chance of developing peptic ulcer disease (see chapter 28). You should consider taking a proton pump inhibitor (table 28.3) regularly to prevent ulcers from occurring. Your doctor can prescribe these types of medicines.

People who have active ulcers at the time they are put on steroids or who have diverticulosis (small pockets sticking out of the large colon) are at increased risk of bowel perforation while on steroids. A perforation is a hole that occurs in the lining of the stomach or intestine that can allow stomach or intestinal contents to leak into the abdomen. This is potentially a life-threatening situation. It is very important to take your anti-ulcer medicine regularly while on the steroids if you have peptic ulcer disease. If you have diverticulosis, you need to pay strict attention to your diet (avoiding corn, nuts, etc.) and take in extra fiber every day. If you develop severe abdominal pain, seek medical attention immediately.

### Immune System

Since steroids suppress the immune system and the immune system is important for fighting off infections, taking steroids can increase the risk for infections. This especially occurs at higher doses such as more than 20 mg a day of prednisone. However, at lower doses of prednisone, increased infections may occur if they have been taken for a long time. It is generally felt that doses of 7 mg a day and lower do not cause infections since this is considered a physiologic dose of steroids. In other words, the adrenal glands of the body normally make this much prednisone. Remember that infections are one of the top three causes of death in people who have lupus. If you have any infection symptoms at all such as a cough, fever, sore throat, painful ears, urinating frequently with discomfort, or having an area of red-hot skin, see your primary care doctor right away to see if you need treatment for an infection. Steroids can also decrease the ability of the body to mount a fever against an infection, so do not make the mistake of thinking that you do not have an infection if you do not have a fever while taking steroids.

While you should stop taking other immunosuppressant medicines during times of infection, it is extremely important not to stop your steroid as this could make you very sick. The body actually makes more steroids (stress steroids) during periods of infection so your rheumatologist may need to have you take a higher dose during times of infection. When you get an infection, in addition to seeing your primary care doctor for treatment of the infection, you should also call your rheumatologist to see if you need to take a higher dose of steroids temporarily as well.

Do everything possible to prevent infections. Refer to table 22.1 to learn how to avoid infections. If you have ever been exposed to tuberculosis (TB), let your doctor know. Most people infected with TB do not get very sick from the infection, and the infection can live in their bodies for the rest of their lives. If a person infected with tuberculosis is put on high doses of steroids, then severe TB can occur. This can be prevented with appropriate antibiotics. Therefore, let your doctor know if you have ever had a positive skin test for TB before or if you have been around someone infected with TB.

If you do everything listed in table 31.4 you should have a much better chance of preventing side effects from your systemic steroid treatment. This list can be quite daunting, but if you are able to get into the habit of following these recommendations, you will come out way ahead as far as preventing or at least greatly decreasing the impact of side effects from the steroids. It can be reassuring to tell yourself that these interventions are under your control, and so you do not have to be completely powerless when it comes to dealing with the potential side effects of the steroids. While these side effects mainly apply to the pills and IV forms of steroids, you can still get them from the other forms of steroids as well.

## Potential Side Effects of High-Dose Pulse IV Steroids

IV pulse steroids are commonly given as 1,000 mg of Solu-medrol (methylprednisolone) a day over a three-day period. Occasionally there can be slight variations of this regimen. In addition to the side effects noted above, there are some other concerns. Since this is a much larger dose of steroids, the chances of people who have diabetes

**Table 31.4** How to Prevent Side Effects from Steroids

- Take your steroid first thing in the morning as soon as you wake up unless directed by your doctor to do otherwise. (Rayos is usually taken at night time.)
- If you are told to take more than one tablet of a steroid a day, take it all in the morning unless directed otherwise by your doctor.
- Never miss a dose of your steroid.
- If you forget a dose, take it as soon as you remember. Take your next dose at the usual scheduled time.
- Do not smoke cigarettes.
- Do not drink any alcohol.
- Take a vitamin D supplement regularly if you have vitamin D deficiency (determined by blood tests). Your goal is a 25-OH vitamin D level of 30 ng/mL or higher.
- If your vitamin D level is normal, take at least an 800 IU vitamin D3 supplement daily.
- Do weight-bearing exercise to stress the bones (to prevent osteoporosis) five days a week, thirty minutes at a time.
- Do strength-training exercises three days a week.
- Do stretching exercises regularly five to seven days a week.
- Do aerobic exercise five days a week, trying to get to thirty minutes each time.
- Get adequate amounts of calcium (chapter 24).
- Take a medication such as a bisphosphonate to prevent osteoporosis.
- Do not taper your dose of steroids or stop them on your own.
- Take a potassium supplement or drink tonic water for muscle spasms.
- Use acne medicines if acne occurs.
- Only use steroid creams as directed by your doctor; consider working closely with a dermatologist to ensure you are using them correctly.
- If you have significant psoriasis, see your dermatologist right away after you start taking steroids and develop a game plan for what to do if your psoriasis worsens as the steroid dose is decreased.
- Eat a low-sodium diet including plenty of fresh fruits, vegetables, and fiber; eat only low-fat meats.
- Consider using a high-potassium salt substitute (if approved by your doctor).
- Consider getting help from a dietician or going to a group such as Weight Watchers to learn proper eating habits.
- If you have high cholesterol, diabetes (or borderline diabetes), or high blood pressure, see your doctor more regularly while you are being treated with steroids. You may need higher doses of your medicines to control these problems.
- Wear a medical alert bracelet or a medical history USB bracelet if you use steroids for more than a month.
- Alert all physicians that you take steroids if you are planning on having surgery.

**Table 31.4** (*Continued*)

- If you are under increased stress (e.g., infection), you may need more steroids temporarily.
- Inform your family members of the potential side effects of steroids. (They may make you moody, depressed, or angry.)
- Ask your family to let you know ASAP if they observe symptoms of moodiness or depression so that you can discuss them with your doctor.
- Avoid caffeine.
- Use good sleep hygiene techniques, as described in table 6.2.
- If you get heartburn, nausea, or an upset stomach, consider taking Tums, Zantac, or Prilosec with your doctor's permission.
- If you take an NSAID as well as steroids, consider taking a PPI daily (table 28.3) to prevent peptic ulcer disease.
- Do everything listed in table 22.1 to avoid infections.
- Tell your doctor if you have been positive for TB in the past or have been exposed to TB.
- If you feel that your lupus is under good control and you are on steroids, always ask your doctor if you can decrease your dose if your doctor forgets to recommend it at your visit.

developing much higher glucose levels is present, so it is important to work closely with your diabetic doctor when you get IV pulse steroids. In addition, during and soon after the IV steroids, there can be elevations of blood pressure and changes in heart rate. The nurse giving the medicine will monitor these closely. After the infusion, the chances for mood changes and insomnia are greatly enhanced as well.

## Potential Side Effects of Topical Steroids

Steroid creams, ointments, and lotions (called topical steroids) can cause side effects on the skin, as discussed above. They can also cause the development of tiny blood vessels under the skin called telangiectasias if used too much or inappropriately. One of the best ways to use the topical steroids is to use them regularly (not just as needed) for two weeks in a row, then stop using them for at least one week to allow the skin to recuperate. Having this rest period also allows the skin to not become used to the medicine and stop responding. When the skin becomes tolerant and stops responding to the topical steroids, doctors call this tachyphylaxis. It is extremely important to use topical steroids only on areas of the skin that actually have active lupus inflammation. A common mistake is that people who have lupus will begin to use these medicines on areas of the skin that have permanent damage (such as on areas that are red from telangiectasias) or on other red areas such as on small red bumps that are actually due to steroid-induced acne instead of the lupus itself. This can be quite a difficult problem to figure out on your own. Make sure to follow up with a dermatologist to ensure that you are using these medications correctly and not on the wrong areas of skin.

## Potential Side Effects of Intra-Articular Joint and Intramuscular Steroid Injections

Injections are generally the safest ways to use steroids as they rarely cause significant side effects. The most common side effect is flushing of the skin, especially the face, where it can become warm and pinkish in color. This is a natural reaction due to dilation of the blood vessels and is not an allergic reaction. It typically comes on during the first twenty-four hours after the injection and can last for a few days in some people. People who have diabetes can have elevations of their glucose (sugar) levels, so it is important to know what to do by checking with your diabetes doctor. Sometimes a joint injection with steroids can cause an inflammatory reaction due to a reaction to the steroid medicine itself. This typically occurs within the first few days after the injection. The best way to try to prevent this from happening is to use an ice pack on the joint for ten minutes as soon as you get home after the injection. Then rest as much as possible during the first few days (i.e., do not use the joint very much), and use an ice pack every hour or two for ten minutes at a time. If this reaction does occur, completely rest the joint and use the ice packs repeatedly. You can also call your doctor to ask what to do for the pain.

Fortunately, getting an infection from a joint injection is very rare, only occurring about once out of every 50,000 injections. If you get a red, hot swollen joint that is very painful to move after the first few days, see your rheumatologist immediately. A joint infection is a very dangerous situation and needs to be identified and treated immediately to prevent permanent joint destruction. If your rheumatologist is not immediately available, go to an emergency room.

One question that commonly comes up is how often intra-articular steroid injections (cortisone joint injections) can safely be given. This has never been studied in lupus patients. It is common practice among rheumatologists not to give injections into any one joint more often than four times a year; however, this is not based on real good medical science. The closest arthritis related to lupus arthritis is rheumatoid arthritis, which is also an inflammatory arthritis. In rheumatoid arthritis, there are actually studies that suggest that cortisone injections performed as often as once a month into the same affected joint can be beneficial and not harmful. The bottom line is that your rheumatologist is the best person to make this decision.

## Steroids

*Generic available*: Yes, except for Rayos, a new delayed-release form of prednisone; this does not have a generic equivalent.

*How steroids work*: Steroids stabilize and calm down the immune system and decrease inflammation.

*What benefits to expect from steroids*: Steroids are the fastest-working medicines of all for lupus. In high doses, beneficial effects, such as decreased joint pain, resolution of fevers, and having an overall feeling of well-being, can be seen within twelve to twenty-four hours.

*How steroids are taken*: Pills, IV, topically, intra-articular injections, or intramuscular injections. However, they can also be used as liquid drops in the eyes, nose, and ears. There are inhaled forms that can help with mild lung inflammation as well.

Oral steroids are best taken immediately after waking up to decrease the risks for side effects. If you are placed on steroids two to three times daily, ask your doctor when you should consolidate your steroids into taking them all in the morning. There are two major exceptions to taking steroids only in the mornings. Rayos, a new delayed-release form of prednisone, is often best to take immediately before going to bed. In addition, sometimes, doctors will have patients who have severe morning pain or stiffness from lupus arthritis take a small dose of steroids immediately before going to bed.

*If you miss a dose of your medicine*: If you miss a dose of your steroid, take your next dose immediately as soon as you remember. It is very important never to miss a day's dose of your steroid. Although it is best to usually take it as soon as you wake up, it is better to not miss a dose at all if you do forget. Then take your next dose first thing when you wake up the next day. This assumes that you are on an every morning dosing schedule of steroids, which is the most common dosing regimen. If you are on a twice-a-day schedule of steroids, take your steroid as soon as you remember, then take your next dose at the usual scheduled time. For example, if you take prednisone at 7:00 AM and 7:00 PM daily and you forget your morning dose of prednisone, if you realized at 1:00 PM that you forgot your morning dose, go ahead and take it right away, then take your next dose at your usual 7:00 PM time. If you completely miss a day's worth of steroids, and you do not realize it until the next day, resume your usual dosing schedule of steroids for that day. Do not try to squeeze in the doses missed from the previous day. Consult with your prescribing doctor to double-check these instructions, but these guidelines will suffice for most people.

*Alcohol/food/herbal interactions with steroids*: Do not drink alcohol if you develop stomach upset.

Taking steroids with food can help to decrease stomach upset. However, calcium supplements should not be taken with steroids as steroids decrease the absorption of calcium. Take calcium supplements at a different time of day. Limit the intake of caffeine or stop caffeine all together as it can increase the risk of developing tremors, moodiness, heart palpitations, and difficulty sleeping. Eat a diet low in fat, calories, and simple carbohydrates. Eat more fresh fruits, vegetables, and fiber. Avoid sodium salt. Consider a potassium salt substitute (after asking your doctor). You may need to take extra calcium, vitamin D, and other vitamins (ask your doctor).

Avoid St. John's wort, which can decrease steroid levels. Avoid Echinacea and cat's claw, which can stimulate the immune system.

*Potential side effects of steroids*: Discussed in detail above.

*What needs to be monitored while taking steroids*: You should see your doctor regularly to make sure you are not getting any side effects from the steroids, to see how your lupus is responding, and to see if your steroid dose needs to be adjusted. Try to decrease the dose of steroids as much as possible and even try to get off them as soon as possible. If you feel that your lupus is in good control and you are still on steroids, always ask your doctor if you can decrease your dose (just in case he or she forgets to recommend doing so). Your blood pressure and blood work for glucose levels and potassium levels should be followed while on steroids. You should also have your cholesterol checked more often with your primary care doctor. If you take a thyroid supplement, your dose may need to be adjusted while on steroids. Make sure to have your levels followed more closely by your thyroid doctor.

*Reasons not to take steroids (contraindications or precautions)*: For life-threatening lupus or lupus affecting the major internal organs there are no absolute contraindications (reasons not to take it).

*While taking steroids*: If you have poorly controlled diabetes, high blood pressure, congestive heart failure, or severe cirrhosis it is very important to see the doctors who treat these conditions more frequently while on steroids. If you have significant psoriasis, work closely with your dermatologist because as the steroid dose is decreased, sometimes psoriasis can become severe. You need to have a game plan in place just in case the psoriasis worsens. If you have ever been positive for a TB skin or blood test or have ever been exposed to someone with TB, make sure to let your doctor know. Do everything possible in tables 22.1 and 31.4.

*Pregnancy and breast-feeding while taking steroids*: Steroids are one of the safest medicines used during pregnancy in women who have lupus; therefore, they are sometimes essential to use during pregnancy. It is much worse for lupus to become active during pregnancy from not taking steroids as it can put the health of both the mother and the fetus at great risk. There are cases of cleft lip and cleft palate occurring in babies when steroids are taken during the first trimester; however, this risk is very low.

If you do get pregnant while taking your steroid, consider contacting the Organization of Teratology Information Specialists (OTIS) Autoimmune Diseases in Pregnancy Project at www.otispregnancy.org or 877-311-8972 or email otisresearch@ucsd.edu so that more can be learned about what happens when women who are on medications used in treating lupus become pregnant.

Although steroids enter breast milk, the American Academy of Pediatrics considers steroids safe to take while breast-feeding. If you are taking high doses of steroids (more than 40 mg a day of prednisone at a time), wait at least four hours before breast-feeding your baby.

*Geriatric use of steroids*: Dosing is no different than for younger adults. However, side effects are more apt to occur, especially osteoporosis, thinning and fragility of the skin, bruising of the skin, muscle atrophy and weakness, glaucoma, cataracts, and infections.

### KEY POINTS TO REMEMBER

1. Steroids continue to be one of the most important medicines to treat moderate to severe lupus. They can be lifesaving medicines for some people.

2. If you take steroids, review table 31.4 several times and do everything it says to decrease your risk of getting side effects.

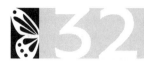

# Immunosuppressants

## From a Weapon to a Life Saver: Chemotherapy

This chapter begins on the night of July 12, 1917, near Ypres, Belgium. It was the middle of World War I and fighting was intense. The Germans attacked the British troops with bombshells containing a chemical developed by the Germans specifically for warfare. It had been shown to cause severe blistering of the skin, lung damage, and death. The effects met their expectations. Its use was devastating, causing 14,278 casualties in the first 3 weeks of its use. The survivors had severe permanent damage to the skin and lungs, and many became blind. The burning sensation it caused on the skin was similar to that caused by the oil from black mustard seeds and subsequently the chemical was named mustard gas.

Autopsies performed at the University of Pennsylvania on soldiers who had died from the effects of mustard gas showed significant decreases in their white blood cell counts. This led to Yale University performing studies on animals using similar substances. Due to dramatic effects on lowering white blood cell counts, nitrogen mustard was then tried on a patient dying from leukemia (a cancer that causes too many white blood cells) in 1942. After receiving the treatment, the dying patient went into temporary remission. The study of medicines to treat cancer, called chemotherapy of neoplasms, was born.

Due to the secrecy of these agents, as they were also intended to be used as warfare agents in World War II at the time, the positive effects were not reported until 1946. A 1947 study showed positive results using nitrogen mustard topically on the skin of patients who had skin cancer. This prompted Dr. Earl D. Osborne and his colleagues at the University of Buffalo School of Medicine to use it on the skin of a patient who had systemic lupus erythematosus (SLE). The results were favorable. The doctors knew that nitrogen mustard decreased the formation of antibodies by the immune system, which is one of the primary problems seen in SLE. Physicians soon used it in other SLE patients with some positive results. Although nitrogen mustard was found to have some positive benefits in treating lupus as well as other diseases (especially cancers such as leukemia, lymphoma, and lung cancer), its side effects were too numerous to be considered a serious long-term therapy. It caused critical decreases in blood counts, vomiting, severe skin rashes, infertility, and even death.

This was a time of great discovery for treatments for SLE. Prior to 1947, there were no good treatments for lupus. Although the anti-malarial quinine helped some people, and gold injections helped others, these agents were ineffective for the vast majority of patients. Lupus patients unresponsive to these were treated with antibiotics (penicillin and sulfa antibiotics), frozen carbon dioxide treatments on the skin, aspirin, cod liver oil, and even tonsillectomies (having their tonsils removed). None of these worked, and a diagnosis of SLE was considered a death sentence. As discussed in chapters 30 and 31, 1949 saw the first SLE patients having dramatic responses to cortisone, and Dr. Francis Page presented his remarkable results using the anti-malarial medicine quinacrine in 1951. Doctors treating lupus were becoming more optimistic about available therapies for lupus.

Nitrogen mustard was too dangerous to consider using regularly in patients so the doors gradually opened up for the development of safer medicines. Other chemotherapy medications, such as chlorambucil and cyclophosphamide, were developed. Chlorambucil had too many side effects. Cyclophosphamide ended up being the best and safest agent out of these three related medicines (nitrogen mustard, chlorambucil, and cyclophosphamide). In 1963, Dr. R. D. Hill and Dr. G. W. Scott at Guy's Hospital in London had a patient from Jamaica who had severe SLE and was developing serious side effects to her steroids. They decided to try the new immunosuppressant cyclophosphamide in treating her. She had a dramatic response to the medicine. In fact, her steroids were stopped and her disease even went into clinical remission (at least for a while). The age of immunosuppressant use in lupus was born. This was followed in 1966 by the use of azathioprine (Imuran), a medicine used to prevent organ transplant rejection (not originally a chemotherapy drug).

The success of cyclophosphamide in the treatment of SLE reached new heights when studies at the National Institutes of Health showed that most patients who had severe lupus nephritis had marked improvements of their kidney disease and many patients even went into remission with the medicine.

Then in the mid-1970s, another chemotherapy used to treat childhood leukemia, methotrexate, was first used in treating SLE with promising results. Additional immunosuppressants followed (see table below).

Chronology of Immunosuppressant Medicines in SLE

| Year of First Use or Reported Use in SLE | Medicine | Initial Use |
| --- | --- | --- |
| 1963 | cyclophosphamide (Cytoxan) | Treat leukemia/lymphoma |
| 1966 | azathioprine (Imuran) | Prevent organ transplant rejection |
| 1975 | methotrexate (Rheumatrex) | Treat childhood leukemia |
| 1986 | cyclosporine (Sandimmune) | Prevent organ transplant rejection |
| 1997 | mycophenolate (CellCept, Myfortic) | Prevent organ transplant rejection |
| 2000 | leflunomide (Arava) | Treat rheumatoid arthritis |

All of these medications are classified as immunosuppressant medicines because they suppress the immune system. So far, I have discussed anti-malarial medicines that calm down the immune system, but do not actually suppress it to the point of causing infections. Immunosuppressant medicines, on the other hand, do suppress the immune system enough that they increase the potential risk for infections. Doctors always hope that anti-malarial medicines are enough to treat lupus in any patient, as they are the safest medicines. However, in patients who have moderate to severe lupus, especially if there is major organ involvement or if the lupus is life threatening, these stronger immunosuppressant medicines are required. It becomes a balancing act with using these medicines. Doctors want to suppress the immune system enough to calm down the severity of the overactive lupus immune system, but not to the point where infections begin to occur.

Steroids also suppress the immune system (causing immunosuppression when used in high doses) and are lifesaving in many lupus patients. However, as chapter 31 points out, almost everyone who takes steroids to treat lupus will get some sort of side effect eventually. Therefore, it is better to try one of these other immunosuppressant medicines to treat moderate to severe lupus to help get people on lower doses of steroids, or hopefully even off steroids.

Immunosuppressants are currently one of the most useful and widely used group of drugs in treating moderate to severe lupus. They can help people get off prednisone, and have saved many lives over the decades. From the original inhumane design of a chemical designed to cause death and suffering in war (mustard gas) to the evolution into a group of lifesaving medicines (immunosuppressants), it is clear that history sometimes takes surprising twists and turns. This chapter goes into more detail about these immunosuppressant medications, including the "chemotherapy" medicine cyclophosphamide.

....

## Cyclophosphamide

*Generic available*: Yes.

*How cyclophosphamide works*: Cyclophosphamide is an alkylating agent chemotherapy medication. It suppresses the immune system strongly.

*What benefits to expect from cyclophosphamide*: Cyclophosphamide is by far the strongest immunosuppressant medication commonly used to treat SLE. It is the drug of choice for severe SLE where there is a chance for major organ damage or life-threatening disease. It is used especially for severe lupus nephritis as well as brain, heart, or lung involvement and for severe vasculitis. It can begin to work as quickly as a couple of weeks after the first dose.

*How cyclophosphamide is taken*: Cyclophosphamide is most commonly used in an intravenous (IV) form in treating SLE. It is usually given as one dose once a month. A common regimen is to give it monthly for six months followed by every three months for up to a total of two years' worth of treatment. However, other dosing regimens are sometimes used as well. For example, it can be given in smaller doses every two weeks for three months, which is then followed by the use of a different immunosuppressant medicine (such as azathioprine or mycophenolate). For membranous lupus nephritis (WHO Class V), it is sometimes given every other month for a year.

While cyclophosphamide can also be taken in pill form, it is not used this way in the United States very often since it causes more side effects than the IV form. However, oral cyclophosphamide is used more often in other countries due to its cheaper cost compared to the IV form.

*If you miss a dose of your medicine*: Set up your cyclophosphamide infusion as soon as you can (as long as there is not a reason you should not get it, such as if you have very low blood counts or infection). Then reset your schedule accordingly. For example, if you are getting your cyclophosphamide once a month and your infusion was scheduled on January 10, but for some reason you had to reschedule it for January 21, get your next infusion scheduled as close to February 21 as you can. Consult with your prescribing doctor to double-check these instructions, but these guidelines will suffice for most people.

*Alcohol/food/herbal interactions with cyclophosphamide*: No alcohol interactions with the IV form.

No food interactions with the IV form.

Do not take Echinacea, which can stimulate the immune system.

*Potential side effects of cyclophosphamide*: Side effects are listed in table 32.1. Thinning of the hair to overt hair loss occurs in some people. The hair begins to grow back three to six weeks after the last infusion. Sometimes it grows back in a different color or texture. Nausea and vomiting typically occur six to ten hours after the infusion. It is very important that you are armed with a good anti-nausea medicine, which should be provided to you by the infusion doctors, and it is extremely important that you take it at any hint at all of nausea. You do not want to wait until you really start to feel sick because it can be much harder to get the nausea under control if you wait too long. If your anti-nausea medicine does not work sufficiently, make sure to let your doctor know so she or he can try a different one or give you a large dose of the anti-nausea medicine.

Although most of the time, I talk about side effects with the medications in this book as being "potential" (they usually do not occur in most people), a low white blood cell count is expected in almost everyone who is treated with cyclophosphamide. Therefore, it is a definite and expected side effect. The white blood cell count decreases predictably after each treatment, with the lowest levels usually reached at around the tenth day after the infusion. Your doctor will use the result of this blood count to figure out if your dose of cyclophosphamide is correct or whether it should be adjusted. For example, if your white blood cell count decreases too much, then usually the dose of cyclophosphamide is decreased for your next infusion.

By far, one of the most common and most serious side effects is infection. The risk for infection correlates with how low the white blood cell count gets. In other words, the lower it is, the higher the chances for getting an infection. If at all possible, try to have all possible immunizations (such as Pneumovax, flu shot, Gardasil, and Zostavax) before you start cyclophosphamide treatment. In addition, most lupus experts recommend that patients take an antibiotic to prevent a lung infection due to *Pneumocystis jirovecii* pneumonia (or *Pneumocystis* pneumonia and PCP for short). The two most commonly used antibiotics are dapsone and Septra.

Cyclophosphamide can cause infertility. The chances of infertility are higher in women who are older. For example, it more commonly occurs in women in their thirties and forties compared to women in their teens and twenties. It may be possible to decrease the risk of infertility by taking hormones (such as Lupron) while you are on cyclophosphamide treatment. If you wish to have children in the future, discuss this possibility with your doctor before starting treatment. It can also cause infertility in men. If you are a man and want to ensure that you can have children in the future, you can look into the possibility of storing your sperm in a sperm bank before you begin treatment. However, since cyclophosphamide typically is used for severe lupus, usually without much advance warning, it is often impractical to take the necessary steps to donate sperm before cyclophosphamide treatment is needed.

There is an increased risk for cancer from using IV cyclophosphamide, especially cancers that are associated with human papilloma virus infection (such as cervical cancer) and cancers of the blood (leukemia and lymphoma). These usually occur many years after treatment and the risk of getting one of these cancers is probably about double that of people who are not treated with this type of medicine. The vast majority of people who are treated with cyclophosphamide do not get cancer from it.

*What needs to be monitored while taking cyclophosphamide*: You need to have a complete blood cell count performed eight to twelve days after each infusion (ten days is optimal). A chemistry panel (to check liver and kidney function) and a urinalysis will also be checked regularly.

*Reasons not to take cyclophosphamide (contraindications or precautions)*: Do not get your infusion if you have an active infection. You should wait until the infection is clear. Your doctor will also hold your infusion if your blood counts are too low. Let your doctor know if you have been exposed to TB before or have ever had a positive TB skin test (PPD) or blood test (QuantiFERON or T-SPOT.TB).

*While taking cyclophosphamide*: Most people should take an antibiotic to prevent PCP (pneumocystis pneumonia). The most commonly used antibiotics are dapsone and Septra. See your primary care doctor or go to an emergency room immediately if you have any symptoms of infection such as fever or chills, cough, painful frequent urination, red painful skin, or a sore throat. Do not get vaccinated with any live vaccines. Always check with your doctor before getting vaccinated. Flu shots and Pneumovax are safe to get. Practice all measures to prevent infections (table 22.1). If you are a woman and want to decrease your chances of developing infertility from cyclophosphamide, ask your doctor about the possibility of taking Lupron.

*Pregnancy and breast-feeding while taking cyclophosphamide*: Both men and women taking cyclophosphamide need to use strict birth control. Life-threatening SLE during the third trimester, however, may be treated with cyclophosphamide. If you decide to become pregnant after stopping cyclophosphamide, it is important to wait at least three months before trying to conceive. If you do get pregnant while taking cyclophosphamide, consider contacting the Organization of Teratology Information Specialists (OTIS) Autoimmune Diseases in Pregnancy Project at www.otispregnancy.org or 877-311-8972 or email otisresearch@ucsd.edu so that more can be learned about what happens when women on medications used in treating lupus become pregnant.

Do not breast-feed while taking cyclophosphamide.

*Geriatric use of cyclophosphamide*: Due to older people usually having reduced kidney function, lower doses are usually used.

*What to do with cyclophosphamide at the time of surgery*: It is always best to double-check with your rheumatologist and surgeon regarding specific instructions. Since

**Table 32.1** Potential Side Effects of Cyclophosphamide

|  | Incidence | Side Effect Therapy |
|---|---|---|
| **Nuisance side effects** | | |
| Nausea, vomiting, loss of appetite, diarrhea | Common | Take anti-nausea or anti-diarrhea medicine. |
| Mouth sores | Common | Reduce dosage. Use prescription mouth rinses and creams from your doctor. |
| Hair loss | Common | Hair grows back after treatment stopped. |
| Rash | Uncommon | Reduce dosage. |
| Runny nose, congestion, watery eyes, sneezing immediately after infusion | Uncommon | Slow down the rate of infusion during subsequent treatments. |
| **Serious side effects** | | |
| Low white blood cell counts | Common | Reduce dosage. Counts can be increased with medicines like Neupogen. |
| Low platelet counts | Uncommon | Reduce dosage. Can be treated with platelet transfusions if severe. |
| Anemia (low red blood cells) | Common | Reduce dosage. Can be treated with erythropoietin medicines such as Epogen and Procrit. |
| Infection | Common | Seek medical attention immediately for any fever or infection symptoms. Do not get infusion during infection. Take prophylactic antibiotics during treatment to prevent lung infections. |
| Cancer, usually years later | Uncommon | Treat the cancer. |
| Lung inflammation (pneumonitis) | Rare | Stop medicine. |
| Liver inflammation (hepatitis) | Rare | Stop medicine. |
| Infertility | Common | May be prevented with hormone treatments (if female) or sperm donation before treatment (if male). |

Side effect incidence key (approximations, as side effects can vary widely study to study): rare < 1% occurrence; uncommon 1%–5% occurrence; common > 5% occurrence

cyclophosphamide is only used for severe, active SLE, elective surgeries should not be done while on cyclophosphamide. For emergency surgeries it would be important not to resume cyclophosphamide treatments until would healing is doing well after surgery and after the dangers of infections from the surgery are minimal.

*Patient assistance program for cyclophosphamide*: See chapter 42.

*Drug helpline for cyclophosphamide*: Unaware of any.

*Website to learn more about cyclophosphamide*: www.rheumatology.org/practice/clinical/patients/medications/cyclophosphamide.asp.

## Azathioprine (Imuran, Azasan)

One of the major strengths of azathioprine is that it is safe to take during pregnancy. In fact, one of the very first lupus patients who ever received azathioprine reported in the medical literature (in 1966) was a woman who had severe SLE who became pregnant while being treated with azathioprine. Although she required a C-section at the thirty-fifth week due to preeclampsia, she had a successful pregnancy. Therefore, it is commonly used in women who have SLE who are interested in becoming pregnant.

*Generic available*: Yes.

*How azathioprine works*: Suppresses the immune system.

*What benefits to expect from azathioprine*: Used for moderate to severe SLE. It may be used immediately in some cases. In others, it may be added to an anti-malarial if the anti-malarial medicine was inadequate when used by itself. It is a slow working medicine. It takes about six weeks to begin to start working and usually takes about three months (but up to six months in some people) to achieve the full effects.

*How azathioprine is taken*: Azathioprine is taken in pill form, which comes in 50 mg tablets. The dosage is based on body weight. Generally up to 2.5 mg per kilogram of body weight are used. In a 180-pound person, that would come to 200 mg a day (100 mg twice a day). It is commonly dosed twice a day. To decrease the risk of stomach upset and nausea, it is helpful to start at a low dose initially and slowly increase the dosage.

*If you miss a dose of your medicine*: If you miss a dose of your azathioprine, take your next dose at the usual time and do not try to squeeze in an extra dose unless it has been just a few hours or less since the missed dose. For example, if you take one tablet of azathioprine after your 8:00 AM breakfast and another dose after a 7:00 PM supper, and you forget your breakfast dose of azathioprine and do not remember until 10:00 AM to 11:00 AM, go ahead and take it. You may want to eat a light snack to make sure there is something in your stomach to help you tolerate it. If you do not remember until 2:00 PM, just skip the dose, wait until your 7:00 PM supper dose, and take your usual one tablet at that time. Consult with your prescribing doctor to double-check these instructions, but these guidelines will suffice for most people.

*Alcohol/food/herbal interactions with azathioprine*: No definite interactions with alcohol except that both can upset the stomach.

Best taken after eating.

Avoid cat's claw and Echinacea, which can stimulate the immune system.

*Potential side effects of azathioprine*: As with the other immunosuppressant medicines, the side effects that are of biggest concern are low blood counts and infections (table 32.2). The risk for infections is especially higher if the white blood cell count is decreased.

There has been some debate in the rheumatologic community for the last couple of decades as to whether azathioprine can cause an increase in cancer (especially lymphoma) or not. This still is not known for 100% sure or not because people who have SLE, Sjögren's syndrome, and rheumatoid arthritis (the other diseases where doctors use a lot of azathioprine) cause increased chances of having lymphoma. So far, after several decades of use, it has not been shown that azathioprine causes more lymphomas than generally seen in people who have these disorders. Fortunately, a large 2013 study showed no relationship between the use of azathioprine and the development of lymphoma in people who have SLE.

Make sure to let your doctor know if you are taking the medicines allopurinol or febuxostat (Uloric), which are prescribed to treat gout, kidney stones, and high uric acid levels. They can cause azathioprine blood levels to become dangerously high, which can cause potentially deadly side effects. Much lower doses of azathioprine must be used when used in combination with these medicines.

*What needs to be monitored while taking azathioprine*: Your doctor will want to check a complete blood cell count and a chemistry panel (to follow liver and kidney function tests) regularly. A common regimen is to follow these once a month initially after starting the medicine, then switching to monitoring the blood tests every two to three months. Before starting on azathioprine, it can be helpful to be checked for a deficiency in thiopurine methyltransferase (TPMT). TPMT is an enzyme in the body that helps to break down (metabolize) azathioprine. This is a simple blood test. If you are deficient in TPMT (missing both genes for TPMT), you should probably not take azathioprine. If you have one of the genes for the enzyme missing, then you are at an increased risk of developing low blood counts from azathioprine and should probably have your blood counts checked more often than usual.

*Reasons not to take azathioprine (contraindications or precautions)*: You should probably not take azathioprine if you are deficient in TPMT. If you have an infection, do not take your azathioprine during the infection. Your doctor will also hold your dose if your blood counts are too low. Let your doctor know if you have been exposed to TB before or have ever had a positive TB skin test (PPD) or blood test (QuantiFERON or T-SPOT.TB).

*While taking azathioprine*: See your primary care doctor or go to an emergency room immediately if you have any symptoms of infection such as fever or chills, cough, painful frequent urination, red painful skin, or a sore throat . Do not get vaccinated with most live vaccines. It is safe to get a Zostavax (shingles vaccine) even though it is a live vaccine. Always check with your doctor before being vaccinated. Flu shots and Pneumovax are safe to get. Practice all measures to prevent infections (table 22.1).

*Pregnancy and breast-feeding while taking azathioprine*: This is one of the few medicines considered safe to take during pregnancy. Although it is classified by the FDA as probably being unsafe during pregnancy (because it is an immunosuppressant), the medical literature and rheumatologists and organ transplant doctors using azathioprine report no increase in congenital malformations. The chances of losing your baby or of becoming very sick from SLE is higher during pregnancy if azathioprine is

**Table 32.2** Potential Side Effects of Azathioprine

| | Incidence | Side Effect Therapy |
|---|---|---|
| **Nuisance side effects** | | |
| Nausea, vomiting, loss of appetite, diarrhea | Common | Take anti-nausea or anti-diarrhea medicine and take after eating. Divide the dose further. Decrease dose if needed. |
| Mouth sores | Rare | Reduce dosage. Use prescription mouth rinses and creams from your doctor. |
| Hair loss | Rare | Stop medicine. Hair grows back after drug stopped. |
| Rash | Uncommon | Reduce dosage or stop drug. |
| **Serious side effects** | | |
| Low white blood cell counts | Common; severe on rare occasions | Reduce dosage. Can be increased with medicines like Neupogen. |
| Low platelet counts | Uncommon; severe on rare occasions | Reduce dosage. Can be treated with platelet transfusions. |
| Anemia (low red blood cells) | Common; severe on rare occasions | Reduce dosage. Can be treated with erythropoietin medicines such as Epogen and Procrit. |
| Infection | Common | Seek medical attention immediately for any fever or infection symptoms. Do not take during infections. |
| Cancer | Rare, may not occur as a true side effect | Treat the cancer. |
| Lung inflammation (pneumonitis) | Rare | Stop medicine. |
| Liver inflammation (hepatitis) | Uncommon | Stop medicine. |
| Pancreatitis (inflammation of pancreas) | Rare | Stop medicine. |

Side effect incidence key (approximations, as side effects can vary widely study to study): rare < 1% occurrence; uncommon 1%–5% occurrence; common > 5% occurrence

stopped compared to any possible side effects that may develop from taking the aza-thioprine. If you do get pregnant while taking azathioprine, consider contacting the Organization of Teratology Information Specialists (OTIS) Autoimmune Diseases in Pregnancy Project at www.otispregnancy.org or 877-311-8972 or email otisresearch@ucsd.edu so that more can be learned about what happens when women on medica-tions used in treating lupus become pregnant.

Although there are reports of no problems in nursing infants, azathioprine does enter breast milk and it is not recommended to use it while breast-feeding.

*Geriatric use of azathioprine*: Dosage is the same as in younger adults.

*What to do with azathioprine at the time of surgery*: It is always best to double-check with your rheumatologist and surgeon regarding specific instructions. A common rec-ommendation is to stop it one week before surgery, then resume taking it after you have healed well after surgery and if there is no evidence for infection.

*Patient assistance program for azathioprine*: www.gskforyou.com.

*Drug helpline for azathioprine*: Call 1-888-825-5249.

*Website to learn more about azathioprine*: You can call 1-888-825-5249 to learn more about Imuran, or go to www.rheumatology.org/practice/clinical/patients/medications/azathioprine.asp.

## Methotrexate (Rheumatrex, Trexall)

*Generic available*: Yes.

*How methotrexate works*: Methotrexate suppresses the immune system; however, it is considered a weak immunosuppressant when used at the doses used in SLE.

*What benefits to expect from methotrexate*: Usually used for moderate to severe SLE. It may be used immediately in some cases. In others, it may be added to an anti-ma-larial if the anti-malarial medicine was inadequate when used by itself. It is a slow-working medicine. It can begin working in a few weeks after starting it, but can take up to three months for the full effects.

*How methotrexate is taken*: Methotrexate is usually taken either orally or by subcu-taneous (under the skin) injection once a week. The maximum number of pills pre-scribed is generally up to 25 mg a week (ten of the 2.5 mg tablets). Usually the tab-lets are taken all at the same time. If someone has problems with side effects (such as stomach upset) from taking it all at once, the dose can be split up over twenty-four hours to make it more tolerable. Since it is not absorbed very well from the gastroin-testinal system at higher doses (15 mg to 25 mg a week) the subcutaneous injection route may work better in some people. When it is injected, 100% of the medicine enters the body. When it is swallowed in pill or liquid form, much of it is actually excreted in the feces.

*If you miss a dose of your medicine*: Take the dosage that you missed right away. Then reset your schedule. For example, if you miss your dose on a Monday and do not realize you missed it until Wednesday of that same week, take your usual dose that you would have taken on that Wednesday. Then do not take your next dose until the following Wednesday.

Everyone who takes methotrexate should also take either Leucovorin or folic acid to decrease the potential for side effects from the methotrexate. If you take the vitamin

Leucovorin (folinic acid), which is usually taken once a week, reset the schedule for your Leucovorin in a similar manner. If you take the vitamin folic acid, continue taking it every day. These instructions suffice for most people taking methotrexate, but make sure to check with your prescribing physician as well.

*Alcohol/food/herbal interactions with methotrexate*: Generally do not drink alcohol while taking methotrexate. However, it is probably safe to drink alcohol in moderation or in small amounts. This decision should be made on a case-by-case basis. Check with your doctor.

Taking the medicine with food can help make it easier on the stomach; however, it also decreases its absorption. If you tolerate taking it without food, it is better to do it that way. Milk especially decreases the absorption of methotrexate. However, if you get stomach upset, take it right after eating something. Some studies suggest that caffeine use may interfere with how well methotrexate works, so it may be a good idea to cut down on caffeine intake or stop it completely on the days that you take methotrexate.

Avoid Echinacea, which increases immune system activity.

*Potential side effects of methotrexate*: As with the other immunosuppressant medicines, the side effects that are of biggest concern are low blood counts and infections (table 32.3). The risk for infections is especially higher if the white blood cell count is decreased.

One of the most common side effects from methotrexate is elevation of liver enzymes (AST and ALT). Actual liver problems with methotrexate are more common in people who have had a history of drinking excessive amounts of alcohol, people who have had hepatitis, and people who have diabetes requiring the use of insulin. In most people, elevated liver enzymes due to methotrexate rarely cause any significant problems. Studies show that as long as the levels of these enzymes remain less than two times the upper limits of normal, liver biopsies generally do not show any damage occurring in the liver. If you get a call from your doctor asking you to lower your methotrexate dose because your liver enzymes are elevated, do not be alarmed. As long as the levels are followed closely and proper adjustments are made to your dose of methotrexate, it should not cause an actual problem. If your liver enzymes are elevated five times or more in a year, you may be asked by your doctor to get a liver biopsy to make sure that everything is OK. Due to there being so many other effective medicines to treat SLE, liver biopsies are rarely done. Most physicians prefer switching patients to a different medicine if the possibility of liver toxicity is present.

It is not uncommon for the blood counts to go down while on methotrexate. This problem is usually very mild and resolves when the dosage is decreased.

If there is thinning of the hair, this is reversible and the hair slowly grows back after the dose is decreased or after the medicine is stopped. Thinning of the hair occurs in less than 10% of people who take methotrexate and is usually noted more by the person affected than by others. If you are taking folic acid to prevent side effects from methotrexate and you notice some thinning of your hair, ask your prescribing doctor if you can switch to the stronger vitamin Leucovorin (folinic acid).

A very important potential side effect is inflammation of the lungs, called pneumonitis. This occurs in approximately 1% of people due to a type of allergic reaction in the lungs called hypersensitivity pneumonitis. The symptoms are similar to those of pneumonia, including cough (often coughing up sputum), fever, and shortness of breath. The chest x-ray can look similar to pneumonia due to infection. Often, it may be impossible to tell if someone who has pneumonia while on methotrexate develops it as an infection or due to hypersensitivity pneumonitis from the methotrexate. Therefore, both possibilities may need treatment with a combination of antibiotics and high doses of steroids. In addition, the methotrexate needs to be stopped. Pneumonitis is more common in people who smoke and in people who have pre-existing lung problems. The bottom line is that both infectious pneumonia and methotrexate-induced hypersensitivity pneumonitis are very dangerous. If you develop these symptoms, it is important to stop methotrexate and seek medical attention immediately.

Be careful when you read the list of side effects from methotrexate given to you by the pharmacy. Methotrexate is given in much higher doses intravenously when used to treat cancer. The doses used in lupus are markedly lower, and many of the side effects do not apply with these low doses. For example, many times the list will instruct patients not to take NSAIDs such as ibuprofen or not to take the methotrexate if they have any kidney problems. Before stopping your medicine, check with your rheumatologist. Doctors commonly are asked even by pharmacists to stop patients' methotrexate based on the side effects seen with the high IV doses. Doctors sometimes have to educate pharmacists, who may be less experienced with the nuances of methotrexate and may not be aware that these precautions do not apply to the very low doses that doctors use in treating lupus.

The side effects of methotrexate can be decreased or prevented by taking either folic acid (1 mg to 5 mg a day) or by taking its metabolite (breakdown product of folic acid) called folinic acid (or Leucovorin; 5 mg to 25 mg a week). If Leucovorin is taken, it is most commonly given the day after taking methotrexate.

*What needs to be monitored while taking methotrexate*: Complete blood cell counts and liver function tests should be checked every four to twelve weeks while taking methotrexate.

*Reasons not to take methotrexate (contraindications or precautions)*: Do not take your methotrexate if you are having an active infection. Do not take methotrexate if you have liver disease. If you have had a history of alcoholism or hepatitis, let your doctor know, as your liver tests may need to be followed more closely.

*While taking methotrexate*: See your primary care doctor or go to an emergency room immediately if you have any symptoms of infection such as fever or chills, cough, painful frequent urination, red painful skin, or a sore throat. Do not get vaccinated with most live vaccines. It is safe to get a Zostavax (shingles vaccine) even though it is a live vaccine. Always check with your doctor before being vaccinated. Flu shots and Pneumovax are safe to get. Practice all measures to prevent infections (table 22.1).

*Pregnancy and breast-feeding while taking methotrexate*: Methotrexate has a high chance of causing miscarriage or congenital abnormalities in the fetus. Strict birth control must be used to prevent pregnancy. Due to theoretical concerns about methotrexate causing abnormalities of the DNA in eggs that are developing in the ovaries before menstruation, it is recommended that if a woman wants to become pregnant while taking methotrexate, she should stop taking methotrexate but continue strict birth control. She can then try to conceive three months after stopping methotrexate. After stopping methotrexate, a woman should take a folic acid supplement every day and then continue taking it throughout pregnancy as well to increase the chances for a

**Table 32.3** Potential Side Effects of Methotrexate

|  | Incidence | Side Effect Therapy |
|---|---|---|
| **Nuisance side effects** | | |
| Nausea, vomiting, loss of appetite, diarrhea | Common | Spread the dose out over twenty-four hours. Take with meals. If you are taking folic acid, Leucovorin may be more helpful. Reduce dosage. Take anti-nausea medicine. |
| Mouth sores | Common | Spread the dose out over twenty-four hours. If you are taking folic acid, Leucovorin may be more helpful. Reduce dosage. Use prescription mouth rinses and creams from your doctor. |
| Hair loss | Common | Taking Leucovorin can prevent it from happening. Hair returns after treatment is stopped or dose is reduced. |
| Headache, dizzy, feeling out of sorts, confused | Common | Spread the dose out over twenty-four hours. If you are taking folic acid, Leucovorin may be more helpful. Reduce dosage. |
| Rash, often sun sensitive | Uncommon | Avoid the sun, use sunscreen regularly (all people who have lupus should be doing this anyway). Reduce dosage or stop medicine. |
| **Serious side effects** | | |
| Low white blood cell counts | Common; rarely severe | Reduce dosage. Counts can be increased with medicines like Neupogen. |
| Low platelet counts | Uncommon; rarely severe | Reduce dosage. Can be treated with platelet transfusions. |
| Anemia (low red blood cells) | Common; rarely severe | Reduce dosage. Can be treated with erythropoietin medicines such as Epogen and Procrit. |
| Infection | Uncommon | Seek medical attention immediately for any fever or infection symptoms. Stop the medicine during any infection. |
| Cancer | Rare | Treat the cancer. |
| Lung inflammation (pneumonitis) | Uncommon | Stop medicine, seek medical attention immediately. |

Side effect incidence key (approximations, as side effects can vary widely study to study):  rare < 1% occurrence; uncommon 1%–5% occurrence;  common > 5% occurrence

successful, safe conception and pregnancy. It is most likely safe for men to take methotrexate while trying to get their partner pregnant. If you do get pregnant while taking methotrexate, consider contacting the Organization of Teratology Information Specialists (OTIS) Autoimmune Diseases in Pregnancy Project at www.otispregnancy.org or 877-311-8972 or email otisresearch@ucsd.edu so that more can be learned about what happens when women on medications used in treating lupus become pregnant.

Methotrexate is excreted in breast milk and is not recommended during breastfeeding.

*Geriatric use of methotrexate*: Lower doses may be used to decrease the potential of side effects.

*What to do with methotrexate at the time of surgery*: It is always best to double-check with your rheumatologist and surgeon regarding specific instructions. However, many experts recommend that methotrexate can be continued up to the time of surgery in people who have normal kidney function. In people who have decreased function, it may be best to stop it two weeks before surgery, then resume it after the surgical wound is healing well and if there is no evidence for infection.

*Patient assistance program for methotrexate*: See chapter 42.

*Drug helpline for methotrexate*: Unaware of any.

*Website to learn more about methotrexate*: www.rheumatrex.info/index.asp?Target =1 and www.rheumatology.org/practice/clinical/patients/medications/methotrexate .asp.

## Cyclosporine (Sandimmune, Neoral, and Gengraf)

Jean-Francois Borel was a microbiologist (bacteria expert) who worked for a pharmaceutical company called Sandoz. Sandoz had a program where it encouraged its employees to bring samples of naturally occurring specimens to its laboratories for testing in the hunt for new medications, especially antibiotics. While vacationing in southern Norway in 1969, Borel took some soil samples containing a fungus called *Tolypocladium inflatum*. While it did not have any antibacterial properties, it was found to have immunosuppressant properties in the lab. After more than a decade of study, its active product cyclosporine was FDA-approved in 1983 to be used to prevent organ transplant rejections. People who get organ transplants can potentially reject the organs due to their own immune systems attacking and destroying the new organs. The immune system senses that the organ does not belong and considers it a "foreign invader." Cyclosporine works by suppressing the immune system to keep that from happening.

Cyclosporine has been used to treat lupus nephritis (kidney inflammation), especially the type called membranous lupus nephritis (or WHO Class V lupus nephritis), as discussed in chapter 12. However, with the increased usage of mycophenolate (discussed below), cyclosporine is being used less often. One reason for this is that it can potentially cause a decrease in kidney function or an elevation in blood pressure. When using cyclosporine, the blood pressure and blood test for kidney function need to be checked as often as every week or two, which makes it very cumbersome to monitor. In addition, cyclosporine tends to cause more side effects compared to some of the other more commonly used immunosuppressants (table 32.4). Cyclosporine is occasionally used to treat other problems with lupus as well, such as cutaneous lupus.

*Generic available*: Yes. However, the body absorbs each brand of cyclosporine (Sandimmune versus Neoral versus generic) differently. Therefore, it is very important to stick with the same brand consistently. In other words, if you start using generic, stay with generic if it is working. If you start with Sandimmune, do not let the pharmacy switch you to Neoral or generic cyclosporine.

*How cyclosporine works*: Cyclosporine suppresses the immune system.

*What benefits to expect from cyclosporine*: Usually used for moderate to severe SLE. It may be used immediately in some cases. In others, it may be added to an anti-malarial if the anti-malarial medicine was inadequate when used by itself. It is a slow working medicine. It takes approximately two to three months until it effectively treats lupus nephritis.

*How cyclosporine is taken*: Cyclosporine is available in both tablet and liquid form. It is usually taken twice a day.

*If you miss a dose of your medicine*: If you miss a dose of your cyclosporine, take your next dose at the usual time and do not try to squeeze in an extra dose unless it has been just a few hours or less since the missed dose. For example, if you take one tablet of cyclosporine at 8:00 AM, and you take another dose at 8:00 PM, if you realize that you forgot your morning dose at 9:00 AM to 11:00 AM, go ahead and take it. If you do not remember until 3:00 PM, just skip the dose, wait until your 8:00 PM dose, and take your usual one tablet at that time. Then continue your usual dosing regimen the next day. Consult with your prescribing doctor to double-check these instructions, but these guidelines will suffice for most people.

*Alcohol/food/herbal interactions with cyclosporine*: No known interactions with alcohol.

Do not drink grapefruit juice or eat grapefruit, which increases the absorption of cyclosporine. Increased absorption could potentially cause an increase in side effects. It can be taken with or without food, but it is best taken at the same time each day and with the same pattern daily as far as timing with meals. This will also help your doctor to adjust your medicine appropriately.

Avoid St. John's wort, which can decrease cyclosporine levels. Avoid cat's claw and Echinacea, which can stimulate the immune system.

*Potential side effects of cyclosporine*: Potential side effects are listed in table 32.4.

*What needs to be monitored while taking cyclosporine*: A blood test for kidney function (serum creatinine and estimated glomerular filtration rate [eGFR]) and blood pressure need to be checked every one to two weeks for three months when the medicine is first started or after dose increases. Then it can be checked every one to three months if doing well after the first few months. A cholesterol panel (includes triglycerides) should be checked periodically.

*Reasons not to take cyclosporine (contraindications or precautions)*: If you are allergic to it or your blood pressure is poorly controlled, you should not take cyclosporine.

*While taking cyclosporine*: Contact your doctor if you develop any of the side effects mentioned above. You should monitor your blood pressure at home periodically and alert your doctor if it begins to increase above your baseline. Do not get live vaccines while you are using cyclosporine. Ask your prescribing doctor before getting any vac-

**Table 32.4**  Potential Side Effects of Cyclosporine

| | Incidence | Side Effect Therapy |
|---|---|---|
| **Nuisance side effects** | | |
| Nausea, vomiting, loss of appetite, diarrhea | Common | Take with food. Decrease dosage or discontinue medicine. |
| Headache | Common | Reduce dosage or stop medicine. |
| Increase in body hair | Common | Reduce dosage or stop medicine. |
| Rash | Common | Reduce dosage or stop medicine. |
| Leg cramps | Common | Reduce dosage or stop medicine. |
| Tremors | Common | Reduce dosage or stop medicine. |
| Tingling in hands and feet | Common | Reduce dosage or stop medicine. |
| Dizziness | Common | Reduce dosage or stop medicine. |
| Fluid retention, swelling of ankles (edema) | Common | Reduce dosage or stop medicine. |
| Swelling of the gums | Common | Reduce dosage or stop medicine. |
| **Serious side effects** | | |
| High blood pressure | Common | Reduce dosage or stop medicine. |
| Decreased kidney function | Common | Reduce dosage if the kidney function decreases more than 25% from baseline. |
| Elevated triglycerides on cholesterol panel | Common | Reduce dosage or stop medicine. |
| Infection | Common | Seek medical attention immediately for any fever or infection symptoms. Do not take during infections. |
| Cancer (lymphoma) | Rare | Treat the cancer. |

Side effect incidence key (approximations, as side effects can vary widely study to study): rare < 1% occurrence; uncommon 1%–5% occurrence; common > 5% occurrence

cines; however, flu shots and Pneumovax are safe. Practice all measures to prevent infections (table 22.1).

*Pregnancy and breast-feeding while taking cyclosporine*: Cyclosporine has been used safely during pregnancy. If you do get pregnant while taking cyclosporine, consider contacting the Organization of Teratology Information Specialists (OTIS) Autoimmune Diseases in Pregnancy Project at www.otispregnancy.org or 877-311-8972 or email otisresearch@ucsd.edu so that more can be learned about what happens when women on medications used in treating lupus become pregnant.

Cyclosporine enters breast milk and should not be used during breast-feeding.

*Geriatric use of cyclosporine*: Usually the same doses are used as in younger adults, but there may be an increased risk for side effects especially high blood pressure and decreased kidney function.

*What to do with cyclosporine at the time of surgery*: It is always best to double-check with your rheumatologist and surgeon regarding specific instructions. A common recommendation is to stop it one week before surgery, then resume taking it after the surgical wound is healing well and if there is no evidence of infection.

*Patient assistance program for cyclosporine*: For Sandimmune and Neoral call 1-800-277-2254. Also see chapter 42.

*Drug helpline for cyclosporine*: Unaware of any.

*Website to learn more about cyclosporine*: www.rheumatology.org/practice/clinical/patients/medications/cyclosporine.asp.

## Mycophenolic Acid (CellCept as Mycophenolate Mofetil and Myfortic as Mycophenolate Sodium)

During the last decade, mycophenolate has become the most popular drug used to treat lupus nephritis. It has been shown to be as effective as cyclophosphamide for many cases of lupus nephritis and may be overall safer. Additional studies have shown it to be helpful for treating other problems from SLE as well. Therefore, many doctors who treat lupus are using it more often. Another advantage over cyclophosphamide is that it does not cause sterility (infertility) in women. Consequently, it is a better option than cyclophosphamide for many young women. Its availability in a pill form instead of taking it intravenously (as is done with cyclophosphamide) is attractive as well. However, it has not been studied for severe cases of lupus nephritis; therefore, cyclophosphamide is usually used in severe kidney disease.

*Generic available*: Yes.

*How mycophenolic acid works*: Mycophenolate suppresses the immune system.

*What benefits to expect from mycophenolic acid*: Usually used for moderate to severe SLE. It may be used immediately in some cases. In others, it may be added to an anti-malarial if the anti-malarial medicine was inadequate when used by itself. It is a slow-working medicine, usually taking several months to work. For lupus nephritis, it may take as long as six months to achieve the full effects.

*How mycophenolic acid is taken*: Mycophenolate mofetil (CellCept) comes in 250 mg and 500 mg tablets or capsules, but it also comes in a liquid preparation as well for people who have difficulty swallowing pills. The extended-release form (Myfortic as mycophenolate sodium) comes in 180 mg and 360 mg tablets. It is most commonly prescribed at 1,000 mg to 1,500 mg taken at a time twice a day (when the immediate-release form is used). African Americans tend to metabolize it (break it down) or not absorb it as well as other ethnicities do. Therefore, 1,500 mg twice a day is most commonly prescribed for people of African American descent. To try to prevent gastrointestinal side effects such as nausea, diarrhea, or stomach upset, it is often initiated at a small dose (such as 500 mg twice a day) and then gradually increased to the maximum prescribed dosage. Taking the enteric-coated delayed-release tablet (Myfortic) may help to decrease GI side effects.

*If you miss a dose of your medicine*: If you miss a dose of your mycophenolate, take your next dose at the usual time and do not try to squeeze in an extra dose unless it has been just a few hours or less since the missed dose. For example, if you take one tablet of mycophenolate at 8:00 AM and you take another dose at 10:00 PM, if you realize that you forgot your morning dose at 9:00 AM to 11:00 AM, go ahead and take it. If you do not remember until 4:00 PM, just skip the dose, wait until your 11:00 PM dose, and take your usual one tablet at that time. If you take the extended-release Myfortic, just take your daily dose as soon as you realize you forgot it that day and resume your usual schedule the following day. Consult with your prescribing doctor to double-check these instructions, but these guidelines will suffice for most people.

*Alcohol/food/herbal interactions with mycophenolic acid*: There are no known interactions with alcohol.

Mycophenolate is absorbed best when taken on an empty stomach. However, if stomach upset or diarrhea occurs, it can be easier to tolerate when taken with food.

Avoid cat's claw and Echinacea, which can stimulate the immune system.

*Potential side effects of mycophenolic acid*: As with the other immunosuppressant medicines, the increased risk for infection is the most significant potential side effect. Generally, the other potential side effects tend to be mild and resolve on their own or if the dose of the medicine is decreased (table 32.5). This particularly pertains to the gastrointestinal tract symptoms that can commonly occur.

Women who can potentially become pregnant are encouraged to enroll in the mycophenolate REMS program. REMS stands for Risk Evaluation and Mitigation Study. The FDA requires that the pharmaceutical companies that produce mycophenolic acid offer this program to healthcare professionals and patients who are involved with mycophenolate prescriptions. Its goals are to educate patients about the potential side effects of mycophenolate and to decrease the risk for pregnancy problems associated with mycophenolate. People who take mycophenolic acid should go to www.mycophenolaterems.com or call 1-800-617-8191 to learn more about and enroll in the program.

*What needs to be monitored while taking mycophenolic acid*: It is recommended that blood tests for blood counts, liver function, and kidney function be checked regularly. The frequency of these tests depends on the particular situation. Usually they are checked anywhere from once a week up to every three months.

*Reasons not to take mycophenolic acid (contraindications or precautions)*: Do not take mycophenolate if you are allergic to it or have an active infection. Do not take it if you have an active ulcer in the gastrointestinal system.

*While taking mycophenolic acid*: Do not get any live vaccines while using mycophenolate. Do not take if you have an active infection. See your primary care doctor or go

**Table 32.5** Potential Side Effects of Mycophenolic Acid

|  | Incidence | Side Effect Therapy |
|---|---|---|
| **Nuisance side effects** | | |
| Nausea, vomiting, loss of appetite, diarrhea, weight loss | Common | Take with food. Reduce the dose or stop the medication. |
| Tremors or anxiety | Uncommon | Reduce dosage or stop medicine. |
| Rash | Uncommon | Reduce dosage or stop medicine. |
| **Serious side effects** | | |
| Low white blood cell counts | Uncommon | Reduce dosage. Can be increased with medicines like Neupogen. |
| Low platelet counts | Uncommon | Reduce dosage. Can be treated with platelet transfusions. |
| Anemia (low red blood cells) | Uncommon | Reduce dosage. Can be treated with erythropoietin medicines such as Epogen and Procrit. |
| Infection | Common | Seek medical attention immediately for any fever or infection symptoms. Do not take during infections. |
| Cancer (lymphoma, skin cancer) | Rare | Treat the cancer. |

Side effect incidence key (approximations, as side effects can vary widely study to study): rare < 1% occurrence; uncommon 1%–5% occurrence; common > 5% occurrence

to the emergency room immediately if you develop any infection symptoms. Practice all measures to prevent infections (table 22.1). Before having surgery, always ask your doctor well in advance if you should stop your medicine in preparation for the surgery or not.

*Pregnancy and breast-feeding while taking mycophenolic acid*: Mycophenolate can cause fetal malformations. Do not take while pregnant, and use strict birth control. Women who are capable of getting pregnant should consider enrolling in the Mycophenolate REMS program; visit the website at www.mycophenolaterems.com or call 1-800-617-8191. If you do get pregnant while taking mycophenolate, consider contacting the Organization of Teratology Information Specialists (OTIS) Autoimmune Diseases in Pregnancy Project at www.otispregnancy.org or 877-311-8972 or email otisresearch@ucsd.edu so that more can be learned about what happens when women on medications used in treating lupus become pregnant.

Safety during breast-feeding is not known. Do not use while breast-feeding.

*Geriatric use of mycophenolic acid*: Usually the same as in younger adults. However, older people tend to have more stomach upset and infections.

*What to do with mycophenolic acid at the time of surgery*: It is always best to double-check with your rheumatologist and surgeon regarding specific instructions. A common recommendation is to stop it one week before surgery, then resume taking it after the surgical wound is healing well and if there is no evidence of infection.

*Patient assistance program for mycophenolic acid*: For CellCept call 1-877-509-2235 for coupons or 1-866-422-2377 for the patient assistance program. For Myfortic call 1-800-245-5356. See chapter 42.

*Drug helpline for mycophenolic acid*: Unaware of any.

*Website to learn more about mycophenolic acid*: www.cellcept.com for CellCept. www.myfortic.com for Myfortic. Also: www.rheumatology.org/practice/clinical/patients/medications/mycophenolate.asp.

## Leflunomide (Arava)

Leflunomide was FDA-approved to treat rheumatoid arthritis in 1998. However, in its earliest stages of development in the late 1980s, it was tested on mice affected by lupus, showing that it could be effective. The first study showing that people who have lupus could benefit from the drug was in 2000, and there have been multiple studies since then showing that it works in treating various problems from lupus. Currently, lupus experts primarily prescribe it for the arthritis of lupus. This most likely is partially a result of its original FDA approval for use in treating rheumatoid arthritis. Its use primarily for lupus arthritis is interesting because there has never really been a large study proving it is better for lupus arthritis compared to the other problems in lupus. During the past few years, there have actually been quite a few studies (primarily from Asia) showing it to be possibly effective in treating lupus nephritis. It appears to be treated as the stepchild drug in treating lupus, primarily being used to treat lupus arthritis when someone does not respond adequately to hydroxychloroquine or methotrexate (the two most commonly used drugs to treat lupus arthritis). However, it is not being used commonly for any other lupus problems. There is much more evidence in the medical literature that it may be helpful for other lupus problems (such as kidney disease), while there is very little information proving it to be effective in lupus arthritis. Currently (as of February 2013), there is a large study comparing the effects of leflunomide and azathioprine in people who have lupus nephritis. This is being conducted at multiple centers in China.

*Generic available*: Yes.

*How leflunomide works*: Leflunomide suppresses the immune system.

*What benefits to expect from leflunomide*: Usually used for moderate to severe SLE. It most commonly is added to an anti-malarial or methotrexate (the medicines most commonly used for lupus arthritis) if either medicine is inadequate alone. It is a slow working medicine. As far as how long it takes to work, it has not been studied extensively in lupus patients. However, in rheumatoid arthritis patients, when it works, it tends to start working several weeks after starting it and takes about three months before the full effects are seen.

*How leflunomide is taken*: Leflunomide comes in 10 mg and 20 mg tablets. Typically, it is started at 100 mg a day (five 20 mg tablets) for the first few days. This is usually done because the medicine works faster compared to starting with only one tablet a day. After the first few days, it is decreased to 20 mg a day. However, if the doctor is worried that a particular patient may be at increased risk for side effects, the initial 100 mg a day "loading dose" may be skipped entirely. In addition, some people may be started off at only 10 mg a day, especially if it is used in combination with methotrexate.

*If you miss a dose of your medicine*: If you miss a dose of your leflunomide, take your next dose as soon as you remember that you forgot it on the same day. For example, if you usually take it at 11:00 AM every day and you realize at 8:00 PM that you forgot to take your medicine, go ahead and take your tablet for that day. Resume taking your next dose of leflunomide at 11:00 AM the next day. However, if you do not remember until the next morning that you forgot your previous day's dose, just wait until 11:00 AM and take your usual dose for that day, totally missing the previous day's dose. Consult with your prescribing doctor to double-check these instructions, but these guidelines will suffice for most people.

*Alcohol/food/herbal interactions with leflunomide*: There are no known alcohol side effects. However, since it can potentially cause inflammation of the liver, you should limit your alcohol intake. Discuss this matter with your physician.

Leflunomide may be taken with or without food. Taking it with food may help to decrease stomach upset.

Do not take Echinacea, which can increase immune system activity.

*Potential side effects of leflunomide*: The most common side effects of leflunomide are mild and reversible (table 32.6). These include stomach upset, diarrhea, and thinning of the hair. If there is thinning of the hair, this is reversible and the hair slowly returns after the dose is decreased or after the medicine is stopped. Thinning of the hair occurs in up to 10% of people who take leflunomide and is usually noted more by the affected person than it is by others. Liver enzymes are the most important blood test to follow while taking leflunomide. The vast majority of the time these are mild elevations. Slightly elevated liver enzyme tests may not even require a lowering of the dose of the medicine. Higher elevations may need a decrease in the dose or even a discontinuation of the medicine.

If any side effects occur that are particularly dangerous, then your doctor will probably have you take a medicine called cholestyramine to absorb the leflunomide. Cholestyramine is a medicine that comes in powder form and is mixed with water and swallowed. It stays in the intestines and absorbs bile salts that enter the intestines from the liver. The binding of the bile to the cholestyramine prevents reabsorption of the bile, allowing it to enter the feces. Leflunomide and its metabolites are found in these bile salts and are removed from the body through this method. The reason this is done is that leflunomide stays in the body and bloodstream for a very long time after it is stopped; taking cholestyramine allows it to be removed much faster. Cholestyramine is usually taken three times a day for eleven days, after which the blood levels for leflunomide can be checked. Medicinal charcoal can also be taken to eliminate leflunomide.

*What needs to be monitored while taking leflunomide*: CBC and chemistry panel blood tests are typically checked monthly for the first three to six months, after which they can be followed every two to three months. Your blood pressure should also be monitored.

*Reasons not to take leflunomide (contraindications or precautions)*: Do not take leflunomide if you have an active infection. Do not take leflunomide if you have liver dis-

**Table 32.6** Potential Side Effects of Leflunomide

|  | Incidence | Side Effect Therapy |
|---|---|---|
| **Nuisance side effects** | | |
| Diarrhea | Common | Usually it resolves if you keep taking leflunomide. If it is too intolerable, decrease the dosage or stop the medicine. |
| Nausea, vomiting, loss of appetite | Common | Take it with food. Reduce dosage or stop the medicine. |
| Hair loss | Common | Reduce dosage or stop the medicine. The hair does grow back. |
| Rash or itchy skin | Common | Reduce the dose or stop taking the medicine. |
| **Serious side effects** | | |
| High blood pressure | Common | Reduce dosage or stop the medicine. |
| Liver inflammation (hepatitis) | Common | If liver enzymes are mildly elevated it can be continued. For higher levels, the dose may need to be lowered or the medicine may need to be stopped. For very high doses, cholestyramine elimination may be needed. |
| Nerve damage (peripheral neuropathy) | Uncommon | Stop leflunomide. Cholestyramine or charcoal elimination procedure may be needed. |
| Infection | Rare | Seek medical attention immediately for any fever or infection symptoms. |

Side effect incidence key (approximations, as side effects can vary widely study to study): rare < 1% occurrence; uncommon 1%–5% occurrence; common > 5% occurrence

ease. If you have had hepatitis or a history of excessive alcohol use, make sure to let your doctor know before starting leflunomide. It is essential not to take it if you are pregnant. A pregnancy test should be done prior to starting leflunomide.

*While taking leflunomide*: Do not get any live vaccines (other than Zostavax) while using leflunomide. The American College of Rheumatology has stated that it is safe to get Zostavax to protect the person from shingles if he or she takes leflunomide. Do not take if you have an infection. See your primary care doctor or go to the emergency room if you develop any infection symptoms. Practice all measures to prevent infections (table 22.1). Contact your doctor if you develop yellow-colored skin and eyes as it may be a sign of jaundice from liver inflammation. If you develop diarrhea or frequent loose feces and it is mild, try to wait it out and see if it resolves or improves after a couple of weeks. If it is intolerable, call your doctor. You must use strict birth control while taking leflunomide. Contact your doctor immediately if you become pregnant so that you can be started on a cholestyramine elimination protocol.

*Pregnancy and breast-feeding while taking leflunomide*: Leflunomide has been shown to cause fetal abnormalities in animals and should not be used if you are pregnant or are considering getting pregnant. If you decide you want to become pregnant and are taking leflunomide, it is important to eliminate it from your body using cholestyramine because leflunomide can stay in the body for a couple of years. The elimination protocol is performed by taking cholestyramine three times a day for eleven days. Then a blood test for leflunomide must be done and repeated fourteen days later. It is important to get two negative results. Cholestyramine may need to be repeated if the blood level is not zero. It is not known whether it is safe for men to take leflunomide while trying to have a baby. Men should also stop leflunomide and follow the elimination procedure as described above.

If you do get pregnant while taking leflunomide, consider contacting the Organization of Teratology Information Specialists (OTIS) Autoimmune Diseases in Pregnancy Project at www.otispregnancy.org or 877-311-8972 or email otisresearch@ucsd.edu so that more can be learned about what happens when women on medications used in treating lupus become pregnant.

It is not recommended to take leflunomide while breast-feeding.

*Geriatric use of leflunomide*: Same dosing as younger adults.

*What to do with leflunomide at the time of surgery*: It is always best to double-check with your rheumatologist and surgeon regarding specific instructions. The best way to deal with leflunomide is not known for certain. Some experts recommend stopping it as far as two months before surgery while others say it can be taken up to the time of surgery. It can be resumed once the surgical wound is healing well and if there is no evidence for infection.

*Patient assistance program for leflunomide*: Call 1-888-847-4877 for assistance with Arava. See chapter 42.

*Drug helpline for leflunomide*: Unaware of any.

*Website to learn more about leflunomide*: www.rheumatology.org/practice/clinical/patients/medications/leflunomide.asp.


## Tacrolimus, Topical Ointment (Protopic)

*Generic available*: No; therefore, it is usually more expensive than topical steroids (creams, lotions, and ointments).

*How tacrolimus works*: Tacrolimus suppresses the immune system. Although it has been used systemically in lupus in pill form, it is more commonly used as an ointment for cutaneous lupus.

*What benefits to expect from tacrolimus*: It is typically used for cutaneous lupus rashes that do not respond adequately to steroid creams or lotions.

*How tacrolimus is taken*: It comes in a 0.03% and a stronger 0.1% ointment. It should be rubbed in completely on areas of active inflammation twice a day regularly (not just as needed). There should be improvement within six weeks. If not, then other therapies should be considered.

*Alcohol/food/herbal interactions with tacrolimus*: Alcohol may cause increased flushing and redness at the application site of the ointment. This is not a dangerous reaction, but something to be aware of.

**Table 32.7** Potential Side Effects of Tacrolimus

|  | *Incidence* | *Side Effect Therapy* |
|---|---|---|
| **Nuisance side effects** | | |
| Burning sensation, itching, redness | Common | Usually mild and resolves the longer you use the ointment. If not, stop using it. |
| **Serious side effects** | | |
| None | | |

Side effect incidence key (approximations, as side effects can vary widely study to study): rare < 1% occurrence; uncommon 1%–5% occurrence; common > 5% occurrence

No interaction with food.

Do not take cat's claw or Echinacea, which can increase the activity of the immune system.

*Potential side effects of tacrolimus*: Potential side effects of tacrolimus are listed in table 32.7.

*What needs to be monitored while taking tacrolimus*: Nothing.

*Reasons not to take tacrolimus (contraindications or precautions)*: Do not use if you are allergic to tacrolimus.

*While taking tacrolimus*: Contact your doctor if the rash worsens while you use the ointment.

*Pregnancy and breast-feeding while taking tacrolimus*: Tacrolimus can be used safely during pregnancy.

Tacrolimus may be used while breast-feeding.

*Geriatric use of tacrolimus*: No special considerations from other adults.

*What to do with tacrolimus at the time of surgery*: Topical tacrolimus can be used up to the time of surgery unless you are using directly over the surgical site. If surgery is going to involve the skin where you are using tacrolimus, ask your prescribing doctor about when you should stop using it.

*Patient assistance program for tacrolimus*: For Protopic call 1-800-477-6472. Also see chapter 42.

*Drug helpline for tacrolimus*: Unaware of any.

*Website to learn more about tacrolimus*: www.protopic.com.

**KEY POINTS TO REMEMBER**

1. The immunosuppressant medications are the most commonly used medications for moderate to severe lupus and they can be lifesaving medicines.

2. Immunosuppressant medications usually take a while to work (weeks to months); therefore, steroids are typically used as well initially as "bridge therapy" while wait-

ing for the immunosuppressant medicine to work, then the steroid dose is usually gradually decreased.

3. Immunosuppressants are also considered steroid-sparing medicines. In other words, they can help to decrease the dose of steroids needed. This is important because virtually everyone will get side effects from steroids, but most people do not get significant side effects to the immunosuppressants when used by experienced lupus doctors.

4. All immunosuppressants cause an increased risk of infection. If you get any infection symptoms at all (fever, cough, sore throat, sinusitis-like headache/congestion, painful/frequent urination, red-hot skin, etc.) stop the immunosuppressant. See your primary care physician or go to the emergency room immediately. Never wait to see if an infection will get better on its own; it is much better to be safe than sorry.

5. Do everything in table 22.1 to prevent infections when taking immunosuppressant medicines.

6. Do not get live vaccines while using these medicines (although you can get a Zostavax to prevent shingles if you take methotrexate, leflunomide, or azathioprine).

7. All of these medicines (except Protopic ointment) have to have labs, especially a complete blood cell count, done regularly. Make sure to see your doctor regularly and have your labs done as often as recommended.

8. Some of these medicines have very strict rules on how they are used or not used in men and women who may want to have a baby. Make sure that you are aware of these recommendations.

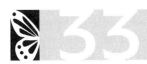

# Biologic Agents

## Biologics . . . Medicines Made by Bacteria

Before describing what biologic medications are, it can be helpful to understand the science that led up to their discovery and use. We can begin in the 1950s when virus experts Alick Isaacs and Jean Lindenmann were working on a concept called virus interference. It had been noted that if cells were exposed to a virus (dead or alive) that those same cells were protected somehow from infection from another virus. Exposure to the first virus somehow "interfered" with infection from the second virus. In the course of their experiments, they exposed chicken eggs to dead influenza (flu) virus. They were able to identify that the dead flu virus caused the eggs to produce particles that protected them from infection when a live influenza virus was then added. The live flu virus was unable to reproduce as normally would have happened. They published their findings in 1957 and named the particles produced by the cells from the chicken egg "interferons." They called it this because the particles "interfered" with the reproduction of virus. This was a big discovery because up to that point there were no known antibiotics effective against viruses, and this was considered an important piece of the puzzle to hopefully find treatments against viruses. It was subsequently shown that these interferons are produced by white blood cells of the immune system and instruct other cells of the immune system to become more active, leading to protection against viruses.

In the late 1960s, it was discovered that a type of white blood cell of the immune system called a macrophage produced a particle that would cause lymphocytes (also important white blood cells involved in the immune system) to become more active. This particle was named "lymphocyte-activating factor."

What these "interferons" and this "lymphocyte-activating factor" have in common is that they are particles produced by cells that communicate a message to other cells, in essence, allowing them to "talk" to each other. The scientists who made these discoveries could not have realized what an avalanche of future discoveries these findings would produce. Cells of the body need to be able to communicate with each other. They need to give commands to each other telling each other to become more active or less active. The term for these communication particles is "cytokines." "Cyto-" comes from the Greek word for cell, while "-kine" comes from the Greek word meaning "to move" or "to stir up." For example, the purpose of the lymphocyte-activating factor is to allow macrophages to tell lymphocytes to become more active. When macrophages of the immune system recognize an invading army of microbes (such as viruses or bacteria), they release lymphocyte-activating factor (now renamed interleukin-1, or IL-1 for short) cytokines. These cytokines tell the lymphocytes and other members of the immune system to reproduce, become "stirred up," and "move" to the area of invasion by the bacteria to destroy the viruses or bacteria and protect the body (see figure below). This IL-1 also causes fever, which is a common symptom seen during bacterial infections.

Research on discovering more cytokines exploded over the next few decades. The need to figure out how different cells of the body talk to each other using these cytokines was felt to be very important not only to understand how the body normally worked, but also to see what their roles were in various diseases as well. While these cytokines especially seemed to be important in the complex immune system, they were also found to be essential in other parts of the body as well. Although many of these cytokines cause other cells to become more active and get "stirred up" (as their Greek-derived name suggests), many cytokines do just the opposite. Some cytokines tell the immune system to become quiet and to decrease inflammation. Some cytokines even tell cells to die when they are not needed any more (a process called apoptosis). A normal functioning immune system requires a fine balancing act of cytokines. Some need to induce inflammation when it is required to attack invading bacteria and viruses, or to get rid of abnormal cells such as tumor cells. On the other hand, other cytokines are needed to decrease the areas of inflammation when it is not required anymore.

Laboratory techniques really took off in the 1970s to 1990s. More and more cytokines were being discovered every year, revealing fascinating secrets into how the body functioned. They received numerous different names, including various interferons, interleukins, colony growth factors, chemokines, and tumor necrosis factors. In the 1970s, a huge obstacle in cytokine research was that these molecules were so complex

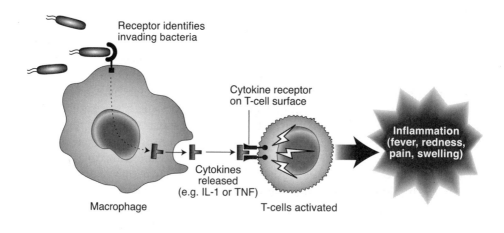

Cytokines causing normal immune response with inflammation

that they could not be produced by ordinary chemical means in a laboratory. In 1980, an interferon-producing gene was inserted into bacteria (which can multiply rapidly), and it was discovered that these bacteria could actually produce the interferon much faster and in much larger quantities than any other laboratory technique used up to that point. The laboratory technique that allowed production of the interferon became known as recombinant DNA technology. This would become a huge revolution in the cytokine research world, allowing the production of cytokines in large quantities for faster and better research.

In autoimmune diseases such as systemic lupus erythematosus (SLE) and rheumatoid arthritis (RA), the immune system is overactive. It was discovered that many of the cytokines that cause inflammation are produced in excess (see figure on the following page), while cytokines that usually calm down inflammation are not being produced as much as they should. Until the 1980s and 1990s, every medicine used to treat lupus was figured out by accident. Anti-malarials were found to decrease inflammation in soldiers in World War II. Immunosuppressants were born out of noting the effects of nitrogen mustard gas causing white blood cells to decrease in affected soldiers. Steroids were found to be effective when a woman with severe rheumatoid arthritis hospitalized at the Mayo Clinic demanded that something be tried experimentally on her to cure her of her crippling disease.

Now, scientists and doctors could actually see at a molecular level what was truly going on in the immune system. Cytokines of all different types were being bounced around from cell to cell, talking with each other, telling each other to become more active or less active. Rheumatoid arthritis and lupus cause an overproduction of the cytokines that cause inflammation. This imbalance causes damage to the organs of the body. Could doctors control these diseases if they could decrease the amounts of cytokines that cause increased inflammation or increase cytokines that decrease inflammation? Could it be possible to design medications that specifically target what is going wrong with specific parts of the immune system instead of suppressing the entire immune system (like the immunosuppressant medications)? The medical community now had a way of producing large quantities of these cytokines through recombinant DNA technology to see what would happen experimentally if levels of individual cytokines were increased or decreased.

In 1975, a cytokine was identified that was produced by macrophages of the immune system, and this cytokine had the ability to actually kill mouse cancer cells. It was named tumor necrosis factor (TNF; illustrated in the figure on page 572). In 1985, using recombinant DNA technology, TNF could be produced in large quantities. It was found that several other previously discovered cytokines (the first one described in the 1960s) were also TNFs and as a group caused numerous inflammatory reactions within the immune system, including increases in white blood cells, fever, loss of appetite, and weight loss. In the mid-1980s it was noted that there was an excessive amount of TNF activity (especially one called TNF alpha) in patients who had rheumatoid arthritis (which is also a systemic autoimmune disease related to SLE).

The next logical step was to try to develop a way to decrease this TNF alpha (also written as TNF-$\alpha$) activity to see what would happen in RA. Recall from chapter 1 that an antibody is a molecule of the immune system that can attach to an antigen protein to remove it from the body. Researchers decided to produce an antibody that could

A

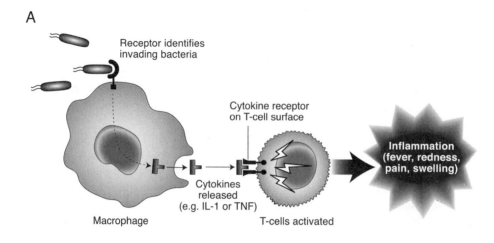

Receptor identifies invading bacteria

Cytokine receptor on T-cell surface

Cytokines released (e.g. IL-1 or TNF)

Macrophage

T-cells activated

Inflammation (fever, redness, pain, swelling)

B

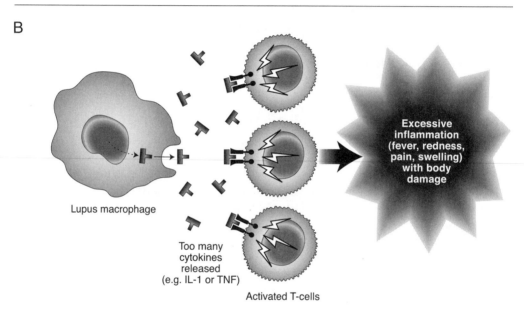

Lupus macrophage

Too many cytokines released (e.g. IL-1 or TNF)

Activated T-cells

Excessive inflammation (fever, redness, pain, swelling) with body damage

(A) Normal inflammation versus (B) inflammation from overproduction of inflammatory cytokines

attach to TNF-α using the recombinant DNA technology. In the early 1990s, it was successful, and antibodies were developed that could attach to TNF-α. It was called anti-TNF (or TNF inhibitor). The technology was sold to a pharmaceutical company called Immunex, and this TNF inhibitor was subsequently called etanercept (Enbrel). Etanercept (Enbrel) was given to people who were crippled with rheumatoid arthritis and not responding to the usual medicines such as steroids and methotrexate. Rapid, miraculous results were noted in these patients, with marked decreases in joint swelling, stiffness, and pain. Etanercept was FDA-approved in 1998 as the first TNF inhibitor. This was soon followed by FDA approval for another TNF inhibitor called infliximab (Remicade). These medicines were used in RA patients who were crippled by their disease, and this seemed like a miracle for these people.

The use of TNF inhibitors to treat RA became more commonplace in the early 2000s. I still remember sitting in a room full of other rheumatologists when we were shown a research slide that showed the effects of the TNF inhibitor infliximab on x-ray changes in a large group of people who had RA. The slide showed a graph demonstrating that infliximab completely stopped the worsening or progression of x-ray deformities occurring over time in a group of patients who had severe RA. The same graph showed another group of RA patients who were not on a TNF inhibitor, but who were taking the usual RA medicines like methotrexate. This group of patients getting methotrexate alone developed the expected progressive crippling effects from their RA. This TNF inhibitor showed that it could stop or at least significantly slow down the crippling effects of this horrible disease. Not only could the TNF inhibitor help patients feel better by decreasing pain, swelling, and stiffness, but there was also hope that these people could possibly be prevented from getting crippled by RA. There was palpable excitement in the room among the rheumatologists because up to this point no medication had ever been shown to stop the crippling effects of RA. Since then three other TNF inhibitors (adalimumab, golimumab, and certolizumab) have also become available and each of these has shown the same effects of stopping or slowing down the crippling effects of RA.

The immune systems of people who have lupus produce too many inflammation-producing cytokines (including TNF-$\alpha$). It was natural for doctors to try using these TNF inhibitors in people who had SLE (see figure on the following page). The first positive studies were published in 2002 and 2003. At the 7th International Congress on SLE held in New York City in 2004, a small study showed infliximab (a TNF inhibitor medicine) as being beneficial in some patients who had lupus nephritis and arthritis. The three patients who had lupus arthritis went into remission after each round of infliximab therapy, and all four patients who had lupus nephritis had significant improvements in the kidney disease. After that, some lupus experts began to recommend the possibility of using TNF inhibitors (such as infliximab) in people who had lupus who were failing other therapies.

These medicines are not easy to produce. The production of medicines can be divided into two main groups (see table on page 573). There are those medicines that have "simple" chemical structures (such as penicillin, prednisone, and methotrexate) and can be produced using "chemical" processes in a laboratory. Chemical processes are ones that you can easily even do yourself. Mixing baking soda and vinegar together and causing foam to occur is a chemical process producing carbon dioxide gas. When a cook bakes a mixture of chocolate, flour, baking soda, baking powder, milk, and eggs in the oven to transform those unrelated ingredients into a delicious chocolate cake, this occurs due to chemical processes. Chemical processes like these are used to produce the vast majority of medicines in the world.

TNF inhibitors are produced using bacteria or mouse cells. This is an example of a "biologic" process to produce the medication. TNF inhibitors are members of a growing group of medicines called biologic agents, or biologics for short. As opposed to

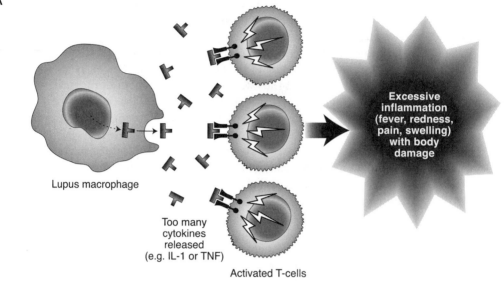

A

Lupus macrophage

Too many
cytokines
released
(e.g. IL-1 or TNF)

Activated T-cells

Excessive
inflammation
(fever, redness,
pain, swelling)
with body
damage

B

TNF inhibitor medicine

Lupus macrophage
releasing TNF

TNF cytokine
blocked by
TNF inhibitor medicine

T-cell not
activated

No
inflammation
occurs

(A) Overproduction of inflammatory cytokines versus (B) the effect of TNF inhibitor treatment

Biologic Agents versus Chemical Agents

| Biologic Agents (examples: infliximab, rituximab, belimumab) | Chemical Agents (examples: prednisone, Plaquenil) |
| --- | --- |
| Made by complex biological processes | Made by simpler chemical processes |
| Very expensive | Less expensive |
| Very large, complex molecules | Smaller, "simpler" molecules |
| Usually given by injection | Many can be taken by mouth |

chemical processes that use simple laboratory techniques, biologic agents require complex biologic processes (such as production of the medicine by living bacteria). The molecules of medicines produced in these ways are usually much larger and complex in structure compared to those of medicines produced by chemical processes. They also tend to be more fragile as well. Due to their large size and complexity, they usually need to be administered by injection (through an IV into a vein, or by using a needle to inject it into muscle or under the skin). Stomach acid contents would destroy these biologic medicines, and therefore they cannot be taken in pill form at the current time.

These biologic techniques are allowing doctors and scientists to produce very specific medications (biologics) that can target a particular function of the body to help treat diseases in ways that are more precise compared to older medications. This can help obtain better results with treatment while also decreasing the risk for side effects. They are not only used for autoimmune disease, but are also revolutionizing the treatments of other disorders as well, including cancers, asthma, neurologic disorders, infections, and even heart disease.

The biologic agents are unfortunately very expensive, ranging from $10,000 to $45,000 a year for just one patient (as far as the ones that doctors use in rheumatologic diseases). Some other biologic agents used to treat cancer are even more expensive. One reason for this expense is the manner in which they have to be produced. The factories that produce these medicines have to be completely sterile at every single step to keep the bacteria or other cell cultures used for reproduction pure and uninfected. Not even one tiny contamination can occur. Everyone who enters the facility must put on a sterile suit. Then each batch of medicine must be tested using expensive biologic systems as opposed to simpler chemical systems. The expense of these medicines is not unprecedented. Recall from the first section in chapter 31 that when cortisone was first produced, new technology was required to produce it. Cortisone initially cost close to $66,000 a year for one patient (factoring in inflation). Its cost was more than one hundred times more expensive than that of a similar amount of gold. Within a year, the cost had decreased to $11,500 a year. Fortunately, the techniques for producing steroids evolved and became easier and cheaper. Today, you can buy a steroid such as prednisone for only four cents a day. Hopefully, this will occur with the biologic agents as well over time, but for now they are incredibly expensive medicines.

In addition to TNF inhibitors, the other biologic agents most commonly used to treat SLE are rituximab (Rituxan) and belimumab (Benlysta). Not all biologics attack cytokines. Some of them interfere with the immune system in other targeted ways. What they share in common is that they must be produced using biologic instead of chemical production processes. It appears that we are currently in the era of biologic therapies for the treatment of SLE, and these biologics are providing additional hope to those not responding to the older medicines. This chapter discusses the TNF inhibitors and rituximab (Rituxan), while chapter 34 covers belimumab (Benlysta). The biologic medications tocilizumab (Actemra) and abatacept (Orencia) also show promise; they are discussed in chapter 37.

. . . .

## TNF Inhibitors

TNF inhibitors were the first biologic agents developed to treat systemic autoimmune rheumatic diseases. They were first FDA-approved to treat rheumatoid arthritis, but subsequently, many of them have been FDA-approved to treat other arthritides such as psoriatic arthritis and ankylosing spondylitis. Five TNF inhibitors (table 33.1) are available to treat rheumatic diseases. Infliximab is only given intravenously (IV), while the other four are given subcutaneously (sub Q or SQ for short). People usually inject the SQ medicine at home.

Out of all of these, infliximab (Remicade) is the only one studied in the treatment of systemic lupus erythematosus. It has shown to be beneficial in lupus nephritis, lupus arthritis, cutaneous lupus, and interstitial lung disease. In a rheumatoid arthritis research study using TNF inhibitors, severe SLE occurred in a couple of patients. At the time, a study looking at the use of etanercept for lupus nephritis had begun, but it was terminated due to the researchers becoming concerned about the potential for possibly making lupus worse (citing the drug-induced lupus cases from the rheumatoid arthritis study). However, it should be pointed out that none of the patients who had lupus got worse when treated with infliximab in the previous studies. Another study using infliximab to treat lupus nephritis in Europe was also terminated, but this time it was due to the researchers not being able to get enough patients to participate in the study.

At this time, the future of the use of TNF inhibitors is uncertain. With many other promising therapies already in use (such as Rituxan and Benlysta) and many more being investigated (see chapter 37), it may be very difficult to get anyone to invest the time and money into conducting a proper large study using TNF inhibitors in people who have SLE.

*Generic available*: No. They may become available in the future and would be called "bioequivalent" instead of "generic."

*How TNF inhibitors work*: Each of them works in a slightly different way to prevent the cytokine TNF-$\alpha$ from attaching to and activating white blood cells. Therefore, the TNF-$\alpha$ molecules cannot cause as much inflammation to occur.

*What benefits to expect from TNF inhibitors*: Lupus arthritis may respond as quickly as a week (but can take up to several months), resulting in decreased pain, swelling, and stiffness. With lupus nephritis, effects have been noted as quickly as within a month of starting infliximab, resulting in significant reductions in the amount of protein spilled by the kidneys into the urine.

**Table 33.1** TNF Inhibitors

| Name | How Given | Typical Dose |
|------|-----------|--------------|
| infliximab (Remicade) | IV | 3–10 mg/kg every 4 to 8 weeks |
| etanercept (Enbrel) | SQ | 50 mg every week |
| adalimumab (Humira) | SQ | 40 mg every 1 to 2 weeks |
| certolizumab pegol (Cimzia) | SQ | 200 mg, 2 injections per month or 1 every 2 weeks |
| golimumab (Simponi) | SQ | 50 mg once a month |

*How TNF inhibitors are taken*: See table 33.1. Infliximab is usually prescribed starting with a "loading" dose consisting of one infusion followed by a second infusion two weeks later, and then a third infusion six weeks after the second. Therefore, the first three infusions are given within the first two months. After that, most people receiving infliximab get their infusions every eight weeks. Infliximab infusions usually take several hours each time.

*If you miss a dose of your medicine*: Give yourself a SQ injection, or have your infusion scheduled as soon as you realize that you forgot a dose. Then you need to reset your schedule from that date. For example, let us say that you get infliximab (Remicade) every eight weeks. You were scheduled for your infliximab on January 4. You had to miss your appointment, and it was rescheduled for January 10. Schedule your next infusion eight weeks after the January 10 infusion. If you inject yourself with adalimumab (Humira) every two weeks on Mondays, and you realize on Wednesday that you forgot your Monday dose, give your SQ injection on that Wednesday and resume your next injections every two weeks on Wednesdays. Consult with your prescribing doctor to double-check these instructions, but these guidelines will suffice for most people.

*Alcohol/food/herbal interactions with TNF inhibitors*: No interactions with alcohol known.

No interactions with food known.

Avoid Echinacea, which can increase the activity of the immune system.

*Potential side effects of TNF inhibitors*: The potential side effects of TNF inhibitors are listed in table 33.2. The most important potential side effect of TNF inhibitors is the potential for increased infections. Therefore, just like with immunosuppressant medicines, if you have any infection symptoms whatsoever, you must see your primary care physician or go to the emergency room immediately. You should also not take your medicine during any infection. The risk for developing infections (other than TB as discussed next) does not appear to be any higher than seen with other immunosuppressant medications.

One type of infection deserves special attention, and that is tuberculosis (TB). Some people infected with TB do not get very sick, but the TB bacteria can live in their bodies for the rest of their lives. If these people start taking a TNF inhibitor (or any other biologic immunosuppressant medication), it can become very dangerous for them as the

TB bacteria can reproduce, causing a severe and sometimes deadly infection. Therefore, those who are treated with biologic immunosuppressant medications (such as TNF inhibitors) must get a TB test before starting the medication.

Both skin tests and blood tests can diagnose TB infections. Sometimes just one or the other is sufficient, but some experts now recommend obtaining both a skin test and a blood test to make sure there has been no previous infection to TB. The skin test uses PPD (purified protein derivative). The test is performed by a small amount of the PPD being injected underneath the skin of the forearm. Then two to five days later, the amount of swelling under the skin (called induration) is measured by a medical professional. In people who are immunosuppressed (this includes many people who have SLE), if this measurement is 5 mm or more, it is considered positive, meaning that they were probably exposed to TB in the past. The blood tests that are used to diagnose infections from TB are called interferon-gamma release assays; one is called the Quanti-FERON-TB Gold In-Tube while the other is the T-SPOT.TB. Neither the skin test nor the blood tests are 100% accurate for diagnosing tuberculosis. When one test misses an infection, doing the other one may catch it. That is why more rheumatologists are starting to do both tests in their patients to ensure that no infections are missed.

If either of these tests are positive, the next step is to make sure there is not an active TB infection by checking a chest x-ray. If people have a positive PPD and a chest x-ray that is negative for active infection, then they are labeled as having "latent TB." This means that they have probably been exposed to TB in the past and could possibly have TB bacteria still living in their bodies, but they do not have an active infection in the lungs. Recommended treatment is a TB antibiotic, such as isoniazid, for nine months. During this period, they can receive the TNF inhibitor medicine as well.

Another test for tuberculosis is now available as a blood test called an interferon-gamma release assay. Neither the skin PPD test nor this blood test is 100% accurate for diagnosing a history of TB infection. Therefore, some experts recommend getting both types of tests done to make sure that a possible history of infection is not missed.

A controversial issue involving these medicines is whether they may cause an increased risk of cancer or not, primarily lymphoma (lymph node cancer) and skin cancer. Solid tumors (such as lung cancer, breast cancer, brain cancer, prostate cancer, etc.) do not appear to occur with these medicines. Lymphoma occurs in people who have RA who are treated with TNF inhibitors more often compared to people who do not have RA. However, the problem with this finding is that people who have autoimmune disorders such as RA and SLE get lymphoma more often because of their abnormal immune systems. TNF inhibitors have been studied most in people who have severe RA. People who have severe RA are twenty-five times more likely to develop lymphoma than people who do not have RA. This occurs due to the effects of the RA itself on the immune system and its subsequent production of cancerous lymphocytes (lymphoma). Thus far, after fifteen years of studying these medications, lower numbers of RA patients have developed lymphoma in the TNF inhibitor studies than would be expected in RA patients, making lymphoma an unlikely side effect. Unfortunately, the FDA mandates that pharmaceutical companies retain this potential side effect in their advertisements that unnecessarily frighten patients.

The other cancer of possible concern is that of skin cancer. So far, the studies are controversial. Rheumatologist Dr. Frederick Wolfe published a study in 2007 that looked at more than 13,000 people who were treated with TNF inhibitors. This particular patient group was 2.3 times more apt to get malignant melanoma (a type of skin cancer) and 1.5 times more likely to get non-melanoma skin cancer (basal cell carcinoma and squamous cell carcinoma). This same study showed no increases in lymphoma or any other type of cancer. Then another study from 2009 followed more than 6,300 people who took TNF inhibitors over at least a 6-year period, and they found no increase in skin cancer, nor any type of cancer.

A 2011 Swedish study looked at 78,483 RA patients and compared the occurrence of cancer in RA patients who received a biologic and those who did not. More severe cancers (stage 4) actually occurred in those who did not receive a biologic compared to those who received a biologic. In addition, a higher percentage of patients died who did not receive a biologic compared to those who were treated with a biologic. When specifically looking at death rates in those who developed cancer, there was no difference between the groups. A 2011 Danish study looked at 5,598 patients who used TNF inhibitors. They found no increases in any types of cancers compared to 13,699 patients who were not using TNF inhibitors. A large 2012 review of this topic surveyed all of the studies that looked at TNF inhibitors and cancer. The authors concluded that there was no sufficient evidence at that time to suggest that these medications cause cancer. An even more recent 2013 study in the United States showed no increases in cancer among 39,708 people who were treated with TNF inhibitors, including skin cancers.

At this point, it really is not known whether TNF inhibitors cause an increase in skin cancer or not. However, to be safe, it is probably a good idea to get your skin checked periodically by your primary care doctor or a dermatologist. Using sunscreen regularly and avoiding sun exposure will also help to decrease this potential risk.

Some of these TNF inhibitors do use latex in the rubber parts of the syringes. These include adalimumab (Humira), etanercept (Enbrel), and golimumab (Simponi). Therefore, if you are latex allergic, it would be best to avoid these three TNF inhibitors in the prefilled syringe forms.

There have been case reports of TNF inhibitors causing drug-induced lupus. However, this has not been observed in patients with SLE treated with TNF inhibitors. In people who develop lupus from a TNF inhibitor, it goes away after the medicine is stopped (similar to other cases of drug-induced lupus, as discussed in chapter 1).

*What needs to be monitored while taking TNF inhibitors*: Your doctor will monitor your lupus labs closely while you are receiving your TNF inhibitor.

*Reasons not to take TNF inhibitors (contraindications or precautions)*: If you have chronic hepatitis B infection, you should not receive a TNF inhibitor. If you have been infected with TB in the past, you should be treated for TB with antibiotics. Everyone should be tested for hepatitis B (a blood test) and TB (a skin test and/or blood test) before starting treatment with a TNF inhibitor. If you have an active infection, do not use a TNF inhibitor.

If you have ever had cancer, check with your oncologist before starting on a TNF inhibitor. The American College of Rheumatology recommends considering another type of biologic, such as Rituxan, instead of a TNF inhibitor, in patients who have had cancer within the previous five years. This recommendation is because patients who had had recent bouts of cancer were not included in the large TNF inhibitor studies, so we really do not know for sure how safe they are in that patient population.

**Table 33.2** Potential Side Effects of TNF Inhibitors

|  | Incidence | Side Effect Therapy |
|---|---|---|
| **Nuisance side effects** | | |
| Injection site reaction (with SQ) | Common | Usually mild and tolerable. Can use ice compresses or over-the-counter cortisone cream on the site. |
| Infusion reaction with infliximab (mild) | Common | Can be prevented or made less severe by taking Benadryl, Tylenol, and steroids before and during the infusion. The rate of the infusion can also be slowed down. |
| Headache | Common | Take Tylenol. |
| Nausea, stomach upset | Common | Usually mild. May need to stop medicine if severe. |
| Rash | Common | Usually mild. May need to stop medicine if significant. |
| Psoriasis rash | Uncommon | Stop medicine and treat psoriasis with cortisone creams. |
| Temporary joint pain | Uncommon | Usually mild. Can treat with Tylenol or temporary increase in steroids. |
| **Serious side effects** | | |
| Infection | Common | See your primary care doctor or go to the emergency room immediately. Do not take medicine during infections. |
| Severe infusion reaction (infliximab) | Uncommon | Stop medicine. |
| Drug-induced lupus | Rare | Stop medicine. |
| Skin cancer | Rare (unknown if truly a side effect or not) | Get skin examined yearly by a dermatologist or your primary care physician. |

Side effect incidence key (approximations, as side effects can vary widely study to study): rare < 1% occurrence; uncommon 1%–5% occurrence; common > 5% occurrence

Do not use TNF inhibitors if you have uncontrolled congestive heart failure, as they can potentially worsen this condition. Do not use the prefilled syringe forms of adalimumab (Humira), etanercept (Enbrel), or golimumab (Simponi) if you are allergic to latex.

*While taking TNF inhibitors*: If you have had skin cancer before, make sure to see your dermatologist for a skin examination more regularly while you are using a TNF inhibitor. If you develop any infection symptoms at all, such as fever, sore throat, cough, red painful skin, sinusitis congestion, or painful frequent urination, see your primary care doctor or go to an emergency room immediately. You should not receive live vaccines, including a Zostavax (for shingles), while being treated with TNF inhibitors. Practice all measures to prevent infections (table 22.1).

*Pregnancy and breast-feeding while taking TNF inhibitors*: The safety of TNF inhibitors in pregnancy is not known. There have been some congenital malformations reported in some babies born to mothers who took TNF inhibitors during pregnancy, but it is not known whether the medicine was the cause or not. It is recommended that you do not use a TNF inhibitor while you are pregnant unless the benefits of using the medicine outweigh the potential risks. This decision should be made on a case-by-case basis. Most women should stop taking their TNF inhibitor when they find out they are pregnant. If you do get pregnant while taking a TNF inhibitor, consider contacting the Organization of Teratology Information Specialists (OTIS) Autoimmune Diseases in Pregnancy Project at www.otispregnancy.org or 877-311-8972 or email otisresearch@ucsd.edu so that more can be learned about what happens when women on medications used in treating lupus become pregnant.

It is not recommended to use TNF inhibitors while breast-feeding.

*Geriatric use of TNF inhibitors*: No differences in dosing are recommended.

*What to do with TNF inhibitors at the time of surgery*: It is always best to double-check with your rheumatologist and surgeon regarding specific instructions. A common recommendation is to not take your medication for several weeks before surgery, then resume it once the surgical wound has healed and if there is no evidence for infection.

*Patient assistance program for TNF inhibitors*: Each medication has its own website. Just type in the name of the brand followed by .com—for example, www.remicade.com and www.enbrel.com. Also see chapter 42.

*Drug helpline for TNF inhibitors*: Each medication has its own website. Just type in the name of the brand followed by .com—for example, www.remicade.com and www.enbrel.com.

*Website to learn more about TNF inhibitors*: www.rheumatology.org/practice/clinical/patients/medications/anti_tnf.asp. In addition, each medication has its own website. Just type in the name of the brand followed by .com—for example, www.remicade.com and www.enbrel.com.

## Rituximab (Rituxan)

Rituximab is biologic agent that decreases the production of B-cell lymphocytes. It was initially FDA-approved in 1997 to treat B-cell lymphoma. However, since autoimmune diseases such as RA and SLE have been noted to have overactive B-cells, rituximab was studied in these disorders as well. It was shown to be highly effective in people affected by RA and was FDA-approved for use in people who have RA in 2006. Its primary use in rheumatology has been in people who have RA who do not adequately respond to TNF inhibitors.

There are numerous studies showing rituximab to also be effective in some people who have SLE as well. In fact, there are many more studies showing it to be effective in SLE than studies looking at TNF inhibitors. Therefore, lupus experts treat SLE more often with rituximab than with TNF inhibitors. A European consensus paper on the treatment of SLE in 2012 specifically recommended that Rituxan be considered to treat various problems from lupus, including difficult cases of nephritis, arthritis, serositis, interstitial lung disease, pulmonary hemorrhage, autoimmune hemolytic anemia, low platelet counts, thrombotic thrombocytopenic purpura, antiphospholipid syndrome, and neuropsychiatric lupus.

*Generic available*: No.

*How rituximab works*: Rituximab binds to a part of B-cells called CD20, and it causes the CD20 labeled B-cells to become inactive or even die. It can be helpful to know how B-cells are produced to understand how the medicine works. This is shown in figure 33.1 in simple terms. There are cells of the immune system that are responsible for producing B-cell lymphocytes; these are pre–B-cells. These cells will produce more mature B-cells that have a molecular structure on their surface called CD20. In easy terms, you can consider CD20 as an identification badge worn by these particular B-cells. When the immune system becomes activated to cause more inflammation, these more mature B-cells reproduce and can cause a special type of B-cell called plasma cells. These plasma cells are the types of B-cells that produce antibodies.

Recall from chapter 1 that one of the primary problems seen in lupus is that the immune system makes too many antibodies that attack the body itself (called autoantibodies). The specialized types of B-cells called plasma cells make these autoantibodies. Rituxan attaches to the CD20 labels on the maturing B-cells and prevents them from producing the antibody-producing plasma cells. This causes less production of the autoantibodies that can attack the body of the person who has lupus (figure 33.1B).

*What benefits to expect from rituximab*: The effects of rituximab can take a few weeks to a few months before they are noted. In addition to helping with many problems from lupus, rituximab may also help increase mouth moisture and saliva flow in people who have Sjögren's syndrome (see chapter 14). Some large studies looking at its use for Sjögren's syndrome were completed in 2012, but the results have not been reported as of this time. A 2013 study showed that Rituxan might also decrease complications from the antiphospholipid syndrome such as low platelet counts, skin ulcers, kidney damage, and memory problems.

*How rituximab is taken*: Rituximab is given as an intravenous (IV) infusion over about six to eight hours. A common dosing schedule is to get 1,000 mg on one day followed by a similar infusion two weeks later. This is often repeated every six months (in other words, four infusions a year). However, there are other dosing schedules used as well. Intravenous steroids are usually given along with the rituximab to decrease the chances of an allergic-type reaction.

*If you miss a dose of your medicine*: Have your infusion scheduled as soon as you realize that you forgot to get your dose. Then you need to reset your schedule from that date. For example, let us say that you realize that you forgot to get your January 10

A

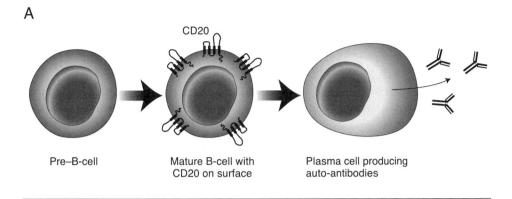

Pre–B-cell

Mature B-cell with
CD20 on surface

Plasma cell producing
auto-antibodies

B

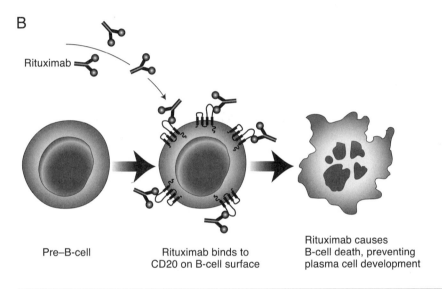

Pre–B-cell

Rituximab binds to
CD20 on B-cell surface

Rituximab causes
B-cell death, preventing
plasma cell development

**Figure 33.1** (A) B-cell production and involvement of CD20 in SLE; (B) how Rituximab works on the immune system in SLE

rituximab (Rituxan) infusion (or it had to be cancelled for some reason), and that you were supposed to get another infusion two weeks after that. You reschedule to have it on January 20. Then you should schedule your next one to occur two weeks after the January 20 infusion. Consult with your prescribing doctor to double-check these instructions, but these guidelines will suffice for most people.

*Alcohol/food/herbal interactions with rituximab*: No interactions with alcohol.

No interactions with food.

Avoid Echinacea, which can stimulate the immune system.

*Potential side effects of rituximab*: Potential side effects of rituximab are listed in table 33.3. The most important potential side effect of rituximab is increased infections. Therefore, just like with immunosuppressant medicines, if you have any infection symptoms whatsoever, you must see your primary care physician or go to the emergency room immediately. You should also not take your medicine during any infection.

One type of infection requires special attention and that is the case of progressive multifocal leukoencephalopathy (PML for short). PML is a brain infection caused by JC virus. JC stands for "John Cunningham," a patient who had PML and in whom the virus was first identified in the early 1970s. Eighty-six percent of all people have been infected with JC virus, most commonly as children, at some point in their lives. It usually does not make you sick, and the immune system is very good at keeping the virus under control. The virus can live inside of people's bodies for the rest of their lives. If the immune system becomes suppressed, then the JC virus can multiply and damage the central nervous system, a condition called PML. This most commonly causes confusion, problems with memory, coordination problems, muscle weakness, difficulty speaking, and double vision. Unfortunately, it is usually deadly if someone gets it. PML has occurred in a few people treated with rituximab. Most of these have been people treated for lymphoma. PML occurs in approximately one out of every 25,000 rheumatoid arthritis patients who receive rituximab, so it is very rare. How often it occurs in SLE is unknown, there have only been a few case reports of its occurring in SLE patients who received rituximab.

Exactly what role rituximab plays in the development of PML is truly not known because PML has been reported in patients who have received most types of immunosuppressant medicines. As far as SLE patients who have developed PML over the years, PML has occurred in lupus patients taking every medicine used to treat SLE. More than 40% of those patients received very little immunosuppression, which suggests that SLE itself may predispose to getting the infection.

To put things into perspective, a 2012 study showed that PML was very rare in people who have autoimmune diseases such as SLE. Only fifty-three total cases had been identified up to that time (out of more than two million patients who had autoimmune disease), and the majority of them who developed PML had coexistent cancer or HIV infection. Only one out of every 500,000 patients who did not have HIV or cancer developed PML, putting it into the very rare category.

At this point, it appears that PML occurs very rarely in RA and SLE patients who receive rituximab, and it really is not even known for sure whether rituximab plays any role in PML occurring. In addition, it may occur simply because of the altered immune systems of the people who have these diseases. The bottom line is that if you develop unusual neurologic symptoms seen with PML, such as difficulty thinking, disorientation, incoordination, muscle weakness, double vision, or difficulty thinking, you should seek immediate medical attention. Since most of these same symptoms also occur in people who have strokes, it is probably best to go to an emergency room for proper evaluation. Of note, this is such a rare infection that most rheumatologists do not consider it a definite side effect of the medicine. The only reason I discuss it in detail is that the FDA requires the pharmaceutical company to include it as a potential side effect in its package insert and when advertising it to the public.

Just as with TNF inhibitors, you should have a TB test performed before starting rituximab therapy. Read the previous section on TNF inhibitors for a full explanation.

Infusion reactions are common with rituximab; however, they are usually mild and temporary. Most doctors treat their patients with an antihistamine, Tylenol, and steroids before and during the infusion to prevent these reactions from happening. The most common symptoms of an infusion reaction include headache, chills, body aches, nausea, upset stomach, and itchy skin. Interestingly, these infusion reactions typically occur with the first infusion in about one-third of people who have RA and become less common after that. More severe allergic infusion reactions are much less common but can potentially cause shortness of breath, swelling in the throat, hives, vomiting, and blood pressure changes. Your infusion center will be prepared to treat this immediately if it occurs.

Since intravenous steroids are usually given along with the rituximab, some of the side effects noted can be from the steroid instead of from Rituxan. These include ankle swelling, elevated glucose levels, and elevated blood pressure.

Rituximab decreases your body's ability to respond to the flu shot and the pneumonia vaccine (Pneumovax). If it is time for you to get either of these, it is best to get them before your first rituximab treatment. While you are on rituximab, plan to get these vaccines about one month before your next scheduled infusion of rituximab.

*What needs to be monitored while taking rituximab*: Your doctor will want to check a blood cell count and a chemistry panel periodically while you are treated with rituximab.

*Reasons not to take rituximab (contraindications or precautions)*: If you have chronic hepatitis B infection, you should not receive rituximab. If you have been infected with TB in the past, you should be treated for TB with antibiotics. Everyone should be tested for hepatitis B (a blood test) and TB (a skin test and/or a blood test) before starting treatment with rituximab. If you have an active infection, do not use rituximab. If you have uncontrolled congestive heart failure or you have a serious heart arrhythmia, you probably should not get rituximab therapy. Discuss this with your prescribing doctor and your cardiologist before getting rituximab therapy.

*While taking rituximab*: If you develop any infection symptoms at all, such as fever, sore throat, cough, red painful skin, sinusitis congestion, or painful frequent urination, see your primary care doctor or go to an emergency room immediately. Do not get your rituximab treatment if you have an active infection. You should not receive live vaccines, including Zostavax (for shingles), while being treated with rituximab. Rituximab decreases your body's ability to respond to the flu shot and the pneumonia vaccine (Pneumovax). Schedule your routine flu shot and pneumococcal vaccine to be given about one month prior to your rituximab treatments. Practice all measures to prevent infections (table 22.1).

*Pregnancy and breast-feeding while taking rituximab*: Rituximab can cause low white blood cell counts in babies. It is recommended to stop rituximab treatments one year before trying to conceive. Use strict birth control during rituximab treatment and continue for one year after you stop using it. If you do get pregnant while taking rituximab, consider contacting the Organization of Teratology Information Specialists (OTIS) Autoimmune Diseases in Pregnancy Project at www.otispregnancy.org or 877-311-8972 or email otisresearch@ucsd.edu so that more can be learned about what happens when women on medications used in treating lupus become pregnant.

Do not get rituximab therapy while breast-feeding.

*Geriatric use of rituximab*: Older people are at increased risk for developing infections, lung problems, and heart problems while using rituximab.

**Table 33.3** Potential Side Effects of Rituximab

|  | Incidence | Side Effect Therapy |
|---|---|---|
| **Nuisance side effects** | | |
| Ankle swelling (edema) | Common | Usually resolves on its own. Avoid salt and salty foods the day before, day of, and day after your infusion. Can use diuretics (fluid pills) if severe. |
| Mild infusion reactions | Common | Taking Benadryl, Tylenol, and steroids before and during the infusion can decrease chances of this happening. Otherwise, they can be treated as needed. |
| Elevated liver enzymes | Uncommon | Usually mild requiring no treatment. |
| Rash | Uncommon | Usually mild and temporary. If persists or is significant, may need to stop therapy. |
| Elevated glucose from the steroids | Common | Usually only lasts a few days. If you have uncontrolled, brittle (unstable or labile) diabetes, track your glucose finger sticks closely and get assistance from your diabetes doctor. |
| **Serious side effects** | | |
| Elevated blood pressure | Common | Usually mild and temporary. Usually does not require treatment. Blood pressure medicines can be used if needed. |
| Severe infusion reaction | Uncommon | Treated by the infusion center. Rituxan treatment most likely would not be repeated. |
| Low white blood cell counts | Common | Usually requires no treatment. Your treatment may be delayed if it persists. Severely low levels may require treatment with Neupogen. |
| Low red blood cells (anemia) and low platelet counts (thrombocytopenia) | Uncommon | Usually mild requiring no treatment. Your treatment may be delayed if they persist. |
| Bowel perforation/ obstruction | Rare | Go to the emergency room if you develop abdominal pain, especially if it is severe or accompanied by fever. |
| Severe rash | Rare | Requires treatment by your doctor. Do not use rituximab anymore. |

Side effect incidence key (approximations, as side effects can vary widely study to study): rare < 1% occurrence; uncommon 1%–5% occurrence; common > 5% occurrence

*What to do with rituximab at the time of surgery*: It is always best to double-check with your rheumatologist and surgeon regarding specific instructions. A common recommendation is to not take rituximab for several weeks before surgery, then resume it once the surgical wound has healed and if there is no evidence for infection.

*Patient assistance program for rituximab*: Call 1-888-MY-RITUXAN as well as 1-866-422-2377. See chapter 42.

*Drug helpline for rituximab*: 1-877-474-8892.

*Website to learn more about rituximab*: www.rituxan.com and www.rheumatology .org/practice/clinical/patients/medications/rituximab.asp.

## KEY POINTS TO REMEMBER

1. Biologics are produced by biological processes (such as produced by living bacteria or mouse cells) instead of by simple chemical processes.

2. Due to this process and the incredible expenses involved, biologics are very expensive medicines.

3. Due to the large size and fragility of the molecules, biologics are usually given by injection (SQ or IV) because the acidity of the stomach would destroy them.

4. The most commonly used biologics to treat SLE are rituximab (Rituxan), and Benlysta (belimumab). TNF inhibitors may be helpful in some people who have SLE but will probably become less popular over time without additional needed research.

5. Just as with the immunosuppressant medicines, there is an increased risk of infections with these medicines.

6. Make sure not to use the medicines during an active infection.

7. See your primary care doctor or go to the emergency room immediately if you have any infection symptoms.

8. Do everything in table 22.1 to prevent infections.

9. Do not get any live vaccines (including a Zostavax for shingles) if you are being treated with a biologic agent.

10. You can learn more about Rituxan at www.rituxan.com.

# Benlysta

*The First FDA-Approved Drug for*
*Lupus in More Than Fifty Years*

## The Miracle Drug for Lupus?

"F.D.A. Approves Drug for Lupus, an Innovation After 50 Years."

That was the headline on March 9, 2011, in the *New York Times*. The first medicine in more than fifty years was finally approved by the FDA to treat lupus, and its name was Benlysta.

The *Washington Post*'s article on Benlysta (pronounced ben-LIST-uh) went on to tell the touching tale of Janice Fitzgibbon, a systemic lupus patient who received Benlysta during its research phase. "Five years ago, when she was 49, her finger and toe joints began to hurt, and then her elbows and neck and knees. 'I was like, "Whoa, what is this?"' she said. Worse than the pain was the crushing fatigue. 'I was always a good sleeper. Now I woke up tired. I felt like a shark: I had to keep moving or I'd fall asleep.' 'Days would go by when I couldn't get out of bed. When I was better, I was constantly afraid because I didn't know when the flares would strike again,' said Fitzgibbon. 'My world was so narrow. Once I spent eight days on the couch, watching Turner Classic Movies. And no one could really understand what was wrong with me'. . . The first time she had severe pain, which eventually spread through her body, leaving her unable to walk up stairs . . . 'The disease is insidious and capricious. You can't make plans; you can't tell what day the flares will happen,' she said. 'It's hard to get people to understand.'

"Two years ago, when she came to the Arthritis Clinic of Northern Virginia to receive her first infusion of an experimental treatment for lupus, she had been in a fog of pain and fear for three years . . . In Fitzgibbon's case, feeling better was also a gradual process. 'After two or three months of infusions [as part of a Benlysta clinical trial], I said, "This isn't working. I must be on the placebo arm." And my husband said, "Are you kidding? You don't look gray anymore. You don't fall asleep at 6 p.m. on the couch." After six months, I knew it was working. I was staying up later, sleeping better. I could take my dog for a walk. Some days I don't remember I have lupus' . . . Today, as far as she can tell, she's a normal 54-year-old woman. 'I walk three miles a day. I lift weights' . . . For Janice Fitzgibbon, this is the story of a miracle drug."

Patients who had lupus, their doctors, and patient advocacy groups had been waiting for a drug like this for a long time. This chapter discusses the drugs that have been FDA-approved to treat lupus and why there has been such a long gap between the previous drugs approved and this recent approval of Benlysta. Is Benlysta a miracle drug to treat lupus? To answer that question, in this chapter I discuss how Benlysta works and what to expect from it in detail.

. . . .

Every person who has lupus should remember what she or he was doing on March 9, 2011, as it was one of the most important days in the history of lupus. Dwight Eisenhower was president when the FDA approved the previous drug to treat lupus. The last couple of decades have seen an explosion of amazing medical and technological advancements. Lupus is not a rare disease (e.g., it affects about one out of two hundred African American women when you include cutaneous lupus). Why did it take so long to get a new medicine for lupus? Is adequate research being done? There are, of course, good answers to these questions, and it can be very helpful to look at the history of the FDA, at how medications are developed, and at how the ever-elusive disease lupus plays a role in this drug development picture to get a better understanding of this long wait. The history of drug regulations is a long one (table 34.1). Due to space limitations, I focus on some of the most important events that shaped this history.

In 1820, eleven doctors met and developed the U.S. Pharmacopeia, which was an officially accepted list of medications felt to be the best understood and truly helpful medications. In addition, it described how they were to be produced. This set up a system of accepted standards and quality control. Any well-respected physician or pharmacist would be expected to use the U.S. Pharmacopeia to help in the treatment of patients. However, things were very different back then. Drugs were sold directly to the public, could be advertised, could contain any ingredients their manufacturers wished, and their manufacturers could make any claims of treatments and "cures" that they desired. In addition, doctors were not required to use only drugs that were included in the U.S. Pharmacopeia.

Up until the early 1900s, drugs not included in the U.S. Pharmacopeia were called patent medicines. The term "patent" is misleading because most did not have patents at all. Many of them made unsubstantiated claims to cure about anything. Advertisements for these drugs promised to cure rheumatism, fatigue, and even cancer. Unfortunately, many of these drugs also contained addictive ingredients such as cocaine, opium, heroin, morphine, cannabis (marijuana), and alcohol. Because of this, many actually did what they advertised to do. For example, some drugs sold as "infant soothers" actually contained highly addictive and sedating opium. These drugs certainly soothed and put babies to sleep, but at the price of using a narcotic unknown to the mothers who used them. Many of these patent medicines became very popular and were quite addictive. Companies sold them legally out in the open. For example, in the 1890s, people could buy a syringe and cocaine from the Sears and Roebuck catalog for $1.50. Even the American icon Coca-Cola got its start during that period as it contained a combination of cocaine (the Coca part of the name) and caffeine (the Cola part of the name since caffeine comes from the Kola plant). Coca-Cola finally removed the cocaine portion of its ingredients in 1903 due to increasing pressure from the media and outcries from the public. You may be surprised to know, though, that up to this day, part of the flavor of Coca-Cola still comes from actual coca plant leaves imported from South America (the cocaine portion is removed).

**Table 34.1** History of U.S. Drug Regulations

| Year | Event |
| --- | --- |
| 1820 | U.S. Pharmacopeia records first list of accepted medicines. |
| 1862 | U.S. Department of Agriculture Division of Chemistry is formed (eventually the FDA). |
| 1800s | Many Americans addicted to uncontrolled "patent medicines"; many deaths occur. |
| 1903 | Coca-Cola voluntarily removes cocaine from formula, keeps caffeine as the primary stimulant. |
| 1905 | American Medical Association allows only medicines with "proven" effects to advertise in its journals. |
| 1906 | The Pure Food and Drug Act is passed demanding that all drugs and medicines list their ingredients. |
| 1912 | Sherley Amendment outlaws fake medical claims by drugs. |
| 1914 | The Harrison Narcotic Act requires prescriptions for narcotics. |
| 1930 | Food and Drug Administration (FDA) name adopted as the final name for the federal food and drug regulatory agency. |
| 1937 | Elixir Sulfanilamide kills 107 people, many of them children. |
| 1938 | The Federal Food, Drug, and Cosmetic (FDC) Act demands that all drugs must be tested on animals, showing safety, before being sold. |
| 1951 | The Durham-Humphrey Amendment requires doctors' prescriptions for any drugs that are habit forming or potentially harmful. |
| 1957 | Thalidomide becomes available. More than 10,000 babies born with deformed limbs. |
| 1962 | The Kefauver-Harris Drug Amendment requires that all drugs must be proven effective and safe in humans before being approved by the FDA. |

Journalists began to write about the dangers of these patent medicines, pointing out their addictive properties. They also noted that people died from taking them. Citizens wrote the White House and Congress about their dissatisfaction with this system, which led to the 1906 Pure Food and Drug Act. This outlawed the sale of mislabeled or tainted drugs. Because drug manufacturers now had to list drug ingredients (such as cocaine), the public voluntarily decreased their use of dangerous substances due to fears of addiction. One year prior to this, the American Medical Association had also made the very important decision of not allowing any drug company to advertise in its journals any medicine that did not show proof of what it claimed to do.

Eventually, events like these led to the formation of the FDA (Food and Drug Administration). It started out as the Division of Chemistry in the U.S. Department of Agriculture in 1862, and it changed names several times until the government named it the FDA in 1930.

The Pure Food and Drug Act only demanded an accurate list of ingredients. Companies could still advertise drugs any way they wished. They could still make unproven claims of cures and treatments in advertisements in the lay press and magazines. For example, the Dr. Johnson Remedy Co. sold "Dr. Johnson's Mild Combination Treatment for Cancer" with its advertisements stating, "Cancer Can be Cured" using their medicine. In 1911, lawyers took the company in front of the U.S. Supreme Court. The Court found the company "not guilty" in the advertising and the selling of their product since the "cure" did show its ingredients and was not breaking the law. The United States did not have any laws prohibiting false advertising at the time. As a response to public outrage, lawmakers passed the Sherley Amendment in 1912 to patch up this loophole of the Pure Food and Drug Act. It outlawed labeling medicines with unproven medical claims.

Although doctors wrote prescriptions for patients to take to their druggists, anyone could buy any drugs without a prescription. Doctors' prescriptions were not necessary. The narcotic problem was huge. Many Americans were addicted to legal cocaine and opium. Fueled as much by racial prejudice as well by the population's safety, Congress passed the Harrison Narcotic Act in 1914. Its proponents in Congress urged its passage to combat "drug-crazed, sex-mad negroes," "degenerate Mexicans smoking marijuana," and "Chinamen seducing white women with drugs [alluding to the opium den problem]." The act required a doctor's prescription for narcotics and the keeping of records of these prescriptions. The practice of prescribing medications (at least for narcotics) was first born in the United States.

Yet, there was still a loophole not addressed. Drug manufacturers had to list the ingredients of drugs, and could not make false advertisement claims. Yet the U.S. legal system had not addressed the drug safety question. The sulfa antibiotics were one of the miracles of modern medicine in the early 1900s. Prior to that, infections such as pneumonia were the most common cause of death. After Germany discovered sulfa antibiotics in 1935, they became the very first widely used antibiotics available. In 1937, S. E. Massengill Co. developed the antibiotic sulfanilamide in liquid form (Elixir Sulfanilamide). Its chief chemist Harold Watkins found that he could dissolve the drug in ethylene glycol (antifreeze) and add some raspberry flavoring, making it more tolerable to consume. The company sold hundreds of bottles. Unfortunately, 107 people (many of them children) died from taking the medicine during the first few months of sales. The drug company had never tested its safety, and ethylene glycol turned out to be poisonous to humans. Watkins, horrified at the consequences, committed suicide before the case even went to court. The public again was enraged. Congress passed the Federal Food, Drug and Cosmetic Act in 1938. Pharmaceutical companies had to perform tests of new medicines on animals and show that they were safe to consume before they could sell them to people. This act also limited the amount of poisonous substances that could be contained in medicines and allowed factory inspections as well.

Up to this point, anyone could still obtain any medicine (other than narcotics) without a doctor's prescription. On the urging of pharmacists in public office, in 1951 Congress passed the Durham-Humphrey Amendment. This law divided drugs into two large categories. The first group was those medicines that were safe enough for the public to purchase without a prescription. These were called over-the-counter drugs. Medicines deemed habit forming or potentially harmful required a prescription from a physician. This was the birth of the current-day U.S. prescription practice.

In 1957, a new drug was marketed as a very effective sleeping pill and pain reliever. It was also found to be very helpful for nausea and was promoted to treat morning sickness. The name of the drug was thalidomide, and many pregnant women around the world took it to help them tolerate their morning sickness. Unfortunately, the drug's bad side effects were quickly noted, but not until more than ten thousand babies were born with missing and deformed legs, arms, fingers, and toes. The drug interfered with the formation of the fetuses' limbs during that critical stage of development. A doctor at the FDA, Dr. Frances Kelsey, even tried to prevent the approval and sale of thalidomide in the United States. Thalidomide's manufacturer distributed it widely among doctors in the United States. Due to huge media attention on the sensitive subject, public outcry again caused Congress to pass the Kefauver-Harris Drug Amendments. This would be some of the most important drug legislation to ever become enacted. Up to this point, drugs only had to be tested on animals. This law required that all drugs had to be proven both effective and safe in humans. In addition, drug companies had to give an accurate list of potential side effects for all medications as well.

Now let us focus our attention on drugs FDA-approved to treat systemic lupus erythematosus (SLE). Up until the passing of this monumental legislation in 1962, there had only been several drugs approved by the FDA to treat lupus (table 34.2). Aspirin still lists SLE as one of its "indications" for use. "Indication" is a medical word meaning "a symptom or disorder for which a therapy is intended to be used for." However, the exact FDA approval date for use in lupus is obscure. Although commonly quoted as being one of the only FDA-approved drugs to treat lupus, and that it was FDA-approved for lupus in "1948" (according to many internet sources), I am not able to confirm this. It is very difficult even for the FDA to find original approval records going back that far before the time of computers. I have contacted both Bayer (the original manufacturer of aspirin) and the FDA and am unable to confirm exactly when it was first FDA-approved. Dr. A. McGehee Harvey, former physician-in-chief of Johns Hopkins Hospital, noted in his textbook on SLE in 1955 that aspirin was "the most useful drug other than the hormones [steroids] in the management of SLE." However, the most comprehensive textbook on drug treatments, Gillman and Goodman's *The Pharmacological Basis of Therapeutics* (second edition, 1955) does not even list aspirin as a treatment for lupus. Nonetheless, the official FDA-approved "Comprehensive Prescribing Information" for aspirin states, "Aspirin is indicated for the relief of the signs and symptoms of . . . arthritis and pleurisy associated with SLE."

The aspirin indication is an interesting one because lupus experts in the United States do not use aspirin to treat either the arthritis or pleurisy of lupus. The doses of aspirin that are required to decrease inflammation sufficiently for these two problems of lupus are very high and can cause high blood pressure, bleeding ulcers, kidney disease, dizziness, and ringing in the ears. This is clearly an "indication" that is still on the books, but that is outdated. There is no way that aspirin could possibly get FDA

Table 34.2 Drugs FDA-Approved to Treat Lupus

| FDA Approval | Name of Drug | Current Status |
| --- | --- | --- |
| ???? | aspirin | Used in low doses to prevent blood clots; not used for arthritis or pleurisy anymore |
| 1949 | chloroquine | Useful, but FDA retracted its formal approval for SLE |
| 1955 | prednisone (Metocorten) | A lifesaving drug for SLE |
| 1955 | hydroxychloroquine (Plaquenil) | Most commonly used drug for SLE |
| 1955 | quinacrine (Triquin) | Available from compounding pharmacists |
| 2011 | belimumab (Benlysta) | Costs about $35,000 a year; used when other lupus drugs fail |

approval to treat SLE today if it were to go through the current channels of approval. Aspirin will most likely continue to be FDA-approved for lupus unless someone puts in the time and legal expense to have its FDA approval revoked.

As discussed at length in chapters 30 and 31, steroids (especially prednisone and methylprednisolone) and hydroxychloroquine (Plaquenil) are the most common medicines prescribed to treat SLE. They continue to live up to their FDA approval expectations. Chloroquine (Aralen) is still used by lupus doctors in special situations, although its FDA approval for lupus has been withdrawn due to its association with retinopathy (eye problems) in 10% of users. After formal complaints (and lawsuits) were filed because of eye damage from chloroquine, the FDA took away its approval for chloroquine to treat SLE. The FDA-approved package insert states that it is indicated to treat malaria, but it does not mention lupus anymore.

Quinacrine is even more interesting. Quinacrine was never FDA-approved for the treatment of lupus by itself. It was FDA-approved when used in combination with hydroxychloroquine and chloroquine in a medicine called Triquin. One Triquin tablet contained 25 mg of quinacrine, 65 mg of chloroquine, and 50 mg of hydroxychloroquine. It was prescribed at a dose of one to two tablets four times a day, which is a much higher dose of each of those different components than what is used today for any one of them individually. Many patients placed on Triquin developed side effects, and it was impossible to figure out which of the three drugs in Triquin may have been the cause in any particular person. Therefore, Triquin was removed from the market in 1972. However, its FDA indication was never withdrawn (according to Dr. Daniel Wallace, a famous lupologist). Quinacrine is still very effective for lupus and prescribed by lupus doctors, but the capsules of quinacrine have be to made by a special kind of pharmacist called a compounding pharmacist. Quinacrine has the unique situation of still being FDA-approved to treat lupus, but only when used in combination with chloroquine and hydroxychloroquine (even though the original combination tablets are not even produced anymore).

It is not a coincidence that there has been no drug approved by the FDA to treat lupus since the 1962 Kefauver-Harris Drug Amendments. There are many reasons why it has been difficult to develop a new drug to treat lupus and obtain FDA approval (table 34.3). According to the law, all drugs must be proven effective in humans for the disease for which the drug is intended before the FDA will approve it. So let us compare systemic lupus erythematosus (SLE) to some other disorders. For a drug to be proven to be effective in treating the disease hypertension (high blood pressure), all that has to be shown is that the average blood pressure in a group of patients who take the medicine must be decreased significantly compared to a group of patients who take a placebo ("sugar pill"). For rheumatoid arthritis (which is also a systemic autoimmune disease and is related to SLE), all that has to be proven is that a group of patients who take the studied medicine end up having a decrease in pain level, swollen joints, and tender joints compared to the group taking a placebo.

SLE is a much more complex disease. It can attack almost every part of the body. Every patient who has SLE is different. You could line up one hundred people who have SLE, and none of them would be the same as far as what is going on. One may have recurrent blood clots in the lungs, and the next one may get a recurrent butterfly rash on the face and joint aches. Another may feel perfectly fine except for a low white blood cell count, another might have Raynaud's and gets recurrent sores in her mouth, and another may have a lot of protein in her urine and high blood pressure due to lupus nephritis.

SLE is associated with problems that fluctuate over time. Even without treatment there can be periods of activity (where SLE gets worse) interspersed with periods of inactivity. Doctors often describe this pattern as having problems that "wax and wane." Even on a placebo, patients can appear to get better if they happen to go through a period where their disease goes into a naturally occurring waning period. This means that the placebo used in lupus research studies could appear to be "working" because of this period of improvement, when in fact the disease itself is not really any better. In fact, placebo groups in lupus studies can have as high as a 50% improvement, meaning

**Table 34.3** Why It Is Difficult to Develop New Drugs for SLE and Get FDA Approval

---

- Most people who have SLE are very different from each other.

- It is hard to come up with a measurable research tool to prove a medicine works in SLE.

- There is up to a 50% placebo effect in lupus drug studies.

- Very large numbers of people are needed in a drug study for SLE. However, SLE is not a common disease, and many people who have SLE are already doing well on the drugs currently available. Therefore, not very many qualified individuals exist to enroll in the studies.

- In lupus nephritis studies, the drug must prove to be superior to cyclophosphamide.

- It is very expensive to develop drugs in the United States and get them FDA-approved.

---

that up to 50% of patients "appear" to get better when they take the placebo. Doctors call this the placebo effect. Since such a large number of placebo patients can appear to be better, it makes it even more difficult to prove that the medicine being studied is working at all, especially when the problem of how to measure improvement in the first place (since every lupus patient is unique) is factored in.

The problem that has eluded scientists and lupus experts is how to prove that a drug works on a disease like lupus in which most patients are very different from each other. The medical community has been trying. The search for effective lupus treatments (and how to prove that they are effective) has been a constant area of intense research for decades. Even more recently, the drugs rituximab (Rituxan) and mycophenolate (CellCept) have not been proved to be effective lupus medications to the FDA. This is counter to what lupus experts have seen in their patients. Many lupus patients who failed other lupus medicines are doing very well on rituximab and mycophenolate.

Because of these problems with each lupus patient being different from each other and with there being such a large placebo effect, it takes a large number of patients in lupus studies to do an adequate research study looking at the effectiveness of medications. It is estimated that SLE (taking out those who only have cutaneous lupus) only affects 0.05% of the population. This means that only one person out of every two thousand people have SLE. Therefore, it is difficult to get enough patients together to do a study on a new medicine. Most patients who have SLE actually are doing very well on existing medicines (such as hydroxychloroquine). The research studies for new medicines are reserved for patients who are not responding to the medicines that are already available.

Then there is even a tougher problem. For a lupus drug to be FDA-approved to treat lupus nephritis (kidney disease), it must be proved that it works better than cyclophosphamide. Recall from chapter 32 that cyclophosphamide is a very strong chemotherapy agent. The FDA calls this a superiority study. A drug company has to prove that its drug is superior or better than cyclophosphamide. At this point, cyclophosphamide is one of the most effective drugs to treat lupus nephritis, especially severe nephritis. Doctors usually like to see drug studies using some sort of placebo to compare the medicine being studied to prove that it works. However, it would be unethical to give people who have severe lupus nephritis a placebo. If patients who have severe lupus nephritis received a fake treatment (a placebo) as part of a research study, a large number of them would end up going on dialysis or even dying. Since doctors consider cyclophosphamide the best drug of choice for treating severe lupus nephritis, it must be used as a comparison in research studies. It just makes no sense at all why the FDA enforces this almost impossible task. Many lupus experts do not support this requirement, but unfortunately, it currently is a huge obstacle in lupus research.

Another part of the equation comes down to money. The FDA approval process is long, complicated, and incredibly expensive for pharmaceutical companies. Of course, this process has developed over the years to satisfy public demands. Doctors do not want any repeats of the thalidomide and sulfanilamide disasters. They want to be sure that the drugs they use are effective and as safe as possible to treat diseases. Yet on the other hand, doctors are also sometimes demanding and want things "now" to treat diseases (like lupus). Finding a balance between these two demands is very difficult, especially when it comes to a complex disorder such as lupus. On average, it takes ten to twenty years from the initial time a potential drug is identified to the time it can become FDA-approved. That period involves an incredible amount of work and money—numerous research studies in the laboratory, on animals, and subsequently in humans—before the stringent requirements of the FDA can be met. After that, there is still all the paperwork and legalities of going through the FDA approval process itself. For a pharmaceutical company to commit itself to develop drugs for any disease, it has to have some glimmer of hope that a successful outcome is possible.

According to the Center for the Study of Drug Development at Tufts University in Boston, drug companies have to spend more than $1 billion for each new medicine that reaches the market (in other words, new drugs that your doctor can prescribe). Only 30% of new drugs that make it to the pharmacy actually end up making enough money to compensate the drug company for all the money it invested into the drug. Along the way, for every five thousand to ten thousand prospective new drugs tested in the laboratory, only a few hundred ever come close to being tested in humans.

The U.S. government cannot be relied on to help with drug development. Although the National Institutes of Health do an incredible amount of good work in research, including giving out money for research, very few drugs ever come directly from government funding. There just is not enough money for the government to do this. Americans are not going to be willing to pay much higher taxes for government-sponsored drug research. Almost all drugs come through the efforts and monies of private investors and pharmaceutical companies. Given the difficulty with proving that a medicine works in lupus and the incredible amount of money needed by drug companies to do research and develop drugs, it is easy to see why there have not been any drugs developed for SLE in a long time.

But then came Benlysta . . .

## What Is Benlysta and How Does It Work?

Benlysta is a biologic medication (see chapter 33). It must be produced using biologic processes (in this case using mouse cells to produce it), which are expensive, and the molecule is very large and fragile. Therefore, like most biologics, Benlysta is very expensive (costing about $35,000 a year for one person) and must be given by injection (intravenously, or IV for short).

Benlysta works by combining with a particular cytokine called B Lymphocyte Stimulator (BLyS for short, pronounced like "bliss"). BLyS is also called B-cell activating factor. BLyS is a very important cytokine that is responsible for increasing the number of mature B-cells to produce antibodies. Recall from the section on rituximab in chapter 33 that rituximab works in a similar manner (it decreases the number of B-cells). The bone marrow is continuously producing B-cells and releasing them into the bloodstream where they can produce antibodies that can protect the body.

Rituximab binds to CD20 on B-cells to stop them from maturing. Benlysta stops the production of B-cells at a slightly later stage of the maturation process, but in essence has a similar result. It decreases the number of antibody-producing B-cells. Recall from chapter 1 that one of the hallmarks of SLE is that lupus causes the immune system to make too many auto-antibodies that end up attacking the body itself (the antinuclear antibodies of lupus that cause the positive ANA test). Therefore, it certainly makes sense that if you can decrease the number of auto-antibodies being made that can attack the body (by decreasing the number of B-cells that produce them), then this sort of medicine should work. And it does!

The studies that were performed leading up to the FDA approval for Benlysta are the largest studies ever done on patients who have SLE. No other studies have ever evaluated such a large number of patients to look at how well the medicine works and what the potential side effects are. In addition, many of the patients from the earlier studies are continuing to be studied to see if there may be any long-term side effects that could potentially have been missed in the shorter initial studies. No other medicine for lupus can make these same claims.

## Benlysta and African Americans, Lupus Nephritis, and Brain Disease

You may have read that Benlysta does not work in black people or in those who have kidney disease or brain disease. This is not necessarily true and deserves some explanation.

The problem with the last two, and most important, Benlysta studies done before it sought FDA approval is that there were not many black people in the studies. Out of 1,684 patients in these 2 studies, only 148 of them were of African descent, which means that less than 9% of the patients were black. The problem with this is that about 25% of all American lupus patients are of African descent. Therefore, African Americans were grossly under-represented in the studies. There were not enough black people in the studies to prove whether the drug worked in them or not.

One of the large studies (called BLISS-52) was primarily conducted in South America, Asia, and Eastern Europe, where the numbers of black patients are relatively very small. The second large study (called BLISS-76) was conducted in North America and Europe. I learned from talking to one of the research investigators in the United States that there was difficulty in getting African Americans to volunteer for the study. This is not surprising as it is a well-documented fact that it is generally difficult to get black Americans to enter research studies due to a distrust of researchers in the black community. A big part of this stems from the horrible treatment that African Americans have received in the past with medical studies. Most notorious and well known is the Tuskegee syphilis experiment. This was an experiment conducted in Macon County, Alabama, between 1932 and 1972. The study was performed on poor, rural black men. Three hundred ninety-nine of them were infected with syphilis before the study started, while 201 men enrolled in the study did not have syphilis (a comparison or control group). The men were only told that they were being treated for "bad blood" and were promised free medical care, meals, and a free burial. The reason for conducting the study was to see what syphilis would do over time. Syphilis is a sexually transmitted disease that if left untreated can cause early death related to brain and heart disease. Babies can be born with severe birth defects if their mother has syphilis.

There were numerous ethical violations, such as not obtaining proper, informed consent from the participants. The worst part, however, was that when penicillin was discovered as a cure for syphilis, the participants were not allowed to be treated with it. By the end of the study in 1972, only seventy-four of the men were still alive. One hundred twenty-eight had died from either syphilis itself or from complications related to syphilis. Forty of their wives became infected, and nineteen of their children were born with birth defects due to syphilis. After the whistle was blown on the study, major laws were enacted to ensure that these ethical violations would not be repeated in the future. However, with this being such a recent event, it makes sense why so many would still harbor distrust.

Recent literature reflects the feelings and beliefs of some in the black community such as the following excerpt from Rebecca Skloot's *The Immortal Life of Henrietta Lacks*:

> "Back then they did things," Sonny said. "Especially to black folks. John Hopkins was known for experimentin on black folks. They'd snatch em off the street . . ."
>
> "That's right!" Bobbette said, appearing in the kitchen door with her coffee. "Everybody knows that."
>
> "They just snatch em off the street," Sonny said.
>
> "Snatchin' people!" Bobbette yelled, her voice growing louder.
>
> "Expermentin' on them!" Sonny yelled.
>
> "You'd be surprised how many people disappeared in East Baltimore when I was a girl," Bobbette said, shaking her head.

Fortunately, with the changes in the laws regulating research ethics, things are very different today. Participants in studies must be given full disclosure on the potential side effects of medicines used for studies, what their rights are in terms of how the study is performed, and what alternatives are available for their medical condition outside of the study, and this must all be put down in writing for the patient's own records.

The bottom line with this issue is that there were not enough black people in the major FDA approval studies to show whether Benlysta works in black people. In the phase II research studies (these are the studies that were done before the final studies) Benlysta did appear to be effective in those of black ethnicity. In fact, 24% of the participants in the phase II earlier study were of African descent. As a group, the black patients in that study overall did better as far as how well they responded to Benlysta. However, there were not enough patients overall in the study for this effect to be considered statistically significant. I believe that it does work in blacks as I have several patients who are African American and who are doing very well on Benlysta after they had failed numerous other medications. I have spoken to physicians involved with the studies who state that they also have many African American patients who have responded well. As a condition for Benlysta's FDA approval, the pharmaceutical company responsible for developing Benlysta, Human Genome Sciences, has agreed to do a study specifically studying patients of black ethnicity. This study is currently being organized as of the time of this writing. I hope that many appropriate SLE patients who are African American seize this opportunity to regain trust in the medical establishment and enter the studies so that doctors can continue to advance their understanding and treatment of SLE.

As far as kidney disease and brain disease, patients who had severe lupus nephritis or those who had significant central nervous system (CNS) involvement were not allowed to enter the initial Benlysta studies. In other words, lupus patients who had severe inflammation of the brain, spinal cord, or kidneys could not volunteer for the study at all. Therefore, it is not that Benlysta does not work for those patients; it is just that it was not studied for these particular conditions when they were particularly severe in nature.

Patients who had mild to moderate cases of lupus nephritis were included in the studies. As long as they did not have more than 6 g/dL of protein per 24 hours in their urine, did not have a serum creatinine greater than 2.5 mg/dL, were not on dialysis, or were not on 100 mg a day of prednisone or more, they could participate in the Benlysta trials. Out of 1,684 total patients in the two phase III studies (BLISS-52 and BLISS-76), 267 of them did have lupus nephritis. In these particular patients, there were some significant improvements noted due to Benlysta. The patients who had kidney disease who received Benlysta had less flares of kidney disease. Remission rates were also higher; 70.5% of the patients who received the full dose of Benlysta achieved remission from their kidney involvement at the end of one year of treatment.

I do not know what the future holds for the possibility of studying Benlysta in patients who have severe nephritis. As long as the FDA demands that medicines be proven to be superior to cyclophosphamide in treating lupus nephritis (as discussed previously), it is going to be very hard to get any pharmaceutical company to do research on medicines for lupus nephritis. Cyclophosphamide is such a strong chemotherapy medicine that it would be very hard to find a drug (including Benlysta) that works significantly better than it does. I hope that leaders in the lupus community can convince the FDA to change its requirements for this particular problem in the future.

Now that Benlysta is available for use, doctors most likely will use it in lupus patients who have severe kidney and brain disease even though these conditions were not studied. For many years, rheumatologists have had to use medicines that are not FDA-approved to treat severe lupus (e.g., cyclophosphamide, methotrexate, mycophenolate, azathioprine, etc.), so this will not stop them from using Benlysta in patients who have these problems if other therapies have not helped them. Doctors who do use Benlysta in these patients, especially doctors who are at large medical centers, will certainly publish their results in the medical journals. This will let other doctors know how their patients do on Benlysta to see if it works or not in severe lupus nephritis and CNS lupus.

## What Did Human Genome Sciences (the Makers of Benlysta) Do Differently to Get FDA Approval?

The FDA approval process for drug development occurs in three phases of research studies. Phase I and phase II studies are the smallest, and are basically looking to see if a medicine may be effective and safe to use in humans and to treat a disorder. Phase III studies are the largest and most important as far as obtaining FDA approval.

The phase II studies using Benlysta to treat SLE actually did not have overall good results. They did not show that it worked any better than placebo. However, Human Genome Sciences (HGS) did a very smart thing. It went through the phase II studies with a fine-tooth comb to figure out which patients responded to Benlysta and which patients did not respond. This makes a lot of sense when you think about it. Some medicines for lupus seem to work better for certain lupus problems than other medicines. For example, quinacrine is a good medicine to try for lupus arthritis, fatigue, and rashes. However, it probably would not work well in a patient who has lupus nephritis. Methotrexate probably works a lot better for lupus arthritis than it would for someone who has lupus lung disease. What Human Genome Sciences figured out was that patients who were positive for antinuclear antibodies and anti-double-stranded DNA antibodies at the time that they entered the study had a much better chance of responding to Benlysta compared to those who were negative for these antibodies. Therefore, they made it a requirement that all patients in the phase III research studies had to be positive for these antibodies. This may have been the answer as to how to do a drug study for SLE properly. It paid off because both large phase III studies showed that Benlysta was effective in treating SLE patients who had previously failed appropriate therapies and who were positive for these autoantibodies.

## How Effective Is Benlysta in Treating SLE?

First, it is important to point out that Benlysta was not used by itself in the studies and compared to a pure placebo "sugar pill." The patients were already on other lupus medications such as prednisone, hydroxychloroquine, or methotrexate, and they continued those medicines during the study. The treated group received Benlysta in addition to those medicines, while the placebo group got an IV infusion of a placebo and stayed on their usual medicines as well. It can be helpful to look at some of the numbers to compare the groups. Although there were two large studies, and various doses of Benlysta were used, I just show the numbers from the longest-run study (called the BLISS-76 study) and compare the placebo group to the group given Benlysta at the 10 mg/kg dose (which is the FDA-approved dose) in table 34.4.

The group that received Benlysta at the dose of 10 mg/kg did better in these measurements compared to the group that did not receive Benlysta (the placebo group). More of them responded, more of them were able to decrease their prednisone to low doses, and fewer of them had flares of their lupus. The SLE Responder Index (SRI) result is especially impressive. Although on the surface it may not look like there is much of a difference between 33.5% and 43.5%, in reality, this is significant. The SRI is a hard standard to meet. For a patient to be considered as having responded (i.e., be counted as meeting the SRI), she had to satisfy four criteria. She had to have a significant decrease in a disease activity scale (called the SELENA/SLEDAI scale), have no worsening of disease as determined by her physician, have no severe flares of her lupus, and only

Table 34.4 Effects of Placebo Group versus Benlysta in BLISS-76 Study

| | SLE Responder Index (%) | Participants Able to Lower Prednisone 7.5 mg/d (%) | Participants Who Flared at Weeks 24–76 (no.) |
|---|---|---|---|
| Placebo group | 33.5 | 17.5 | 21.8 |
| Benlysta group | 43.5 | 25.8 | 15.7 |

have had one moderate flare of her lupus during the study. It is very hard to find patients who have severe lupus (the ones who participated in the studies) who satisfy all of those requirements. In addition, 43.5% of the Benlysta group achieving an SRI actually represents a 33% higher number of patients relatively compared to the placebo group.

Benlysta especially seemed to be helpful for arthritis, cutaneous lupus, and fatigue in the studies. A 2012 report from Dr. Ronald van Vollenhoven of Sweden and other international lupus experts actually showed that the patients who did best on Benlysta were those who had the worst disease activity. Especially those with positive ds-DNA levels, those with low complement levels, and those who required steroids seemed to have a better chance of responding to Benlysta. Yet Benlysta certainly did not help everyone. A significant number of SLE patients did not respond to the medicine. However, it is important to keep in mind that these were people not responding to the usual lupus medicines. A significant number of people did respond very well to Benlysta.

In 2011, results were presented at the American College of Rheumatology scientific meeting in Chicago on the six-year data in the patients receiving Benlysta. These results were very exciting. Lupus experts examined the data year by year; it appears that patients continued to improve over time. As a baseline, during the first year of treatment, 85% of patients who received placebo had a flare of their lupus. During the third year of treatment with Benlysta, this number fell to 55%, and by the sixth year, it was down to 42%. During the six years, most lab values improved significantly, and steroid doses decreased by an average of 55%. These numbers are even more impressive because these results occurred in patients who had failed the usual therapies for SLE before they entered the study. So far, the future of Benlysta as an important treatment for lupus looks very promising.

## So, Is Benlysta the Miracle Drug for Lupus?

Since Benlysta does not cure lupus, and some patients still do not respond to the medicine, Benlysta is not a miracle drug as far as how well it treats lupus. It also has not been shown to be any better than the medicines doctors already use. (So definitely do not consider stopping medicines you are currently taking if they are helping you.) However, it does offer hope for some people who are not responding to the usual medicines (just as it helped Janice Fitzgibbon whose real life story was mentioned in the first section of this chapter).

I would argue, though, that Benlysta is a miracle drug for lupus in another sense. Human Genome Sciences has done what was considered the impossible. They were able to prove that a new medicine could be developed, could be safe, could be proven to work, and could get approved by the FDA to treat lupus. I suspect that this success will do a lot to encourage other pharmaceutical companies to take the chance and to invest in more research to try to find better treatments for lupus. Therefore, Benlysta may in fact be the miracle drug doctors have been waiting for in this respect.

*Generic available*: No.

*How Benlysta works*: See previous discussion. Benlysta decreases the number of B-cells that end up producing auto-antibodies that can attack the person's body.

*What benefits to expect from Benlysta*: Benlysta is a slow working medication, usually taking three to six months to work, although there are some people who notice benefits within one to two months.

*How Benlysta is taken*: Benlysta is given at a dose of 10 mg per kilogram of patient's body weight. It is infused into a vein (intravenous infusion, or IV). Three infusions are given during the first month at two-week intervals. This is followed by one IV infusion every four weeks. It takes about one hour for the infusion of the medicine itself. Currently, a subcutaneous (SQ) version of belimumab is being studied.

*If you miss a dose of your medicine*: Have your infusion scheduled as soon as you realize that you forgot to get your dose. Then you need to reset your schedule from that date. For example, let us say that you realize you forgot to get your January 10 Benlysta infusion (or it had to be cancelled for some reason), and that you were supposed to get another infusion four weeks after that. You reschedule to have it on January 20. You should schedule your next one to occur four weeks after the January 20 infusion. Consult with your prescribing doctor to double-check these instructions, but these guidelines will suffice for most people.

*Alcohol/food/herbal interactions with Benlysta*: No known alcohol interactions.

No known food interactions.

Do not take Echinacea, which can stimulate the immune system.

*Potential side effects of Benlysta*: One interesting thing about Benlysta is that there was no statistically significant difference for any side effects in the Benlysta group compared to the placebo group (table 34.5). Some of the main potential side effects that concern the FDA are listed in table 34.5. You can review chapter 29 to get a better idea of how to evaluate side effects of research studies. These numbers come from the FDA-approved drug package insert for Benlysta and include all the side effects noted in all 2,133 patients who were in the phase II study and both phase III studies. Although there was no difference statistically, there was a slight trend of more patients who took Benlysta having some of these side effects compared to those who received placebo. Whether these truly represent an increase in side effects or not is not known. Potential side effects from Benlysta are listed in table 34.6.

The lupus patients who entered these studies for the most part had failed the usual drugs used to treat lupus. They had significant, uncontrolled disease and were taking other immunomodulating medicines (such as steroids, hydroxychloroquine, methotrexate, mycophenolate, or azathioprine) at the same time as the placebo and Benlysta. Therefore, some of these medicines and the lupus disease itself certainly contributed to the number of "side effects" noted in these numbers.

The three primary areas of concern with Benlysta, as with any biologic that calms down the immune system, are infections, cancer, and allergic reactions. Although these did not occur any more often with Benlysta compared to placebo as far as reaching statistical significance, there were slightly more infections and allergic reactions occurring in patients who received Benlysta compared to those who did not receive it. Another area of potential concern is that of depression and psychiatric problems. Most of the people in both the placebo group and the Benlysta group who developed

**Table 34.5** Side Effects (SE) Reported in the Major Benlysta Studies Used for FDA Approval

| Side Effect | Placebo Groups (% with SE) | Benlysta Groups (% with SE) |
|---|---|---|
| Any type of infection | 67 | 71 |
| Serious infection | 5.2 | 6.0 |
| Death due to infection | 0.1 (1 out of 675) | 0.3 (4 out of 1458) |
| Depression | 4.7 | 6.3 |
| Severe depression | 0.1 | 0.4 |
| Suicide | 0 | 0.15 (2 out of 1458) |
| Severe allergy (anaphylaxis) | 0.4 | 0.6 |
| Low white blood cells | 2 | 4 |
| Cancer | 0.4 | 0.4 |
| Died | 0.4 (3 out of 675) | 0.75 (11 out of 1458) |
| Nausea | 12 | 15 |
| Diarrhea | 9 | 12 |
| Difficulty sleeping | 5 | 7 |
| Pain in the arms and legs | 4 | 6 |

**Table 34.6** Potential Side Effects of Benlysta

| | Incidence | Side Effect Therapy |
|---|---|---|
| **Nuisance side effects** | | |
| Nausea/diarrhea | Uncommon | Treat as needed. |
| Difficulty sleeping | Uncommon | Consider a sleeping aid. |
| Pain in the arms and legs | Uncommon | Take pain medicines. |
| **Serious side effects** | | |
| Infection | Uncommon | Treat infection. Do not use during infections. |
| Worsening of depression | Uncommon | Treat depression or stop medicine. |
| Allergic reaction, anaphylaxis | Uncommon | Treat allergic reaction. May need to stop medicine. |
| Low white blood cell count | Uncommon | Medicine stopped or dose decrease. |

Side effect incidence key (approximations, as side effects can vary widely study to study): rare < 1% occurrence; uncommon 1%–5% occurrence; common > 5% occurrence

depression had pre-existing depression and most were on medications for it. We cannot say that Benlysta worsens depression from this data, but it is something that has to be watched on the medicine. Two of the patients (out of 1,458 patients) who took Benlysta did commit suicide, but again, this number is far too small to draw any conclusions. Both of these patients had significant depression before they even entered the study. Benlysta has been studied for six years, and with this data, there have actually been a similar percentage of suicides in the placebo group as well as in the Benlysta group, which raises some doubt as to whether Benlysta causes suicide.

As far as patients who died, more patients who died during the studies were in the Benlysta group. This number did not reach statistical significance. The causes of death in these patients included infection and cardiovascular disease (the most common causes of death in SLE patients); as noted above, two patients committed suicide. Since the deaths did not occur for the same reasons, it is difficult to blame them particularly on Benlysta.

Whenever doctors use a medication to suppress the immune system, they are always theoretically worried about the possibility of causing more cancer since the immune system is important in protecting the body from cancer. Cancer did not occur more commonly in the Benlysta patients. However, this possibility will be closely studied and monitored over time. The pharmaceutical company (currently manufactured by GlaxoSmithKline) has committed itself to study the medicine on as many patients as it can for many years to come.

With medicines that calm down the immune system, doctors are always worried about the possibilities of infections. The numbers in table 34.5 are derived from the earlier studies on Benlysta for it to receive its FDA approval. There are now more recent data on the patients as they have now been treated with Benlysta for up to six years. There are no differences in the numbers of infections between the placebo patients and the Benlysta patients. In fact, data presented in 2011 at the American College of Rheumatology meeting showed that 6.8% of placebo patients had had a serious or severe infection while only 6.1% of those who had the full dose of Benlysta had. This does not mean that placebo causes more infections, by the way. This simply illustrates that there are no statistically significant differences in the numbers of infections between the two groups.

There were also some nuisance types of side effects that were seen with Benlysta (but again without achieving statistical significance). These included a slight increase in the numbers of patients who experienced nausea, diarrhea, fever, difficulty sleeping, and pain in the arms and legs.

In 2012, Dr. Joan Merrill and other lupus experts reported on the long-term side effects of Benlysta. They followed the patients from the original studies over time and found that after four years of taking Benlysta, severe side effects, including infections, infusion reactions, and bad lab abnormalities, actually improved over time. These results are reassuring regarding the overall safety of using Benlysta in people who have SLE.

In 2013, Dr. Daniel Wallace and other lupus experts combined the data from all phase II and phase III clinical trials on Benlysta. They actually showed that more infections and cancers occurred in the placebo group than in the Benlysta group when these studies were combined (a total of 1,458 patients). Of course, this does not mean by any means that placebo is more apt to cause infections and cancer. It just emphasizes the point about how few major side effects appear to occur with Benlysta. This is a very exciting concept: to think that there is an effective yet safe medicine to use in patients who have severe SLE.

I have a few final thoughts on potential side effects with Benlysta. There were no differences statistically between Benlysta and placebo. However, there were more infections, depression, allergic reactions, deaths, and some nuisance type reactions among Benlysta patients compared to the placebo patients. Doctors do not know whether these are true side effects of Benlysta or not. There is some comfort knowing that Benlysta was studied using the best current research methods, using the largest numbers of lupus patients ever, and for the longest time of any medicine studied in SLE patients up to this point. Based upon how the medicine works (it calms down the immune system), it may increase the chances of having an infection (although this risk fortunately appears to be very low), and there most likely are some patients who will be allergic to the medicine (which can happen with any medication). Doctors will get a better handle as to whether these side effects truly exist or not over time as we use the medicine in more people.

*What needs to be monitored while taking Benlysta*: Your doctor will check the usual labs used to follow lupus patients (especially a CBC) while you are on the treatment.

*Reasons not to take Benlysta (contraindications or precautions)*: Do not take Benlysta if you have an active infection.

*While taking Benlysta*: If you develop any infection symptoms at all, such as fever, sore throat, cough, red painful skin, sinusitis congestion, or painful frequent urination, see your primary care doctor or go to an emergency room immediately. Do not get your Benlysta treatment if you have an active infection. You should not receive live vaccines, including a Zostavax (for shingles), while being treated with Benlysta. If you feel more depressed than usual while taking Benlysta, and especially if you develop any suicidal thoughts, let your prescribing doctor know as soon as possible.

*Pregnancy and breast-feeding while taking Benlysta*: Do not use Benlysta while pregnant. If you want to become pregnant and you are using Benlysta, use birth control for four months after you stop Benlysta before you try to get pregnant.

If you do get pregnant while taking your medicine, consider contacting the Organization of Teratology Information Specialists (OTIS) Autoimmune Diseases in Pregnancy Project at www.otispregnancy.org or 877-311-8972 or email otisresearch@ucsd .edu so that more can be learned about what happens when women on medications used in treating lupus become pregnant. Also, contact the Benlysta pregnancy register at 877-681-6296 if you become pregnant while you are using Benlysta.

Some pregnancies occurred in the phase II and phase III Benlysta studies. Six placebo patients got pregnant, and unfortunately, all of them ended in either miscarriage or abortion. There have been fifty-four pregnancies in the women who were on Benlysta. Four of those patients were lost to follow-up, but of the fifty remaining patients, twenty-one resulted in live births and six were ongoing (representing 54% of those fifty pregnancies). Ten of the fifty women decided to have an abortion, while thirteen ended in miscarriage or stillbirth. The take home point from these numbers, for me, is that it underscores the importance of planning for pregnancy appropriately (see chapter 41), not becoming pregnant until lupus disease is under excellent control, and then holding medications (such as belimumab) appropriately in preparation for pregnancy.

Benlysta does enter the breast milk. It is not known whether it is safe to use while breast-feeding or not.

*Geriatric use of Benlysta*: Benlysta has not been studied in a large number of older people. There may be an increased risk of side effects such as infections as may occur with other immunosuppressant medicines.

*What to do with Benlysta at the time of surgery*: It is always best to double-check with your rheumatologist and surgeon regarding specific instructions. A common recommendation is to not take Benlysta for several weeks before surgery, then resume it once the surgical wound has healed and if there is no evidence for infection.

*Patient assistance program for Benlysta*: Call 1-877-423-6597. Also see chapter 42.

*Drug helpline for Benlysta*: 1-877-423-6597.

*Website to learn more about Benlysta*: www.benlysta.com .

### KEY POINTS TO REMEMBER

1. Benlysta is the first medicine FDA-approved for lupus that was specifically developed for lupus.

2. Benlysta was FDA-approved March 9, 2011, more than fifty years after the previous FDA-approved medicine for lupus.

3. Benlysta is the best-studied medicine to treat SLE (studied on larger numbers of patients and over a longer amount of time than any other lupus medication).

4. Benlysta is a biologic agent; therefore, it is expensive and must be given by injection (IV).

5. Benlysta was not tested in patients who have severe lupus nephritis nor in those who have active CNS lupus. However, patients who had mild to moderate kidney disease had significant improvements (70% went into remission).

6. Just as with the immunosuppressant medicines, there may be an increased risk of infections with Benlysta; however, thus far the numbers are no different from placebo.

7. Make sure not to use Benlysta during an active infection.

8. Do everything listed in table 22.1 to prevent infections.

9. Do not get any live vaccines (including a Zostavax for shingles) if you are being treated with Benlysta.

10. See your primary care doctor or go to the emergency room immediately if you have any infection symptoms, increased depression, or suicidal thoughts.

11. You can learn more about Benlysta at www.benlysta.com.

# Other Therapies for SLE

## Thalidomide to Treat Lupus?

Recall from chapter 34 that thalidomide was a medicine that caused severe birth defects. It is one of the major reasons that the current FDA laws are in place stipulating that drugs have to be proven safe and effective before becoming FDA-approved. Interestingly, the same medicine that greatly contributed to the difficulty of lupus medicines receiving FDA approval during the past fifty years is also used to treat lupus. An Israeli doctor used thalidomide on his patients who had an infection called leprosy in the early 1960s. He was using it to help them sleep (as it is a very effective sleeping medicine). Some people who have leprosy develop an inflammatory condition of the skin called erythema nodosum leprosum. Some of his patients who had this leprosy problem who took thalidomide had remarkable improvements of their skin disease. Subsequently, it was found to be useful in people who had other inflammatory skin diseases such as cutaneous lupus. It is primarily used in people who have severe chronic cutaneous lupus (such as severe discoid lupus; see chapter 8) when the other usual treatments have not worked. However, it also has many potential side effects; therefore, it is not used very often.

Although anti-malarial medications, steroids, immunosuppressants, and biologic agents are the most commonly used medicines to treat systemic lupus erythematosus (SLE), there are other therapies, such as thalidomide, which do not fall into one of these categories. Some were found to be helpful "accidentally" to treat lupus (such as thalidomide), while others were tried based on their known effects on the immune system. These therapies represent a hodgepodge group of medicines, most of which are not related to each other at all. Because they do not fit in the previous chapters about anti-malarials, immunosuppressants, steroids, and biologics, this chapter discusses them separately. The chapter is not intended to be exhaustive. It includes medicines that continue to have current benefits to treat lupus, but does not discuss rarely used medicines that may have been used more frequently in the past (such as gold).

## Dapsone (Diamino-Diphenyl Sulfone)

*Generic available*: Yes.

*How dapsone works*: Decreases inflammation in the immune system in several different ways. Dapsone is an antibiotic used to treat leprosy.

*What benefits to expect from dapsone*: Dapsone is most commonly used to treat bullous lupus. Bullous lupus is a type of cutaneous lupus that causes fluid-filled blisters to occur on the skin. Dapsone is also used in some people who have lupus to prevent severe lung infections (specifically an infection called pneumocystis pneumonia). It is primarily used for this purpose in people who are treated with high doses of steroids along with immunosuppressant medicines such as cyclophosphamide.

*How dapsone is taken*: Dapsone comes in 25 mg and 100 mg tablets. A common dosing regimen is 100 mg a day.

*If you miss a dose of your medicine*: Take your dapsone dose during the same day that you forgot to take it, then resume your normal schedule the next day. Do not take extra doses of dapsone in a day if you forgot to take it the preceding day. Consult with your prescribing doctor to double-check these instructions, but these guidelines will suffice for most people.

*Alcohol/food/herbal interactions with dapsone*: No interactions with alcohol noted. Taken with or without food.

Avoid St. John's wort, which can decrease dapsone levels in the body. Taking vitamin E daily may decrease the risk of getting anemia from dapsone.

*Potential side effects of dapsone*: One of the most important potential side effects of dapsone is anemia, specifically a certain type of anemia called hemolytic anemia (table 35.1). It especially can be severe in someone who is deficient in an enzyme called G6PD (short for glucose-6-phosphate dehydrogenase). Therefore, everyone should have a blood test for G6PD before being treated with dapsone. People who are deficient in G6PD should probably not take dapsone. Taking 800 IU of vitamin E a day may decrease the risk of getting anemia.

*What needs to be monitored while taking dapsone*: A complete blood cell count and chemistry panel should be checked regularly.

*Reasons not to take dapsone (contraindications or precautions)*: If you are deficient in the enzyme G6PD, you should probably not take dapsone. If you do take it, your blood counts should be followed more closely than normal.

*While taking dapsone*: Let your doctor know if you become short of breath, are fatigued, develop a rash, have numb feet, or develop yellow eyes (jaundice).

*Pregnancy and breast-feeding while taking dapsone*: There is an increased risk of the fetus developing abnormalities during pregnancy. It can be used during pregnancy if the potential benefits outweigh the risks.

Do not use while breast-feeding.

*Geriatric use of dapsone*: No special considerations.

*What to do with dapsone at the time of surgery*: It is always best to double-check with your rheumatologist and surgeon regarding specific instructions. However, dapsone is probably safe to take up to the time of surgery.

*Patient assistance program for dapsone*: See chapter 42.

*Drug helpline for dapsone*: Unaware of any.

*Website to learn more about dapsone*: Unaware of any.

Table 35.1  Potential Side Effects of Dapsone

|  | Incidence | Side Effect Therapy |
|---|---|---|
| **Nuisance side effects** | | |
| Stomach upset, nausea | Common | Decrease dose or stop medicine. |
| Elevated liver enzymes | Uncommon | Decrease dose or stop medicine. |
| Rash | Uncommon | Decrease dose or stop medicine. |
| **Serious side effects** | | |
| Anemia | Common | Decrease dose or stop medicine. |
| Low white blood cell count | Uncommon | Decrease dose or stop medicine. |
| Hepatitis (liver inflammation) | Uncommon | Stop medicine. |
| Nerve damage | Uncommon | Stop medicine |

Side effect incidence key (approximations, as side effects can vary widely study to study): rare < 1% occurrence; uncommon 1%–5% occurrence; common > 5% occurrence

## Thalidomide (Thalomid)

Read the first section of this chapter to learn more about thalidomide.

*Generic available*: No.

*How thalidomide works*: Thalidomide decreases inflammation in the immune system through several different ways. It is FDA-approved to treat a complication of leprosy called erythema nodosum leprosum.

*What benefits to expect from thalidomide*: Ninety percent of people who have severe discoid lupus that does not respond to anti-malarial medicines have a good response to thalidomide. It can also increase hair growth on the scalp.

*How thalidomide is taken*: Thalidomide comes in capsules ranging from 50 mg to 200 mg. It is best taken at nighttime before bed at least one hour after eating.

*If you miss a dose of your medicine*: Since thalidomide is best taken before bed, if you realize you missed your dose the day after, skip the dose that you missed. Consult with your prescribing doctor to double-check these instructions, but these guidelines will suffice for most people.

*Alcohol/food/herbal interactions with thalidomide*: Alcohol increases the drowsiness effects of thalidomide and should be used with caution.

Take at least one hour after eating anything.

Avoid cat's claw and Echinacea, which can stimulate the immune system.

*Potential side effects of thalidomide*: Thalidomide has a high rate of side effects (table 35.2). Most people get drowsy from the medicine (it was first developed as a sleeping medicine), and approximately 25% of people can get nerve damage (called peripheral neuropathy). Peripheral neuropathy typically causes numbness in the feet and hands, but sometimes will just cause a burning sensation or a feeling like bugs crawling on the skin. Sometimes the nerve damage can be permanent even after thalidomide is discontinued.

The most dreaded side effects are the malformations of the limbs that can occur in the fetus. Due to this, thalidomide users must be enrolled in the S.T.E.P.S. program by their prescribing physician. S.T.E.P.S. stands for System for Thalidomide Education and Prescribing Safety and is run by Celgene Corporation, the pharmaceutical company that makes thalidomide. This program ensures that the person prescribed thalidomide has thoroughly read the information on its potential side effects; he or she must take and pass a questionnaire over the telephone regularly to get the prescription filled. Prescriptions can only be written for twenty-eight days' worth at a time with no refills to ensure that both doctor and patient are monitoring for side effects and preventing pregnancy as much as possible.

Another serious potential side effect is that of blood clots, which most commonly can cause deep venous thrombosis causing swelling and pain in the legs, pulmonary embolism of the lungs causing shortness of breath and chest pain, or a stroke if it occurs in the brain.

*What needs to be monitored while taking thalidomide*: You must be active in the S.T.E.P.S. program while on the medicine. You can enroll by calling 1-888-423-5436, or by going to www.thalomid.com. Information on how to participate in the program must be provided to you by your prescribing physician. You must answer a questionnaire regularly over the telephone while you are taking thalidomide to receive your prescription every twenty-eight days. If you are able to have children, then you must have a regular pregnancy test. Your blood counts and chemistry blood panel should be checked periodically.

*Reasons not to take thalidomide (contraindications or precautions)*: If you are able to have children (i.e., have not had a hysterectomy or have had a menstrual cycle within the previous two years), you must have a negative pregnancy test. You must promise to use at least two types of pregnancy prevention at the same time. The partners of men taking thalidomide must use birth control as well. If you have a pre-existing nerve disease, seizures, or heart disease, or have a history of having blood clots, then thalidomide may not be a good option.

*While taking thalidomide*: You must be active in the S.T.E.P.S. program while on the medicine. You can enroll by calling 1-888-423-5436, or by going to www.thalomid.com. See your doctor regularly for a checkup and labs. Let your doctor know immediately if you are pregnant or miss a period. Let your doctor know immediately if you get numbness or burning sensations in the feet or hands; dizziness; a red, swollen, painful leg; shortness of breath; chest pain; weakness in an arm or leg; slurred speech; or a rash.

*Pregnancy and breast-feeding while taking thalidomide*: If you are a woman taking Thalomid or if you are the female partner of a man taking Thalomid, you must use at least two forms of effective contraception while taking the medicine. Women must have a periodic pregnancy test.

Do not use while breast-feeding.

*Geriatric use of thalidomide*: Drowsiness and other side effects may be more common.

*What to do with thalidomide at the time of surgery*: It is always best to double-check with your rheumatologist and surgeon regarding specific instructions. Since thalidomide can potentially cause blood clots (which is a dangerous complication of surgery),

**Table 35.2** Potential Side Effects of Thalidomide

|  | Incidence | Side Effect Therapy |
|---|---|---|
| **Nuisance side effects** | | |
| Drowsiness | Common | Take at bedtime. |
| Weight gain, edema, fluid retention | Common | Decrease dose or stop medicine. |
| Fatigue | Common | Decrease dose or stop medicine. |
| Dizziness | Common | Decrease dose or stop medicine. |
| Dry mouth | Common | Decrease dose or stop medicine. |
| Constipation, diarrhea, stomach upset, nausea | Common | Decrease dose or stop medicine. |
| Increased sweating | Common | Decrease dose or stop medicine. |
| Low calcium levels | Common | Decrease dose or stop medicine. |
| **Serious side effects** | | |
| Blood clots | Common | Seek medical attention immediately and stop medicine. |
| Severe fetal malformations | Definite | Must use two forms of contraception simultaneously. |
| Nerve damage | Common | Stop medicine. |
| Rash, which can sometimes be severe | Common | Decrease dose or stop medicine. |
| Low red blood cell and white blood cell counts | Common | Decrease dose or stop medicine. |

Side effect incidence key (approximations, as side effects can vary widely study to study): rare < 1% occurrence; uncommon 1%–5% occurrence; common > 5% occurrence

it is probably best to stop thalidomide at least a few days before surgery, then not resume taking it until you are able to walk normally and are active.

*Patient assistance program for thalidomide*: Call 1-800-931-8691. Also see chapter 42.

*Drug helpline for thalidomide*: Call 1-888-423-5436.

*Website to learn more about thalidomide*: www.thalomid.com.

## Danazol

Danazol is an androgen, meaning that it is related to the male hormone testosterone. How it works in SLE is unknown. However, its primary use is to treat low platelet counts (thrombocytopenia) in lupus.

*Generic available*: Yes.

*How danazol works*: How danazol works in SLE is not fully understood.

*What benefits to expect from danazol*: About two-thirds of lupus patients who have low platelet counts can expect to have a significant increase in their platelets. It is primarily used to treat thrombocytopenia, but it has also been reported to help some lupus patients who have lupus flares around the time of their menstrual cycle; it is also used to treat discoid lupus, mouth sores, and hemolytic anemia.

*How danazol is taken*: Danazol comes in 50 mg, 100 mg, and 200 mg capsules. Doses as high as 800 mg a day are sometimes needed. It is usually taken two to three times a day.

*If you miss a dose of your medicine*: Skip the dose you missed and resume at your next regularly scheduled dose. Consult with your prescribing doctor to double-check these instructions, but these guidelines will suffice for most people.

*Alcohol/food/herbal interactions with danazol*: No interactions with alcohol noted. Taken with or without food. Fatty meals, though, increase its absorption.

Avoid Echinacea, which can stimulate the immune system.

*Potential side effects of danazol*: Since it is a male type hormone, some of the potential side effects are directly related to this (table 35.3). Acne, hair growth on the body (such as the face), decreased breast size, enlargement of the clitoris, and deepening of the voice may occur. Women may also stop menstruating, which can sometimes persist even after the medicine is stopped.

**Table 35.3**  Potential Side Effects of Danazol

|  | Incidence | Side Effect Therapy |
|---|---|---|
| **Nuisance side effects** | | |
| Stomach upset | Not noted | Reduce dose or stop medicine. |
| Elevated liver enzyme blood tests | Not noted | Reduce dose or stop medicine. |
| Acne | Not noted | Reduce dose or stop medicine. |
| Elevated cholesterol levels | Not noted | Reduce dose or stop medicine. |
| **Serious side effects** | | |
| Worsening of SLE itself | Not noted | Stop medicine. |
| Loss of menstrual cycles | Not noted | Stop medicine. |
| Breast size reduction | Not noted | Stop medicine. |
| Enlargement of the clitoris | Not noted | Stop medicine. |
| Deepening of the voice | Not noted | Stop medicine. |
| Male pattern hair growth | Not noted | Stop medicine. |

Side effect incidence key (approximations, as side effects can vary widely study to study): rare < 1% occurrence;  uncommon 1%–5% occurrence;  common > 5% occurrence

*What needs to be monitored while taking danazol*: Liver enzymes and a cholesterol panel should be checked periodically.

*Reasons not to take danazol (contraindications or precautions)*: Do not take if you have severe kidney, liver, or heart disease. Do not take if you have a disease called porphyria. Do not take if you have abnormal vaginal bleeding.

*While taking danazol*: Let your doctor know if you develop any of the side effects due to the male hormone influence (extra body hair, deepening of the voice, smaller breasts, larger clitoris, decreasing menstrual cycles).

*Pregnancy and breast-feeding while taking danazol*: Do not take while pregnant. Must use effective birth control while using danazol.

Do not use while breast-feeding.

*Geriatric use of danazol*: No special problems.

*What to do with danazol at the time of surgery*: It is always best to double-check with your rheumatologist and surgeon regarding specific instructions. Since there is an increased risk for developing blood clots on danazol (which is a potential complication of surgery), it may be best to stop danazol one week before surgery.

*Patient assistance program for danazol*: See chapter 42.

*Drug helpline for danazol*: Unaware of any.

*Website to learn more about danazol*: Unaware of any.

## Dehydroepiandrosterone (DHEA)

DHEA is also related to androgen (male-type) hormones. It is actually a type of steroid that is produced by the adrenal glands, and it is converted into male androgen sex hormones. People who have SLE have lower levels of DHEA on average compared to people who do not have SLE. Studies showed that DHEA may improve energy levels ("global well-being"), can help with mild lupus symptoms, may help decrease the doses of steroids needed, and tends to increase bone density levels. It was attempted to get the drug FDA-approved to treat SLE, but as with so many other medicines, FDA approval was not achieved. However, as noted in chapter 34, this does not mean that it does not help some lupus patients.

*Generic available*: DHEA is available in two forms. One is over the counter. However, studies show that most brands do not have the correct dose of DHEA in them; in fact, some even have no DHEA at all. This occurs because the FDA does not regulate over-the-counter food supplements, herbs, and nutritional supplements. If you decide to take DHEA, it is best to get it as a prescription from your doctor and obtain the medicine from a compounding pharmacist who can ensure that you are getting a pure product at the correct dose.

*How DHEA works*: Unknown.

*What benefits to expect from DHEA*: Some people may develop improvement in energy levels, memory abilities, and mild lupus symptoms, and may be able to reduce their prednisone dose. It may also improve bone density.

*How DHEA is taken*: Most lupus studies used 200 mg a day. However, it may be beneficial at lower doses as well.

*If you miss a dose of your medicine*: If you realize you did not take your dose during the day it was intended, you can take it later that day. However, do not double up on the

611

dose if you forgot your medicine the day before. Consult with your prescribing doctor to double-check these instructions, but these guidelines will suffice for most people.

*Alcohol/food/herbal interactions with DHEA*: Do not drink alcohol.

May be taken with or without food.

Do not take cat's claw or Echinacea, which can stimulate the immune system. There may be interactions with soy products, flavonoids, fiber supplements, and vitamin E.

*Potential side effects of DHEA*: Potential side effects of DHEA are listed in table 35.4.

*What needs to be monitored while taking DHEA*: Blood pressure, cholesterol levels, and liver function tests (blood tests) should be monitored while taking DHEA.

*Reasons not to take DHEA (contraindications or precautions)*: Caution should be used if you have significant liver disease. Avoid if you have polycystic ovarian syndrome.

*While taking DHEA*: If you have insulin-requiring diabetes, your insulin dose may need to be adjusted while taking DHEA. Inform your doctor if you develop increased hair growth or acne.

*Pregnancy and breast-feeding while taking DHEA*: Avoid during pregnancy.

Do not use while breast-feeding.

*Geriatric use of DHEA*: Older people have lower levels of DHEA. Therefore, the higher range of doses is often used in older individuals.

*What to do with DHEA at the time of surgery*: There are not definite known surgical risks with taking DHEA. It may be safe to take DHEA up to the time of surgery. Check with your rheumatologist.

*Patient assistance program for DHEA*: See chapter 42.

*Drug helpline for DHEA*: Unaware of any.

*Website to learn more about DHEA*: Unaware of any.

Table 35.4  Potential Side Effects of DHEA

|  | Incidence | Side Effect Therapy |
| --- | --- | --- |
| **Nuisance side effects** | | |
| Acne | Common | Decrease dose or stop medicine. |
| Increased hair growth on the face and other body areas | Common | Decrease dose or stop medicine. |
| Decrease in HDL (good) cholesterol | Uncommon | Decrease dose or stop medicine. |
| Elevated liver enzymes | Uncommon | Decrease dose or stop medicine. |
| **Serious side effects** | | |
| Elevated blood pressure | Uncommon | Decrease dose or stop medicine. |
| Increased psychiatric problems | Rare | Decrease dose or stop medicine. |

Side effect incidence key (approximations, as side effects can vary widely study to study): rare < 1% occurrence; uncommon 1%–5% occurrence; common > 5% occurrence

## Intravenous Immune Globulin (IVIG)

Immune globulins (also called immunoglobulins) are antibodies. A large number of antibodies given in the form of IVIG may help in some autoimmune disorders such as polymyositis and dermatomyositis, but IVIG is not commonly used for SLE. However, there are two situations where it is used. It is useful in people who have a deficiency in IgG immune globulins (medically known as hypogammaglobulinemia) and have recurrent infections due to this deficiency. A person with hypogammaglobulinemia can benefit greatly from IVIG therapy because it replaces the absent IgG globulins, which are beneficial for fighting off infections. IVIG therapy is also useful for a type of autoimmune disorder of the nerves called chronic inflammatory demyelinating poly-neuropathy (CIDP), which can cause significant muscle weakness as well as numbness of the arms and legs. This is a rarely seen nerve problem in lupus.

There have been recent studies looking at the use of IVIG to treat lupus nephritis, low platelet counts, arthritis, anemia, severe antiphospholipid syndrome, and central nervous system involvement with some preliminary encouraging results. A small 2012 study also suggested that it may be helpful in preventing congenital heart block in women who have lupus who are SSA or SSB antibody positive. However, larger studies will be needed to see if IVIG should be used more often to treat lupus. Unless larger studies are done, IVIG will continue to be used primarily for IgG globulin deficiency and CIDP in SLE.

*Generic available*: No.

*How IVIG works*: IVIG can decrease immune system overactivity.

*What benefits to expect from IVIG*: IVIG can help to decrease the numbers of infec-tions in people who have low levels of IgG globulins. It can help decrease the amount of numbness and weakness due to CIDP.

*How IVIG is taken*: Usually given as an intravenous (IV) infusion once or twice a month.

*If you miss a dose of your medicine*: Reschedule as soon as you realize that you missed your dose, then reset your schedule from that point. Consult with your prescribing doctor to double-check these instructions, but these guidelines will suffice for most people.

*Alcohol/food/herbal interactions with IVIG*: No interactions with alcohol.

No interactions with food.

Avoid cat's claw and Echinacea, which can stimulate the immune system.

*Potential side effects of IVIG*: Potential side effects of IVIG are listed in table 35.5.

*What needs to be monitored while taking IVIG*: You will need to have periodic lab tests, including blood cell counts and kidney function tests.

*Reasons not to take IVIG (contraindications or precautions)*: Many brands of IVIG are unsafe to receive if you have a deficiency in IgA globulins. Your IgA globulin level can be measured using a blood test similar to the one that measures IgG globulin levels. Gammagard S/D and Polygam brands of IVIG are generally safe to use if you are IgA deficient. Pre-existing heart disease, kidney disease, and a history of blood clots may increase your risk of having these sorts of problems on IVIG. Discuss these possibili-ties with your doctor.

**Table 35.5** Potential Side Effects of IVIG

|  | Incidence | Side Effect Therapy |
|---|---|---|
| **Nuisance side effects** | | |
| Mild infusion reactions (headache, muscle aches, fever, hives) | Common | Slow down rate of infusion. |
| Mild headaches | Common | Treat with headache medicines. |
| **Serious side effects** | | |
| Severe allergic reaction (anaphylaxis) | Uncommon | Stop medicine. |
| Severe headache, aseptic meningitis | Uncommon | May be prevented with antihistamines, steroids, and pain medicines. May need to stop medicine. |
| Kidney failure | Rare | Stop medicine. |
| Increase in lupus flares | Uncommon | Stop medicine. |
| Low blood pressure | Uncommon | Stop medicine. |
| Skin vasculitis | Uncommon | Stop medicine. |
| Blood clots | Uncommon | Seek immediate medical attention. Stop medicine. |
| Low red blood cell and white blood cell counts | Uncommon | Lower dose or stop medicine. |

Side effect incidence key (approximations, as side effects can vary widely study to study): rare < 1% occurrence; uncommon 1%–5% occurrence; common > 5% occurrence

*While taking IVIG*: See your doctor regularly for appropriate blood tests. Seek medical attention immediately if you develop a red, painful, swollen leg; shortness of breath; chest pain; slurred speech; or arm or leg weakness.

*Pregnancy and breast-feeding while taking IVIG*: IVIG has been used to treat certain fetal problems. Discuss use with your obstetrician and prescribing doctor. If you do get pregnant while taking your medicine, consider contacting the Organization of Teratology Information Specialists (OTIS) Autoimmune Diseases in Pregnancy Project at www.otispregnancy.org or 877-311-8972 or email otisresearch@ucsd.edu so that more can be learned about what happens when women on medications used in treating lupus become pregnant.

Safety during breast-feeding is unknown.

*Geriatric use of IVIG*: There may be an increased risk for side effects such as kidney problems, heart problems, and blood clots.

*What to do with IVIG at the time of surgery*: I am not aware of any specific recommendations on stopping IVIG before surgery. However, since IVIG can potentially increase the risk for blood clots, it may be best not to receive IVIG immediately before surgery. Check with the prescribing rheumatologist and infusion doctor for more information.

*Patient assistance program for IVIG*: There are numerous brands and manufacturers. Ask your infusion center for contact information. See chapter 42.

*Drug helpline for IVIG*: There are numerous brands and manufacturers. Ask your infusion center for contact information.

*Website to learn more about IVIG*: There are numerous brands and manufacturers. Ask your infusion center for contact information.

## Plasmapheresis (Therapeutic Plasma Exchange)

Plasmapheresis is a medical treatment where blood is removed from a person's vein. The blood goes through some sterile tubing and into a machine that filters out the largest molecules from the blood. The machine removes antibodies, which are very large molecules, in various amounts as determined by the doctor. Since the hallmark of lupus is the production of auto-antibodies that attack the body, this can be helpful in some people who have SLE. However, it is a very expensive therapy, and it is invasive (requiring the actual removal of blood from the body, filtering the blood, and then returning the filtered blood back into the body). Doctors prescribe it for rare complications of lupus where very large antibody molecules are causing problems. Cryoglobulinemia is a problem where large antibodies can clot up the blood and cause vasculitis (see chapter 11). Plasmapheresis is one of the best treatments for cryoglobulinemia as it can actually remove the dangerous cryoglobulin molecules from the person's body. Thrombotic thrombocytopenic purpura (see chapter 9) is another dangerous problem in lupus that can cause severe kidney and brain damage. Plasmapheresis is the treatment of choice for this condition. It may also be useful for pulmonary hemorrhage (see chapter 10), which can be a deadly complication from lupus. Small studies suggest it may be helpful in cases of severe antiphospholipid syndrome and neuropsychiatric lupus. A small 2012 study suggested that it may also be helpful in preventing congenital heart block in women who have lupus who are SSA or SSB antibody positive. Otherwise it is used rarely.

*Generic available*: Not applicable.

*How plasmapheresis works*: Plasmapheresis removes antibodies (including lupus auto-antibodies) and other large molecules from the blood, including dangerous substances such as cryoglobulins.

*What benefits to expect from plasmapheresis*: Can be lifesaving for people who have cryoglobulinemia, thrombotic thrombocytopenic purpura, or pulmonary hemorrhage.

*How plasmapheresis is performed*: Blood is removed using a thin, sterile rubber tube from a vein; the blood circulates through a machine that filters the blood, then it is returned back through another vein.

*If you miss a dose of your medicine*: Not applicable.

*Alcohol/food/herbal interactions with plasmapheresis*: Not applicable.

*Potential side effects of plasmapheresis*: Plasmapheresis is given to very sick lupus patients who are in the hospital. Doctors and nurses monitor the patient very closely during the treatment. Potential side effects are looked for by the staff and dealt with appropriately if they occur (table 35.6). Plasmapheresis removes many medicines from the body (such as azathioprine and cyclophosphamide). Therefore, many lupus medicines should be given to the patient again soon after the procedure is done. Prednisone and other steroids (which are smaller molecules) are not affected.

*What needs to be monitored while getting plasmapheresis*: Blood pressure and a chemistry panel.

*Reasons not to take plasmapheresis (contraindications or precautions)*: If your blood pressure is low.

*While taking plasmapheresis*: You will be monitored very closely by the plasmapheresis personnel.

*Pregnancy and breast-feeding while taking plasmapheresis*: May be needed during pregnancy for life-threatening lupus conditions. It may increase the risk for premature delivery and other pregnancy complications; however, severe SLE is usually more dangerous for the pregnancy than the plasmapheresis is.

Breast-feeding is not a concern.

*Geriatric use of plasmapheresis*: No different from other age groups.

**Table 35.6**  Potential Side Effects of Plasmapheresis

|  | *Incidence* | *Side Effect Therapy* |
|---|---|---|
| **Nuisance side effects** | | |
| Mild infusion reactions | Common | Dealt with by the infusion staff. |
| Removal of some medicines out of your system | Common | Some of your medicines are dosed again after plasmapheresis. |
| **Serious side effects** | | |
| Low blood pressure | Common | Dealt with by the infusion staff. |
| Shortness of breath | Common | Dealt with by the infusion staff. |
| Low calcium and potassium levels | Common | Dealt with by the infusion staff. |
| Increased bleeding | Uncommon | Dealt with by the infusion staff. |
| Increased infections | Uncommon | Treat infection. |
| Severe allergy (anaphylaxis) | Uncommon | Dealt with by the infusion staff. |

Side effect incidence key (approximations, as side effects can vary widely study to study): rare < 1% occurrence; uncommon 1%–5% occurrence; common > 5% occurrence

1. Dapsone is a medication used to treat leprosy that can sometimes be useful in some people who have lupus, especially those who have the cutaneous lupus called bullous lupus.

2. Dapsone can also be used as an antibiotic to prevent pneumocystis pneumonia in lupus patients who receive very strong immunosuppressant medicines such as cyclophosphamide.

3. Dapsone can potentially cause hemolytic anemia; therefore, a complete blood cell count must be checked regularly while taking it.

4. Thalidomide can help severe cases of cutaneous lupus that do not respond to the usual therapies.

5. Thalidomide can potentially cause severe birth defects. Two simultaneous forms of birth control must be used while taking thalidomide if you have not gone through menopause.

6. The prescribing of thalidomide is very tightly controlled through a program called S.T.E.P.S., which is run by the drug company Celgene Corporation.

7. Danazol is a male-type hormone (androgen) that can be helpful for some lupus problems, especially low platelet counts.

8. Danazol can potentially cause male characteristics such as a deep voice, acne, excessive hair growth on the face, and decreased menstruation.

9. DHEA is a type of steroid converted in the body to male sex hormones. SLE patients typically have low levels of DHEA in their bodies.

10. DHEA therapy can potentially increase energy levels, help with mild lupus problems, and increase bone density. It can help decrease the need for prednisone.

11. DHEA bought off the shelf is unreliable as far as quality. It is best to get it from a compounding pharmacist using a prescription from your doctor.

12. IVIG is rarely used in lupus, but may be used to prevent infections in those who are deficient in IgG immunoglobulins (called hypogammaglobulinemia) and in those who have a severe nerve problem called chronic inflammatory demyelinating polyneuropathy, or CIDP.

13. Plasmapheresis is a very complicated treatment where large molecules are filtered from the blood.

14. Plasmapheresis is reserved for critically ill lupus patients, especially those who have cryoglobulinemia, thrombotic thrombocytopenic purpura, or pulmonary hemorrhage.

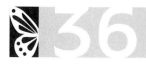

# Prescription Pain Medicines

### Use of Pain Killers in SLE

Most people who have systemic lupus erythematosus (SLE) have joint pain or arthritis. Chapter 7 provides numerous recommendations on how people can help their own aches and pains. Reread that chapter if pain is a significant problem for you. However, sometimes these measures are not enough, and some people need stronger, prescription pain relievers. This chapter discusses the stronger pain medicines that doctors prescribe to help decrease pain.

### Non-Steroidal Anti-Inflammatory Drugs (NSAIDs)

NSAIDs (pronounced IN-saydz or IN-sĕdz) comprise the largest group of medications used for the aches and pains of SLE. They are also used to treat the inflammation and pain of serositis (such as pleurisy and pericarditis). There are many different NSAIDs available by prescription (table 36.1). Some of the NSAIDs have slight advantages and disadvantages compared to the others, so the pros and cons of each NSAID are also listed where appropriate.

*Generic available*: Yes, for many.

*How NSAIDs work*: NSAIDs are weak anti-inflammatory medications. In other words, they appear to decrease inflammation but only slightly. They inhibit an enzyme in the body that is responsible for producing chemical substances called prostaglandins; therefore, less prostaglandins are formed. Prostaglandins are important in causing inflammation, but they also have essential roles in keeping the body healthy (such as protecting the stomach, stabilizing blood pressure, regulating kidney function, helping the platelets of the blood work normally, and many others). Due to most NSAIDs decreasing the production of many different types of prostaglandins (good and bad), not only can they help with pain and inflammation but they can also cause side effects (such as stomach ulcers, high blood pressure, kidney failure, bleeding, and many others).

The low doses of NSAIDs obtained over the counter probably have minimal, if any, anti-inflammatory effects. NSAIDs have two closely related effects. They have analgesic (pain-relieving) properties, which occur even in smaller doses. The amount of analgesic effect tends to parallel the dose taken. In other words, high doses tend to decrease pain more than lower doses. For pain relief, it is better to take the lowest dose needed to decrease the potential of side effects that are more apt to occur at higher doses. However, to help with inflammation (the anti-inflammatory effects of NSAIDs), they need to be taken at high doses on a regular basis. They tend to take anywhere between one to three weeks (when taken at a high dose regularly) to achieve their full anti-inflammatory effects. Therefore, for pain due to significant lupus inflammation (such as pleurisy or inflammatory arthritis), your doctor will probably ask you to take your NSAID at a high dose on a regular basis (instead of just as needed).

Not all NSAIDs work in everyone. One NSAID may work very well in one person, and not at all in another. Therefore, your doctor may need to have you try more than one NSAID to figure out which one is best for you. In addition, NSAIDS need to be used regularly for a few weeks before you know if a particular NSAID will work or not. Just trying an NSAID as needed or just for a few days is insufficient.

*What benefits to expect from NSAIDS*: Decreased pain and fever.

*How NSAIDs are taken*: NSAIDs come in pill, capsule, liquid, and topical forms. They all come in different doses and different dosing schedules. Some can conveniently be taken once a day (e.g., Celebrex, meloxicam, piroxicam, etodolac extended release, Naprelan, EC-Naprosyn, Voltaren-XR, ketoprofen extended release), which can help a lot with compliance (i.e., not missing any doses when compared to a two- or three-times-a-day NSAID).

If you take a daily aspirin to prevent heart attacks and strokes, check with your doctor, as the combination of aspirin and an NSAID increases the risk for ulcers. If you are given permission to take them together, make sure to take the aspirin first thing in the morning, and wait at least two hours before you take either naproxen or ibuprofen. If you take the NSAID earlier than that, it negates the blood-thinning properties of the aspirin. You want the aspirin to thin the blood to prevent heart attacks and strokes. Doctors have studied this so far only with naproxen and ibuprofen; it is probably a good idea to take all NSAIDs at least two hours after your daily aspirin due to this possible interaction.

*If you miss a dose of your medicine*: If you miss a dose of your NSAID, in general, skip that dose and take the next regularly scheduled dose. However, since the NSAIDs come in so many different dose forms, this may not apply to all of them. Check with your prescribing physician.

*Alcohol/food/herbal interactions with NSAIDs*: Avoid alcohol with NSAIDs, as it can increase the risk for developing stomach ulcers.

NSAIDs are best taken with food to decrease stomach upset.

Avoid alfalfa, anise, bilberry, bladderwrack, bromelain, cat's claw, celery, chamomile, coleus, cordyceps, dong quai, evening primrose, fenugreek, feverfew, garlic, ginger, ginkgo biloba, ginseng (American, Panax, Siberian), grape seed, green tea, guggul, horse chestnut seed, horseradish, licorice, meadowsweet, motherwort, prickly ash, red clover, reishi, SAMe (S-adenosylmethionine), sweet clover, tamarind, turmeric, and white willow (all have additional anti-platelet activity).

*Potential side effects of NSAIDs*: In general, NSAIDs are safe to take by most people. However, in people who are at increased risk for stomach ulcers, kidney problems, heart problems, and strokes, there can be an increased chance of these problems occurring (table 36.2). NSAIDs should not be taken by people who have some forms of kidney disease, uncontrolled high blood pressure, active stomach ulcers, a history of recurrent strokes and heart attacks, severe liver disease, or congestive heart failure.

Table 36.1  Prescription NSAIDs

*Non-Acetylated Salicylates*

diflunisal

Pros: Less likely to cause stomach ulcers than other NSAIDs. Does not inhibit platelet function. Generic available.

Cons: Weaker pain relief and anti-inflammatory properties than other NSAIDs.

choline magnesium trisalicylate

Pros: Less likely to cause stomach ulcers than other NSAIDs. Does not inhibit platelet function. Generic available. Available in liquid form.

Cons: Weaker pain relief and anti-inflammatory properties than other NSAIDs.

salsalate

Pros: Less likely to cause stomach ulcers than other NSAIDs. Does not inhibit platelet function. Generic available.

Cons: Weaker pain relief and anti-inflammatory properties than other NSAIDs.

*COX-2 Inhibitors*

celecoxib (Celebrex)

Pros: Less chances for stomach ulcers. Does not inhibit platelet function. Safer than other NSAIDs when taken with blood thinners. May be taken once a day.

Cons: 50% of people who are allergic to sulfa antibiotics may get a rash. No generic form as of 2013.

meloxicam (Mobic)

Pros: The 7.5-mg tablet has much less chance of causing stomach ulcers. Does not inhibit platelet function. Available in liquid form. Taken once a day. Inexpensive generic form is available.

Cons: Otherwise similar to other NSAIDs.

*Nonspecific (COX-1 and COX-2) NSAIDs*

diclofenac (Voltaren-XR, Cambia, Cataflam, Zipsor, Arthrotec, Voltaren gel, Pennsaid, Flector patch)

Pros: Comes in tablets, capsules, oral liquid, rectal suppository, topical gel, topical patch, and topical drops forms. Generic available. Arthrotec contains the anti-ulcer medicine misoprostol to decrease the chances of getting ulcers. Voltaren-XR is taken once daily. Cambia is a powder that can be mixed in water to drink; it is flavored with mint and black licorice (anise).

Cons: Increased risk of liver inflammation. Liver blood tests (AST/ALT) should be checked every three months. The topical forms (gel and liquid drops) must be used four times a day regularly to be effective.

etodolac

Pros: Available only as generic.

Cons: Similar to other NSAIDs.

fenoprofen (Nalfon)

Pros: Generic is available.

Cons: Usually needs to be taken three to four times daily.

ibuprofen (Motrin, Duexis)

Pros: Generic is available. Low doses available over the counter (Advil, Midol, Motrin IB). Available as tablet, capsule, caplet, gelcap, oral liquid.

Cons: Must be taken three to four times a day for full anti-inflammatory effects. Can interfere with the stroke and heart attack protection effects of low-dose aspirin. Should be timed to take at least two hours after your daily aspirin.

indomethacin (Indocin)
> Pros: Comes in oral liquid; available as generic.
> Cons: Has an increased risk for side effects compared to many other NSAIDs. Should be avoided by older individuals. More commonly causes headaches and difficulty with thinking compared to other NSAIDs.

flurbiprofen
> Pros: Comes in generic form.
> Cons: Otherwise similar to other NSAIDs.

ketoprofen
> Pros: Available as a once-a-day extended-release form.
> Cons: Must be taken three to four times a day for its full anti-inflammatory effects when it is not the extended-release form tablet.

ketorolac
> Pros: Given by injection for fast pain relief followed by oral tablets.
> Cons: Otherwise similar to other NSAIDs.

meclofenamate
> Pros: Available only as generic.
> Cons: Otherwise similar to other NSAIDs.

mefenamic acid (Ponstel)
> Pros: Generic form available.
> Cons: Must be taken every four hours for full effect. Usually only prescribed for one week.

nabumetone (Relafen)
> Pros: Available only as generic. Can be taken once a day. Causes less platelet dysfunction than many other NSAIDs. There may be fewer ulcers compared to some NSAIDs.
> Cons: Otherwise similar to other NSAIDs.

naproxen (Naprosyn, EC-Naprosyn, Naprelan, Anaprox, Vimovo)
> Pros: Available as generic. Available in lower doses over the counter (Aleve, Midol Extended Relief, Pamprin ALL DAY). Available in an enteric-coated form that may be easier on the stomach. Comes in caplet, capsule, oral liquid, gelcap, and tablet forms. Available in slow-release forms (EC-Naprosyn and Naprelan). Vimovo contains the anti-ulcer medication esomeprazole (a proton pump inhibitor) that decreases the risk for stomach ulcers.
> Cons: Interferes with the heart attack and stroke protection benefits of aspirin. Should be taken two hours after your daily aspirin dose to minimize this effect. Vimovo, Naprelan, and EC-Naprosyn do not come in a generic form as of 2013.

oxaprozin (Daypro)
> Pros: Can be taken once a day.
> Cons: Otherwise similar to other NSAIDs.

piroxicam (Feldene)
> Pros: Taken once a day.
> Cons: Otherwise similar to other NSAIDs.

sulindac (Clinoril)
> Pros: Similar to other NSAIDs.
> Cons: Similar to other NSAIDs.

tolmetin
> Pros: Available only as generic.
> Cons: Must be taken three times a day for its full anti-inflammatory effects.

Other people should be monitored more carefully when they take these medicines, including those who have high blood pressure, those who have a history of a heart attack or stroke, those who have diabetes, those who have had stomach ulcers, and older people.

Some potential problems from NSAIDs can be dealt with to decrease their chances from occurring. For example, people who are at increased risk for stomach ulcers (table 28.4) can do things to avoid ulcers from NSAIDs (table 28.5). If you are at increased risk of having an ulcer, then you should discuss these options with your doctor.

*What needs to be monitored while taking NSAIDs*:

- Blood tests for kidney function, liver function tests, and blood counts
- Blood pressure

*Reasons not to take NSAIDs (contraindications or precautions)*:

- If you have decreased kidney function.
- If you have severe liver disease with decreased liver function.
- If your blood pressure is not under good control.
- If you have ever had congestive heart failure.
- If you have an active stomach ulcer. If you have had an ulcer in the past, you should take an anti-ulcer medicine with it to decrease stomach acidity.
- If you have an upcoming surgery (so that you do not bleed too much during surgery). Celebrex, meloxicam, and non-acetylated salicylates, however, do not interfere with platelet function.
- If you have had severe allergic reactions to other NSAIDs or aspirin products.
- If you have a type of aspirin sensitivity that causes nasal polyps and asthma.
- Check with your doctor first, especially if you have high blood pressure, diabetes, heart problems, or a history of stroke or heart attacks, or if you are on blood thinners (such as Plavix, Coumadin, or heparin).

*While taking NSAIDs*:

- Contact your physician immediately if you throw up blood, develop abdominal pain, have bloody stools, or develop black tarry stools (melena). These could be warning signs for a bleeding ulcer. Remember, though, that most people have no preceding stomach upset or pain from a bleeding ulcer from NSAIDs.
- Contact your doctor if you develop heartburn, diarrhea, constipation, rash, elevated blood pressure, shortness of breath, yellowish-colored whites of eyes (jaundice), or swelling of the ankles.
- Let any dentist or surgeon know you are on an NSAID before a dental procedure or surgery. You may need to stop the NSAID beforehand. Celebrex, meloxicam, and the non-acetylated salicylates do not prevent platelets from working properly.
- Let any doctor know you are on an NSAID before prescribing something for pain. The doctor needs to ensure the new pain medicine does not contain an NSAID.

**Table 36.2**  Potential Side Effects of NSAIDs

| | Incidence | Side Effect Therapy |
|---|---|---|
| **Nuisance side effects** | | |
| Heartburn, nausea, and stomach pain | Common | Take with food, or discuss with your doctor to either try a different NSAID or take a medicine to decrease stomach acidity. |
| Cramping or diarrhea | Common | Take with food, reduce dosage, or switch to a different NSAID. |
| Increased bleeding and bruising | Common | Usually no treatment needed for bruises; stop NSAID for actual bleeding. |
| Fluid retention, ankle swelling (edema), weight gain | Common | Decrease salt intake, take a fluid pill (diuretic), or stop medicine. Contact your doctor. |
| Headache, drowsiness, dizziness, difficulty concentrating | Common | Try a different NSAID. Occur more commonly with indomethacin. |
| Elevated liver enzyme blood tests | Common | Usually minimal problems. Your doctor may continue NSAID, decrease dose, or change to a different NSAID. |
| Ringing in the ears or decreased hearing | Uncommon | Discontinue NSAID. |
| Rash | Uncommon | Stop NSAID. |
| **Serious side effects** | | |
| Elevated blood pressure | Common | Stop NSAID, lower dose, or change to a different NSAID. |
| Gastritis, esophagitis, stomach ulcers | Common | Stop NSAID and take medicine to decrease stomach acidity. |
| Bleeding ulcers (bloody stools, vomit blood, or have black tarry stools) | Common | Seek medical attention immediately. Discontinue NSAID and take medicine to decrease stomach acidity. |
| Decreased kidney function | Common | Discontinue NSAID. |
| Allergic reaction, anaphylaxis | Rare | Seek medical attention immediately. |
| Hepatitis (liver inflammation, damage) | Rare | Stop NSAID. |
| Worsening of aspirin-sensitive asthma | Uncommon | Treat asthma. Stop medicine. |
| Decreased blood counts | Rare | Discontinue NSAID. |

Side effect incidence key (approximations, as side effects can vary widely study to study): rare < 1% occurrence; uncommon 1%–5% occurrence; common > 5% occurrence

• Let any doctor know you are on an NSAID before prescribing anything to ensure there are no drug interactions.

• Do not take two or more NSAIDs. The only exception is if your doctor gives you approval to take an NSAID with low-dose aspirin (used to prevent heart attacks and strokes). Make sure to ask your doctor to consider giving you a medicine to decrease acidity of the stomach if you take aspirin plus another NSAID to prevent stomach ulcers. Take your NSAID at least two hours after you take your daily aspirin to ensure the NSAID does not interfere with the helpful effects of the aspirin.

*Pregnancy and breast-feeding while taking NSAIDs*: It is reassuring that a 2012 report showed no increased risks of major fetal malformation from NSAIDs. This study looked at a total of 109,544 pregnancies between 1998 and 2009 of which 5,267 women were taking NSAIDs.

If you have trouble getting pregnant (infertility), consider not taking NSAIDs, which may decrease fertility. There was a 2011 report from Canada that suggested that NSAIDs might increase the risk for miscarriage if taken during the first twenty weeks of pregnancy. However, an editorial about the study criticized the study's findings and pointed out some important flaws of the study. Until known for sure, if you do not absolutely need to take an NSAID during the first twenty weeks, it is probably best not to do so.

NSAIDs should not be taken at week 30 of pregnancy or later to prevent a problem called patent ductus arteriosus (a problem where a very important blood vessel does not close properly in the baby's heart and lung circulation). Many doctors recommend not taking NSAIDs during the third trimester entirely.

Diflunisal, salsalate, ketoprofen, flurbiprofen, oxaprozin (Daypro), diclofenac (Cataflam, Cambia, Zipsor, Voltaren-XR, Arthrotec), etodolac, sulindac (Clinoril), meloxicam (Mobic), meclofenamate, or nabumetone should not be taken while breast-feeding.

Caution is recommended when breast-feeding while taking choline magnesium trisalicylate or celecoxib (Celebrex) by their manufacturers.

Ibuprofen (Advil, Motrin, and Nuprin), indomethacin (Indocin), ketorolac, mefenamic acid (Ponstel), naproxen (Naprosyn, EC-Naprosyn, Naprelan, and Aleve), tolmetin, and piroxicam (Feldene) are considered by the American Academy of Pediatrics to be safe and "compatible" for use while breast-feeding.

*Geriatric use of NSAIDs*: Older people have a much higher chance for side effects such as elevated blood pressure, ulcers, kidney failure, heart failure, and heart attacks from NSAIDs and should not take them unless approved by their physician.

*What to do with NSAIDs at the time of surgery*: It is always best to double-check with your rheumatologist and surgeon regarding specific instructions. Most people should stop their NSAID before surgery. In general, they should be stopped around three days before surgery. One exception is ibuprofen (Motrin, Advil), which is usually safe to stop twenty-four hours before surgery.

Theoretically, the non-acetylated salicylates (such as salsalate and choline magnesium trisalicylate) as well as the COX-2 inhibitors (Celebrex and meloxicam) can be continued up to the day before surgery, as they do not cause increased bleeding (they do not inhibit platelet function). However, they can potentially raise blood pressure and decrease kidney function (which would be undesirable during surgery). Therefore, many surgeons would rather have them stopped before surgery. One exception is that if these NSAIDs provide profound pain relief and if there is the chance of your having severe pain if you stop it, then it may be worth taking it up to the day of surgery. You should discuss this with your rheumatologist and surgeon.

Aspirin is a more complicated issue. If you are taking aspirin to prevent strokes, heart attacks, and blocked arteries and if you are at very high risk for this occurring during surgery, it may be better to continue taking aspirin up to the time of surgery. It is important to discuss this with your cardiologist, neurologist, or vascular doctor. On the other hand, some surgeries (such as brain, spine, inner ear, and retina surgery) have such a high risk for bleeding that aspirin should always be stopped. Aspirin usually does not have to be stopped for cataract or dental procedures. If you are told to stop aspirin, you should stop taking it seven to ten days before surgery to prevent excessive bleeding during and after surgery.

*Patient assistance program for NSAIDs*: For Celebrex www.celebrex.com. For Vimovo www.vimovo.com. For Duexis www.duexis.com. For Arthrotec www.arthrotec.com. Also see chapter 42.

*Drug helpline for NSAIDs*: Unaware of any.

*Website to learn more about NSAIDs*: For Celebrex www.celebrex.com. For Vimovo www.vimovo.com. For Duexis www.duexis.com. For Arthrotec www.arthrotec.com. Also: www.rheumatology.org/practice/clinical/patients/medications/nsaids.asp.

### KEY POINTS TO REMEMBER

1. Non-steroidal anti-inflammatory drugs are often called NSAIDs for short.

2. NSAIDs can be helpful to treat the arthritis and serositis problems of SLE.

3. Lower doses can help with mild and moderate discomfort.

4. To help with severe pain, or pain due to inflammation, NSAIDs usually do better when taken regularly on a set schedule; they can take one to three weeks to work.

5. Often one NSAID will work better in any particular person compared to another. Therefore, it can be helpful to try different ones until the best one is found. There is no way to predict ahead of time what NSAID will help which person.

6. Potential side effects of NSAIDs include stomach ulcers, high blood pressure, kidney problems, heart attacks, and strokes.

7. You should never take NSAIDs if your kidneys do not work properly, if you have had congestive heart failure, if you have an active stomach ulcer, if you have uncontrolled high blood pressure, or if you have severe liver damage (cirrhosis).

8. If you are at increased risk of having stomach ulcers (table 28.4), then you should do one of the things mentioned in table 28.5 to prevent ulcers from occurring.

9. You should get blood work done regularly for blood counts, kidney function tests, and liver function tests; you should also have your blood pressure checked regularly while taking an NSAID.

### Tramadol (Ultracet, Ultram, Ultram ER, Ryzolt, Rybix, and ConZip)

Tramadol is a pain reliever (analgesic) that does not have anti-inflammatory properties.

*Generic available*: Yes.

*How tramadol works*: Tramadol is an opioid pain reliever. Opioids work by attaching to opioid receptors on pain nerves, decreasing the pain messages sent to the brain. "Opioid" may sound familiar, as it comes from the word "opium," which is made from poppies. Opioids include narcotics such as heroin, morphine, hydrocodone, and oxycodone. However, tramadol is rarely ever addictive. There have been rare cases of addiction in people with previous addiction problems but this is uncommon. Tramadol also blocks the reuptake of both serotonin and norepinephrine, which helps to decrease pain (see the section on dual uptake inhibitors in chapter 27).

*What benefits to expect from tramadol*: A decrease in pain severity.

*How tramadol is taken*: The immediate-release forms (generic tramadol, Ultracet, Ultram, and Rybix) are generally taken three to four times a day. The extended-release forms (tramadol ER, Ultram ER, Conzip, and Ryzolt) are generally taken once a day. Rybix is an orally disintegrating form; therefore, it may be more desirable in people who have difficulty swallowing pills. Do not crush or bite tramadol ER or Ultram ER as these are extended-release forms. They would be absorbed too quickly and could potentially cause significant side effects if you crush or chew them. If you take the extended-release form, make sure to take it on a regular schedule and not just as needed.

*If you miss a dose of your medicine*: If you miss a dose of your tramadol immediate release, take the dose you missed as soon as you realize you missed taking it. Usually immediate-release tramadol is taken a similar number of hours apart from each other while you are awake, for example, you may take one or two tablets every six hours while you are awake (e.g., 8:00 AM, 2:00 PM, and 8:00 PM). If you realize at 10:00 AM that you missed your morning dose, take your next dose six hours later at 4:00 PM and then the last dose of the day six hours later at 10:00 PM. If it is too late in the day and past your bedtime to take the last dose, just skip the last dose and resume your regular dosing schedule the next day.

If you take the extended-release form tramadol ER or Ultram ER, take your dose as soon as you remember you missed it that day, then resume your usual dosing schedule the next day. If you do not realize you missed your dose until the next morning, do not try to make up for it by taking an extra dose. Just resume your usual dosing schedule. Consult with your prescribing physician as well to make sure these instructions apply to you, but these guidelines will suffice for most people taking tramadol.

*Alcohol/food/herbal interactions with tramadol*: Avoid alcohol, which can increase the side effects of tramadol.

The extended-release forms (tramadol ER, Ryzolt, and Ultram ER) are absorbed faster if taken with fatty food. Therefore, it is best to take them on an empty stomach to decrease the risk for side effects. The immediate-release forms and ConZip (a combination of immediate-release and extended-release in one capsule) are not affected by food.

Avoid chamomile, valerian, St. John's wort, kava kava, and gotu kola.

*Potential side effects of tramadol*: Potential side effects of tramadol are listed in

626

table 36.3. If you are taking the extended-release forms (tramadol extended release, Ultram XR, or Ryzolt), it is best to take the medicine on an empty stomach and avoid fatty foods after taking it to decrease the risk of side effects. Some people can develop withdrawal symptoms if they miss a dose or take a dose later than their usual scheduled time. Withdrawal symptoms include moodiness, depression, restlessness, difficulty sleeping, runny nose, teary eyes, chills, flu-like symptoms, joint and muscle pain, stomach upset, nausea, vomiting, diarrhea, repetitive yawning, and having goose bumps. If you develop withdrawal symptoms, it does not mean that you have a psy-

**Table 36.3** Potential Side Effects of Tramadol

|  | Incidence | Side Effect Therapy |
|---|---|---|
| **Nuisance side effects** | | |
| Drowsiness | Common | Decrease dose or stop it. Try taking it later in the day. |
| Insomnia | Common | Take your last dosage earlier in the day. |
| Nausea | Common | Decrease dose or stop it. |
| Itchiness | Common | Decrease dose or stop it. Can try an antihistamine such as Claritin or Alavert daily. |
| Constipation | Common | Consider taking something for constipation every day such as over-the-counter MiraLAX, Colace, or senna (Senekot). Decrease dose or stop it. |
| Dizziness | Common | Decrease dose or stop it. |
| Headaches | Common | Decrease dose or stop it. |
| Withdrawal symptoms if stopped abruptly (anxiety, stomach upset, pain, sweating, insomnia) | Common | Taper off tramadol slowly if you plan to stop taking it. Do not miss any doses or be late on any doses. |
| **Serious side effects** | | |
| Seizures | Rare | Seek immediate medical attention. |
| Serotonin syndrome (anxiety, agitation, difficulty thinking, increased sweating, feeling hot, increased heart rate, stomach upset, and muscle spasms) | Rare | Seek immediate medical attention. |

Side effect incidence key (approximations, as side effects can vary widely study to study): rare < 1% occurrence; uncommon 1%–5% occurrence; common > 5% occurrence

chological addiction, which is a different matter. Make sure not to miss any doses or be late on your doses if you develop withdrawal symptoms. If you develop withdrawal symptoms and you decide to come off the medicine, it is important to work with your doctor to taper off the medicine gradually.

All opioids can potentially cause insomnia because they can interrupt the brain's natural sleep cycle. If you develop a restless night's sleep after taking the immediate-release forms of tramadol, adjust your schedule to take the last dosage earlier in the day (e.g., no later than 5:00 PM if you go to bed at 10:00 PM).

*What needs to be monitored while taking tramadol*: No labs need to be monitored.

*Reasons not to take tramadol (contraindications or precautions)*:

- If you have a history of drug or alcohol abuse let your doctor know as you may have an increased risk for addiction.

- Should generally be avoided if you have ever had seizures.

- Usually lower doses are taken by people who have decreased kidney or liver function.

- Inform your doctor if you have been diagnosed with increased intracranial pressure (such as pseudotumor cerebri) or have had a brain injury.

*While taking tramadol*:

- Let your doctor know if you develop any side effects.

- Do not stop the medicine abruptly to avoid withdrawal symptoms.

*Pregnancy and breast-feeding while taking tramadol*: Crosses the placenta during labor and can cause seizures, withdrawal, and even death in the baby. Do not take during pregnancy.

Enters breast milk. Do not use while breast-feeding.

*Geriatric use of tramadol*: Causes increased side effects in older patients; therefore, usually lower doses are used.

*What to do with tramadol at the time of surgery*: It is important to get specific instructions from your surgeon and anesthesiologist. When tramadol is stopped, there is the risk for developing withdrawal symptoms. Your surgical team may need to give you an alternative around the time of surgery to prevent withdrawal symptoms and pain.

*Patient assistance program for tramadol*: www.access2wellness.com for Ultram and Ultracet. Also see chapter 42.

*Drug helpline for tramadol*: Unaware of any.

*Website to learn more about tramadol*: Unaware of any.

### KEY POINTS TO REMEMBER

1. Tramadol is an opioid that very rarely becomes addictive.

2. Tramadol should not be taken if you have had seizures before.

3. Drowsiness, nausea, itching, and constipation are the most common side effects.

4. Make sure to take the extended-release forms on an empty stomach to decrease the chances of side effects.

5. The extended-release forms need to be taken regularly on a set schedule and not just as needed.

## Scheduled Opioids

Opioids are drugs that have morphine-like activity. They can be extracted naturally from the opium poppy plant, or they can be produced synthetically in a laboratory. There are numerous opioid medications that are considered "scheduled" by the DEA (Drug Enforcement Administration) section of the U.S. Department of Justice. These are commonly called narcotics in non-technical language, and all of them can possibly cause addiction. However, in people who have risk factors for having bad side effects to other pain relievers (such as the NSAIDs and tramadol) they can be some of the safest pain relievers available when prescribed by an experienced physician. The most commonly prescribed scheduled opioids are listed in table 36.4.

Scheduled drugs are divided into five lists by the DEA, with schedule I drugs deemed the most addictive. The scheduled drugs with the higher numbers have decreasing addictive capabilities relative to their list number (i.e., schedule V drugs are the least addictive). Schedule I drugs are not felt to have any proven medical benefits and are commonly used recreationally (and illegally). These include drugs such as heroin, marijuana, Ecstasy, crack cocaine, PCP (angel dust), LSD, hallucinogenic mushrooms, and methamphetamine (crystal meth). While some of these may be approved for medical use by some physicians (including marijuana and Ecstasy), they are generally not felt by the U.S. government to be more beneficial than the side effects that they cause. Schedule II opioids are highly addictive and when taken regularly cause both physical and mental dependency. Schedule III drugs are less addictive (although they still carry that risk). No schedule IV or V opioid drugs are used to treat pain.

*Generic available*: Yes.

*How opioids work*: Opioids work by attaching to opioid receptors on pain nerves, decreasing the pain messages sent to the brain.

*What benefits to expect from opioids*: Opioids are generally potent pain relievers. The schedule II opioids (like morphine, oxycodone, and fentanyl) are the strongest pain relievers available to doctors to help with pain. Their pain-relieving properties are dependent on the dose, with higher doses relieving pain better than lower doses. The opioids that do not contain other medicines (such as Tylenol) can be used at any dose. However, the higher the dose, the higher the chances for side effects as well. Therefore, these medications are typically started out with a small dose. Doctors can slowly increase the dose over time if the medicine helps the person with pain without causing side effects. Some of the opioids work faster than others do. If side effects are encountered without significant pain relief, then it is better to gradually taper off the medication and try something different.

*How opioids are taken*: Opioids come in pill, oral liquid, oral dissolving, injectable, and topical patch forms. They are available in both immediate-release forms and

**Table 36.4** Scheduled Opioid Drugs

---

**Schedule II drugs**

codeine: Codeine by itself (as opposed to acetaminophen with codeine, such as Tylenol No. 3) is not recommended for long-term pain relief use because side effects often outweigh its potential pain-relieving properties.

fentanyl (Abstral, Actiq, Duragesic, Fentora, Onsolis, Lazanda, Subsys)

hydromorphone (Dilaudid-HP, Dilaudid, Exalgo)

levorphanol

meperidine hydrochloride (pethidine, Demerol)

methadone (Dolophine, Methadone Diskets, Methadone Intensol, Methadose)

morphine (Astramorph/PF, Avinza, Duramorph, Infumorph 200, Infumorph 500, Kadian, MS Contin)

oxycodone (Oxecta, OxyCONTIN, Roxicodone, Endocet, Magnacet, Percocet, Primlev, Roxicet, Tylox)

oxymorphone (Opana, Opana ER)

tapentadol (Nucynta, Nucynta ER)

**Schedule III drugs**

buprenorphine (Buprenex, Butrans)

codeine (Tylenol with Codeine No. 3, Tylenol with Codeine No. 4)

dihydrocodeine, acetaminophen, and caffeine (Trezix)

dihydrocodeine, aspirin, and caffeine (Synalgos-DC)

hydrocodone and acetaminophen (hycet, Lorcet, Lorcet Plus, Lortab, Margesic H, Maxidone, Norco, Stagesic, Vicodin, Vicodin ES, Vicodin HP, Xodol, Zamicet, Zolvit, Zydone)

hydrocodone and ibuprofen (Ibudone, Reprexain, Vicoprofen)

---

extended-release forms. People who have permanent joint or nerve damage who are expected to have persistent, chronic pain are often treated with an extended-release form (e.g., MS Contin, Avinza, Kadian, fentanyl patch, and OxyCONTIN) on a regular basis. Many pain specialists feel this approach is better than taking numerous doses of immediate-release forms of opioids in the setting of chronic pain. Doctors may prescribe immediate-release forms to take for "break-through" pain in addition to the extended-release forms.

The topical patch forms (such as fentanyl patch and Duragesic) can be applied anywhere on the body, with the upper chest wall and upper arms being the preferred areas. They do not need to be placed directly on the area of pain. In fact, the patches often are less effective if applied to an area of the body with thicker skin such as the back or knees. The opioid medicine in the patch is absorbed into the skin where it can dissolve into the blood vessels. The bloodstream then carries the opioids to the central nervous system (brain and spinal cord) where they help to decrease pain. Therefore, they work better when applied over thinner-skinned areas such as the chest and upper arms.

Never crush or chew the slow-release forms such as OxyCONTIN, Kadian, or Avinza; otherwise, you could develop severe, life-threatening side effects since a larger amount of the medicine would be absorbed at once.

*If you miss a dose of your medicine*: The immediate-release forms can be taken as needed if you are not physically addicted to the medicine. If you use an extended-release form (such as MS Contin, Avinza, Kadian, fentanyl patch, Duragesic, or OxyCONTIN), it is very important to take the medicine regularly as prescribed and never miss a dose. If you miss a dose, you are at risk of developing withdrawal side effects as discussed below. Check with your prescribing doctor for further instructions.

*Alcohol/food/herbal interactions with opioids*: Do not drink alcohol, which increases the risk of side effects such as drowsiness, accidents, respiratory depression (where you stop breathing), and even death. If you do elect to drink alcohol, make sure not to drink more than two servings within any twenty-four-hour period if your opioid also contains acetaminophen to decrease the risk of liver damage. See chapter 38 for the definition for one serving of alcohol.

Avoid taking immediate-release forms of morphine and oxycodone with fatty meals, which can increase the rate at which they are absorbed. The extended-release forms (Kadian, Avinza, MS Contin, and OxyCONTIN) as well as the other opioids are not affected by food.

Avoid chamomile, valerian, St. John's wort, kava kava, and gotu kola. These can increase the side effects of opioids.

*Potential side effects of opioids*: Common and important potential side effects of opioids are listed in table 36.5. Drowsiness, dizziness, difficulty thinking, moodiness, nausea, increased sweating, and difficulty urinating tend to be dose-related side effects, meaning they are more apt to occur at higher doses, and less so at lower doses. In addition, if they occur and are mild and tolerable when the medicine is first started and the person continues taking the medicine, these side effects often improve and can potentially resolve completely with continued use. Sometimes people can get itchy skin when they take opioids due to the release of histamine in the skin as a reaction to the medicine. Taking an antihistamine such as over-the-counter Claritin or Alavert daily can help to decrease this side effect. People with lung disease, especially emphysema, can have difficulty breathing; therefore, opioids need to be used with caution in this group of people.

Constipation can be a particularly difficult side effect. Constipation can even become severe, causing complete bowel obstruction and abdominal pain with nausea and vomiting. Constipation tends to affect those who have had a history of constipation and the elderly most often. This side effect usually does not improve over time with taking the opioid (as opposed to the other side effects listed previously). If you are prone to getting constipation, it is generally best to take something every day (such as over-the-counter senna, Colace, docusate, or MiraLAX) to prevent constipation in the first place instead of waiting for it to occur. If you develop constipation at all while taking opioids, you should also take something daily to prevent it. Other measures that are helpful in keeping constipation under control include exercising daily, staying active, drinking plenty of water to stay hydrated, and making sure to have a lot of fiber in

631

**Table 36.5** Potential Side Effects of Opioids

| | Incidence | Side Effect Therapy |
|---|---|---|
| **Nuisance side effects** | | |
| Constipation, bloating, stomach upset | Common | May need to take a daily anti-constipation medicine such as over-the-counter senna, Colace, or MiraLAX. Exercise regularly, eat extra amounts of roughage and fiber (fruits and vegetables), and drink plenty of water. |
| Nausea, vomiting | Common | May need to take an anti-nausea medicine or decrease the dose. |
| Itching | Common | Decrease the dose or take an antihistamine (Claritin, Alavert, Benadryl) regularly. |
| Muscle spasms | Uncommon | Reduce the dose of medicine or take muscle relaxants. |
| **Serious side effects** | | |
| Drowsiness and difficulty thinking | Common | Decrease the dose. |
| Withdrawal symptoms (discussed below) | Common | Do not be late on taking your medicine. Take your medicine as soon as you notice the symptoms. |
| Decreased production of sex hormones causing infertility, decreased libido, fatigue | Uncommon | Decrease the dose. |
| Difficulty breathing (respiratory depression) | Uncommon | Mainly a concern in the elderly or in those who have severe lung disease, especially COPD. Opioids need to be started in very low doses in these individuals. |

Side effect incidence key (approximations, as side effects can vary widely study to study): rare < 1% occurrence; uncommon 1%–5% occurrence; common > 5% occurrence

the diet from vegetables and fruits. If the constipation is uncontrollable on your own using these measures, make sure to see your physician as there is a prescription medication called Relistor (methylnaltrexone) that is used specifically for opioid-induced constipation.

Some of the most important potential side effects of the scheduled opioid medications are physical dependency and psychological addiction. These two terms mean very different things and should be differentiated from each other. Physical dependency is an expected side effect of these medications. Since physical dependency is a known and expected part of taking opioids, it is not a reason to stop the medicine when it develops. What it means is that the body becomes used to having the medication inside of it. If the medicine is stopped abruptly, the person goes through withdrawal symptoms. While withdrawal symptoms are very uncomfortable, they are usually not a dangerous thing for most people as long as they are not doing important activities (such as driving, using machinery, caring for others, etc.). However, in people who have heart problems, withdrawal symptoms can potentially be dangerous. Physical dependency usually occurs in people who are taking a medication such as an opioid on a regular basis. People who take one or two tablets infrequently usually do not become physically dependent.

The symptoms of withdrawal due to physical dependency include moodiness, depression, restlessness, difficulty sleeping, runny nose, teary eyes, chills, flu-like symptoms, joint and muscle pain, stomach upset, nausea, vomiting, diarrhea, repetitive yawning, and having goose bumps. Withdrawal can occur even if you are just slightly late in taking your medication. It is expected to occur if you abruptly stop your medicine. If you are trying to come off your medicine, it is very important to work very closely with your doctor and slowly decrease the dose of your medicine to reduce the chances of developing withdrawal symptoms. Some withdrawal symptoms can be decreased by taking other medications such as clonidine, diazepam, promethazine, or loperamide. These options can be discussed with your doctor as well.

When people describe their fear of taking an opioid because they are afraid of addiction, they are usually referring to psychological addiction. It is very important to understand that psychological addiction (which doctors do not want to occur) is very different from physical dependency (which is expected to occur). Psychological addiction is continuing to take the opioid despite the presence of opioid-induced problems and side effects. This includes the presence of what doctors call euphoria. Euphoria occurs when the medicine causes the person to feel an increased amount of excitement and happiness. This feeling can cause many people to develop the uncontrollable desire to keep taking the medication as an "escape" from the real world, including having to deal with a disease such as lupus. The opioid medications differ in how often they produce euphoria. The schedule II opioids are much more likely to cause it, and therefore are much more likely to cause addiction than are the schedule III opioids. However, they all can do it; there are many people who are addicted to schedule III medicines such as Vicodin, Lortab, or Lorcet. In January 2013, the FDA's Drug Safety and Risk Management Advisory Committee recommended that hydrocodone (Vicodin, Lortab, and Lorcet) be rescheduled as schedule II drugs. The FDA will most likely make this recommendation to the DEA, which will then decide whether to make this change or not.

People addicted to opioids lose their control over their use of the drugs. They may start to take extra doses (above what is prescribed); they may begin to use the drugs compulsively, crave them, or continue to use them even though they are causing side effects. Some signs of addiction include hoarding medicine while continuing to get the prescription filled (to use later), and getting into arguments with others over use of the opioid. Addicted people may neglect house/work/school responsibilities due to taking the medicine, or stop enjoyable activities or hobbies to take the medicine. They may become preoccupied with taking the medicine or use the medication up faster than prescribed. Addiction to opioids can often occur without people even realizing it. They may even convince themselves that they "need" the medicine for their health and pain, while they are really using it because of psychological addiction. This use of the drug due to addiction will often lead to problems with relationships with others who note the addiction, and this includes problems with their treating physicians who are trying to get them off the medication. Many do not realize they are even addicted until they are successfully taken off the medicine (they realize their addiction only retrospectively).

The potential for becoming psychologically addicted to opioids varies between people. People who have depression, bipolar disorder, post-traumatic stress disorder, anxiety, or who have suffered major trauma (such as having a history of sexual, physical, and mental abuse) can become addicted to opioids when they begin to use them to escape from their problems. Doctors often say the person is "self-medicating" when taken for these reasons. Another common way to become addicted is when people who began to use drugs (including tobacco and alcohol) while preteens or teens are prescribed opioids. It is felt that young people who smoke cigarettes, drink alcohol, and use other drugs before they are psychologically mature miss out on very important social milestones and do not learn proper social skills. Instead, they become reliant on drugs (such as tobacco, alcohol, illegal drugs, and opioids) to escape life or to "handle" problems in their life in an abnormal way.

Addiction also more commonly occurs in people who have a family history of alcoholism, drug addiction, depression, bipolar disorder, and other psychiatric disorders. This may represent learning the behavior socially from their family, or could potentially represent a genetic predisposition to drug dependency. In addition, addiction is more common in younger people (such as those age 45 years old and younger) compared to someone who is older and takes an opioid for the very first time. It is important that if you have any risk factors (table 36.6) for potentially becoming psychologically addicted to opioid medications that you inform your doctor before they are prescribed. In fact, the more of these risk factors that apply to you, the higher are your chances of becoming addicted to opioid medications. You can still get the medication if it is medically indicated. However, you and your doctor need to discuss ahead of time boundaries and warning signs to look out for so that addiction can be identified and dealt with early if it occurs.

One way to try to prevent side effects from taking opioids and to learn how to take them properly is to ask your doctor to give you a "pain contract" to read and sign. A good "pain contract" will list the side effects that opioids can cause, the withdrawal symptoms, and the rules you must follow to get your prescriptions. It should also spell out what the steps would be if psychological addiction were to occur. Reading the contract, signing it, and having a copy put into your chart (as well as your getting a copy to keep at home) can be very informative to you and help protect both you and your prescribing doctor from the potential problems that these medications can cause. If you do develop any warning signs of psychological addiction (table 36.7), it is very important that you discuss it with your doctor sooner rather than later. The longer you allow addiction to go on unrecognized and untreated, the harder it is to overcome. In addition, if your doctor, a family member, or a friend mentions the possibility that you are addicted, instead of becoming angry and denying it, look at this table and see if any of these things apply to you. If they do, then you most likely are addicted and just

**Table 36.6** Risk Factors for Developing Psychological Addiction to Opioid Medications

- Age 45 years old or younger

- A history of smoking cigarettes or drinking alcohol while still a teenager

- Any history of excessive alcohol use (including weekend binging or having a blackout)

- Any history of illegal drug use

- Any history of abusing any type of prescription medication

- A family history of psychiatric disorders, alcoholism, or drug abuse

- A history of sexual abuse

- A history of physical abuse or mental abuse

- A history of depression, bipolar disorder, or other psychiatric disorders

- A stressful or chaotic life

had not realized it. If you do become psychologically addicted, you can be treated with medications that can help you get off the medicine. In addition, psychological treatment is sometimes needed to help with other addictive issues (such as dealing with stress and past traumatic events).

Many opioid preparations include acetaminophen (Tylenol). Sometimes you can tell if an opioid has acetaminophen in it by the abbreviation APAP occurring in the name, for example, hydrocodone/APAP contains the opioid hydrocodone as well as acetaminophen. APAP is the abbreviation for N-acetyl-para-aminophenol, which is the chemical name of acetaminophen. However, some preparations with a brand name, such as Vicodin, Lorcet, Lortab, and Percocet, are not as easy to figure out. It is important to know whether an opioid contains acetaminophen or not to ensure that you do not take too much acetaminophen (over the counter) for pain when taken along with the opioid prescription. Most people should restrict their total daily use of acetaminophen to no more than 4,000 mg a day, while some (the elderly and those who have severe kidney disease) may need to take 3,000 mg a day or less. You can tell how much acetaminophen is contained in each tablet of your opioid as follows: if it says hydrocodone/APAP or oxycodone/APAP (for example) and the dose is 5/325 mg, the first number is the number of mg of the hydrocodone or oxycodone (5 mg), while the second number is the amount of APAP (acetaminophen) in each tablet (325 mg). Currently, the amount of acetaminophen used in combination with opioids varies widely, and is as high as 750 mg in some tablet forms. However, beginning in 2014, the FDA has mandated that all opioids containing more than 325 mg of acetaminophen per tablet be removed from the market. After January 14, 2014, all opioid/APAP combinations will contain 325 mg of acetaminophen or less per dose to decrease the risks for side effects and overdosage.

Although the potential for addiction is a very real possibility with opioids, it is very important to remember that they can also be some of the safest medications to use in some people for their pain. In people who are at high risk for side effects to the NSAIDs

**Table 36.7**  Signs of Psychological Addiction to Opioid Medications

- Craving the medication
- Becoming preoccupied about when you are going to take your next dose or get your next prescription
- Taking more of the medication than is prescribed
- Losing control in taking the drug
- Giving up previously enjoyable activities or hobbies to use the drug
- Neglecting work, home, or school responsibilities
- Arguing with others about using the medicine
- Having legal troubles related to using the drug
- Wanting to use the drug even though it is causing side effects
- Using up your medicine faster than prescribed
- Using the medication recreationally to "feel good"
- Using the medicine to escape from stress or to help you sleep
- Getting opioids filled by more than one doctor
- Using more than one pharmacy to fill your opioids
- Altering the prescription to get a higher dose or more tablets
- Hoarding some of your pills to use at a later time

and other pain relievers, they can be very helpful and safe. This includes older people and people who have problems such as kidney disease, liver disease, active stomach ulcers, heart disease, or uncontrolled high blood pressure.

*What needs to be monitored while taking opioids*: See your doctor frequently to make sure you are not having any of the side effects or evidence of addiction, as discussed above. Occasionally read over table 36.7 to ensure you are not developing any signs of psychological addiction.

*Reasons not to take opioids (contraindications or precautions)*: If you are at high risk of developing addiction (table 36.6). If you have severe lung disease such as COPD (chronic obstructive pulmonary disease), it is important to start off at very low doses. Do not drive, use machinery, or work in high places when you initially start the medicine. After a while, when your body becomes used to the medicine, then it usually is safe to do these things as long as you are not having side effects (discuss with your doctor). If you cannot stop drinking alcohol, do not take opioids.

*While taking opioids*: Tell your doctor if you develop any of the side effects or signs of addiction discussed above. Before having surgery, always inform your surgeon and anesthesiologist that you take the opioid so that proper precautions are taken to prevent withdrawal.

*Pregnancy and breast-feeding while taking opioids*: It is best to avoid opioids during pregnancy as they can cause physical dependency in newborns and even cause them to not breathe when they are born. The baby can develop withdrawal side effects such as crying, diarrhea, fever, irritability, tremors, vomiting, and even stroke.

The American Academy of Pediatrics lists codeine (Tylenol No. 3, Tylenol No. 4), fentanyl (Abstral, Actiq, Duragesic, Fentora, Onsolis), morphine (Astramorph/PF, Avinza, Duramorph, Infumorph 200, Infumorph 500, Kadian, MS Contin), meperidine (Demerol), and methadone (Dolophine, Methadone Diskets, Methadone Intensol, Methadose) as being safe and "compatible" with breast-feeding. The other opioids should be avoided while breast-feeding.

*Geriatric use of opioids*: Opioids can be some of the safest medicines to use for pain in older people due to their increased chances of developing kidney problems, stomach ulcers, high blood pressure, heart attacks, and strokes if they take an NSAID for pain. However, they are also at increased risk of side effects of opioids such as difficulty thinking, drowsiness, falls, and constipation. It is best to start out with a very small dose to decrease the chances for side effects.

*What to do with opioids at the time of surgery*: It is important to get specific instructions from your surgeon and anesthesiologist. When your opioid is stopped, there is the risk for developing withdrawal symptoms. Your surgical team may need to give you an alternative around the time of surgery to prevent withdrawal symptoms and pain.

*Patient assistance program for opioids*: See chapter 42.

*Drug helpline for opioids*: Unaware of any.

*Website to learn more about opioids*: Unaware of any.

### KEY POINTS TO REMEMBER

1. Scheduled opioid medications are called narcotics; they work like morphine.

2. These drugs can potentially become habit forming. They are therefore "scheduled" by the DEA.

3. When taken regularly, scheduled opioids are expected to cause physical dependence where the person goes through withdrawal if the medicine is stopped abruptly or if a dose is not taken on time.

4. Symptoms of withdrawal due to physical dependence include moodiness, depression, restlessness, difficulty sleeping, runny nose, teary eyes, chills, flu-like symptoms, joint and muscle pain, stomach upset, nausea, vomiting, diarrhea, repetitive yawning, and having goose bumps.

5. If you have risk factors for developing psychological addiction (table 36.6), make sure to bring this up with your doctor before starting one of these medicines so that you can work together to ensure that you do not become addicted.

6. Make sure to ask your doctor for a "pain contract" before starting an opioid so that you know what the rules are for getting opioid prescriptions and what the steps are if addiction occurs.

7. If you develop any signs of addiction in table 36.7, make sure to let your doctor know right away so that the proper treatments for addiction can be started. The quicker this is done the easier it is to overcome.

8. If you develop constipation due to an opioid, it is generally best to take something every day (such as over-the-counter senna, Colace, docusate, or MiraLAX) to prevent constipation. Also make sure to exercise daily, stay active, drink plenty of water, and eat a diet containing lots of vegetables and fruits to control constipation.

9. The long-acting opioids (such as MS Contin, Avinza, Kadian, and fentanyl patch) need to be taken on a regular basis and on a set schedule. If they are stopped abruptly or a dose is taken late, withdrawal symptoms may occur.

10. Do not crush or chew long-acting opioids such as OxyCONTIN, MS Contin, Avinza, and Kadian.

11. Make sure to find out if your opioid contains acetaminophen (APAP). If it does, make sure that you do not take too much over-the-counter acetaminophen (Tylenol) along with your prescription opioid.

## Other Pain Medications

There are many other medications used to treat pain in people who have lupus. It is important to remember that the way we feel pain is by the pain nerves of the body sending messages up to the brain. Therefore, many medications that decrease the activity of nerves can also be effective pain relievers. Medications designed to treat depression and seizures are included in this category. They include antidepressants such as the tricyclic antidepressants, venlafaxine, and duloxetine (Cymbalta). In fact, Cymbalta has gone through the expensive hoops and necessary research to get its FDA-approved indication to treat chronic pain. The anti-seizure medicines pregabalin (Lyrica) and gabapentin (Neurontin) can also be helpful to treat pain. These medicines typically take longer to work than other pain medicines (such as NSAIDs and opioids). They generally need to be taken three to eight weeks to provide significant pain relief at any particular dose. If you do not feel that the medicine is working, do not stop taking it because your doctor may want to increase your dose when he or she sees you back at your next visit. These medicines are especially useful in lupus patients who have pain due to nerve damage or fibromyalgia. Since these medicines are also commonly used to treat the pain of fibromyalgia, they are discussed in detail in chapter 27.

### KEY POINTS TO REMEMBER

1. Some pain medicines are classified as antidepressants or anti-seizure medicines.

2. They work by decreasing the overactivity of the pain nerves of the body.

3. They usually take three to eight weeks to work.

4. They are often started at a low dose and increased slowly in dosage over time; therefore, do not stop the medicine if you think it is not working unless discussed with your doctor first.

# Future Treatments for SLE

## A Cure for Lupus Soon?

Down the line, we will be able to fashion new immune environments that may eliminate lupus. Not only will people who carry lupus genes be vaccinated to prevent the disease's activation, but gene therapies will become important . . . We may hope that, by the year 2020, some lupus can be prevented, no one will die from it, and treatment will be both effective and safe.

—Dr. Daniel Wallace, *The Lupus Book*, 5th edition

We are entering an era of unparalleled potential advancements in the treatment of lupus and similar disorders. The FDA approval of Benlysta in March 2011 showed that it is possible to do successful research on a lupus treatment and have it subsequently FDA-approved. This should open the doors for other companies and investors to try to do the same. There are multiple possible ways for doctors to try to control lupus better, and this chapter discusses those possibilities.

I would like to dedicate this chapter to LC and a few of my other lupus patients who are not responding to currently available lupus medicines, hoping that someday soon a therapy will be discovered that will work for them. I would also like to dedicate it to everyone who has lupus alive now and who will be born with the genes that can cause it in the future. I hope that a cure or preventative therapy will truly become available soon. I hope this book can someday just be sitting somewhere as a medical curiosity during a time when people who have lupus do not have to take medicines, do not have to get labs, and are able to live their lives to their fullest not having to worry about lupus at all.

••••

To understand what therapies may potentially treat or prevent or even (can we dare to hope?) cure lupus in the future, it is helpful to go over the current understanding of what causes lupus. A simplified version of the causes and problems of lupus is outlined in figure 37.1 (see also chapters 1, 3, and 4).

1. Lupus occurs in someone who is born with the genes that can cause the immune system to become overactive and cause lupus in the first place.

2. Research shows that factors (such as UVA-2 and UVB light, hormones, vitamin D deficiency, smoking, or a viral infection) must then act on the person to turn on these genes and cause the person to develop lupus.

3. Then members of the immune system (such as macrophages, B-cells, and T-cells) communicate with each other using cytokine messages to talk to each other and tell each other to become more active than normal.

4. The activated B-cells turn into more mature plasma cells that make the antibodies that attack the body (auto-antibodies).

Any of these areas can be potential targets in the treatment of lupus.

Therapies that are currently used to treat lupus and in which areas they exert their benefits are shown in figure 37.2. All people who have lupus should be using sunscreen regularly and protecting themselves from UVB and UVA-2 light. They should also not smoke cigarettes, and they should ensure that their vitamin D levels are normal by taking vitamin supplements. Taking the steroid (hormone precursor) DHEA may also help to decrease lupus activity. All people who have lupus should be taking an anti-malarial medication, such as hydroxychloroquine (Plaquenil); anti-malarials are the safest medicines to calm down the immune system and try to prevent severe lupus from attacking the internal organs. In people who have moderate to severe lupus, steroids, stronger immunosuppressants, and/or biologic agents may be needed.

Figure 37.3 shows the areas where future therapies could potentially be helpful. These include medications that are currently available for other disorders (e.g., abatacept and tocilizumab), therapies that are currently in the research stages (e.g., epratuzumab), as well as therapies that have a potential to help in the future (e.g., Dr. Wallace's wish for a vaccine to prevent lupus as mentioned in the epigraph to this chapter). This chapter discusses these therapies grouped into three categories (therapies currently available, therapies currently in studies seeking possible FDA approval, and therapies possible in the future).

Since I will be alluding to the different types of research studies (called clinical trials), I describe them briefly here. As mentioned in chapter 34, research studies for medicines seeking FDA approval for treating diseases go through three stages of clinical trials. Phase I trials look at side effects of the medication in humans as well as how it is dealt with by the body. Phase II trials look at how effective the medication is to treat the disease at various doses (while also looking at side effects). If the phase II clinical trials show promise, then much larger phase III studies are done with many more patients involved than were in the previous studies. The results of the phase III studies must show that the medication does help the disease for which it is being studied with the least amount of side effects possible.

## Therapies Currently Available and Being Studied for SLE

### Abatacept (Orencia)

Abatacept (pronounced AB-uh-TA-sept) is a biologic agent that was FDA-approved in December 2005 for the treatment of rheumatoid arthritis. As with other biologic agents (see chapter 33), it is expensive and is given by injection. In a 2012 report, a European group of lupus experts recommended using abatacept for difficult to treat arthritis and serositis in SLE patients.

Abatacept has been studied in several phase II clinical trials in the treatment of SLE. The first one was finished in 2010; 118 SLE patients were given abatacept and 57

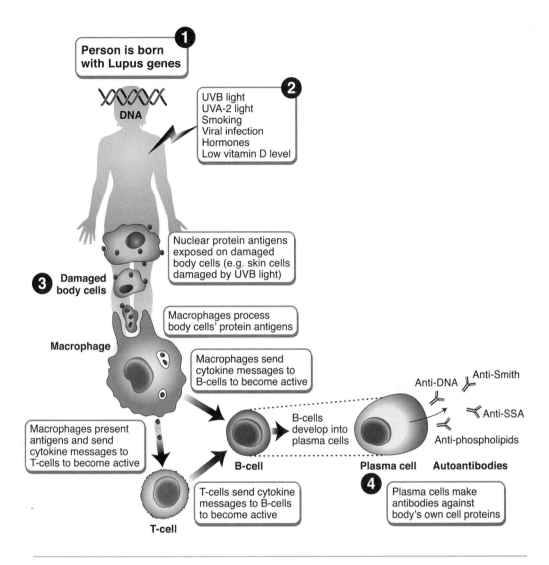

Figure 37.1 How lupus occurs

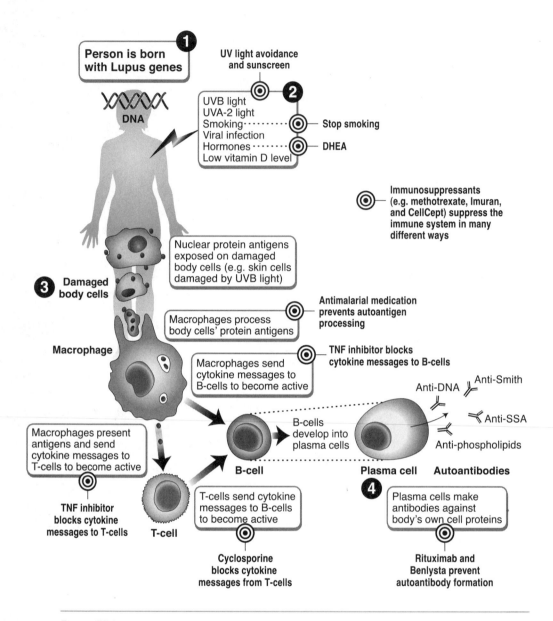

Figure 37.2 Current therapies to treat lupus

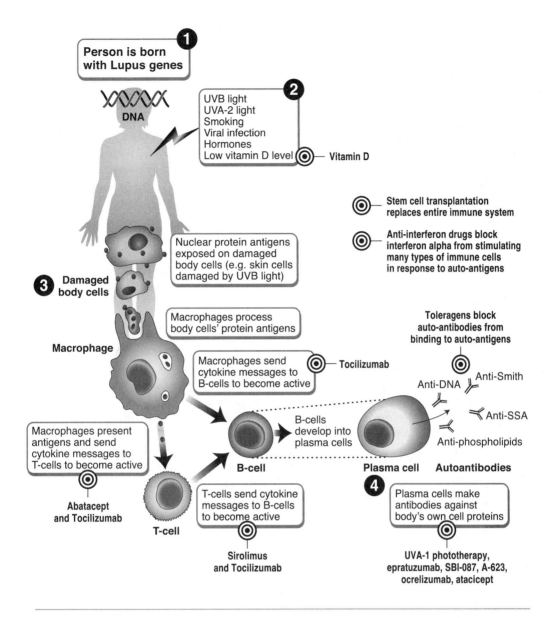

Figure 37.3 Where future therapies may help lupus

received placebo. The patients were treated with 30 mg a day of prednisone for one month while they received abatacept. Then the prednisone was tapered down while the research doctors looked at what percentage of patients flared during the following year. It primarily looked at patients who had pleurisy, arthritis, and cutaneous lupus.

The effects of abatacept did not show any significant difference set up by the very strict standards of the study. However, there was a trend for less severe flares in the group who took abatacept, especially in those who had arthritis. For example, when the doctors were asked which lupus patients had a flare at each visit, over the course of a year, 83% of the patients who took placebo had a flare, while only 64% of those who were treated with abatacept had a flare.

Currently (as of February 2013), there is one phase II study using abatacept in combination with cyclophosphamide in the treatment of lupus nephritis, and there are plans to begin a phase III trial using it in combination with mycophenolate mofetil (CellCept). In 2012, a phase II study using it with CellCept for lupus nephritis was terminated early due to the medication not being shown to be effective. However, as we learned in chapter 34, this does not necessarily mean that abatacept does not work in SLE. Doctors are still waiting to find out exactly what the results showed as well as the reasons that it was felt to be ineffective.

*Generic available*: No.

*How abatacept works*: Abatacept interferes with how white blood cells of the immune system, called antigen-presenting cells, interact with T-cells. Macrophages are one example of antigen-presenting cells (figure 37.3). Abatacept stops the macrophages from telling the T-cells to become more active. Therefore, it can help decrease how many B-cells are told to make more lupus auto-antibodies to attack the body.

*What benefits to expect from abatacept*: Unknown yet. May possibly be helpful with lupus arthritis and serositis (such as pleurisy).

*How abatacept is taken*: Abatacept is given by IV (intravenous) and under the skin (subcutaneous or SQ) injections. One method is to receive an IV infusion of abatacept every two weeks three times in a row followed by an IV infusion every four weeks after the first three infusions. Each infusion takes about thirty minutes. Another method is to receive just one IV infusion followed by a SQ injection the following day and then a SQ injection weekly after that. The patient can learn how to do the injection at home. Another method is to skip the IV infusions totally and just do one SQ injection a week; however, it may take longer for abatacept to work if done this way.

*If you miss a dose of your medicine*: Reschedule your missed dose as soon as possible, then reset your infusion schedule starting from that date. For example, if you are scheduled to get your monthly (every four weeks) IV infusion on January 2 and it has to be cancelled, if you reschedule it for January 10, then your next infusion should be 4 weeks after January 10. Consult with your prescribing doctor to double-check these instructions, but these guidelines will suffice for most people.

*Alcohol/food/herbal interactions with abatacept:* No known interaction with alcohol. No known interaction with food.

Avoid Echinacea, which can increase immune system activity.

*Potential side effects of abatacept*: Just like with other biologic medications, the increased risk of infections is the most important potential side effect (table 37.1). It is important to be tested for TB infection before starting treatment with abatacept.

This can be done using the skin test (PPD) and/or a blood test (QuantiFERON and T-SPOT.TB).

In the SLE phase II clinical trial published in 2010, there was a significant increase in side effects in those who took abatacept (19.8% of patients) compared to only 6.8% of patients who received placebo. This potential higher rate of side effects in lupus patients needs to be considered. However, this was only one study; additional studies are needed.

In the rheumatoid arthritis studies using abatacept, patients who had chronic obstructive pulmonary disease (COPD) such as emphysema and chronic bronchitis appeared to have a higher chance for developing an exacerbation of their COPD, with increased coughing and shortness of breath.

As with all immunosuppressant medications, the possibility of developing cancer on abatacept must be considered. However, thus far, there has not been a statistically increased number of cancers compared to other people who have SLE and rheumatoid arthritis. This will need further long-term studies.

*What needs to be monitored while taking abatacept*: Nothing other than making sure you do not develop an infection.

**Table 37.1** Potential Side Effects of Abatacept

|  | *Incidence* | *Side Effect Therapy* |
|---|---|---|
| **Nuisance side effects** | | |
| Headache | Common | Take pain medicine. |
| Nausea | Uncommon | Take anti-nausea medicine. |
| Rash | Uncommon | Stop medicine. |
| Dizziness | Uncommon | Slow down infusion or stop medicine. |
| **Serious side effects** | | |
| Infection | Common | Treat infection. |
| Elevated blood pressure | Uncommon | Slow down infusion, treat with blood pressure medicine. |
| Infusion allergic reaction | Uncommon | Slow down infusion. Treat with appropriate medicines prescribed by your doctor. |
| COPD exacerbation | Uncommon | Treat COPD exacerbation. |
| Bowel perforation | Rare | Seek immediate medical attention. |

Side effect incidence key (approximations, as side effects can vary widely study to study): rare < 1% occurrence; uncommon 1%–5% occurrence; common > 5% occurrence

*Reasons not to take abatacept (contraindications or precautions)*: If you have chronic hepatitis B or have an active infection, you should not receive abatacept. You need to have a skin and/or blood test for tuberculosis (TB) prior to starting abatacept. If you have had TB in the past or have tested positive for TB, you need to let your doctor know before you start abatacept.

*While taking abatacept*: Practice all measures to prevent infections (table 22.1). Before having surgery, always ask your doctor well in advance if you should stop your medicine in preparation for the surgery or not. Do not get any live vaccines, including FluMist and Zostavax, while using abatacept.

*Pregnancy and breast-feeding while taking abatacept*: Do not get pregnant while using abatacept.

If you do get pregnant while taking your medicine, consider contacting the Organization of Teratology Information Specialists (OTIS) Autoimmune Diseases in Pregnancy Project at www.otispregnancy.org or 877-311-8972 or email otisresearch@ucsd.edu so that more can be learned about what happens when women on medications used in treating lupus become pregnant.

Do not use abatacept while breast-feeding.

*Geriatric use of abatacept*: Older patients appear to be at increased risk of developing infections with abatacept compared to younger patients.

*What to do with abatacept at the time of surgery*: It is always best to double-check with your rheumatologist and surgeon regarding specific instructions. A common recommendation is to not take abatacept for several weeks before surgery, then resume it once the surgical wound has healed and if there is no evidence for infection.

*Patient assistance program for abatacept*: Call 1-800-ORENCIA or go to www.Orencia.com. See chapter 42.

*Drug helpline for abatacept*: 1-800-ORENCIA.

*Website to learn more about abatacept*: www.Orencia.com and www.rheumatology.org/practice/clinical/patients/medications/abatacept.asp.

## Cholecalciferol (Vitamin D-3)

As mentioned in chapter 3, it appears that vitamin D is essential for proper functioning of the immune system. Vitamin D deficiency has been associated with the development of autoimmune diseases, including SLE. Studies have shown that patients who have severe SLE tend to have lower levels of vitamin D than patients who have milder disease. Currently there is one active phase II clinical trial looking at the effectiveness of vitamin D-3 in treating SLE. They are also testing the participants to see how it may affect interferon alpha levels in lupus patients. Interferon alpha is a cytokine in the immune system that increases inflammation and is found at higher levels in people who have SLE. Another study has recently been completed, but the results have not been reported yet; another one is being planned to look at its use in children who have SLE. Doctors look forward to learning these results.

*Generic available*: Yes, commonly found over the counter. However, a 2013 study showed that the quality of over-the-counter vitamin D-3 varies tremendously.

*How cholecalciferol works*: How vitamin D is important for proper immune system functioning is being investigated. The current active study is looking at its effects on the cytokine interferon alpha.

*What benefits to expect from cholecalciferol*: Normalization of vitamin D levels if you were low in vitamin D before starting it. This will increase your body's ability to absorb calcium and help to keep your bones strong. It is unknown if it decreases lupus disease activity or not.

*How cholecalciferol is taken*: In the phase II clinical trial it is being tested at 2,000 IU and 4,000 IU a day taken orally. It is commonly found over the counter in numerous doses, including 400 IU, 1,000 IU, 2,000 IU, 5,000 IU, 10,000 IU, and even 50,000 IU capsules. However, the quality of the over-the-counter brands varies a lot since the FDA does not regulate quality in these preparations.

*If you miss a dose of your medicine*: If you forget to take your dose, take it the same day.

*Alcohol/food/herbal interactions with cholecalciferol*: No known interactions with alcohol.

No known interactions with food.

Do not take Echinacea, which increases immune system activity.

*Potential side effects of cholecalciferol*: Significant side effects from taking cholecalciferol are rare (table 37.2). It is best to have your vitamin D levels monitored by your doctor while you take the supplement to ensure your levels do not go too high.

*What needs to be monitored while taking cholecalciferol*: Your calcium level and vitamin D level should be checked periodically.

*Reasons not to take cholecalciferol (contraindications or precautions)*: Do not take cholecalciferol if you have elevated vitamin D levels.

*While taking cholecalciferol*: Tell your doctor if you get abdominal pain in case this could be related to kidney stones. However, getting kidney stones from taking vitamin D-3 would be rare.

*Pregnancy and breast-feeding while taking cholecalciferol*: Only take during pregnancy if you have low vitamin D levels and are being monitored by your doctor.

Do not use during breast-feeding unless you have low vitamin D levels and are being monitored by your doctor.

**Table 37.2** Potential Side Effects of Cholecalciferol

|  | Incidence | Side Effect Therapy |
|---|---|---|
| **Nuisance side effects** | | |
| Nausea, stomach upset | Uncommon | Decrease your dose. |
| **Serious side effects** | | |
| High calcium levels | Uncommon | Decrease your dose. |
| High vitamin D levels | Uncommon | Decrease your dose. |

Side effect incidence key (approximations, as side effects can vary widely study to study): rare < 1% occurrence; uncommon 1%–5% occurrence; common > 5% occurrence

*Geriatric use of cholecalciferol*: Used commonly in older people due to their having a higher chance of being vitamin D deficient and as part of the treatment of osteoporosis (see chapter 24).

*What to do with cholecalciferol at the time of surgery*: Can be taken up to the day before surgery.

*Patient assistance program for cholecalciferol*: This can be obtained at low costs especially when bought in bulk at large discount stores.

*Drug helpline for cholecalciferol*: None.

*Website to learn more about cholecalciferol*: None I am aware of.

## Sirolimus (Rapamycin, Rapamune)

Sirolimus is an FDA-approved medication to prevent organ transplant rejection. Three other medications commonly used to treat SLE were also originally designed as medications to prevent organ transplant rejection: azathioprine (Imuran), cyclosporine (Sandimmune, Neoral), and mycophenolate mofetil (CellCept).

Sirolimus is manufactured by Pfizer and there are currently two active phase II clinical trials using it in SLE. A phase II trial was completed in 2012 assessing how well it works for membranous lupus nephritis (WHO V nephritis), but these results have not been reported yet.

*Generic available*: No.

*How sirolimus works*: Sirolimus inhibits the activation of T-cells of the immune system.

*What benefits to expect from sirolimus*: Hopefully to decrease lupus disease activity.

*How sirolimus is taken*: Sirolimus is being studied at the dose of 2 mg orally a day in two of the studies, while using blood drug levels to help adjust the dose in another trial.

*Alcohol/food/herbal interactions with sirolimus*: No interactions with alcohol known.

Do not eat grapefruit or drink grapefruit juice. High-fat meals change the way it is absorbed; therefore, it is best to take it consistently either with or without food (depending on which you tolerate best) to get a consistent result and to minimize variability.

Avoid St. John's wort (it decreases sirolimus's blood levels); cat's claw and Echinacea (they stimulate the immune system); alfalfa, aloe, bilberry, bitter melon, burdock, celery, damiana, fenugreek, garcinia, garlic, ginger, ginseng (American), gymnema, marshmallow, and stinging nettle (they can potentially cause low glucose [sugar] levels when taken with sirolimus).

*Potential side effects of sirolimus*: Sirolimus is an immunosuppressant medication (just like the other transplant rejection medicines); therefore, increased infections or malignancies as well as decreased blood counts are some of the potential side effects (table 37.3). Just as with cyclosporine, it can increase the blood pressure.

*What needs to be monitored while taking sirolimus*: You will need regular blood tests for blood counts, kidney function tests, and liver function tests. Your blood pressure will also need regular monitoring. Sometimes drug levels are checked as well.

*Reasons not to take sirolimus (contraindications or precautions)*: Do not take sirolimus if you have an active infection, open sore, open surgical wound, or elevated blood pressure, or if your kidneys do not work normally.

**Table 37.3** Potential Side Effects of Sirolimus

|  | Incidence | Side Effect Therapy |
|---|---|---|
| **Nuisance side effects** | | |
| Edema | Common | To be determined by the research doctors. |
| Acne | Common | To be determined by the research doctors. |
| Headache | Common | To be determined by the research doctors. |
| Insomnia | Common | To be determined by the research doctors. |
| Pain | Common | To be determined by the research doctors. |
| High cholesterol levels | Common | To be determined by the research doctors. |
| Stomach upset, constipation, diarrhea, nausea | Common | To be determined by the research doctors. |
| Elevated liver enzymes | Uncommon | To be determined by the research doctors. |
| **Serious side effects** | | |
| High blood pressure | Common | To be determined by the research doctors. |
| Infections | Common | To be determined by the research doctors. |
| Anemia, low platelet counts, low white blood cell counts | Common | To be determined by the research doctors. |
| Decreased kidney function | Common | To be determined by the research doctors. |

Side effect incidence key (approximations, as side effects can vary widely study to study): rare < 1% occurrence; uncommon 1%–5% occurrence; common > 5% occurrence

*While taking sirolimus*: Do not take your sirolimus if you have an active infection. See your doctor or go to an emergency room immediately if you have any symptoms of possible infection such as fever, pain with urination, increased urinary frequency, cough, a sore throat, or painful red skin. Practice all measures to prevent infections (table 22.1).Do not get live vaccines such as FluMist or Zostavax while taking sirolimus.

*Pregnancy and breast-feeding while taking sirolimus*: Do not get pregnant while taking sirolimus. Continue using effective birth control measures for three months after stopping sirolimus.

If you do get pregnant while taking your medicine, consider contacting the Organization of Teratology Information Specialists (OTIS) Autoimmune Diseases in Pregnancy Project at www.otispregnancy.org or 877-311-8972 or email otisresearch@ucsd .edu so that more can be learned about what happens when women on medications used in treating lupus become pregnant.

Do not breast-feed while taking sirolimus.

*Geriatric use of sirolimus*: Older people are probably at increased risk for getting side effects such as infections and decreased kidney function while taking sirolimus.

*What to do with sirolimus at the time of surgery*: It is always best to double-check with your rheumatologist and surgeon regarding specific instructions. A common recommendation is to not take sirolimus for several weeks before surgery, then resume it once the surgical wound has healed and if there is no evidence for infection.

*Patient assistance program for sirolimus*: Call 1-866-364-1297 or go to www.Rapamune .com. Also see chapter 42.

*Drug helpline for sirolimus*: None.

*Website to learn more about sirolimus*: www.Rapamune.com.

## Stem Cell Transplant after High-Dose Cyclophosphamide

This is a very aggressive, radical form of treatment and is only performed in highly specialized medical centers. This has generally been tried on people who had very severe SLE who had failed the usual treatments, including cyclophosphamide. One form of treatment is where the doctors remove cells from the person's bone marrow that are able to develop into mature immune cells. These cells are called stem cells. Then the person receives high doses of chemotherapy in the form of cyclophosphamide (other studies have used rituximab and fludarabine) that are intended to completely kill all mature cells of the immune system. The person's original stem cells are returned to the bone marrow so that they can multiply and make a brand new immune system. The doctors hope that the new immune system cells will not make the lupus auto-antibodies that attack the body. Approximately 40% of the patients did go into remission; however, there were high rates of infections and death. The patients who died in the studies were already very sick with multiple organs doing poorly.

Another related type of treatment used stem cells (immature cells that can produce mature immune system cells) obtained from umbilical cords (from newborn babies). Researchers call these cells umbilical mesenchymal stem cells. Some early case reports show some satisfactory early results when used in patients who had severe lupus who did not respond to usual treatments such as cyclophosphamide.

There are currently several stem cell transplant studies being done in patients who have SLE using these various methods.

*Generic available*: Not applicable.

*How stem cell transplantation works*: Completely obliterates the person's immune system in the hopes that a brand new one can take over where the lupus is not active and does not make auto-antibodies to attack the person's body.

*What benefits to expect from stem cell transplantation*: Improvement of the lupus and hopefully remission.

*How stem cell transplantation is taken*: Discussed above.

*If you miss a dose of your medicine*: Not applicable.

*Alcohol/food/herbal interactions with stem cell transplantation*: Alcohol and food not applicable.

Do not take Echinacea, which can increase immune system activity.

*Potential side effects of stem cell transplantation*: Potential side effects of stem cell transplantation are listed in table 37.4.

Table 37.4  Potential Side Effects of Stem Cell Transplantation

|  | Incidence | Side Effect Therapy |
| --- | --- | --- |
| **Serious side effects** | | |
| Infection | Common | Treat infection. |
| Death | Common | Not applicable. |

Side effect incidence key (approximations, as side effects can vary widely study to study):
rare < 1% occurrence; uncommon 1%–5% occurrence; common > 5% occurrence

*What needs to be monitored while taking stem cell transplantation*: Only done in specialized centers. Patients stay in the hospital for a long time in special areas using highly sophisticated anti-infection techniques.

*Reasons not to take stem cell transplantation (contraindications or precautions)*: If you do not have severe, life-threatening lupus not responding to other available therapies.

*While taking stem cell transplantation*: Patients are monitored very closely in all aspects by hospital staff.

*Pregnancy and breast-feeding while taking stem cell transplantation*: Do not get pregnant.

Do not breast-feed.

*Geriatric use of stem cell transplantation*: Not studied.

## Tocilizumab (Actemra)

Tocilizumab (pronounced toe-sĭ-LĬZ-ooh-mab) is a biologic agent FDA-approved to treat rheumatoid arthritis in January 2010. It works by preventing the cytokine (a chemical message given off by immune cells to talk to each other) called interleukin-6 (IL-6 for short). IL-6 is released by macrophage cells and T-cells of the immune system to cause more inflammation and more immune system activity. SLE patients have higher levels of IL-6 than normal; therefore, a very early phase I clinical trial was performed in sixteen patients who had SLE. Tocilizumab showed significant improvements in the patients who had SLE and decreases in their anti-DNA levels (anti-DNA levels tend to correlate with lupus disease activity). All seven patients who had lupus arthritis had significant improvements in their arthritis. These are very encouraging results. Although these results suggest that further studies should be done, to my knowledge, there are no current active studies looking at the use of tocilizumab in SLE.

*Generic available*: No.

*How tocilizumab works*: Tocilizumab prevents IL-6 (an inflammatory cytokine) from stimulating cells of the immune system.

*What benefits to expect from tocilizumab*: Decreased lupus activity. May particularly be helpful in people who have lupus arthritis.

*How tocilizumab is taken*: In the phase I trial it was given intravenously (IV) every two weeks. However, for rheumatoid arthritis it is given every four weeks.

*If you miss a dose of your medicine*: Reschedule your missed dose as soon as possible, then reset your infusion schedule starting from that date. For example, if you are scheduled to get your monthly (every four weeks) IV infusion on January 2 and it has to be cancelled, if you reschedule it for January 10, then your next infusion should be four weeks after January 10. Consult with your prescribing doctor to double-check these instructions, but these guidelines will suffice for most people.

*Alcohol/food/herbal interactions with tocilizumab*: Alcohol and food not applicable. Do not take Echinacea.

*Potential side effects of tocilizumab*: The most common side effects are low white blood cell counts, elevated cholesterol levels, and elevated liver enzymes (ALT and AST) on the blood work (table 37.5). It is important to be tested for TB infection before starting treatment with tocilizumab. This can be done using the skin test (PPD) and/or a blood test (QuantiFERON and T-SPOT.TB).

*What needs to be monitored while taking tocilizumab*: Blood counts, liver enzyme blood tests, and cholesterol are checked frequently.

*Reasons not to take tocilizumab (contraindications or precautions)*: If you have had a demyelinating neurological disease such as Guillain-Barré syndrome, multiple sclerosis, optic neuritis, or chronic inflammatory demyelinating polyneuropathy (CIDP), do not take tocilizumab, which may worsen these conditions. If you have chronic hepatitis B or have an active infection, you should not receive tocilizumab. You need to have

**Table 37.5** Potential Side Effects of Tocilizumab

|  | *Incidence* | *Side Effect Therapy* |
|---|---|---|
| **Nuisance side effects** | | |
| Elevated cholesterol levels | Common | Treat with cholesterol-lowering medicines. |
| Elevated liver enzymes | Common | Decrease dose or stop medicine. |
| **Serious side effects** | | |
| Low white blood cell count | Common | Decrease the dose or stop if severe. |
| Infections | Common | Treat infection. |
| Infusion allergic reaction | Common | Treat the reaction. Slow down the rate of infusion. May need to stop medicine if severe. |
| Low platelet counts | Uncommon | Decrease dose or stop medicine if severe. |
| Intestinal perforation | Rare | Seek emergency medical attention for severe abdominal pain. |

Side effect incidence key (approximations, as side effects can vary widely study to study): rare < 1% occurrence; uncommon 1%–5% occurrence; common > 5% occurrence

a skin and/or blood test for tuberculosis (TB) prior to starting tocilizumab. If you have had TB in the past or have tested positive for TB, you need to let your doctor know before you start tocilizumab.

*While taking tocilizumab*: Do not take tocilizumab if you have an active infection. Practice all measures to prevent infections (table 22.1). Before having surgery, always ask your doctor well in advance if you should stop your medicine in preparation for the surgery or not. Do not receive live vaccines such as FluMist or Zostavax while using tocilizumab. If you develop severe abdominal pain, seek medical attention immediately as intestinal perforation has been reported rarely.

*Pregnancy and breast-feeding while taking tocilizumab*: Do not get pregnant.

If you do get pregnant while taking your medicine, consider contacting the Organization of Teratology Information Specialists (OTIS) Autoimmune Diseases in Pregnancy Project at www.otispregnancy.org or 877-311-8972 or email otisresearch@ucsd .edu so that more can be learned about what happens when women on medications used in treating lupus become pregnant.

Do not breast-feed.

*Geriatric use of tocilizumab*: Older patients have a higher chance of developing infections while using tocilizumab.

*What to do with tocilizumab at the time of surgery*: It is always best to double-check with your rheumatologist and surgeon regarding specific instructions. A common recommendation is to not take tocilizumab for several weeks before surgery, then resume it once the surgical wound has healed and if there is no evidence of infection.

*Patient assistance program for tocilizumab*: Call 1-866-681-3261 or go to www.Actemra .com. See chapter 42.

*Drug helpline for tocilizumab*: 1-800-228-3672.

*Website to learn more about tocilizumab*: www.Actemra.com and www.rheumatology .org/practice/clinical/patients/medications/tocilizumab.asp.

## UVA-1 Phototherapy

No one who has lupus should ever sunbathe outdoors or use a sun-tanning booth. Ultraviolet B (UVB) and ultraviolet A-2 (UVA-2) light activates the immune system in people who have lupus and can potentially cause severe disease activity, including kidney disease and brain disease. However, it appears that a small section of ultraviolet light called ultraviolet A-1 (UVA-1) may be beneficial for lupus (figure 38.1). This was initially discovered by Dr. Hugh McGrath Jr., a rheumatologist, who after experimenting with UV light on lupus cells in Petri dishes, noted that mice that had lupus that were exposed to UVA-1 light did better (i.e., lived longer) compared to mice that had lupus exposed to other parts of UV light. Subsequent U.S. and European studies in humans who had lupus showed disease activity decreased substantially without any significant side effects. In particular, UVA-1 light alleviated one of the more common and difficult problems that people who have lupus face: fatigue. Studies have also shown decreased levels of some auto-antibodies. Amazingly, every study using UVA-1 phototherapy on lupus patients has shown beneficial results.

There are several theories why UVA-1 light may help people who have lupus even though UVA-2 and UVB light are dangerous. UVA-2 and UVB light have similar effects on the body. They interact with the DNA and other proteins inside of cells close to the skin surface. This causes the skin cells to release DNA, proteins, and antigens from within their nuclei to the outer surfaces of the membrane of the cells where they can interact with the autoantibodies of lupus. This exposure causes the immune system to become more active. UVA-1 light, however, does not interact harmfully with the cells of the skin. Instead, it penetrates deeper into the tissues of the skin along with the deep blood vessels they contain to affect the white blood cells of the immune system itself.

One big problem with the immune system is some immune cells appear to live on for much longer periods than they should. Normally in the body, when any cell has completed its mission (whether it is a cell of the skin, muscle, kidney, immune system, etc.) it dies through a process called apoptosis. In apoptosis, the cell is internally programmed to "die" when it has completed its job. UVA-1 light appears to encourage this process naturally in such a way that it simply "kills off" the older, unneeded immune cells. Other cells of the body neatly dismantle and reuse individual parts of these "killed" cells for regeneration of other cells and for energy use.

In SLE, there is a problem with apoptosis. Many immune system cells, such as the B-cells that make the bad auto-antibodies that attack the body in lupus, lack this ability for apoptosis. They continue to live and continue to make dangerous auto-antibodies that encourage disease activity. Because lupus immune cells have receptors for the UVA-1 light's photons (which carry the wavelengths' energy), it appears UVA-1 light may actually encourage apoptosis in immune system cells, causing them to appropriately quiet down, stop working, and be broken down and neatly packaged for reuse elsewhere. The result is a quieter, less dangerous immune system.

UVA-1 light also appears to stimulate DNA repair inside of cells. This is opposite of what occurs with UVA-2 and UVB light, which actually damages DNA inside of cells. UVA-1 light has also been shown to decrease cytokines known to cause inflammation such as interferon-alpha, interferon-gamma, tumor necrosis factor-alpha, and ICAM-I. Due to this multitude of beneficial effects, UVA-1 light is already used to treat some skin diseases such as morphea, scleroderma, mastocytosis, and mycosis fungoides.

So if this therapy appears to be so effective and so safe, why isn't it being used and why don't most rheumatologists know about it? First, most doctors who treat lupus have an immediate negative gut reaction to the term "ultraviolet light." Very few, if any, rheumatologists are well versed in the field of physics and light chemistry. They do not know or understand the differences between different wavelengths of ultraviolet light. Rheumatologists are conditioned early in their training to keep their patients away from all UV light.

Second, no one knows what the potential long-term effects are. For example, could long-term exposure to even pure UVA-1 light cause an increase in skin cancer? Only long-term studies could adequately answer this question. Many who study UVA-1 light feel that it may not cause skin cancer, and there has never been a case of skin cancer reported from exposure to UVA-1 light, despite its use at much higher doses to treat certain autoimmune skin disorders than is required to treat lupus. Still, UVA-1's role, if any, in the development of melanoma or other cancers in humans is unknown. Lastly, few pure UVA-1 phototherapy machines are available for clinical use in the United States. Some of those available emit higher doses of UVA-1 light than is recommended for the treatment of lupus. They are also very expensive (and large) pieces of equipment to buy. At the current time, insurance does not pay for this type of treatment for lupus patients. Therefore, for a doctor to own a UVA-1 phototherapy unit and use it on patients, he or she would have to have a lot of patients who are willing to pay out of pocket for the treatment to come close to covering the office's cost of purchasing, operating, and maintaining the equipment.

Still, some people who have lupus have actually developed their own home UVA-1 phototherapy equipment (as described in the book *Lupus Underground* by Anthony DeBartolo). UVA-1 light is composed of a short wavelength spectrum of light that is directly adjacent to those of UVA-2 and UVB light. It is essential to ensure the equipment uses only UVA-1 light to prevent severe flares of lupus. Such home equipment is not yet commercially available.

By the way, if you are interested in UVA-1 phototherapy, please do not attempt to do so without professional help. For example, do not use a black light (which contains both UVA-1 and UVA-2 waves) or a commercial UVA light unless proven to only have UVA-1 light. Also, do not use sunblock that only blocks UVB rays (in the hopes that you will only get UVA light exposure) because sunblock creams still allow all types of UV light to contact the skin (including UVB light). In addition, if you are fortunate enough to be close to a medical facility that offers UVA-1 phototherapy, make sure that you work with someone who has experience with lupus. UVA-1 light therapy should be done in very small doses, as opposed to the high doses used for other skin diseases.

Currently, the Department of Dermatology at the University of Texas Southwestern Medical Center in Dallas, Texas, is performing a clinical trial using UVA-1 phototherapy for cutaneous lupus.

*Generic available*: Not applicable.

*How UVA-1 phototherapy works*: See above.

*What benefits to expect from UVA-1 phototherapy*: Overall decreased lupus activity, including reduced joint pain, reduced inflammation, reduced fever, reduced morning stiffness, improved cognitive function, and decreased photosensitivity. Improvements in fatigue and energy level may particularly be noted.

*How UVA-1 phototherapy is taken*: The current study at Southwestern Medical Center is using a low dose of 20 J/cm2 UVA-1 three times a week for less than thirty minutes at a time.

*Alcohol/food/herbal interactions with UVA-1 phototherapy*: No known interactions with food or alcohol.

Herbal supplements that contain photosensitizing substances, such as St. John's wort, if taken at high doses may promote minor skin burning and damage. Avoid Echinacea, which can increase immune system activity.

*Potential side effects of UVA-1 phototherapy*: The only side effect noted in lupus studies is transient, mild pink coloration of the skin (table 37.6). The primary medical concern would be long-term effects, especially as to whether it could increase the chances for developing skin cancer. Any patient who uses UVA-1 phototherapy should have yearly skin exams by a dermatologist.

*What needs to be monitored while taking UVA-1 phototherapy*: Your physical exam and lupus labs should be monitored frequently by your doctor. You should see a dermatologist yearly for skin examinations to ensure no skin cancer occurs.

**Table 37.6** Potential Side Effects of UVA-1 Phototherapy

|  | Incidence | Side Effect Therapy |
|---|---|---|
| **Nuisance side effects** | | |
| Pink skin coloration | Common | No treatment needed. |

Side effect incidence key (approximations, as side effects can vary widely study to study): rare < 1% occurrence; uncommon 1%–5% occurrence; common > 5% occurrence

*Reasons not to take UVA-1 phototherapy*: Do not use if you have a history of skin cancer.
*While taking UVA-1 phototherapy*: See your lupus doctor regularly.
*Pregnancy and breast-feeding while taking UVA-1 phototherapy*: No known effect.
*Geriatric use of UVA-1 phototherapy*: Unknown.

## Therapies Currently in Studies Seeking Possible FDA Approval for SLE

The following are some of the medications that are currently being studied in patients with SLE. They are listed by the way in which they work.

### B-Cell Depleters and Modulators

B-cells are the cells of the immune system that make the auto-antibodies that attack the person's own body in lupus. These drugs either decrease the number of B-cells in the immune system or decrease their activity. Drugs currently available that work in this manner include belimumab (Benlysta) and rituximab (Rituxan).

*Epratuzumab.* Epratuzumab finished phase II clinical trials in 2010 with impressive results. It is given by IV infusion every one to two weeks and is manufactured by the pharmaceutical company UCB, Inc. It showed decreased disease activity, less flares, improvements in quality of life, and the ability to decrease steroid doses. It was particularly helpful in patients who had lupus involvement of the heart, lungs, brain, and nerves. This is exciting because especially brain and nerve involvement from SLE can be some of the most challenging aspects of the disease to treat. As with other biologic agents, infusion allergic reactions and infections were the most common side effects observed, but they were not much more numerous than those that occurred with placebo. Phase III clinical trials are currently being conducted. Epratuzumab may become one of the next approved medications for SLE if the preliminary trial results are reproduced in the phase III trials.

*SBI-087.* This medication is manufactured by Pfizer and completed phase I clinical trials primarily focusing on side effects in 2012. It is given by subcutaneous injection. Pfizer has not released the results of this trial yet.

*Ocrelizumab.* Ocrelizumab by Genentech works similarly to rituximab (Rituxan). In 2009, the largest studies on this drug were discontinued due to significant infections occurring in patients. However, some patients who had lupus nephritis who were also receiving mycophenolate mofetil (CellCept) responded well and tolerated it. There is currently a phase III trial using ocrelizumab in treating lupus nephritis.

*Atacicept.* Atacicept by EMD Serono decreases the activity levels of mature B-cells, therefore decreasing the production of antibodies (and therefore hopefully the production of the dangerous auto-antibodies of lupus). A phase II study using it in combination with mycophenolate mofetil (CellCept) to treat lupus nephritis was terminated due to increased problems with infections. In contrast, the earlier phase I study showed that it was well tolerated when used without mycophenolate mofetil. Phase II and phase III clinical trials using it in SLE patients who did not have severe kidney or nervous system disease to evaluate its effect on lupus flares were completed in 2012. The results have not been disclosed as of February 2013.

*Tabalumab (LY2127399).* Tabalumab neutralizes B-cell activating factor (BAFF) to decrease the activation of B-cells. It is produced by Eli Lilly & Company. Initial studies have shown that it decreases the number of B-cells and appears to decrease lupus activity. It is currently in phase III studies.

*Blisibimod.* Blisibimod is being studied by Anthera Pharmaceuticals. A phase II trial has been completed and a phase III trial has been planned. It interferes with the maturation of B-cells in the hopes that they will produce less lupus autoantibodies. It is administered subcutaneously (SQ) either once a week or once a month in the studies.

## Anti-Cytokine Therapies

These biologic medications prevent cytokines (the chemical messages that immune cells send to each other to make each other more active or less active) from influencing cells of the immune system. The goal is to decrease the activity of the cytokines that cause increased immune activity and inflammation. Examples of anti-cytokine therapies that have already been discussed are the tumor necrosis factor (TNF) inhibitors (see chapter 33) and Actemra (mentioned previously in this chapter). Currently interferon (especially interferon alpha) appears to be an exciting, potentially promising cytokine to block. People who have more lupus disease activity have higher amounts of interferon alpha, which leads to increased inflammation and tissue damage in the body. Since interferons are important for protecting the body from viral infections and cancers, these possible side effects (viral infections and cancer) will require close monitoring during the studies.

*Rontalizumab (NNC 0152).* This anti-interferon biologic agent is produced by Genentech and is currently in phase II clinical trials for moderate to severe SLE. It is being studied as a subcutaneous (SQ) as well as an intravenous (IV) medication.

*Sifalimumab (MEDI-545).* This anti-interferon biologic agent is produced by MedImmune and is currently in phase II studies for SLE. It is given intravenously (IV).

*MEDI-546 (Anti-Interferon).* This is another anti-interferon biologic agent produced by MedImmune in partnership with AstraZeneca and is currently in phase II studies for SLE. Instead of directly binding to interferon, as Sifalimumab does, MEDI-546 binds to the interferon receptors of white blood cells to prevent the overproduced interferon molecules of SLE from causing the immune system to become overactive. Both subcutaneous and intravenous forms are being investigated.

*AMG 811 (Anti-Interferon).* This anti-interferon biologic agent is produced by Amgen and is currently in very early phase I clinical trials for SLE, lupus nephritis, and discoid lupus. It is in early phase I studies.

*PF-04236921 (Anti-IL6).* This potential therapy acts by inhibiting IL-6 (similar to tocilizumab discussed earlier in this chapter). It is produced by Pfizer and the name of the study is aptly called the BUTTERFLY study.

*Anti-Macrophage Migration Inhibitory Factor (Anti-MIF).* This potential therapy blocks the activity of macrophages and monocytes (types of white blood cells) that help to cause inflammation and body damage in patients who have SLE. It is produced by Baxter Healthcare Corporation and is currently in phase I trials.

*PD-0360324 (Anti-Macrophage Colony-Stimulating Factor).* This potential therapy also blocks the activity of macrophages and monocytes to see if it can decrease inflammation in lupus. It is being studied in people who have discoid lupus and subacute cutaneous lupus who have failed anti-malarial therapies (such as Plaquenil). It is given intravenously every two weeks, is in phase I trials, and is produced by Pfizer.

*BIIB023 (Anti-TWEAK, Anti-Tumor Necrosis Factor-Like Weak Inducer of Apoptosis).* This potential therapy is being investigated by Biogen Idec in the treatment of lupus nephritis in phase II trials. Preliminary studies show that there is an excess of TWEAK involved in the inflammation of lupus nephritis. Therefore, if TWEAK can be blocked by a medication, there is the possibility that it could protect the kidneys in lupus nephritis.

## Tolerogens

Tolerogens are substances that interact with antibodies of the immune system (like antigens do), but they do so in such a way as to cause the immune system to not become more active. The theory is that tolerogens bind to the lupus auto-antibodies that normally bind to the nuclear antigens of the lupus person's body. If the auto-antibodies of the immune system in the person with lupus are bombarded by these tolerogens, then they may keep the nuclear antigens of the person's body from binding to the lupus auto-antibodies. This could prevent the immune system from attacking the body of the person who has lupus. They do not suppress the immune system; therefore, theoretically, they should not increase the risk of infections.

*Rigerimod (Lupuzor, CEP-33457).* Rigerimod is a very small protein and therefore is not a biologic medication. It is administered once a month by subcutaneous (SQ) injection and is manufactured by Teva Pharmaceutical Industries, which acquired it through its acquisition of Cephalon. It has completed a phase II trial and is currently looking for a financial partner to proceed to its phase III trial plans. This potential therapy may show some promise, and it illustrates the difficulties with getting large sums of money to conduct proper research for lupus medications.

*Laquinimod.* This tolerogen is being studied by Teva Pharmaceutical Industries to treat lupus nephritis and lupus arthritis. Phase II studies were completed in September 2012, but the results have not been disclosed as of February 2013. An advantage of this medication is that it is available in oral pill form instead of having to be injected.

*Paquinimod (ABR-215757).* This drug is also categorized as a tolerogen and has completed a phase II clinical trial in patients who have skin disease, oral ulcers, and arthritis due to SLE. The results have not been disclosed as of this writing. It is manufactured by Active Biotech Research.

## Investigational Lupus Therapies That Work through Other Mechanisms

*ABT-199 (a Selective BCL-2 Inhibitor).* Recall in earlier chapters (33 and 37) the discussion regarding the topic of apoptosis. Apoptosis is a process where cells are programmed to die as they become older and less useful. It is a safety mechanism by which the body can ensure that new cells continuously replace older, less effective cells, and that these older cells do not live forever and become out of control. One problem in SLE is that the B-cells that produce auto-bodies lose their ability to undergo normal apoptosis. ABT-199 inhibits a protein made inside of our cells called BCL-2 protein (short for B-cell lymphoma 2 protein). BCL-2 protein causes cells to survive, continue to live on and on, and not undergo natural programmed cell death (apoptosis). The theory is to try to get the overactive B-cells of lupus that continue to live too long to die quicker and therefore stop producing the auto-antibodies that attack the body. It is produced by Abbott and is in early phase I studies.

*CDP7657 (CD40L Inhibitor).* CDP7657 is a fragment of an antibody that prevents a protein on T-cells (called CD40L) from activating B-cells in the hopes that there will be less B-cell activation. It is produced by UCB and is in very early phase I trials.

*AMG 557 (MEDI-5872 or Anti-B7RP1 MAb).* This medication is produced and is being investigated in collaboration between MedImmune and Amgen. It binds a molecule called B7 related protein (B7RP-1) to decrease the activation of T-cells in the immune system. It is currently in phase I studies.

*Omalizumab (Xolair).* This medication is already used to treat asthma. It decreases the production of certain antibodies that can also be produced in abundance in SLE. It is given subcutaneously every two to four weeks. It is in early phase I trials.

*KRP203.* KRP203 is produced by Novartis Pharmaceuticals primarily as a potential therapy to prevent organ transplant rejection by suppressing the immune system in the hopes that it will be safer than current therapies. Remember that azathioprine (Imuran) and mycophenolic acid (CellCept and Myfortic) were also originally used to prevent organ transplant rejection and are now commonly used to treat SLE. KRP203 is in phase II trials assessing whether it helps subacute cutaneous lupus.

*CC-11050 (PDE4 Inhibitor, Phosphodiesterase Type 4 Inhibitor).* CC-11050 is taken orally twice a day and is produced by Celgene Corporation. It blocks an enzyme called PDE4, which is abundant in cells of the immune system. It appears to decrease numerous inflammatory compounds. It currently is being tested in people who have discoid lupus and subacute cutaneous lupus in phase II trials.

*Valcade (Bortezomib).* Valcade is already a medication FDA-approved to treat multiple myeloma, which is a cancer of mature B-cells called plasma cells. It works by preventing proteasomes from working correctly. Proteasomes are important enzymes that clean up unneeded proteins from cells and help them live longer. Therefore, a proteasome inhibitor, such as Valcade, can cause the overactive mature B-cells that are living too long to die earlier. Studies show that patients who have SLE have higher levels of proteasome activity. A small study was presented at the European Union League Against Rheumatism in 2012 where thirteen patients who had lupus nephritis (who had failed standard therapies) were treated with IV Valcade. All of them had significant improvement in their nephritis. The lead investigator of the study, Dr. Reinhard Voll of Germany, hopes that the maker of the drug, Millennium Pharmaceuticals, will proceed with larger studies.

## Other Investigational Therapies

In the 1800s, arsenic (a well-known poison) was used to treat lupus. Today, a safer version called arsenic trioxide is being investigated in its IV (intravenous) form at the Nantes University Hospital in France to assess its safety and possible usefulness in patients who have SLE.

Statins are a group of medications used to lower cholesterol levels, and as mentioned in chapter 21, some lupus experts believe that most, if not all, patients who have SLE should be on a statin to reduce their chances of developing strokes and heart attacks. The statins also appear to have anti-inflammatory properties, therefore, the Buddhist Tzu Chi General Hospital in Taiwan is investigating the use of atorvastatin (Lipitor) in the treatment of SLE to see if it decreases disease activity. They also want to see if it makes a difference in the severity of Raynaud's phenomenon or not.

Dipyridamole (Persantine) is used to decrease blood clots in people who have had artificial heart valve surgery and to prevent strokes in other people when used along with aspirin. It has been shown to inhibit overactive lymphocyte blood cells in SLE and has been shown to be beneficial in lupus mice. The Oklahoma Medical Research Foundation is currently studying its use to see if it can decrease flares of SLE in humans.

Retinoids are chemicals related to vitamin A. They have been found helpful in regulating the growth of epithelial cells of the skin and have mostly been used for conditions such as acne. However, the kidneys also have epithelial cells in multiple sections. Therefore, Kinki University in Japan is performing a study using the retinoid tamibarotene to see if it can help people who have lupus nephritis.

Studies show that T-cells in lupus patients have lower amounts of an antioxidant substance called glutathione. One theory is that the lack of this important antioxidant may cause early inflammatory death in the T-cells of lupus patients, adding to their imbalanced immune system problems. N-acetylcysteine (NAC) is converted in the body into glutathione. If NAC is given to SLE patients, it is hypothesized that it may help to increase T-cell glutathione levels and prevent them from dying prematurely. State University of New York–Upstate Medical University is studying two different doses in SLE patients to see how well it is tolerated and what its effects are on the immune system and steroid needs of lupus patients.

## Therapies Possible for SLE in the Future

Of course, future therapies that are not currently being studied are only limited by the human mind and the technology that is available to try to turn human ideas into actual treatments. During the past couple of decades, we have seen enormous advances in medicine that appear to be increasing exponentially. As I have mentioned several times before, the FDA approval of Benlysta will most likely open the doors for other therapies to be investigated to treat lupus in the future. I hope that investors and pharmaceutical companies will realize that their money will not be wasted in developing newer and better treatments for lupus. Researchers and doctors will not be fully happy though, until either effective preventative therapies are developed or a possible cure is found for lupus. Dr. Wallace's dream of a vaccine to prevent lupus (as mentioned in the lead to this chapter) may one day be a reality: keeping those people who are born with the genes that can cause lupus from ever developing it.

**KEY POINTS TO REMEMBER**

1. We are entering a new, exciting period in the treatment of lupus with numerous potential therapies being studied.

2. Some medications being studied as potential treatments for lupus are currently available to treat other diseases. These include abatacept, cholecalciferol, sirolimus, stem cell transplantation, tocilizumab, and UVA-1 phototherapy.

3. There are numerous medications in the research pipeline for lupus treatment.

4. Researchers, doctors, and especially patients will not be satisfied until a safe cure for lupus or a preventative therapy (such as a vaccine) is discovered.

# Nonmedical Therapies for Lupus

### Getting Lupus from a Xerox Machine

A 34-year-old woman who had systemic lupus erythematosus (SLE) had problems with arthritis, low platelet counts, and low complement levels. She began to develop a burning red rash on the backs of her hands and on her palms. It then spread to her arms, neck, and face. Her doctor treated her with anti-malarial medications, steroid creams, and steroid pills, and she would wear her sunscreen when she would go outside. None of these kept the rash under control. Astutely, she noted that her rash got much better after being away from work for a week, and then it recurred within a week or two of returning to work. She worked as a photocopy technician at a law firm, and part of the time when she would photocopy materials, she would do so with the lid of the photocopier open while holding the books she was copying flat on the copy surface. The machine she used was an Eastman Kodak model (generically called a Xerox machine). She quit her job and within four weeks her rash became markedly better.

The photocopy machine was subsequently tested for its ultraviolet (UV) light output and was found to emit UVA light but no UVB light. Other photocopy machines (such as Xerox, Sharp, Konica, and Mita) were also tested and were also found to emit UVA light. Although the amount of UVA light emitted was very small (compared to that received from sunlight), the repetitive exposure to these small amounts was enough to cause her lupus to become more active. Another person, a research biologist, appears in the medical literature; this biologist developed discoid lupus on her forearm from simply using a fluorescence microscope.

Using ultraviolet light protection all the time, not just when outside in the sun, is one of the important measures to take when managing lupus. It is just as important as taking the medication pills, and is one of the standard treatments of lupus (just as taking Plaquenil is). Other nonmedical therapies are also very important for people who have lupus to abide by to help them live a long, normal life. This chapter goes into detail about these important aspects. I consider this chapter to be one of the most important in the book. Most patients easily recognize the importance of taking their medications. Unfortunately, it can be more difficult to convince them to wear sunscreen religiously every day (even in the winter), eat properly, exercise regularly, get enough sleep, and avoid stress.

It is early spring here in Washington, DC as I am writing this. In the past couple of weeks, I have seen several patients who were having flares of their lupus in our office. Each of them had a faint pink coloration to their forearms and backs of the hands, the telltale sign of their not using their sunscreen daily. They did not realize (or forgot about) the importance of using sunscreen daily, wearing a wide-brimmed hat while outside, wearing clothing with an increased SPF (sun protection factor), as well as the other important UV protection matters. After further education and convincing, they do much better when they put UV light protection into practice. These typical flares of lupus in the spring rarely occur in my patients who practice the measures discussed in this chapter. If you can do everything in this chapter along with being compliant with taking your medications, you will have a much better chance of controlling lupus.

····

## Ultraviolet Light Protection

Protection from ultraviolet light (specifically UVA-2 and UVB light) is one of the most important things for people who have lupus to do regularly. It needs to become a reflexive, automatic part of life. The reason for this is clear. Unless you live in a dark hole or cave, ultraviolet light bombards your exposed skin almost constantly. Light is made up of electromagnetic waves that are categorized based on their wavelengths and how they affect living things (figure 38.1). Note that some electromagnetic waves are also responsible for x-rays used to image the body, microwaves used for cooking, and radio waves used to communicate. Visible light is made up of the colors of the rainbow. As the light wave frequencies start from lower to higher they go from red to orange to yellow to green to blue to indigo to violet (as per the popular school mnemonic ROY G. BIV). "Ultra" is derived from Latin and means "beyond"; therefore, the ultraviolet spectrum of light is composed of wave frequencies beyond the color violet. This is in contrast to infrared, where "infra" is Latin for "below," and the infrared spectrum of light comprises light waves that are below those of the color red on the visible light scale.

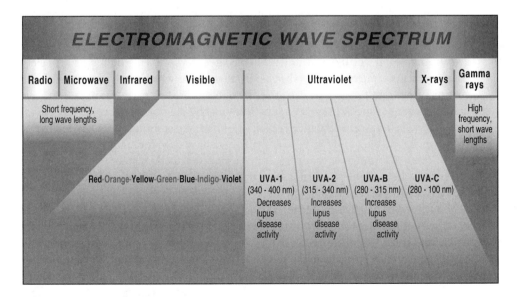

Figure 38.1  Electromagnetic wave spectrum

Scientists divide ultraviolet light into ultraviolet A (UVA), then UVB, then UVC light. The sun emits all three types, but the atmosphere filters out the UVC light; therefore, only UVA and UVB light reach the earth. The UVA light is further divided into UVA-1 and UVA-2 light. These divisions are based on the biologic effects of the light. UVA-2 light is more similar to UVB than UVA-1 light in regards to how it reacts with living things. In fact, UVA-2 and UVB light both make lupus worse while UVA-1 light does not. When UVA-2 and UVB light contact the skin, even in small amounts, they cause chemical reactions with the proteins and DNA of the skin cells that actually damage the cells. Proteins deep within the cells migrate from the damaged nuclei up to the cell surface where they attach on the outside of the cell surface. The lupus immune system recognizes them by way of its antinuclear antibodies (those of the famous ANA test of lupus), which in turn cause the immune system to become more active, causing inflammation and damage throughout the body. This increased lupus activity sometimes occurs as a rash on the skin, but often occurs inside deeper organs of the body.

The amount of damage done by these UVA-2 and UVB light waves is proportionate to the amount of light exposure. Since the sun is the major source of UV light, being out in the sun especially in the middle of the day, causes the most interaction with the cells of the skin and increased lupus activity. Many people who have lupus quickly learn to stay out of the sun because they may develop red rashes on the skin due to sun exposure. Others may not feel well, develop fever, or feel a burning discomfort on the skin when they go out in the sun.

It is just as important to realize that you undergo UV light exposure even when you are not outside in the sun. There are three major types of light bulbs used inside of homes and businesses. The one invented by Edison is the incandescent light bulb. This is the screw-in bulb-shaped light bulbs that are so familiar to most of us. It emits light by electricity heating up a metal filament inside of the bulb, which then glows brightly, producing not just light, but also a lot of heat. These emit much heat and visible light, but only a small amount of ultraviolet light. However, they do emit some ultraviolet light.

Fluorescent bulbs are the other major type of light bulbs. These are the ones that are commonly long, cylindrical, and usually coated in white. They light up due to electrical reactions occurring within the gas inside the tube, which then interacts with the coating on the white tube. They are also the light bulbs that are recommended to cut down on energy consumption as a substitute for the older incandescent light bulbs. These newer, energy-efficient fluorescent bulbs have the commonly recognized metal screw tip, but instead of the usual bulb shape we have used for many years, they have the white coated thin tubes that are spiraled around each other. Fluorescent bulbs give off more UV light than the incandescent bulbs but much less than sunlight. Although they are better for the environment, they are not as good in regards to lupus.

The third type of light bulb is the halogen light bulb. These emit the largest amounts of ultraviolet light and should be avoided as much as possible by people who have lupus. These are not used as often in homes, but are commercially available. People who have lupus should especially make sure that their desk lamps at home and work do not contain halogen bulbs. They are more commonly found in situations that need a lot of light, for example, garages, factories, and stages. Therefore, people in these occupational situations (such as actors, stage entertainers, factory workers, and mechanics) need to pay special mind to this hazard. Ensuring that halogen lights are covered with a glass/heat filter can greatly reduce the amount of ultraviolet light emission.

Although incandescent and fluorescent bulbs give off just a fraction of the amount of ultraviolet light as the sun, they still cause skin to be continuously exposed to UVA and UVB light where it can interact with the cells of the skin. The total amount of ultraviolet light exposure is dependent on both the strength of the UV light as well as the total amount of time exposed. For example, although indoor lighting may have a much smaller strength of UV light emission compared to sunlight, people are generally exposed to this for great lengths of time every day and therefore can receive high doses of ultraviolet light exposure and subsequent damage to skin cells and subsequent activation of the immune system in lupus over time. Therefore, it is truly important that people who have lupus learn to apply sunscreen on all exposed skin surfaces, even if they do not go outside.

Another common misconception by some people who have lupus is that they do not think they need to avoid the sun if it is winter or if it is cloudy. This is a natural reaction since we automatically associate sunburns and the need for sunscreen with the beach and hot, sunny summer days. It is true that the dose of ultraviolet light that we encounter is highest when the sun is high in the sky (such as noon on a summer day) when there are no clouds. However, up to 80% of ultraviolet light penetrates the clouds on cloudy days, and is still very much present during wintertime; it is just in slightly smaller doses. In addition, sand (think beach), snow, concrete, and water reflect UV light. Therefore, if you are outside at the beach, surrounded by snow, near water, or in an urban area, you are exposed to higher amounts of UV light than from the sun itself. For example, snow reflects about 85% of sunlight, nearly doubling the UV exposure. Concrete reflects only 15%, but it still increases exposure, making outdoor exposure in the city higher than normal.

Just as the photocopy technician using the Xerox machine and the biologist using the microscope, mentioned in the first section of this chapter, had worsening lupus related to their occupations, there are other occupations that expose people to increased ultraviolet radiation (table 38.1). In addition, some artificial light sources emit UV radiation at higher amounts than other sources (table 38.2).

Therefore, learning to protect your skin from being exposed to even the smaller amounts of ultraviolet light while inside as well as outside on winter and cloudy and stormy days is just as important as avoiding the sun at noon in the summertime. Table 38.3 lists suggested measures to decrease exposure of your body to the damaging effects of UV light.

Sunscreen lotions need to be a part of your daily routine. People who have lupus need to consider these as one of their medications to treat their lupus. It is incorrect to think that you do not need sunscreen if you do not develop a rash from lupus. While 30% to 50% of people who have lupus will develop a rash due to light exposure, others do not. However, the lupus inside the body still becomes more active due to ultraviolet radiation exposure. As mentioned above, all of us are constantly exposed to UV light (unless you are in a dark room or if it is nighttime outside).

It is best to use a sunscreen (or a sunblock) with the highest SPF tolerable. Currently, they are available with SPFs well above 100. Sunscreens with higher SPF values provide more protection from UV radiation. However, the higher SPFs tend to be thicker

**Table 38.1** Occupations at Potentially Increased Risk of UV Light Exposure

- People who use photocopier machines with the lid open
- Food and drink irradiators
- Hairdressers
- Nail technicians (use UV drying lamps)
- Laboratory workers
- Lighting technicians
- Lithographic and printing workers
- Police
- Outdoor workers (construction workers, farmers, etc.)
- Paint and resin curers
- Physiotherapists
- Plasma torch operators
- Metal factory workers
- Welders
- Navy and Coastguard personnel
- Stage entertainers
- Office workers with halogen-light desk lamps
- Anyone working around water, snow, glass, and concrete reflecting sunlight

**Table 38.2** Devices Emitting Higher Amounts of UV Radiation

- Bactericidal lamps
- Black light lamps
- Halogen lamps
- Spot lights
- Stage lighting
- Movie projector lighting
- Carbon, xenon, and other arcs
- Dental polymerizing equipment
- Fingernail-drying lamps
- Fluorescence equipment
- Hydrogen and deuterium lamps
- Metal halide lamps
- Mercury lamps
- Plasma torches
- Phototherapy lamps
- Printing ink polymerizing equipment
- Welding equipment

**Table 38.3** Ultraviolet Light Protection Measures

- Wear sunblock on all exposed skin areas every day, even if you do not go outside.

  Use the highest SPF tolerable (SPF 30 or higher is preferable).

  Should be UVA and UVB protective.

  Avoid the ingredient PABA if you are sensitive to sunscreens.

  Should be waterproof or water resistant. Waterproof lasts longer.

  Apply thirty minutes before going outside.

  Apply a lot; most people apply about one-third the recommended amount.

  Do not forget to apply on lips, ears, nose, neck, hands, feet. Consider sunblock sticks to use on the lips, ears, and around the eyes.

  Sunscreen gel may be best for oily skin, while lotions may work best with dry skin.

  When going outside, reapply again during the day.

- Avoid the sun as much as you can between 10:00 AM and 4:00 PM. (A good rule of thumb is avoid outdoor activities if your shadow is shorter than your height.)

- Wear a wide-brimmed hat when outside.

- Consider wearing additional loose-fitting pants and long-sleeve shirts.

- Tightly woven, dark, dry fabrics keep out UV rays best.

- Wear sun-protective clothing. Coolibar, Solumbra, Sunday Afternoons, Solartex, Eclipse Couture, and SunGrubbies are some brands to consider.

- Consider using Rit Sun Guard when you wash your clothes to increase their SPF.

- Do not use UV drying lamps when you get your nails done.

- *Never* tan! If you become tan, you did not protect yourself adequately from UV light.

- Instead of a natural tan, consider artificial tanning sprays, lotions, and gels.

- Wear UV-protective glasses when outside.

- Always drive with the windows up.

- Consider additional UV tinting for car and home windows. UV tinting does not need to be dark. Some brands to consider include Sunscape, SunTek, and UVShield.

- Consider putting plastic covers on inside lighting (especially fluorescent and halogen lamps) to block UV light.

- Ask employers if they can tint windows with UV protection.

- Ask employers if they can cover fluorescent and halogen lights with protectant plastic covers.

in consistency, and some people have difficulty tolerating them. If you can tolerate the thicker, higher SPFs, then that is good. If you find you cannot, then try a lower SPF. It may take some experimentation with different brands and SPFs until you find one that is a good fit for you. Some people prefer the spray-on types while others prefer the lotions. A nice thing about skin care products these days is that there is a large variety of products. Many popular moisturizers (such as Neutrogena brands) also contain sunscreen. There are also easy-to-use sunblock sticks that make application on the lips, nose, and ears easy to do repetitively throughout the day. Make sure that your brand blocks both UVA and UVB rays and that it is water resistant or waterproof. If you have difficulty tolerating off-the-shelf sunscreen products and skin care products due to allergies, consider seeing a dermatologist to help you find one that you can tolerate.

There is a difference between a sunscreen and a sunblock. Sunscreens absorb UV radiation while sunblocks reflect the UV radiation. Whether one is better than the other is not certain. Currently two forms of sunblock reflect both UVA and UVB rays. These are Mexoryl and Helioplex. Therefore, if you prefer using a sunblock, make sure it contains one of these products.

Many people do not use sunscreens adequately. It is important to use a thicker instead of a thinner amount on the skin. Studies show that most people do not apply enough to the skin. Make sure to apply it as early in the morning as possible (remember, it is important to wear it even if you do not go outside). If you do go outside, make sure to reapply it thirty minutes before going outside to allow it to penetrate the skin and exert its effects. Additional information on how to properly protect yourself from UV radiation can be obtained from the American Academy of Dermatology at www.aad.org.

Some people develop an allergic reaction or intolerance to some sunscreens and sunblocks. If you develop an unusual reaction to a sunscreen, such as a rash or itching, the first step to take is to try a sunscreen that does not contain para-aminobenzoic acid (PABA), which is a common cause of sunscreen intolerances. However, sunscreens contain numerous other potential chemical causes of allergies. If you still do not tolerate a PABA-free sunscreen, then you should see a dermatologist to help you find one that you can tolerate.

Wearing UV protectant clothing and sunglasses while outside can also be helpful. Most clothing only has an SPF of 5 or 6. There are companies that make special UV protectant clothing, however, these can sometimes be expensive. An easy way to make your clothing more UV protectant is by adding a protectant such as Rit Sun Guard powder to your clothing in the washing machine. It increases the SPF of the clothes up to as high as 30. The manufacturer states that it lasts for up to twenty washings; therefore, using it in the wash several times a year would suffice for most people.

Nail manicures and pedicures are becoming more popular in the past few years, especially the use of gel nails. The lamps used to dry the nails emit significant UV light. I had not realized this until one of my patients developed a severe flare of her lupus nephritis (kidney inflammation) soon after she started getting gel nails put on her fingers. My very observant nurse fortunately obtained this important piece of history for me from the patient. As a man who never gets manicures, I may never otherwise have found this out. Please do not get manicures or pedicures that require the use of these

UV nail drying lamps. Also, be very careful if you enter an establishment that uses them to ensure you are not exposed to them accidentally.

Fortunately, car windshields and windows have UV protection, preventing most UV light from entering the car. Therefore, you should drive with the windows up whenever you are in the car to decrease the amount of UV light contacting your skin. You can add additional UV tinting to your car for better UV protection. UV protectant window tinting does not need to be dark in color. The same thing can be done for windows in the home as well. It is important to note that some localities do not allow car window tinting. However, a note from your doctor stating that the window tinting is "medically necessary" usually satisfies local requirements.

## No Smoking Cigarettes

Doctors tend to become a broken record (if they are doing their job) by telling patients about the dangers of smoking. In people who have lupus, it is even truer for several reasons (table 38.4). First, it is important to realize that tobacco and the additives placed in them contain hundreds of potentially harmful chemicals. Not only do some of them cause cancer and permanent lung damage, but they have other far-reaching effects as well. For example, people who smoke develop autoimmune diseases more commonly and of a more severe nature compared to people who do not smoke. This has been demonstrated not only in people who have SLE, but also in other autoimmune diseases such as rheumatoid arthritis. Their disease also tends to be more difficult to control. Why this occurs, we do not know, but some of the chemicals inside the cigarettes in some way must interact with the immune system causing increased immune system activity. One lupus-causing chemical identified in cigarettes is hydrazine. Hydrazine is known to make lupus worse and can even cause lupus. Cigarette smoking also decreases the effectiveness of anti-malarial medicines such as hydroxychloroquine (Plaquenil). It is not known why this occurs. This is especially troublesome to doctors who treat people who have lupus because hydroxychloroquine is by far the safest medication to treat lupus. If someone is unable to stop smoking while taking hydroxychloroquine, she or he has a higher chance of it not working properly. This may require the doctor to add a stronger immunosuppressant medication and/or steroid to the medical regimen. These medications have many more potential side effects compared to hydroxychloroquine.

**Table 38.4** Why Cigarette Smoking Is Bad for Lupus

- Cigarettes contain hydrazine, which increases lupus activity.
- Smoking decreases the effectiveness of hydroxychloroquine (Plaquenil).
- Smoking increases cardiovascular complications (most common cause of death in people who have lupus).
- Smoking increases the risk for cancer, especially lung cancer, in lupus.

As discussed in chapter 21, the number one cause of death of people who have lupus in the United States is cardiovascular disease causing strokes, heart attacks, and blood clots. People who smoke cigarettes are at much higher risk for getting these complications compared to people who do not smoke. The tobacco chemicals cause the blood vessels of the body to become thickened, hard, and clogged up with plaque. Then the nicotine from the cigarettes causes the arteries to constrict (clamp down) causing even further loss of blood flow to vital organs such as the brain and heart. The fourth most common cause of death in people who have lupus is cancer. They get cancer more often than people who do not have lupus. When doctors studied cancer in lupus, cigarette smoking was proven one of the primary risk factors for developing cancer, especially for those who developed lung cancer.

It is clear that people who have lupus who continue to smoke are sabotaging their care from many different directions causing increased disease activity, keeping their safest medicine (Plaquenil) from working, and increasing their chances of getting heart attacks, strokes, blood clots, and cancer. Doctors certainly also recognize the incredible addictiveness of cigarette smoking. The addictive aspects of smoking not only include the highly addictive nature of the nicotine itself, but also the obsessive/compulsive ritual of smoking as well. In addition, people who smoke, on average, have been doing this for many years: most since they were teenagers. Some people are fortunate and are able to stop cold turkey when they learn of the health dangers they are putting themselves in. Unfortunately, most smokers have great difficulty stopping due to these addictive properties. It is very important for this latter group to put everything they can into stopping smoking. Most primary care physicians can help by recommending smoking cessation groups, classes, and even using prescription medications that can decrease the urge to smoke. In addition, the U.S. government supplies services free of charge to help people stop smoking. You can go to www.smokefree.gov or call 1-800-QUIT-NOW or 1-877-44U-QUIT to get help.

## Diet

While there is no diet that has been proven effective for lupus, some things are probably beneficial from a theoretical perspective (table 38.5). It is important to avoid alfalfa sprouts and mung bean sprouts in your diet (such as in salads). These sprouts contain elevated amounts of the amino acid L-canavanine, which stimulates the immune system to become more active (just what doctors do not want in lupus patients). At least two studies have shown this to cause lupus-like changes in the immune system in monkeys. In one of these studies, three of five macaque monkeys fed ground alfalfa sprouts developed symptoms of lupus as well as abnormal lupus blood test results with positive ANA, double-stranded DNA, low complement levels, and even hemolytic anemia and lupus nephritis. This does not appear to be isolated to monkeys; an environmental study in Baltimore showed an association of the ingestion of alfalfa sprouts with an increased risk of developing lupus as well.

Some doctors advocate staying away from garlic, which contains substances (allicin, ajoene, and thiosulfinates) that can potentially increase immune activity. However, I do not see enough evidence to make this recommendation myself. In fact, gar-

**Table 38.5** Recommended Diet in Lupus

- Avoid alfalfa sprouts and mung bean sprouts.
- Eat a diet low in fat, calories, and simple carbohydrates.
- Consume foods that are higher in vitamin D (table 24.8).
- Eat foods rich in omega-3 fatty acids (flaxseed, coldwater fish, walnuts, etc.).
- Use more olive oil in your diet.
- Use alcohol in moderation.
- Follow the guidelines in table 38.6.

lic is actually used by some alternative and complementary medical practitioners to decrease inflammation. In addition, there is no medical evidence showing increased lupus activity due to eating garlic.

Calorie-restrictive diets in mice with lupus increase their lifespan as well as decrease lupus nephritis and inflammation of the salivary glands (as seen in Sjögren's syndrome). Lupus mice fed high-fat diets develop increased activity of the immune system, including increased production of auto-antibodies (such as anti-DNA and antiphospholipid antibodies) as well as increased lupus nephritis activity. Weight gain appears to increase activity of the immune system. While these studies have not been repeated in humans, most people who have lupus are overweight or obese (chapter 21). Theoretically, this weight gain with fat increases activity of the immune system, subsequently requiring increased needs for medications such as steroids, which in turn causes even more fat weight gain. It is easy to see that this could become a vicious cycle. Being overweight also increases the chances of developing cardiovascular complications such as strokes, heart attacks, and blood clots; this as a group is the most common cause of death in people who have lupus.

To further add evidence in choosing a low-calorie diet and losing weight, a 2010 study showed that SLE patients who lost weight through low-calorie as well as low-carbohydrate diets ended up having improved energy levels. Fatigue is one of the most difficult problems in many people who have SLE. To add evidence that avoiding too many carbohydrates is important, a 2012 study showed that patients who had SLE who ate diets high in carbohydrates had higher disease activity and higher cholesterol levels than SLE patients who did not eat a lot of carbohydrates. Interestingly, calorie-restricted diets have also been associated with longer longevity in people who do not have lupus. Therefore, dieting to lose weight (if starting out overweight) should be a dietary goal of anyone who has SLE. It appears that diets that are low in calories and in simple carbohydrates (sugars, breads, pastas, sweets, juices) both may be beneficial.

As discussed in chapter 3, most people who develop SLE are deficient in vitamin D levels. Vitamin D is essential for proper function of the immune system, and more severe cases of SLE have been associated with lower vitamin D levels. A 2012 study even showed that people who have antiphospholipid syndrome (causing recurrent blood clots in lupus patients) also have lower vitamin D levels than other people. Although most people require vitamin D supplements in the form of capsules, people who have lupus should also strongly consider consuming foods that are higher in vitamin D, as listed in table 24.8.

So what level of vitamin D should people who have SLE aim for? When you look at your lab results for vitamin D, the only result that is important is the 25-hydroxy vitamin D (25-OH Vit D). I prefer to accept the recommendations of the Institute of Medicine. After reviewing the world's literature regarding vitamin D levels and optimum health, and only including the best studies, they concluded that a 25-OH vitamin D level of 20 ng/mL or higher was adequate for optimal health. It is reassuring that a large 2012 report followed 1,621 people over 11 years and also came to the same independent conclusion that a level of 20 ng/mL was adequate in regards to avoiding problems such as broken bones, cancer, heart attacks, and death. Therefore, I aim for a level of 20 ng/mL and higher in most patients. The main exception is patients who take steroids. Steroids, such as prednisone and methylprednisolone, decrease the absorption of calcium, while higher vitamin D levels improve the absorption of calcium. Therefore, the American College of Rheumatology recommends a goal of at least 30 ng/mL in this group of patients. However, if I have a patient seeing another doctor who wants to achieve a higher level (e.g., many doctors aim for a level of 50 ng/mL) I do not object to this goal as it certainly will not cause any side effects.

A special note about vitamin D supplements needs to be mentioned. Although I have had success using both prescription vitamin D (ergocalciferol, vitamin D-2) as well as over-the-counter vitamin D (cholecalciferol, vitamin D-3) in normalizing vitamin D levels, there are large variations in the quality of the over-the-counter (OTC) preparations. A 2013 study in the *Journal of the American Medical Association* tested a number of OTC brands and found that they contained anywhere from 52% to 135% of the expected dose. This is not acceptable in the terms of quality, but unfortunately, the way that the current laws are written, the FDA does not have the authority to step in to enforce better-quality controls. In light of this information, my best recommendation is that if you do use an OTC brand of vitamin D-3 to normalize your vitamin D level, always stick with the same brand, and make sure to have your levels checked regularly. This way, if you were taking the brand that only had 52% of what it should have in it, if I find that it normalized your vitamin D level, then that particular brand should be adequate at that particular dosage. However, my concern is that if quality is poor enough that there is only 52% of the stated active vitamin, then that company's quality control may not be good enough to ensure that the same amount will occur in capsules from different bottles and different lots. Therefore, it is very important to have your blood levels checked regularly to ensure they stay normal. The other alternative would be to ask your doctor to prescribe the prescription-strength ergocalciferol instead. This can end up being more expensive for some people, but at least you know you are getting a good-quality product.

Certain fats appear to be more beneficial to health than others are. Especially a group of fats called omega-3 fatty acids appear to have beneficial effects on cholesterol levels and inflammation. American diets tend to be relatively deficient in omega-3 fatty acids and higher in omega-6 fatty acids that are common in meats and protein sources other than fish. Omega-6 fatty acids tend to increase inflammation and cholesterol. Omega-3 fatty acids are abundant in certain foods, including cold-water fish (such as salmon, halibut, snapper, mackerel, albacore tuna, and sardines), flax seeds (the food with one of the highest concentrations of omega-3 fatty acids), walnuts, tofu, shrimp, and scallops. Lupus mice fed diets high in omega-3 fatty acids develop less immune system activity, less autoantibody production (such as anti-DNA and antiphospholipid antibodies), and less lupus nephritis activity with decreased protein in the urine and less kidney damage.

There have been several diet studies using omega-3 fatty acids in people who have lupus. One study looked at twelve patients with lupus nephritis. For five weeks, they took 6 g of fish oil a day followed by five weeks of a normal diet, then followed by five more weeks of 18 g of fish oil a day. The higher dose of fish oil significantly improved their cholesterol studies, but had no measurable effects on their lupus labs, including the activity of their lupus nephritis. Another study looked at twenty-six patients who had lupus nephritis who were evaluated for two years. Part of the time they were on a high fish oil diet while the rest of the time they were on a "normal" diet. Again, their cholesterol improved but their lupus nephritis did not improve.

Although these two studies did not have promising results, several other studies have shown good results. One study put twenty-seven patients who had SLE on a diet rich in alpha-linolenic acid (a type of omega-3 fatty acid) in the form of olive oil (20 g a day). Only seventeen of the patients completed the thirty-four-week study, but they had improvements in their lupus activity. In another study, a group of patients was placed on a diet with increased fish oils; they had decreased lupus activity and improvements in their blood work compared to a placebo control group. Another study assessed twenty-two pregnant women who had the antiphospholipid antibody syndrome and previously had had recurrent miscarriages (see chapters 9 and 18). They took omega-3 fatty acids daily. There was only one premature fetal death among the twenty-two pregnancies, much lower than would have been expected.

The lupus mice studies showing benefits from a diet rich in omega-3 fatty acids is encouraging, while the human studies have had mixed results. The disappointing results have generally occurred in the studies that included the lupus patients with more severe disease (lupus nephritis). This does not prove that a diet rich in these healthy oils does not help lupus patients. For example, it could be possible that these anti-inflammatory fats may benefit patients who have less severe lupus disease. The proper studies to answer these questions have not been done yet, and there is a great need to have them done.

Looking at this issue from another aspect, a 2012 study looked at the eating habits of 114 SLE patients. They found that those who had a diet low in omega-3 fatty acids had worse lupus disease activity as well as higher levels of cholesterol and atherosclerosis (which can cause heart attacks and strokes). Therefore, it is important for people who have lupus to supplement their diet with foods rich in omega-3 fatty acids, olive oil, or supplements containing these oils. Not only may this possibly improve lupus disease activity, but it may also improve cholesterol levels, which would be possibly a good way to decrease the risk of getting heart attacks, strokes, and blood clots.

Personally, I am not a fish lover. I have found it very easy to increase the amount of omega-3 fatty acids in my diet by drinking protein shakes every day with walnuts and flax seeds mixed in. Added to a chocolate protein powder mix, low-sugar soymilk, and some ice, it produces a very tasty, healthy milk shake–like drink. Using my Magic Bullet, this is quick and easy, and cleanup is a breeze. Various brands of flax seed snacks and crackers are also readily available, and many of them are quite tasty. These provide high levels of omega-3 fatty acids.

A 2012 study showed a correlation between the types of fats eaten in the diet and memory decline. Since problems with memory, called cognitive dysfunction, is such a common problem in people who have SLE, this is an important study to mention. This study showed that women who ate a diet high in "unhealthy fats" (saturated fats) had worse memory problems over a four-year period than those who ate a diet higher in "healthy fats" (monosaturated fats). In fact, those with the highest levels of intake of the saturated fats were 70% more likely to develop cognition (memory, math, verbal) problems compared to those with the lowest intakes. Examples of foods high in saturated fats include most meat products (beef, pork, poultry, all processed meats), whole milk, cheese, butter, coconut oil, and palm oil. Therefore, it is wise to decrease the intake of these food products and substitute foods higher in monosaturated fats such as legumes (lentils, beans, peas, peanuts), fish, nuts, skim milk, and monosaturated oils (olive, canola, safflower, sesame, corn, soybean). When you do eat meats, make sure to choose the leanest cuts; trim off the visible fat; broil, grill, or bake them (instead of frying); and remove the skin from poultry.

In addition to eating low-calorie diets that are rich in omega-3 fatty acids, one of the most important things with respect to eating is to eat a balanced, healthy diet. The typical American diet is very unhealthy, loaded with high amounts of bad fat, simple sugars, high-fructose corn syrup, and salt while being deficient in vitamin-rich, healthy foods such as whole grains, fruits, vegetables, and nuts. America is in the midst of an obesity epidemic. Many nutrition experts link this epidemic to "fast food" and the abundance of foods rich in high-fructose corn syrup. Fructose sugar is associated with increased fat production (and therefore obesity), increased rates of heart disease, and the increase in other medical conditions such as gout. It is important to learn to read product ingredient labels and avoid those products that list fructose corn syrup in the first few ingredients. Most people are surprised at how many of their favorite foods are actually very unhealthy due to the amount of fructose corn syrup that the food contains. In fact, many "low fat" foods are just as unhealthy, even less healthy, than their high-fat counterparts are because of the fructose corn syrup taking the place of the fat.

Table 38.6 lists the recommendations of the USDA for a proper, healthy daily diet. In addition, the USDA has alternative diet recommendations for people with special dietary needs and desires, including children, older people, overweight people, vegetarians, Mediterranean peoples, Asian peoples, Hispanics, and Native Americans. I would encourage people who desire a proper diet in any one of these categories (to include the average recommended diet) to visit www.usda.gov for further information. The USDA has also replaced its previous food pyramid recommendations with an easier to use MyPlate recommendation, which shows the food recommendations as well as relative quantities on a simple food plate design (figure 38.2). It can also be viewed at www.choosemyplate.gov.

Eating a proper diet can become quite complicated in some people who have lupus. For example, people who have certain forms of kidney disease, diabetes, and high blood pressure should make specific dietary changes. Knowing the proper things to

**Table 38.6** Recommended Daily Diet by the U.S. Department of Agriculture

- Grains (at least half of which are whole grains), 6 ounces a day.

- Vegetables, 2½ cups a day. The more colors (dark green, orange, red, yellow) the better. More beans and legumes should be included.

- Fruit, 2 cups a day; mainly from fresh, frozen, canned, and dried. Avoid too much fruit juice, which is high in sugar and low in fiber.

- Milk, 3 cups a day, primarily low-fat and fat-free products (milk, cheese, and yogurt). Lactose-intolerant people can choose lactose-free calcium-rich products.

- Meat and beans (protein) 5½ ounces a day.

- Make sure that fat sources primarily come from fish, nuts, and vegetable oils (less from other meats).

- Limit solid, unhealthy fats such as butter, margarine, shortening, and lard.

- Read nutrition labels and limit foods high in sodium, saturated fats, and trans-fatty acids.

- Read ingredient lists and avoid foods with added sugar such as high-fructose corn syrup.

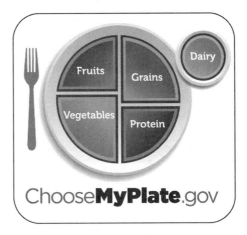

**Figure 38.2** MyPlate recommendations of a proper diet by the USDA

do can become quite daunting, especially when adding the above recommendations for diet. Those who have difficulty in eating a proper diet should strongly consider asking their doctors to send them to an experienced dietician for assistance. Many insurance companies will help cover the cost of seeing a dietician when it can improve health as prescribed by a doctor.

As far as the question of alcohol and lupus, the jury is still out whether it is protective against lupus or not. There have certainly been no studies showing that drinking alcohol increases the risks for developing lupus. However, there have been studies showing either a decreased risk of lupus or no increased risk in those who drink alcohol. A 2012 Japanese study showed that a light to moderate intake of alcohol appeared to be protective against developing SLE. Of course, there were patients who drank alcohol who developed SLE in the study, but the light or moderate drinkers were overall less likely to develop SLE compared to those who drank no alcohol and those who drank too much alcohol.

Numerous studies suggest that moderate intake of alcohol may decrease the risks for developing cardiovascular disease problems (which is the number one cause of death in people who have lupus), increases HDL good cholesterol levels, and may even decrease certain cancers. Before drinking alcohol, first double-check with your doctor to make sure it is not forbidden with your medicines. Prednisone, non-steroidal anti-inflammatory drugs (NSAIDs), acetaminophen, antidepressants, opioids, and methotrexate can potentially have more side effects if taken with alcohol. If you do drink alcohol, it is very important to drink a moderate amount of it. If you drink more than that, then the alcohol becomes toxic to various organs of the body such as the liver, brain, nerves, heart, and bones. Women should generally not drink more than one serving of alcohol within any twenty-four-hour period, while men should not drink more than two servings. One serving is approximately 12 ounces of beer, 8 ounces of malt liquor, 5 ounces of wine, 3 to 4 ounces of fortified wine (such as sherry and port), 2.5 ounces of 24% alcohol liqueur, or 1.5 ounces of 80-proof liquor. There is some evidence that red wine may have more health benefits than other forms of alcohol due to its containing antioxidants.

One word of caution is that there is a suggestion that regular alcohol consumption may increase the risk for breast cancer. It appears that a daily folic acid supplement may offset this potential risk. A woman's genes may also increase or decrease the risk of breast cancer from wine consumption. A 2011 study showed that women who carried a gene called BRCA1 actually had a much lower chance of getting breast cancer if they drank wine in moderation, while those who had a gene called BRCA2 mutation had a higher chance for getting breast cancer. These studies will need to be replicated, but it points out what the future may hold as to the importance of knowing exactly what genes we carry and how they affect our healthcare.

## Exercise

Just as Americans in general do not eat proper diets, we also do not exercise enough. In people who have lupus, regular exercise is important for many reasons (table 38.7). As mentioned numerous times in this book, the most common cause of death in people who have lupus is cardiovascular disease (heart attacks, strokes, and blood clots). Regular exercise (see chapter 7 for more detail on exercise), especially aerobic exercise, decreases the chances of developing these complications by improving cardiovascular health, decreasing bad cholesterol (LDL), increasing good cholesterol (HDL), decreasing blood pressure, improving diabetes control, and decreasing fat weight.

Most people who have lupus are overweight or obese (as mentioned in chapter 21) due to numerous reasons, including the use of steroids and decreased activity levels as a natural response of trying to deal with pain and fatigue. Obesity increases the chances of dying prematurely due to cardiovascular complications. Obesity also increases the activity of the immune system and inflammation, which can result in the need

**Table 38.7** Benefits of Regular Exercise in Lupus

- Decreases risk for heart attacks, strokes, and blood clots
- Decreases bad cholesterol (LDL) while increases good cholesterol (HDL)
- Decreases pro-inflammatory HDL cholesterol levels
- Improves high blood pressure control
- Improves diabetes control
- Decreases fat weight
- Increases muscle mass
- Increases bone density to fight osteoporosis
- Improves sleep quality
- Increases energy levels
- Decreases depression and anxiety
- Improves memory
- Improves quality of life, self-esteem, and one's sense of well-being

to use more steroids, which can in turn cause more fat weight gain. This vicious cycle of fat weight in lupus must be fought against with a concerted effort to lose weight through a combination of diet and exercise. Aerobic exercise (such as bicycling, brisk walking, jogging, treadmill, elliptical machine, or swimming) helps to burn up calories, while toning exercises (weight and strength training) can increase the amount of calorie-burning muscle mass. The USDA recommends a minimum of thirty minutes a day of physical activity to prevent weight gain. To lose appreciable weight, sixty minutes a day of physical exercise may be needed.

People who have lupus are at increased risk for brittle bones (osteoporosis) especially because of the use of steroids. The bones must "learn" to become strong by feeling stress through weight-bearing activities such as weight training, walking, and low-impact aerobics. People who are at high risk of osteoporosis should perform thirty minutes of a weight bearing–type exercise five days a week.

People who have lupus have more problems with sleep than do people who do not have lupus. This most likely is due to numerous reasons, including dealing with pain, medications that cause trouble sleeping, depression, fibromyalgia, and stress. Regular exercise helps to improve sleep quality (chapter 6). Exercise should be done at least a couple of hours before going to bed; otherwise the mind may be too active from all the activity from the exercise, making it more difficult to sleep.

Fatigue is by far one of the most common problems in lupus and one of the most difficult to manage. Regular exercise helps to improve energy levels. This can at first be difficult in someone who feels too tired to exercise. It is best to start on an exercise program gradually, increasing the amount of exercise slowly over time. Start with just a few minutes at a time, five days a week. Then every week or so increase the number of minutes until you get to thirty minutes or more of exercise a day.

Another good benefit of regular exercise is improved quality of life. Having a poor quality of life is a common denominator in studies on lupus patients. Regular exercise has been shown in lupus patients to significantly improve quality of life beyond just improving sleep and energy levels. It can help to decrease the amount of depression and anxiety, improve self-esteem, improve memory abilities, and increase one's sense of well-being.

Many people are not used to exercising, having grown up in families where exercise was not a priority or at a time before exercise became a focus in society. In addition, some people who have lupus have physical and mental difficulties that could place them at increased risk of injury if they were to exercise incorrectly. In these situations, it is best to get some professional help in learning to exercise properly. Getting a referral to a physical therapist from your doctor or getting assistance from a good personal trainer at a fitness center can be very helpful in these situations. In addition, there are community exercise classes specifically geared for people who have arthritis and other physical impairments. Water exercise classes are a good option for many people as well as exercise classes for seniors. The Arthritis Foundation is another good source to find out more information on exercise programs for people who have physical difficulties.

## Stress Reduction

Numerous studies have suggested that lupus can flare during times of stress. This has been shown to occur with major stressful events such as divorce or the death of a loved one as well as with intermittent normal stress (such as "daily hassles"). In addition, certain problems from lupus, such as having difficulty with memory, have been associated with increased amounts of stress as well. One study showed that increased stress was associated with an increase in memory problems in lupus patients. This association was independent from problems with depression and anxiety (both of which cause memory problems and are worse with stress).

The immune system becomes more active during stressful periods. This certainly is an interesting theory on why lupus may flare or become more active during stressful periods. A study in 2006 found a very interesting relationship to a gene that predisposes to stress. There are certain genes that people can be born with that make it more difficult to produce important chemicals in the brain such as serotonin (which is important for mood stabilization and pain relief). This report in 2006 showed that lupus patients who had this gene abnormality had increased lupus nephritis flares when they were exposed to increased stressful situations.

Experiencing stress while having a chronic disease, such as lupus, can become a vicious circle. People who have lupus and who are predisposed to stress can develop increased flares of their lupus. A lupus flare of course is an additional stressful event itself. Therefore, it would seem important that people who have lupus should learn important stress reduction techniques as an important part of treating their lupus. A study in 2010 attempted to answer this question by teaching a group of lupus patients how to handle stress by way of cognitive behavioral therapy (see chapter 27). They found that the group of patients who learned proper ways of dealing with stress ended up with decreased depression, anxiety, daily stress, and symptoms such as pain. They also had an overall better quality of life compared to the lupus patients who did not learn how to deal with stress. Therefore, it is important to learn to manage stress appropriately as part of your treatment.

Table 38.8 lists some strategies for decreasing stress. However, if you find that you are not able to cope and learn these techniques on your own, it can be a good idea to work with someone who can help. Professionals who can help you learn to deal with stress include counselors, psychologists, and sociologists.

An often-overlooked aspect of dealing with stress is that of how we deal with others in our lives. How we interact with our family, loved ones, and co-workers plays a much larger role in how we deal with medical illnesses and stress than we realize. It is a big mistake if you feel and act as if you are in this alone. People who have a good, thoughtful support structure are much better equipped for dealing with their medical problems and stressors compared to people who are isolated. It is very important not to isolate yourself. Instead, work on making interpersonal connections with other people; you never know when you will need their help. Getting involved in social events such as at church, other religious activities, groups that do hobbies you are interested in, or volunteering can all help in this aspect.

It is especially important to get your partner involved in what is going on with you. Some of the best supportive relationships I have witnessed have been those where the spouse or significant other accompanies the person to doctor visits. That way they can learn more about their loved one's disorder and understand more about what they are going through medically. If your loved one works during the periods that you see your doctor, you can consider other activities such as attending educational lupus seminars together, or at least provide him or her with educational material to read. If your relationship unfortunately was already not on very good grounds, then inserting a chronic medical condition such as lupus can make things even more difficult for you. In that type of situation, professional help such as counseling may be needed to learn proper communication skills for reconnecting in a loving, giving two-way relationship.

## Adequate Sleep

Most Americans do not get enough sleep. Inadequate sleep is linked to numerous medical conditions, including obesity, body pain, fibromyalgia, depression, diabetes, and migraines. Although inadequate sleep does not cause lupus, people who have SLE have been shown to have worse sleep patterns compared to people who do not have lupus. Inadequate sleep in people who have SLE has been associated with an increased amount of depression, difficulties with memory, fatigue, and fibromyalgia. In addition, increased disease activity disrupts normal sleep. Getting inadequate sleep increases the chances of developing these common problems in lupus (fatigue, memory problems, depression, fibromyalgia, and obesity) and therefore needs to be taken seriously. All people who have lupus need to learn to purposefully schedule in at least eight hours of sleep a night and practice good sleep hygiene (see table 6.2).

**Table 38.8** Stress Reduction Techniques

- Learn to say "no" to increased amounts of work and duties.
- When you have children, it is even more important to learn to say "no" to additional activities other than what is immediately important for your family and your health.
- Learn to ask for help in doing activities.
- Proactively lighten your load.
- Prioritize the important things in your life; cut out activities that are less important.
- Do yoga and/or tai chi.
- Get biofeedback training from a professional to learn to decrease anxiety and stress.
- Do deep breathing exercises and perform "mental imagery" exercises.
- Pray frequently.
- Meditate.
- Prepare well ahead of time for any major activity.
- Learn to practice good time management.
- Plan specifically for periods of rest and relaxation in your routine *every day*.
- Learn to say positive things to yourself and compliment yourself for doing things well.
- Do not think negative things about yourself.
- When running errands or going to appointments, always get ready early and give yourself more time than you think you need; always plan on arriving early for any occasion.
- Schedule appointments and errands during less busy times such as early Saturday mornings. This can greatly decrease stress due to traffic, waiting in long lines, and the like.
- Learn not to argue with others. Learning and accepting that everyone has differing opinions or ways of doing things and that many conflicts are not very important is essential. Learn to take a deep breath, relax, leave before an argument begins or before you say something you may regret.
- Learn to live at or below your means. Too many people in America try to keep up with the "Joneses" or other family members and friends. Learning to stay out of debt can greatly decrease stress. Always ask yourself "is this something I truly need, or just something I want?" before you buy it.
- Whenever you feel stressed, put it into perspective compared to the important things in life (health, family, religion). Learn to "not sweat the small stuff."
- Exercise regularly.
- Schedule in at least eight hours of planned sleep a night.
- Do not skip healthy, planned meals.
- Avoid unhealthy foods such as sweets, carbohydrates, greasy foods, and "fast food."
- Consider counseling to learn better communication skills if you have difficulties with relationships.
- Consider attending lupus or chronic illness support groups to learn techniques for dealing with lupus, stress, and relationships.

## Brief Summary

The importance of these non-drug therapies in lupus cannot be overemphasized. Although this chapter dealt with these measures specifically in regards to how they are important in people who have SLE, many of these measures are very important in people who do not have lupus as well. A 2011 study by the Centers for Disease Control and Prevention showed this poignantly. The study showed that four health risk behaviors were responsible for most early deaths. These were poor nutrition, not exercising, drinking excessive amounts of alcohol, and smoking cigarettes. Not smoking cigarettes provided the best protection from dying from all causes. In people who eat a proper diet, exercise, drink alcohol in moderation (as defined previously in the chapter), and do not smoke cigarettes, there was a 63% overall reduction in death rate. There was a 66% reduction in cancer deaths, and 65% reduction in cardiovascular deaths (heart attacks and strokes). Interestingly, moderate alcohol consumption showed the largest single benefit on lowering cardiovascular death (which is the most common cause of death of people who have SLE in the United States). Many people get tired of their doctors telling them to "eat right, exercise regularly, don't drink too much, and don't smoke!" This study showed that what physicians tell their patients is true. The people in this study who did all four of these healthy habits added more than a decade (11.1 additional years) to their lifespan on average simply from following these recommendations. Therefore, it really is imperative that people who have SLE learn to do and put into practice the lifestyle changes presented in this chapter. It takes a lot of work, but in the end, it is worth it.

### KEY POINTS TO REMEMBER

1. The treatment of lupus should include non-drug measures in addition to just taking medicines.

2. All people who have lupus (whether they get lupus rashes or not) need to abide by strict UV light protection (table 38.3), including wearing sunscreen religiously every day.

3. There are numerous reasons people who have lupus should not smoke. If you do smoke, get help to stop smoking ASAP.

4. If you are unable to stop smoking on your own, go to www.smokefree.gov or call 1-800-QUIT-NOW.

5. Do not eat alfalfa or mung bean sprouts, which can cause lupus to flare.

6. Eat a low-calorie, low-fat diet.

7. Include foods rich in omega-3 fatty acids in your daily diet.

8. Include olive oil in your diet.

9. Eat a diet rich in vegetables, fruits, whole grains, nuts, and low-fat dairy.

10. Limit the amounts of non-fish meat proteins, high-fructose corn syrup, sugar, salt, and fat in your diet.

11. Thirty minutes or more of physical activity should be done daily.

12. Up to sixty minutes of physical activity a day may be needed to help with weight loss.

13. Learn and practice stress reduction techniques regularly (table 38.8).

14. Schedule in at least eight hours of sleep a day and abide by good sleep hygiene (table 6.2).

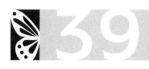

# Complementary and Alternative Medicine

## Complementary Medicine Can Be Good;
## Alternative Medicine Is Bad

Ms. DC has had systemic lupus erythematosus (SLE) for quite a few years. She has had arthritis, rash, and Raynaud's phenomenon from her lupus. However, her biggest problem is severe lung disease. In the past, she had severe inflammation of the lungs (pneumonitis) that ended up causing permanent, severe lung damage. As you may recall from chapter 10, lupus pneumonitis is a very dangerous problem. In Ms. DC's case, she survived the active inflammatory part of her lung disease, but her lungs have permanent scarring that leaves her dependent on the use of oxygen and that has given her significant pulmonary hypertension. I have cared for Ms. DC for more than ten years, and she continues to do as well as when I first met her. She has defied the odds as far as doing so well while having such severe lupus. So what sets her apart from other patients who have lupus? I believe it is due to how she lives her life outside of taking the medicines I have prescribed for lupus.

Ms. DC is practicing what is termed "complementary medicine" (more recently, "integrative medicine"). In other words, she uses these other forms of therapies along with the medical therapies that I recommend that she use. The natural therapies (nutrition, supplements, and exercise) "complement" her prescribed lupus therapies. She is fully committed to eating properly. She only eats organic food, includes lots of vegetables and fruits in her diet, and avoids milk "because it increases mucus." She prefers to see a holistic or naturopathic primary care doctor who treats her with dietary supplements and guides her medical care with dietary recommendations. She is very much into taking dietary supplements and she exercises regularly. She always has a smile on her face and is optimistic about her life and her future. Although I do not fully understand everything about her "natural" diet, such as why avoiding milk is so important in decreasing mucus . . . it works for her. I cannot deny the success of her lifestyle. In fact, it makes me very happy because it is so hard to get patients to eat a proper diet, exercise regularly, and take their medications. I am perfectly fine if she takes dietary supplements as long as she checks with me first to ensure that they are not harmful for her lupus.

An opposing example would be Ms. AK. She was another woman who had SLE whom I met while I was learning rheumatology as a rheumatology fellow. I got to know her best during my time on the rheumatology hospital service. She was severely ill in the intensive care unit. I reviewed her clinic records and talked with her primary rheumatologist. Like Ms. DC, she also strongly believed in herbal and holistic medicine. However, what sets her apart from Ms. DC is that she continuously refused to take any of the medications for lupus, saying that she was "afraid of the side effects." Her use of these other therapies is what doctors call "alternative medicine." In other words, she preferred to use non-conventional, non-medical therapies by themselves (as an "alternative") without using the treatments that her rheumatologist recommended.

Sadly, Ms. AK passed away quickly while on an artificial respirator due to severe, untreated lupus. Since treating Ms. AK, I have had to watch several additional lupus patients die from their disease due to their being "afraid of the side effects" of medicines and preferring to take herbal, holistic products instead. In contrast, I have not had any patients die from any of the medicines I have used to treat their lupus, including strong ones such as cyclophosphamide. Now, whenever I hear patients say they do not want to take their medicine because they are "afraid of the side effects" and would rather take herbal, holistic therapies . . . I cringe inside. I know what can and most likely will happen. I educate them about their lupus, about what happens when it is not treated appropriately. I teach them about how important it is to realize that "side effects" do not happen in most patients who take the medicines doctors prescribe (other than with prednisone), and that the vast majority of side effects can be dealt with safely if they do occur. The expected consequences of untreated lupus far outweigh the possibility of side effects from the medications. I do not mind at all if patients want to incorporate holistic and complementary medicine along with their medical therapy (i.e., use them as "complementary medicine" or "integrative medicine"). However, I strongly believe it is bad to use these non-conventional medical therapies as an alternative to the proven medical therapies for SLE.

This chapter discusses in detail the views of doctors when it comes to alternative forms of therapies. It explains why many doctors do not embrace them as much as patients and how herbal and "natural" products can be just as unsafe as prescribed medicines. However, people who have SLE can safely combine "complementary medicine" or "integrative medicine" with the therapies prescribed by their physician, and this chapter provides some guidance. In fact, some of these therapies can be greatly helpful, especially if they help someone to become better with their diet, exercise, and lifestyle habits.

. . . .

Alternative medicine is a group of therapies that do not fall under the realm of conventional, Western medicine. They are often based on cultural and historical traditions instead of scientific proof. "Alternative medicine" is the term applied when these therapies are used by themselves. "Complementary medicine" and "integrative medicine" are the terms used when they are practiced in conjunction with conventional, Western medicine. So why are so many doctors skeptical about these non-conventional medical therapies and herbal medicines?

Doctors always want to do what is best for their patients (contrary to what some people may think). They want to help prevent bad things from happening (hence, their soapbox lectures on eating right, exercising, not smoking, etc.), plus diagnose and treat any illnesses based on the best available research. Doctors want to use therapies proven to work and that have been shown to be safer than other forms of treatments. First, let us look at the real-life results of a real research study to help illustrate how doctors evaluate treatments.

Figure 39.1 shows the results of a study looking at the effects of a pill to treat rheumatoid arthritis. The measurement used for this study was something called an ACR-20 score. This measurement counts patients as having a significant response to a treatment for rheumatoid arthritis only if they have at least a 20% reduction in several different measurements (such as at least a 20% decrease in pain severity and a 20% decrease in the number of tender joints). This bar graph shows the results in the patients who took one of the therapies in the study. Thirty-five percent of the patients who took this treatment reached an ACR-20 response or higher at the end of the study. This means that 35% of the patients had at least a 20% improvement in several measurements such as at least a 20% decrease in pain and at least a 20% decrease in the number of tender, painful joints. Thirty-five percent of the patients thought, "This medicine is really helping my arthritis!"

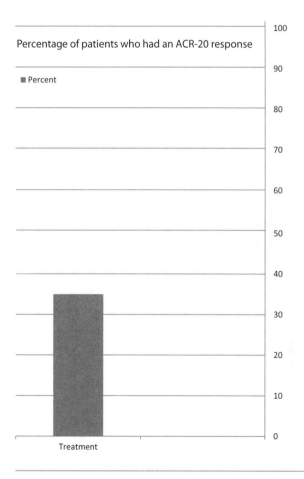

Figure 39.1 ACR-20 response in people who have rheumatoid arthritis

Next, look at figure 39.2. This shows the full results of the study. The "therapy" that those 35% of patients were taking was no therapy at all. It was actually a placebo ("sugar pill"). In this particular study, the placebo group was being compared to a group of patients taking a non-steroidal anti-inflammatory drug (NSAID) called rofecoxib. Forty-nine percent of the patients who took rofecoxib at a dosage of 25 mg a day also reached an ACR-20 response. Statisticians (mathematical experts) determined that there was a statistically significant difference between the placebo and the medication being studied (rofecoxib).

What this illustrates is what doctors call the placebo effect. Especially with arthritis problems, there is typically a significant placebo effect. Placebos repeatedly have about a 35% response rate in arthritis studies. There are numerous potential reasons for this. One is that the pain of arthritis tends to fluctuate over time even without treatment. If someone's arthritis is doing poorly at the beginning of the research study,

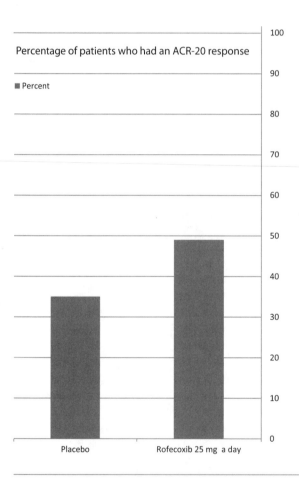

Percentage of patients who had an ACR-20 response

■ Percent

**Figure 39.2** ACR-20 response in people who have rheumatoid arthritis: typical placebo effect

then improves on its own at the end of the study (since it just happens to be in its particular cycle of improvement), then that person will appear to have gotten better, even if she or he took a fake medicine (the placebo). Another reason is what you could call the power of suggestion or the power of the mind. It is amazing how the brain can decrease pain on its own. For example, think about times when you had some sort of discomfort such as back pain and then "something came up" that made your mind start thinking about something else. Before you knew it, your back stopped hurting because your mind and thoughts focused on something other than the pain. The opposite also happens. For example, think about times when you had a little bit of back soreness, and then something happens that really stresses you. All at once, your back pain is unbearable. This is most likely not because your back problem actually got worse, but because the stress caused an increased amount of muscle spasms and pain in your back. The effect of the mind can be very strong when it comes to arthritis and pain. In studies with SLE, the placebo effect can be as high as 50%.

For any treatment to be considered truly effective, it must be proven to be better than a placebo in a research study conducted in such a way that neither the doctors nor the patients know if they are taking the treatment or the placebo (fake medicine). Both the doctors and the patients are "blind" as to what treatment they are actually getting (the study therapy versus the placebo therapy). If both the doctors and the patients do not know what the treatments are, then it is a "double-blind" study. At the end of the study, statisticians calculate whether the treatment being tested (whether it is a drug, exercise, an herb, acupuncture, etc.) worked better than the placebo. The best studies to show whether a therapy works or not are double-blind, placebo-controlled studies. Research studies that do not use some sort of placebo or where the doctors and patients know what therapy they are taking (and therefore, not a double-blind, placebo-controlled study) are considered inferior studies. This is one of many potential reasons a doctor may say, "This was not a very well done study" when evaluating studies of lower quality.

One reason for bringing up the placebo effect is that when people decide to try anything to help them with a medical condition, there is always the chance that they could feel that the therapy helped them simply from either the condition getting better on its own, or their feeling better through the power of the mind. For example, let us say someone sees an advertisement in a magazine (or on late night television) for a copper bracelet touted as a cure for arthritis pain. Along with the ad are numerous testimonials from people who used it and claim that it got rid of their arthritis pain. Therefore, the person sends away a check for the bracelet (e.g., three low monthly payments of only $19.99 per month) and starts to wear it immediately after it arrives. A week or so later, the hand pains start to feel better. The person cannot help but think, "Wow, this really works." She or he tells friends and relatives, and maybe a couple of them end up buying one as well. Therefore, did the bracelet really work, or is this person simply one of the 35% of arthritis patients who were destined to feel better because of the placebo effect? More than likely, it is the latter. Studies on copper bracelets and arthritis show that they do not work any better than placebo. If you were my patient and asked me about it, I would give you my typical answer, "If you can afford it, and you like the way it looks, and it helps you feel better, I think it is a good idea for you to use it; however, it has not been proven to be effective for arthritis."

That is my standard thought on complementary and alternative therapies that have not been proven through good, double-blind, placebo-controlled studies. Even if I do not think something may work, if it is not too expensive for the person, is not going to be harmful, and does not interact with other medicines, then it is fine to do. In fact, anything that helps my patients feel better about themselves and about their condition is good. I can never underestimate the power of the mind-body connection. I do object, though, if patients want to abandon their medical therapy for unproven alternative therapies. In that case, they are putting their health and their lives at risk. Otherwise, there is no reason why someone cannot use both the proven medical therapies and the complementary therapies.

The problem with many alternative and complementary studies is that many of them (if not most of them) have not passed the stringent tests of well-done research studies (proving them more effective than a placebo). Therefore, many doctors are reluctant to recommend them to patients. However, this way of thinking must also be tempered by the fact that it can be very difficult to get the proper studies done in the first place. It takes a lot of money to do large, proper research studies. Without major investments from large pharmaceutical companies and rich investors, it is very difficult to fund such studies.

Fortunately, the National Institutes of Health established the National Center for Complementary and Alternative Medicine (NCCAM) in 1998. NCCAM promotes and funds exactly this type of research. A list of its active research studies can be viewed at www.nccam.nih.gov/research/clinicaltrials/alltrials.htm. Unfortunately, there currently are no complementary therapy trials studying lupus, but there are numerous studies being done on other types of arthritis and pain (table 39.1). You can check to see if any of these studies are recruiting patients to participate and even join a study if you are close to the center that is conducting it. As the results of these studies become published and known to physicians, it will make it easier for them to advise patients on the potential benefits and risks of using these forms of therapies.

The process of picking and choosing between the different available complementary therapies can be quite daunting since many different forms of therapies exist. I briefly discuss some of the facts about them to give some guidance from a medical doctor's point of view. When considering complementary therapies, weigh the potential pros and cons of each therapy. Ask yourself if it is truly worth your time and money to consider the therapy if it has not been proven to work. Always ask your doctor whether it is safe for you to participate in the therapy in regards to your medical condition and medications. If you see a complementary or alternative therapy provider, ask him or her to send notes with diagnoses and therapy recommendations to your medical doctor (and vice versa) so that open communication exists to give you the best overall, coordinated medical care. The rest of this chapter is divided into large categories of complementary medicine as delineated by the NCCAM. Some therapies overlap between these major categories and some therapies use a combination of various different categories.

**Table 39.1** Complementary Therapy Research Sponsored by the NCCAM

- Acupuncture (osteoarthritis, back pain, carpal tunnel syndrome, fibromyalgia)
- Aerobic exercise (fibromyalgia)
- Biofeedback (fibromyalgia)
- Black cohosh (osteoporosis)
- Borage seed oil (rheumatoid arthritis)
- Chinese herbs (rheumatoid arthritis)
- Chiropractic and spinal manipulation (back pain, neck pain, temporomandibular joint disorder [TMJ])
- Fish oil (rheumatoid arthritis)
- Glucosamine and chondroitin (osteoarthritis)
- Green tea (osteoporosis)
- Homeopathy (fibromyalgia)
- Isoflavones (osteoporosis)
- Magnetic therapy (rheumatoid arthritis, carpal tunnel syndrome)
- Marine and botanical oils (rheumatoid arthritis)
- Massage (back and neck pain, headaches, knee arthritis)
- Mind-body interventions (fibromyalgia, back pain, knee osteoarthritis)
- Phytoestrogens (osteoporosis)
- Prolotherapy (osteoarthritis, tennis elbow)
- Qigong (osteoarthritis)
- Relaxation therapy (rheumatoid arthritis, back pain)
- Reiki (fibromyalgia)
- Shamanic healing (temporomandibular joint disease [TMJ])
- Tai chi (rheumatoid arthritis, osteoarthritis, back pain, fibromyalgia, osteoporosis)
- Therapeutic touch (wrist fractures, knee arthritis, low back pain, chronic neck pain, fibromyalgia)
- Yoga (arthritis in general, osteoarthritis, back pain, insomnia, smoking cessation)

## Whole Medical Systems

Whole medical systems are complete systems of diagnosis and medical practice that focus on a particular philosophy such as the power of nature or the presence of energy in the body. Traditional Chinese medicine is one of the most widely recognized systems, but several others exist as well and are discussed in this section.

### Traditional Chinese Medicine

Traditional Chinese medicine has been around for thousands of years. It is based on the theory that disease and illness result from improper flows of energy through the body. A proper balance of the opposing forces of yin and yang is felt to be important. Traditional Chinese medicine uses a combination of diet, Chinese herbs, massage, meditation, and acupuncture. Most medical doctors (including myself) are opposed to the use of Chinese herbs. They are not standardized; may contain harmful drugs, metals, and chemicals; and have been reported to cause significant health problems, including kidney failure. However, there are some interesting study results using Chinese herbs in the treatment of lupus.

Lupus nephritis (kidney inflammation) is treated as a deficiency of "kidney yin" or "liver-kidney yin" in traditional Chinese medicine. There have been at least eight studies showing that traditional Chinese medicine helps lupus nephritis when it is added to conventional medical therapies. In addition, these studies reported fewer side effects in those who took the herbs with their medicines compared to the patients who did not take the herbal products. However, the vast majority of these studies were published in Chinese medical journals without the scrutiny and evaluation of worldwide lupus experts. Doctors like to see studies published in what are called peer-reviewed journals. This means that they are evaluated very carefully by experts in the medical journal's specialty, often from different countries. These particular studies using Chinese herbs came from Chinese journals, so their reproducibility and accuracy cannot be verified. However, it is clear that these herbal products deserve closer attention and more in-depth studies. The studies need to be repeated using standardized dosing of the herbs (as discussed below) in the setting of proper large, placebo-controlled studies. One thing to keep in mind is that herbal therapies are indeed medicines and are not without the potential for side effects. There have been cases of severe kidney disease, anemia, and heart problems from taking Chinese herbal products.

Acupuncture is one of the most familiar forms of traditional Chinese medicine. It consists of the insertion of very tiny needles into the skin at various points of the body. This is felt to affect the flow of energy (called qi) of different parts of the body and to restore a balance of yin and yang forces. This form of Chinese medicine is becoming more widely accepted and used by medical doctors. It may be useful for some medical conditions, including decreasing the severity of pain. A 2012 report in the Archives of Internal Medicine reviewed the largest and best studies using acupuncture for chronic pain and found that it can be helpful. There are drawbacks: it usually entails getting treatment several times a week, most insurance companies do not cover it, and it can get quite expensive over time. In addition, unwarranted claims are sometimes made such as it being able to cure conditions or help the immune system. These claims have absolutely no basis and should make you think twice before seeing a practitioner who makes such exaggerated claims. Also, make sure that you see an acupuncturist who has proper credentials and training to do acupuncture.

There have been no well-done studies in lupus to look at the usefulness of acupuncture. One small 2008 study using acupuncture showed no difference between the acupuncture group and the placebo acupuncture group as far as pain or fatigue improvement in lupus patients. Another Chinese study suggested that acupuncture of the earlobes improved discoid lupus rashes and "well-being" in fifteen patients. However, there was no placebo control group. For rheumatoid arthritis (which is closely related to lupus), there are a few published trials. The best-done study showed no significant benefit. Based on these results, I cannot recommend its use for SLE.

## Ayurveda

Ayurveda comes from India and may be a couple of thousand years older than even Chinese medicine. It also is based on the belief that illness comes from an imbalance of the body's life force. Its practitioners use a combination of diet, herbs, massage, meditation, yoga, fasting, and internal cleansing. Just as with Chinese herbs, there are no standard controls with Ayurvedic herbs and they should be avoided. Yoga (which is practiced in Ayurvedic medicine) has been shown to be helpful for some medical conditions such as fibromyalgia.

## Witchcraft

Witchcraft, the use of magical and supernatural powers to heal disease, is practiced in many cultures around the world. There is one case of a lupus patient being "cured" by a Filipino witch doctor. She was 28 years old and had severe lupus nephritis. When she was not able to tolerate prednisone, she returned to her village in the Philippines where the local witch doctor removed a curse placed on her by a previous suitor. Her Western doctor documented no evidence of active SLE at a follow-up visit a few weeks later. Other than this case report (which, by the way, does not prove that witchcraft works in SLE), there are no other cases of witchcraft in the medical literature being used in SLE.

## Homeopathy

"Homeo-" comes from the Greek word for "like" while "-opathy" comes from the Greek word for "disease." It is based on the principle that "like cures like." If something causes problems or a disease when given in large doses, then it is felt that it may cure that disease when given in very tiny doses. The father of homeopathy was Christian Friedrich Samuel Hahnemann, a German physician. Its origins actually share a path similar to that of lupus treatments. Hahnemann was interested in cinchona bark, which was being touted as useful to treat malaria. (Remember, quinine derived from the cinchona bark has some similarities to anti-malarials used to treat lupus.) He decided to take some of the bark medicine himself. He developed symptoms that he felt were similar to the problems seen from malaria (fever, changes in blood flow, feeling poorly, etc.), coming up with his "like cures like" hypothesis.

Practitioners of homeopathy base treatments not only on the symptoms of a disease, but also on a person's personality and lifestyle. No homeopathic therapies have been proven to be helpful for any rheumatologic condition. In addition, a 2012 review found a total of 1,159 reported side effects occurring from homeopathic remedies with allergic reactions and intoxications being the most common. Four fatalities were included. Due to there being no evidence of homeopathy being helpful in lupus, yet a significant number of side effects being reported, homeopathy should not be used by people who have SLE.

## Naturopathy

Naturopathy emphasizes prevention and treatment of disease through a healthy lifestyle. Treatment of the whole person is emphasized and trying to find the root cause of a disease and addressing the cause becomes a focus of treatment instead of just treating symptoms. It can use a combination of therapies, including herbs, homeopathy, physical therapy, mind-body therapy, exercise, diet, stress reduction, and hydrotherapy. Naturopathic doctors can employ a combination of many different forms of complementary medicine. Naturopathic doctors may also go by the term "integrative medicine doctors" as they "integrate" complementary therapies into standard medical regimens.

Since they often emphasize diet, exercise, stress reduction, and other healthy lifestyle choices, naturopathic therapies can be a good choice for many people. Just as it is important to choose a medical doctor with proper credentials and expertise, it is just as important to do the same with a naturopathic doctor (table 39.2). Choose a doctor who fulfills the recommendations listed in table 39.2. Make sure that you do not replace your medical doctor's therapies with the naturopathic therapies, but use them in conjunction with each other. You should also always check with your medical doctor before beginning any naturopathic therapies to ensure that they will not be bad for your lupus or have any untoward interactions with your medications.

## Mind-Body Medicine

These techniques are based on the theory that mental and emotional factors influence physical health and well-being. They use behavioral, social, psychological, and spiritual methods. Many of these techniques (such as biofeedback, hypnosis, and relaxation techniques) are a part of mainstream medicine to treat some problems. These therapies are most commonly used for problems such as pain, anxiety, panic disorder, problems with sleeping, headaches, and depression.

### Biofeedback

Biofeedback is a fascinating type of therapy where you can teach your brain to control biologic processes that are not under conscious control. The biofeedback therapist monitors various biologic functions such as blood pressure, brain waves, heart rate,

**Table 39.2**  How to Choose a Naturopathic Doctor

- Graduated with a degree, ND (doctor of naturopathy) or NMD (doctor of naturopathic medicine), from a recognized institution
- Has a current license recognized by the ruling state or national agency
- Carries malpractice insurance
- Is a member in good standing with a professional organization for naturopathic doctors
- The office staff's and doctor's manners are professional
- The doctor provides diagnoses and treatments, and has reasonable expectations of results and side effects of the treatments
- Keeps accurate records
- Is willing to send notes to your rheumatologist and other physicians

muscle tension, and temperature and guides the person undergoing the therapy to learn how to change these conditions. It can be used to treat pain, stress, and sleep problems. In SLE, it particularly has a potential role in treating Raynaud's phenomenon. I have actually participated in biofeedback, and I was amazed at my ability to decrease my own blood pressure and to increase the temperature of my own hands. Unfortunately, many health plans do not pay for it, and I have found very few patients willing to consider it in the treatment of their Raynaud's (although I would much prefer trying this over my giving them a medication).

## Prayer

The power of prayer has not been formally studied in lupus, but it has been studied in other medical conditions. A 2000 review of medical prayer studies showed that 57% of the studies had a positive treatment effect. Therefore, prayer should be encouraged in people who use prayer in their religious beliefs. I personally use prayer daily in my own practice for my patients.

## Meditation

Meditation refers to a large group of practices used in religion as well as for secular (non-religious) purposes to change a person's inward mode of consciousness. Prayer is one type of meditation. It often involves resting quietly, often with the eyes closed, concentrating on breathing, and sometimes involves saying words repeatedly (called a mantra). In complementary medicine, it is used to increase calmness and physical relaxation, to improve psychological balance, to cope with illness, or to enhance overall health and well-being. There are no studies using meditation for lupus, however, two studies have shown its usefulness for the pain and tenderness of rheumatoid arthritis.

## Relaxation, Aromatherapy, and Art Therapies

Relaxation therapies comprise a very large group of interventions, including meditation, prayer, and many other techniques such as hypnosis to help decrease pain and anxiety. Doctors and nurses practice it daily by teaching patients breathing techniques, guided/mental imagery, and other strategies to take the person's mind off potentially painful procedures as well as for other uses.

Hypnotherapy (hypnosis) can be included as a type of relaxation therapy where the hypnotherapist guides the individual into a heightened state of relaxation along with an increased focus in attention. It has been used for anxiety, smoking cessation, weight control, and to help decrease pain.

Aromatherapy uses the inhalation of essential oils from trees, herbs, and flowers to promote health and well-being. Examples of oils used include chamomile, lavender, geranium, cedar, and lemon. Proponents of this form of therapy suggest that they can help with mood, sleep, decrease stress, and possibly help with pain and nausea. Research suggests that lavender and chamomile may help with sleep. There are no studies proving their use in lupus.

Art therapy is a type of psychotherapy where the patient uses art to communicate. Patients do not need to have any art experience at all. It can especially be helpful to try to deal with the emotional stresses of illness. You can find a practitioner of art therapy by contacting the American Association of Art Therapists at www.arttherapy.org.

## Biologically Based Practices

### Dietary Supplements

Some dietary supplements may be useful in treating SLE (table 39.3). DHEA is a pre-steroid hormone (see chapter 35). Many people who have lupus have lower DHEA levels than normal. Several studies suggest that taking DHEA regularly can improve mild lupus symptoms, including increase energy levels, help with mental clarity, and allow doctors to decrease steroid doses. It also may improve bone density, which can be helpful in people who have osteoporosis. The studies were impressive enough that an attempt was made to get DHEA FDA-approved to treat SLE. This attempt failed, as has occurred with many other medications useful for lupus, due to the difficulties involved in proving that medicines for lupus are effective. The most common side effects seen were acne and increased hair growth.

A downside of dietary supplements is that currently in the United States, there is no purity regulation for the supplements that you can buy over the counter. The government exerts its power by removing and policing items that are unsafe for the public; other than that, a lot of the time you do not know what you are truly buying. For example, studies show that a large number of DHEA products that you can buy over the counter are inferior. Many contain a much smaller amount of DHEA (and even no DHEA in some cases) than what is listed on the label. This even goes for minerals and vitamins that you buy. A 2013 study showed that vitamin D-3 supplements vary widely regarding how much vitamin D they actually contain. Therefore, it is always better to try to get as much as you can (vitamins and minerals) from the foods you eat, as discussed in chapter 38. For other supplements such as DHEA, it is actually better to ask your doctor to write you a prescription and then have it filled by a compounding pharmacist to ensure that you get a superior product.

Another type of supplement that may potentially be helpful in lupus (but not proven) is the anti-inflammatory fats (eicosapentaenoic acids, or omega-3 fatty acids), as discussed in chapter 38. In addition, they may also be helpful for the dry eyes of Sjögren's syndrome, as discussed in chapter 14. However, highly processed capsules that you buy over the counter may not be as trustworthy as foods rich in these oils. Try to get these fats naturally by eating more fish, flaxseed, olive oil, and walnuts instead of through supplements (as they may help to decrease inflammation from SLE).

**Table 39.3** Dietary Supplements Possibly Helpful in Some People Who Have SLE

- DHEA
- Omega-3 fatty acids (fish oil and flaxseed oil)
- Multiple vitamin
- Calcium supplements
- Vitamin D

Avoid taking mega-doses of vitamins. Doctors really do not know how safe they are, and some studies have shown surprising results with increased side effects with some vitamins. It is much better to eat lots of fruits and vegetables, as well as whole grains in place of simple carbohydrates (wheat flour, pasta, etc.), instead of taking high doses of vitamins (refer to chapter 38). If you cannot force yourself to eat enough daily whole grains, fruits, and vegetables, then you probably should be taking a daily multi-vitamin tablet.

Most people who have lupus are deficient in vitamin D and should be taking a vitamin D supplement (see chapter 24). Vitamin D is essential for proper functioning of the immune system and its deficiency has been associated with more severe cases of SLE. Therefore, it is essential that all people who have lupus have their vitamin D levels checked regularly and that they take a supplement if they are low in vitamin D.

Anyone who is taking a medication to lower stomach acidity should consider taking a calcium citrate supplement as these stomach acid lowering medicines prevent you from absorbing most forms of calcium from food as well as calcium carbonate (the calcium found in products such as OsCal and Caltrate). Many people of African ancestry are lactose intolerant and cannot eat or drink enough dairy products daily to get enough calcium, so they should also take a daily calcium supplement. Again, refer to chapter 24 for more in-depth instructions.

There is some controversy over the use of melatonin by people who have lupus. Melatonin is a hormone released by the pineal gland of the brain. It signals the brain to prepare for sleep when it senses decreased light in the evening. Therefore, melatonin can be helpful as a sleep aid. There are some theoretical concerns that it may also increase activity of the immune system. Therefore, some doctors recommend that lupus patients not take it. However, medical studies do not support this concern. In fact, female mice that had SLE in a couple of studies have actually shown that their lupus improved when they took melatonin. However, male mice that had SLE got worse. The only use of melatonin in humans with systemic autoimmune disease was done in patients who had rheumatoid arthritis. Taking melatonin neither worsened nor improved their disease. If melatonin were to make autoimmune diseases worse, you would expect it to cause rheumatoid arthritis to be worse. Based on this evidence, I would caution men who have lupus not to take melatonin (based on the lupus mouse studies), but there is no evidence to dissuade women who have lupus from taking it.

## Herbal Therapies

Other than Chinese herbal therapies mentioned previously, the other most commonly studied herb to treat lupus is *Tripterygium wilfordii hook F* (TwHF). TwHF is a Chinese herb that has been used for more than two thousand years. There have been no large, well-designed studies looking at the use TwHF in lupus. However, there have been 5 uncontrolled studies in a total of 249 lupus patients. These studies suggested improvements in some lupus symptoms such as fatigue, joint pain, fever, rash, lupus nephritis activity, and low platelet counts. There may actually be some theoretical reasons TwHF may potentially help with inflammatory diseases, as it does appear to have some anti-inflammatory effects in research studies. However, it is not without its potential risks. Side effects of taking TwHF include intestinal problems (diarrhea, nausea, vomiting), hair loss, dry mouth, headaches, rash, mouth sores, changes in weight, and elevated blood pressure. Infertility has been reported with its use, and there is a case of a young man who died from heart toxicity from the use of TwHF. It is also not safe to take during pregnancy as fetal abnormalities have been reported.

Another herbal supplement called pycnogenol phytotherapy was used in one small study. It suggested that it may be useful in lupus patients. However, there were only eleven SLE patients in this study.

Chinese herbs as a part of traditional Chinese medicine have been the most studied herbs used to treat lupus, as noted previously. Almost all of the studies showed significant improvements in SLE patients, especially when the herbs were used in conjunction with Western medicines (such as prednisone and cyclophosphamide). However, these studies are limited to some Chinese medical journals and no significant studies have been reported in Western medical journals. The safety of Chinese herbal medications cannot even be assured in China itself. One study obtained 430 different samples of Chinese herbs in Taiwan from local hospitals, medical centers, and herb stands. The study found that one-third of the herbal products were contaminated with Western medicines, including phenylbutazone, which is no longer used in the United States because of its severe side effects.

Some important reservations exist regarding the use of herbal products in treating people who have lupus. "Natural herbs" are medications. Just because something is "natural" does not at all mean that it is "safe." Some of the most powerful and potentially toxic medicines (when not dosed and monitored correctly) have come directly from plants. These include the use of colchicine for gout (from the Autumn crocus), digoxin for heart disease (originating from the digitalis plant), quinidine for heart disease and quinine for malaria (both from the cinchona tree bark), and Taxol for cancer (from the Pacific yew tree). *Tripterygium wilfordii hook F* is another good example. It appears to have medicinal qualities and may help with inflammatory diseases (not just lupus, but also rheumatoid arthritis); however, it also has potential side effects as well.

There are other numerous accounts in the medical literature of herbal products causing bad side effects. This has especially been noted for some Chinese herbal supplements causing kidney disease. Chinese herbal preparations made from the plants of the Aristolochia family have repeatedly been connected with reports of kidney failure and even cancer of the urinary tract.

Echinacea deserves special mention. It is touted as boosting the immune system and theoretically could cause autoimmune diseases to become more active. Dr. Michelle Petri, medical director of the Lupus Clinic at Johns Hopkins, reports that they have had a series of patients who developed significant flares of their SLE while taking Echinacea. Unfortunately, two patients even required the use of the strong chemotherapy agent cyclophosphamide for severe lupus nephritis flares due to taking Echinacea. I had one teenage boy who came to our pediatric rheumatology clinic with new-onset scleroderma (a systemic autoimmune disease related to lupus) who had been taking large doses of Echinacea on the advice of his parents who were into natural supplements. Patients who have SLE should not take Echinacea.

Since herbal therapies are chemical compounds that react with the body, they can also interact with other medications. It is very important to ensure that an herbal medicine does not have a bad interaction with the medicines that you take. I have listed some of these interactions throughout this book under each medicine used for lupus. Pay particular attention if you are on blood thinners when taking some herbs. Some herbs can even react with foods. For example, St. John's wort (used by some people for depression) can cause very high blood pressure when consumed with aged cheeses or with red wine.

A big problem with herbal products is that you do not know exactly how much of the active ingredients you are getting in the herbal supplement. Concentrations of active ingredients from a natural product can vary greatly, depending on numerous factors such as how much rain and sun the plant received, what type of soil it grew in and what nutrients it received, how it was harvested, at what stage of maturity it was harvested, and how it was processed. Each of these variables can greatly change the concentration of the active ingredients. For example, if the plant received a lot of water and little sunshine while growing, the active ingredients may potentially be less concentrated (diluted by the water) compared to if there was a dry growing season with lots of sunshine.

In addition, the FDA does not regulate herbal products; so again, you really do not know what you are getting in an herbal product. The bottom line is that herbal products that have medicinal qualities should be considered the same as unregulated medications. They probably do have significant effects on the body. Anything that can have a health effect on the body can potentially have a bad effect on the body. Researchers need to do the proper studies to figure out what the active ingredients are, standardize the amounts, and do the proper studies in people to prove that herbal products are effective and also safe. The bottom line is that the current medical evidence surrounding herbal products shows that they have both beneficial and toxic effects on the human body. At this time, most are not standardized (in relation to safe amounts), and I cannot recommend their use in patients who have lupus.

## Folk Medicine Biological Therapies

In addition to herbs, other biological substances are sometimes used as medicine. For example, Mexican botanicas (stores that sell Mexican folk medicine supplies) sell many types of folk remedies to treat various illnesses. There have been reports of lupus patients getting Salmonella poisoning from ingesting capsules containing powdered rattlesnake meat in the hopes that they could find a cure. There have been repeated cases of deaths in Americans from ingestion of rattlesnake capsules to treat other conditions as well. In people who have SLE, who have compromised immune systems, this infection can be deadly and these treatments should be avoided.

Another recent example is a product called Reumofan-Plus, which is used to treat arthritis pain and rheumatism and is widely available on the internet. It contains shark cartilage and medicinal roots as its main ingredients. However, after the FDA received reports of deaths, stroke, intestinal bleeding, dizziness, and problems with liver and kidney tests, this product was investigated. It was found that some lots contained the prescription medications methocarbamol (a muscle relaxant) and diclofenac (an NSAID). Diclofenac can be especially dangerous in people who have kidney problems, ulcers, and high blood pressure. The FDA issued a consumer alert recommending that people avoid using it, and the manufacturer recalled the suspected contaminated lots from the market. It is important to consider avoiding all "dietary supplements" (such as Rheumofan) as they are not regulated very well for safety and purity. What may sound like it should be safe because it is "natural" does not in any way guarantee that it is truly safe.

## Manipulative and Body-Based Practices

These therapies treat medical conditions through various forms of manipulation of parts of the body.

### Chiropractic Therapy

Chiropractors believe that misalignment of the spine is a major source of some medical problems, especially involving spine pain and health of the nervous system. They use spinal manipulation and other techniques to relieve the problems from misalignment. In addition, they may use other techniques such as massage, acupressure, electrical stimulation, heat, cold, and exercise. There are no studies looking at the use of chiropractic therapies in lupus. Since lupus does not affect the spine, and chiropractic care is not useful for autoimmune problems, it most likely has no significant role in the treatment of SLE. In addition, be careful if you have osteoporosis (brittle bones), a history of stroke, or hardening of the arteries, or have had previous spine surgery. Spinal manipulation could potentially be dangerous if you have any of these problems.

Some chiropractors recommend their services for fibromyalgia. Since 20% of people who have SLE also suffer from fibromyalgia, it may be tempting to try chiropractic for the pain and fatigue of fibromyalgia. However, a study in the journal *Clinical Rheumatology* in 2012 looked at the largest and best studies on this question, and they could not find sufficient evidence for chiropractic therapies helping with fibromyalgia.

### Massage

Massage involves the physical manipulation of body tissues by a massage therapist to decrease pain, anxiety, stress, and to improve "circulation." Massage therapy has not been studied formally in people who have SLE. However, there is some emerging evidence that it may be beneficial for depression, anxiety disorders, and to help decrease pain severity. Since these problems occur commonly in people who have SLE, massage therapy may possibly help some people feel better. Make sure that your massage therapist has a state license. Be aware that most insurance companies do not cover massage therapy.

### Colonic Irrigation and Cleansing

This is a form of therapy where fluids are used to clean out the colon. Its proponents believe that "toxins" in the colon can be unhealthy and cause disease. First, there are no studies to show this therapy helps any disease. Second, there are potential risks to doing this procedure, including its possibly causing dehydration, bowel perforation, and an increased risk for infection. In addition, it can cause a shift in electrolytes (calcium, sodium, potassium, and magnesium levels) that can potentially be dangerous in people who have heart disease, who have kidney or liver problems, or who take certain medications. In particular, steroids can thin out the bowel wall, making people who have taken prednisone and methylprednisolone at particularly increased risk for bowel perforation. People who have SLE should not get colonic irrigation or cleansing treatments.

## Energy Medicine

This group of therapies attempts to manipulate the energy fields in and around the body. They attempt to affect the energy field of the person in such a way as to improve health.

### Qi Gong (or Qigong)

Qi gong is a Chinese approach to pain treatment using slow movements and breathing exercises. Studies show that Qi gong may help decrease painful disorders such as neck pain. Therefore, it may potentially be helpful in people who have lupus who have pain. No studies have been done in lupus patients.

### Reiki

Reiki is a Japanese healing art developed in the 1920s by a Japanese Buddhist. Its proponents believe that an invisible healing energy can be transmitted from the healer to the patient through intuition by placing the hands on certain parts of the patient's body. It can also be practiced at a distance from the patient as well. There are no studies of its use in lupus. A 2011 study in cancer patients suggested that it might be helpful for pain, sleep, relaxation, anxiety, and improving one's sense of overall well-being. Since these problems are common in people who have SLE, and Reiki is very safe, I would not object to its use.

### Therapeutic Touch

Therapeutic touch was developed in the 1970s by a nursing professor, Dolores Krieger, and is commonly referred to as "the laying on of hands." It shares some principles similar to those of Reiki. It usually does not entail actually touching the patient, but instead the hands are held one to three inches away from the patient and are swept downward from the head to the lower part of the body. Practitioners state that they are able to sense a person's energy field (aura) and manipulate it. Its purpose is to restore the person's mind and "energy" to a peaceful state. There are some studies suggesting its use in fibromyalgia, osteoarthritis, pain, and anxiety disorders. However, the studies are small and none of them are large, well-done, placebo-controlled studies. There are no lupus studies using therapeutic touch. However, since people who have SLE often have fibromyalgia, pain, and anxiety disorders, it may potentially be helpful in people who believe in its use and who have these problems. It certainly is safe without any known side effects. Some nursing schools that incorporate holistic forms of nursing teach therapeutic touch.

### Magnetic Therapy

The use of magnets and magnetic fields has been a huge marketing success for many businesses touting their use for arthritis. However, there are no well-done studies using placebos to prove that magnets work. They are no more effective than using a placebo to help with arthritic conditions. In fact, there are studies showing them not to be helpful for back pain, carpal tunnel syndrome, or osteoarthritis pain of the knees and hips. There is one Russian medical article from 1995 suggesting the use of pulsed magnetic fields to treat lupus, but again, this study did not use a placebo control group at all. I cannot advocate the use of magnetic therapy in people who have lupus. Whenever patients ask me if they should use magnets for their arthritis pain, I tell them that it is safe (as long as they do not have a pacemaker or other implanted electrical medical device). As long as it is not too expensive and they can afford it, there is no harm in using it. They will probably have about a 35% chance of feeling better (the placebo effect that doctors see in pain treatments).

## The Current Status of Complementary and Alternative Therapies in American Medicine

Complementary and alternative therapies are becoming incorporated to a greater extent in American medicine. As new and better quality studies suggest that some of them are helpful, more physicians are using them along with conventional Western medicine. More than half of all medical schools in the United States offer courses on the use of integrative/complementary medicine. Some insurance companies are even paying for complementary therapies such as massage therapy, chiropractic therapy, and acupuncture.

### KEY POINTS TO REMEMBER

1. Complementary medicine therapies are being used increasingly along with mainstream medicine.

2. Just as with the medications prescribed to you by your doctor, complementary medicines need to pass the test of being proven effective and safe by properly done research studies that include a large number of patients and use placebo control groups.

3. The National Institutes of Health has a special section 100% committed to the study of complementary and alternative therapies called the National Center for Complementary and Alternative Medicine.

4. Having a naturopathic doctor (or integrative medicine doctor) in addition to your traditional doctors (such as your rheumatologist) could be beneficial for integrating complementary therapies into your usual lupus therapies. Just follow the advice in table 39.2, especially ensuring that he or she communicates with your rheumatologist about your naturopathic therapies to ensure there are not dangerous conflicts with your SLE therapies or with lupus itself.

5. I cannot recommend that any lupus patients take herbal therapies internally because they do have effects on the body. They are not regulated and significant side effects have been seen with some herbal products. They also can have important interactions with many medications as well.

6. Some very interesting studies have come out of China suggesting that the addition of traditional Chinese medicine (including the use of Chinese herbs) to the usual Western medication regimen (prednisone and cyclophosphamide) may have better results compared to taking the Western medications alone. However, these studies need to be repeated using standardized techniques with evaluation by Western medicine peer-reviewed journals before I can recommend their use.

7. Do not take the herbal supplement Echinacea, which can potentially worsen SLE.

8. Many people who have SLE should consider taking a multiple vitamin, vitamin D, and calcium supplements.

9. DHEA and omega-3 fatty acid supplements could potentially be beneficial for people who have SLE. It is probably better to get DHEA from a compounding pharmacist to ensure high quality. It is probably better to eat a diet that is rich in fish, flax seed, walnuts, olive oil, and other omega-3 fatty acid rich foods instead of taking unregulated over-the-counter supplements.

10. Biofeedback can be helpful for Raynaud's phenomenon, pain, and anxiety disorders.

11. Complementary therapies that may be useful in certain situations (such as for pain, relaxation, and anxiety) are probably safe. These include the use of acupuncture, prayer, meditation, relaxation techniques, art therapy, massage therapy, Qi gong, Reiki, and therapeutic touch.

12. There is no evidence that either colonic cleansings or magnets work for any medical condition. Do not get a colonic cleaning if you have been treated with steroids, immunosuppressant medicines (which increase the risk of infection), or if you have heart or kidney disease.

13. Although spinal manipulation (such as from chiropractors) may be useful for some spinal disorders, it has no role in the treatment of systemic autoimmune diseases such as SLE.

14. If you decide to use any of these therapies for your SLE, use complementary medicine as a supplement to conventional, Western medicine instead of an alternative therapy (which is where these are practiced alone without getting any conventional, Western medical help).

# PART V

# Practical Matters

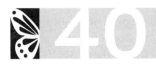

# Talking to Your Doctor and Deciphering Symptoms

## What Is Wrong? . . . How to Talk to Your Doctor

What should you do when you notice something that concerns you? How do you know if it may be important to see a doctor about it right away or not? How do you know if it is due to your lupus or something else? While it would be impossible to go over every possible situation, this chapter addresses some of the most common symptoms that can occur in people who have lupus, and gives you some guidance as far as what you can do about them.

Healthcare providers use the term "symptoms" to refer to what patients are feeling, what problems they are having, and how they communicate these problems to healthcare providers. The first thing physicians do when evaluating patients is to ask them to describe what symptoms or problems they may be having. This is actually one of the most important parts of the evaluation by physicians. Often, the symptoms alone, if well described, are enough to make an accurate diagnosis without even doing a physical examination or doing any tests. The physical exam and tests can help narrow down the possibilities of what is going on, though, if there are many possible causes for a problem. Being able to communicate to your doctor in a succinct, yet orderly way can go very far in making sure that a correct diagnosis is made and that the correct tests are done. This chapter gives you the tools to be able to do this the best way that you can.

## How to Talk to Your Doctor

One of the most powerful and effective tools you can master is to know how to talk to someone in their profession in such a way that improves their ability to help you. When talking to a doctor this does not mean that you need to know big medical words. Any good physician should be able to communicate to you in such a way as to make what is being said easily understandable. The purpose of the first part of this chapter is to give you some tools to use to make the most of your doctor visits and to be able to tell your doctor what is wrong so that you can get the very best results.

First, it can be helpful to understand a little bit about the doctor's world. Individual doctors of course do things a little bit differently from each other, but many things are done commonly. Start with the fact that they only have a certain amount of time allotted to each patient appointment. The amount of time allotted depends a lot on the doctor, the specialty, the types of insurance that are accepted, the types of problems the doctor sees, and the average amount of time most problems take to address. During the rest of this discussion, I will be talking from the standpoint of a typical rheumatologist who sees people who have lupus in a private practice setting. An initial, new patient visit on average takes about twenty-five to forty-five minutes. After that initial visit, subsequent visits are considered "follow-up" visits, and on average may take ten to twenty minutes. These times are averages. If someone comes into the office and is very ill, requiring an extensive evaluation and possibly needing to be prepared to be sent to the emergency room, such a visit can easily take up an hour. Someone who comes in whose lupus is doing very well, has no problems or complaints, and mainly needs a medicine refill and labs may only require five minutes of the doctor's time. There is no way the doctor can figure these time requirements out ahead of time. If the doctor sees several sick patients in a row, then all of the patients scheduled afterward may end up having long wait times. I know that in my own clinic, the most common reason for patients having unexpected long wait times is due to an unusually large number of complicated patient visits. This is important to realize, as it can be frustrating if you have to wait a long time for your scheduled visit. In a well-run office, this should not happen frequently. If you find that you have long waits all of the time, then it is most likely more of a problem with how the office runs. Most likely, too many patients are being scheduled in too short of time slots. This is one measurement you can use as far as deciding what doctor you want to stay with as your regular doctor. I believe that a patient's time is just as valuable as my own, so personally I like to schedule patient visits appropriately so that they do not have long wait times.

Another thing to realize is that the doctor's time is not spent just seeing the patient in the examination room. During the allotted office visit time, the doctor reviews the patient's chart; reviews the labs, x-rays, and other tests done since the last visit; calls and gets missing test results (if they have not made it into the chart yet); reviews the medication list for appropriateness, accuracy, and potential drug interactions; and reads any consultation notes from any other doctors. I review all of these things before I even enter the examination room; that way I am completely prepared to take the best care of my patient. After the patient leaves the room, the visit has not ended. The doctor needs to document the visit. These days it must be done through a system called electronic medical records (EMR; also called electronic health records or EHR) where the doctor has to accurately record the history, physical exam, test findings, diagnoses, and what plan (therapy and tests) the doctor intends to do. There is a huge amount of work that goes on at the patient's office visit that begins before the doctor enters the examination room, and does not end until after the office visit is recorded in the records. The doctor is usually on a very tight schedule in doing all of these things, while at the same time making sure to give the patient the best quality of care possible.

In the middle of all of this, other things happen unexpectedly, of course. These things include needing to answer phone calls from other doctors and hospitals about sick patients, tending to an emergency other than the patient who is being seen in the exam room, the computer system going down, being put on hold on the telephone by another doctor's office, and any number of unintended interruptions. If your doctor ever appears to be in a rush, or overworked, or frazzled . . . it is probably a hectic day with lots of things going on. However, on most days it is not like that. In my own office, I do my best to try to schedule in extra time to allow for these situations, but it is not always possible to cover all bases.

Why might it help you to know how your doctor spends his or her time? For one thing, you can easily see that your doctor's time (just like your time) is very valuable. Understanding this, there are many things you can do to maximize your visit with your doctor (table 40.1). First, make sure that you arrive early for your visit. Schedule enough time to be at your doctor's office at least fifteen minutes before your appointment time. This means leaving plenty early from wherever you have to travel from to allow for the possibility of extra heavy traffic. If you arrive early, you will be calm and your blood pressure will be reliable when measured. You can fill out the necessary paperwork for your office visit and do the necessary things required by your insurance carrier for the visit as well.

If you have an HMO and are required to have referrals from your primary care doctor, it is your responsibility to ensure that your referral is current and up to date. People who have chronic disorders such as SLE (which require frequent visits to specialists) should consider having an insurance (such as a PPO) that does not require referrals. Being required to have a referral to see a specialist automatically throws a roadblock

**Table 40.1** How to Make the Most of Your Doctor Visits

- Arrive at least fifteen minutes early for your appointment.
- If you require a referral to see a specialist, make sure you have a current up-to-date referral before your appointment day. Do not wait until the last minute to check.
- Find out from the staff what office visit times are usually least busy.
- Keep some abbreviated medical records with you.
- Keep a complete list of your medications or bring all your pill bottles to every visit; never assume that the medication list in your chart is correct.
- Dress appropriately for the doctor visit to allow an examination.
- Write down a list of your main concerns and questions.

    Write down your three most important concerns.

    Do not make the questions long.

    Hand the list to your doctor as soon as he or she enters the exam room.

    Realize that one doctor cannot solve all problems.

    You may need to make more than one appointment for numerous problems.

    Let your doctor know what your concerns are about your problem, but do not overly insist on a self-diagnosis.

- Give 100% true answers to all questions.
- Be courteous to the staff.
- Discuss staff and billing issues with the office manager instead of with the doctor.
- Ask the doctor to write down his or her instructions for you.
- Always say "I don't understand" if your doctor says something that does not make sense.

between the specialist and the patient. It is an attempt on the part of the insurance company to decrease the amount of specialist visits by the patient. However, in the case of a disorder such as lupus, this can lead to the patient not getting the best possible medical care. Some people have jobs (such as in the federal government) where they can choose what insurance to get. If you have this option, it is better not to have an HMO if you have SLE.

If you do have an HMO, then you are usually required to have a referral to see your rheumatologist. It is too much work for most doctors' offices to keep track of referrals from multiple patients using different insurance companies. Therefore, most doctors' offices put the burden on patients to ensure that their referrals are up to date for each office visit. Try not to get angry with your specialist over the office's referral policy. You have to realize that specialists are required by your insurance carrier to see you only if your referral is up to date. Most insurance contracts specifically state that the patient has the responsibility to ensure the referral from the primary care doctor is current and properly filled out.

Every physician's office has different appointment times and days that are least likely to be busy. Having an appointment during these particular periods can allow you the best chances of not having to wait very long. Often these tend to be the first appointments in the morning or afternoon. However, some doctors double book these particular office times, so these times may not be best in some offices. In my own practice, if you have the very first appointment in the morning or in the afternoon, you will be seen promptly on or even before your appointment time. In fact, most of the time if the first patient of the morning or afternoon arrives early, I will see that patient as quickly as possible because it helps me be on time for the patients scheduled afterward. If your appointment is toward the end of the morning or afternoon, you run a much higher risk of earlier patients with very difficult medical problems or who required medical procedures that may take longer than expected. These obstacles can cause you to be seen later than your scheduled time.

It can be very helpful to keep a shortened version of your medical records with you and to bring it to each visit. In today's era of computers, this has become even easier. You can keep your medical information on your computer and simply make changes as they occur. An example of an abbreviated medical record would only be one to two pages listing the names and contact numbers of your doctors, what medical problems you have, what surgeries you have had, and what your allergies are. You should also note if there have been any changes in any medicines by any other doctors, or if you have had any new medical problems at all since your last doctor's visit. You can easily print this out and bring it in to each doctor's visit. I have many patients who do this, and it really helps keep track of their medical care more easily.

Just as important is to keep an up-to-date medication list with you at all times (see chapter 29). It is amazing how often patients are taking medicines in a very different way than how doctors think they are taking them. If people bring a medicine list to every visit, it makes it much easier for doctors to ensure that they are taking their medicines correctly. Another alternative is to bring all pill bottles to the visit. However, if you do this but you are not taking all your medicines regularly as the bottle labels state, it is very important to point this out to your doctor.

Plan to wear appropriate clothing to the office visit. As an arthritis doctor, I often need to examine parts of the body that are covered with clothing such as the hips, knees, ankles, feet, and shoulders. It is quite surprising when patients come in knowing that they are there for a problem with a particular body part, then they have on numerous layers of clothing that take a long time to remove (suspenders, long underwear, stockings that go up to the hips, several different shirts/sweaters, etc.). Although you should always dress appropriately for the weather, this should be balanced by wearing clothing that is not too time consuming to remove to make the evaluation easier. For example, I have many patients who have bad knee arthritis who get knee injections regularly. Most of them get into the habit of wearing loose-fitting shorts and pants with no stockings, which makes it much easier to evaluate and treat their condition.

Before your visit, you should already have in mind what your goals are for the visit. Maybe you have a new problem that you want to discuss. Maybe you want to know if you can cut back on some of your medicines. Maybe you want to know what to do to prepare for an upcoming surgery. Often, the goals of the doctor for the visit may be different from what your goals are, yet both goals are equally important. Hand the doctor your questions and concerns at the very beginning of the visit. (Remember, your doctor is on a very tight schedule.) One of the worst things you can possibly do at a doctor's visit is at the very end of the visit, hand your doctor a list of ten questions while there are three more patients waiting in exam rooms, and he or she thought your visit was over.

It is also important not to write down every single problem you can think of. It makes me laugh when I get five pages of incredibly detailed problems that a patient has written down and hands it to me. It could take fifteen to twenty full minutes just to read it all. Patients like this think that they are doing the proper thing, trying to convey to their doctors as accurately as possible what has been going on. However, it also points out his or her lack of insight as to what is a practical amount of time the doctor has to spend on each patient. Keep in mind that the doctor may not have time to answer all of your questions and solve every single problem that you have. Pick out your top three most important concerns and write them down. Be brief in writing down the questions as well. Hand your doctor this list at the very start of the visit to allow him or her time to read them and plan them into the visit. If you do this, your doctor will be most appreciative and you will get the best results and answers to your questions.

Specialists should handle primarily the problems in which they are trained. Briefly tell each doctor if any new medical problems have occurred. Nevertheless, do not think that any one doctor is going to be able to solve all of your problems. For example, although your rheumatologist (your lupus doctor) is very important for taking care of your lupus, and lupus can affect every part of the body, it is very important not to overwhelm him or her with everything that may be going on. Do not go into great detail about your stress, depression, heart bypass surgery, moles that were removed, the diarrhea and constipation problems you are having, the problems you are having with your teenagers, problems with being the caregiver of older relatives, and every single area of your body that hurts and how it hurts. The list can get quite daunting in some cases, and your doctor is only human and can handle only so much at one time. So pick out just a few of the most important problems, and make sure that they are problems that this particular specialist can handle. Your lupus doctor can usually sort out what may be related to your lupus and what may not when presented in a brief format. If you do have numerous medical problems such as with the lungs, heart, skin, and kidneys, it is best to address these individual areas with the respective specialists. Then insist that they send notes to each other and communicate with each other about your medical problems and how they are being handled. I feel very strongly that all doctors treating a patient with SLE should be sending each other notes regularly, especially when any new problems arise or when changes in therapy occur. It is your right to insist that this occur as well. If your doctors do not do this, you should be seeking out a different doctor. The only doctor who usually is not expected to send out notes, by the way, is the primary care provider. Primary care doctors are the ones, though, who should be getting notes from all of the specialists.

Because of the Internet, patients are much more educated today than they have ever been before. However, the Internet is also a double-edged sword as there is a lot of medical misinformation out there as well. It is very easy to find questionnaires on the Internet that can convince people that they have a disease that they do not have at all. Becoming focused on one possible diagnosis without allowing your doctor to consider all the possibilities can be detrimental if you do not have an open mind. A better approach is to let your doctor know what your worry is instead of insisting that you have a particular disease. For example, instead of saying, "Doctor, I know I have chronic Lyme disease. I took this questionnaire on the Internet and all the answers applied to me. I also read on the internet that most doctors do not believe in chronic Lyme disease and that those doctors just don't know what they are talking about." Instead, it is better to state what your concern is in a more open way such as, "Doctor, five years ago, I was bitten by a tick, and ever since then I have felt badly with a lot of pain and fatigue. Could you check and see if I may have Lyme disease or not? I was reading about chronic Lyme disease on the Internet, but I am interested in your opinion and expertise."

It is perfectly human and normal to be worried about your medical condition when you compare it to bad things that you have personally witnessed in other people. For example, if you had an aunt who died from Alzheimer's disease, and you remember it as being very traumatic for her and your whole family, it is normal for you to worry about the same thing if you begin to have some forgetfulness. Make sure to tell your doctor that you are worried about the possibility of Alzheimer's disease since your aunt had it and you are getting forgetful. It is very common for people to get forgetful as they get older, and most do not have Alzheimer's disease. Not only is it important for your doctor to know that this may run in your family, but it is equally important for your doctor to relieve your fears if you do not actually have Alzheimer's disease or to advise you appropriately if you do.

It is in your best interest to answer all questions asked by all staff and the doctor completely and truthfully. Even what seem to be very personal questions may be very important for your medical condition. For example, questions about sex, alcohol, and drugs may make many patients uncomfortable and they may even consider it not to be anyone's business but their own. If you do feel that way, just be honest and say so, but do not give a false answer. Also, let the doctor know if you are not taking your medications exactly as prescribed. If you take something just as needed, or you are not taking it because you cannot afford it, it is extremely important to let your doctor know that. Many times, I have wondered why patients were not doing well only to find out that although they always answered "yes" to taking an important medicine regularly, they actually were not taking it at all. Doctors do not want to know what patients should be doing; doctors need to know exactly what patients are actually doing. For example, if you have been prescribed a medicine to be taken three times a day, but you usually only remember to take it twice a day, it is important to let the medical assistant or nurse know this while reviewing your medication list. Your doctor can then try to find a medicine that can be taken twice a day to take the place of the medicine that you keep missing.

As far as difficulty affording medicines, these are very hard times for many people. The economy has been rough, many people or their family members have lost jobs, and many people are on fixed incomes and very tight budgets. If you cannot afford your medicine, let your doctor know. Doctors do realize the difficulties that patients are having financially as they also have family members who are struggling during these hard times. My own family is in rural Ohio where many factories have closed down and family members cannot get jobs and do not have good healthcare. So I can relate to what is happening to you, as can so many other doctors. Never be ashamed to let your doctor know your problems. Sometimes doctors can come up with alternate, less expensive treatments than the ones they have patients on. Sometimes doctors may have samples of medicines that they may be able to provide. However, doctors will not be able to do this unless patients let them know. Also, if a medicine is too expensive for you, ask your pharmacist what alternative medicines your insurance plan will cover and let your doctor know. It is usually too difficult for the doctor to know what medicines every insurance plan covers, as they vary widely. The patient-doctor relationship is extremely important. You should feel comfortable enough with your doctor to be 100% truthful and forthcoming with every aspect of your medical care so that your doctor can provide the best guidance possible.

An overlooked part of getting good results from an office visit is to be courteous to the staff. To start with, I would like to point out that the vast majority of patients in my experience are wonderful people and very nice to everyone. However, some patients quickly build up a bad reputation with the staff. Although they will be very nice to me and in front of me, I will be told by various members of the staff (receptionists, nurses, office manager, medical assistants, and others) that they are not nice or are rude to them. Although I think that my staff overall is very professional and courteous, it is human nature to not treat someone who is rude in the best way possible. It is important to remember that your medical care does not begin and end with the doctor. Rather, your medical care begins at the time you pick up the phone to call the office or the time you walk through the door. Your path to and from the doctor is paved with other members of the healthcare team. If you do not treat them with respect and politeness, you may find it more difficult to reach the doctor to your full satisfaction. On the other hand, patients who come in smiling, who say "hello" to everyone, and who are courteous in person and on the phone are usually treated with a "red carpet" treatment by all members of the staff. That, too, is human nature. For some reason, chocolate and homemade cookies seem to be favorite bribes.

On the other side of things, doctors also want to surround themselves with the best possible staff to provide the best quality of service possible to their patients. If you find that a particular staff member repeatedly gives you subpar service, then it is very important to let someone know. The best person to inform is actually the office manager.

Most doctors' offices have an office manager who is actually in charge of ensuring that the staff is the very best that they can be. While you can tell the doctor what is going on, it is usually more effective (both time-wise and results-wise) to go directly to the office manager about this matter. It is best to reserve the time with your doctor for your medical problems. You do not want your office visit with the doctor to be filled with ten minutes of discussing a staff issue when the time could be better spent on a more important medical issue.

When your doctor gives you instructions such as medicine changes, what your diagnosis or problem is, what possible problems could be causing a symptom, or what tests are needed, ask for a written list or recommended literature to read on the subjects. It can be overwhelming to be told to do many different things at a doctor's visit. What may seem simple and straightforward to a physician may actually be quite complex to a nonmedical person. Also, always make sure that you leave the encounter understanding what is going on. While it is not necessary (nor possible in many circumstances) to know everything (such as what every single lab result means), it is important to understand the big picture. It is very easy for doctors to forget how to say things in understandable, everyday language. Doctors spend much of their time talking to other doctors and nurses, and the complex language of medicine becomes second nature. However, very few nonmedical people understand it. Never be afraid to say, "I don't understand . . . can you explain that or write it down in simpler terms for me?" You are not being stupid or ignorant if you say this. Most good doctors realize that most laypeople do not understand medical jargon. Doctors want patients to understand what is truly going on with them and sometimes just need to be reminded of this. Also, do not wait to do this until the very end when the doctor is mentally preparing to end the visit and see the next patient. Make sure to let your doctor know early on in the discussion that you do not understand what is being said. I highly respect any patient who tells me this. Personally, I am never afraid to say this myself when I am talking to the computer tech, air conditioning/heating person, mechanic, electrician, lawyer, TV repairperson, or administrative person. All jobs and professions have languages and jargons all their own, and often I have no idea what they are talking about. It is worse to nod "yes," pretending to know what they are saying. I would much rather plead "dumb" so that I can better understand them.

The first part of any doctor's visit is known as the history portion of the visit. This typically is followed by the physical examination and then by the part where the doctor says how you are doing, what is wrong, and what the plan is as far as tests or medicine changes. Knowing this order can be helpful to you as far as what to expect. The initial history portion of the evaluation is very important. This usually starts with a key phrase from the doctor such as "How have you been doing?" or "How can I help you today?" or "What brings you here today?" This is when it is your turn to tell the doctor anything wrong or worrisome that has happened to you. You should bring up what you want addressed at the visit.

In the history portion of the visit, you want to express what has been happening as succinctly as possible. It is usually best to do this chronologically (i.e., start from the beginning). "Doctor, I was doing really well until about two weeks ago when . . ." While describing to your doctor what has been happening, do not include a bunch of unrelated information. Try to stick to the story and not branch off on sidetracks. For example, if you have been having chest pain, describe the chest pain to your doctor, what you were doing at the time it happened, and what things made it worse or better. However, do not go into a long story about how your Aunt Mabel was making cookies for your husband's birthday at her house. However, she ran out of brown sugar, which makes the best cookies in the world as she uses a recipe handed down from your great-grandmother who was an incredible cook. Your great-grandmother came over from Germany where her family always used this recipe back in the days when sugar was expensive and hard to get. Then you started to have chest pain. You get the point. If you notice your doctor's eyes starting to glaze over or roll, you are probably getting off track (remember, you only have so much time to spend with your doctor).

Learning how to state what your problem is in a useful, succinct way is one of the secrets in learning to talk to your doctor. The more useful information you give your doctor in the shortest amount of time will do the best for you in the end. Table 40.2 gives some recommendations on how to tell your doctor a problem, story, or symptoms of a problem succinctly. If you get into the habit of using this system, it can help you not to forget important aspects of your problem, provide valuable information, not get side tracked, and get the best results possible.

**Table 40.2** How to Describe a Medical Problem to Your Doctor

- Start at the very beginning of when the problem began and relay what has happened to you in chronological order.
- What were you doing when you first noticed the problem?
- Did it start gradually or abruptly?
- Describe how it made you feel; use adjectives.
- In what part of your body is the problem occurring?
- Is the problem constant (never a second without it), or does it come and go in a particular pattern?
- How often does it occur?
- What things make the problem worse (certain times of day, certain activities, certain body positions)?
- Is there anything that makes the problem better (times of day, body positions, any medicines taken)?
- Is it getting worse, getting better, or staying about the same?
- How severe is the problem using a scale such as mild, moderate, or severe. Or use a scale of 1–10 where 10 would be the worst ever in your whole life and a 1 would be hardly noticeable.
- Are there any associated problems or symptoms?
- How has the problem interfered with any activities in your life?
- Has anyone else (family, friends, or co-workers) had similar symptoms?
- Have you ever had this problem before?
- What is your biggest concern about what may be going on or what is your biggest fear?

It can be very helpful to write your problem down in words first answering the above questions to help you get organized. Here is an example.

"Doctor, about two months ago, right after you saw me and after I started taking the new medicine, naproxen, I began to get stomach upset. This came on slowly and infrequently, but now occurs more often, about five times a day. It occurs at the top of my stomach and feels like a mild achy, gnawing feeling that sometimes goes up into my chest. When I eat food or take some Tums it seems to get better. When I lay down it gets worse, and I will often get heartburn with it when I lay down. I occasionally also feel mild nausea, but I don't vomit; and I will sometimes cough. I can do anything I want without problems, and no one else I know has similar problems. I am worried that this could be pancreatic cancer as my cousin had similar problems and died from it." This account is very succinct, but it is loaded with information. This patient is describing gastroesophageal reflux disease perfectly, brought on by taking naproxen, which is a non-steroidal anti-inflammatory drug (NSAID; see chapter 36). However, the doctor will also realize that an ulcer in the stomach is another possibility. The doctor would next do a physical examination and may order a blood count to ensure there is no anemia due to bleeding from an ulcer. Yet, there is enough information in this detailed story to stop the naproxen, give the patient advice on dietary changes for GERD (see table 15.1), and to prescribe a medication to calm down the acidity of the stomach (see table 28.3). In addition, and possibly most importantly, the doctor can reassure the patient that she or he probably does not have pancreatic cancer, but if things do not get better quickly, additional tests can be done. Here is another example.

"This morning while I was sitting watching television I developed the abrupt onset of a sharp, stabbing pain in the middle of my chest under my breast bone. Every time I try to breathe deeply it gets more intense and will spread to the left side of my chest. During normal breathing it feels like a tolerable 2 to 3 out of 10 scale of pain, but when I breathe real deep it really takes me back and is about 8 out of 10. The only thing that seems to make it feel better is if I don't try to breathe too deeply. If I try to do too much strenuous work it is difficult to breathe, and I feel hot and sweaty. I took my temperature a few times and it ranges from 99.6°F to 100.2°F. I have difficulty walking very fast due to shortness of breath and the chest pain; I basically have to sit still to feel the most comfortable. I have never had this before, but it seems to be getting worse throughout the day. No one in my family has been sick." This also describes very nicely a problem for the doctor that has many possibilities. The increased pain with deep breathing suggests the possibility of pleurisy from SLE; however, the fever and shortness of breath add the possibilities of a blood clot in the lung (pulmonary embolism) or infection (such as pneumonia). Other possibilities such as a heart attack certainly have to be considered as well. Nonetheless, all of these are serious possibilities and will require an extensive workup with x-rays, ECG, and blood work that can only be done at a hospital. Yet the story is told in such a way that the doctor will know exactly what to look for. Using these questions as a guide makes it much easier to evaluate, allowing you the best chances for your doctor to arrive at a proper diagnosis and management plan. Use this approach for all problems from very mild to severe.

Describe your problem using words that are more descriptive instead of nonspecific terms. For example, if you say you are "tired," what exactly do you mean? There are many different ways to feel tired and all of them can point to something different.

Feeling tired can refer to mental exhaustion, being overworked, being stressed, being sleepy, having shortness of breath, or having muscle weakness. One person may be referring to mental fatigue while another may mean physical fatigue. You may feel sleepy all the time, and fall asleep easily while driving or watching television. This description would make your doctor think of the possibility of a sleep disorder such as sleep apnea, insomnia, or narcolepsy. Do you feel drained of energy and not feel like doing anything? Do you often wake up in the middle of the night, or do you wake up in the mornings feeling like you did not sleep well? Have you lost the desire to do many activities that you once enjoyed doing, but you are now so exhausted all the time that you stay in bed? This could point to problems such as depression. Your feeling tired may mean that you normally feel OK, but when you try to exert yourself such as walking upstairs or briskly, you may feel short of breath and exhausted at the same time. This could suggest problems such as anemia (low red blood cell count), being overweight, or even having a lung or heart problem. Does your sense of feeling tired mean that your muscles feel weak and you have great difficulty standing up from a chair or have trouble lifting your arms up to brush your hair? This could point to inflammation of the muscles (myositis) as a possibility. Even though "tired" can fit all of these situations, simply by using words that are more descriptive to describe it (think of writing it down in a book, like a story, for others to read and understand) in detail and describing how it interferes with your life, you can really help narrow down the cause of your tiredness.

Another example that can have multiple meanings is dizziness. If it feels like the room is moving and you have trouble walking it could point to vertigo, which is a problem with the inner ear or with the nerve that goes to the ear. If you get light-headed when you try to stand up, this could mean that a blood pressure medicine is making your blood pressure too low, or you could be dehydrated, you could be anemic (low red blood count), or you could have a nerve or heart problem causing problems with your blood pressure. Although both vertigo and light-headedness make people feel dizzy, the possible causes are immensely different, and it is easier to figure out when you describe it in more detail. Note that describing your symptoms using table 40.2 should be done in simple, everyday language. Just say exactly how you feel; you do not need to know any medical jargon at all to adequately describe your problem.

The next section goes into more detail about some symptoms or problems that can occur in people who have lupus. Knowing what the possibilities are and how urgent the problems can potentially be can help you know how to respond to these when they occur.

## Deciphering What Your Doctor Tells You

Many times doctors tell patients things that mean something in medical terms, but that can be easily misunderstood by nonmedical people. A couple of terms deserve special attention, as they are used frequently and are a common source of misunderstanding. The first is the term "differential diagnosis." Whenever a doctor is confronted with a medical problem in someone, there is usually a list of possible things that can cause that problem. Let us take the example of anemia, which is the medical term used when the red blood cell count (measured by the blood tests hemoglobin and hematocrit) is low. There are many possible reasons for a person to have anemia. Finding the exact cause is very important in making sure it is treated properly. Most people quickly jump to the conclusion that they must be low in iron and should take an iron supplement, but that is only one possibility. Taking iron supplements do not help with any of the other causes of anemia. Therefore, usually additional tests are required to figure out why someone is anemic (has anemia).

Before ordering any tests, though, the doctor comes up with a list of possible causes for the anemia. This list is called the "differential diagnosis." The doctor may list iron deficiency, stomach ulcers, intestinal bleeding (such as from colon cancer), vitamin B-12 deficiency, folic acid deficiency, anemia of chronic disease (due to lupus inflammation), and hemolytic anemia (from the immune system attacking the red blood cells) as all being in the differential diagnosis. Therefore, the doctor will order the appropriate studies, including blood tests, feces testing, and even a colonoscopy and upper endoscopy (to look into the stomach and intestines) as the most important investigations. Usually the doctor puts one or two possibilities at the top of the list as being the most probable causes of the anemia and says that those are "at the top of the differential diagnosis." For example, anemia of chronic disease may be the most likely explanation based on the size of the red blood cells on the complete blood cell count. No additional treatment may be needed if it proves to be mild anemia of chronic disease.

When your doctor tells you that you need tests to figure out what is causing a problem, it never hurts to ask what the most likely problem is out of the list of possibilities. This can help greatly in relieving any fears when possibilities that are more dangerous are being investigated as well. For example, this patient with anemia may be sent for a colonoscopy to make sure there is no evidence of colon cancer, which can cause anemia due to slow bleeding from the intestines. Too many times, I hear a patient of mine in this type of situation say something like, "my doctor thinks I have colon cancer." The person jumps to the conclusion that it could be the most dangerous thing being investigated, when in reality that particular problem may not be very likely, but would be very dangerous if missed by the doctor (and therefore, the test is very much needed).

Another common term used in this type of situation is the medical term "rule out." When a doctor comes up with a differential diagnosis and one or two things are placed at the top of possibilities, often it is important to do all of the tests to ensure that the less likely, but possibly more dangerous problems do not exist. These other tests are done to rule out these other possibilities. When someone hears a doctor say that he or she wants to do a test to rule something out, it is frequently a mistake to jump to the conclusion that the doctor actually thinks she or he has that problem. While it certainly could be a possibility, often, the doctor thinks it is unlikely (e.g., getting the colonoscopy for anemia to rule out colon cancer), but it would be a very dangerous (yet very treatable) problem if the test were not performed and the actual cause of the anemia was missed.

In this particular instance of anemia, the doctor may accidentally say in medical terms (forgetting to use nonmedical language), "The *differential diagnosis* for the cause of your anemia is anemia of chronic disease from your lupus inflammation, hemolytic anemia, iron deficiency, stomach ulcers, colon cancer, vitamin B-12 deficiency, and folic acid deficiency. However, I would place anemia of chronic disease *at the top of the differential diagnosis* for which no additional treatment would be required. I will need some blood tests, a stool sample, an upper endoscopy, and a colonoscopy to *rule out* these possibilities." If you did not understand how to interpret what is meant by something being at "the top of the differential diagnosis" or what "rule out" means, it is easy to become scared, feeling that your doctor thinks that you have colon cancer from this explanation. However, if this same explanation were put in nonmedical terms, it would be best to say, "Your red blood cell count is slightly low. I think that it is most likely due to the inflammation of your lupus, or what we call, 'anemia of chronic disease.' It is so mild that no additional treatment is needed if this is what it turns to be. However, it is very important that we make sure that there is not another reason for your anemia. Although I think these other possibilities are unlikely, we must make sure that you do not have hemolytic anemia from your lupus, any vitamin deficiencies, or bleeding from the stomach or intestines which can sometimes occur from problems such as bleeding ulcers or, even worse, colon cancer."

The bottom line is that "differential diagnosis" refers to a list of possible causes of a medical problem. Various medical studies or tests may be required to "rule out" many of those possibilities. The only possibilities that the doctor thinks are probably the real cause of the problem are what he or she places "at the top of the differential diagnosis." Always ask your doctor to repeat things in nonmedical terms if you do not completely understand something. In addition, if something dangerous is being considered as a possibility, ask the doctor to tell you directly how likely it is for you to have that particular problem (i.e., if you are the type of person who prefers to know something like this up front).

## Symptoms

This section lists some of the problems and symptoms that can occur in people who have lupus. Many possible problems exist as a potential cause of the same symptom. (For example, totally unrelated problems such as pleurisy, a heart attack, acid reflux, blood clot in the lung, and fibromyalgia can all cause chest pain.) Only a thorough evaluation from your doctor along with a proper management plan can arrive at a proper diagnosis. However, the purpose of this section is to give you information that can help you figure out whether the problem is an emergency that should alert you to seek immediate medical attention, whether you can wait to see your doctor later for the problem, and what the possible causes could be. Table 40.3 is a comprehensive list to refer to for knowing when you need to seek immediate medical attention. In a medical emergency, call 911.

## Fever

The basic approach to fever in people who have lupus is "it is an infection until proven otherwise." The reason for this is that infection is one of the most common causes of death in people who have lupus and a prompt diagnosis and treatment are needed to prevent something bad from happening. As explained in chapter 6, you can consider yourself as having a fever if your temperature taken by mouth is above 98.9°F in the morning (when normal body temperature is lower) or above 99.9°F in the afternoon (when normal body temperature is higher). Keep a working thermometer in your home at all times. If you feel like you are hot or feverish, or if you are sweating as if you may

**Table 40.3** If You Have Lupus and You Develop One of These Symptoms, When Do You Need to Seek Immediate Medical Attention?

For Fever
Always seek immediate medical attention for any fever by contacting your primary care physician, going to an urgent care clinic, or going to the emergency room.

For Fatigue
Seek immediate medical attention:
- If you have shortness of breath or chest pain
- If you have stomach pain
- If you have difficulty thinking
- If you have a fever
- If you develop muscle weakness or numbness in an arm or leg
- If you are losing weight
- If you have a new-onset headache

For Joint and Muscle Pain
Seek immediate medical attention:
- If you have a fever
- If you feel it is due to a flare of your lupus

Rash
Seek immediate medical attention:
- If you are getting a new rash or increase in your lupus rash
- If it occurs soon after starting a new medicine (call the doctor who prescribed it)
- If you develop a burning, painful area of skin, especially if it has blisters (possible shingles)
- If you develop an area of red, hot, painful skin (possible cellulitis)
- If you notice any new spot or mole, especially if it is enlarging or if it is a sore that is not healing well

Raynaud's Phenomenon
Seek immediate medical attention:
- If a finger or toe becomes dark purple, black, and very painful without returning to normal while warming the body up
- If open sores develop on your fingertips or toes

Chest Pain
Seek immediate medical attention for a first episode of chest pain or any new type of chest pain

Trouble Breathing
Seek immediate medical attention for any new episode of shortness of breath

Difficulty Urinating
Seek immediate medical attention:
- If you have a fever

- If you have classic urinary tract infection symptoms with increased frequency of urination, a feeling of urgency to urinate, or discomfort when you urinate
- If you are unable to urinate and develop a sensation of building pressure in the lower abdomen
- If you develop weakness or loss of sensation in your legs
- If you develop back pain

Numbness
Seek immediate medical attention:

- For sudden onset of loss of sensation in an arm, leg, or face
- If it is associated with arm or leg weakness
- If other symptoms such as fever, weight loss, and leg bruising are occurring

Muscle Weakness
Seek immediate medical attention if you develop:

- Weakness in an arm or leg
- Weakness in the facial muscles (droopy face)
- Double vision, difficulty talking, slurred speech
- Difficulty raising the arms to brush your hair and difficulty standing from a chair without using your arms to push yourself up

Headache
Seek immediate medical attention:

- If you develop a fever
- If the headache is accompanied by sinus congestion or thick nasal secretions
- For a new type of headache, especially if "the worst headache I've ever had in my life"
- If the headache is accompanied by nausea and vomiting (unless it is a classic, recurrent migraine that has been evaluated and diagnosed before)
- If the headache worsens in different body positions
- If the headache is accompanied by arm or leg muscle weakness, numbness, or visual changes (unless it is your recurrent migraine that has already been evaluated and diagnosed before)

Stomach Upset
Seek immediate medical attention:

- If accompanied by fever, nausea, or vomiting
- If accompanied by black, tarry feces, or if there is blood in the feces
- If severe

Blurred Vision
Seek immediate medical attention if accompanied by fever, red eyes, eye pain, headache, or double vision

have a fever, you want to check your temperature. Sometimes you can feel feverish yet not truly have a fever. If you have a fever, it is very important to contact your doctor right away and get a proper evaluation. Try to figure out if you have any other problems or symptoms that could potentially point to an infection. If you develop a lot of sweating with the fever or you develop chills or keep shivering, this can potentially mean a bacterial infection and urgent medical attention is needed. Some examples of infection symptoms include cough (pneumonia or bronchitis), pain while urinating or increased frequency of urination (urinary tract infection), red and painful skin (cellulitis, skin infection), headache and congestion (sinusitis), runny nose with sneezing (upper respiratory tract infection), and diarrhea (intestinal infection). Some medicines used to treat lupus such as steroids (prednisone and methylprednisolone) as well as the NSAIDs (such as ibuprofen and naproxen) can decrease the ability of the body to cause a fever. You need to take even a mild fever seriously when you are on these medications.

Certainly, lupus itself can cause fever, which may require the use of anti-inflammatory drugs, acetaminophen (Tylenol), or even steroids in severe cases. You should never assume that lupus is the cause without ruling out infection first. If you have had a fever before with lupus flares, then often it can be accompanied by other lupus problems such as hair loss; chest pain when you take in a deep breath (pleurisy); joint pain and swelling (arthritis); red rash on the cheeks, upper chest, and arms (sun-sensitive rash); or other lupus problems such as sores in the mouth. However, sometimes a fever can also occur with more severe, dangerous problems such as a blood clot in the lungs, which can also cause chest pain and shortness of breath.

I recommend that my patients call and see their primary care doctor right away, or if it is the evening or on a weekend, they should go to an emergency room or to an urgent care center for proper evaluation by a healthcare provider if they develop a fever. A telephone call is not sufficient to evaluate a fever properly. Sometimes, even after a thorough evaluation, it can be difficult to tell whether a fever is due to an infection or due to lupus. In this case, the doctor evaluating you should contact your rheumatologist, as it may be best to treat you for both possibilities at the same time.

## Tiredness and Fatigue

Feeling tired and fatigued is one of the most common problems in society. Even in people who are not "sick" or who do not have a chronic illness such as lupus, about 20% of the population admit to having significant fatigue. In people who have lupus, the percentage is much higher and fatigue can be one of the most frustrating and life-altering problems that can occur.

Fatigue and tiredness can refer to very different problems. Fatigue is defined as having a sense of a loss of energy. This can refer to both mental energy and physical energy. Sleepiness can be interpreted as fatigue, but can have other potential causes. If you find yourself sleepy, or if you fall asleep easily during the day while at rest (sitting, driving), this could point to a sleep disorder such as sleep apnea. Having muscle weakness can also be interpreted as fatigue. If you have difficulty raising your arms up to brush your hair or have trouble standing up from a chair without having to use your arms to push you up, this could point to a problem with the muscles such as myositis from lupus, or even other causes of muscle problems such as thyroid disease. If you

720

have actual muscle weakness, you should make an appointment with your doctor for proper evaluation.

Shortness of breath could indicate the possibilities of a low red blood cell count (anemia), or even lung or heart problems. If you have shortness of breath with your fatigue, then you need to seek immediate medical attention.

If you are tired, ask yourself how many hours of sleep you get each night. If you get less than eight hours of sleep a night, have trouble falling asleep, wake up throughout the night, or feel exhausted when you wake up (as if you did not get a good night's sleep), all of these point to a possible sleep disorder. It could simply mean that you are sabotaging your sleep quality by making poor lifestyle choices (not scheduling enough sleep, not exercising, smoking cigarettes, drinking alcohol too close to bedtime, etc.), or you could have a disorder that is interrupting your sleep cycle such as depression, anxiety, fibromyalgia, or sleep apnea. You should take the tests in table 6.3 (sleep apnea), the beginning of chapter 27 (fibromyalgia), table 13.2 (anxiety disorder), and table 13.4 (depression). If you score positive on these tests, then you may have one of these problems. You should show the results to your doctor. If you are not getting eight hours of sleep every night or you identify a problem with sleep, then you really need to adhere strictly to the sleep hygiene recommendations listed in table 6.2. You should also try the suggestions listed in table 6.1 to try to help with your fatigue as well. If you do all of these things but still have trouble with sleep and fatigue, then you should see your doctor for further evaluation.

Of course, sometimes fatigue can point to a more urgent medical problem. If you develop new-onset fatigue accompanied by shortness of breath, chest pain, stomach pain, trouble thinking, or numbness or weakness in an arm or leg, have difficulty talking, have a fever, have a headache, or are losing weight, then you should seek medical attention.

Sometimes medications can cause fatigue. Some medicines that can cause fatigue include blood pressure medicines, antidepressants, anti-histamines for allergies, immunosuppressant medicines, pain medicines, muscle relaxants, and even steroids. If the fatigue occurs soon after you start taking a new medicine, it is important to call your doctor, as he or she most likely will want to change the dose or try something different. Fatigue can also be a symptom while coming down or off a medicine. For example, decreasing the dose of steroids too quickly may cause adrenal insufficiency (see chapter 26) which can cause fatigue. Therefore, you should let your doctor know if fatigue occurs while your steroid dose is lowered.

## Joint and Muscle Pain

Ninety percent of all people who have SLE will get joint and muscle pain due to their lupus. If there is actual arthritis (inflammation inside of the joint) from lupus, there may be notable swelling of the joint itself or increased morning stiffness. The muscle and joint pain of lupus can improve with anti-inflammatory medicines, pain medicines such as acetaminophen (Tylenol), or even steroids or immunosuppressant medicines if the pain is severe.

However, not all joint and muscle pain is due to the inflammation of lupus. About 20% of all people who have lupus will develop a condition called fibromyalgia (see chapter 27). Fibromyalgia is due to a chemical imbalance problem of the pain nerves of the body instead of being due to inflammation of the lupus. The treatment of fibromyalgia is completely different from the treatment of lupus arthritis. Instead of using anti-inflammatory medicines, doctors use medicines that reverse the chemical imbalances (such as antidepressants and anti-seizure medicines). Exercise and improving sleep are also important in the treatment of fibromyalgia. Some common symptoms that can point to the possibility of fibromyalgia include having pain "all over"; having tenderness of the muscles, bones, and skin; having headaches; waking up in the mornings feeling like you did not get much sleep; and feeling tired and fatigued. You can take the self-test at the beginning of chapter 27 to see if fibromyalgia is a possibility or not. It is extremely important to identify it as a cause of pain when it occurs. Unfortunately, I have seen many patients treated inappropriately with steroids by other doctors when their pain was actually due to fibromyalgia instead of lupus arthritis.

Depression and anxiety disorders can also cause pain. It can be difficult to convince someone that these disorders can cause pain. People can be resistant to the notion of taking an antidepressant or an anti-anxiety medicine to treat their joint or muscle pain. However, in depression and anxiety disorders, body pain is a very common problem. The treatment of choice is to use medicines that reverse the chemical imbalances that are causing the depression, anxiety, and pain. Pain medicines, anti-inflammatory medicines, and steroids should not be used in these cases. Taking the self-tests in tables 13.2 and 13.4 can help you figure out if these are possible problems. If you can be open to these other possible causes of pain (fibromyalgia, depression, anxiety), you can spare yourself the possibility of inappropriate overuse of steroids and other immunosuppressant medicines, which may not be the right ways to treat your pain.

Viral infections can also cause joint and muscle pain. If you get a fever and have a lot of achiness, it certainly could be due to lupus, but you need to see a doctor right away and be evaluated to make sure it is not an infection as well.

## Rash

Of course, having a rash is one of the most common problems that people who have lupus can have. If you do get a rash from your lupus, it can be a very helpful sign that your lupus is more active whenever it occurs. If you had been doing well for a while, but then your lupus rash recurs or gets worse, it is important to contact your rheumatologist for an evaluation to make sure that your lupus is not causing any problems in any other parts of your body such as the kidneys or blood counts.

A couple of the lupus rashes deserve special attention. First are the sun-sensitive rashes. If you develop a pink discoloration or redness on the sun-exposed areas of your body, such as the tops of the hands and arms, cheeks, forehead, nose, and upper chest area, this is a sign that your lupus is most likely becoming more active. In particular, it also means that you are not protecting yourself from ultraviolet light adequately. It is important to protect yourself from ultraviolet light as discussed in chapter 38. If you develop a rash, you need to evaluate your daily habits and determine if you are exposing yourself to the sun, whether you have been using your sunscreen religiously every day (or even several times a day), and if you are wearing a wide brimmed hat and clothing that has ultraviolet protection. If you are getting the skin reaction on sun-exposed areas, it means that you need to improve your ultraviolet light protection habits.

Another rash that needs special attention is the discoid lupus rash. Discoid lupus can unfortunately cause permanent scarring and hair loss when it occurs. The rash usually starts as a small red- or dark-colored area of the skin and then spreads outward in a disc- or round-shaped pattern. Often it is slightly tender as well. If you have discoid lupus and you have been under good control, it is important to recognize when it becomes active and seek immediate help from your dermatologist (skin doctor) as well as your rheumatologist. The longer you wait to get help, the greater the possibility of developing permanent damage to the skin. Signs that discoid lupus is becoming more active include if it appears pinkish or red in color and if it is tender. Areas of previous discoid lupus involvement may have permanent color changes, loss of hair, or indentations in the skin. However, if these same areas become pink or tender, that is when you want to see your doctor right away. The quicker the rash is treated, the lower your chances of worsening skin damage.

Certainly, people who have lupus can develop rashes from things other than their lupus as well. Drugs are a common cause of rashes. An allergic reaction to a drug typically will cause a rash to occur on average seven to ten days after starting the medication. Especially if you develop hives or a diffuse red rash soon after starting a new drug, you should contact the prescribing doctor right away for an evaluation. The anti-malarial medicines commonly can cause color changes to the skin. Both hydroxychloroquine and quinacrine can cause increased dark-colored areas to the skin. This will often occur on the fronts of the legs, forehead, or neck, typically after many years of use. These color changes occur very slowly. They may get better when the doses of these medicines are decreased; therefore, it is important to let your doctor know if they occur. Dark areas of skin also occur in areas of previous lupus inflammation as a part of the healing process. For example, they are commonly seen on the cheeks from previous sun inflammation or on the ears from previous discoid lupus. Some doctors prescribe lightening creams, but they usually do not work very well.

Shingles is a very painful skin rash that occurs due to the chicken pox virus. When people are young and infected with chicken pox, the chicken pox virus ends up living inside of the body in the nerves of the spine. Over the years, the immune system is very good at keeping the virus under control. However, when the immune system stops working properly, such as when people get older or if they develop problems with the immune system (such as SLE), the virus can become active again. When it becomes active and begins reproducing, it travels down the nerves that lead away from that particular area of the spine, infecting the nerves that go to the skin. This can potentially cause severe pain, often described as a burning sensation. The skin that the nerves lead to will usually develop red bumps and blisters due to the infection and this is called shingles (or herpes zoster in medical terminology). It is very important to seek medical attention immediately. If the doctor can prescribe an anti-viral medication quickly, the outcome is much better. If you wait too long to get treatment, severe damage to the nerves may occur. This can cause severe permanent nerve pain in that area of the body.

An area of red, hot, tender skin can also potentially be a sign of a skin infection called cellulitis. This most commonly occurs on the feet and lower legs. If this occurs, it is important to see a doctor right away for antibiotic treatment. A blood clot in the leg, called deep venous thrombosis, can also cause red, painful swelling of the lower leg. This also requires immediate treatment to prevent it from going to the lungs where it can become dangerous and even deadly. Gout (a disease caused by too much uric acid in the body) can also cause red, painful swelling of the foot.

People who have lupus are also at increased risk for getting certain forms of cancer. Recent studies suggest that they are especially at increased risk to get cancers associated with a viral infection called human papilloma virus, which may cause non-melanoma skin cancers. If you develop any new spot or mole, point it out to your doctor, especially if it is growing in size. A sore on the skin that is not healing properly is also suspicious and should be pointed out as well.

### Fingers or Toes Turn Colors and Become Cold with Stress and Cold

Many people who have SLE will have a problem called Raynaud's phenomenon (see chapter 11). This occurs when lupus causes the arteries in the hands and feet to be smaller than normal. The blood vessels constrict when a person becomes cold or stressed. Raynaud's causes decreased blood flow to the fingers and toes causing them to first turn pale, followed by a bluish color during which they sometimes can feel uncomfortable. After warming up, the fingers and toes may turn reddish. Some people only develop the pale or bluish discoloration alone. Table 11.1 gives helpful advice on how Raynaud's is treated. It is rarely a severe problem, but occasionally it can cause open sores on the fingertips. In the most severe cases, it can cause total loss of blood flow to the fingers or toes causing infection such as gangrene and even the potential loss of a finger or toe. It is important to seek immediate medical attention if a finger or toe loses blood flow and does not improve after rewarming the body. If there is severe pain and the toe or finger turns dark purple or even black in color, you need to seek medical attention immediately.

### Chest Pain

If you ever call up a doctor's office complaining of chest pain, you will almost always be told to call 911 and/or go directly to an emergency room. Although chest pain can be something as simple as indigestion, gastroesophageal reflux, or a muscle spasm, some causes of chest pain (think heart attack, pulmonary embolism, or aneurysm) are potentially deadly and require prompt medical evaluation. As stated repeatedly in this book, the number one cause of death in people who have lupus is cardiovascular disease causing heart attacks, strokes, and blood clots. Therefore, if you ever get chest pain for the first time, never wait and see if it will go away or schedule an appointment to see your doctor later. Instead, seek immediate medical attention. This is especially true of women. For reasons that are not entirely clear, women often will have unusual symptoms during a heart attack. While the typical heart attack causes severe, crushing pain under the breastbone, often radiating down the arm or into the jaw, some people, especially women, may have very different symptoms. They may have symptoms such as nausea, fatigue, indigestion, dizziness, or light-headedness as predominant symptoms with just some minor chest discomfort. Therefore, never try to brush it off or try to diagnose the problem yourself.

Some people get recurrent chest pain from a previously diagnosed cause that does not require immediate medical attention. In those cases, it is OK not to go to the emergency room as long as you have been thoroughly evaluated before, have a definite diagnosis, and have been told how to handle it. However, if you develop chest pain that is at all different from your usual chest discomfort, you need to have it immediately evaluated to make sure it is not something more serious. Some causes of chest pain and what they feel like are listed below.

### Heart Attacks (Myocardial Infarctions)

A heart attack (myocardial infarction) occurs when there is a blockage in an artery of the heart, which causes a part of the heart muscle to die. Pain that "comes and goes" can be due to milder decreases in heart muscle blood flow; this is called angina. This should be treated as a medical emergency to prevent permanent heart damage or even death. The typical symptoms are severe, crushing pressure–like chest pain under the breastbone that may radiate to the jaw, neck, or left arm. It is usually worse with exertion and is better with rest.

### Blood Clot in the Lungs (Pulmonary Embolism)

A blood clot in the lungs (pulmonary embolism) occurs when a blood clot blocks a blood vessel in the lungs. This can also be life threatening. Sometimes it is preceded by symptoms of a blood clot in the leg (deep venous thrombosis), which may cause pain and swelling in one of the calf muscles sometimes accompanied by red-colored, warm skin. This may occur after sitting for a long time in one spot such as a long car trip or plane trip. Pulmonary embolism can cause various symptoms, including rapid-onset stabbing chest pain with shortness of breath. The chest pain may be pleuritic (like pleurisy) where it gets worse by taking in a deep breath. Sometimes the person may cough up blood. Other symptoms such as light-headedness, dizziness, fever, and a feeling of dread or anxiety may also occur. You should seek immediate medical attention for any of these problems when they occur with chest pain.

### Thoracic Aortic Aneurysm

A thoracic aortic aneurysm occurs when a portion of the largest artery, called the aorta, enlarges and is in danger of rupturing. This can be a medical emergency requiring emergency lifesaving surgery in some cases. This aneurysm will typically cause a deep, throbbing chest pain or back pain that may also cause shortness of breath, cough, or hoarseness.

### Gastroesophageal Reflux Disease (GERD)

Gastroesophageal reflux disease (GERD; see chapter 28) is due to acidic contents from the stomach traveling up into the esophagus (which is located in the chest cavity under the breast bone). Although many people will feel heartburn, sometimes chest pain may be the primary or only symptom. It can also cause a dry, nagging cough. Often the chest pain gets worse with lying down because it is easier for stomach contents to enter the esophagus, and then improves after the person takes an antacid like Tums or Maalox. Other esophagus problems, such as esophageal muscle spasms, can also cause chest pain.

### Musculoskeletal (MS) Chest Wall Pain

Musculoskeletal (MS) chest wall pain occurs when any of the ligaments, tendons, muscles, ribs, or cartilage of the chest wall is the source of pain. This is a common cause of chest pain in people who have lupus, but other causes should always be ruled out. Costochondritis is one example of MS chest wall pain where there will be exquisite tenderness over the area where the ribs connect to the breastbone at the area of cartilage connections. This most commonly occurs at the left lower side of the breastbone but may occur anywhere in the front part of the chest. Fibromyalgia is also a common cause of chest wall pain causing tenderness and pain of the muscles, ribs, and cartilage of the chest wall. After dangerous causes have been ruled out (such as heart conditions), MS chest wall pain can usually be identified by noting areas of tenderness when you push down on the muscles and ribs of the chest area.

### Trouble Breathing

Just as with chest pain, any new episode of shortness of breath is a medical emergency. The affected person should seek medical attention, most preferably at the emergency room of a hospital. It is most important to make sure that there are no problems going on with the heart or lungs. A low red blood cell count (anemia) can also cause shortness of breath. If the onset of shortness of breath is gradual, then other possibilities may be the cause, especially conditions that affect the lungs and heart. Interstitial lung disease and pulmonary hypertension from lupus (see chapter 10) especially need to be considered by your doctor. Certainly, other possibilities such as weight gain or lack of exercise are common causes of gradually increasing shortness of breath with activity, but they are usually considered after other dangerous causes are first ruled out.

### Difficulty Urinating

Urinary tract infections (UTIs) are one of the most common reasons for having problems with urination in people who have lupus. People who have lupus have abnormal immune systems, putting them at increased risk for infections such as UTIs. In addition, women (90% of SLE patients) have a very short urethra (the tube that empties urine from the bladder). Bacteria continuously enter the short urethra of women from the vaginal and anal areas. This makes it easier for bacteria to get up into the bladder and cause an infection. Sexual intercourse further increases this risk by applying repeated pressure and trauma to the urethra. If bacteria infect the bladder (a type of UTI), it is common to have irritation of the bladder wall from the infection, and the bladder can contract uncontrollably. This will often cause people to feel an urgency to urinate and cause them to have to urinate more frequently than normal. A burning discomfort or even pain may also accompany urination. An early UTI may or may not have fever associated with it. It is very important to let your doctor know right away if you develop UTI symptoms such as increased urinary frequency with urgency as well as discomfort while urinating. If you wait too long, the infection could travel up to the kidneys where it can become severe, or it could even enter the blood causing a severe and potentially life-threatening infection called sepsis.

Some medicines can interfere with how the bladder muscles are able to squeeze out the urine. This can happen with some pain medicines such as tramadol or with some antidepressants. If you have trouble urinating and begin to feel pressure building up in the lower abdominal area where the bladder is located, this could be a sign of this type of problem. If you have recently started a new medicine, make sure to call your doctor immediately.

As men get older, they can develop a problem called benign prostatic hypertrophy (BPH). The prostate is a round organ that encircles the urethra at the lower part of the urinary bladder. It helps to keep the bladder closed until it is time to urinate. As many men get older, their prostates enlarge. This can squeeze abnormally on the urethra causing difficulty with urinating. They may develop smaller urinary streams, they may have difficulty initiating their urination, it may take them longer to urinate, and they may not be able to empty their bladders completely. This can cause them to have to urinate more frequently than normal (including having to get up throughout the night to urinate). This is rarely a medical emergency unless it occurs abruptly.

A rare problem in lupus occurs when the nerves that go to the urinary bladder are compromised, causing the bladder not to be able to contract. One potential cause of this in SLE is transverse myelitis. The spinal cord is attacked by lupus causing paralysis and loss of sensation in the legs as well causing difficulties with urination and defecating. Sometimes the opposite can occur with there being no control over urination and urinating when you do not want to. Other problems such as herniated disks or broken bones in the back (see the opening section of chapter 24), spinal cord tumors, and infections can also do these same things. If you find that you are not able to urinate and feel pressure building up in the lower abdominal area (where the bladder is), you need to seek immediate medical attention.

Along with urinary tract infections, the most common cause of urination problems in women is incontinence, especially stress incontinence. This occurs in some women when they get older due to the muscles of the pelvic region not working normally. This is often related to having had children in the past (causing weakness of the pelvic muscles) and losing the beneficial female hormones after menopause. Women can also develop an overactive bladder as well. These women typically experience problems with frequent urination or bladder incontinence that comes on gradually and gets worse with time unless proper medical attention is sought. It is best to see your primary care provider, your gynecologist, or a urologist (bladder specialist) for these problems.

## Numbness

Having a decreased amount of sensation in a part of the body is called numbness. It is most commonly a problem with the nerves although sometimes it can be due to other problems such as arthritis or fibromyalgia. Some nerve problems are considered medical emergencies, the best known of which are strokes. A stroke occurs when there is a loss of blood flow to a part of the brain causing that part of the brain to die. Strokes are sometimes referred to as "heart attacks of the brain." Sudden loss of sensation to any part of the body, especially an arm, leg, or one side of the face, should prompt people to seek immediate medical care. If doctors diagnose a stroke within the first couple of hours, they can provide blood thinners that can potentially reverse the stroke and prevent permanent brain damage.

Numbness can also occur due to other nerve problems. Transverse myelitis was mentioned above. This occurs when lupus attacks the spinal cord and usually causes paralysis of both legs as well as loss of sensation in both legs. This is a severe problem that requires immediate medical treatment at an emergency room.

Vasculitis from lupus can sometimes cause a nerve problem called mononeuritis multiplex. This occurs when inflammation of the blood vessels (vasculitis) decreases blood flow to many different nerves of the arms and legs. Areas of the hands and feet may get numb, sometimes accompanied by a painful, burning sensation. Areas of muscle weakness may also occur, especially something called foot drop where the person is unable to raise a foot up. Most people with vasculitis are usually very sick, often having other symptoms such as fever, weight loss, and bruising on the legs.

Peripheral neuropathy is a common nerve problem due to damage of small nerves of the legs and arms. It most commonly causes a gradual onset of decreased sensation in the feet sometimes followed by similar problems in the hands. Sometimes the person will notice a burning sensation or a feeling of "pins and needles" in the feet. The problems may be worse while in bed at night. This is usually not an emergency, but is addressed by treating the lupus more aggressively and using pain medicines specifically for nerve pain.

Various types of peripheral neuropathy can occur in the hands. One of the best known is carpal tunnel syndrome (CTS). The carpal tunnel is a very narrow tunnel in the wrist where the tendons that curl the fingers go through along with a nerve called the median nerve. SLE can sometimes cause swelling in the carpal tunnel, which compresses the median nerve. Usually this causes numbness in the thumb through ring fingers, clumsiness and hand weakness, and often a burning discomfort in the hands. It is not uncommon for it to be worse when someone first wakes up in the morning or for it to wake someone up in the middle of the night because it is common to sleep with the hands curled up, which scrunches the nerve, causing it to be more problematic.

A condition related to carpal tunnel syndrome is cubital tunnel syndrome. The cubital tunnel is located at the bone on the inner side of the elbow where the ulnar nerve travels. When you hit your "funny bone" and get severe, electrical shock–like pain that runs into the pinky and ring finger, this is due to hitting the ulnar nerve in the cubital tunnel. If there is compression of the ulnar nerve in the cubital tunnel, then a person can develop numbness as well as burning discomfort in the pinky and ring finger. This is usually worse when the elbow is bent. Important aspects of treatment of cubital tunnel syndrome include keeping the elbows straight and not resting the elbows on tables and arm supports.

## Muscle Weakness

Muscle weakness refers to actual weakness of a particular muscle or group of muscles instead of generalized fatigue. An abrupt onset of weakness of an arm and leg can potentially mean a stroke, while abrupt onset of weakness of both legs could mean spinal cord damage from lupus or other emergency conditions such as Guillain-Barré syndrome. These problems should prompt a person to seek immediate medical attention. A stroke can sometimes cause problems with the muscles of the face causing one side of the face to look very different from the other side, or cause problems with double vision, talking, smiling, or opening and closing the eyes.

Lupus can affect muscles and nerves in ways other than strokes (see chapter 13). Sometimes it can affect just one nerve at a time. For example, if it attacks the facial nerve that is responsible for the muscle tone in the face, it can cause half of the face to droop, and cause difficulty with smiling, raising the eyebrow, and closing the eye on the affected side of the face. This condition is often called Bell's palsy, but SLE can also cause it. Prompt treatment with strong immunosuppressant medicines is needed to prevent permanent nerve damage.

If you have difficulty raising your arms up to brush your hair or difficulty standing up from a chair without using your hands, this can sometimes be due to inflammation of the muscles of the shoulders and hips (myositis). This condition should be assessed and treated quickly to prevent severe muscle weakness problems. Generally, it can be assumed that any form of muscle weakness is a medical emergency requiring immediate medical attention.

## Headache

Muscle tension headaches are the most common headaches; they typically cause pain on both sides of the head or neck. People often describe tension headaches as a steady pressing or tightening sensation. Physical activity usually does not make them worse.

Migraine headaches are the second most common type of headache. They are related to abnormal activity of the nerves and blood vessels of the head and brain. Migraines tend to be more severe than muscle tension headaches and are more apt to occur on one side of the head with a throbbing quality. They can sometimes be accompanied by nausea and vomiting or sensitivity to light and noise. They usually get worse with physical activity. Sometimes they can be preceded by an aura with visual changes, skin numbness, or difficulty speaking. Both tension headaches and migraines are treated in lupus the same way as headaches are in people who do not have lupus.

Sinusitis is due to an infection of the sinuses of the bones of the face. The sinuses are air-filled cavities that lighten the weight of the skull and transmit sound waves. If the sinus passages are blocked, fluid can build up inside of the sinuses and lead to infection. This typically causes pain of the face associated with a sense of fullness or congestion. The headache may feel worse when the head is lowered or if pressure is applied to the bones of the face. Fever and thick nasal secretions are other important symptoms. Infections such as sinusitis can potentially be very dangerous in people who have lupus and need to be identified and treated rapidly.

Any type of new headache, especially if it is severe, needs to be taken seriously. Ruptured brain aneurysms classically cause abrupt onset of a severe headache that most people describe as "the worst headache I've ever had in my life." A ruptured aneurysm is a life-threatening situation usually requiring emergency surgery.

Brain tumors are an uncommon cause of headache; however, 50% of people who have a brain tumor develop headaches due to it. Headaches associated with a brain tumor may cause nausea and vomiting (just as a migraine can), and worsen with body positions (similar to sinusitis headache).

One interesting type of headache is known as a "medication overuse headache." This usually occurs in someone who actually has recurrent problems with either migraine headaches or tension headaches and uses pain relievers such as opioids or NSAIDs to treat the headache. Over time, these pain relievers may actually cause the headaches to worsen. Proper treatment for this type of headache is to stop all pain medicines.

The evaluation and treatment of chronic headaches can become very complex. A headache expert, most commonly a neurologist, best handles these sorts of situations.

## Stomach Upset

The most common reason for stomach upset in people who have SLE is due to medications. Even taking a multiple vitamin or a calcium supplement can potentially cause stomach upset. If you develop stomach upset soon after starting a new medicine, make sure to call your doctor for instructions. Usually this involves stopping the medicine or taking a lower dosage. Sometimes medicines to calm down the acidity of the stomach may be needed to help you tolerate an important medicine. GERD and ulcers can also certainly cause stomach upset (see chapter 28).

Mesenteric vasculitis is one of the most devastating potential complications of lupus (see chapter 15), but fortunately it is rare. It occurs when lupus causes inflammation in the arteries going to the intestines causing decreased blood flow and subsequent death to part of the intestines. It causes severe abdominal pain, nausea, and vomiting. Usually people are very sick and have other symptoms such as fever and weight loss. These problems are usually so severe that they force someone to seek emergency medical care.

Serositis in the form of pleurisy is one of the most common problems in lupus causing chest pain that is worse when taking in a deep breath. However, serositis can also affect the tissue lining the abdominal cavity (called the peritoneal cavity). If it becomes inflamed from lupus it is called peritonitis. Peritonitis may cause abdominal pain and fever along with tenderness of the abdomen.

Pancreatitis is due to inflammation of the pancreas. It can be a life-threatening situation. It typically causes upper abdominal pain usually with nausea and vomiting. Sometimes the pain will radiate to the back.

## Blurred Vision

The bottom line is that you need to see an eye doctor if any type of blurred vision occurs. Interestingly, many people who have lupus are quick to blame their hydroxychloroquine (Plaquenil) for blurred vision and want to stop taking it. Please do not do this, as Plaquenil is the safest medicine used to treat lupus. The vast majority of the time, blurred vision is due to something other than Plaquenil such as cataracts (clouding of the lens) or presbyopia (the eyes getting older causing problems with reading). Actual Plaquenil retina problems are rare. It is best left to your eye doctor to figure these out. If you develop blurred vision associated with eye pain, red eye, headache, or double vision, this could be a sign of something more dangerous such as an eye infection, glaucoma, vasculitis, uveitis, nerve damage, or stroke. If these symptoms occur, seek immediate medical attention instead of waiting for an appointment with your eye doctor.

## Is the Problem Lupus or Not?

SLE is an incredibly complex disorder. It can be confusing for many doctors to figure out. Since SLE can affect nearly every part of the body, it is not uncommon for doctors to "blame" the lupus for many things even when lupus may not be the culprit. Your best defense is that if anything ever happens and you are told by a doctor that it is due to your lupus, make sure to make an appointment with your rheumatologist to find out for sure. If you are in the hospital at the time, ask the doctors in the hospital to consult a rheumatologist who works in the hospital to evaluate you as well. If the hospital does not have a rheumatologist, ask if you can be transferred to a hospital that does have one available. If these are not possible, the doctors should at least make a courtesy phone call to your regular rheumatologist to discuss what is going on with you.

If you are ever admitted to the hospital for anything (other than a planned surgery or procedure), always ask the admitting physician to have the hospital rheumatologist look at you as well, even if the admission problem is not felt to be related to lupus. Too many times, I have had patients admitted to the hospital for something not felt to be due to their lupus, when it was actually their lupus that was causing the problems. For example, lupus pneumonitis (see chapter 10) can appear just like bacterial pneumonia, but the treatment would be to use immunosuppressant medicines instead of antibiotics (or use both). A stroke or heart attack may need special treatment in regards to SLE instead of the standard care for people who do not have lupus. It is usually in your best medical interests for a rheumatologist to evaluate you while you are in the hospital if you are sick enough to be there in the first place.

## KEY POINTS TO REMEMBER

1. Strive to make your doctor visits as productive as possible using table 40.1.

2. Learn to describe problems to your doctor using the points in table 40.2; you will increase your chances of getting an accurate diagnosis and treatment.

3. Some problems and symptoms occurring in lupus require immediate medical attention (such as going to an emergency room). Use the recommendations in table 40.3 to help guide you.

4. Some problems are common in people who have lupus (such as headache and fatigue). This chapter discusses some of these problems, and can help you help your doctor figure out what may be going on.

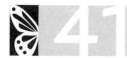

# Becoming Pregnant, Breast-Feeding, and Using Contraception

### Prepare . . . Have a Successful Pregnancy

> For most women with lupus, a successful pregnancy is possible . . .
> For nearly all mothers, a happy outcome is possible.
>
> —Michelle Petri, MD, MPH; Co-Director of the Hopkins Lupus Pregnancy Center

With proper preparation and monitoring during pregnancy, the vast majority of women who have lupus will have a good outcome with a healthy baby from their pregnancy. This is a huge change compared to previous decades. As recently as the 1970s, most women who had lupus were asked not to get pregnant by their rheumatologists.

However, the risks for potentially having more flares of lupus and having complications during the pregnancy such as a miscarriage are still real. At a large medical center, such as at the Johns Hopkins Lupus Pregnancy Center in Baltimore, Maryland, where in general more complex lupus patients are followed, there is a 7% chance for a severe complication during pregnancy and the risk for the mother dying is about one out of 150. Using the advice in this chapter, I have not had a patient, yet, have a bad outcome during pregnancy in my nearly twenty years of practice as a rheumatologist. It does take some work, however, on the part of the mother to ensure the best chances possible in having a good outcome. It is important to understand what the potential problems during pregnancy are. Therefore, I encourage the woman who has lupus who is interested in becoming pregnant to read chapter 18 first. If you desire to breast-feed, this chapter also gives advice on what medications are safe to take. In addition, it is important to know how to prevent an unintended pregnancy. You should not become pregnant until you have thoroughly planned for it, and some medications require strict birth control while they are being taken. This chapter gives you the necessary tools to prevent pregnancy when your doctor advises you to avoid it, as well as how to become pregnant and have a successful pregnancy when desired.

### How to Have a Successful Pregnancy

The first step to having a successful pregnancy is to assess what your risk for having a difficult pregnancy is. There are certainly women who have a higher chance for having difficulties during pregnancy compared to others, and you can figure this out ahead of time. You certainly do not have to do this to prepare for your pregnancy. If you are the type of person who becomes very anxious or too worried about things, skip this section of the chapter. If you are the type of person who likes to have all the information possible to maximize your healthcare, then read on. In table 41.1, put a check next to each item that pertains to you. You can ask your rheumatologist for assistance in answering some of these questions. If any of these lab tests have not been done, you can ask your rheumatologist to do them. Some of these, such as anti-SSA, anti-SSB, and the antiphospholipid antibodies, are essential.

As far as estimating your risk of having a complicated pregnancy, add up how many checkmarks you put down. The higher you score on a 1 to 13 scale, the higher your chances are of having complications such as preeclampsia, miscarriage, or preterm delivery. If you score 0, however, do not think you are completely out of the woods; it is still very important to plan appropriately for your pregnancy.

The items in table 41.1 are the major risk factors for having complications, and some of them you have absolutely no control over (such as being African American or being positive for anti-thyroid antibodies). On the other hand, many of these risk factors can be and should be dealt with to maximize your chances of having a good pregnancy outcome. This section gives you the proper advice to do just that.

**Table 41.1** Calculating Risk for Pregnancy Complications during Pregnancy

- Have you had any active lupus problems within the previous six months?
- Have you ever had lupus nephritis or been told that your kidneys had inflammation in them due to lupus?
- Do you have severe lupus, such as having problems with myocarditis, CNS lupus, interstitial lung disease, and pulmonary hypertension?
- Do you currently have an increased amount of protein in your urine?
- Are your C3 or C4 complement levels currently lower than normal?
- Is your platelet count lower than normal?
- Is your anti-ds DNA currently elevated?
- Are you positive for anti-thyroid antibodies? Do you have autoimmune thyroid disease such as Hashimoto's thyroiditis or a history of Graves' disease?
- Have you been positive for anti-SSA or anti-SSB antibodies in the past?
- Have you been positive for any of the tests that identify antiphospholipid antibodies such as false positive syphilis tests, anticardiolipin antibodies, lupus anticoagulant, beta-2 glycoprotein I antibodies, or antiphosphatidyl serine antibodies? (Lupus anticoagulant may be the most important of these tests.)
- Are you of African descent?
- Is your blood pressure currently elevated?
- Are you not taking an anti-malarial medication such as hydroxychloroquine (Plaquenil)?

1. *Ensure that your lupus is under excellent control for at least six months before trying to become pregnant.* This is the most important initial thing to do before even considering pregnancy. Please do not have an unplanned pregnancy if you have lupus. You should be using birth control measures. If you and your partner decide that you would like to have a baby, begin this discussion with your rheumatologist, asking if it is OK for you to become pregnant. You also need to find out how you should begin preparing for pregnancy. One of the first things to find out is if your lupus has been under good control for at least six months. If it has not, then that should be your first goal. After six months of good lupus control, then it is safer to try to get pregnant. To illustrate this importance, a study of 275 pregnancies showed that if a woman who has SLE had active disease within three months of getting pregnant, she was four times more likely to lose her baby. If SLE is under excellent control for the six months prior to pregnancy, the chances of having a normal outcome from pregnancy approach that of someone who does not have SLE.

Some of the risk factors in table 41.1 are signs of having active lupus disease. These include having an elevation of protein in the urine, low complement levels, elevated anti-ds DNA, and a low platelet count. While it is optimal to try to get all of these tests within normal ranges in preparation for pregnancy, this is not possible in everyone. For example, if you have permanent kidney damage from previous episodes of lupus nephritis or have had other kidney problems in the past, then you may always have an elevation of protein in your urine.

Although complement levels can be low as a sign of active lupus inflammation, some people always have low levels even when their lupus is doing well. Some people who have lupus have complement level deficiencies due to a genetic disorder where their bodies cannot make normal amounts of complements (especially C4 and C2). In these people, the complement levels will never be normal. Anti-ds DNA levels can be elevated in some people as a reflection of active lupus inflammation while in others it may always be elevated and not correlate with disease activity. In this latter group, aggressive treatment will probably not lower the anti-ds DNA level.

In regards to the platelet count, doctors generally do not use stronger medicines to increase the platelet count as long as it remains above a level of $50,000/\mu L$ (normal values are considered as being greater than $140,000/\mu L$). One reason for this is that it is rare to have a bleeding problem as long as the platelet count remains above $50,000/\mu L$. Although bleeding naturally occurs during all vaginal and cesarean deliveries, as long as the platelet count stays above $50,000/\mu L$, blood experts consider it safe to go ahead with the delivery without any additional treatments for the low platelet count. The potential side effects of using stronger immunosuppressant medicines or steroids are not worth the risks as long as the platelet count is above this number. Although having a low platelet count during pregnancy is associated with more pregnancy complications, the potential risks from side effects of taking a stronger medicine to try to increase the platelet count is probably greater.

If you have abnormalities in any of these blood tests, ask your rheumatologist if these levels (elevated urine protein, low complement levels, elevated anti-ds DNA, and low platelet counts) can be improved on with treating your lupus, or whether they are as good as they can be expected to be. Doctors want to treat lupus in the safest way possible, but without overtreating it as well. Your rheumatologist is the best judge of this.

*2. If you have hypertension (high blood pressure) make sure that your blood pressure is under perfect control.* If you have hypertension, make sure your blood pressure is under excellent control. In most people this means making sure the top number (systolic blood pressure) remains less than 140 and that the bottom number (diastolic blood pressure) remains below 90. You may need to see your primary care physician (or cardiologist or nephrologist) frequently for medication adjustments to achieve this goal. If you have kidney problems, you may need to have an even lower blood pressure for optimal control. Paying close attention to diet, weight loss, and exercise can also help with controlling blood pressure. Staying away from caffeine and foods that are high in sodium can help to control blood pressure levels. Make sure that you have a home blood pressure machine so that you can monitor your blood pressure at home. If you find that your blood pressure is consistently higher than the recommended levels, see your primary care doctor right away for medication adjustments. Also, make sure that your machine is accurate. Take it with you to one of your doctor appointments so that you can compare its results with the result that your doctor's machine gets. Many blood pressure medicines cannot be used during pregnancy. For example, ACE (angiotensin-converting-enzyme) inhibitors and ARBs (angiotensin receptor blockers), which are commonly used in people who have lupus nephritis, should not be used during pregnancy. Some blood pressure medicines that are safe to use during pregnancy include hydrochlorothiazide (HCTZ), methyldopa, hydralazine, and labetalol. You may want to consider planning ahead of time for pregnancy and ask your primary care doctor if you can switch your blood pressure medicines to those that are safe to take during pregnancy.

*3. Make sure you are taking your anti-malarial medication (such as hydroxychloroquine) regularly.* Whatever you do, *do not stop taking your Plaquenil (hydroxychloroquine).* Even if an obstetrician tells you to stop your Plaquenil, do not do so. If your OB/GYN doctor asks you to stop taking Plaquenil, politely (and tactfully) ask her or him to call your rheumatologist to discuss this matter. Unfortunately, not all doctors realize how important it is for lupus patients to continue taking Plaquenil during pregnancy. One of the worst things that can happen during pregnancy is if your lupus were to flare. Plaquenil helps to prevent lupus from flaring during pregnancy.

Taking Plaquenil also decreases the possibility of having miscarriages due to being positive with antiphospholipid antibodies, which are a major cause of miscarriage in women who have SLE. In fact, Plaquenil decreases the levels of these antiphospholipid antibodies. In addition, there is evidence that it also decreases the chances of having a baby with neonatal lupus if a woman is positive for SSA or SSB antibodies from her lupus. Plaquenil is safe to take during pregnancy and does not cause any problems with the baby at all.

*4. If you are taking an immunomodulating medication that should not be taken during pregnancy and you are ready to become pregnant, ask your rheumatologist if it can be changed to a medicine that is safer to take during pregnancy.* Table 41.2 lists the medicines that are used to treat lupus as well as special recommendations on their safety during pregnancy. Substituting most lupus medicines should not be done until after a six-month waiting period of ensuring that your lupus is under control. Once you get past the six-month mark, then you can discuss with your doctor the possibility of adjusting your medications. Some medications must be stopped for a period of time before getting pregnant. During the time you are waiting, it is important to use safe birth control measures. Medications that should be stopped followed by a waiting period before getting pregnant include mycophenolate (six weeks), cyclophosphamide (three months), methotrexate (three months), belimumab (four months), bisphosphonates such as alendronate (six months), and rituximab (one year). Most other medications can be stopped at the time that you find out you are pregnant. This list includes abatacept, adalimumab, certolizumab, etanercept, golimumab, infliximab, and tocilizumab.

Leflunomide (Arava) is a special case. After stopping leflunomide, it stays in the body for a very long time, and it can potentially cause problems with the fetus. It is important to do an elimination protocol using cholestyramine or charcoal to remove the leflunomide from your body before trying to get pregnant. It is also important to have two negative blood level results for leflunomide before trying to get pregnant. Chapter 32 describes the elimination process.

Your doctor needs to replace an immunosuppressant medicine that is stopped for one that can be safely used during pregnancy. If a woman has severe enough lupus that she requires a medicine such as methotrexate or mycophenolate, then another medicine should take its place. Azathioprine is the most common substitution. Since it can take up to three months for azathioprine to work, it is advised to keep this in mind when planning for the pregnancy.

Not using some of these medicines during pregnancy is not 100% set in stone. Remember that one of the absolute worst things that can occur is if you have a severe lupus flare during pregnancy. If you are on some medications, your rheumatologist may decide that it is safer to stay on that particular medicine to keep your lupus under control. In addition, if you were to have a particularly severe lupus flare, then some medications, such as cyclophosphamide, may be needed during pregnancy. Certainly, this would increase the risk of not being able to complete the pregnancy, but in reality, a flare that is severe enough to require cyclophosphamide would most likely terminate the pregnancy anyway.

These medication planning recommendations can be quite complex. Make sure that your rheumatologist writes down the recommendations so that you clearly know what to do. At the end of this section, we will look at an example of a lupus patient who is planning her pregnancy.

5. *If you are taking a non-steroidal anti-inflammatory drug (NSAID) or low-dose aspirin, make sure to stop it during your third trimester.* It is common to use an NSAID (such as ibuprofen or naproxen) to help decrease the inflammation and pain of lupus arthritis during pregnancy. In addition, taking low-dose aspirin, 81 mg a day can decrease the chances of having a miscarriage, getting a blood clot, or having preeclampsia if you are positive for antiphospholipid antibodies. However, it is important to stop these medicines during the third trimester. If they are not stopped, there is the potential that a blood vessel could remain open in the baby's heart and lung circulation causing significant oxygenation problems (in other words, blood could flow through the baby's body that has a dangerously low oxygen content). Patent ductus arteriosus is the name for this condition. However, if the NSAID is stopped before delivery (and hence the "stop during the third trimester" recommendation) this should not occur.

6. *Make sure you have your proper vaccinations.* Hopefully you have been a good lupus patient and have already had your proper vaccinations: a Pneumovax (done twice

**Table 41.2** Medications Used to Treat Lupus and How They Are Managed during Pregnancy

| Drug | Use in Pregnancy |
| --- | --- |
| abatacept (Orencia) | Do not generally use during pregnancy |
| adalimumab (Humira) | Do not generally use during pregnancy |
| aspirin | Stop during the third trimester |
| azathioprine (Imuran) | Generally safe to take during pregnancy |
| belimumab (Benlysta) | Do not get pregnant for four months after stopping |
| bisphosphonates for osteoporosis | Do not get pregnant for six months after stopping (table 24.10) |
| certolizumab pegol (Cimzia) | Do not generally use during pregnancy |
| chloroquine | Generally safe to take during pregnancy |
| cyclophosphamide | Do not get pregnant for three months after stopping |
| cyclosporine (Sandimmune, Neoral) | Generally safe to take during pregnancy |
| etanercept (Enbrel) | Do not generally use during pregnancy |
| golimumab (Simponi) | Do not generally use during pregnancy |
| hydroxychloroquine (Plaquenil) | *Safe!* Absolutely continue during pregnancy |
| infliximab (Remicade) | Do not generally use during pregnancy |
| intravenous immunoglobulin (IVIG) | Generally safe to take during pregnancy |
| leflunomide (Arava) | Must do an elimination protocol (chapter 32) |
| methotrexate | Do not get pregnant for three months after stopping |
| methylprednisolone | Generally safe to take during pregnancy |
| mycophenolic acid (CellCept, Myfortic) | Do not get pregnant for six weeks after stopping |
| non-steroidal anti-inflammatory drugs | Stop during the third trimester (table 36.1) |
| prednisone | Generally safe to take during pregnancy |
| rituximab (Rituxan) | Do not get pregnant for one year after stopping |
| sulfasalazine (Azulfidine) | Generally safe to take during pregnancy |
| tacrolimus | Generally safe to take during pregnancy |
| tocilizumab (Actemra) | Do not generally use during pregnancy |

five years apart), a flu shot yearly in the fall, as well as other maintenance vaccines for all adults, including a tetanus vaccine (see chapter 22). If not, then these need done not only to protect you, but also to protect your baby.

7. *Do not take any medications during pregnancy unless approved by your rheumatologist and obstetrician.* There are other medications not listed here that may not be good to take during pregnancy. Although your rheumatologist can usually address those that are specifically used to treat your lupus, you may need to check with your obstetrician about your other medicines. This should be planned ahead of time before you get pregnant.

8. *Do not smoke cigarettes.* As explained numerous times throughout this book, there are many reasons people who have lupus should not smoke. It is even more important during pregnancy because not only are you putting your life in danger; you are endangering the life of your unborn baby. Smoking during pregnancy increases the risk of preeclampsia, death of the baby, congenital malformations, preterm delivery, and having a baby born who is smaller than normal. In addition, exposure to second-hand smoke has been associated with an increased risk of having a stillbirth (death of the baby), congenital malformations, and having a baby born who is smaller than normal. It is a good time for the entire family to stop smoking together. Think of all the money you will save in addition to the improved health of your family.

9. *Do not drink alcohol.* Drinking alcohol during pregnancy increases the chances for stillbirth and congenital malformations related to fetal alcohol syndrome. There is currently no level of safe alcohol consumption known not to cause problems during pregnancy; therefore, complete abstinence from any alcohol during pregnancy is recommended.

10. *Exercise regularly during pregnancy unless told otherwise.* Regular exercise generally is important during pregnancy as it decreases the chances for some complications, including diabetes and preeclampsia. However, physical activity restrictions are recommended for some pregnant women depending on their medical condition, including decreasing the amount of activity if there is a risk for a baby with low birth weight. It is very important to ask your obstetrician to advise you on what exercises you can safely do during pregnancy.

11. *Eat a healthy diet.* Remember that you are eating for two during pregnancy; however, this does not mean that you should be overeating. Consider seeing a dietician during pregnancy to learn what foods (and amounts of food) are best to eat in regards to your lupus and your pregnancy. Extra precautions need to be taken to ensure that you decrease the risk of getting any food-borne illnesses (such as hepatitis A, listeria, toxoplasmosis, or brucellosis). You can get a list of foods to avoid from your dietician or obstetrician. In general, if you eat a healthy diet full of whole grains, vegetables, and fruit along with an adequate amount of protein and dairy products, you may not need to take any vitamin supplements at all (except for folic acid, as discussed below).

12. *Take supplements as directed by your obstetrician.* Unfortunately, most Americans do not eat a healthy diet and most women do need to take extra vitamins and minerals during pregnancy. These options should be discussed with your obstetrician, dietician, and rheumatologist. If you are at increased risk of osteoporosis (see chapter 24), then you may need to take calcium and vitamin D supplements. The calcium requirement increases to 1,000 mg a day during pregnancy to allow for the in-

creased calcium requirements of the developing baby's skeleton. All pregnant women should take a supplement that contains at least 0.4 mg of folic acid daily one month before conception and then continue it for the first several months to prevent problems with development of the baby's spinal cord (spina bifida).

13. *Make sure that you are seeing a high-risk obstetrician.* All pregnancies in women who have SLE are considered to be possibly high-risk. I recommend that all of my lupus patients see a high-risk obstetrician in consultation at least once before pregnancy. Women who do have increased risk factors for pregnancy complications (i.e., if you checked off any of the items in table 41.1) should see a high-risk obstetrician regularly throughout pregnancy as well.

14. *If you have any major organ involvement from lupus, make sure to see a specialist for that organ system during pregnancy.* This is especially true for certain complications such as heart disease, lung disease, kidney disease, central nervous system involvement, or if you have pulmonary hypertension. If you have had lupus nephritis before, but it is in remission when you get pregnant, you do not have to see a kidney doctor (nephrologist) if you do not have permanent kidney damage, as long as your rheumatologist feels comfortable monitoring your kidneys.

15. *Follow up with your rheumatologist at least monthly.* If lupus were to flare, such as lupus nephritis, there may be no symptoms whatsoever until severe disease has become rampant, at which time it can endanger the baby and the mother. However, if increased lupus activity is identified early, it can be treated while in a mild stage, which can greatly increase the chances of having a successful outcome for everyone.

16. *If you are positive for anti-SSA and/or anti-SSB antibodies, have your baby's heart monitored regularly.* When the mother is positive for anti-SSA or anti-SSB antibodies, these antibodies can potentially cross the placenta and attack the baby's heart, causing permanent heart block. This means that the baby may require a pacemaker at the time of delivery. This complication occurs in 2% to 3% of women who are positive for these antibodies overall. However, the probability jumps to a 15% chance of recurrence in a woman who has already had one baby born with congenital heart block.

With early diagnosis, treatment with steroids may be able to decrease this risk. Therefore, have your baby's heart monitored using pulsed Doppler fetal echocardiography (which safely uses sound waves to monitor the heart). This should be done weekly beginning around the eighteenth week of pregnancy through the twenty-sixth week. After that, once every two weeks is usually sufficient. This study should be set up ahead of time by the high-risk obstetrician.

17. *If you are positive for antiphospholipid antibodies, ask your rheumatologist if you should be taking aspirin or other blood thinners during and after pregnancy.* Antiphospholipid antibodies (especially lupus anticoagulant) increase the risk for blood clots occurring in the placenta, which can increase the risks for miscarriage, stillbirth, preeclampsia, and other pregnancy complications. It is generally recommended that women take 81 mg of aspirin a day during the first two trimesters (hoping to prevent these complications), then stop it during the third trimester (to prevent patent ductus arteriosus). Taking hydroxychloroquine (Plaquenil) also decreases the chances for these complications from happening. However, if you have had recurrent early miscarriages in the past, have had a late pregnancy loss or stillbirth, or have ever had a blood clot of any kind, you should probably be taking a stronger blood thinner such as hepa-

rin during pregnancy. Discuss this important option with your rheumatologist. If you need to take heparin during pregnancy, it is important to take enough calcium and vitamin D and to do regular weight-bearing exercise to prevent getting broken bones due to heparin-induced osteoporosis.

One area of controversy is whether blood thinners should be continued after delivery of the baby. The problem is that there is an increased risk of getting blood clots during the first four to six weeks after delivery. Therefore, the American College of Chest Physicians Evidence-Based Clinical Practice Guidelines recommend that blood thinners (such as heparin or Coumadin) be used during the first four to six weeks after delivery of the baby if you required heparin during your pregnancy. This possibility as well as the potential risks of taking or not taking the blood thinners should be discussed with your rheumatologist and obstetrician.

18. *If you are on thyroid medications, make sure your thyroid blood tests are being monitored during pregnancy and that they are kept normal by proper adjustments of your medication.* Approximately one out of every twenty women who have SLE will also have autoimmune thyroid disease. Often this requires the use of thyroid hormone supplements or other medications to control the thyroid problem. There is an increased risk of preterm delivery in women who have autoimmune thyroid disease, and it is important to make sure that your thyroid status is monitored closely during pregnancy. This is simple to do through regular blood tests. Currently the Lupus Center at Johns Hopkins Hospital in Baltimore is doing a study looking at the effects of thyroid disease in pregnancy and the utility of thyroid hormones during pregnancy.

19. *If you have been on steroids such as prednisone for a significant amount of time, alert your obstetrician as you may need to have "stress doses" of steroids at the time of delivery.* Delivery is a very stressful event for the body, and normally the adrenal glands secrete a large amount of steroids during the event to help the body handle the stress appropriately. However, people who have taken steroids in high enough doses or for a long time are at increased risk of the adrenal glands not working properly and not being able to provide these essential increases in steroids. This condition is called adrenal insufficiency (see chapter 26). It is very important that women who may have adrenal insufficiency take additional doses of steroids at the time of delivery to compensate for this problem. Make sure to alert your OB/GYN and high-risk obstetrician ahead of time to ensure that the appropriate increase in steroids is given at delivery. Wear a medical alert bracelet stating that you may have adrenal insufficiency or have been on chronic steroids as well. If you were to go into labor prematurely in an area where the doctors do not know you, they need to be able to recognize that you need the steroids. A recent additional option is to wear a medical history bracelet. This contains a memory chip with a USB port that can be connected to any computer. Your entire medical history, including what medications that you take, can be easily seen by the medical personnel. Wearing a medical alert bracelet or a medical history bracelet can be the extra insurance that you need.

20. *Consider asking your rheumatologist if you can either get a shot of steroids, or take some extra steroids ten to fourteen days after your delivery to prevent a postpartum flare of lupus.* The fetal side of the placenta produces extra steroids during pregnancy. This can actually be helpful in some women in decreasing the activity of their lupus during pregnancy, especially during the third trimester. After delivery, this source of steroids

abruptly halts, major hormonal changes occur, and there is a lot of stress. All of these factors increase the possibility of having a flare of lupus after delivery of the baby. There is especially a drop in steroids during the first two to eight weeks after delivery. Therefore, some lupus experts recommend taking extra doses of steroids ten to fourteen days after delivery. This can either be done by taking extra steroids by mouth, or by getting a shot of steroids in the muscle of the buttock in your rheumatologist's office.

## Pregnancy Case Example

BG is a young woman who developed SLE right before getting married. She had severe disease with significant arthritis and lupus nephritis as her major problems. She is positive for anti-SSA, anti-SSB antibodies, and antiphospholipid antibodies. She is a very compliant patient and is very fortunate to have a supportive husband who comes in with her at many of her office visits so that he keeps informed about his wife's progress. She responded very well to treatment (as most compliant patients do), and was taking CellCept, Plaquenil, low-dose prednisone, and low-dose aspirin (to prevent blood clots from her antiphospholipid antibodies). She and her husband had been very much looking forward to having a baby and had the appropriate discussion with me about planning for it. After six months of being under control with no elevation in her urine protein and no flares of her lupus, she stopped taking her CellCept (which should be stopped six weeks before trying to conceive), and I replaced it with azathioprine (which is safe to take during pregnancy). Since it takes three months for azathioprine to work, I recommended that we wait another three months just to make sure that it was going to be enough to control her lupus nephritis before getting pregnant. Therefore, her total waiting time would be nine months (six months for good disease control plus the three months for making sure the azathioprine was going to work).

Three months later, her labs looked fantastic and her lupus was still under excellent control. She continued the hydroxychloroquine (Plaquenil) and azathioprine (Imuran) throughout her pregnancy. I also continued the low-dose aspirin in the hopes that it might possibly decrease the risk of having a miscarriage related to her positive antiphospholipid antibodies. However, knowing that aspirin (like other NSAIDs) can cause patent ductus arteriosus, I stopped it during her third trimester.

As instructed, she increased her rheumatology visits to once a month throughout pregnancy to ensure that her lupus (especially the lupus nephritis) did not flare during pregnancy. She was also seeing a high-risk obstetrician in addition to her regular OB/GYN doctor throughout pregnancy. All doctors communicated with each other with notes and lab results throughout her pregnancy to ensure the optimal amount of perinatal care.

Since she was positive for anti-SSA and anti-SSB antibodies, there was a very small, but real, increased risk of congenital heart block occurring in the baby. Therefore, during her eighteenth week of pregnancy, she began to have the baby's heart monitored, which was set up by the high-risk obstetrician. Her baby's heart never developed congenital heart block.

She had previously let her OB/GYN and high-risk obstetrician know that she had been on steroids for a long time, and she was told to get "stress doses" of steroids at the time of delivery. During labor, the increased steroids were given as planned, and she had a very healthy baby through vaginal delivery. As previously planned with her rheumatologist, she took extra doses of steroids ten days after delivery to prevent a postpartum (after pregnancy) flare of her SLE.

## Assisted Reproduction and IVF

Although SLE itself does not appear to cause infertility, infertility is not uncommon in women who have SLE. In addition, women who have received cyclophosphamide can develop infertility due to its permanent effects on the eggs in the ovaries. In these situations, other alternatives need to be considered in regards to having children, which can include assisted reproduction techniques such as in vitro fertilization (IVF) as well as other alternatives such as donating sperm and eggs to a surrogate mother. In some cases, adoption of children may be the only practical solution to having a family.

One of the methods used to help produce pregnancies in women who have fertility problems is called ovarian stimulation. This is a medical technique where women receive hormones to cause the production of increased numbers of eggs. These eggs are then fertilized with the father's sperm (in vitro fertilization), which is then followed by placement of embryos into the woman's uterus. A potential problem with ovarian stimulation is that certain hormones, especially a group called gonadotropins, have an increased chance of causing lupus flares. In fact, even in women without a history of lupus, about 2% of women who have this procedure develop a complication called ovarian hyperstimulation syndrome, which can mimic flares of lupus. To decrease the risks of developing flares of lupus in women who have SLE, and of decreasing complications during assisted reproduction, it is recommended that the guidelines in table 41.3 be followed.

## Breast-Feeding

Breast-feeding your newborn baby can potentially provide significant health benefits to your baby as well as to you (table 41.4). Many women who have SLE are able to breast-feed their newborn babies.

**Table 41.3** Decreasing the Risk of Lupus Flares and Pregnancy Complications during Assisted Reproduction, Ovarian Stimulation, and IVF

- SLE should be in remission for at least twelve months prior to ovarian stimulation.
- People who have pulmonary hypertension, severe kidney disease, or severe heart disease, or who have had significant blood clots in the past should not undergo assisted reproduction.
- Hypertension (high blood pressure) should be brought under excellent control prior to beginning ovarian stimulation.
- Medications that are less likely to cause ovarian hyperstimulation syndrome should be used.
- Only one embryo should be implanted at a time.

**Table 41.4** Potential Benefits of Breast-Feeding for Babies and Their Mothers

Potential benefits of breast-feeding for the baby

- Decreased infections
- Improved health of the stomach and intestines
- Decreased risk of maternal neglect and child abuse
- Less obesity, cancer, cardiovascular disease, allergies, and diabetes later in life
- Improved intelligence, vision, and hearing
- Less stress

Benefits of breast-feeding for the mother

- Speeds up recovery from childbirth
- Decreases stress in the mother
- Better weight loss after childbirth
- Reduces the risk of breast and ovarian cancer
- Decreases the risk of cardiovascular disease
- Saves money (conservative estimate of $1,000 savings in formula per year as of 2011)

The primary concern in mothers who have lupus and breast-feeding is that some medications can enter the breast milk (table 41.5). This can potentially cause problems in the baby. The medications used to treat moderate to severe lupus (the immunosuppressants) should not be used during breast-feeding. This creates quite a problem in the mother who has moderate to severe lupus because the only medicines that can safely be used are the anti-malarial medicines (which are not sufficient to treat moderate to severe lupus by themselves) and steroids. If a woman is on an immunosuppressant medicine for her lupus and decides to stop it to be able to breast-feed, she places herself at increased risk of her lupus flaring. Certainly, there are many health benefits in breast-feeding your baby, but these potential benefits should be weighed against what could happen if you were to get very sick with SLE. This is a choice that only you can make, but you need to think about it long and hard because it is very important to have a healthy mother to take care of the baby in the future and to be able to see that baby grow up into an adult over time.

## Contraception (Preventing Pregnancy)

### Oral Contraceptive Pills (OCPs)

The most effective oral contraceptive pills (birth control pills) are those that contain a combination of the female hormones estrogen and progestin. In addition to helping to prevent pregnancy, they can also lower the risks of getting certain gynecological cancers, including uterine, endometrial, and ovarian cancers. However, they can potentially cause blood clots, worsen migraines, worsen liver disease, or increase the risk of developing breast cancer. Studies since the 1970s have shown that the "newer"

**Table 41.5** Medications Used to Treat Lupus during Breast-Feeding

| Drug | Use in Pregnancy |
| --- | --- |
| abatacept (Orencia) | Safety during breast-feeding is unknown |
| adalimumab (Humira) | Safety during breast-feeding is unknown |
| aspirin (low dose) | Safe during breast-feeding |
| azathioprine (Imuran) | Do not use during breast-feeding |
| belimumab (Benlysta) | Safety during breast-feeding is unknown |
| bisphosphonates for osteoporosis | Safety during breast-feeding is unknown (table 24.10) |
| certolizumab pegol (Cimzia) | Safety during breast-feeding is unknown |
| chloroquine | Safe during breast-feeding |
| cyclophosphamide | Do not use during breast-feeding |
| cyclosporine (Sandimmune, Neoral) | Do not use during breast-feeding |
| etanercept (Enbrel) | Safety during breast-feeding is unknown |
| golimumab (Simponi) | Safety during breast-feeding is unknown |
| hydroxychloroquine (Plaquenil) | Safe during breast-feeding |
| infliximab (Remicade) | Safety during breast-feeding is unknown |
| intravenous immunoglobulin (IVIG) | Safe to use during breast-feeding |
| leflunomide (Arava) | Do not use during breast-feeding |
| methotrexate | Do not use during breast-feeding |
| methylprednisolone | No problems at doses $\leq$ 16 mg a day; if taking more than 16 mg a day, wait four hours after taking this medicine before you breast-feed |
| mycophenolic acid (CellCept, Myfortic) | Do not use while breast-feeding |
| non-steroidal anti-inflammatory drugs | Diclofenac, ibuprofen, indomethacin, ketorolac, mefenamic acid, naproxen, and piroxicam are OK |
| prednisone | No problems at doses $\leq$ 20 mg a day; if taking more than 20 mg a day, wait four hours after taking prednisone before you breast-feed |
| rituximab (Rituxan) | Safety during breast-feeding is unknown |
| sulfasalazine (Azulfidine) | Safe for full-term infants |
| tacrolimus | Safe to use during breast-feeding |
| tocilizumab (Actemra) | Safety during breast-feeding is unknown |

OCPs that contain lower amounts of estrogen are generally safe in most women who have well-controlled lupus without increasing the risk for lupus flares. However, they can increase the risk of getting blood clots in lupus patients (who already have a higher risk of getting clots). Women who have lupus and who should not take OCPs are listed in table 41.6.

## Progestin Only Pills

These may be an alternative for women who cannot take estrogen-containing OCPs. However, they are less effective and must be taken at exactly the same time every day to prevent pregnancy.

## Depo-Provera Shots

Depo-Provera can be administered by injection. It can also be used in women who cannot take estrogen-containing OCPs and it lasts for three to four months after the injection. Potential side effects include osteoporosis, weight gain, and vaginal bleeding.

## Implanon

Implanon is a tiny, plastic rod containing the female hormone progestin. It is inserted under the skin of the inner upper arm where it continuously releases progestin into the bloodstream where it can prevent pregnancy for three years. It may also be a good alternative for women who are unable to take OCPs.

Table 41.6 Women Who Have Lupus Who Should Not Take Oral Contraceptive Pills

- Those who have active moderate to severe lupus
- Those who are positive for antiphospholipid antibodies
- Those who have had blood clots in the past
- Those who have had a stroke before
- Those with poorly controlled hypertension (high blood pressure)
- Those with pulmonary hypertension
- Those with atrial fibrillation
- Those who have coronary artery disease or have had a heart attack before
- Those who have migraine headaches
- Possibly those with Raynaud's phenomenon (although this is not for certain)
- Those who smoke (have a higher risk for blood clots)
- Those who have nephrotic syndrome (a complication of lupus nephritis that increases the risk of getting blood clots)
- Those who have had breast cancer in the past
- Those who have very high cholesterol (increases the chances for blood clots)
- Those who have cirrhosis of the liver or liver cancer (to include hepatic adenoma)

## Intrauterine device (IUD)

An IUD is a device inserted into the uterus by a gynecologist. It releases the female hormone progestin to prevent pregnancy. The biggest danger with IUDs is the increased risk of infection, especially sexually transmitted diseases. It may be a good choice in someone who is in a stable, monogamous relationship and who is not taking immunosuppressant medications.

### KEY POINTS TO REMEMBER

1. Before getting pregnant, make sure that your lupus has been under excellent control for at least six months and that you have discussed getting pregnant with your rheumatologist.

2. If you are positive for anti-SSA or anti-SSB antibodies, make sure that you have your baby's heart monitored regularly starting at week 18.

3. If you are positive for antiphospholipid antibodies, make sure that you are taking aspirin or a stronger blood thinner during pregnancy.

4. Review the medicines that are safe to take during pregnancy (table 41.2) and breast-feeding (table 41.5).

5. Continue Plaquenil throughout pregnancy.

6. See your rheumatologist monthly during pregnancy.

7. See a high-risk obstetrician if you get pregnant.

8. If you are at increased risk of adrenal insufficiency, wear a medical alert bracelet or a medical history bracelet, and ensure that you get extra steroids at the time of delivery.

9. Do not take OCPs if you have any of the problems listed in table 41.6.

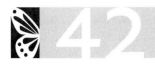

# Health Insurance and Affording Healthcare

## Lupus, an Expensive and Potentially Disabling Disease

Dealing with a chronic disorder that requires making frequent doctor visits, taking medications, and getting regular studies (such as labs and x-rays) done can become an expensive hardship for many. A study in 2009 showed that the medical costs for a person who had systemic lupus erythematosus (SLE) averaged $18,940 per year. For a person who had lupus nephritis requiring dialysis treatments, this average jumped to an astonishing $67,969 per year. Yet these numbers do not really tell the whole story. This is only the direct cost of medical treatment itself to pay for doctors, nurses, lab tests, x-rays, medical equipment, and hospital costs. The other part of the equation is the indirect cost of dealing with SLE, which includes the loss of wages from time missed from work when having to deal with these medical issues. A study in 2008 showed that this averaged $8,659 per year per patient just for missing work and missing wages.

Although many people who have SLE are fortunate to have excellent jobs with good sick-day benefits as well as excellent health benefits requiring relatively low out-of-pocket payments, others are not so fortunate. Some have to pay high co-pays to see doctors, to get necessary tests done, and to pay for their medicines. Others are even much less fortunate, and have no benefits at all, having to pay everything out of pocket or having to rely 100% on government aid.

It is impossible to separate the financial problems of lupus from dealing with the disease. The number one cause of not doing well with SLE (such as having more severe disease and higher death rates) is noncompliance. If someone does not have the means to be able to afford the best medical care and is not able to take the medications required to treat lupus, it automatically makes them noncompliant against their will. This places them at high risk of not doing very well.

In addition, although most people who have SLE do very well, live long, normal lives, and are able to work with no problems at all, some people are not able to continue working and they become disabled. The process of becoming disabled, losing your job, and dealing with the necessary bureaucracy and paperwork to get the assistance you need can be overwhelming. This chapter goes over some of the details about financial issues, insurance, and affording medications, while chapter 43 deals with disability. I must preface these chapters with the reality that currently the country is going through a large number of changes in insurance, healthcare, and disability benefits as a result of the global economic recession that began in December 2007. Although the recession ended by definition in mid-2009, unemployment is still high in the United

States (and worldwide), and the political arguments continue as to how to deal with the economic difficulties in the United States. These political differences in how to deal with economic problems will play a huge role in how healthcare and disability are eventually dealt with. Therefore, some of the things that I talk about in chapters 42 and 43 may be true at this time, but they could very well change in the future. Consider getting proper professional help with many of these matters to make sure that you are dealing with your own situation to the best of your abilities.

However, much of this advice will be usable for many years; much of it is universal in its concepts. If you are struggling financially or are wrestling with the prospects of disability, the tools in these chapters can at least give you some guidance on some of the things that you can do to improve your situation.

## Healthcare Insurance: Private and Public

There are numerous ways that people get their healthcare in the United States. This section discusses some of those aspects and gives some advice for those who have choices in what healthcare they can have and how to deal effectively with their particular healthcare situation. Dealing with healthcare benefits can be overwhelming, as the terms and systems involved vary widely depending on which healthcare benefits one has.

Healthcare benefits can be divided into large categories. There are those who have private insurance healthcare provided for them by their employers or from buying it individually, and there are people who get their healthcare through government-run programs such as Medicare and Medicaid. Lastly, there are people who are uninsured who must pay everything out of pocket. If you fall into this latter category, I provide some strategies to help you navigate the healthcare system.

### Private Healthcare Insurance

There are two major types of private healthcare insurance: group plans and individual plans. Most Americans who have private healthcare insurance are covered under group insurance plans that are offered by their employers. Most of the time, the employees have very little to say about which healthcare plan they get or the terms of the healthcare plan. Generally, the larger the company that you work for, the greater your chances are of having better healthcare benefits. The reason for this is that a very large company can buy a very large number of policies for a large group of people. Through having a large number of healthy individuals in that plan, it can be advantageous to the insurance company itself as well as your employer to bargain for better benefits at reduced costs. On the other hand, smaller companies tend to have lower bargaining power with the insurance companies and may have more difficulty getting better rates for better insurance coverage. If they do get better insurance coverage benefits for their employees, it may come at the cost of having to pay higher insurance rates. Some people who get group health insurance do have the advantage of being able to choose from a number of different plans offered by their employers. The federal government is a good example of this type of system. In this situation, the employee has the choice of paying different costs out of pocket for different plans. I offer some advice in this section for people who have SLE on these choices as what may appear as the least expensive healthcare plan choice may actually end up being more expensive in the long run.

The second major way of getting private insurance is through an individual health insurance plan. This is an insurance plan paid for completely by an individual where an employer is not involved. This may need to be done by people who have jobs where no group insurance is offered or for people who are self-employed. Since an individual does not have the luxury of the risks of healthcare being spread out among a large number of people (as occurs with group health insurance), individual plans tend to cost more and offer fewer benefits compared to the better group insurance plans offered by larger companies to their employees. People purchasing individual health insurance must choose very carefully, depending on what their personal health situation is and what their potential medical needs may be, to get the best plan possible. I give some advice on these decisions as well. Another disadvantage of individual health insurance is the problem of having a pre-existing medical condition. Many plans do not accept individuals who have pre-existing health conditions (such as SLE). However, one good thing for the near future is that the Patient Protection and Affordable Care Act was signed into law in March 2010. This act mandated that children with pre-existing conditions could not be excluded from their parents' healthcare plans because of a pre-existing condition (including SLE) beginning in September 2010. For adults over age 19 years old, this law will become valid in 2014.

Until this law comes into effect, people need to understand that they still do have some protection even though they have a pre-existing condition such as SLE. If you have had at least a full year of health insurance, but you find that you need to change health plans (such as switching jobs) for any reason, if you have not had a break of sixty-three days or more without health insurance, you cannot be discriminated against for having a pre-existing health condition. It is extremely important to keep your health care insurance going for as long as you can and to obtain your new health care insurance as quickly as you can to make sure that the amount of time between those two plans is less than sixty-three days. In a disorder such as SLE where disease flares can occur suddenly without warning, it is better to be safe and plan for no lapse in healthcare at all.

Starting January 1, 2014, when the Patient Protection and Affordable Care Act takes effect for adults, people who have pre-existing medical conditions cannot be discriminated against. They must be offered healthcare without being charged higher rates. This is wonderful news for those who have lupus and other chronic medical disorders, and the lupus community should congratulate the politicians who worked so hard to make this happen.

Several types of private medical plans are available. As mentioned above, you may not have a choice in which one you get, but sometimes (as with some government employees) you do have a choice. The major players include Health Maintenance Organizations (HMOs), Point-of-Service (POS) plans, Preferred Provider Organizations (PPOs), and Indemnity Plans.

*Health Maintenance Organization (HMO).* HMOs require you to have a primary care provider, called a PCP for short (such as a family practice or an internal medicine physician) who acts as a "gate keeper." You are required to see your PCP for all medical conditions and care. When a specialist is needed, such as a rheumatologist for SLE, then you must obtain a referral from the PCP to see the specialist. The referral may be good for only one visit or may be good for multiple visits. There are advantages to an HMO. It is often one of the least expensive forms of private healthcare insurance since it figures that the PCP (working as a "gate keeper") can decrease overall healthcare costs for the insurance plan by limiting the amount of specialist visits by its members. Usually the total premium (amount of money that you pay for the plan) is one of the lowest, and the co-pays (shortened form of co-payments) that the individual pays for each doctor's visit are usually lower than in other plans. In fact, some plans do not charge any co-pay when seeing a PCP.

There are downsides to using an HMO. One downside is that it can be a hardship when someone must see a specialist frequently (such as someone who has SLE needing to see a rheumatologist frequently) plus having to get a referral for each visit. This often forces members to see their PCPs more regularly than they normally would need to, just to keep up with the referrals.

In addition, most HMO plans stipulate that it is the individual's responsibility to keep up with the referrals to ensure that they are up to date. A referral to a specialist usually has a timed limit on it and expires after a certain date. It is up to the individual to ensure that the referral is good for the appointment time scheduled with the specialist. In addition, the specialist is not allowed (by her or his contract with the HMO) to see the patient unless that individual has an up-to-date referral. One example of where this can be problematic is in the case of when an appointment with a specialist needs to be rescheduled for any reason. Of course, this could occur due to many possible reasons, including weather closures of the office, the patient being unable to make the appointment, or illness on the specialist's part. It is up to the individual to get a new referral if that new appointment occurs after the expiration date of the initial referral. Due to the numerous and often complicated requirements of HMOs on these referrals, most specialists in turn stipulate that it is the patient's responsibility to keep up with referrals (even those that may have more than one appointment included on one referral). It is usually too much work for a doctor's office to keep track of. In addition, patients participating in HMOs must see specialists who are members of the HMO. This can also potentially cause problems if a patient's regular rheumatologist is not a member of the HMO.

In addition, the PCP usually must also give the person a referral for any special procedures or tests ordered by the specialist. For example, an HMO may require that the person obtain a referral even for a simple x-ray ordered by the specialist.

Although many people may decide that it is advantageous to participate in an HMO due to its lower cost, they must take into account the potential downsides of the referral system. The referral system can be very difficult to maneuver. For example, you may find yourself having to see your PCP more often than you thought you would need to just to keep up with your referrals. It can be quite a challenge to keep up with the dates of expiration on the referrals and the number of appointments allowed on each referral as well. An HMO can be a fantastic, low-cost alternative for people who rarely need to see a specialist. However, it can quickly become a huge burden to those who have chronic illnesses. In SLE, for example, not only do people need to see their rheumatologist at least four times a year, but they usually must also see an ophthalmologist (eye doctor) once a year to monitor their hydroxychloroquine (Plaquenil) therapy, and may need to see other specialists regularly as well. So if you do have a choice, think twice about the cost because it can actually become more costly in the long run when you need to miss additional days of work just to keep up on the referrals from your PCP.

Another potential downside of an HMO occurs in situations where you may need to see a doctor who does not participate in the HMO plan. For example, if you are visiting another city and have a medical emergency, if you see doctors who are not in your particular HMO, you may not be covered at all and you may face large medical bills. However, some HMOs do offer emergency benefits to cover these sorts of situations, but this varies from plan to plan.

Cost is also not the only issue. The referral system sometimes inserts a wedge in the patient-doctor relationship. It is human nature to blame the doctor (specialist) and his staff for problems when referrals prevent the patient from being able to see the specialist, or when the patient ends up paying out of pocket because of expired referrals. All of these headaches (financial and professional) can be prevented by avoiding an HMO in the first place. If you are the type of person who is incredibly well organized, is very comfortable with the HMO system, and does not get frazzled when you need to get new up-to-date referrals when required, then an HMO may be the best affordable plan for you.

*Point-of-Service Plan (POS).* A POS is a hybrid sort of HMO plan. You can utilize doctors and specialists who participate in the plan using referrals as outlined above, but then you also have the choice of using doctors and specialists outside of the plan (called out-of-network providers). When you use doctors who are in the network of the plan, you can expect to pay lower co-pays to see those doctors, but you also usually need to have an up-to-date referral when you see a specialist in the plan. When you use an out-of-network provider, you pay a higher amount of money to see that doctor by paying either a high deductible or a co-insurance charge. These plans generally are more expensive than the traditional HMO as they do provide greater flexibility in terms of the doctors you can see. This is a good option for people who want some of the financial benefits of an HMO when electing to see specialists who participate in the plan, while providing the flexibility to see a specialist who is outside of the plan also. This type of plan can especially be good if you have been seeing a rheumatologist whom you like for a long time, and then need to change insurance plans. If you switch to a plan your rheumatologist does not belong to, but it is a POS, then it allows you to continue your long-term patient-physician relationship.

*Preferred Provider Organization (PPO).* A PPO tends to cost more than the two plans described above, yet it offers much more flexibility. You are not required to have any referrals to see specialists. This makes it much easier for people who have chronic disorders that must see specialists. Most PPOs have provisions where you can see doctors who are not part of the PPO plan as well; however, this is more expensive. For example, a PPO may pay for 90% of the cost of seeing a specialist who participates in the plan, but only 70% of the costs of a specialist who does not. This gives you some added flexibility in seeing doctors both in the plan and outside of the plan, realizing that it is more expensive to do the latter.

*Indemnity Plan (also called Fee for Service and Traditional Plan).* This is the least restrictive type of plan to have. The person with this sort of plan does not have to see any particular doctor and is not required to have any type of referral at all. There may be a high deductible where the person is responsible for paying a certain amount of money out of pocket before the insurance plan starts to pay for medical expenses. If there is a high deductible, then usually the yearly premium paid is lower compared to those of other types of plans. A typical plan may pay for 80% of healthcare costs, after the yearly deductible is met, leaving the member to pay the other 20% of the costs. Most plans also usually have a maximum yearly amount that the policyholder must pay for medical costs. Once that maximum amount is met, the indemnity plan may pay for up to 100% of the additional costs. Although these are the least restrictive plans, they still usually require pre-authorizations for certain medical procedures and tests. A pre-authorization (often shortened to "pre-auth") is a process where a doctor must fill out paperwork to prove to an insurance company that a particular test or procedure is needed for a particular situation for a particular patient. A pre-auth tries to decrease the number of unneeded expensive medical procedures from being performed.

*High-Deductible Health Plan (HDHP).* An HDHP is considered a type of a "consumer-driven health plan" where the person pays a small yearly premium for the health coverage compared to other plans such as HMOs and PPOs, but at the expense of a high deductible that must be met yearly. These plans also supply something called catastrophic coverage where the member of the plan pays up to a maximum amount of money per year for healthcare costs. HDHPs are usually used in conjunction with tax-advantaged programs such as health savings accounts and medical savings accounts. These are accounts set up by participating people. Money is put into the account to only be used for medical expenses. This money is not subject to payroll income taxes, therefore, lowering the income taxes taken out of the person's paycheck. In addition, the money builds up over time and does not have to be used up every year (as occurs with flexible spending accounts, as discussed below). These accounts must be used to cover medical expenses such as doctor visits, hospital bills, prescription drugs, and medical devices prescribed by a doctor. Even over-the-counter medicines can be covered as long as a doctor writes a prescription for it. Another advantage of these plans is that if monies are still in the plan at retirement, they can be used for nonmedical uses provided certain requirements are met. These plans tend to be more beneficial to people who are healthy and younger.

## Government Insurance Programs

By far, the largest two government healthcare programs are Medicare and Medicaid. There are other government healthcare systems in addition to these two, including the Indian Health Service, Military Health System, TRICARE (the civilian component of the Military Health System), the State Children's Health Insurance Program (SCHIP), and the Veteran's Health Administration (VA). I do not discuss these other systems, but I encourage you to use these to the utmost of your abilities if you qualify for any of these programs. While most people who qualify for these programs (such as the Indian Health Service and the VA) are aware of their eligibility, many are not that familiar with SCHIP. It provides medical care to the children (18 years old and younger) of families who have difficulty affording medical care (even if they are not eligible for other programs such as Medicaid). All states offer SCHIP with federal support, but each state runs its particular plan individually and often very differently than other states may do. If you have children and are unable to afford healthcare, you can call 1-877-KIDS-NOW (1-877-543-7669) to learn more about the program and to try to enroll your children in the program.

*Medicare.* Medicare is a social insurance program run by the U.S. federal government that provides medical care assistance to people over 65 years old, those who are blind, those who are disabled, and those who have permanent kidney failure. The Medicare system has four different parts (A, B, C, and D).

*Medicare Part A (Hospital Insurance).* Everyone who is eligible and enrolled in Medicare gets Part A benefits, and it does not cost anything. Medicare Part A covers the costs of overnight hospital stays, including the costs of food and medical tests. It can also cover some of the costs of being in a skilled nursing facility up to a hundred-day stay if it occurs after a three-night hospitalization and if skilled nursing services are required for the reason that the person was in the hospital.

*Medicare Part B (Medical Insurance).* Medicare Part B is an optional service in that it can be deferred if the person is still working or if the spouse is still working. However, if not working, the person is subjected to a monetary penalty if not enrolled in Part B. What this means is that you are required to enroll in Part B within a certain time around your 65th birthday (unless exempt due to having certain work-related health insurances). If you do not enroll within the deadline, usually within three months of your birthday, then it may cost you more to have Medicare Part B. The premium costs for Medicare Part B are automatically deducted from your Social Security check. Part B covers expenses not covered by Part A, including outpatient doctor visits, labs, x-rays, vaccinations, medications given by doctors in their offices, and dialysis. It can also cover the costs of medical equipment such as canes, walkers, wheelchairs, motorized scooters, and home oxygen equipment. After a necessary out-of-pocket yearly deductible is met, Medicare generally pays 80% of these medical expenses while the participant pays the remaining 20% of the costs.

*Medicare Part C (Medicare Advantage Plans).* The Medicare Advantage Plans are private insurance plans that take the place of traditional Medicare. If you subscribe to one of these plans, then you forfeit your usual Medicare benefits (and this is a very important point that many do not know about when they sign up for these plans), and you use the private plan instead. You also still must pay your Medicare Part B premiums that are automatically deducted out of your Social Security checks. There are three major types of Medicare Advantage Plans. They can be grouped similarly to the private insurance plans discussed previously. HMOs can be quite inexpensive, even cheaper than traditional Medicare when it comes to how much money you pay for hospitalizations, doctor visits, and the like. However, they are usually very restrictive, requiring you to only use doctors and facilities within the plans and they usually require the use of referrals as with all HMOs. One of the biggest complaints about these plans is the difficulty with getting necessary medical care due to the many restrictions employed within the plans. Most HMO plans still allow the Medicare Part D Prescription Plan, as discussed below.

There are also PPO plans that cost more than the HMO plans, but you can go out of network to see other doctors and specialists. Referrals to specialists are not required, which can be of benefit to patients who must see specialists frequently (such as lupus patients), and most allow the use of Medicare Part D. Although you can go out of network to see doctors and go to hospitals out of network, it is more expensive compared to using services supplied within the network.

The third type of Medical Advantage Plan consists of the Private Fee-For-Service plans. These plans are very flexible in terms of which doctors you can see, and therefore, the costs for the plans are generally higher than for the PPO plans. A major disadvantage of these plans, though, is that you must contact the doctor's office and hospital before each appointment to ensure that they will abide by the terms of the insurance. If a doctor sees you the first time under your plan, but then realizes later that the plan did not pay appropriately, she or he can refuse to see you a second time. Never assume that a doctor will see you using this plan if she or he has seen you once before; always call ahead of your appointment to check on this.

Choosing between traditional Medicare and a Medicare Advantage Plan can be a difficult decision. One word of advice is to be very careful of the sales pitches on these plans. Make sure to do your homework before applying for one of these plans. Check with other people (friends, family); research internet resources before buying into a sales pitch. While some of these plans can be excellent, many people become disillusioned when they find that they have more difficulty getting the medical care that they need due to the restrictions in their plan when it comes to which doctors they can see, which medical services they can get, and which medicines they can take.

There are several potential advantages of Medicare Advantage Plans. They can sometimes be cheaper overall than traditional Medicare, and they may offer services not offered by traditional Medicare such as free wellness exams with your PCP, eyeglasses, and hearing aids. Some also offer emergency medical services outside of the United States, which traditional Medicare does not offer. These advantages must be weighed very carefully against their potential disadvantages, which mainly include the increased restrictions on which doctors, hospitals, and services will be covered. In addition, many people are very surprised to find out that their overall costs for their doctors and tests end up being even more than what they would have been if they had kept their traditional Medicare. Therefore, be a smart "shopper"; investigate a plan very closely, and factor in all the potential cost possibilities before considering one of these plans over your traditional Medicare.

*Medicare Part D (Prescription Drug Plans).* Anyone who is eligible for either Medicare Part A or Part B is eligible for Medicare Part D. Since traditional Medicare (Parts A and B) does not cover medications outside of a doctor's office, this plan is specifically designed to help cover costs of prescription medicines. This is a voluntary plan and requires that the person apply for the plan through private insurance companies that run the plans. The plans vary a lot from company to company, and therefore it is very important to do your homework and compare the benefits of plans that you are eligible to join. The plans charge various amounts of monthly premiums, have different required deductibles, and have different medication co-payment amounts. In addition, they usually have formularies, which are lists of medicines that they will cover and which medicines they will not cover. If a plan sounds good to you on the surface, but the medicines you require for your health are not in its formulary, it would not be a good choice for you.

One disadvantage of the Medicare Part D for people who have disorders such as lupus is the "donut hole" gap. The amount of the donut hole changes from year to year. In 2013, once an individual reaches a limit of $2,970 for prescription drugs, she or he is responsible for the costs of 47.5% of brand-name medications and up to 79% of the costs of generic medications. Subsequently, after spending $4,750 for medications, the "donut hole" ends. The person then enters the "Catastrophic Coverage" portion of the plan where the drug costs go down significantly. A major problem with the donut hole is that some people who have SLE are required to take large numbers of medications that can easily put them into this donut hole. Many people are on fixed incomes where they are not able to afford the medicines while in the donut hole portion of the plan.

*Medigap (Medicare Supplemental Insurance).* These insurance plans may be purchased, usually by paying a monthly premium. They pay for healthcare services not paid for by Medicare. For example, Medicare recipients must pay for 20% of their healthcare benefits after they meet their yearly deductible. Many Medigap policies will cover these 20% payments as well as the Medicare deductible payments that usually the individual is responsible for paying. These plans can be very helpful, especially for people with high medical costs who can afford to pay the premiums for the plans. You can learn more about these plans at www.medicare.gov. It is important to note that Medigap cannot be used in conjunction with the Medicare Advantage Plans of Medicare Part C.

*Medicaid.* Medicaid is a welfare program for people with low incomes to help with their healthcare costs. The states administer these programs in conjunction with the federal government. Since the states run the programs, eligibility and the services provided vary a lot from state to state. If you have significantly limited income and have very little assets (savings and property, not counting your primary home and car), then you should contact your state Medicaid department to see if you may be eligible. By the way, you can participate in both Medicare and Medicaid.

## What to Do If You Are Uninsured, Underinsured, or Cannot Afford Your Healthcare

With the economic crisis beginning in 2007, a large number of Americans have become uninsured through the loss of jobs, or they have less income and find it very difficult to pay for their healthcare even using insurance. Being without health insurance or not having enough money for healthcare can be catastrophic to someone who has lupus. While the best solution is to keep searching for a good job with good health benefits, there are other options available to help get through such a crisis. In addition, some people have insurance, but still have difficulty affording their healthcare. Some of these tips may be useful in those situations as well.

*If you are laid off or lose your health insurance, get good advice.* In addition to working hard to try to find a job as quickly as possible, it is also important for you to try to find health coverage as soon as possible. Some places that may help include Healthcare

Advocates (www.healthcareadvocates.com), the Patient Advocate Foundation (www
.patientadvocate.org), and Patient Services Incorporated (www.patientservicesinc
.org). Find out immediately if you are eligible to extend your health insurance through
COBRA (discussed later in this chapter). This is a program where you can pay the premiums of your health insurance after you lose your job. Unfortunately, only about 9%
of people are able to continue getting insurance through COBRA due to the expense
of paying for it.

*Be honest and forthcoming about not having the money to pay for healthcare.* These
are tough times, and your healthcare providers understand that. However, doctors will
not know to help you out financially if they do not know the troubles you are having.
When making any of the requests listed below, be honest about your tough financial
situation. Your doctors' offices can try to help in some ways if they know what a rough
time you are having. Find out at your doctor's office if there is an office manager or
practice manager. The office manager is the person you want to speak to when making special financial arrangements with your doctor. Keep your visits with your doctor strictly focused on your medical condition. However, some doctors who are in solo
practice may not have an office manager. In those cases, speak to the doctor.

*Ask for discounts from doctors' offices and hospitals.* Most doctors' offices and hospitals will give discounts to people who have to pay out of pocket and have no insurance.
The best person to speak to is the office manager of the practice. Let him or her know
your financial problem and ask for discounted rates. If you do have insurance that requires co-pays, usually the doctor's office cannot help. The doctor is required to collect a co-pay from you as part of the arrangement with your insurance plan. The same
goes with your hospital. Make an appointment with the billing department manager
or a hospital social worker to help. With a large hospital, be prepared to show your
financial hardship. If you go prepared with information such as family income, bills
(utilities), and proof of residency in the state, age, and U.S. citizenship, it can help your
plan of getting the help that you need.

*Set up an interest-free payment plan with your doctor or hospital.* If you do owe money, the worst thing you can do is to ignore the situation and not pay. Even if you can pay
a small amount each month, it is better than paying nothing. Make an appointment
with the office manager or with a social worker at the hospital to explain your situation. See if you can get the amount of money that you owe cut down and work out a
payment plan that you know you can afford. Never agree to a plan that is beyond your
budget. It is better to pay a smaller amount every month and stand behind your word
with making the payments compared to coming up with a plan that you are unable
to afford. A doctor's office would much rather you pay a little bit at a time over an extended amount of time instead of paying little to none of your bill owed. In addition,
if you work out a plan ahead of time, it saves the doctor's office money because office
staff will not have to keep calling you on the phone, will not have to keep sending you
letters asking for payment, and will not need to hire a collection agency to try to get
the money from you. You can keep your credit score from becoming affected if you do
these things before you begin to run behind on your bills. Again, doctors understand
people are going through tough times, and they would much rather see someone be
honest and try to work with them from the start instead of ignoring the problem.

*Ask your doctor if generics are available in place of expensive brand-name medicines.*

Many times doctors prescribe newer brand-name medicines that do not have generic equivalents because they may be better than older medicines for several reasons. For example, a newer version of a medicine may be a slow-release, once-a-day form while the older generic form may have to be taken three to four times a day. It is much easier for a patient to be compliant with taking a once-a-day medicine compared to taking a medicine more often throughout the day. Whenever you are prescribed a new medicine, or if you are already on an expensive medicine, ask your doctor if there is a cheaper, generic medicine that can potentially take its place. Realize that this may be difficult for your physician to do. For example, there may be no way to know exactly how to convert a person from one medicine in a class of drugs to a completely different medicine, so it may take some trial and error on your doctor's part to try to do this. There also may be no possible generic equivalent for some medicines, but it never hurts to ask. If a medicine has no generic equivalents, ask if your doctor has samples of the medicine or any coupons. If you do not want to bother the doctor, ask the receptionist, nurse, or medical assistant for samples. I do not even mind if patients call the office just to ask for samples as long as they are keeping up with the necessary labs and appointments to monitor the medicine in question. Another option is to contact the pharmaceutical company that makes the medicine and see if it has a patient assistance program in which you can participate. These are usually based on household income, so you may need to send in proof of income for these programs. Almost all brand-name medicines have easy-to-find websites using the name of the medicine. For example, the new lupus medicine Benlysta's website is www.Benlysta.com. Many brand-name medicines have coupons available at their websites. Many of the medications used to treat lupus are discussed in detail in preceding chapters, and most of these discussions include information regarding the pertinent patient assistance programs.

*Apply for patient drug assistance programs.* Table 42.1 lists agencies that can potentially help you with prescription medications.

**Table 42.1** Prescription Drug Assistance Organizations

| | |
|---|---|
| - Partnership for Prescription Assistance | www.pparx.org<br>(888-477-2669) |
| - HealthWell Foundation | healthwellfoundation.org |
| - FamilyWize Discount Drug Card | www.familywize.org |
| - Needy Meds | www.needymeds.org |
| - Rx Assist | www.rxassist.org |
| - Rx Hope | www.rxhope.com |
| - Chronic Disease Fund | www.cdfund.org |
| - The Access Project | www.accessproject.org |
| - United Networks of America | www.unitednetworksofamerica.com<br>(click on "important links") |

*Ask for medicines covered in $4 generic drug lists.* Many pharmacies have low-cost generic drug lists. Get a copy of this list from each pharmacy in your area and keep them with you. Check the lists for the types of medicines you are taking. If there are any alternative medicines on the lists that could potentially replace a more expensive medicine, ask your doctor if this is possible. Take the lists with you to doctor appointments, and if you are prescribed a new medicine ask your doctor to check to see if he or she can put you on a medicine that is on the list.

*Ask your government representatives for help.* Many government agencies exist that can provide help with healthcare. This can vary a lot between cities, counties, and states. Contact your local city councilperson, mayor's office, state-level representative and senator, as well as your federal-level representative and senator. Be honest about your financial situation, and explain that you have a potentially very dangerous medical situation that requires treatment that you cannot afford. They may be able to direct you to organizations that offer help in your area that you may have never known existed. I did not realize that this method was an option until one of my patients who fell on hard times told me that by doing this, she received more help than through any other method she tried.

*Contact your closest Lupus Foundation of America chapter as well as other patient advocacy groups.* They usually have a list of local and national organizations that are available to help with the healthcare of people who do not have insurance or the financial means to get adequate healthcare. Our local DC/MD/VA chapter has a "Patient Navigator" whom patients can contact to help answer their questions and steer them in the right direction for obtaining help. It even has an Emergency Assistance Fund that can help as well.

*Go to a publicly funded clinic and local health department.* Many healthcare benefits can be received at publically funded health clinics, including PAP smears, immunizations, pelvic exams, mammograms, cholesterol levels, blood pressure checks, glucose (sugar) checks, and ECGs. You can get information for clinics in your area by contacting the Health Resources and Services Administration at 877-464-4772 or by going to findahealthcenter.hrsa.gov on the internet. Additional low-cost healthcare clinics not run by the federal government may also be available in your community. Make sure you find them, make an appointment, and take advantage of all the services you can get. There are even clinics specifically for people who have SLE. You can call the National Institute of Arthritis and Musculoskeletal and Skin Diseases at 1-877-226-4267 to see if there is an available clinic close to where you live.

*Contact a teaching hospital rheumatology clinic.* Some rheumatology clinics at large teaching hospitals may be able to see patients who have no insurance to help with their healthcare. This may especially be true if they have any active research studies going on in lupus. In fact, volunteering to participate in a lupus research study is a good way to get your foot in the door of a lupus clinic at a teaching hospital. Call the clinic; be straightforward and explain that you have no money or insurance and that you desperately need healthcare for your lupus. Ask them if they can provide any care and ask them if they have any research studies that you could potentially benefit from.

*Go to health fairs for free services.* Health fairs sometimes offer free services such as mammograms, bone density measurements, cholesterol levels, blood counts, chemistry tests (kidney, sugar, and liver function tests), blood pressure, hearing tests, and vision screenings. Make sure to keep copies of your results and keep them organized in your home personal health records.

*Ask your doctor to only order absolutely essential tests.* SLE is a complex disease, and to follow it closely and completely involves numerous tests, some of which can be quite expensive (e.g., anti-ds DNA, C3 complement and C4 complement levels). Ask your doctor to order only the bare necessities at each visit. The absolute minimum requirements are a CBC (complete blood cell count), urinalysis (then a random urine protein/creatinine if any protein shows up positive on this test), and a chemistry panel that includes ALT (liver enzyme), and a serum creatinine with a calculated eGFR (estimated glomerular filtration rate). All of these are discussed in chapter 4.

*Ask x-ray and blood drawing offices for a special discount and compare prices.* When you need to get x-rays and labs, call all the offices available in your area. Ask to speak to the office manager or billing department. Explain over the telephone that you will be paying out of pocket and that you do not have very much money and really need some help. Ask for a discounted rate and promise to pay before you get the test done with cash. Tell them exactly what tests you need. Call up several different offices and then choose the one that gives you the best rate. If your rheumatologist does lab tests inside the office, ask the office manager how much the office would charge; again, do not be ashamed to say that you need financial help to get a good rate. In fact, your rheumatologist is more apt to give you a better rate compared to an independent outside company since you already have a relationship with your doctor, who has a stake in your personal health. As long as you pay upfront with cash, you should get a good price. For example, in our clinic, all we would ask for is what it would cost for the supplies needed to do the test and the time and work spent by the technician (not expecting any profit from doing the test).

*Choose a cheaper hospital.* When you have to go to the hospital, choose a nonprofit hospital, a teaching hospital, a charity hospital, or a public hospital instead of a for-profit hospital. Call the billing departments or social work departments ahead of time to find out if your local hospitals fall into one of the above categories. Ask for a hospital discount. An advantage of teaching hospitals is that the hospitals pay the doctors directly, and you can include the doctors' fees under your discount. Other hospitals (including nonprofit hospitals, public hospitals, and charity hospitals) have doctors whose fees are paid separately from the hospital. Do not be afraid of going to a teaching hospital, fearing that you will be taken care of by a young intern or resident. The way teaching hospitals are set up is that patients are seen by an intern (first-year resident), possibly a medical student, plus a senior resident, plus a senior staff member as well. Some of the best rheumatology programs in the country (such as Johns Hopkins in Baltimore, UCLA Medical Center in California, and the Mayo Clinic in Minnesota) are teaching hospitals. They tend to have some of the most modern equipment and keep up on the latest in therapies. It may also be a good way to get plugged into their lupus clinic as a patient (just make sure that you ask them to consult rheumatology while you are in the hospital and then ask the rheumatologists if that is a possibility).

*Avoid duplicate tests; keep copies of all test results.* A big downfall of the current medical system is that there is not a good way to centralize the results of tests (blood, urine, x-rays, etc.). Due to this, unfortunately, it is common to have to repeat tests because the doctors do not have the results of each other's tests. A way to get around this is to take things into your own hands. Every time you get a test done, contact your doctor's office to get a copy of the test. Make sure to give the office staff enough time to get the result back and filed into your chart; if you call too soon for a test result, it can just be more difficult to get the result. Ask the front desk or receptionist to mail you a copy or arrange to stop by the office for a copy for your own personal records. Keep these copies well organized in your own personal home records. If you need to see another doctor, and you think he or she may need the result, just photocopy it, and take it in with you to your next visit. Also, always carry your records and results with you; you may circumvent having an unnecessary test done.

*Do research on resources on transportation to doctors' offices and hospitals.* If you cannot get to the doctor due to not having transportation, then that can be a huge obstacle to your medical care. It is essential that you investigate your area to find out what resources are available. Contact your local public servants (town councilperson, state-level as well as federal-level senators and representatives), senior citizens' center, free medical clinic, and hospital social worker's office to find out what services you may have available. If you have Medicaid, there are often free transportation services available, so contact your local Medicaid office to find out.

*Look for bargains on medical equipment.* Go to Goodwill, the Salvation Army, yard sales, thrift shops, auctions, and www.craigslist.com to find good deals on medical equipment such as wheelchairs, canes, scooters, crutches, walkers, hospital beds, bedside commodes, shower chairs, lift chairs, and electric stair climbers.

*Learn to budget.* When you are strapped for money, it is even more important than ever to learn to keep a budget and stay on it. Before buying anything, ask yourself, "Is this something I really need, or something that I just want?" Be honest. If it is the latter, skip it.

*Save all medically related tax receipts for tax purposes.* Even if you do not think that you can deduct your medical expenses from your income tax, still save all receipts throughout the year and keep them organized. This includes all doctor co-pays, prescription co-pays, over-the-counter medicines (with a doctor's prescription showing need), physical therapy costs, health insurance premiums, eyeglasses, dental expenses, medical equipment, and stop-smoking classes. Save the receipt for anything medically related. If your medical expenses exceed a certain amount of your adjusted gross income on your taxes (this amount is currently set at 7.5% or higher), then this could save you money on your income tax. Even if you usually are not qualified to use this deduction, still keep track of your expenditures. You never know beforehand if you will have a more difficult year than normal. It is much easier to have everything filed away for easy access compared to having to backtrack and try to find the information later. A tax advisor can then be helpful in figuring out which expenses you can deduct and which ones you cannot deduct. For anything that you need to get that is medically necessary, always ask your doctor to write it on a prescription pad for you to help with your documentation as well.

*Eat healthy and cheaply.* Eating healthy will help your lupus and decrease healthcare costs in the end. Eating healthy is less expensive than eating unhealthy (think fast food, chips, and soda pop). Drink lots of water instead of soda pop. Tap water is generally safe and markedly cheaper than bottled water. Fill up a water bottle and drink it throughout the day. Learn to "shop the perimeter" of the store where fresh fruits and vegetables, dairy, and fresh meats are located instead of the central aisles where more expensive canned goods and bagged foods are sold. Large bags of frozen vegetables can be quite inexpensive. Buy large amounts of chicken on sale; make sure to prepare it broiled or baked (not fried) and remove the skin before eating it. Do not eat junk food and do not eat out (which is always more expensive than preparing food yourself). Learn to buy in bulk, look for sales, and learn to use coupons as well. Buy generic brands instead of the more expensive brand names. Learn to eat smaller portions; Americans unfortunately are used to consuming oversized servings, which greatly contribute to the obesity epidemic.

*Exercise.* Exercise can be free (brisk walking on a track, free arthritis class exercise groups, seniors groups, or doing them yourself at home). Lupus patients who exercise regularly tend to overall be healthier, and require less medical care (think "therefore cheaper and pay less money") overall compared to patients who do not exercise. You do not have to have an expensive membership at a health club to exercise. Check out what is available in your community. One of my favorite cartoons by Randy Glasbergen that I have hanging up in my office shows a doctor asking a patient, "What fits your busy schedule better, exercising one hour a day or being dead 24 hours a day?" This is so true.

*Stop smoking.* One of the most frustrating things for doctors is to have patients sitting in front of them who complain about having to pay money for their medicines, doctor visits, and other healthcare costs, yet they smell like a chimney from all the cigarettes that they smoke. Smoking is expensive. Plus it worsens your health, which in turn increases your healthcare costs. It is a losing battle if you keep smoking. As mentioned multiple times in the book, smoking increases the severity of SLE, keeps Plaquenil (hydroxychloroquine) from working, and causes early heart attacks and strokes, in addition to all the other horrible things it does (cancer, emphysema, etc.). Just do the math on how much money you would save if you stopped smoking. However, do not stop there. Your future healthcare costs would be lower if you stopped smoking, your lupus got under better control, and you did not develop heart disease, strokes, or cancer at an earlier age. You can contact your local free health care clinic for free smoking cessation assistance.

*Learn to treat some conditions on your own.* Throughout this book there are numerous recommendations on how to treat some conditions on your own without using medications. Put these suggestions to use. This includes things such as gastroesophageal reflux disease, insomnia, fatigue, and joint pain. Many people can control many of these problems adequately by simply eating properly, exercising adequately, getting rid of bad lifestyle habits, and doing the non-drug recommendations discussed. I am not at all trying to minimize the effects and complications of lupus, by the way. It is just a common practice for people to want to take a little purple pill for something over doing the harder work of trying to control things on their own. Even if you are not able to get rid of your problems by doing all of the suggestions, often you can decrease their severity enough so that less expensive medications can be used to help you out.

*Consider working a part-time job that has good health insurance.* Some people may find it "demeaning" to become a barista making cappuccinos when they used to have a very important managerial job in the workplace. However, it can potentially make a huge difference in the quality of your healthcare if you are fortunate enough to find any job that offers good healthcare. This is the time to throw your ego out the window. Here are some examples of companies that offer health insurance to part-time employees: Aerotek, Costco, 5/3 Bank, Staples, U-Haul, Caribou Coffee, Publix, The Fresh Market, Kaplan, Starbucks, Whole Foods Market, REI, Barnes & Noble, Nordstrom, Lowes, Lands' End, Nike, JCPenney, JP Morgan Chase, Trader Joe's, FedEx, DHL, UPS, Sam's Club, Home Depot, Macy's, Safeway, Kroger, Wegman's, Target, and Cost Plus World Market. However, this list may shrink in the future, depending on the healthcare reform situation. Local hospitals and local governments also often offer part-time employee health benefits. Other part-time jobs such as working as a teacher's aide may also offer good benefits such as healthcare insurance in some areas. Make sure that there is not a time lapse between insurances to avoid being denied insurance due to your pre-existing condition of lupus. However, this problem will become moot in 2014 when the new healthcare laws go into effect on pre-existing conditions in adults.

*If you are disabled and cannot work due to SLE, apply for disability ASAP.* Although it is better for your health and finances to keep working a job (even part-time) that has good health benefits, if you are unable to work, it is best to apply for disability as soon as possible. Consider getting help from a lawyer who specializes in Social Security Disability (see chapter 43).

*Apply for Supplemental Security Income (SSI).* If you have limited income and have very little assets, apply for SSI, which is a welfare program aimed at helping people with the lowest incomes in society. The requirements for SSI are very stringent, but if you satisfy these requirements, it can add a little bit to your income benefits.

*Get your child on the State Children's Health Insurance Program (SCHIP).* This is a state-by-state-run welfare program dedicated to giving medical care to children from lower-income families. Even if you do not meet the stringent requirements for SSI or Medicaid, you may still be able to get your child help with this program. Just call 1-877-KIDS-NOW or go to www.insurekidsnow.gov to learn more about the program.

*Read* 101 Ways to Save Money on Healthcare *by Cynthia J. Koelker, MD.* This excellent book has many good ideas on how to save money when it comes to healthcare. You may be able to find it at your local library or purchase an inexpensive, used copy on the internet.

## Additional Healthcare Considerations

### Flexible Spending Accounts (FSA)

An FSA is a financial account that people can set up through their employers that allows them to save money to use for medical expenses. An advantage of these plans is that the money is not subject to income payroll taxes. The amount is deducted from people's gross income, therefore lowering the total amount of income tax they are required to pay out of their paychecks. They may use that money to pay for medical expenses such as doctors' co-pays, prescription costs, medical devices, and even for over-the-counter medications (as long as they have a prescription from a doctor for the items). Dental and eye expenses (including LASIK surgery) can be covered as well. FSAs can generally be used in conjunction with any type of medical insurance. People who have chronic illnesses such as lupus would be well advised to take advantage of this type of plan if their employers offer it as it saves money in the end.

One potential downside is that if you do not use up the money you put into your FSA in a year, you do lose the money at the end of the year. For example, if you decide to put $2,000 a year into your FSA, but at the end of the year, you spent $1,500 in qualified medical expenses, then you lose the $500 that you did not spend for that year. Most people who have lupus, however, can calculate a minimum amount of money that they spend every year for medical expenses. If you generally pay $2,000 a year or more for your healthcare (medical, dental, eyes, and over-the-counter medications) and you put $2,000 a year into an FSA it can be a very good bargain. For example, if you are in a 30% income tax bracket, it is like having a coupon for 30% off. If you use up all $2,000 that year, it is like having an extra $600 in your pocket to pay for whatever you like, instead of that $600 going to the Internal Revenue Service as income tax. Some FSA plans require you to fill out paperwork for each medical cost (providing adequate proof such as receipts and doctor prescriptions). Other plans use an FSA debit card, similar to a bank account debit card, which withdraws the money from your account for your medical services.

## Premiums

A healthcare insurance premium is the amount of money that you must pay (usually monthly) for your insurance. Be careful when choosing a healthcare plan. Often, a cheaper plan with lower premiums may not actually be the cheapest. This can be apparent after you factor in your out-of-pocket costs for the medications, doctor co-pays, hospitalization costs, and the hassles you may have to go through to get referrals and pre-authorizations for various aspects of your healthcare. Putting in that extra time to research these issues before deciding can make a big difference for you in the end.

## Deductibles

A deductible is the amount of money you must pay before your insurance starts to pay for something. For example, if your deductible for the year is $500 for healthcare costs (such as your x-rays, labs, doctor visits) before your insurance kicks in, then you have to pay $500 yourself out of pocket to the provider of service (such as the doctor, hospital, x-ray office, laboratory, etc.) before your insurance begins to pay. Many people who have SLE find that they end up paying their full deductible every year. Healthcare costs for the rest of the year are usually markedly cheaper after the person reaches the deductible amount. After that happens, then it is often to your advantage to get the tests done that you need (such as your Plaquenil eye exam, x-rays, mammogram, etc.). If you have some tests that are due in January, try to see if you can schedule them in December instead. They will likely be cheaper compared to waiting until January when you have to pay it yourself since the deductible starts all over again.

## Annual Out-of-Pocket Maximum Payments

Some people are fortunate to have a maximum annual out-of-pocket expense clause with their insurance. This can be a godsend for catastrophic health problems. For example, if you are unfortunate and have a year requiring numerous specialist visits, numerous tests, medicines, hospitalizations, or an unexpected surgery, if you have this clause as part of your insurance, you may get to a point where all of your medical care is taken care of after a certain dollar amount. If this happens, take advantage of it. In

December, try to do as much as you can that you would normally do the following January (doctor visits, fill medications, get tests done, etc.).

## Pre-Certification for Medications and Procedures

"Pre-certifications" also go by the terms "pre-authorizations," "pre-auths," and "prior authorizations" depending on the health plan. Unfortunately, this is a fact of life for today's medical care. A pre-certification is a process where your doctor has to fill out paperwork to prove to your insurance company that a particular medication or procedure is required before your insurance will pay for it. This is one reason why some doctors are actually refusing to participate in any insurance plans at all, as it often requires hiring extra staff just simply to handle all of the pre-certification paperwork.

Every doctor's office will handle "pre-auths" (short for pre-authorizations) differently. In my office, we have people whose sole jobs are to do pre-auths. I ask that patients call us up immediately if they require a pre-auth for a medicine or x-ray and tell them to ask to speak to the person who handles pre-auths so that we can do it as expeditiously as possible. Doing pre-auths can be quite a complex process; it is important to remember that the whole reason your insurance company is requiring it is that it does not want to pay the money for whatever it is that you need. Due to the complexity of the process and its not wanting to pay for it, it is not uncommon for pre-auths to be tied up somewhere in the system. It is virtually impossible for the doctor's office to keep track of pre-auths after they are submitted to the insurance company. Whenever you ask for a pre-auth, call your pharmacy or x-ray office a couple of days later to see if the pre-auth went through. If not, call the doctor's office and talk to the pre-auth person again; kindly ask her or him to look into it for you. Keep doing this (follow through with the pre-auth person) until the process is complete. Also, always be very nice to the person who does pre-auths. It can be a very stressful job dealing with all of the paperwork, insurance companies, pharmacies, x-ray offices, and patients (some of whom can be impatient and release their frustrations on the poor pre-auth staff person).

## COBRA

COBRA stands for Consolidated OmniBus Reconciliation Act. This law allows people to keep their health insurance when they lose their jobs. It applies to companies that have twenty or more employees and usually lasts for eighteen months. One of the worst things that can happen to people who have SLE is to lose their insurance, so keeping good health insurance should always be a priority. If you become one of the many unfortunate Americans who end up losing their jobs, make sure to apply for COBRA as soon as you can to keep your insurance while you look for a new job. You will get the same group rate that your employer was paying along with an additional administrative fee. Paying for your own insurance can be quite costly, but being without it and potentially dealing with significant healthcare costs if your lupus flares could be more costly.

Do your best not to be without any insurance for more than any sixty-three-day period. HIPAA (Health Insurance Portability and Accountability Act) is a law that protects people with pre-existing conditions from being denied insurance. As long as you do not go for more than sixty-three days without health insurance, you cannot be discriminated against for health insurance due to having a pre-existing condition such as lupus. Be very careful with this rule, though. Never try to cut it close to the sixty-three-day mark. Never assume that when you get a new job that you will get health insurance quickly. Plan on keeping your insurance with COBRA until you know for sure that your new healthcare plan has started. If you cannot afford COBRA, at least get some inexpensive private healthcare insurance. It may not be very good or come close to the quality of healthcare insurance that you had with your previous job, but any insurance at all is better than having none.

### KEY POINTS TO REMEMBER

1. People who have SLE need to do everything they can to get the best healthcare insurance possible.

2. If you have the luxury of being able to choose between different healthcare plans, do not automatically choose the least expensive plan. What appears to be cheaper may actually cost you more in the long run with higher doctor co-pays, more expensive medicine co-pays, more restrictive medication formularies, and the headaches that can come with keeping up with referrals to see specialists.

3. If you are having difficulty affording your healthcare or do not have insurance, use the strategies under the heading "What to Do If You Are Uninsured, Underinsured, or Cannot Afford Your Health Care."

4. If you lose your job and are disabled due to your SLE, apply for Social Security Disability immediately as discussed in chapter 43 and get help from a lawyer who specializes in Social Security.

5. If you have private short-term or long-term disability insurance, apply for disability immediately as well. You can take advantage of both your private insurance and Social Security at the same time.

6. If you lose your job and are at risk of losing your health insurance, do everything you can to keep some sort of insurance plan (COBRA or a private insurance plan). Do not go longer than sixty-three days without insurance. Otherwise, you run the risk of being denied insurance in the future due to having a pre-existing condition (lupus).

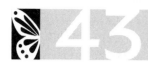

# Working and Dealing with Disability

## Lupus, Working, and Disability

LC has had SLE for many years. Her biggest problems are severe arthritis of the wrists and fibromyalgia, which cause her to have severe pain in her muscles and joints as well as profound fatigue and depression. LC is a model patient. She keeps all of her appointments, she takes her medications as prescribed, she does her exercises as prescribed, and she does not smoke cigarettes. However, she is one of a small percentage of patients where none of the medications has been able to prevent her lupus arthritis from getting worse. She has literally been on everything, and still she has severe inflammation of the wrists, which has caused her to lose most of the use of her wrists as well as causing daily severe pain. It is amazing how perseverant she is. Even though she has such severe disease, she has insisted on continuing to work throughout the entire ordeal. She is like many of my SLE patients. They constantly amaze me at how resilient they can be through all of their hardships. It would have been so easy for her to have received disability a long time ago, but she had refused to do so even with her doctors recommending it to her. At some point, though, I think she will need to apply for disability.

Although people who have chronic diseases should work as long as they can to have better incomes and to keep better insurance, there comes a point where the job itself can become detrimental to the disease. LC has a job that requires repetitive activities with her hands and involves lifting packages; her job will most likely worsen her arthritis unless she stops working.

Choosing to apply for disability can be a very stressful decision process. If you are not prepared for the application process, you have a high chance of failing to get disability benefits the first time around, being forced to go through an appeals process. Nationwide, only about one-third of initial applications for Social Security Disability are approved. This chapter gives you the tools to navigate the system and have a better chance of getting what you deserve. If you read and do everything in this chapter, you will greatly increase the chances of getting disability. Even if you are not planning on going on disability, this chapter contains some important information on how to maximize the quality of your medical records so that if you ever do decide to apply for disability, it will be a smoother process for you. This chapter is dedicated to LC and my other wonderful patients who have been so strong yet ended up facing the realities of disability.

## Chronic Disease and the Workplace

Continuing to work and deal with a chronic disorder such as lupus can become very difficult. In addition to the usual stress of working you are also dealing with doctors' appointments, taking medications, using your sunscreen regularly, avoiding cold temperatures that could upset Raynaud's phenomenon, avoiding ultraviolet light exposure, minimizing your stress level, eating a proper diet and exercising, while scheduling in that much needed eight hours of sleep every night. You must make your health a priority because if your lupus gets worse, it could potentially cause you not to be able to work, which can lead to the loss of income and the loss of good healthcare. You can work with your employer to improve your work environment.

### Americans with Disabilities Act

The Americans with Disabilities Act is a federal law that prohibits employers from discriminating against people who have disabilities. It is intended to help people who want to continue working but who may have some difficulties in the workplace because of a disability or illness. It also requires employers to make "reasonable accommodations" for people who have disabilities unless those accommodations would cause "undue hardship." Some examples of types of requests that can be made of your employer are listed in table 43.1. A doctor's note saying that it is medically necessary for your medical condition often suffices for these recommendations. It may be helpful for you to ask your doctor to refer you to an occupational therapist (OT). An OT can assess your working situation and determine what changes or aids are appropriate to request for the workplace as well as determine if they fall under the entitlements of the Americans with Disabilities Act. Having formal recommendations from an occupational therapist can greatly increase the strength of your requests.

The language used in the act itself can be problematic. How do you exactly define "reasonable accommodations" and "undue hardship"? There certainly is a point where requests to an employer go beyond what is reasonable to expect, and many court cases have tried to answer those questions. You can get more information and recommendations on how the Americans with Disabilities Act may apply to you and for advice on how you can work with your employer by contacting the Job Accommodation Network (www.askjan.org), the Patient Advocate Foundation (www.patientadvocate.org), Hire Disability Solutions (www.hireds.com), and Disability.gov (www.disability.gov).

### Choosing the Right Job

Having the right employer can make all the difference in the world as far as your ability to continue to work and deal with SLE. I have seen some patients who had severe SLE who had wonderful, understanding employers and supervisors who did everything they could to ensure that they could continue working. I have also seen others who had much milder SLE who found the workplace intolerable. Employing assistance using the ADA as well as other protections such as the Federal and Medical Leave Act (FMLA), described below, can help make working in a tough environment easier. However, sometimes many things are out of your control. Sometimes it is better to try to find a different position or workplace instead of trying to deal with an unwilling employer who makes working too stressful.

**Table 43.1** Potential Requests of Employers to Ensure a Better Work Environment

Cognitive Impairment:
- Ask for written job instructions when possible instead of verbal ones.
- Ask that your job assignments be prioritized.
- Ask for flexible work hours.
- Allow periodic rest periods to reorient.
- Ask for memory aids such as schedulers or organizers.
- Minimize distractions.
- Allow for a self-paced workload.
- Reduce job stress.
- Provide more structure.

Fatigue/Weakness:
- Reduce or eliminate physical exertion and workplace stress.
- Schedule periodic rest breaks from the workstation.
- Allow a flexible work schedule and use of leave time.
- Allow work from home (telecommuting).
- Implement ergonomic workstation design.
- Provide a scooter or other mobility aid if demanded to travel long distances.

Motor Impairments:
- Use an ergonomic workstation design.
- Provide alternative computer and telephone access.
- Provide arm supports.
- Provide writing and grip aids.
- Provide a page-turner and a book holder.
- Provide a note taker.
- Modify the worksite to make it accessible.
- Provide parking close to the worksite (make sure that you yourself have handicapped tags from your local department of motor vehicles to assist in getting this privilege).
- Provide an accessible entrance.
- Install automatic door openers.
- Provide an accessible restroom and break room.
- Provide an accessible route of travel to other work areas used by the employee.
- Adjust desk height for wheelchair or scooter if used.
- Make sure materials and equipment are within range.
- Move workstation close to other work areas, office equipment, and break rooms.

Photosensitivity (applies to everyone with lupus):
- Minimize outdoor activities between 10:00 AM and 4:00 PM.
- Avoid reflective surfaces outside such as sand, snow, and concrete.
- Provide clothing to block UV rays if required to be outdoors.

- Provide "waterproof" sun-protective agents such as sunblocks and sunscreens.
- Install low-wattage overhead lights (non-fluorescent and non-halogen if possible).
- Install adjustable window blinds and UV light filters.

Breathing Difficulties:
- Provide adequate ventilation.
- Keep work environment free from dust, smoke, odor, and fumes.
- Implement a "fragrance-free" workplace policy and a "smoke-free" building policy.
- Avoid temperature extremes.
- Allow fan-air-conditioner or heater at workstation.
- Redirect air conditioning and heating vents.
- Provide adequate exhaust systems to remove fumes from office machines.
- Allow individual to wear a respirator mask.
- Allow work from home.

Raynaud's Phenomenon:
- Modify worksite temperature.
- Modify dress code (allowing layers of clothes, long sleeves, hat while inside).
- Allow heater at workstation.
- Allow work from home during cold weather.
- Redirect air-conditioning vents.
- Provide an office with separate temperature control.

---

Portions of this list come from the Job Accommodation Network.

In addition, it is very important to look at the benefits of a job. Good health insurance is critical when you are dealing with such a complex disorder as lupus. Planning ahead of time for adequate retirement benefits is also paramount as you never know what the future will hold, and you should think well ahead of time about the importance of saving up for retirement and having a job that has a good retirement plan. Sometimes it is much smarter to choose a job with great benefits compared to a job that pays more but that has worse benefits. Along these same lines, it is probably better to choose a workplace that offers less stress and hourly demands compared to a high-stress job that pays a lot more.

Many businesses and jobs offer their employees ongoing, additional job training. It is often best to take advantage of these offers as much as possible. The more workplace skills you develop, the more open doors and flexibility you have in the job market. If you get to a place where you need to consider getting a less strenuous or stressful job, having these extra skills can make all the difference in finding the right job.

Of course, it is not easy to leave a job at any time and find a job suitable for a particular medical condition. Not everyone has the luxury of having the perfect job with the perfect employer with the perfect supervisor. There are other things that you should do to help your situation if you are not able to change jobs. Of course, your medical condition does not need to be made public to anyone. However, if you feel that it is in your best interest to educate your supervisor and co-workers, you can give them educational pamphlets to learn more about your situation. However, be careful about doing this. Most people are too busy to spend a lot of time reading about something that does not pertain to them. It is probably better to do this in small steps, such as providing a short, easy-to-read pamphlet from your doctor's office. Keep in mind that you cannot force people to learn about something that they do not want to learn. These issues are even more difficult with a disorder such as lupus where most people do not have outward signs of being ill. The person can appear to be perfectly normal, and it can be all too easy for other people to think that the person is exaggerating her or his problems. This "invisibility" aspect of lupus is another reason it may be a good idea to attempt to educate your supervisor, or at least protect yourself through measures such as the FMLA, discussed below.

Be realistic about your limitations. Do not accept work activities that are not required if there is a chance that you may not be able to follow through due to fatigue, pain, or difficulty thinking. A supervisor is much more apt to remember when you did not get something done that you volunteered to do compared to a time when you "saved the day." Also, try to keep in mind what your supervisor's goals are when you are doing your work. If you do your job with those goals in mind, then you are more apt to make your supervisor happy. In fact, if you come up with doable ways to achieve those goals, then it makes you an even more valuable employee.

### Federal and Medical Leave Act (FMLA)

The Federal and Medical Leave Act (FMLA) is a law designed to allow employees the ability to juggle their work and family responsibilities by permitting them to take up to twelve weeks of unpaid leave per year for various reasons, including medical leave "because of a serious health issue." FMLA applies to all public agencies, all public and private elementary and secondary schools, and companies with fifty or more employees. You must have worked for your employer at least 1,250 hours during the previous 12 months to qualify. Having SLE, taking your medications to treat it, and having to see your doctor regularly satisfies the medical criteria for being eligible for FMLA. To protect themselves, people who have SLE should have their doctors fill out FMLA paperwork. This can cover their required absences from work for when they must see their doctors and fulfill other requirements for their healthcare. If you become ill from lupus and require additional time off, then this would need to be added to your FMLA paperwork. FMLA paperwork can usually be obtained from your employer's personnel department. You can learn more about FMLA from the Department of Labor at www.dol.gov.

### Disability

The decision to go on disability is one of the hardest decisions that there is. In my experience, people who have SLE tend to be some of the hardest-working people there are. I am frequently impressed with the drive to continue to work in some patients who clearly should consider disability. While the vast majority of people who have SLE are under excellent control and doing well on their medications, some patients unfortunately have severe enough problems from their lupus that they are unable to do their jobs anymore. Considering the possibility of applying for disability is a complex, long, and often painful process. People who have to stop working due to the severity of their lupus face many obstacles. Although the difficulties and stresses that their jobs caused may be gone, these are replaced with a different set of problems (table 43.2).

These problems include the loss of income. People who stop working and end up relying on disability checks usually end up making much less money than while they were working. In addition to worrying about and caring for their medical health, they are also faced with the difficulties of how to make ends meet financially and have to learn how to live a more frugal lifestyle. The amount of money that people get from disability is usually barely enough to survive on at all. The amount of money you get from Social Security Disability is determined by your average lifetime income. In 2011, it ranged from a low of $500 per month up to a maximum of $1,800 per month for an individual. Many people face the extra burden of downsizing simply to survive. They may end up having to sell their homes and move into much smaller places in less desirable areas. They may have to sell their vehicles and rely on others for transportation. The required changes can be devastating.

How we feel about ourselves (called self-esteem) often depends a lot on our work. Although most of us have stressful jobs, and we may complain a lot about our work, most people spend more time working than on any other activity in their lives. According to the Bureau of Labor Statistics, Americans spend an average of 8.7 hours per day of their working lives performing their work and doing work-related activities and 7.7 hours sleeping; the rest of the time is divided up into everything else they do in life. We spend more time around those we work with than we do with our closest loved ones. It is not surprising that when that environment is removed, it creates a huge vacuum. Even if people have jobs that they consciously think are unimportant, mundane, and stressful, every job is important. While working, we are contributing to society, which adds to our self-esteem. When that is taken away, if it is not replaced with other important activities, it can quickly cause problems related to self-esteem issues, including depression and feelings of isolation.

Some people who become disabled state that they seem to be treated differently by friends and family. Whether this is simply a self-perception or a reality varies from person to person. However, due to this possibility along with the loss of finances and the loss of self-esteem, people who have disabilities often find that their circle of friends

**Table 43.2** Difficulties Facing People Who Must Go on Disability

- Loss of income
- Lowered self-esteem
- Isolation; less contact with friends and family
- Loss of good-quality health insurance

changes or disappears. They may also not see family as frequently either. A problem of isolation may set in.

A huge potential problem for the disabled is the loss of insurance. As I have stressed numerous times in this book, the number one cause of not doing well with SLE is not being compliant with all aspects of treatment, including taking the medications, using sunscreen daily, not smoking, seeing doctors regularly, and getting the appropriate medical tests done as directed. Although the quality of health insurance varies a lot from job to job, it is usually better than what can be afforded when you go on disability. When you are disabled, you must wait twenty-five months before you can even get Medicare—that is potentially more than two years of not having any healthcare insurance at all. For someone who has severe enough lupus to go on disability, this could potentially be catastrophic. If someone gets Medicaid, the medical care available is usually inferior to that available to the person who has good insurance. The reason I am pointing out these downsides of disability is that it is very important that you consider all the potential ramifications of going on disability.

When you become disabled and are unable to work, it is essential that you apply for disability as soon as possible. The process can take a long time, and it is in your best interest to do so immediately. If you need to apply for disability, then please read and follow the instructions in the remainder of this chapter very carefully to increase your chances of getting the disability you deserve. However, if there is any chance that you can keep working, then do everything you can to do so, especially if you have good health insurance with your job.

Even if you find that you cannot adequately perform the job that you are currently doing, it is better to try to find a job that you are able to do. For example, consider the possibilities of getting a job with less stress and less physically demanding work. There are even companies that offer healthcare insurance to people who work part-time. Working part-time in a job with good health insurance can be a lot better than relying on a very small amount of disability income with inferior health benefits. Some companies that offer health insurance to part-time employees as of 2013 are listed in table 43.3. Other part-time jobs such as working as a teacher's aide may also offer good benefits such as healthcare insurance in some areas. Recall from chapter 42: it is extremely important that you make sure there is not a time lapse between insurances to avoid being denied insurance due to your pre-existing condition of lupus. However, this problem will become moot in 2014 when the new health care laws go into effect on pre-existing conditions in adults.

## Private Disability Insurance

If you have private disability insurance or have it available through your workplace, it is very important that you apply for this in addition to Social Security Disability. Every private disability insurance plan is different when it comes to the definition of disability and the process for getting the disability. However, in general, the requirements for disability tend to be more difficult with Social Security than for private disability in many cases. Therefore, if you follow all of the steps for Social Security Disability outlined below, it should make it easier for you to qualify for your private disability.

**Table 43.3** Companies That Offer Health Insurance to Part-Time Employees

| | |
|---|---|
| - 5/3 Bank (Fifth Third Bank) | - Macy's |
| - Aerotek | - Nike |
| - Barnes & Noble | - Nordstrom |
| - Caribou Coffee | - Publix |
| - Cost Plus World Market | - REI |
| - Costco | - Safeway |
| - DHL | - Sam's Club |
| - FedEx | - Staples |
| - The Fresh Market | - Starbucks |
| - Home Depot | - Target |
| - JCPenney | - Trader Joe's |
| - JP Morgan Chase | - U-Haul |
| - Kaplan | - UPS |
| - Kroger | - WalMart |
| - Lands' End | - Wegman's |
| - Lowes | - Whole Foods |

## Social Security Disability

Understanding how the Social Security Disability process works can make it easier to fulfill all the requirements of applying for disability and help you determine whether it is a possibility for you to get Social Security Disability. Although this is a federally funded program, the decision as to whether you are disabled is made at a state-level Disability Determination Service and through your local Social Security office; however, all states must go by the same federal rules and guidelines in making these decisions.

The very first step in applying for disability is to obtain an "Adult Disability Starter Kit" from Social Security. You can get one by calling Social Security at 1-800-772-1213 or online at www.ssa.gov/disability/disability_starter_kits.htm. You can fill out the information yourself at home on paper or fill them out online. An advantage of doing it at home is that you can complete the paperwork at your own pace. However, it can be more advantageous to begin this process by making an appointment with a claims representative at your local Social Security office. The representative can then notice if you have difficulties such as walking, thinking, or using your hands; he or she can also make sure that you fill out all the forms correctly. Just make sure to go in prepared with all of the information listed in table 43.4. After you apply for your Social Security Disability, the next step is for the claims representative to determine if you meet certain administrative requirements or not. These administrative requirements look at your work history and your financial eligibility, and confirm that you are a U.S. citizen. The first step is making sure that you meet these administrative eligibility requirements.

**Table 43.4** Documents Required When Applying for Social Security Disability

- Social Security number (yours and your dependents')
- Proof of age such as birth certificate (for you and your dependents)
- Names, addresses, phone numbers of all doctors, hospitals, clinics, physical therapists, psychologists, social workers, chiropractors, and any other medical professionals you have seen
- All copies of medical records that you have collected
- A list of every place you have worked and description of that work during the fifteen years before the date your disability started
- A copy of your past year's W-2 forms or your last federal income tax form
- All dates of military service
- Information about any other disability payments you are receiving or that you are applying for
- If your spouse is applying as a dependent, the dates of any prior marriages (certified copy of divorce papers)
- If you are applying as a disabled widow or widower, your dead spouse's Social Security number and a copy of the death certificate
- If you are applying as a disabled surviving divorced husband or wife and were married for at least ten years, certified copies of your marriage and divorce papers

As soon as it is determined that you do, the claim's representative sends your application to the disability examiner. This is a state employee (who may be hundreds of miles away from your location) who actually makes the medical decision as to whether you are medically disabled or not. The disability examiner will review your application and then send out requests for your medical records to the doctors and hospitals that you listed on your application to help make the determination for disability. The disability examiner will probably send you more questionnaires to fill out as well. These additional questionnaires vary from case to case. For someone who has SLE, they may include things such as forms to assess Activities of Daily Living, Exertional Daily Activities, fatigue, and pain. Filling out these forms completely and honestly and sending them back in as soon as possible is extremely important for your application process. The disability examiner may also request records from other sources such as employers, psychologists, physical therapists, and chiropractors.

After receiving all of this information, the disability examiner will summarize these findings and give them to the medical consultant. The medical consultant can be a medical doctor (MD or DO) or a licensed clinical psychologist (PhD or PsyD). The medical consultant will review all of the information as well as the disability examiner's summary and recommendations to determine whether you have physical and/or medical limitations in working. The medical consultant will then give this assessment back to the disability examiner who will then determine whether you are able to do any job based on this determination.

The entire process takes an average of sixty days. In clear-cut cases of disability, it may take just a few days, while in others it may take many months. How complex your case is, how thorough your doctor's evaluations are, and how quickly each source sends back the requested materials determines how quickly a decision can be made. There is a high fail rate for acceptance of Social Security Disability. In 2012, the application success rate for first-time applicants nationwide was only 35%, but it varies a lot from state to state. The lowest success rate in 2008 was in Mississippi, with only 24.5% being determined as disabled, while 52.6% of Hawaiian residents met disability requirements. After a denial for disability, most people go through an appeals process for reconsideration of disability status. These numbers are even lower, with only 13.8% of people nationwide getting disability on appeals. The lowest rates of 6.8% and 6.9% were in Indiana and Mississippi, respectively, while New Yorkers led the pack on appeals with a whopping 51.2% success rate.

In my experience, people who have SLE who are truly disabled usually get disability the first time around; however, this takes a lot of work on the patient's and doctor's parts. For example, you can clearly be disabled from your lupus, but if your doctor does not keep very good notes in your chart on your condition, you may not have a sound enough case to convince Social Security of your disability. The following section goes into detail about some important strategies you can take to ensure that you end up having a strong case to support your disability application. In addition to understanding the process of applying for Social Security Disability (outlined above), it is also important to understand what the definition of disability is, how the medical decision for disability is made, and what role your physician has in the process.

*Requirements and Definition of Social Security Disability.* Determining disability through Social Security generally follows a series of steps, beginning at step 1 and proceeding to the last step. You must meet the requirement of an earlier step before proceeding to the next step. If your application claim does not meet the requirements of step 1, 2, or 3, then your claim does not go any farther in the process and it is denied. It is also possible (and should occur for people who are disabled from SLE) to be approved at step 4 and not have to go any farther in the process.

1. *You must have enough work credits.* This is a very important administrative decision made by the claims representative soon after you submit your claims application at your local Social Security office. Throughout life, people get "work credits" through the Social Security system. The amount of work credits that people get are based on income and numbers of hours worked. The amount of work credits required to get Social Security disability varies by age with less required in the very young (such as those less than 24 years old), while those who are 62 years old or older require the most. Most people who work full-time will get four work credits per year of working. Only six work credits are required if you are less than 24 years old, while 40 credits are required if you are 62 years old or older. You also must have had at least 20 credits earned in the 10 years before you became disabled. You can think of this requirement as having had worked full-time and paid FICA (Federal Insurance Contributions Act) taxes for five of the previous ten years before your disability. (FICA taxes are the taxes taken out of your paycheck for Social Security and Medicare.) However, if you are 31 years old or younger, the work credit requirements are less due to it being more difficult in building up work

credits at such a young age. There are exceptions to these rules, including the blind, widows, and widowers, which is beyond the scope of this book.

2. *You cannot be working a substantial, gainful job.* If you are working a "substantial, gainful" job, then the Social Security Administration assumes that you are not disabled. As of 2011, if your income is an average of $1,000 or more per month, then you are usually considered as having "substantial, gainful" employment. Some benefits with a job may be counted toward this $1,000 a month. This includes things such as health insurance, dental insurance, and employee benefits plans. The very day that you stop working "substantial, gainful" work is the day that you can begin to file for Social Security Disability. However, if you start working again, then you cannot be considered disabled.

3. *Your physical and/or mental condition must be severe.* This does not mean that the disease is potentially a severe disease. It means that it is severe in your case. For example, although SLE can potentially be a severe disease, the vast majority of people who have SLE are not considered disabled. I have met a few people who assumed that since they have a diagnosis of SLE, they should automatically get disability. This is incorrect. Your condition must prevent you from being able to work at all, and your doctor must classify your SLE as severe before your lupus is considered a disabling disorder. The definition of severe, of course, is very subjective, but it can be considered to mean that your condition is substantial enough to prevent you from working.

4. *You must have a physical and/or mental disability that will last or has lasted at least one year or is expected to result in death.* This decision is the one made by the disability examiner using the information from your treating physician. People who have SLE are at an advantage when it comes to applying for Social Security Disability because systemic lupus is one of the recognized "listed conditions" by Social Security. You can see the list at www.socialsecurity.gov/disability/professionals/bluebook/14.00 -Immune-Adult.htm#14_02. The actual listing of SLE by the Social Security Administration is as follows:

**Systemic lupus erythematosus (14.02).**

**a. General.** Systemic lupus erythematosus (SLE) is a chronic inflammatory disease that can affect any organ or body system. It is frequently, but not always, accompanied by constitutional symptoms or signs (severe fatigue, fever, malaise, involuntary weight loss). Major organ or body system involvement can include: Respiratory (pleuritis, pneumonitis), cardiovascular (endocarditis, myocarditis, pericarditis, vasculitis), renal (glomerulonephritis), hematologic (anemia, leukopenia, thrombocytopenia), skin (photosensitivity), neurologic (seizures), mental (anxiety, fluctuating cognition ["lupus fog"], mood disorders, organic brain syndrome, and psychosis), or immune system disorders (inflammatory arthritis). Immunologically, there is an array of circulating serum auto-antibodies and pro- and anti-coagulant proteins that may occur in a highly variable pattern.

**b. Documentation of SLE.** Generally, but not always, the medical evidence will show that your SLE satisfies the criteria in the current "Criteria for the Classification of Systemic Lupus Erythematosus" by the American College of Rheumatology found in the most recent edition of the Primer on the Rheumatic Diseases published by the Arthritis Foundation.

Before being determined as disabled, the person who has SLE must have at least two out of the following symptoms: severe fatigue, fever, malaise, or involuntary weight loss. In addition to this, there must be at least two organ systems involved, with at least one of them to a moderate severity, or the person must have severe limitations in daily activities, social functioning, or in "completing tasks in a timely manner due to deficiencies in concentration, persistence, or pace."

The advantage of having an illness on this list is that it can potentially satisfy the requirements of disability without any further steps. However, this requirement hinges completely on how well your doctor (rheumatologist) has documented how your lupus was diagnosed, how severe your condition is, and what difficulties it causes you. As of the writing of this book, the Social Security Administration suggests that SLE be diagnosed using the older American College of Rheumatology's classification criteria for SLE (as opposed to the criteria presented in chapter 1). This set of criteria can be found at www.rheumatology.org/practice/clinical/classification/SLE/1997_update_of_the_1982_acr_revised_criteria_for_classification_of_sle.pdf. If you satisfy the first three disability requirements, and your doctor has documented your diagnosis of SLE using these criteria in his or her medical notes as well as the severity of your lupus, then you may be qualified for Social Security Disability without going through the following steps. That is one reason why it is so important that you ask your doctor to make sure that this is done in the notes (as recommended in the following sections of this chapter).

5. *You must be unable to do work you did during the previous fifteen years.* If the disability examiner considers that you do have some medical and/or mental impairments, but you do not automatically qualify for one of the listed medical requirements in step 4 above, additional steps are required. The disability examiner will list your impairments (i.e., what you can and cannot do) and give them back to the claims representative at the local Social Security office to determine if there are any jobs that you are physically and mentally able to perform with these impairments. On your application claim, you must list every single job you have had in the previous fifteen years. If you can do any of those jobs with your medical condition impairments, then you will most likely not be qualified for Social Security Disability. This can be very difficult for people to accept. If you recently had a high-paying job that you can no longer do, but in the past you had a sedentary low-paying job, you may be ineligible for disability since you can do the latter job with your lupus.

6. *You must be unable to do any work in the American economy.* If you are unable to do jobs that you previously had done within the previous fifteen years, the claims representative will then review the job demands of occupations determined by the Department of Labor using the list of your impairments provided by the disability examiner. The claims representative will also keep in mind your age, education, past work experience, and what your potential is as far as being able to learn a new vocation. For example, if you have been a carpenter for fifteen years and now, have back problems, you could be trained to work on an assembly line (while seated) and not be considered

disabled. If you are a physician and have severe SLE rendering you unable to take care of patients, yet you are able to do consultant work for $1,200 a month (compared to your previous $8,000 a month), you would be ineligible for Social Security Disability. The drastic reduction in pay would make no difference in this determination.

*How to Increase Your Chances of Getting Social Security Disability.* There are things that you can do to ensure the best possibility of having your Social Security Disability claim accepted the first time around. If you do the things that I suggest here and you satisfy the requirements of disability as outlined in the previous section, you will greatly increase your chances of getting disability.

1. *Consider getting another job first.* If you are unable to do your job due to your SLE, consider the option of changing jobs. A job that pays less or even a part-time job that has good healthcare benefits can often be better than disability. Remember that Social Security Disability barely pays enough money to get by on at all. In addition, medical health benefits do not kick in until the twenty-fifth month after your disability begins. Few people who have SLE can afford to be without healthcare for two years. Table 43.3 lists employers who provide health insurance to part-time employees. Of course, if working in a different job is not an option for you, then proceed ASAP with the disability application process. If you are not sure which you can do (work a lower-paying or part-time job versus going on disability), work on doing both at the same time. If you find an adequate job with good healthcare benefits, you can always stop the disability application process.

2. *Apply early.* As soon as you are unable to work "substantial, gainful" employment, as discussed in step 2 above, and you are expected not to be able to work for the next year due to your lupus, then you should apply immediately. If you are found disabled by Social Security, you will not be paid any disability benefits until you have been disabled for six full months beginning the first full month after you became disabled. It can take a few months (average of two to six months) for the disability process to be completed and that time can become incredibly stressful due to the loss of income. The faster you apply, the quicker you can get your disability and begin to receive your benefit payments.

3. *Apply for private disability insurance as well.* You are permitted to collect both private disability insurance and Social Security Disability. Make sure to check with your recent employer to see if you are eligible to apply for disability through your workplace.

4. *Hire a lawyer who specializes in Social Security Disability right away.* It can greatly increase your chances for having a successful outcome. The fees for the lawyer are the same everywhere since the government sets these rates. The lawyer would get 25% of your back benefits or $6,000 (whichever is less). You would not be required to pay any of your future benefits. You can find names of Social Security lawyers at www.NOSSCR .org, which is the website for the National Organization of Social Security Claimants' Representatives.

5. *Gather all necessary documents as soon as possible.* These are listed in table 43.4.

6. *See your doctor regularly.* You must have a diagnosis of SLE by a medical doctor documented in your medical records. It is also assumed that if you are sick enough to get disability, then you should be seeing a doctor regularly. If you are not seeing a doctor regularly, then the severity of your disease is in question. Prepare ahead of time for your disability. Ask your doctor to make a notation in your progress note (the written note that the doctor makes of each visit in your medical record at the doctor's office) of *your physical and mental limitations.* For example, if you are having difficulty in doing any tasks such as working, dressing, or doing household chores, make sure to ask that they are included in the note. However, do not overwhelm your doctor with these things all at once as he or she will be more interested in focusing on your medical care instead of satisfying disability requirements.

As soon as your medical condition has reached the point that it interferes with your ability to work, there are things that your doctor can include in your progress notes that can greatly increase the chances of your having your disability claim approved. Ask your doctor to include a statement in the progress note that *your SLE is severe enough to interfere with your ability to work and that this difficulty is expected to last for at least a year.* Ask that it be noted on each progress note after that as well. In addition, ask your doctor to *state how your diagnosis of SLE was made in each note.* Most rheumatologists tend to write just "SLE" as the diagnosis on a note, but that notation can be insufficient for Social Security Disability. You want it to state how the diagnosis of SLE meets the diagnostic criteria for SLE. Ask how your doctor diagnosed your SLE. If it is because you have had a butterfly rash, arthritis, a positive ANA, and a positive Smith antibody, then instead of just putting "SLE" in the note as your diagnosis, your doctor should state "SLE manifested by butterfly rash, arthritis, positive ANA, and positive Smith antibody." If these things (physical and mental *limitations*, SLE is "*severe,*" the condition will *last at least a year*, and how your SLE was *diagnosed*) are done for each note from here on out, you greatly increase your chances of satisfying step 4 of the disability process, which can expedite approval of your disability claim.

Your doctor's notes and opinions (based on the medical facts) are the heart of a medical disability claim. However, do not ask your doctor if you are disabled. Your doctor actually has no say as to whether you are disabled or not. Your doctor's responsibility is to state your medical diagnosis, prove how your SLE was diagnosed, and state what functional limitations your medical condition causes inside and outside of the workplace. Social Security determines whether you are disabled using this information.

7. *If you cannot afford to see a doctor, go to a free clinic regularly.* Unfortunately, Social Security does not care if you have insurance or cannot afford to see a doctor regularly on your own. It needs to confirm that SLE is your diagnosis, and that you have significant functional limitations documented by a medical doctor. If you cannot afford to see a doctor, go to a free clinic regularly to get basic care. Make sure to remind the clinic doctor to list SLE as a diagnosis (how it was diagnosed), and keep copies of your labs and notes from the free clinic as well for your own personal records. Ask the doctor at the free medical clinic to include in your notes the same items discussed in point 6 above (your functional limitations that will last at least a year due to severe SLE and how your SLE was diagnosed). Remember that very few doctors know Social Security Disability requirements, so it can be very helpful for you to make this request specifically.

8. *If you have significant depression, anxiety, or other mental health problems, make sure you see a psychiatrist regularly.* A large number of people who have SLE have mental disorders such as depression and anxiety (e.g., panic disorder) that can also limit the amount of work that they can do. If this applies to you, then it is in your best interest to see a psychiatrist regularly. Psychiatrists are the experts when using the medications to treat these disorders, and people who have SLE typically do better if they see a psychiatrist to help with their treatment. In addition, it makes a huge difference in increasing your chances of successfully getting disability.

Be honest with your psychiatrist. I am frequently amazed at how patients will tell me that their psychiatrists told them how well they are doing while they are crying uncontrollably in my exam room due to their depression. I think that this is because they have a longer, more comfortable relationship with me compared to their psychiatrists, or maybe they are afraid of appearing "crazy" to their psychiatrists. One of my SLE patients told me how she stayed in her house for an entire month due to her severe depression, yet when she saw her psychiatrist, she told him that everything was fine. Your psychiatrist cannot help with your medical condition or your disability unless you are completely honest.

Social Security does not accept psychiatric diagnoses (e.g., depression) from your rheumatologist or from your primary care doctor. Social Security will only accept these diagnoses and their associated impairments from a licensed psychiatrist. The best person to come to your defense is a psychiatrist who knows you very well. Otherwise, you will most likely be required to see a psychiatrist chosen by Social Security for an independent examination where there is an increased likelihood of something being missed and potentially not getting approved for disability.

9. *Make a special disability appointment with your doctor.* Social Security requires certain items be commented on specifically for people to be found eligible for Social Security Disability. The vast majority of doctors do not know what these items are because most of them receive no training in disability.

a. Arrange a special visit to your doctor solely for making sure that the proper remarks are placed in your records. Do not expect your doctor to do this during one of your routine medical visits. If your SLE is severe enough to require disability, then your routine visits with your doctor will usually focus on your medical care (history, physical examination, lab results, adjustments to your therapy, etc.). If you try to ask that the visit include a disability evaluation, this will be too much for your doctor to handle and can only result in a less than optimal result. Instead, schedule an extra appointment with your doctor before your scheduled routine appointment. Let your doctor know ahead of time that it is solely for the benefit of applying for disability. Of course, if there is a pressing issue about your health, your doctor will include that at the visit as well, but do not expect non-urgent issues to be addressed.

Go to this visit with a list of what needs to be included in the note for that day (table 43.5). Give your doctor this short list and ask that it be included in the note. Also, make sure to give your doctor a concise, short list of functional limitations to include in the note (the last part in table 43.5). Examples include difficulties with dressing, bathing, doing bills, doing housework, driving, taking public transportation, completing tasks at work promptly, forgetting tasks at work, work tasks caus-

**Table 43.5** What Items Need to Be Added to Your Disability Note by Your Doctor

- Medical history
- Clinical findings (physical exam, mental status exam if psychiatrist note)
- Diagnoses (along with how your SLE meets the American College of Rheumatology's classification criteria)
- Treatments prescribed with responses and prognosis (include previous treatments)
- A statement as to what limitations you have at work and away from work
- A statement saying that the limitations in your ability to work are expected to last a year or longer

ing increased pain, or your depression causing repetitive conflicts with co-workers and supervisors. Make sure to give specific examples, but do not overburden your doctor with multiple pages of examples.

Realize that this is asking for a lot, because it is a lot more to add to the typical progress note usually done at appointments. This is one reason that you should plan to request that only disability be addressed during this visit (including not asking for medication refills or anything else). A typical routine doctor's progress note will not suffice for disability purposes.

In addition, a note from the doctor stating, "Mrs. So-And-So is medically disabled and cannot nor should not work because she has SLE" will not work either. Social Security does not care if your doctor thinks you are disabled or not; it wants to know what your diagnoses are from your doctor, how they were diagnosed, how severe they are, and what functional limitations are based on medical information. The actual decision for disability is up to Social Security.

Certainly, you may very well be strapped for cash during such a difficult time in your life. Social Security will usually pay for a disability examination from your doctor because it saves them the expense of having to schedule and pay for an independent medical examination from another doctor plus it speeds up the process. Make sure to talk to your claims representative and the disability examiner at Social Security to get this approved appointment ahead of time. If either one of them tell you there are insufficient funds, ask to talk to their supervisor to make the request as that person usually has the ability to do so (and press your case that if they do this, it will save them time and money from not having to get an additional independent medical evaluation).

b. In addition to bringing the list of things that you want included in the progress note (table 43.5), make sure to also bring in a blank copy of a Medical Source Statement (MSS) to the disability appointment with your doctor. This is also referred to as a Residual Functional Capacity (RFC) form. This special form lists what you are not able to do because of your SLE. This form is essential (in conjunction with your doctor's disability exam note and medical records) in the disability process. You can download a copy of the form (make sure it is the physical MSS or RFC form instead of the mental health MSS or RFC form) from the Social Security Administration's website, or you can call your Social Security office to get a copy of the form.

Most doctors are not comfortable at filling out this form, by the way, and few of them have received any training at all in how to fill it out appropriately. One way you can help is to fill out a sample form yourself and give it to your doctor. Explain to your doctor that you filled out a form as a suggestion as to how you feel your lupus affects your ability to work and that you are giving it to him or her to potentially help out. In addition, make sure to fill out as much of the blank form as you can (such as your name, address, and personal information), as the less information your doctor has to put on the form, the more willing he or she will be to fill it out. If your doctor's office requires that a fee be paid for filling out forms, volunteer to do this yourself. Doctors are being asked to fill out more nonmedical paperwork every year. Therefore, most doctors now charge their patients a fee to fill out these forms since they are not covered by insurance. These forms place additional burdens on the doctor. If you fill out all your personal information yourself on the form, give a copy of a form that you fill out as an example, and pay the form fee upfront, you will have a much better chance of your doctor expediting and completing the process to your benefit.

Do not exaggerate when you fill out your copy of the MSS form. Doctors are constantly sorting through the problems of patients who exaggerate their symptoms and requests for disability. It can become quite frustrating. One example to illustrate this point is where the form asks the frequency of being able to perform certain activities. One of these activities is "reach down to waist level." The three choices are "rarely," "frequently," and "consistently." It is not uncommon for people seeking disability to want to mark the least amount in every category, but this can be tricky and can appear exaggerated. The definition of "rarely" is "very little up to one third of an 8 hour work day." If you answer this particular question "rarely," then you have to be able to explain this clearly in the comments section. Most people, even those who are severely disabled, are able to "reach down to waist level" at least frequently. Therefore, it is in your best interest to be as honest as you can and mark the appropriate boxes.

There are other sections of the MSS where you can easily answer "never" as an answer. Sometimes these can be accepted as not being exaggerations. For example, if you have bad arthritis in your knees then you should not "kneel" as a job requirement as it could damage your knee joints more, and you should answer this as "never." If you have rotator cuff tendonitis or shoulder arthritis, then you should answer "never" to reaching above the shoulders. Read the instructions on this form very carefully, and answer the questions as truthfully as possible. Do not answer the questions as far as "what you want to do and do not want to do," but rather, "how your lupus realistically prevents or allows you to do these things."

10. *Make a special appointment with your psychiatrist for the disability application.* All of the recommendations above for seeing your rheumatologist also apply for seeing your psychiatrist. If this applies to you, then it is in your best interest to do this instead of relying on an evaluation by someone chosen by Social Security. However, when you take in a copy of the MSS or RFC to your psychiatrist visit, make sure that it is the

one specifically labeled as "mental." When discussing your mental functional limitations with your psychiatrist, make sure to include things such as "make mistakes paying bills due to problems concentrating," "have difficulty adequately doing my job, and can't keep up the pace because of memory problems and fatigue," "continuously have conflicts with my neighbors and co-workers due to my moodiness," "my job is too stressful and I feel like I'm having a nervous breakdown," or "I often will stay in the house for long lengths of time avoiding contact with others." These are just examples, but anything where your mood, concentration, memory, or difficulties with keeping up the pace at work or at home can be important to your psychiatrist in terms of your mental function.

11. *Be compliant with your therapy.* Make sure that you do what your doctor recommends. This includes keeping your doctors' appointments, taking your medicines, seeing specialists as recommended, and getting the tests done as asked to do. These days it is getting easier for doctors to know when patients are not taking their medicines. Doctors regularly get notes from insurance companies and pharmacies letting them know when patients are not filling their prescriptions as prescribed, and these forms become a permanent part of medical records. You could be denied medical disability by Social Security if you are noncompliant with your recommended treatment. Social Security will assume that you are disabled and doing poorly due to your own fault, and society should not have to pay for your rejection of proper treatment. There are a few exceptions to this rule of compliance. These include having a severe mental illness that prevents compliance, having below normal intelligence preventing compliance, or having religious beliefs that prohibit you from receiving medical therapy.

One of the most common reasons for people not to be compliant with their treatment is not having the money to afford the treatments. This is where my recommendation of always being honest with your doctor comes into play. If you are not taking your medicine because you cannot afford to do so, it is very important that you let your doctor know and have it documented each visit. First, your doctor may be able to help you out or give you advice on how to get around this. Furthermore, you can ask your doctor to make sure and document this difficulty in your medical record as a way to support why you are not taking your medicine. Be careful with this, though. If you are spending money on other unhealthy things (such as cigarettes and alcohol), your inability to afford medicine will most likely become a moot issue.

12. *Keep copies of your medical records.* This is a good habit to get into anyway. Every time you see a doctor ask the receptionist or another office staff person for a copy of the latest note, lab results, x-rays, or consultation notes from other doctors. You have the legal right to have these copies yourself. Keep them well organized in a three-ring binder; it can become invaluable in the future. For example, you could potentially have enough medical evidence to get disability simply by giving copies of all your medical records to Social Security when you initially apply. In addition, your doctor usually will not charge you for these copies if you ask for them at each visit. However, if you ask for your records to be copied for you all at once, you will most likely have to pay a fee.

13. *Keep copies of all paperwork turned in to Social Security.* Every time you turn in filled out paperwork or medical records to Social Security, always keep a copy. You never

know if something may become lost as they handle hundreds to thousands of cases at a time. The same goes for your doctor. Make sure that you keep a copy of all filled out forms and blank forms that you give to your doctor to fill out. This way if something gets lost, you will easily be able to supply another copy.

14. *Be organized*. Keeping copies of your medical records and forms can become a lot to keep track of. Come up with a system to keep everything organized. For example, have a file or section of a folder to file your labs in chronologic order. The same goes for doctor's notes, x-rays, hospital notes, and the like. The more organized you are, the easier it is to find what you need when you need it.

15. *Be cordial and polite with everyone working on your case*. This goes for every single person, from the receptionist in your doctor's office, to the medical assistant who puts you in the examination room, to the person whom you talk to on the telephone at the Social Security office. There is no faster way to cause someone to put your needs on the bottom of the priority list than to be rude to him or her. Even if you feel that your case has been handled inappropriately, or that there was mismanagement, it is always best to smile and have good relations with everyone involved. You will find that in the end, things run smoother and quicker.

16. *Be prompt in filling out all forms and replying to questions and appeals*. The faster you do your part in the process, the faster things will happen. In addition, there are time limits on some things.

17. *Keep in contact with Social Security on the status of your claim*. Your claim will be at one of two different places as explained at the beginning of this chapter. Initially it goes to the claims representative at your local Social Security office, then it goes to the disability examiner at the Disability Determination Services for your state (which could be far away), then it returns back to your claims representative. After each step of the process, it can be helpful for you to monitor the process. Make sure things are running smoothly and see if you can help in any way with the process.

It is best to speak directly to your claims representative or disability examiner personally instead of whoever answers the phone at the 1-800 number. Let them know (very politely) that you would like to help in any way possible to make their job easier. One of the most common holdups in the process is waiting for copies of your medical records to arrive from your doctors and hospitals. A clue that your doctors have probably received requests for copies of your records is at the time you receive additional questionnaires through the mail from the disability examiner. The disability examiner usually sends these out at the same time. Some examples of questionnaires include those on Activities of Daily Living, Pain, and Fatigue. You should fill these questionnaires out completely as soon as possible and send them back immediately. (These questionnaires are very important for your disability case, by the way.)

A couple of weeks later, call the disability examiner to find out if there are any outstanding medical records. If the disability examiner is still waiting for some, ask if the office would cover the costs of your getting the records yourself (often they will). You can go to the doctor's office, let them know it is an important timely matter for you to get a copy of all of your medical records, pay the doctor's office fee for the records, then send them yourself to the medical director (keeping a copy for yourself, of course, just in case). Calling your disability examiner every couple of weeks and saying, "I am willing to do anything I can to help" is not out of line. In addition, a good question to ask is, "If this were your own claim what would you do now?"

18. *Keep a disability journal.* While you are disabled, keep a journal of what difficulties you have in your daily life due to your medical problems. Be thorough. Include when you fill out certain forms for your disability claim, when you talk to anyone on the phone at Social Security, what you talked about, whom you talked to, etc. This journal can especially become very important if you have to appeal your disability request.

It can become a full-time job keeping up with your disability, but it is an incredibly important matter. If you are diligent and compulsive in going through all of these steps, your efforts will usually be rewarded.

## What to Do after You Get Disability

*Continue to see your doctor regularly and be compliant with treatment.* The Social Security Administration (and private disability companies as well) reviews disability eligibility periodically. If you go on disability and then stop seeing your doctors, Social Security will assume that your health has improved and that you can return to the workplace.

*Make your health your new job.* Before you became disabled, your workdays were filled with your work requirements. When you become disabled, there is often a large void. Make it a priority to work on your health as your "new job." Work at exercising, eating healthy, and making sure that you take advantage of all the health benefits that you can find. Research as much as you can about SLE and your condition, always striving to improve in some aspect of your physical and mental health. Consider volunteering at your local hospital, at the seniors' center, or for a charitable organization such as the Lupus Foundation. Giving back to the community in this manner can greatly increase one's self-esteem and improve the quality of life.

*Pursue one or more of your passions.* Even if it is just for fifteen minutes a day, work on a hobby, volunteer, or learn to cook something new. Whatever you do, do not sit in front of the TV all day. It is important to do things to improve your self-esteem.

*Stop negative thinking.* When you are not working due to disability, it can become easy to blame yourself and feel depressed. Instead, learn to focus on problem solving. Try to get as much under your control as possible instead of letting life and your disability control you. If there is something that depresses you or gets you down, write it down as a problem. Then come up with some solutions and actions that you can do that can solve the problem or decrease the severity of the problem. Then reward yourself when you conquer any problem. Learn to praise yourself and compliment yourself.

*Take advantage of the nine-month "work trial period."* You are allowed to work nine total months within any five-year period while you receive full Social Security Disability benefits. This is a good way to test out the job market waters to see if there is a job you are able to do with your medical condition. These nine months do not have to be consecutive, so you can work a job for a month or two to test it out, and if it does not work out, try another at another time. You also still have to be considered as having a disabling impairment during this period; therefore, it is in your best interests to check with your Social Security office on the exact rules for this nine-month "work trial period." You also must openly report the work to your Social Security claims representative. Just inform the claims representative that you want to take advantage of the "work trial period" and make sure that you know all of the rules of doing so.

After nine months of working this "work trial period," if you decide you want to continue working, you can enter an additional thirty-six-month trial work period (an "extended period of eligibility"). During this stage, you can make as much income as you are able to make, but you do not receive your Social Security Disability benefits during this time. At any point during this period, if you are unable to make more than $1,000 a month (including benefits), you can get your full disability benefits for that month during the trial period. This trial period allows you to see if you are able to get back into the workforce without penalizing yourself. During this thirty-six-month trial period, if you find that you are not able to keep up with the job, you immediately get your Social Security Disability benefits and payments started back up. Another benefit during the "extended period of eligibility" and beyond is that your Medicare benefits continue for another ninety-three months if you were getting Medicare before you entered this period.

After this additional thirty-six-month trial of work, if you are still working, then you do lose your disability benefits. However, for five additional years after your benefits stop, if at any point your lupus becomes severe again, keeping you from being able to work, you can fill out a simple Social Security application form requesting a "resumption of benefits." Your request will be reviewed similar to the initial review process, and you must still meet the same requirements. However, a good benefit is that your disability benefits, including your check payments, begin the first of the month following the submission of your request. You do not have to wait for the review to be completed.

The take home message from this is that after you become disabled, you can still attempt to enter the workplace (which is to your benefit due to the possibilities of better income and better health insurance) without penalties of losing your disability as long as you know what the time lines are and what the restrictions are. It is important to note that currently the healthcare system is undergoing significant changes, so any of these "rules" could change at any time. Always make sure to contact your claims representative to double-check on the current rules. In addition, the "Patient's Resources" at the end of this book lists two excellent books (especially *Social Security, Medicare & Government Pensions*) that are very useful for the person seeking disability. I would encourage you to read those books as well if this pertains to you.

### KEY POINTS TO REMEMBER

1. It is usually to your advantage for numerous reasons to keep working instead of going on disability (better income, better health insurance, better self-esteem, etc.).

2. If you are having difficulties at work due to your lupus, check and see if some adjustments are possible to continue working as per the Americans with Disabilities Act (table 43.1).

3. Using a note from your doctor and recommendations from an occupational therapist can help strengthen your work accommodation requests.

4. Organizations that can give you advice on appropriate work accommodations include the Job Accommodation Network (www.askjan.org), the Patient Advocate Foundation (www.patientadvocate.org), Hire Disability Solutions (www.hireds.com), and Disability.gov at www.disability.gov.

5. If your SLE is severe and prevents you from doing your current job as well as any job you have held during the previous fifteen years, and this disabling condition is expected to last at least one year, apply for Social Security immediately.

6. Get the help of a lawyer who specializes in Social Security Disability.

7. Follow the guidelines in this chapter to ensure that your disability application has the best chances for approval the first time that it is submitted.

8. Good luck, and remember, you can make it happen!

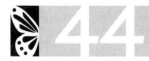

# The Lupus Secrets Checklist

This book contains a lot of important information. In my experience, patients who learn as much as they can about lupus seem to do best in the end in terms of their health. However, it can be very challenging to remember most of this material. There are certain things, though, that are important for all lupus patients to follow to maximize their health. The following list summarizes these important issues. Although I call them the Lupus Secrets, they are not secrets at all; they are things that all lupus patients should know. Most physicians and nurses unfortunately do not have time to go over all of these with their patients, even though they are important. I recommend that you go through this list on a regular basis and work on whichever sections you are not practicing or have forgotten about. You should also double-check any of these recommendations with your doctor, as your particular situation may need to be addressed differently.

» Avoid sulfa antibiotics (Septra and Bactrim); include them in your allergy list (chapters 1 and 3).

» Keep a personal record of your labs, biopsy results, x-rays, and doctor's notes (especially those that established your diagnosis of SLE) (chapter 1).

» See a rheumatologist or other lupus specialist regularly, commonly every three months, even if you feel great. Kidney inflammation occurs in around 50% of SLE patients and doctors can identify it at early stages (by way of a urine sample) when it is easy to treat. It causes no symptoms until it becomes severe (chapter 12).

» Take 81 mg of aspirin a day if you are at increased risk for heart attacks or strokes or if you are positive for antiphospholipid antibodies (check with your doctor first) (chapters 4, 9, 11, and 21).

» If you are fatigued and tired, do everything in table 6.1.

» Get eight hours of quality sleep a day (table 6.2 and chapter 38).

» If you have trouble sleeping, do tables 6.2 and 6.3.

» For aches and pains of lupus do everything listed in tables 7.1–7.3.

» If you have troubles with memory, try the measures in table 13.3.

» Tell your doctor if you feel depressed or down in the dumps, especially if you have thoughts about hurting yourself. Do the questionnaire in table 13.4.

» If you have problems with dryness, practice the suggestions listed in tables 14.3–14.10.

» If you have heartburn, do the measures listed in table 15.1 regularly.

» Keep blood pressure consistently < 140/90 mm/Hg (chapter 21).
    < 130/80 mm/Hg if you have had a heart attack or stroke, or have chronic kidney disease (chapter 21). Keep cholesterol normal (chapter 21).

» Do not smoke cigarettes. Smoking causes lupus to be more active, keeps hydroxy-chloroquine from working, increases strokes and heart attacks (which are the most common causes of death in lupus patients), increases the risk for lung cancer (which occurs more commonly in lupus patients), and causes broken bones from osteoporosis (chapters 3, 21, 23, 24, and 38).

» If you are unable to stop smoking on your own, go to www.smokefree.gov or call 1-800-QUIT-NOW (chapter 38).

» Exercise regularly (chapters 7 and 21, and table 38.7).

» Maintain normal weight (chapters 21 and 38, figure 21.2, and table 21.2).

» If you get a fever, call/see your primary care doctor ASAP (chapters 22 and 40).

» Get an influenza vaccination yearly in the fall (table 22.1).

» Get a Pneumovax and PCV-13 pneumonia vaccines if you are on immunosuppressant medicines (table 22.1).

» Keep up to date on all vaccinations to prevent infections (chapter 22).

» Have screening tests done regularly for cancers (e.g., breast, cervical, colon, etc.) (table 23.2).

» Consider getting the human papilloma virus vaccine (Gardasil) series to prevent HPV-associated cancers if you are not in a permanent, monogamous relationship (chapters 22 and 23).

» Get adequate calcium (chapter 24).

» If you are on any stomach acid–lowering medicines, consider taking calcium citrate (chapters 24, 28, 29, and 39).

» Get adequate vitamin D. If you are vitamin D deficient, you may need vitamin D supplements for the rest of your life (chapters 24, 38, and 39). Your 25-OH vitamin D level should be at least 20 ng/mL; at least 30 ng/mL if you take steroids.

» If you take steroids (such as prednisone) regularly, make sure you are taking a medicine to prevent osteoporosis if it is appropriate; check with your doctor (chapter 24).

» If you take steroids regularly, consider wearing a medical alert bracelet (chapters 26 and 31).

» If you take steroids, practice everything in table 31.4 to minimize side effects.

» Learn to take your medications regularly (table 29.8).

» Take a completed medication list (table 29.9) or a bag of all your medicines to every doctor's visit.

» Take Plaquenil (hydroxychloroquine) as one of your medications (chapters 22, 29, and 30).

» Double-check your dose of hydroxychloroquine (tables 30.2 and 30.3).

» Practice measures in table 30.3 to prevent side effects from hydroxychloroquine.

» Use an Amsler grid monthly when taking Plaquenil (hydroxychloroquine) or chloroquine (figure 30.2).

» Use sunscreen every day and regularly avoid UV light (chapter 3 and table 38.3).

» Avoid alfalfa and mung bean sprouts (chapter 3 and table 38.5).

» Eat a well-balanced diet with plenty of fruits and vegetables (table 38.6 and figure 38.2).

» Include fish, walnuts, and flax seed rich in omega-3 fatty acids in your diet (table 38.5).

» Include more olive oil in your diet (table 38.5).

» Decrease stress (table 38.8).

» Do not take Echinacea (herbal supplement promoted to treat colds) (chapters 3 and 39).

» Consider taking DHEA and other supplements if approved by your rheumatologist (chapter 35 and table 39.3).

» Do not get pregnant until cleared by your rheumatologist (chapters 18 and 41).

» If you are anti-SSA or anti-SSB positive and get pregnant, alert your OB/GYN so you can get fetal heart monitoring beginning at sixteen to eighteen weeks of pregnancy (chapters 18 and 41).

» If you get pregnant, see your rheumatologist more often and consider seeing a high-risk obstetrician (chapters 18 and 41).

» If you run into financial problems, read chapter 42 and contact the organizations listed in table 42.1.

» Ensure your work environment is conducive for your SLE (table 43.1).

» If your SLE is severe and you can no longer do your job, read chapter 43 completely.

» Continue to educate yourself about lupus; consider joining a lupus educational organization (see "Patient Resources" at the back of this book).

» Every day tell yourself it is going to be a good day, that there is a lot in your power to do well, and remember that knowledge is power.

This book cannot cover every aspect of subjects of interest to people who have lupus or to their family members or friends. The following represents only a small percentage of the vast amount of information that is available through organizations, in print, and on the internet. I have included those sources that I feel are helpful and up to date and those with which I am familiar. These sources are professional and accurate, and give good advice and services to people who have lupus and other problems. I have tried to mainly include printed sources that are most recent (within the past ten years). There are other important, excellent sources that I may not know about and that may not be listed here; however, it does not mean that they are any less valuable than those that are. Please note that organization addresses, websites, emails, and telephone numbers may change over time.

Following are some guidelines about accessing medical information not listed here (including Internet sources, organizations, books, and healthcare providers):

Avoid any source promising a cure. In this same light, be skeptical of any treatment that promises "quick," "dramatic," or "miraculous" results.

Avoid sources stating that mainstream medicine and doctors are not to be trusted and are wrong in their advice.

Be skeptical of sources that appear to try to sell something. This includes those that routinely sell vitamins or other dietary supplements as part of their practice.

Be wary of sources that use words such as "toxins," "detoxify," "purify," "revitalize," "rejuvenate," "support," and "boost." These nonmedical terms are often used to sell unproven therapies and supplements.

Be skeptical of sources that offer a treatment and primarily cite individuals' personal experiences (called anecdotes or testimonials) instead of proving the treatment works through major research studies. Studies involving large numbers of patients using a placebo to compare a potential treatment to are the best ones to trust.

Be skeptical of a treatment that only mentions good benefits without listing any possible adverse effects. It is rare for a truly effective treatment to have only good results without possible side effects, especially for a complex disorder such as lupus.

Be skeptical of any therapy that states that it treats lupus along with a large number of other disorders (especially if they are unrelated diseases such as AIDS, cancer, etc.).

Sources endorsed by professional and patient advocacy organizations such as the Arthritis Foundation, the Lupus Foundation of America, and the Sjögren's Syndrome Foundation, as well as others, tend to be reviewed by experts and can usually be trusted.

Read books that have a recent publishing date. Medical information and knowledge increases and improves dramatically from year to year. A source that was produced within the past five years is best. Sources more than ten years old probably have too much outdated information to be completely trusted, even if they were the best sources of information at the time.

Be wary of information and sources written by doctors who use superlatives such as "America's leading . . ." or "the world's foremost expert in . . .", and the like unless this is written by a third party about the doctor or person. People who are selling themselves with their own agenda in mind often use these phrases. Most experts in medicine whom I know tend to be quite unassuming and modest, and rarely need to sell themselves.

Be skeptical of any source stating that mainstream medicine is incorrect, that the doctors in mainstream medicine persecute them, or that their work is suppressed because it is controversial. In medicine, there are always controversies. Controversies are actually good and desired by mainstream medicine as they push the medical community to formally evaluate these controversies, accept those proven correct, and continue to improve over time. The physicians who believe in their controversial ideas rarely try to sell their ideas to the public or to patients prior to their being proven. They work on proving their ideas through the proper research avenues instead.

Be skeptical if a source tells you not to trust your doctor. A truly professional healthcare provider would not say this unless she or he personally knows that another healthcare provider is inept or is not to be trusted.

You cannot assume that everything written by a medical doctor (MD or DO) is accurate. Unfortunately, not all doctors ascribe to the highest levels of medical knowledge and integrity. Be very skeptical of anything that does not satisfy the above recommendations (even if written by a doctor). If a medical source appears suspicious, ask your personal doctor for his or her opinion.

## Patient Advocacy Organizations (U.S.)

Patient advocacy organizations generally have patients, friends, family members, and medical professionals as members. As a group, they tend to focus on patient education while also striving for public education, encouraging research, and advocating for patients with governmental issues. You may want to consider joining some of these groups. You can obtain additional self-education while also having opportunities to participate in volunteer work and social advocacy.

American Association of Kidney Patients
www.aakp.org

American Autoimmune Related Diseases
  Association
www.aarda.org; 800-598-4668
22100 Gratiot Ave., Detroit, MI 48021
750 17th St., NW, Ste. 1100, Washington,
  DC 20006

American Chronic Pain Association
www.theacpa.org; 800-533-3231
PO Box 850, Rocklin, CA 95677

American Diabetes Association
www.diabetes.org; 800-342-2383

American Kidney Fund
www.kidneyfund.org

American Liver Foundation
www.liverfoundation.org; 800-GO-LIVER
39 Broadway, Ste. 2700, New York, NY 10006

American Lung Association
www.lungusa.org; 800-548-8252
1301 Pennsylvania Ave., NW, Washington,
  DC 20004

American Pain Foundation
www.painfoundation.org; 888-615-7246
201 North Charles Street, Ste. 710,
  Baltimore, MD 21201-4111

Antiphospholipid Syndrome Foundation of
  America
www.apsfa.org

Arthritis Foundation
www.arthritis.org; 800-283-7800
PO Box 7669, Atlanta, GA 30357-0669

Family Caregiver Alliance
www.caregiver.org

Fibromyalgia Network
www.fmnetnews.com; 800-853-2929
PO Box 31750, Tucson, AZ 85751-1750

Lupus Alliance of America
www.lupusalliance.org; 866-415-8787
3871 Harlem Rd., Buffalo, NY 14215

Lupus Foundation of America, Inc.
www.lupus.org; 800-558-0121, 202-349-1155
2000 L St., NW, Ste. 410, Washington, DC
  20036

The Myositis Association
www.myositis.org; 800-821-7356

National Alliance for Caregiving
www.caregiving.org

National Fibromyalgia Association
www.fmaware.org

National Health Council
www.nationalhealthcouncil.org

National Kidney Foundation
www.kidney.org; 800-622-9010
30 East 33rd Street, New York, NY 10016

National Organization for Rare Disorders
www.rarediseases.org; 800-999-6673

National Osteoporosis Foundation
www.nof.org; 800-223-9994

National Stroke Association
www.stroke.org; 800-787-6537
9707 E. Easter Lane, Ste. B, Centennial, CO
  80112

Pulmonary Hypertension Association
www.phassociation.org; 800-748-7274
801 Roeder Road, Ste. 1000, Silver Spring,
  MD 20910

Raynaud's Association
www.raynauds.org; 800-280-8055

Scleroderma Foundation
www.scleroderma.org; 800-722-4673
300 Rosewood Dr., #105, Danvers, MA
  01923

Sjögren's Syndrome Foundation
www.sjogrens.org; 800-475-6473
6707 Democracy Blvd., #325, Bethesda, MD
20817

SLE Lupus Foundation
www.lupusny.org; 212-685-4118
300 Seventh Ave, #1701, New York, NY
10001

The Vasculitis Foundation
www.vasculitisfoundation.org;
800-277-9474

Well Spouse Association
www.wellspouse.org
Offers support to spousal caregivers

## Patient Advocacy (Worldwide)

European Lupus Erythematosus
Federation
www.lupus-support.org.uk

Hughes Syndrome Foundation
www.hughes-syndrome.org; 0207-188-8217
Conybeare House, Guy's Hospital, London,
SE1 9RT, England
Hughes syndrome = antiphospholipid
antibody syndrome

International Sjögren's Network
www.sjogrens.org/home/get-connected/isn

Irish Lupus Support Group
www.lupus.ie

Lupus Association of Tasmania
www.lupustas.bigpondhosting.com

Lupus Australia, Queensland, Inc.
www.lupus.com.au

Lupus Canada
www.lupuscanada.org; 800-661-1468
3555 14th Ave., Unit #3, Markham, ON L3R
0H5

Lupus Care & Support, Inc. (New Zealand)
www.lupussupport.org.nz

Lupus Europe
www.lupus-europe.org

The Lupus Group of Western Australia
www.lupuswa.com.au

Lupus Groups Around The World
http://www.lupus.org/resources/
international-resources
Lists lupus support groups alphabetically
by country

Lupus New South Wales
www.lupusnsw.org.au

Lupus Patients Understanding & Support
(United Kingdom)
www.lupus-support.org.uk

Lupus Trust of New Zealand
www.lupus.org.nz

Lupus UK
www.lupusuk.org.uk

## Other Sources of Patient Education

About.com
www.lupus.about.com

About Herbs, Botanicals & Other Products
www.mskcc.org/mskcc/html/11570.cfm
Website of Memorial Sloan Kettering

Acupuncture.com
www.acupuncture.com

American Academy of Medical Acupuncture
www.medicalacupuncture.org

American Chiropractic Association
www.acatoday.org

American College of Physicians Online
www.acponline.org/patients_families

American Massage Therapy Association
www.amtamassage.org

Association for Applied Psychophysiology
and Biofeedback
www.aapb.org

Be MedWise
www.bemedwise.org
Website of the National Council on Patient
Information and Education

Brigham and Women's Hospital Lupus
Center: Facts About Lupus
www.brighamandwomens.org/
Departments_and_Services/medicine/
services/rheumatology/lupus/
forpatients_quickfacts.aspx

Centers for Disease Control and Prevention
(CDC)
www.cdc.gov

ConsumerLab.com
www.consumerlab.com
Tests over-the-counter supplements

Drug Guide (Arthritis Today)
www.arthritistoday.org/treatments/drug-
guide/index.php

Drugs.com
www.drugs.com

Dry.Org
www.dry.org
Internet resources for Sjögren's syndrome

DxLupus.org
www.dxlupus.org

Healingwell.com
www.healingwell.com

Health A to Z
www.healthatoz.com

Health Information
www.niams.nih.gov/health_info
Information on various diseases by the
National Institutes of Health (NIH)

The Johns Hopkins Lupus Center
www.hopkinslupus.org

The Johns Hopkins Vasculitis Center
www.hopkinsvasculitis.org

LabTests Online
www.labtestsonline.org

Learn About Prescription Safety
www.learnaboutrxsafety.org
Website of the National Council on Patient
Information and Education

Living with Dryness
www.livingwithdryness.com
Website for people who have Sjögren's
syndrome

Lupus Center of Excellence at West Penn
Allegheny Health System: Interactive
Health Library
www.wpahs.org/health-information
-library?search_topicTB=lupus

Lupus Links
www.sblupus.org/lupuslinks.html

The Lupus Site
www.thelupussite.com

Mayo Clinic
www.mayoclinic.com/health/lupus/
DS00115

Med Help International
www.medhelp.org

MedicineNet.com
www.medicinenet.com

MedlinePlus (National Library of Medicine)
www.nlm.nih.gov/medlineplus
www.medlineplus.gov

MedlinePlus Patient Education Tutorial on
  Lupus
www.nlm.nih.gov/medlineplus/tutorials/
  lupus/htm/_no_50_no_0.htm
Excellent interactive slide show regarding
  many aspects of lupus and its treatment

Medscape
www.emedicine.com

The Merck Manual: Home Health
  Handbook
www.merckmanuals.com/home/index
  .html

The Moisture Seekers Newsletter
www.sjogrens.org
Focuses on Sjögren's syndrome

National Center for Complementary
  and Alternative Medicine, National
  Institutes of Health
www.nccam.nih.gov

National Center for Homeopathy
www.homeopathic.org

The National Center on Physical Activity
  and Disability
www.ncpad.org

National Certification Commission for
  Acupuncture and Oriental Medicine
www.nccaom.org

National Institute of Arthritis and
  Musculoskeletal and Skin Diseases
  (NIAMS)
www.niams.nih.gov
Bldg. 31, Room 4C05, 31 Center Dr., MSC
  2350, Bethesda, MD 20892-2350

Office on Women's Health
www.womenshealth.gov; 202-690-7650
200 Independence Ave, SW, Washington
  DC 20201

RxList (The Internet Drug Index)
www.rxlist.com

SafeMedication
www.safemedication.com
Website of the American Society of Health-
  System Pharmacists

Sjögren's Forum: Living Well With
  Sjögren's
www.sjogrensforum.com

Sjögren's Syndrome Clinic, National
  Institute of Dental and Craniofacial
  Research
301-435-8528
Building 10, Room 1N113, 10 Center Drive
  MSC 1190
Bethesda, MD 20892-1190

Sjögren's Syndrome Internet Resources
www.dry.org

Sjögren's World
www.sjsworld.org

UpToDate
www.uptodate.com/home/uptodate
  -benefits-patients

U.S. Food and Drug Administration (FDA)
www.fda.gov; 888-463-6332
10903 New Hampshire Ave., Silver Spring,
  MD 20993

WebMD
www.lupus.webmd.com

Whole Health MD
www.wholehealthmd.com

## Additional Resources

But You Don't Look Sick.com
www.butyoudontlooksick.com

CaringBridge
www.caringbridge.org/partner/lupus
Create your own website on your personal
    journey living with lupus

Charla de Lupus
866-812-4494
Talk to counselors in Spanish about lupus

Daily Strength: Lupus Forum
www.dailystrength.org/c/Lupus/forum

E-Health Forum: Lupus Forum
www.ehealthforum.com/health/lupus
    .html

Friends Health Connection.org
www.friendshealthconnection.org
Online support for medical problems

HealthBoards: Lupus Message Boards
www.healthboards.com/boards/lupus

LifeWithLupus.org
www.lifewithlupus.org
Forum for people who have lupus

LupusLine
866-375-1427
Talk to counselors about lupus

MD Junction: Lupus Forum
www.mdjunction.com/forums/lupus
    -discussions

MedHelp: Lupus Forum
www.medhelp.org/forums/Lupus/show/149

Sjögren's World
www.sjogrensworld.org/forum
Forum for people who have Sjögren's
    syndrome

Wehavelupus.com
forum.wehavelupus.com
Forum for people who have lupus

## Clinical Trials (Research Studies)

Center for Clinical Trials Education (Lupus
    Foundation of America)
www.lupus.org/clinicaltrials

Center for Information and Study on
    Clinical Research Participation
www.ciscrp.org

Center Watch
www.centerwatch.com

National Data Bank for Rheumatic
    Diseases
www.arthritis-research.org

National Institutes of Health
www.clinicaltrials.gov
clinicalstudies.info.nih.gov

Search Clinical Trials
www.searchclinicaltrials.org

## Patient Registries

Lupus Family Registry and Repository
lupus.omrf.org

Multiple Autoimmune Disease Genetics
    Consortium
www.madgc.org; 877-698-9467; email =
    madgc@nshs.edu
Includes families that have at least
    four family members who have an
    autoimmune disease

National Databank for Rheumatic Diseases
    (Arthritis Research Center Foundation)
www.arthritis-research.org; 800-323-5871

National Institute of Arthritis and Musculoskeletal and Skin Diseases Lupus Registry (NIH)
www.niams.nih.gov/Funding/Funded_Research/registries.asp

Neonatal Lupus Research Registry (New York University School of Medicine)
www.neonatallupus.com; 212-263-2255

Oklahoma Medical Research Foundation
www.omrf.org; 405-271-2534; email = clinic@omrf.org

The SICCA International Registry (Sjögren's Syndrome, Johns Hopkins Hospital)
www.hopkinssjogrens.org/research/sicca-project; 410-550-1887; email = sjogrens@jhmi.edu

Sjögren's International Collaborative Clinical Alliance (University of California, San Francisco)
sicca.ucsf.edu; 415-476-0535; email = sicca@dentistry.ucsf.edu

## Organizations Focused on Research

Alliance for Lupus Research
www.lupusresearch.org
28 W. 44th St., Ste. 501, New York, NY 10036

Lupus Research Institute
www.lupusresearchinstitute.org; 212-812-9881
330 Seventh Ave., #1701, New York, NY 10001

Rheumatology Research Foundation of the American College of Rheumatology
http://www.rheumatology.org/foundation/default.aspx; 404-633-3777
2200 Lake Boulevard NE, Atlanta, GA 30319

## Disability and Employment Assistance

Americans with Disabilities Act
www.ada.gov

Benefits.gov
www.benefits.gov

The Council for Disability Rights
www.disabilityrights.org

Disability & Business Technical Assistance Centers
800-949-4232

Disability.gov
www.disability.gov

Disability Rights Education & Defense Fund
www.dredf.org; 510-644-2555

*Disability Workbook for Social Security Applicants*. D. M. Smith and B. W. Smith. Demos Medical Publishing, 2008.

Disabled Online
www.disabledonline.com
Internet portal for people who have special needs

Employee Rights: Disability Discrimination
employment.findlaw.com/employment-discrimination/disability-discrimination
Website by findlaw.com

Hire Disability Solutions
www.hireds.com; 800-238-5373

*How to Get SSI & Social Security Disability: An Insider's Step by Step Guide*. M. Davis, iUniverse, 2000.

Invisible Disabilities Association
www.invisibledisabilities.org

Job Accommodation Network
www.askjan.org; 800-526-7234

National Organization of Social Security
　　Claimants' Representatives
www.nosscr.org; 800-431-2804

Patient Advocate Foundation
www.patientadvocate.org; 800-532-5274

Social Security Administration
www.socialsecurity.gov/applyfordisability;
　　800-772-1213
Disability application

Social Security Administration (The Work
　　Site)
www.ssa.gov/work; 800-772-1213
Employment support

Social Security Disability and Disability
　　Resource Center
www.ssdrc.com

U.S. Department of Health and Human
　　Services
www.hhs.gov; 877-696-6775
200 Independence Ave, SW, Washington,
　　DC 20201

U.S. Equal Employment Opportunity
　　Commission
www.eeoc.gov; 800-669-4000

U.S. Equal Employment Opportunity
　　Commission
www.eeoc.gov/facts/ada18.html
Americans with Disabilities Act; Your
　　Employment Rights

## Financial Assistance
## (Prescriptions, Insurance)

Access2wellness
www.access2wellness.com

Benefits.gov
www.benefits.gov

Centers for Medicare and Medicaid
　　Services
www.cms.hhs.gov
7500 Security Blvd., Baltimore, MD 21244

Giant Eagle Pharmacy
www.gianteagle.com/Save/Health-Savings
　　-Programs/4-10-Dollar-Drug-Program/
　　Discount-Drugs/
Generic drug program

High Risk Health Insurance Pools
　　(National Association of Health
　　Underwriters)
www.nahu.org/consumer/HRPGuide.cfm

Kroger
https://www.kroger.com/topic/save-on
　　-generic-prescriptions
$4 and $10 generic prescriptions

ModestNeeds.org
www.modestneeds.org/intro

National Association of State
　　Comprehensive Health Insurance Plans
www.naschip.org; 919-783-5766
Health Insurance Risk Sharing Plan

NeedyMeds, Inc.
www.needymeds.org
PO Box 219, Gloucester, MA 01931

Partnership for Prescription Assistance
www.pparx.org; 888-477-2669

Patient Advocate Foundation
www.patientadvocate.org; 800-532-5274

Pre-Existing Condition Insurance Plan
www.healthcare.gov/law/features/choices/
　　pre-existing-condition-insurance-plan/
　　index.html

Publix Pharmacy
www.publix.com/pharmacy/Free
　　-Medications.do
Free antibiotics, lisinopril, and metformin

RxAssist Patient Assistance Program
Center
www.rxassist.org

RxHope
www.rxhope.com; 877-267-0517

Target
www.target.com/pharmacy/generics
$4 and $10 generic prescriptions

Together Rx Access Prescription Savings
Program
www.togetherrxaccess.com; 800-444-4106

WalMart Prescriptions
www.walmart.com/cp/1078664
$4 and $10 prescriptions

## Pharmaceutical (Drug) Company Patient Assistance Programs

Find out from your pharmacist what
pharmaceutical companies produce your
medications. Then contact their individual
patient assistance programs to find out
whether you qualify for help in obtaining
your medications.

Abbott Patient Assistance Program
800-222-6885

AbbVie Patient Assistance Program
800-222-6885
This section of Abbott supplies
medications such as Humira and
Gengraf

AstraZeneca patient assistance programs
800-292-6363

Bristol-Myers Squibb
www.bms.com/products/Pages/programs
.aspx

Eli Lilly & Company (Lilly TruAssist
Program)
www.lillytruassist.com; 855-559-8783

Genentech Patient Access Programs
866-4ACCESS

GlaxoSmithKline (Bridges to ACCESS)
www.bridgestoaccess.com; 866-728-4368
PO Box 29038, Phoenix, AZ 85038-9038

Johnson & Johnson Patient Assistance
(Access2Wellness)
www.access2wellness.com; 800-652-6227

Lilly TruAssist Program
www.lillytruassist.com; 855-559-8783

Merck Helps
www.merck.com/merckhelps; 800-727-5400

Novartis Patient Assistance Now
www.patientassistancenow.com;
800-245-5356

Ortho-McNeil-Janssen Patient Assistance
Program (Johnson & Johnson Patient
Assistance)
www.access2wellness.com; 800-652-6227

Pfizer Helpful Answers
www.pfizerhelpfulanswers.com;
866-706-2400

Roche U.S. Pharmaceuticals Assistance
Program
http://www.gene.com/patients/patient
-access; 866-4ACCESS
Same as Genentech program

Schering-Plough
www.merck.com/merckhelps; 800-727-5400
Uses Merck program

Wyeth
www.pfizerhelpfulanswers.com;
866-706-2400
Uses Pfizer program

## Professional Medical Organizations

These groups mainly have medical professionals as members, but they are also sources to obtain additional patient education as well.

Academy of Nutrition and Dietetics
www.eatright.org

African League of Associations for
    Rheumatology
www.aflar.net

American Academy of Dermatology
www.aad.org

American Academy of Neurology
www.aan.com

American Academy of Ophthalmology
www.aao.org

American Academy of Orthopaedic
    Surgeons
www.aaos.org

American Academy of Pediatrics
www.aap.org

American Board of Medical Specialties
www.certificationmatters.org
How to tell if your doctor is board certified

American College of Pediatricians
www.acpeds.org

American College of Physicians
www.acponline.org

American College of Rheumatology
www.rheumatology.org/
2200 Lake Boulevard NE, Atlanta, GA 30319

American Medical Association
www.ama-assn.org

American Psychological Association
www.apa.org/helpcenter

American Society of Nephrology
www.asn-online.org

Asia Pacific League of Associations for
    Rheumatology
www.aplar.org

Canadian Rheumatology Association
www.rheum.ca

European Union League Against
    Rheumatism
www.eular.org

National Medical Association
www.nmanet.org
Largest and oldest organization
    representing African American health
    professionals in the United States

National Sleep Association
www.sleepfoundation.org

Pan-American League of Associations for
    Rheumatology
www.panlar.org

## Medical Textbooks

These are in-depth, highly technical textbooks written for doctors, especially rheumatologists. They may be of interest to anyone who wishes to obtain a much higher level of scientific understanding of lupus and the rheumatologic disorders related to it.

*Dubois' Lupus Erythematosus and Related Syndromes*. 8th edition. D. J. Wallace and B. H. Hahn. Saunders, 2012.

*Kelley's Textbook of Rheumatology*. 9th edition. G. S. Firestein, R. C. Budd, S. E. Gabriel, I. B. McInnes, and J. R. O'Dell. W. B. Saunders, 2012.

*Rheumatology*. M. C. Hochberg, A. J. Silman, J. S. Smollen, M. E. Weinblatt, and M. H. Weisman. Mosby, 2012.

*Systemic Lupus Erythematosus*. 5th edition. G. Tsokos, J. P. Buyon, T. Koike, and R. G. Lahita (eds.). Academic Press, 2010.

## Miscellaneous Reading

These are other resources that can be useful for some problems that may occur in people who have SLE. These books provide additional educational material.

*The Autoimmune Connection: Essential Information for Women on Diagnosis, Treatment, and Getting on with Your Life*. R. Baron-Faust and J. P. Buyon, MD. McGraw-Hill, 2004.

*The Balance Within: The Science Connecting Health and Emotions*. E. M. Sternberg. W. H. Freeman, 2001.

*A Body out of Balance: Understanding and Treating Sjögren's Syndrome*. N. Carteron and R. Fremes. Avery Trade, 2003. (Written by a woman who has Sjögren's syndrome and her doctor. It contains many useful coping strategies.)

*The Chronic Illness Workbook: Strategies and Solutions for Taking Back Your Life*. Revised edition. P. A. Fennell. Albany Health Management Publishing, 2012.

*Chronic Pain for Dummies*. S. S. Kassan, C. J. Vierck, and E. Vierck. For Dummies, 2008.

*Coping with Lupus: A Practical Guide to Alleviating the Challenges of Systemic Lupus Erythematosus*. R. H. Phillips. Avery, 2012. (This new, revised edition gives lots of practical advice on how to cope and live with lupus.)

*Dancing at the River's Edge: A Patient and Her Doctor Negotiate Life with Chronic Illness*. 3rd edition. A. Brill and M. D. Lockshin. Schaffner Press, Inc., 2010. (An excellent read for patients, family members, and medical professionals. This book explores the personal difficulties of dealing with chronic disease from both the patient's as well as her doctor's perspectives. A must read for anyone looking for more in how to deal with the emotional consequences of illness, and learning how to appreciate both doctor and patient perspectives.)

*A Delicate Balance: Living Successfully with Chronic Illness*. S. M. Wells. Da Capo Press, 2000.

*Despite Lupus: How to Live Well with a Chronic Illness*. S. Gorman. Four Legged Press, 2009. (This book is especially excellent for the person who is having difficulty coping with her or his diagnosis and treatment. It is the personal story of a woman who has SLE and her journey through the difficult times and how she was finally able to overcome those problems. It is a motivational story with excellent recommendations on how to live with SLE.)

*Dry Mouth, The Malevolent Symptom: A Clinical Guide*. L. M. Sreebny and A. Vissink. Wiley-Blackwell, 2010. (This book is primarily written for health professionals caring for people suffering from dry mouth. However, people who have a dry mouth from Sjögren's syndrome who are seeking more advanced information will find this resource helpful.)

*Fibromyalgia: An Essential Guide for Patients and Their Families.* D. J. Wallace and J. B. Wallace. Oxford University Press, 2003. (This book supplies much needed practical information for the 20% of lupus patients who also have fibromyalgia as well as the science behind the disorder.)

*The First Year—Lupus: An Essential Guide for the Newly Diagnosed.* N. C. Hanger. Da Capo Press, 2003. (This book gives practical advice on how to live with and cope with lupus and its associated problems such as fatigue and fibromyalgia written from the perspective of someone who has lupus.)

*If You Have to Wear an Ugly Dress, Learn to Accessorize: Guidance, Inspiration, and Hope for Women with Lupus, Scleroderma, and Other Autoimmune Illnesses.* L. McNamara and K. Kemper. Wheatmark, 2011. (This book is written by authors who have SLE and scleroderma. They describe their own journeys living with these disorders and provide valuable tools of self-empowerment to help others learn to manage their own lives.)

*Living Well with Autoimmune Disease: What Your Doctor Doesn't Tell You . . . That You Need to Know.* M. J. Shomon. William Morrow Paperbacks, 2002.

*Living with Coronary Heart Disease: A Guide for Patients and Family.* J. E. Granato, MD, FACP. A Johns Hopkins Press Health Book, 2008.

*Living with Lupus: The Complete Guide.* 2nd edition. S. P. Blau and D. Schultz. Da Capo Press, 2004. (This book also provides a lot of practical information for people who have lupus.)

*Living with Rheumatoid Arthritis.* 2nd edition. J. L. McGuire and T. L. Shlotzhauer. Johns Hopkins University Press, 2003.

*Lupus: Alternative Therapies That Work.* S. Moore. Healing Arts Press, 2000.

*Lupus: A Patient's Guide to Diagnosis, Treatment, and Lifestyle.* A. I. Quintero Del Rio. Hilton Publishing, 2007.

*The Lupus Book: A Guide for Patients and Their Families.* 5th edition. D. J. Wallace. Oxford University Press, 2012. (Long regarded as one of the best books about lupus. Dr. Wallace is one of the world's leading experts in lupus after taking over Dr. Dubois's very large lupus practice in California. It has a lot of excellent information, and is regularly updated.)

*Lupus: Everything You Need to Know (Your Personal Health).* S. Bernatsky and J.-L. Senécal. Firefly Books, 2005. (Doctors Bernatsky and Senécal are leading lupus experts who provide much practical information in their book for people who have lupus, giving advice on how to cope with many aspects of the disorder. They give a lot of useful information in an easy-to-read format.)

*Lupus (Facts).* 2nd edition. D. Isenberg and S. Manzi. Oxford University Press, 2008. (Dr. Isenberg and Manzi are world famous lupologists who do an excellent job in giving concise information about lupus. This book is very short and easy to read, cutting to the chase but with a load of information about SLE.)

*A Lupus Handbook: These Are The Faces of Lupus.* A. G. Moore. CreateSpace, 2012. (This is an interesting book presenting information about some famous people who have had lupus, as well as an account of the author's journey with lupus. There are chapters devoted to advice on sun protection, finance, insurance, and treatments for lupus as well.)

*Lupus, My Doctor and Me: A Sacred Dialogue.* A. A. Fricklas and S. S. Kassan. Astute Press LLC, 2010. (The authors are a woman who has lupus and her rheumatologist. It gives a wealth of helpful information on the types of conversations patients should have with their doctors. It includes a lot of useful advice on how to manage and cope with lupus.)

*Lupus Q + A: Everything You Need to Know.* Revised edition. R. G. Lahita and R. H. Phillips. Avery Trade, 2004. (I like this interesting presentation. Dr. Lahita is one of the world's leading lupus experts who provides, with the help of Dr. Phillips, a lot of information and facts about lupus in a question-and-answer format. This is perfect for the person who likes to read a little bit at a time without a long dialogue.)

*Lupus Underground: A Patient's Case for a Long-Ignored, Drug-Free, Non-Patentable, Counter-Intuitive Therapy That Actually Works.* A. DeBartolo. Hyde Park Media, 2004. (Mr. DeBartolo is a champion in spreading the word about the use of UVA-1 therapy in treating lupus. He is dedicated to getting the word out to the lupus community. This book goes deeply into the science behind it as well as offers information on how to use UVA-1 therapy. Hopefully the rheumatologic community will start to do larger studies to further investigate its usefulness.)

*The Memory Bible: An Innovative Strategy for Keeping Your Brain Young.* G. W. Small. Hyperion, 2003. (Large numbers of lupus patients suffer from memory problems, called cognitive dysfunction. This book gives practical advice on how to improve one's memory.)

*New Hope for People with Lupus: Your Friendly, Authoritative Guide to the Latest in Traditional and Complementary Solutions.* T. F. DiGeronimo. Prima, 2002. (This book provides a lot of excellent, practical advice on many aspects of complementary therapies in lupus such as UV protection, diet, and exercise. I do not agree with some of the conclusions about how effective many of the treatments are because some poor-quality studies are listed to support use of some therapies. However, it goes into detail about many complementary therapies beyond what chapter 39 in this book deals with. The vast majority of these therapies are safe for people who have lupus. Please read chapter 39, which covers more stringent medical views on complementary therapies, and ask your doctor if any of these therapies are safe for your particular situation before using them. I think it is important to list a book about complementary medicine for people who have lupus and who wish to know more about this subject. I find this one to be overall very well done.)

*Nuances of Nasal and Sinus Self-Help.* S. F. Rudy. Trafford Publishing, 2003. (This book provides extensive self-help advice for people who have lupus and Sjögren's syndrome suffering from dry, irritated, sore noses and recurrent sinus problems.)

*Peripheral Neuropathy: When the Numbness, Weakness, and Pain Won't Stop.* N. Latov. Demos Medical Publishing, 2006.

*The Scleroderma Book: A Guide for Patients and Families.* M. D. Mayes. Oxford University Press, 2005.

*Sick and Tired of Feeling Sick and Tired: Living with Invisible Chronic Illness.* 2nd edition. P. J. Donoghue and M. E. Siegel. W. W. Norton & Company, 2000. (This book, written by two psychologists, contains lots of self-help strategies useful in living with a chronic illness.)

*The Sjögren's Book.* 4th edition. D. J. Wallace. Oxford University Press, 2011. (This book is excellent, and is certainly the most comprehensive book written about Sjögren's syndrome. However, it is written for both health professionals and patients. Therefore, much of the information is highly technical and written at a physician level. This book is for those who want to know as much as they can and who can read at a postgraduate level. An easier-to-read book is *A Body out of Balance,* listed above.)

*The Sjögren's Syndrome Survival Guide.* T. P. Rumpf and K. M. Hammitt. New Harbinger Publications, 2003. (This book includes many self-help strategies in dealing with Sjögren's syndrome.)

*Social Security, Medicare and Government Pensions: Get the Most Out of Your Retirement and Medical Benefits.* 16th ed. D. M. Berman and J. Matthews. Nolo, 2011.

*Taking Charge of Lupus: How to Manage the Disease and Make the Most of Your Life.* D. Hallegua and M. Pratt. New American Library, 2002. (This book contains a lot of practical advice on what people who have lupus can do to cope with the disease in their daily life.)

*Thriving with Your Autoimmune Disorder: A Woman's Mind-Body Guide.* S. Ravicz. New Harbinger Publications, 2000. (This book is written by a psychologist with chapters addressing SLE, Sjögren's syndrome, as well as other disorders commonly seen in people who have lupus. This book's strength lies in its addressing psychological coping mechanisms to include mind-body techniques.)

*The Vulvodynia Survival Guide: How to Overcome Painful Vaginal Symptoms and Enjoy an Active Lifestyle.* H. I. Glazer and G. M. Rodke. New Harbinger Publications, 2002. (Many women who have SLE do not realize how Sjögren's syndrome may play a role in some of their problems. If you note vaginal dryness problems accompanied by its associated difficulties, this is an excellent source of information.)

*The Woman's Book of Sleep: A Complete Resource Guide.* A. Wolfson and K. A. Lee. New Harbinger Publications, 2001. (A large percentage of people who have SLE have insomnia with accompanied fatigue. Getting a good night's sleep is essential, and this book provides a lot of good advice for improving one's sleep habits.)

*Women, Work, and Autoimmune Disease: Keep Working, Girlfriend!* J. Friedlander and R. Joffe. Demos Health, 2008.

*You Can Cope with Peripheral Neuropathy: 365 Tips for Living a Full Life.* M. Cushing. ReadHowYouWant, 2012.

# BIBLIOGRAPHY

## GENERAL

Aringer M, Burkhardt H, Burmester GR, Fischer-Betz R, Fleck M, et al. Current state of evidence on "off-label" therapeutic options for systemic lupus erythematosus, including biological immunosuppressive agents, in Germany, Austria and Switzerland—a consensus report. *Lupus*. April 2012;21(4):386–401.

Petri M, Abuav R, Boumpas D, Goldblatt F, Isenberg I, Anhalt GJ, et al. Systemic lupus erythematosus. In: Stone JH, ed. *A Clinician's Pearls and Myths in Rheumatology*. New York: Springer Science+Business Media; 2009:131–155.

Tsokos G, Buyon JP, Koike T, Lahita RG, eds. *Systemic Lupus Erythematosus*. 5th ed. San Diego, Ca: Elsevier Academic Press; 2010.

Wallace DJ. *The Lupus Book*. 5th ed. New York, NY: Oxford University Press, Inc.; 2012.

Wallace DJ, Hahn BH, eds. *Dubois' Lupus Erythematosus*. 7th ed. Philadelphia, Pa: Lippincott Williams & Wilkins; 2007.

*UpToDate, Inc.* Retrieved August 1, 2010–August 31, 2011, from www.uptodate.com.

## CHAPTER 1

Allison MJ, Gerszten E, Martinez AJ, Klurfeld DM. Generalized connective tissue disease in a mummy from the Huari culture (Peru). *Bulletin of the New York Academy of Medicine*. April 1977;53(3):292–301.

Bateman T. *A Practical Synopsis of Cutaneous Diseases, According to the Arrangements of Dr. Willan*. Thomas AT, ed. 8th ed. London: Longman, Rees, Orme, Brown, Green and Longman, Paternoster-Row; 1936:298–299.

Du Cange. *Glossarium medie et infimelatinitatis*. Carpenterii DP, Henschel GAL, Favre L, eds. Niort [France]; 1885: *tomusquintus, col. 155b*.

Farmer S. *Communities of Saint Martin: Legend and Ritual in Medieval Tours*. Ithaca, NY: Cornell University Press; 1991:271–276.

Guigonis de Caulhiaco (Guy de Chauliac). *Inventariumsive Chirurgia Magna*. Vol. 2: Commentary. McVaugh M, Ogden MS, eds. Leiden, The Netherlands: Koninklyke Brill; 1997:183.

Hebernus (Archbishop of Tours). Miracula B. Martini [The Miracles of St. Martin]. AD 855. In: *Anastasius (the Librarian). Patrologiae Cursus Completus Sive Bibliotheca Universalis, Integra, Uniformis, Commoda, Oeconomica, Omnium SS Patrum, Doctorum Scriptorum que Ecclesiasticorum, patrologiae tomus CXXIX*. Paris: J.-P. Migne; 1853: col. 1036. Translated from the Latin into English courtesy of Darrel W. Amundsen, professor emeritus of Classics, Western Washington University, Bellingham, Wa.

Hebra F, Kaposi M. *On Diseases of the Skin Including the Exanthemata*. London: The New Sydenham Society; 1875:50.

Kaposi M. *Lupus Vulgaris*. In: Virchow RLK, ed. *Handbuch der speciellenpathologie und therapie*. Vol. 3, part 2: *Lehrbuch der hautkrankheiten*. Stuttgart: Verlag von Ferdinand Enke; 1876:325. Translated from the German and Latin by Gary E. O'Connor.

*La vie et les miracles de Monseigneur Saint Martin* [The life and miracles of Saint Martin (of Tours)]. May 7, 1496. Translated from Latin to French by Mathieu Latheron. Obtained from Paris, Bibliotèque Nationale. La Réserve (shelf mark) vélin 1159: L1 v°.

Makol A, Petri M. Pancreatitis in systemic lupus erythematosus: frequency and associated factors—a review of the Hopkins Lupus Cohort. *Journal of Rheumatology*. 2010;37:341–345.

Merrill JT. The rarity of antinuclear antibody negativity in systemic lupus erythematosus: comment on the article by Merrill et al. [Reply to letter to the editor]. *Arthritis & Rheumatism*. March 2011;63(4):1157–1158.

Petri, M, Systemic Lupus International Collaborating Clinic (SLICC). SLICC revision of the ACR classification criteria for SLE [Abstract]. *Arthritis & Rheumatism*. 2009;60(suppl 10):895.

Sacks JJ, Luo YH, Helmick CG. Prevalence of specific types of arthritis and other rheumatic conditions in the ambulatory health care system in the United States, 2001–2005. *Arthritis Care & Research*. April 2010;62(4):460–464.

Smith CD, Cyr M. The history of lupus erythematosus: from Hippocrates to Osler. *Rheumatic Disease Clinics of North America*. 1988;14:1–14.

## CHAPTER 2

Burgio GR, Martini A. Immunological features of diffuse connective tissue diseases. *European Journal of Pediatrics*. January 1990;149:224–231.

Connor SK. Systemic lupus erythematosus: a report on twelve cases treated with quinacrine (Atabrine) and chloroquine (Aralen). *Annals of Rheumatic Diseases*. 1957;16:76–81.

Dubois EL. The effect of the L. E. Cell test on the clinical picture of systemic lupus erythematosus. *Annals of Internal Medicine*. June 1953;38(6):1265–1294.

Friou GJ. Proceedings of the forty-ninth annual meeting of the American Society for Clinical Investigation held in Atlantic City, N. J., May 6, 1957: Clinical application of lupus serum-nucleoprotein reaction using fluorescent antibody technique. *Journal of Clinical Investigation*. June 1957;36(6):890–898.

Hargraves MM. Discovery of the LE cell and its morphology. *Mayo Clinic Proceedings*. September 1969;44(9):579–599.

Hargraves MM. Presentation of two bone marrow elements: the "Tart" Cell and the "L.E." Cell. *Staff Meetings of the Mayo Clinic*. January 1948;23(2):25–28.

Hepburn AL. Heberden historical series: the LE Cell. *Rheumatology*. 2001;40:826–827.

Holman H. The discovery of autoantibody to deoxyribonucleic acid. *Lupus*. 2011;20:441–442.

Klemperer P, Pollack AD, Baehr G. Diffuse collagen disease: acute disseminated erythematosus and diffuse scleroderma. *Journal of the American Medical Association*. May 1942;119:331–332.

Mosca M, Tani C, Talarico R, Bombardieri S. Undifferentiated connective tissue diseases (UCTD): simplified systemic autoimmune diseases. *Autoimmunity Reviews*. September 2010 [Epub ahead of print].

Wallace DJ, ed. *The Sjögren's Book*. New York: Oxford University Press; 2012.

CHAPTER 3

Alarcón-Segovia D, Alarcón-Riquelme M, Cardiel MH, Caeiro F, Massardo L, et al. Familial aggregation of systemic lupus erythematosus, rheumatoid arthritis, and other autoimmune diseases in 1,177 lupus patients from the GLADEL cohort. *Arthritis & Rheumatism*. April 2005;52(4):1138–1147.

Andreoli L, Piantoni S, Fall'Ara F, et al. Vitamin D and antiphospholipid syndrome. *Lupus*. June 2012;21(7):736–740.

Birmingham DJ, Hebert LA, Song H, Noonan WT, Rovin BH, et al. Evidence that abnormally large seasonal declines in vitamin D status may trigger SLE flare in non-African Americans. *Lupus*. July 2012;21(8):855–864.

Boeckler P, Cosnes A, Francès C, Hedelin G, Lipsker D. Association of cigarette smoking but not alcohol consumption with cutaneous lupus erythematosus. *Archives of Dermatology*. September 2009;145(9):1012–1016.

Bonakdar ZS, Jahanshahifar L, Jahanshahifar F, Gholamrezaei A. Vitamin D deficiency and its association with disease activity in new cases of systemic lupus erythematosus. *Lupus*. 2011;20:1155–1160.

Cervera R. "ASIA": a new systemic autoimmune syndrome? *Lupus*. 2010;20:665–666.

Chou C-T. Alternative therapies: what role do they have in the management of lupus? *Lupus*. 2010;19:1425–1429.

Cooper G, Gilbert K, Greidinger E, James J, Pfau J, et al. Avanços e oportunidades atuais na pesquisa sobre lupus: influências ambientais e mecanismos da doença [Recent advances and opportunities in research on lupus: environmental influences and mechanisms of disease]. *Ciência & Saúde Coletiva*. November/December 2009;14(5):1865–1876.

Cooper G, Wither J, Bernatsky S, Claudio JO, Clarke A, et al. Occupational and environmental exposures and risk of systemic lupus erythematosus: silica, sunlight, solvents. *Rheumatology* (Oxford). November 2010;49(11):2172–2180.

Cooper GS, Dooley MA, Treadwell EL, St. Clair EW, Parks CG, et. al. Hormonal, environmental, and infectious risk factors for developing systemic lupus erythematosus. *Arthritis & Rheumatism*. October 1998;41(10):1714–1724.

Criswell LA. Genome-wide association studies of SLE. *The Rheumatologist*. February 2011;5(2):1, 26, 27, 31–32.

Deapen D, Escalante A, Weinrib L, Horwitz D, Bachman B, et al. A revised estimate of twin concordance in systemic lupus erythematosus. *Arthritis & Rheumatism*. March 1992;35(3):311–318.

Harley JB, James JA. Everyone comes from somewhere: systemic lupus erythematosus and Epstein-Barr virus induction of host interferon and humoral anti-Epstein-Barr nuclear antigen 1 immunity. *Arthritis & Rheumatism*. June 2010;62(6):1571–1575.

Hession MT, Au SC, Gottlieb AB. Parvovirus B 19-associated systemic lupus erythematosus: clinical mimicry or autoimmune induction? *Journal of Rheumatology*. 2010;37:2430–2432.

Hutchinson J. Harveian lectures on lupus. *British Medical Journal*. January 1888;1(1412):58–63.

Jimenez-Caliani A, Jimenez-Jorge S, Molinero P, Rubio A, Guerrero JM, Osuna C. Treatment with testosterone or estradiol in melatonin treated females and males MRL/MpJ-Fas[lpr] mice induces negative effects in developing systemic lupus erythematosus. *Journal of Pineal Research*. September 2008; 45(2):204–211.

Johnson KL, McAlindon TE, Mulcahy E, Bianchi DW. Microchimerism in a female patient with systemic lupus erythematosus. *Arthritis & Rheumatism*. September 2001;44(9):2107–2111.

Kamen DL. Vitamin D: new kid on the block? *Bulletin of the NYU Hospital for Joint Diseases*. 2010;68(3):218–222.

Kaufman M. Pancytopenia following use of hydralazine ("Apresoline"): report of a case. *Journal of the American Medical Association*. 1953;151(17):1488–1490.

Kremer Hovinga ICL, Koopmans M, Baelde HJ, van der Wal AM, Sijpkens YWJ, et al. Chimerism occurs twice as often in lupus nephritis as in normal kidneys. *Arthritis & Rheumatism*. September 2006;54(9):2944–2950.

Lim S-Y, Ghosh SK. Autoreactive responses to an environmental factor: 1. Phthalate induces antibodies exhibiting anti-DNA specificity. *Immunology*. December 2003;110(4):482–492.

Lupus Foundation of America, Inc. Complex genetics of lupus. Retrieved January 1, 2011, from www.lupus.org/webmodules/webarticlesnet/templates/new_aboutdiagnosis.aspx ?articleid=413&zoneid=15.

Maestroni GJ, Otsa K, Cutolo M. Melatonin treatment does not improve rheumatoid arthritis. *British Journal of Clinical Pharmacology*. May 2008;65(5):797–798.

Mok CC, Birmingham DJ, Ho LY, Hebert LA, Song H, Rovin BH. Vitamin D deficiency as marker for disease activity and damage in systemic lupus erythematosus: a comparison with anti-ds DNA and anti-C1q. *Lupus*. 2012;21:36–42.

Moser KL, Kelly JA, Lessard CJ, Harley JB. Recent insights into the genetic basis of systemic lupus erythematosus. *Genes & Immunity*. May 2009;10(5):373–379.

Murashima A, Fukazawa T, Hirashima M, Takasaki Y, Oonishi M, et al. Long term prognosis of children born to lupus patients. *Annals of Rheumatic Diseases*. January 2004;63(1):50–53.

Perry H, Schroeder H. Syndrome simulating collagen disease caused by hydralazine (Apresoline). *Journal of the American Medical Association*. February 1954;154(8):670–673.

Pertea M, Salzberg SL. Between a chicken and a grape: estimating the number of human genes. *Genome Biology*. May 2010;11:206:1–7. Retrieved January 1, 2011, from www .genomebiology.com/2010/11/5/206.

Petri M. Diet and systemic lupus erythematosus: from mouse and monkey to woman? *Lupus*. 2001;10:775–777.

Ruiz-Irastorza G, Gordo S, Olivares N, Egurbide M-V, Aguirre C. Changes in vitamin D levels in patients with systemic lupus erythematosus: effects on fatigue, disease activity, and damage. *Arthritis Care & Research*. August 2010;62(8):1160–1165.

Schonfeld AR. Insecticides linked to autoimmune diseases. *Rheumatology News*. November 2009;8(11):12.

Scofield RH, Bruner GR, Namjou B, Kimberly RP, Ramsey-Goldman R, et al. Klinefelter's syndrome (47,XXY) in male systemic lupus erythematosus patients: support for the notion of a gene-dose effect from the X chromosome. *Arthritis & Rheumatism*. August 2008;58(8):2511–2517.

Tsokos GC. Mechanisms of disease: systemic lupus erythematosus. *New England Journal of Medicine*. December 2011;365(22):2110–2121.

Zhou L-l, Wei W, Si J-F, Yuan D-P. Regulatory effect of melatonin on cytokine disturbances in the pristine-induced lupus mice. *Mediators of Inflammation*. Vol. 2010, article ID 951210, 7 pages, 2010. doi:10.1155/2010/951210. Retrieved July 4, 2011, from www.hindawi.com/ journals/mi/2010/951210/cta/.

Zandman-Goddard G, Solomon M, Rosman Z, Peeva E, Shoenfeld Y. Environment and lupus-related diseases. *Lupus*. 2012;21:241–250.

Zulian F, Pluchinotta FR, Martini G, Da Dalt L, Zachello G. Severe clinical course of systemic lupus erythematosus in the first year of life. *Lupus*. 2008;17:780–786.

### CHAPTER 4

Aggarwal R, Liao K, Nair R, Ringold S, Costenbader KH. Anti-citrullinated peptide antibody assays and their role in the diagnosis of rheumatoid arthritis. *Arthritis & Rheumatism*. November 2009;61(11):1472–1483.

Aldar H, Lapa AT, Bellini B, Siknicato NA, Postal M, et al. Prevalence and clinical significance of anti-ribosomal P antibody in childhood-onset systemic lupus erythematosus. *Lupus*. 2012;21:1225–1231.

American College of Rheumatology. *Position Statement: Methodology of Testing for Antinuclear Antibodies*. Retrieved August 24, 2011, from www.rheumatology.org/practice/clinical/position/ana_position_stmt.pdf.

Amezcua-Guerra LM. High-sensitivity C-reactive protein is not a good indicator of infection in patients with systemic lupus erythematosus [Letter to the editor]. *Lupus*. 2011;20:1567–1568.

Cervera R, Vinas O, Ramos-Casals M, Font J, Garcia-Carrasco M, Siso A, et al. Anti-chromatin antibodies in systemic lupus erythematosus: a useful marker for lupus nephropathy. *Annals of Rheumatic Diseases*. May 2003;62(5):431–434.

Firooz N, Albert DA, Wallace DJ, Ishimori M, Berel D, Weisman MH. High-sensitivity C-reactive protein and erythrocyte sedimentation rate in systemic lupus erythematosus. *Lupus*. 2011;20:588–597.

Gerli R, Caponi L, Tincani A, Scorza R, Sabbadini MG, et al. Clinical and serological associations of ribosomal P autoantibodies in systemic lupus erythematosus: prospective evaluation in a large cohort of Italian patients. *Rheumatology* (Oxford). 2002;41(12):1357–1366.

Haserick JR, Long R. Systemic lupus erythematosus preceded by false-positive serologic tests for syphilis: presentation of five cases. *Annals of Internal Medicine*. September 1952;37(3):559–565.

Kakumanu P, Sobel ES, Narain S, Li Y, Akaogi J, Yamasaki Y, et al. Citrulline dependence of anti-cyclic citrullinated peptide antibodies in systemic lupus erythematosus as a marker of deforming/erosive arthritis. *Journal of Rheumatology*. November 2009;36(12):2682–2690.

Karassa FB, Aleltra A, Ambrozic A, Chang DM, De Keyser F, et al. Accuracy of anti-ribosomal P protein antibody testing for the diagnosis of neuropsychiatric systemic lupus erythematosus: an international meta-analysis. *Arthritis & Rheumatism*. 2006;54(1):312–324.

Kavanaugh A, Tomar R, Reveille J, Solomon DH, Homburger HA. Guidelines for clinical use of the antinuclear antibody test and tests for specific autoantibodies to nuclear antigens. *Archives of Pathology & Laboratory Medicine*. January 2000;124(1):71–81.

Kim H-A, Jeon J-Y, An J-M, Koh G-R, Suh C-H. C-reactive protein is a more sensitive and specific marker for diagnosing bacterial infections in systemic lupus erythematosus compared to S100A8/A9 and procalcitonin. *Journal of Rheumatology*. 2012;39(4):728–734.

Merrill JT. The rarity of antinuclear antibody negativity in systemic lupus erythematosus: comment on the article by Merrill et al. [Reply to letter to the editor]. *Arthritis & Rheumatism*. March 2011;63(4):1157–1158.

Moore JE, Shulman LE, Scott JT. The natural history of systemic lupus erythematosus—an approach to its study through chronic biologic false positive reactors: interim report. *Transactions of the American and Climatological Association*. 1957;68:59–68.

Murphy FT, George R, Kubota K, Fears M, Pope V, Howard RS, Dennis G. The use of western blotting as the confirmatory test for syphilis in patients with rheumatic disease. *Journal of Rheumatology*. 1999;26:2448–2453.

Rensch MJ, Szyjkowski R, Shaffer RT, Fink S, Kopecky C, Grissmer L, Enzenhauer R, Kadakia S. The prevalence of celiac disease autoantibodies in patients with systemic lupus erythematosus. *American Journal of Gastroenterology*. 2001;96:1113–1115.

Respaldiza N, Wichmann I, Ocaña C, Garcia-Hernandez FJ, Castillo MJ, Magariño MI, et al. Anti-centromere antibodies in patients with systemic lupus erythematosus. *Scandinavian Journal of Rheumatology*. July 2006;35(4):290–294.

Rezaieyazdi Z, Sahebari M, Hatef MR, Abbasi B, Rafatpanah H, et al. Is there any correlation between high sensitive CRP and disease activity in systemic lupus erythematosus? *Lupus*. 2011;20:1494–1500.

Ruiz-Irastorza G, Gordo S, Olivares N, Egurbide M-V, Aguirre C. Changes in vitamin D levels in patients with systemic lupus erythematosus: effects on fatigue, disease activity, and damage. *Arthritis Care & Research*. August 2010;62(8):1160–1165.

Ruperto N, Hanrahan LM, Alarcón GS, Belmont HM, Brey RL, et al. International consensus for a definition of disease flare in lupus. *Lupus*. April 2005;20(5):453–462.

Villalta D, Bizzaro N, Tonutti E, Tozzoli R. IgG Anti-transglutaminase autoantibodies in systemic lupus erythematosus and Sjögren Syndrome [Letter to the editor]. *Clinical Chemistry*. 2002;48:1133.

VonMühlen CA, Tan EM. Autoantibodies in the diagnosis of systemic rheumatic diseases. *Seminars in Arthritis and Rheumatism*. April 1995;24(5):323–358.

CHAPTER 5

Duarte-García A, Fang H, To CH, Magder LS, Petri M. Seasonal variation in the activity of systemic lupus erythematosus. *Journal of Rheumatology*. 2012;39(7):1392–1398.

Hebra F, Kaposi M. *Lupus Erythematosus*. Tray W, ed. and trans. *On Diseases of the Skin, Including Exanthemata*. London: The New Sydenham Society; 1875.

CHAPTER 6

Chung F, Yegneswaran B, Liao P, Chung SA, Vairavanathan S, Islam S, et al. STOP questionnaire: a tool to screen patients for obstructive sleep apnea. *Anesthesiology*. 2008;108:812–822.

Davies RJ, Lomer MCE, Yeo SI, et al. Weight loss and improvements in fatigue in systemic lupus erythematosus: a controlled trial of a low glycaemic index diet versus a calorie restricted diet in patients treated with corticosteroids. *Lupus*. May 2012;21(6):649–655.

Mackowiak PA, Wasserman SS, Levine MM. A critical appraisal of 98.6 degrees F, the upper limit of the normal body temperature, and other legacies of Carl Reinhold August Wunderlich. *Journal of the American Medical Association*. 1992;268(12):1578–1580.

Mishra R, Vivino FB. Diagnosis and management of fatigue. In: Wallace DJ, ed. *The Sjögren's Book*. New York: Oxford University Press; 2012:228–234.

O'Malley PG, Jackson JL, Santoro J, Tomkins G, Balden E, Kroenke K. Antidepressant therapy for unexplained symptoms and symptom syndromes. *Journal of Family Practice*. 1999;48(12):980–990.

Sheon RP, Moskowitz RW. *Soft Tissue Rheumatic Pain*. 3rd ed. Philadelphia, Pa: Lippincott Williams & Wilkins; 1996.

Stockton KA, Kandiah DA, Paratz JD, Bennell KL. Fatigue, muscle strength and vitamin D status in women with systemic lupus erythematosus compared with healthy controls. *Lupus.* March 2012;21(3):271–278.

Yuen HK, Holthaus, Kamen DL, Sword DO, Breland HL. Using Wii Fit to reduce fatigue among African American women with systemic lupus erythematosus: a pilot study. *Lupus.* 2011;20:1293–1299.


CHAPTER 7

Abebe W. Herbal medication: potential for adverse interactions with analgesic drugs. *Journal of Pharmacy and Therapeutics.* December 2002;27(6):391–401.

Guillaume de Baillou. Retrieved May 7, 2011, from www.en.wikipedia.org/wiki/Guillaume_Baillou.

Kaufman MB. Drug updates: information on new approvals and medication safety. *The Rheumatologist.* September 2011. Retrieved October 1, 2011, from www.the-rheumatologist.org/details/article/1332713/Drug_Updates.html.

Lawrence JS. What we know and need to know about rheumatism. *New Scientist.* January 1964;219:202–205.

Longstreth M. *Rheumatism, Gout, and Some Allied Disorders.* New York: William Wood & Co; 1882.

Nakhai-Pour HR, Broy P, Sheehy O, Bérard A. Use of nonaspirin nonsteroidal anti-inflammatory drugs during pregnancy and the risk of spontaneous abortion. *Canadian Medical Association Journal.* 2011;183:1713.

Rheumatism. Retrieved May 7, 2011, from www.inform.com/health/rheumatism-2646230a.

Saketkoo LA, Quinet R. Revisiting Jaccoud arthropathy as an ultrasound diagnosed erosive arthropathy in systemic lupus erythematosus. *Journal of Clinical Rheumatology.* December 2007;13(6):322–327.

Sheon RP, Moskowitz RW, Goldberg VM. *Soft Tissue Rheumatic Pain: Recognition, Management, and Prevention.* 3rd ed. Philadelphia, Pa: Lippincott Williams & Wilkins.

Shlotzhauer TL, McGuire JL. *Living with Rheumatoid Arthritis.* 2nd ed. Baltimore, Md: Johns Hopkins University Press; 2003.

Wright S, Filippucci E, Grassi W, Grey A, Bell A. Hand arthritis in systemic lupus erythematosus: an ultrasound pictorial essay. *Lupus.* August 2006;15(8):501–506.


CHAPTER 8

Grönhagen CM, Gunnarsson I, Svenungsson E, Nyberg F. Cutaneous manifestations and serological findings in 260 patients with systemic lupus erythematosus. *Lupus.* 2010;19:1187–1194.

Jancin B. Cutaneous LE likely to progress to SLE early. *Rheumatology News.* November 2011;9(11):12.

La Placa M, Passarini B. Subacute cutaneous lupus erythematosus after a tattoo. *Clinical and Experimental Dermatology.* July 2009;34(5):632–633.


CHAPTER 9

Ali YM, Urowitz MB, Ibañez D, Gladman DD. Monoclonal gammopathy in systemic lupus erythematosus. *Lupus.* 2007;16:426–429.

Angles-Cano E, Sultan Y, Clauvel J-P. Predisposing factors to thrombosis in systemic lupus erythematosus: possible relation to endothelial cell damage. *Journal of Laboratory Clinical Medicine*. August 1979;94(2):312–323.

Baehr G, Klemperer P, Schifrin A. A diffuse disease of the peripheral circulation (usually associated with lupus erythematosus and endocarditis). *American Journal of Medicine*. November 1952;13(5):591–596.

Beaumont JL. [Acquired hemorrhagic syndrome caused by a circulatin anticoagulant; inhibition of the thromboplastic function of the blood platelets; description of a specific test]. *Sang* 1954;25(1):1–15.

Bertero MT. Primary prevention in antiphospholipid antibody carriers. *Lupus*. 2012;21:751–754.

Bowie EJW, Thompson Jr JH, Pascuzzi CA, Owen Jr CA. Thrombosis in systemic lupus erythematosus despite circulatin anticoagulants. *Journal of Laboratory and Clinical Medicine*. September 1963;62:416–430.

Castillo-Martínez D, Amezcua-Guerra LM, Bojalil R. Neutropenia and the risk of infections in ambulatory patients with systemic lupus erythematosus: a three-year prospective study cohort [Letter to the editor]. *Lupus*. 2011;20:998–1000.

Conley CL, Rathbun HK, et al. Circulating anticoagulant as a cause of hemorrhagic diathesis in man. *Bulletin of the Johns Hopkins Hospital*. October 1948;83(4):288–296.

Feinstein DI, Rapaport SI. Acquired inhibitors of blood circulation. *Progress in Hemostasis and Thrombosis*. 1972;1:75–95.

Hughes GRV. Connective tissue disease and the skin [The Prosser-White Oration 1983]. *Clinical and Experimental Dermatology*. 1984;9:535–544.

Ley AB, Reader GG, Sorensen CW, Overman RS. Idiopathic hypoprothrombinemia associated with hemorrhagic diathesis, and the effect of vitamin K. *Blood*. 1951;6(8):740–755.

Pengo V, Denas G, Banzato A, Bison E, Bracco A, et al. Secondary prevention in thrombotic antiphospholipid syndrome. *Lupus*. June 2012;21(7):734–735.

CHAPTER 10

Badshaa H, Cheng LT, Konga KO, Liana TY, Chnga HH. Pulmonary hemorrhage in systemic lupus erythematosus. *Seminars in Arthritis and Rheumatism*. June 2004;33(6):414–421.

Minai OA. An update in pulmonary hypertension in systemic lupus erythematosus—do we need to know about it? [Letter to the editor]. *Lupus*. 2009;18:92.

Santiago-Casas Y, Vila LM. Pulmonary hemorrhage in patients with systemic lupus erythematosus. *Current Respiratory Medicine Reviews*. February 2009;5(1):49–54.

CHAPTER 11

Apte M, McGwin Jr G, Vilá LM, Kaslow RA, Alarcón GS, Reveille JD, et al. Associated factors and impact of myocarditis in patients with SLE from LUMINA, a multiethnic US cohort. *Rheumatology* (Oxford). 2008;47(3):362–367.

Borenstein DG, Fye WB, Arnett FC, Stevens MB. The myocarditis of systemic lupus erythematosus: association with myositis. *Annals of Internal Medicine*. 1978;89:619–624.

Bourré-Tessier J, Huynh T, Clarke AE, Bernatsky S, Joseph L, et al. Features associated with cardiac abnormalities in systemic lupus erythematosus. *Lupus*. December 2011;20(14):1518–1525.

Mavrogeni S, Bratis K, Markussis V, Spargias C, Papadopoulou E, et al. The diagnostic role of cardiac magnetic resonance imaging in detecting myocardial inflammation in systemic lupus erythematosus. Differentiation from viral myocarditis. *Lupus*. January 2013;22(1):34–43.

Suri V, Varma S, Joshi K, Malhotra P, Kumari S, Jain S. Lupus myocarditis improvement in cardiac function after intravenous immunoglobulin therapy. *Rheumatology International*. 2010;30(11):1503–1505.

Your heart and blood vessels. Retrieved April 23, 2011, from www.my.clevelandclinic.org/heart/heartworks/heartfacts.aspx.

Zawadowski GM, Klarich KW, Moder KG, Edwards WD, Cooper Jr. LT. A contemporary case series of lupus myocarditis. *Lupus*. October 2012;21:1378–1384.


CHAPTER 12

Alarcon GS. The LUMINA Study: impact beyond lupus in U.S. Hispanics. *The Rheumatologist*. April 2011;5(4):1+.

Castro-Santana LE, Colón M, Molina M, Rodríguez VE, Mayor AM, Vilá LM. Efficacy of two cyclophosphamide regimens for the treatment of lupus nephritis in Puerto Ricans: low vs standard dose. *Ethnicity & Disease*. Spring 2010(suppl 1);20:116–121.

Dooley MA, Houssiau F, Aranow C, et al. Effect of belimumab treatment on renal outcomes: results from the phase 3 belimumab clinical trials in patients with SLE. *Lupus*. January 2013;22(1):63–72.

Hahn BH, McMahon MA, Wilkinson A, Wallace WD, Daikh DI, et al. American College of Rheumatology guidelines for screening, treatment, and management of lupus nephritis. *Arthritis Care & Research*. June 2012;64(6):797–808.

Norby GE, Leivestad T, Mjøen G, Hartmann A, Midtvedt K, Gran JT, et al. Premature cardiovascular disease in patients with systemic lupus erythematosus influences survival after renal transplantation. *Arthritis & Rheumatism*. March 2011;63(3):733–737.

Shimiau A, Tamura A, Tago O, Abe M, Nagai Y, Ishikawa O. Lupus cystitis: a case and review of the literature. *Lupus*. 2009;18:655–658.

Tornatore KM, Sudchada P, Dole K, DiFrancesco R, Leca N, Gundroo AC, et al. Mycophenolic acid pharmacokinetics during maintenance immunosuppression in African American and Caucasian renal transplant recipients. *Journal of Clinical Pharmacology*. January 2011. Retrieved April 10, 2011, from www.jcp.sagepub.com/content/early/2011/01/05/00912700 10382909.abstract.

Wakasugi D, Gono T, Kawaguchi Y, Hara M, Koseki Y, et al. Frequency of class III and IV nephritis in systemic lupus erythematosus without clinical renal involvement: an analysis of predictive measures. *Journal of Rheumatology*. 2012;39:79–85.

Weening JJ, D'Agati VD, Schwartz MM, Seshan SV, Alpers CE, Appel GB, et al. The classification of glomerulonephritis in systemic lupus erythematosus revisited. *Journal of the American Society of Nephrology*. 2004;15:241–250.

Zhang G, Li H, Huang W, Li X, Li X. Clinical features of lupus cystitis complicated with hydroureteronephrosis in a Chinese population. *Journal of Rheumatology*. 2011;38:667–671.


CHAPTER 13

ACR Ad Hoc Committee on Neuropsychiatric Lupus Nomenclature. The American College of Rheumatology nomenclature and case definitions for neuropsychiatric lupus syndromes. *Arthritis & Rheumatism*. April 1999;42(4):599–608.

Antonchak MA, Saoudian M, Khan AR, Brunner HI, Luggen ME. Cognitive dysfunction in patients with systemic lupus erythematosus: a controlled study. *Journal of Rheumatology.* 2011;38:1020–1025.

Buća A, Perković D, Martinović D, Vlastelica M, Titlić M. Neuropsychiatric systemic lupus erythematosus: diagnostic and clinical features according to revised ACR criteria. *Collegium Antropologicum.* March 2009;33(1):281–288.

Dave S, Longmuir R, Shah VA, Wall M, Lee AG. Intracranial hypertension in systemic lupus erythematosus. *Seminars in Ophthalmology.* 2008;23(2):127–133.

Hanly JG. ACR classification criteria for systemic lupus erythematosus: limitations and revisions to neuropsychiatric variables. *Lupus.* 2004;13:861–864.

Katz P, Julian L, Tonner MC, Yazdany J, Trupin L, et al. Physical activity, obesity, and cognitive impairment among women with systemic lupus erythematosus. *Arthritis Care & Research.* 2012;64(4):502–510.

Kozora E, Hanly JG, Lapteva L, Filley CM. Cognitive dysfunction in systemic lupus erythematosus: past, present, and future. *Arthritis & Rheumatism.* November 2008;58(11):3286–3298.

Kroenke K, Spitzer RL, Williams JB. The PHQ-9: validity of a brief depression severity measure. *Journal of General Internal Medicine.* 2001;16(9):606–613.

Lorayne H, Lucas J. *The Memory Book: The Classic Guide to Improving Your Memory at Work, at School, and at Play.* New York: Ballantine Books; 1996.

Migraines are not a lupus symptom: study. *Reuters.* August 30, 2011. Retrieved September 11, 2011, from www.reuters.com/article/2011/08/30us-migranes-lupus-idUSTRE77T51K2 0110830.

Moldovan I, Katsaros E, Carr FN, Cooray D, Torralba K, Shinada S, et al. The patient reported outcomes in lupus (PATROL) study: role of depression in health-related quality of life in a Southern California lupus cohort. *Lupus.* 2011;20:1285–1292.

Murray SG, Yazdany J, Kaiser R, Criswell LA, Trupin L, et al. Cardiovascular disease and cognitive dysfunction in systemic lupus erythematosus. *Arthritis Care & Research.* September 2012;64(9):1328–1333.

Otto MA. Guidelines address neuropsychiatric issues in SLE. *Rheumatology News.* October 2010;9(10),26.

Petri M, Naqibuddin M, Carson KA, Wallace DJ, Weisman MH, Holliday SL, et al. Depression and cognitive impairment in newly diagnosed systemic lupus erythematosus. *Journal of Rheumatology.* 2010;37(10):2032–2038.

Spitzer RL, Kroenke K, Williams JB, Lowe B. A brief measure for assessing generalized anxiety disorder: the GAD-7. *Archives of Internal Medicine.* 2006;166(10):1092–1097.

Unterman A, Nolte JES, Boaz M, Abady M, Shoenfeld Y, Zandman-Goddard G. Neuropsychiatric systemic lupus erythematosus: a meta-analysis. *Seminars in Arthritis and Rheumatism.* October 2010. Retrieved on April 17, 2011, from www.sciencedirect.com/science?_ob=ArticleURL&_udi=B6WWX-518VXJW-2&_user=10&_coverDate=10%2F20%2F2010&_rdoc=1&_fmt=high&_orig=gateway&_origin=gateway&_sort=d&_docanchor=&view=c&_searchStrId=1729238940&_rerunOrigin=scholar.google&_acct=C000050221&_version=1&_urlVersion=0&_userid=10&md5=748aec1e383e8be1d0252af89eda56ba&searchtype=a.

CHAPTER 14

Macsai MS. The role of omega-3 dietary supplementation in blepharitis and Meibomian gland dysfunction [AOS thesis]. *Transactions of the American Ophthalmological Society.* December 2008;106:336–356.

Sjögren H. Zur kenntnis der keratoconjunctivitis sicca (keratitis filiformis bei hypofunction der tranendrusen). *Acta Ophthalmologica, Copenhagen*. 1933;(suppl 2):1–151.

Wallace DJ, ed. *The Sjögren's Book*. New York: Oxford University Press; 2012.


## CHAPTER 15

Dhir V, Misra R, Agarwal V, Lawrence A, Aggarwal A. Lupus pancreatitis—early manifestation of active disease. *Lupus*. 2011;20:547–548.

Freeman HJ. Adult celiac disease followed by onset of systemic lupus erythematosus. *Journal of Clinical Gastroenterology*. March 2008;42(3):252–255.

Hoffman BI, Katz WA. The gastrointestinal manifestations of systemic lupus erythematosus: a review of the literature. *Seminars in Arthritis and Rheumatism*. 1980;9(4):237–247.

Irving KS, Sen D, Tahir H, Pilkington C, Isenberg DA. A comparison of autoimmune liver disease in juvenile and adult populations with systemic lupus erythematosus—a retrospective review of cases. *Rheumatology* (Oxford). 2007;46(7):1171–1173.

Ludvigsson JF, Rubio-Tapia A, Chowdhary V, Murray JA, Simard JF. Increased risk of systemic lupus erythematosus in 29,000 patients with biopsy-verified celiac disease. *Journal of Rheumatology*. October 2012;39(10):1964–1970.

Nesher G, Breuer GS, Temprano K, Moore TL, Dahan D, Baer A, Alberton J, et al. Lupus-associated pancreatitis. *Seminars in Arthritis and Rheumatism*. 2006;35(4):260–267.

Nitzan O, Elias M, Saliba WR. Systemic lupus erythematosus and inflammatory bowel disease. *European Journal of Internal Medicine*. 2006:313–318.

Pascual-Ramos V, Duarte-Rojo A, Villa AR, et al. Systemic lupus erythematosus as a cause and prognostic factor of acute pancreatitis. *Journal of Rheumatology*. 2004;31(4):707–712.

Piga M, Vacca A, Porru G, Caulia A, Mathieu A. Liver involvement in systemic lupus erythematosus: incidence, clinical course and outcome of lupus hepatitis. *Clinical and Experimental Rheumatology*. 2010;28(4):504–510.

Piga M, Vacca A, Porru G, Garau P, Caulia A, Mathieu A. Two different clinical subsets of lupus hepatitis exist: mimicking primary autoimmune liver diseases or part of their spectrum? *Lupus*. 2011;20:1450–1451.

Sultan SM, Ioannou Y, Isenberg DA. A review of gastrointestinal manifestations of systemic lupus erythematosus. *Rheumatology* (Oxford). 1999;38(10):917–932.

Wang CH, Yao TC, Huang YL, Ou LS, Yeh KW, Huang JL. Acute pancreatitis in pediatric and adult-onset systemic lupus erythematosus: a comparison and review of the literature. *Lupus*. 2011;20:443–452.

Zizic TM, Shulman LE, Stevens MB. Systemic lupus erythematosus. *Medicine* (Baltimore). 1975;54(5):411–426.


## CHAPTER 16

Brydak-Godowska J. [Ocular changes and general condition in lupus erythematosus (SLE)—own observation.] *Klinika Oczna*. 2007;109(1–3):11–14.

Frigui M, Frikha F, Sellemi D, Chouayakh F, Feki J, Bahlou Z. Optic neuropathy as a presenting feature of systemic lupus erythematosus: two case reports and literature review. *Lupus*. 2011;20:1214–1218.

Santosa A, Vasoo S. Orbital myositis as manifestation of systemic lupus erythematosus—a case report. *Postgraduate Medical Journal Online First*. September 11, 2012. Retrieved January 29, 2013 from http://pmj.bmj.com/articleusage?rid=postgradmedj-2012-130974v1.

## CHAPTER 17

Hijmans W, Doniach D, Roitt IM, Holborow EJ. Serological overlap between lupus erythematosus, rheumatoid arthritis, and auto-immune thyroid disease. *British Medical Journal.* October 1961;2:909–914.

Tagoe CE, Zezon A, Khattri S. Rheumatic manifestations of autoimmune thyroid disease: the other autoimmune disease. *Journal of Rheumatology.* 2012;39(6):1125–1129.

## CHAPTER 18

Bates SM, Greer IA, Pablinger I, Sofaer S, Hirsh J. Venous thromboembolism, thrombophilia, antithrombotic therapy, and pregnancy: American College of Chest Physicians evidence-based clinical practice guidelines (8th edition). *Chest.* 2008;133(6 suppl):S844.

Clowse MEB, Magder LS, Petri M. The clinical utility of measuring complement and anti-ds-DNA antibodies during pregnancy in patients with systemic lupus erythematosus. *Journal of Rheumatology.* 2011;38:1012–1016.

Clowse MEB, Magder LS, Petri M. Cyclophosphamide for lupus during pregnancy. *Lupus.* 2005;14(8):593–597.

Clowse MEB, Magder LS, Witter F, Petri M. Early risk factors for pregnancy loss in lupus. *Obstetrics & Gynecology.* February 2006;107(2):293–299.

Clowse MEB, Magder LS, Witter F, Petri M. Hydroxychloroquine in lupus pregnancy. *Arthritis & Rheumatism.* November 2006;54(11):3640–3647.

Izmirly PM, Kim MY, Llanos C, Le PU, Guerra MM, Askanase AD, et al. Evaluation of the risk of anti-SSA/Ro-anti-SSB/La antibody-associated cardiac manifestations of neonatal lupus in fetuses of mothers with systemic lupus erythematosus exposed to hydroxychloroquine. *Annals of the Rheumatic Diseases.* 2010;69:1827–1830.

Izmirly PM, Llanos C, Lee LA, Askanase A, Kim MY, Buyon JP. Cutaneous manifestations of neonatal lupus and risk of subsequent congenital heart block. *Arthritis & Rheumatism.* April 2010;62(4):1153–1157.

Jancin B. Managing rheumatologic diseases in pregnancy. *Rheumatology News.* April 2010;9(4):28.

Kubetin SK. Risk of neonatal lupus in next baby less than 20%. *Rheumatology News.* May 2010;9(5):2.

Kubetin SK. Use of echocardiograms in fetal heart block. *Rheumatology News.* May 2010;9(5):13.

Ofori B, Oraichi D, Blais L, Rey E, Bérard A. Risk of congenital abnormalities in pregnant users of non-steroidal anti-inflammatory drugs: a nested case-control study. *Birth Defects Research* (Part B). August 2006;77(4):268–279.

Otto MA. Tips for predicting high-risk pregnancies in SLE. *Rheumatology News.* August 2010;9(8):42.

Pasoto SG, Mendonça BB, Bonfá E. Menstrual disturbances in patients with systemic lupus erythematosus without alkylating therapy: clinical, humoral and therapeutic associations. *Lupus.* March 2002;11(3):175–180.

Petri M. The Hopkins Lupus Pregnancy Center: ten key issues in management. *Rheumatic Disease Clinics of North America.* May 2007;33(2):227–235.

Ruffatti A, Milanesi O, Chiandetti L, Cerutti A, Gervasi MT, et al. A combination therapy to treat second-degree anti-Ro/La-related congenital heart block. A strategy to avoid stable third-degree heart block? *Lupus.* 2012;21:666–671.

Stagnaro-Green A, Akhter E, Yim C, Davie TF, Magder LS, Petri M. Thyroid disease in pregnant women with systemic lupus erythematosus: increased preterm delivery. *Lupus.* 2011;20:690–699.

CHAPTER 19

Alarcon GS. The LUMINA Study: impact beyond lupus in U.S. Hispanics. *The Rheumatologist.* April 2011;5(4):1+.

Alonso MD, Martinez-Vazquez F, Diaz de Teran T, Miranda-Filloy JA, Dierssen T, et al. Late-onset systemic lupus erythematosus in Northwestern Spain: differences with early-onset systemic lupus erythematosus and literature review. *Lupus.* September 2012; 21(10):1135–1148.

Ang-Lee MK, Moss J, Yuan CS. Herbal medicines and perioperative care. *Journal of the American Medical Association.* July 2001;286(2):208–216.

Boumpas DT, Bertsias G. Immunosuppressive treatment for lupus in the next decade: it's time for a new strategy. *The Rheumatologist.* April 2011;5(4):1+.

Dang Do N, Umoren RA, Tarvin SE, Heilbrunn BR, Mahajerin A, Bowyer SL. Systemic lupus erythematosus in a 3-month-old male presenting as thrombocytopenia. *Lupus.* 2011;20:527–530.

Dáran S, Apte M, Alarcón GS. Poverty, not ethnicity, accounts for the differential mortality rates among lupus patients of various ethnic groups. *Journal of the National Medical Association.* October 2007;99(10):1196–1198.

De Carolis S, Botta A, Santucci S, Salvi S, Moresi S, et al. Complementemia and obstetric outcome in pregnancy with antiphospholipid syndrome. *Lupus.* June 2012;21(7):776–778.

Freire de Carvalho J, Patrícia do Nascimento A, Testagrossa LA, Barros RT, Bonfá E. Male gender results in more severe lupus nephritis. *Rheumatology International.* 2010;30(10):1311–1315.

Fernández M, Alarcón GS, Calvo-Alén J, Andrade R, McGwin Jr G, Vilá LM, et al. A multiethnic, multicenter cohort of patients with systemic lupus erythematosus (SLE) as a model for the study of ethnic disparities in SLE. *Arthritis & Rheumatism.* 2007;57(4):576.

Isenberg DA. Male lupus and the Loch Ness syndrome. *British Journal of Rheumatology.* 1994;33(4):307–308.

Jiménez-Alonso J, Jiménez-Jáimez J, Almazán MV. Pollen allergies in patients with systemic lupus erythematosus. *Journal of Rheumatology.* September 2004;31(9):1873.

Johnson K. Hallucinations common in pediatric lupus. *Rheumatology News.* March 2010;9(3):22–23.

Lalani S, Pope J, deLeon F, Peschken C. Clinical features and prognosis of late-onset systemic lupus erythematosus: results from the 1000 faces of lupus study. *Journal of Rheumatology.* 2010;37(1):38–44.

Livingston B, Bonner A, Pope J. Differences in clinical manifestations between childhood-onset lupus and adult-onset lupus: a meta-analysis. *Lupus.* 2011;20:1345–1355.

Lu L-J, Wallace DJ, Ishimori ML, Scofield RH, Weisman MH. Male systemic lupus erythematosus: a review of sex disparities in this disease. *Lupus.* 2010;19:119–129.

Peschken CA, Katz SJ, Silverman E, Pope JE, Fortin PR, Pineau C, et al. The 1000 Canadian faces of lupus: determinants of disease outcome in a large multiethnic cohort. *Journal of Rheumatology.* 2009;36(6):1200–1208.

Pope J, Jerome D, Fenlon D, Krizova A, Ouimet J. Frequency of adverse drug reactions in patients with systemic lupus erythematosus. *Journal of Rheumatology.* 2003;30:480–484.

Renau AI, Isenberg DA. Male versus female lupus: a comparison of ethnicity, clinical features, serology and outcome over a 30 year period. *Lupus*. September 2012;21(10):1041–1048.

Resende AL, Titan SM, Barros RT, Woronik V. Worse renal outcome of lupus nephritis in male patients: a case-control study. *Lupus*. 2011;20:561–567.

Sekigawa I, Yoshiike T, Iida N, Hashimoto H, Ogawa H. Allergic diseases in systemic lupus erythematosus: prevalence and immunological considerations. *Clinical and Experimental Rheumatology*. 2003;21(1):117–121.

Silva CAA, Bonfá E, Borba EF, Braga AP, Moraes AJP, Saito O, Cocuzza M. Saúde reprodutiva em homens com lupus eritematoso sistemico [Reproductive health in male systemic lupus erythematosus]. *Revista Brasileira de Reumatologia*. May/June 2009;49(3).

Tan TC, Fang H, Magder LS, Petri MA. Differences between male and female systemic lupus erythematosus in a multiethnic population. *Journal of Rheumatology*. 2012;39(4):759–769.

Thompson RA. Current status of allergen immunotherapy: shortened version of a World Health Organisation-International Union of Immunological Societies Working Group report. *Lancet*. 1989;1(8632):259–261.

Zulian F, Pluchinotta FR, Martini G, Da Dalt L, Zachello G. Severe clinical course of systemic lupus erythematosus in the first year of life. *Lupus*. 2008;17:780–786.

## CHAPTER 20

Dubois E, ed. (1966). *Lupus Erythematosus: A Review of the Current Status of Discoid and Systemic Lupus Erythematosus and Their Variants*. New York: McGraw-Hill Book Company; 1966.

Gilbert S. "Blood don't lie": The diseased family in Flannery O'Connor's *Everything that rises must converge*. *Literature and Medicine*. 1999,18(1):114–131.

Hsu C-Y, Chiu W-C, Yang T-S, Chen C-J, Chen Y-C, Lai H-M, et al. Age- and gender-related long-term renal outcome in patients with lupus nephritis. *Lupus*. 2011;20:1135-1141.

Kang KY, Kwok S-K, Ju JH, Park K-S, Cho C-S, Kim H-Y, et al. The causes of death in Korean patients with systemic lupus erythematosus over 11 years. *Lupus*. 2011;20:989–997.

Koneru S, Kocharla L, Higgins GC, Ware A, Passo M, Farhey Y, et al. Adherence to medications in systemic lupus erythematosus. *Journal of Clinical Rheumatology*. August 2008;14(4):195–201.

Mok CC. Epidemiology and survival of systemic lupus erythematosus in Hong Kong, China. *Lupus*. 2011;20:767–771.

O'Connor, F. *The Habit of Being: Letters of Flannery O'Connor*. Fitzgerald S, ed. New York: Farrar, Straus and Giroux; 1988.

Posnick J. Systemic lupus erythematosus: the effect of corticotropin and adrenocorticoid therapy on survival rate. *California Medicine*. June 1963;98(6):308–312.

Styles MM, Moccia P. *On Nursing: A Literary Celebration (an Anthology)*. Evans N, ed. New York: National League for Nursing; 1993:50–52.

## CHAPTER 21

Bengtsson C, Öhman M-L, Nived O, Rantapää Dahlqvist S. Cardiovascular event in systemic lupus erythematosus in northern Sweden: incidence and predictors in a 7-year follow-up study. *Lupus*. April 2012;21(4):452–459.

Bernatsky S, Boivin JF, Joseph L, Manzi S, Ginzler E, Gladman DD, et al. Mortality in systemic lupus erythematosus. *Arthritis & Rheumatism*. August 2006;54(8):2550–2557.

Cairoli E, Rebella M, Danese N, Garra V, Borba EF. Hydroxychloroquine reduces low-density lipoprotein cholesterol levels in systemic lupus erythematosus: a longitudinal evaluation of the lipid-lowering effect. *Lupus*. October 2012;21(11):1178–1182.

Durán S, Apte M, Alarcón GS. Poverty, not ethnicity, accounts for the differential mortality rates among lupus patients of various ethnic groups. *Journal of the National Medical Association*. October 2007;99(10):1196–1198.

Endocrinology Today. DXA more accurately predicts obesity compared with BMI. *Diabetes and Metabolism*. April 23, 2010. Retrieved May 22, 2011, from www.endocrinetoday.com/view.aspx?rid=63584.

Fessler BJ, McGwin Jr G, Alarcón GS, Roseman JM, Bastian HM, Friedman AW, et al. Hydroxychloroquine (HCQ) usage is associated with decreased renal and cardiovascular damage in patients with systemic lupus erythematosus (SLE). *Arthritis & Rheumatism*. September 2001;44(S9):S201.

Gabriel IU. Obesity. *Medscape*. April 19, 2011. Retrieved May 22, 2011, from www.emedicine.medscape.com/article/123702-overview.

Graham L. ADA releases updated recommendations on standards of medical care in diabetes. *American Family Physician*. July 2010;82(2):206.

Hahn BH, Grossman J, Ansell BJ, Skaggs BJ, McMahon M. Altered lipoprotein metabolism in chronic inflammatory states: proinflammatory high-density lipoprotein and accelerated atherosclerosis in systemic lupus erythematosus and rheumatoid arthritis. *Arthritis Research & Therapy*. 2008;10:213–225.

Hersh AO, Trupin L, Yazdany J, Panopalis P, Julian L, Katz P, et al. Childhood-onset disease as a predictor of mortality in an adult cohort of patients with systemic lupus erythematosus. *Arthritis & Rheumatism*. August 2010;62(8):1152–1159.

Ippolito A, Petri M. An update on mortality in systemic lupus erythematosus. *Clinical and Experimental Rheumatology*. 2008;26(suppl 51):S72–S79.

Jafar TH, Stark PC, Schmid CH, Landa M, Maschio G, de Jong PE, et al. Progression of chronic kidney disease: the role of blood pressure control, proteinuria, and angiotensin-converting enzyme inhibition: a patient-level meta-analysis. *Annals of Internal Medicine*. 2003;139(4):244–252.

Johnson K. Clinically quiescent lupus does not progress. *Rheumatology News*. March 2010;9(3):20.

Jung H, Bobba R, Su J, Shariati-Sarabi Z, Gladman DD, Urowitz M, Lou W, et al. The protective effect of antimalarial drugs on thrombovascular events in systemic lupus erythematosus. *Arthritis & Rheumatism*. March 2010;62(3):863–868.

Karp I, Abrahamowicz M, Fortin PR, Pilote L, Neville C, et al. Longitudinal evolution of risk of coronary heart disease in systemic lupus erythematosus. *Journal of Rheumatology*. 2012;39(5):36–41.

Kasitanon N, Magder LS, Petri M. Predictors of survival in systemic lupus erythematosus. *Medicine*. May 2006;85(3):147–156.

Katz P, Gregorich S, Yazdany J, Trupin L, Julian L, Yelin E, et al. Obesity and its measurement in a community-based sample of women with systemic lupus erythematosus. *Arthritis Care & Research*. February 2011;63(2):261–268.

Kaul MS, Rao SV, Shaw LK, Honeycutt E, Ardoin SP, St. Clair EW. Association of systemic lupus erythematosus with angiographically defined coronary artery disease: a retrospective cohort study. *Arthritis Care & Research*. 65(2):266–273.

Mancia G, De Backer G, Dominiczak A, Cifkova R, Fagard R, Germano G, et al. 2007 Guidelines for the management of arterial hypertension: the Task Force of the Management of

Arterial Hypertension of the European Society of Hypertension (ESH) and of the European Society of Cardiology (ESG). *European Heart*. 2007;28(12):1462–1536.

Mok CC, Kwok CL, Ho LY, Chan PT, Yip SF. Life expectancy, standardized mortality ratios, and causes of death in six rheumatic diseases in Hong Kong, China. *Arthritis & Rheumatism*. May 2011;63(5):1182–1189.

Rosendorff C, Black HR, Cannon CP, Gersh BJ, Gore J, Izzo Jr JL, et al. Treatment of hypertension in the prevention and management of ischemic heart disease: a scientific statement from the American Heart Association Council for High Blood Pressure Research and the Councils on Clinical Cardiology and Epidemiology and Prevention. *Circulation*. 2007;115(21):2761–2788.

Steiman AJ, Gladman DD, Ibañez D, Urowitz MB. Prolonged serologically active clinically quiescent systemic lupus erythematosus: frequency and outcome. *Journal of Rheumatology*. 2010;37:1822–1827.

Uribe AG, Alarcón GS, Sanchez ML, McGwin Jr G, Sandoval R, Fessler BJ, et al. Systemic lupus erythematosus in three ethnic groups. XVIII. Factors predictive of poor compliance with study visits. *Arthritis & Rheumatism*. April 2004;51(2):258–263.

Vokmann ER, Grossman JM, Sahakian LJ, Skaggs BJ, FitzGerald J, et al. Low physical activity is associated with proinflammatory high-density lipoprotein and increased subclinical atherosclerosis in women with systemic lupus erythematosus. *Arthritis Care & Research*. February 2010;62(2):258–265.

Wallace DJ. Does hydroxychloroquine sulfate prevent clot formation in systemic lupus erythematosus? [Letter]. *Arthritis & Rheumatism*. 1987;30:1435–1436.

Walsh SJ, Gilchrist A. Geographical clustering of mortality from systemic lupus erythematosus in the United States: contributions of poverty, Hispanic ethnicity and solar radiation. *Lupus*. 2006;15:662–670.

Wilhelmsson C, Vedin JA, Elmfeldt D, Tibblin G, Wilhelmsen L. Smoking and myocardial infarction. *Lancet*. 1975;1(7904):415–420.

CHAPTER 22

American College of Rheumatology. Herpes zoster (shingles) vaccine guidelines for immunosuppressed patients in *Hotline*. August 1, 2008. Retrieved May 30, 2011, from American College of Rheumatology website, www.rheumatology.org/publications/hotline/2008_08_01_shingles.asp.

Bridges CB. Recommended adult immunization schedule: United States, 2013. *Annals of Internal Medicine*. February 2013;158(3):191–199.

Dao K, Cush JJ. A vaccination primer for rheumatologists. *Drug Safety Quarterly*. 2012;4(1):1.

Dubois E, ed. *Lupus Erythematosus: A Review of the Current Status of Discoid and Systemic Lupus Erythematosus and Their Variants*. New York: McGraw-Hill Book Company; 1966.

Ghaussy NO, Sibbitt Jr WL, Bankhurst AD, Qualls CR. Cigarette smoking and disease activity in systemic lupus erythematosus. *Journal of Rheumatology*. 2003;30:1215–1221.

Gilliland WR, Tsokos GC. Prophylactic use of antibiotics and immunisations in patients with SLE. *Annals of the Rheumatic Diseases*. 2002;61:191–192.

Jewell ML, McCauliffe DP. Patients with cutaneous lupus erythematosus who smoke are less responsive to antimalarial treatment. *Journal of the American Academy of Dermatology*. June 2000;42:983–987.

Kang KY, Kwok S-K, Ju JH, Park K-S, Cho C-S, Kim H-Y, et al. The causes of death in Korean patients with systemic lupus erythematosus over 11 years. *Lupus*. 2011;20:989–997.

Mahoney D. Immunizations should precede rituximab. *Rheumatology News*. August 2008;8(8):28.

Mok CC. Epidemiology and survival of systemic lupus erythematosus in Hong Kong, China. *Lupus*. 2011;20:767–771.

Rahman P, Gladman DD, Urowitz MD. Smoking interferes with efficacy of antimalarial therapy in cutaneous lupus. *Journal of Rheumatology*. September 1998;25(0):1716–1719.

Science M, Johnstone J, Roth DE, Guyatt G, Loeb M. Zinc for the treatment of the common cold: a systematic review and meta-analysis of randomized controlled trials. *Canadian Medical Association Journal*. July 2012;184:E551–E561.

Singh JA, Furst DE, Bharat A, Curtis JR, Kavanaugh AF, et al. 2012 update of the 2008 American College of Rheumatology recommendations for the use of disease-modifying antirheumatic drugs and biologic agents in the treatment of rheumatoid arthritis. *Arthritis Care & Research*. May 2012;64(5):625–639.

Wang C-H, Fang C-C, Chen N-C, Liu S S-H, Yu P-H, et al. Cranberry-containing products for prevention of urinary tract infections in susceptible populations: a systematic review and meta-analysis of randomized controlled trials. *Archives of Internal Medicine*. July 2012;172(13):988–996.

Wilson W, Taubert KA, Gewitz M, Lockhart PB, Baddour LM, Levison M, et al. Prevention of infective endocarditis: guidelines from the American Heart Association: a guideline from the American Heart Association Rheumatic Fever, Endocarditis, and Kawasaki Disease Committee, Council on Cardiovascular Disease in the Young, and the Council on Clinical Cardiology, Council on Cardiovascular Surgery and Anesthesia, and the Quality of Care and Outcomes Research Interdisciplinary Working Group. *Circulation*. 2007;116(15):1736–1754.

### CHAPTER 23

Bernatsky S, Boivin JF, Joseph L, Manzi S, Ginzler E, Urowitz M, et al. Race/ethnicity and cancer occurrence in systemic lupus erythematosus. *Arthritis Care & Research*. October 2005;53(5):781–784.

Bernatsky S, Boivin JF, Joseph L, Rajan R, Zoma A, Manzi S, et al. An international cohort study of cancer in systemic lupus erythematosus. *Arthritis & Rheumatism*. May 2005;52(5):1481–1490.

Bernatsky S, Easton DF, Dunning A, Michailidou K, Ramsey-Goldman R, et al. Decreased breast cancer risk in systemic lupus erythematosus: the search for a genetic basis continues. *Lupus*. July 2012;21(8):896–899.

Bernatsky S, Joseph L, Boivin J-F, Gordon C, Urowitz M, Gladman D, et al. The relationship between cancer and medication exposures in systemic lupus erythematosus: a case-cohort study. *Annals of Rheumatic Diseases*. 2008;67:74–79.

Bernatsky S, Clarke AE, Ramsey-Goldman R. Cancer in systemic lupus: what drives the risk? *Cancer Causes Control*. 2008;19:1413–1414.

Bernatsky S, Ramsey-Goldman R, Foulkes WD, Gordon C, Clarke AE. Breast, ovarian, and endometrial malignancies in systemic lupus erythematosus: a meta-analysis. *British Journal of Cancer*. 2011;104:1478–1481.

Bernatsky S, Ramsey-Goldman R, Joseph L, Boivin J-F, Costenbader KH, et al. Lymphoma risk in systemic lupus: effects of disease activity versus treatment. *Annals of the Rheumatic Diseases*. (Published online January 2013.) Retrieved February 22, 2013, from http://ard.bmj.com/content/early/2013/01/08/annrheumdis-2012-202099.abstract.

Bin J, Bernatsky S, Gordon C, Boivin J-F, Ginzler E, Gladman D, et al. Lung cancer in systemic lupus erythematosus. *Lung Cancer*. June 2007;56(3):303–306.

Dreyer L, Faurschou M, Mogensen M, Jacobsen S. High incidence of potentially virus-induced malignancies in systemic lupus erythematosus. *Arthritis & Rheumatism*. October 2011;63(10):3032–3037.

Lin A, Abu-Isa E, Griffith KA, Ben-Josef E. Toxicity of radiotherapy in patients with collagen vascular disease. *Cancer*. 2008;113(3)648–653.

Löfström B, Backlin C, Sundström C, Ekbom A, Lundberg IE. A closer look at non-Hodgkin's lymphoma cases in a national Swedish systemic lupus erythematosus cohort: a nested case-control study. *Annals of Rheumatic Diseases*. 2007;66:1627–1632.

Parikh-Patel A, White RH, Allen M, Cress R. Cancer risk in a cohort of patients with systemic lupus erythematosus (SLE) in California. *Cancer Causes Control*. 2008;19:887–894.

Pinn ME, Gold DG, Petersen IA, Osborn TG, Brown PD, Miller RC. Systemic lupus erythematosus, radiotherapy, and the risk of acute and chronic toxicity: the Mayo Clinic experience. *International Journal of Radiation Oncology • Biology • Physics*. June 2008;71(2):498–506.

Ragnarsson O, Gröndal G, Steinsson K. Risk of malignancy in an unselected cohort of Icelandic patients with systemic lupus erythematosus. *Lupus*. 2003;12(9):687–691.

Tam S-S, Chan PKS, Ho SC, Yu M-Y, Yim S-F, Cheung T-H, et al. Risk factors for squamous intraepithelial lesions in systemic lupus erythematosus: a prospective cohort study. *Arthritis Care & Research*. February 2011;63(2):269–276.

The Johns Hopkins Lupus Center. Lupus and cancer. Retrieved June 4, 2011, from the Johns Hopkins Lupus Center website, www.hopkinslupus.org/lupus-info/lifestyle-additional-information/lupus-cancer/.

## CHAPTER 24

Abrahmsen B, Eiken P, Eastell R. Subtrochanteric and diaphyseal femur fractures in patients treated with alendronate: a register-based national cohort study. *Journal of Bone and Mineral Research*. 2009;24(6):1095–1102.

Bonakdar ZS, Jahanshahifar L, Jahanshahifar F, Gholamrezaei A. Vitamin D deficiency and its association with disease activity in new cases of systemic lupus erythematosus. *Lupus*. 2011;20:1155–1160.

Bultink IE. Osteoporosis and fractures in systemic lupus erythematosus. *Arthritis Care & Research*. 2012;64(1):2–8.

Drug Safety Quarterly. *The American College of Rheumatology*. October 2011;3(2).

Grossman JM, Gordon R, Ranganath VK, Deal C, Caplan L, Chen W, et al. American College of Rheumatology 2010 recommendations for the prevention and treatment of glucocorticoid-induced osteoporosis. *Arthritis Care & Research*. 2010;62:1515–1526.

*Health Information. Office of Dietary Supplements, National Institutes of Health*. Dietary supplemental fact sheet: Vitamin D: Health Professional. February 25, 2011. Retrieved June 5, 2011, from www.ods.od.nih.gov/factsheets/vitamind/.

Hetény S, Ohlsson C, Carlsten H, Forsblad-d'Elia H. Prevalence and risk factors of vertebral compression fractures in female SLE patients. *Arthritis Research & Therapy*. August 2010;12(4):R153.

Holliman K. Glucocotricoids: a fracture risk at any dose. *The Rheumatologist*. March 2011; 43–54.

Kamen DL. Vitamin D: new kid on the block? *Bulletin of the NYU Hospital for Joint Diseases*. 2010;68(3):218–222.

Khan AA, Rios LP, Sándor GKB, Khan N, Peters E, Rahman MO, et al. Bisphosphonate-associated osteonecrosis of the jaw in Ontario: a survey of oral and maxillofacial surgeons. *Journal of Rheumatology.* 2011;38(7):1396–1402.

Levis S, Strickman-Stein N, Ganjei-Azar P, Xu P, Doerge DR, Krischer J. Soy isoflavones in the prevention of menopausal bone loss and menopausal symptoms: a randomized, double-blind trial. *Archives of Internal Medicine.* August 2011;171(15):1363–1369.

Lewiecki EM, Bilezikian JP, Khosla S, Marcus R, McClung MR, Miller PD, et al. Osteoporosis update from the 2010 Santa Fe Bone Symposium. *Journal of Clinical Densitometry: Assessment of Skeletal Health.* 2011;14(1):1–21.

Meier RPH, Perneger TV, Stern R, Rizzoli R, Pete RE. Increasing occurrence of atypical femoral fractures associated with bisphosphonate use. *Archives of Internal Medicine.* 2012;172:930–936.

National Osteoporosis Foundation. 25 calcium-rich foods. Retrieved June 5, 2011, from www.bones.nof.org/site/PageServer?pagename=NOF_25th_Anniversary_CalciumRich_Foods.

Østensen M, Khamashta M, Lockshin M, Parke A, Brucato A, Carp H, et al. Anti-inflammatory and immunosuppressive drugs and reproduction [Review]. *Arthritis Research & Therapy.* May 2006;8:209–227.

Rosen CJ, Gallagher JC. The 2011 IOM report on vitamin D and calcium requirements for North America: clinical implications for providers treating patients with low bone mineral density. *Journal of Clinical Densitometry: Assessment of Skeletal Health.* 2011;14(2):79–84.

Ruiz-Irastorza G, Gordo S, Olivares N, Egurbide M-V, Aguirre C. Changes in vitamin D levels in patients with systemic lupus erythematosus: effects on fatigue, disease activity, and damage. *Arthritis Care & Research.* August 2010;62(8):1160–1165.


CHAPTER 25

Agarwala S, Shah S, Joshi VR. The use of alendronate in the treatment of avascular necrosis of the femoral head: follow-up to eight years. *Journal of Bone and Joint Surgery* (British Volume). 2009;91(8):1013–1018.

Dubois EL, ed. *Dubois' Lupus Erythematosus.* New York: McGraw Hill; 1966:229–239.

Dubois EL, Cozen L. Avascular (aseptic) necrosis associated with systemic lupus erythematosus. *Journal of the American Medical Association.* 1960;174(8):966–971.

Mont MA, Carbone JJ, Fairbank AC. Core decompression versus nonoperative management for osteonecrosis of the hip. *Clinical Orthopaedics and Related Research.* 1996;324:169–178.

Nagasawa K, Tada Y, Koarada S, Tsukamoto H, Horiuchi T, Yoshizawa S, et al. Prevention of steroid-induced osteonecrosis of femoral head in systemic lupus erythematosus by anticoagulant. *Lupus.* 2006;15(6):354–357.

Nagasawa K, Tsukamoto H, Tada Y, Mayumi T, Satoh H, Onitsuka H, et al. Imaging study on the mode of development and changes in avascular necrosis of the femoral head in systemic lupus erythematosus: long-term observations. *British Journal of Rheumatology.* 1994;33(4):343–347.

Prasad R, Ibanez D, Gladman D, Urowitz M. The role of non-corticosteroid related factors in osteonecrosis (ON) in systemic lupus erythematosus: a nested case-control study of inception patients. *Lupus.* 2007;16:157–162.

Zizic TM. Avascular necrosis of bone. *Current Opinion in Rheumatology.* 1990;2:26–37.

## CHAPTER 26

Faure L, Kolenc M. [Comatous form of acute adrenal insufficiency caused by sudden interruption of cortisone therapy of long duration in persistent asthma; cure by an extracted adrenal cortex hormone]. *Journal de Medecine de Bordeaux et du Sud-Ouest*. October 1954;131(10):1196–1199.

Lewis L, Robinson RF, Yee J, Hacker LA, Eisen G. Fatal adrenal cortical insufficiency precipitated by surgery during prolonged continuous cortisone treatment. *Annals of Internal Medicine*. July 1953;39(1):116–126.

Salem M, Tainsh Jr RE, Bromberg J, Loriaux DL, Chernow B. Perioperative glucocorticoid coverage: a reassessment 42 years after emergence of a problem. *Annals of Surgery*. 1994;219(4):416–425.


## CHAPTER 27

Abebe W. Herbal medication: potential for adverse interactions with analgesic drugs. *Journal of Clinical Pharmacy and Therapeutics*. December 2002;27(6):391–401.

Carson JW, Carson KM, Jones KD, Bennett RM, Wright CL, Mist SD. A pilot randomized controlled trial of the Yoga of Awareness program in the management of fibromyalgia. *Pain*. 2010;151(2):530–539.

Goldenberg DL, Burckhardt C, Crofford L. Management of fibromyalgia syndrome. *Journal of the American Medical Association*. 2004;292(19):2388–2395.

Gupta A, Silman AJ. Psychological stress and fibromyalgia: a review of the evidence suggesting a neuroendocrine link. *Arthritis Research & Therapy*. April 2004;6(3):98–106.

Häuser W, Petzke F, Sommer C. Comparative efficacy and harms of duloxetine, milnacipran, and pregabalin in fibromyalgia syndrome. *Journal of Pain*. 2010;11(6):505–521.

Häuser W, Petzke F, Uçeyler N, Sommer C. Comparative efficacy and acceptability of amitriptyline, duloxetine and milnacipran in fibromyalgia syndrome: a systematic review with meta-analysis. *Rheumatology* (Oxford). 2010;50(3):532–543.

Mayhew E, Ernst E. Acupuncture for fibromyalgia—a systematic review of randomized clinical trials. *Rheumatology* (Oxford). 2007;46(5):801–804.

Nishikai M, Akiya K. Fluvoxamine therapy for fibromyalgia. *Journal of Rheumatology*. 2010;30(5):1124–1125.

Sewitch MJ, Dobkin PL, Bernatsky S, Baron M, Starr M, Cohen M, Fitzcharles MA. Medication non-adherence in women with fibromyalgia. *Rheumatology* (Oxford). 2004;43(5):648–654.

Wang C, Schmid CH, Rones R, Kalish R, Yinh J, Goldenberg DL, et al. A randomized trial of tai chi for fibromyalgia. *New England Journal of Medicine*. 2010;363(8):743–754.

Wolfe F, Clauw DJ, Fitzcharles M-A, Goldenberg DL, Katz RS, Mease P, et al. The American College of Rheumatology preliminary diagnostic criteria for fibromyalgia and measurement of symptom severity. *Arthritis Care & Research*. May 2010;62(5):600–610.

Wolfe F, Smythe HA, Yunus MB, Bennett RM, Bombardier C, Goldenberg DL, et al. The American College of Rheumatology 1990 criteria for the classification of fibromyalgia. Report of the Multicenter Criteria Committee. *Arthritis & Rheumatism*. 1990;33(2):160–172.


## CHAPTER 28

Graham DY, Agrawal NM, Campbell DR, Haber MM, Collis C, Lukasik NL, et al. Ulcer prevention in long-term users of nonsteroidal anti-inflammatory drugs: results of a double-blind, randomized, multicenter, active- and placebo-controlled study of misoprostol vs lansoprazole. *Archives of Internal Medicine.* 2002;162(2):169–175.

Kidd M, Modlin IM. A century of helicobacter pylori: paradigms lost—paradigms regained. *Digestion.* 1998;59(1):1–15.

Lanza FL, Chan FK, Quigley EM, Practice Parameters Committee of the American College of Gastroenterology. Guidelines for prevention of NSAID-related ulcer complications. *American Journal of Gastroenterology.* 2009;104(3):728–738.

Lynch RG. Helicobacter pylori and ulcers. *ASIP Bulletin.* February 2005;8(1):15–16.

Marshall B. *Helicobacter Pioneers: Firsthand Accounts from the Scientists Who Discovered Helicobacters, 1892–1982.* Oxford: Blackwell; 2002.

## CHAPTER 29

Callaway JL, Stokes JH. Relapse in lupus erythematosus after treatment with sodium gold thiosulfate. *Archives of Dermatology and Syphilology.* 1938;37(4):627–630.

Farmer S. *Communities of Saint Martin: Legend and Ritual in Medieval Tours.* Ithaca, NY: Cornell University Press; 1991:272–276.

Federal Drug Administration. How to dispose of unused medicines. Retrieved August 7, 2011, from www.fda.gov/downloads/Drugs/ResourcesForYou/Consumers/BuyingUsingMedicine Safely/UnderstandingOver-the-CounterMedicines/ucm107163.pdf.

Feng X, Zou Y, Pan W, Wang W, Wu M, Zhang M, et al. Prognostic indicators of hospitalized patients with systemic lupus erythematosus: a large retrospective multicenter study in China. *Journal of Rheumatology.* 2011;38:1289–1295.

Fox T. Tuberculae, or degenerations. In: *Skin Diseases; Their Description, Pathology, Diagnosis, and Treatment. With a Copious Formulary.* London: Robert Hardwicke; 1864:200–205.

Green, J. Lupus. In: *A Practical Compendium of the Diseases of the Skin with Cases including Consideration of the More Frequent and Intractable Forms of These Affections.* London: Whittaker and Co; 1835:241–254.

Hebernus (Archbishop of Tours), Miracula B. Martini [The Miracles of St. Martin]. AD 855. In: *Anastasius (the Librarian). Patrologiae Cursus Completus Sive Bibliotheca Universalis, Integra, Uniformis, Commoda, Oeconomica, Omnium SS Patrum, Doctorum Scriptorum que Ecclesiasticorum, patrologiae tomus CXXIX.* Paris: J.-P. Migne; 1853: col. 1036. Translated from the Latin into English courtesy of Darrel W. Amundsen, professor of classics at Western Washington University, Bellingham, Wa.

Hunt T. Lupus. In: *A Guide to the Treatment of Diseases of the Skin: With Suggestions for Their Prevention.* 8th ed. London: T. Richards; 1865:159–172.

Hunt T. On the arrangement and treatment of cutaneous diseases. *The Provincial Medical and Surgical Journal* (now *British Medical Journal*). March 1846;145–146.

Koneru S, Kocharla L, Higgins G, Ware A, Passo M, Farhey Y, et al. Adherence to medications in systemic lupus erythematosus. *Journal of Clinical Rheumatology.* August 2008;14(4):195–201.

Miller HE. Gold and sodium thiosulphate in the treatment of lupus erythematosus. *California and Western Medicine.* October 1928;29(4):243–246.

Neugut AI, Ghatak AT, Miller RL. Anaphylaxis in the United States: an investigation into its epidemiology. *Archives of Internal Medicine.* January 2001;161(1):15–21.

Norton S. A brief history of potable gold. *Molecular Interventions.* June 2008;8(3):120–123.

Pfizer, Inc. Celebrex highlights of prescribing information. Retrieved on August 7, 2011, from www.pfizer.com/files/products/uspi_celebrex.pdf.

Rowell NR. Some historical aspects of skin disease in lupus erythematosus. *Lupus*. 1997;6:76–83.

Safe disposal of used needles and other "sharps." *Drug Safety Quarterly*. 2012;4(1):3.

Squire B. On the treatment of lupus by linear scarification. *British Medical Journal*. May 1880;1(1009):654.


## CHAPTER 30

*Basko v. Sterling Drug, Inc.*, 416 F.2d 417 (2d Cir. 1969) (n.d.). Retrieved August 24, 2011, from www.ftp.resource.org/c/F2/416/416.F2d.417.578.32669_1.html.

Bauer F. Quinacrine hydrochloride drug eruption (tropical lichenoid dermatitis): its early and late sequelae and its malignant potential: a review. *Journal of the American Academy of Dermatology*. 1981;4:239–248.

Broder A, Putterman C. Hydroxychloroquine use is associated with lower odds of persistently positive antiphospholipid antibodies and/or lupus anticoagulant in systemic lupus erythematosus. *Journal of Rheumatology*. 2013;40(1):30–33.

Browning DJ. Bull's-eye maculopathy associated with quinacrine therapy for malaria. *American Journal of Ophthalmology*. March 2004;137(3):577–579.

Carr RE, Henkind P, Rothfield N, Siegel IM. Ocular toxicity of antimalarial drugs: long-term follow-up. *American Journal of Ophthalmology*. October 1968;66(4):738–744.

Devine BJ. Gentamycin therapy. *Drug Intelligence and Clinical Pharmacology*. 1974;8:650–655.

Evans J. Antimalarials remain essential for lupus. *Rheumatology News*. November 2009; 8(11):1, 31.

Fine SD. Winthrop Laboratories: combination drug containing quinacrine hydrochloride, chloroquine phosphate, and hydroxychloroquine sulfate; notice of opportunity for hearing on proposal to withdraw approval of new drug application [Notices]. *Federal Register*. November 1972;37(221):24209–24210.

Harvey AM, Shulman LE, Tumulty PA, Conley CL, Schoenrich EH. *Systemic Lupus Erythematosus: Review of the Literature and Clinical Analysis of 138 Cases*. Baltimore, Md: Williams & Wilkins Company; 1955.

Hobbs HE, Sorsby A, Freedman A. Retinopathy following chloroquine therapy. *Lancet*. 1950; 2(7101):478–480.

Jung H, Bobba R, Su J, Shariati-Sarabi Z, Bladman DD, Urowitz M, et al. The protective effect of antimalarial drugs on thrombovascular events in systemic lupus erythematosus. *Arthritis & Rheumatism*. March 2010;62(3):863–868.

Keeble TW. A cure for the ague: the contribution of Robert Talbor (1642–81). *Journal of the Royal Society of Medicine*. May 1997;90:285–290.

Kersley GD, Glyn J. *A Concise International History of Rheumatology and Rehabilitation: Friends and Foes*. London. Royal Society of Medicine Services Limited; 1991:88–89.

Leden I. Antimalarial drugs—350 years. *Scandinavian Journal of Rheumatology*. 1981;10:307–312.

Marmor MF. Hydroxychloroquine retinopathy still alive and well: how rheumatologists are affected by new guidelines from ophthalmology. *The Rheumatologist*. May 2011;1, 51, 56.

Marmor MF, Kellner U, Lai TYY, Lyons JS, Mieler WF. Revised recommendations on screening for chloroquine and hydroxychloroquine retinopathy. *Ophthalmology*. February 2011;118(2):415–422.

Østensen M, Khamashta M, Lockshin M, Parke A, Brucato A, Carp H, et al. Anti-inflammatory and immunosuppressive drugs and reproduction [Review]. *Arthritis Research & Therapy*. May 2006;8:209–227.

Page F. Treatment of lupus erythematosus with Mepacrine. *The Lancet*. October 1951;2(6687):755–758.

Payne JF. A post-graduate lecture on lupus erythematosus. *The Clinical Journal*. August 1894;4:223–229.

Peponis V, Kyttaris VC, Chalkiadakis SE, Bonovas S, Sitaras NM. Ocular side effects of anti-rheumatic medications: what a rheumatologist should know [Review]. *Lupus*. 2010;19:675–682.

Ruiz-Irastorza G, Khamashta MA. Hydroxychloroquine: the cornerstone of lupus therapy [Editorial]. *Lupus*. 2008;17:271–273.

Shee JC. Lupus erythematosus treated with chloroquine. *Lancet*. July 1953;265(6778):201–202.

Shinjo SK, Bonfá E, Wojdyla D, Borba EF, Ramirez LA, Scherbarth HR, et al. Antimalarial treatment may have a time-dependent effect on lupus survival: data from a multinational Latin American inception cohort. *Arthritis & Rheumatism*. March 2010;62(3):855–862.

Thomas WE. *Hahnemann's allergy to quinine*. March 4, 2002. Retrieved August 24, 2011, from www.angelfire.com/mb2/quinine/allergy.html.

Wallace DJ. The history of antimalarials. *Lupus*. 1996;5(suppl 1):S2–S3.

Wallace DJ. Is there a role for quinacrine (Atabrine) in the new millennium? [Editorial]. *Lupus*. 2000;9:81–82.

Wallace DJ. The use of quinacrine (Atabrine) in rheumatic disease: a reexamination. *Seminars in Arthritis and Rheumatism*. 1989;18(4):282–297.

Wallace DJ. Thrombovascular events in systemic lupus erythematosus: comment on the article by Jung et al. [Letter to the editor]. *Arthritis & Rheumatism*. September 2010;62(9):2824–2825.

CHAPTER 31

Baehr G, Soffer LJ. Treatment of disseminated lupus erythematosus with cortisone and adrenocorticotropin. *The Bulletin of the New York Academy of Medicine*. April 1950;26(4):229–234.

Danowski A, Magder L, Petri M. Flares in lupus: outcome assessment trial (FLOAT), a comparison between oral methylprednisolone and intramuscular triamcinolone. *Journal of Rheumatology*. 2006;33(1):57–60.

Dubois EL, Commons RR, Starr P, Stein Jr CS, Morrison R. Corticotropin and cortisone treatment for systemic lupus erythematosus. *Journal of the American Medical Association*. July 1952;149(11):995–1002.

Gray RG, Tenenbaum J, Gottlieb NL. Local corticosteroid injection treatment in rheumatic disorders. *Seminars in Arthritis and Rheumatism*. May 1981;10(4):231–254.

Hench PS, Kendall EC, Slocumb CH, Polley HF. The effect of the adrenal cortex (17-hydroxy-11-dehydrocorticosterone: compound E) and of pituitary adrenocorticotrophic hormone on rheumatoid arthritis: preliminary report. *Annals of the Rheumatic Diseases*. 1949;8:97–104.

Hillier SG. Diamonds are forever: the cortisone legacy [Review]. *Journal of Endocrinology*. 2007;195:1–6.

Kendall EC. The development of cortisone as a therapeutic agent [Nobel lecture]. *Les Prix Nobel*. December 1951.

Moghadam-Kia S, Werth V. Prevention and treatment of systemic glucocorticoid side effects [Review]. *International Journal of Dermatology*. 2010;49:239–248.

Orr H. Acute disseminated lupus erythematosus. *Canadian Medical Association Journal*. May 1950;62:432–437.

Østensen M, Khamashta M, Lockshin M, Parke A, Brucato A, Carp H, et al. Anti-inflammatory and immunosuppressive drugs and reproduction [Review]. *Arthritis Research & Therapy*. May 2006;8:209–227.

Roberts WN, Babcock EA, Breitbach SA, Owen DS, Irby WR. Corticosteroid injection in rheumatoid arthritis does not increase rate of total joint arthroplasty. *Journal of Rheumatology*. 1996;23(6):1001–1004.

Werth B. *The Billion Dollar Molecule: One Company's Quest for the Perfect Drug*. 1st Touchstone Edition. New York: Simon & Schuster, 1995:129.

### CHAPTER 32

Barthel HR. Leflunomide for the treatment of systemic lupus erythematosus: comment on the article by McMurray [Letter to the editor]. *Arthritis Care & Research*. 2001;45:472.

Bartlett RR, Popovic S, Raiss RX. Development of autoimmunity in MRL/lpr mice and the effects of drugs on this murine disease. *Scandinavian Journal of Rheumatology Supplement*. 1988;75:290–299.

Corley CC, Lessner HE, Larsen WE. Azathioprine therapy of "autoimmune" diseases. *American Journal of Medicine*. September 1966;41(3):404–412.

Dubois EL. Nitrogen mustard in treatment of systemic lupus erythematosus. *Archives of Internal Medicine*. May 1954;93(5):667–672.

Erickson AR, Reddy V, Vogelgesang SA, West SG. Usefulness of the American College of Rheumatology recommendations for liver biopsy in methotrexate-treated rheumatoid arthritis patients. *Arthritis & Rheumatism*. August 1995;38(8):1115–1119.

Fox, RI. Can methotrexate be given safely to men with RA and planning to have children? *Medscape*. June 5, 2006. Retrieved September 5, 2011, from www.medscape.com/viewarticle/533259.

Gillibrand PN. Systemic lupus erythematosus in pregnancy treated with azathioprine. *Proceedings of the Royal Society of Medicine*. September 1966;59(9):834.

Goodman LS, Gilman A. *The Pharmacological Basis of Therapeutics*. 2nd ed. New York: The MacMillan Co; 2009:1414–1425.

Henstell HH, Tober JN, Newman BA. The influence of nitrogen mustard on mycosis fungoides: observations relating its effect to the reticuloendothelial system. *Blood*. 1947;2(6):564–577.

Hill RD, Scott GW. Cytotoxic drugs for systemic lupus. *British Medical Journal*. February 1964;1(5379):370.

Medical discoveries. *Cyclosporine*. Retrieved September 3, 2011, from www.discoveriesinmedicine.com/Com-En/Cyclosporine.html.

Osborne ED, Jordon JW, Hoak FC, Pschierer FJ. Nitrogen mustard therapy in cutaneous blastomatous disease. *Journal of the American Medical Association*. 1947;135(17):1123–1128.

Østensen M, Khamashta M, Lockshin M, Parke A, Brucato A, Carp H, et al. Anti-inflammatory and immunosuppressive drugs and reproduction [Review]. *Arthritis Research & Therapy*. May 2006;8:209–227.

Pisoni CN, Sanchez FJ, Karim Y, Cuadrado MJ, D'Cruz DP, Abbs IC, et al. Mycophenolate mofetil in systemic lupus erythematosus: efficacy and tolerability in 86 patients. *Journal of Rheumatology*. 2005;32:1047–1052.

Rahier J-F, Moutschen M, Gompet AV, Ranst MV, Louis E, Segaert S, et al. Vaccinations in patients with immune-mediated inflammatory diseases [Review]. *Rheumatology*. 2010;49:1815–1827.

Rohn RJ, Bond WH. Some effects of nitrogen mustard and triethylene melamine in acute disseminated lupus erythematosus. *American Journal of the Medical Sciences*. August 1953;226(2):179–190.

Rothenberg RJ, Graziano FM, Grandone JT, Goldberg JW, Bjarnason DF, Finesilver AG. The use of methotrexate in steroid-resistant systemic lupus erythematosus. *Arthritis & Rheumatism*. May 1988;31(5):612–615.

Seah CS, Wong KH, Chew AGK, Jayaratnam FJ. Cyclophosphamide in the treatment of systemic lupus erythematosus [Research article]. *British Medical Journal*. February 1966;1:333–335.

Tam L-S, Li EK, Wong C-K, Lam CWK, Szeto C-C. Double-blind, randomized, placebo-controlled pilot study of leflunomide in systemic lupus erythematosus [Concise report]. *Lupus*. 2004;13:601–604.

Wang HY, Cui TG, Hou FF, Ni ZH, Chen XM, Lu FM, et al. Induction treatment of proliferative lupus nephritis with leflunomide combined with prednisone: a prospective multi-centre observational study [Paper]. *Lupus*. 2008;17:638–644.

Zhang FS, Nie YK, Jin XM, Yu HM, Li YN, Sun Y. The efficacy and safety of leflunomide therapy in lupus nephritis by repeat kidney biopsy. *Rheumatology International*. 2009;29(11):1331–1335.

## CHAPTER 33

Aringer M, Houssiau F, Gordon C, Graninger WB, Voll RE, et al. Adverse events and efficacy of TNF-alpha blockade with infliximab in patients with systemic lupus erythematosus: long-term follow-up of 13 patients. *Rheumatology (Oxford)*. November 2009;48(11):1451–1454.

Bharat A, Xie F, Baddley JW, Beukelman T, Chen L, et al. Incidence and risk factors for progressive multifocal leukoencephalopathy among patients with selected rheumatic diseases. *Arthritis & Care Research*. 2012;64(4):612–615.

Chambers CD. Biologics in pregnancy: an update on everything you are too afraid your patients are going to ask. American College of Rheumatology 2009 Annual Scientific Meeting, Philadelphia, Pa.

Clifford DB, Ances B, Costello C, Rosen-Schmidt S, Andersson M, Parkds D, et al. Rituximab-associated progressive multifocal leukoencephalopathy in rheumatoid arthritis. *Archives of Neurology*. May 2011. Retrieved September 4, 2011, from www.archneur.ama-assn.org/cgi/content/abstract/archneurol.2011.103.

Coico R, Sunshine G. *Immunology: A Short Course*. Hoboken, NJ: Wiley-Blackwell; 2009.

Drug Safety Quarterly. *The American College of Rheumatology*. October 2011;3(2).

Erkan D, Vega J, Ramón G, Kozora E, Lockshin M. A pilot open-label phase II trial of rituximab for non-criteria manifestations of antiphospholipid syndrome. *Arthritis & Rheumatism*. February 2013;65(3):464–471.

Fernández-Nebro A, Marenco de la Fuente LJ, Carreño L, Galindo Izquierdo M, Tomero E, et al. Multicenter longitudinal study of B-lymphocyte depletion in refractory systemic lupus erythematosus: the LESIMAB study. *Lupus*. September 2012;21(10):1063–1076.

Haynes K, Beukelman T, Curtis JR, Newcomb C, Herrinton LJ, et al. Tumor necrosis factor α inhibitor therapy and cancer risk in chronic immune-mediated diseases. *Arthritis & Rheumatism*. January 2013;65(1):48–58.

Interferon. Retrieved September 4, 2011, from www.wikipedia.org/wiki/Interferon.

Isaacs A, Lindenmann J. Virus interference. I. The interferon. *Proceedings of the Royal Society B: Biological Sciences*. September 1957;147(927):258–267.

Katz R. Polyarthritis in systemic lupus erythematosus treated with infliximab. Rush University Medical Center. Retrieved September 4, 2011, from www.drrobertkatz.com/wp-content/uploads/2011/04/polyarthritis.pdf.

Kendall EC. The development of cortisone as a therapeutic agent [Nobel lecture]. *Les Prix Nobel*. December 1951.

Mariette X, Matucci-Cerinic M, Pavelka K, Taylor P, van Vollenhoven R, Heatley R, et al. Malignancies associated with tumour necrosis factor inhibitors in registries and prospective observational studies: a systematic review and meta-analysis. *Annals of Rheumatic Diseases*. September 2011. Retrieved September 24, 2011, from www.ard.bmj.com/content/early/2011/07/29/ard.2010.149419.short.

Molloy ES, Calabrese LH. Progressive multifocal leukoencephalopathy: a national estimate of frequency in systemic lupus erythematosus and other rheumatoid diseases. *Arthritis & Rheumatism*. December 2009;60(12):3761–3765.

Molloy ES, Calabrese LH. Progressive multifocal leukoencephalopathy in patients with rheumatic disease: are patients with systemic lupus erythematosus at particular risk? *Autoimmunity Review*. December 2008;8(2):144–146.

Østensen M, Förger F. Management of RA medications in pregnant patients. *Nature Reviews Rheumatology*. July 2009;5:382–390.

Pinto LF, Velásquez CJ, Prieto C, Mestra L, Forero E, Márquez JD. Rituximab induces a rapid and sustained remission in Colombian patients with severe and refractory systemic lupus erythematosus. *Lupus*. 2011;20:1219–1226.

Raaschou P, Simard JF, Neovius M, Askling J. Does cancer that occurs during or after anti-tumor necrosis factor therapy have a worse prognosis? *Arthritis & Rheumatism*. July 2011;63(7):1812–1822.

Ramos-Casals M, Soto MJ, Cuadrado MJ, Khamashta MA. Rituximab in systemic lupus erythematosus: a systematic review of off-label use in 188 cases. *Lupus*. 2009;18:767–776.

Sawsen JH, Uppal SS, Narayanan Nampoory MR, Johny KV, Gupta R, Al-Oun M. Safety and efficacy of infliximab in a patient with active WHO class IV lupus nephritis [Case report]. *Clinical Rheumatology*. 2007;26(6):973–975.

Smolen JS. Slide presentation and abstract. Blocking proinflammatory cytokines in lupus. Poster session at the 7th International Congress on SLE and Related Conditions, May 9–13, 2004, New York, NY.

Solomon DH, Mercer E, Kavanaugh A. Observational studies on the risk of cancer associated with tumor necrosis factor inhibitors in rheumatoid arthritis: a review of their methodologies and results. *Arthritis & Rheumatism*. 2012;64(1):21–32.

Thompson AE, Rieder SW, Pope JE. Tumor necrosis factor therapy and the risk of serious infection and malignancy in patients with early rheumatoid arthritis: a meta-analysis of randomized controlled trials. *Arthritis & Rheumatism*. June 2011;63(6):1479–1485.

Tumor necrosis factor-alpha. Retrieved September 4, 2011, from www.en.wikipedia.org/wiki/Tumor_necrosis-factor-alpha.

Weckerle CE, Mangale D, Franek BS, Kelly JA, Kumabe M, et al. Large-scale analysis of tumor necrosis factor α levels in systemic lupus erythematosus. *Arthritis & Rheumatism*. September 2012;64(9):2947–2952.

Wolfe F, Michaud K. Biologic treatment of rheumatoid arthritis and the risk of malignancy: analyses from a large US observational study. *Arthritis & Rheumatism*. 2007;56(9):2886–2895.

Zhu L-J, Yang X, Yu X-Q. Anti-TNF-α therapies in systemic lupus erythematosus [Review article]. *Journal of Biomedicine and Biotechnology*. Vol. 2010, Article ID 465898, 8 pages, 2010. doi:10.1155/2010/465898. Retrieved September 4, 2011, from www.hindawi.com/journals/jbb/2010/465898/cta/.


**CHAPTER 34**

Allen A. New lupus drug gets only mixed reactions from patients, experts. *Washington Post*. June 13, 2011. Retrieved September 4, 2011, from www.washingtonpost.com/national/health/new-lupus-drug-gets-only-mixed-reactions-from-patients-experts/2011/05/31/AGRffcTH_story.html.

Braunstein JB, Sherber NS, Schulman SP, Ding EL, Powe NR. Race, medical researcher distrust, perceived harm, and willingness to participate in cardiovascular prevention trials. *Medicine*. January 2008;87(1):1–9.

Dooley MA, Houssiau F, Aranow C, D'Cruz DP, Askanase A, et al. Effect of belimumab treatment on renal outcomes: results from phase 3 belimumab clinical trials in patients with systemic lupus erythematosus. *Lupus*. January 2013;22:63–72.

Elixir Sulfanilamide. Retrieved September 4, 2011, from www.en.wikipedia.org/wiki/Elixir_sulfanilamide.

Freimuth VS, Quinn SC, Thomas SB, Cole G, Zook E, Duncan T. African Americans' views on research and the Tuskegee Syphilis Study. *Social Science and Medicine*. 2001;52:797–808.

GlaxoSmithKline. Response rates of black/African-Americans systemic lupus erythematosus (SLE) patients in the clinical trials with Benlysta. Research Triangle Park, NC; June 28, 2011.

Janssen WF. Cancer quackery: past and present. *Cancer Treatment Watch*. Retrieved September 11, 2011, from www.cancertreatmentwatch.org/q/janssen.shtml.

Lipsky PE, Dörner T. The red wolf remains a wily foe [Editorial]. *Nature Reviews Rheumatology*. June 2010;6:307–308.

Mahoney D. Expert outlines drug-development obstacles in lupus. *Rheumatology News*. Retrieved September 11, 2011, from www.rheumatologynews.epubxpress.com/wps/portal/rhu/c0/04_SB8K8xLLM9MSSzPy8xBz9CP0os3iLkCAPEzcPIwMLTwNTAyM3f1NTs1AvQwN_A_1I_ShzhLy_ha-zgadnkKWXu4m_sYGJgX4IyMRM_UgzMyMDELNYPxJMF-hHQgXyS4uSU_Uji1MTi5Iz9AuyE5OqUpOqHB0VFQHG32yz/.

Manzi S, Sanchez-Guerrero J, Merrill JT, Furie R, Gladman D, et al. Effects of belimumab, a B lymphocyte stimulator-specific inhibitor, on disease activity across multiple organ domains in patients with systemic lupus erythematosus: combined results from two phase III trials. *Annals of the Rheumatic Diseases*. 2012;71:1833–1838.

Mechcatie E. BLISS-76 yields data on belimumab in SLE. *Rheumatology News*. July 2010. Retrieved September 22, 2011, from www.rheumatologynews.epubxpress.com/wps/portal/rhu/c0/04_SB8K8xLLM9MSSzPy8xBz9CP0os3iLkCAPEzcPIwMLTwNTAyM3f1NTs1AvQwN_A_1I_ShzhLy_ha-zgadnkKWXu4m_sYGJgX4IyMRM_UhzA2MjELNYP9IARBfoRxqbggXyS4uSU_Uji1MTi5Iz9AuyE5OqUpOqHB0VFQHGzuf8/.

Mechcatie E. FDA panel backs belimumab for lupus. *Rheumatology News*. December 2010;9(12):1,7.

Merrill JT, Furie RA, Wallace DJ, Stohl W, Chatham W, et al. Sustained disease improvement and safety profile over the 1500 patient-year experience (6 years) with belimumab in patients with systemic lupus erythematosus: phase 2 long-term extension. ACR/ARHP Annual Scientific Meeting, November 4–9, 2011.

Merrill JT, Ginzler EM, Wallace DJ, McKay JD, Lisse JR, et al. Long-term safety profile of belimumab plus standard therapy in patients with systemic lupus erythematosus. *Arthritis & Rheumatism*. October 2012;64(10):3364–3373.

Patent medicine. Retrieved September 4, 2011, from www.en.wikipedia.org/wiki/Patent_medicine.

Peirce A, Lipsky P, Schwartz BD. Mitigate risk and increase success of lupus clinical trials: design strategies from a Lupus Research Institute conference. *The Rheumatologist*. August 2010. Retrieved September 11, 2011, http://www.the-rheumatologist.org/details/article/863303/Mitigate_Risk_and_Increase_Success_of_Lupus_Clinical_Trials.html.

Pollack A. F.D.A. Approves Drug for Lupus, an Innovation After 50 Years. *New York Times*. March 9, 2011. Retrieved September 4, 2011, from www.nytimes.com/2011/03/10/health/10drug.html.

Stohl W, Hiepe F, Latinis KM, Thomas M, Scheinberg MA, et al. Belimumab reduces autoantibodies, normalizes low complement levels, and reduces select B cell populations in patients with systemic lupus erythematosus. *Arthritis & Rheumatism*. July 2012;64(7):2328–2337.

Stork A. The long, winding road to a new drug. *National Psoriasis Foundation Psoriasis Advance*. Summer 2010. Retrieved September 22, 2011, from www.psoriasis.org/publications/psoriasis-advance/2010/summer/drug-development.

Swann JP. About FDA: FDA's origin. Retrieved September 11, 2011, from U.S. Food and Drug Administration website: www.fda.gov/AboutFDA/WhatWeDo/History/ProductRegulation/SulfanilamideDisaster/default.htm.

Thalidomide. Retrieved September 11, 2011, from www.en.wikipedia.org/wiki/Thalidomide.

Tuskegee Syphilis Experiment. Retrieved September 4, 2011, from www.en.wikipedia.org/wiki/Tuskegee_syphilis_experiment.

U.S. Food and Drug Administration. About FDA: milestones of drug regulation in the United States. Retrieved September 11, 2011, from www.fda.gov/AboutFDA/WhatWeDo/History/FOrgsHistory/CDER/CenterforDrugEvaluationandResearchBrochureandChronology/ucm114463.htm.

U.S. Food and Drug Administration. About FDA: sulfanilamide disaster. June 1981. Retrieved September 11, 2011, from www.fda.gov/AboutFDA/WhatWeDo/History/ProductRegulation/SulfanilamideDisaster/default.htm.

U.S. Food and Drug Administration. Aspirin comprehensive prescribing information. Retrieved September 11, 2011, from www.fda.gov/ohrms/dockets/ac/03/briefing/4012B1_03_Appd%201-Professional%20Labeling.pdf.

van Vollenhoven RF, Petri MA, Cervera R, Roth DA, Ji BN, et al. Belimumab in the treatment of systemic lupus erythematosus: high disease activity predictors of response. *Annals of the Rheumatic Diseases*. 2012;71:1343–1349.

Wallace DJ. The use of quinacrine (Atabrine) in rheumatic disease: a reexamination. *Seminars in Arthritis and Rheumatism*. 1989;18(4):282–297.

Wallace DJ, Navarra S, Petri MA, Gallacher A, Thomas M, et al. Safety profile of belimumab:

pooled data from placebo-controlled phase 2 and 3 studies in patients with systemic lupus erythematosus. *Lupus.* January 2013;22(1):144–154.

Walsh N. New lupus drugs remain elusive after 50 years. *Internal Medicine News.* March 15, 2009. Retrieved September 11, 2011, from www.imn.gcnpublishing.com/fileadmin/content_pdf/imn/archive_pdf/vol42iss6/70206_main.pdf.

Zoler ML. Belimumab reduced SLE activity in phase III study. *Rheumatology News.* November 2009;8(11):28.


CHAPTER 35

Karim MY, Ruiz-Irastorza G, Khamashta MA, Hughes GRV. Update on therapy—thalidomide in the treatment of lupus. *Lupus.* 2001;10:188–192.

Perri AJ, Hsu S. A review of thalidomide's history and current dermatological applications. *Dermatology Online Journal* 9(3):5. Retrieved September 21, 2011, from www.dermatology.cdlib.org/93/reviews/thalidomide/hsu.html.


CHAPTER 36

Abebe W. Herbal medication: potential for adverse interactions with analgesic drugs. *Journal of Clinical Pharmacy and Therapeutics.* December 2002;27(6):391–401.

American Academy of Pediatrics. Maternal medication usually compatible with breast-feeding. Retrieved September 25, 2011, from www.aappolicy.aappublications.org/cgi/content-nw/full/pediatrics;108/3/776/T6.

Daniel S, Matok I, Gorodischer R, Koren G, Uziel E, et al. Major malformations following exposure to nonsteroidal anti-inflammatory drugs during the first trimester of pregnancy. *Journal of Rheumatology.* 2012;39:2163–2169.

Nakhai-Pour HR, Broy P, Sheehy O, Bérard A. Use of nonaspirin nonsteroidal anti-inflammatory drugs during pregnancy and the risk of spontaneous abortion. *Canadian Medical Association Journal.* 2011;183:1713.

U.S. Department of Justice, Drug Enforcement Administration, Office of Diversion Control. Code of regulations, section 1308, schedules of controlled substances. Retrieved September 25, 2011, from www.deadiversion.usdoj.gov/21cfr/cfr/2108cfrt.htm.


CHAPTER 37

Breuckmann F, Gambichler T, Altmeyer P, Kreuter A. UVA/UVA1 phototherapy and PUVA photochemotherapy in connective tissue diseases and related disorders: a research based review. *BMC Dermatology.* 2004;(1):11.

Comte C, Bessis D, Picot E, Peyron JL, Guillot B, Dereure O. [Treatment of connective tissue disorder-related acral syndromes using UVA-1 phototherapy: an open study of 11 cases]. *Annales de Dermatologie et de Venereologie.* April 2009;136(4):323–329.

Dall'Era M, Chakravarty E, Wallace D, et al. Reduced B lymphocyte and immunoglobulin levels after Atacicept treatment in patients with systemic lupus erythematosus: results of a multicenter, phase Ib, double-blind, placebo-controlled, dose-escalation trial. *Arthritis & Rheumatism.* 2007;56:4142–4150.

D'Andrea Denise (senior director, clinical research, for Cephalon, Inc.). Lupuzor(tm) being studied for treatment of systemic lupus erythematosus [Youtube video]. October 31,

2010. Lupus Foundation of America. Retrieved October 1, 2011, from www.youtube.com/watch?v=Tg1BwAB86Jg.

DeBartolo A. *Lupus Underground: A Patient's Case for a Long-ignored, Drug-free, Non-patentable, Counter-intuitive Therapy That Actually Works.* Chicago: Hyde Park Media; 2004.

DrugLib.com. Drug information portal. Retrieved October 1, 2011, from www.druglib.com/.

Fanouriakis A, Boumpas DT, Bertsias GK. Balancing efficacy and toxicity of novel therapies in systemic lupus erythematosus. *Expert Review of Clinical Pharmacology.* 2011;4(4):437–451.

Hawk D. Cancer drug shows promise in treating lupus. *Value-Based Care in Rheumatology.* August 2012;1(3):1,15.

Illei GG, Shirota Y, Yarboro CH, Daruwalla J, Tackey E, Takada K, et al. Tocilizumab in systemic lupus erythematosus: data on safety, preliminary efficacy, and impact on circulating plasma cells from an open-label phase I dosage-escalation study. *Arthritis & Rheumatism.* February 2010;62(2):542–552.

Kaufman MB. Drug updates: information on new approvals and medication safety. *The Rheumatologist.* March 2010. Retrieved October 1, 2011, from www.the-rheumatologist.org/details/article/865867/Drug_Updates.html.

Kaufman MB. Drug updates: information on new approvals and medication safety. *The Rheumatologist.* September 2011. Retrieved October 1, 2011, from www.the-rheumatologist.org/details/article/1332713/Drug_Updates.html.

McBride JM, Jiang J, Abbas AR, Morimoto A, Li J, et al. Safety and pharmacodynamics of rontalizumab in patients with systemic lupus erythematosus: results of a phase I, placebo-controlled, double-blind, dose-escalation study. *Arthritis & Rheumatism.* November 2012;64(11):3666–3676.

McGrath H, Bell JM, Hayne MR, Martinez-Osuna P. Ultraviolet-a irradiation therapy for patients with systemic lupus erythematosus: a pilot study. *Current Therapeutic Research.* April 1994;55(4):373–381.

Merrill JT, Burgos-Vargas R, Westhovens R, Chalmers A, D'Cruz D, Wallace DJ, et al. The efficacy and safety of abatacept in patients with non-life-threatening manifestation of systemic lupus erythematosus: results of a twelve-month, multicenter, exploratory, phase IIb, randomized, double-blind, placebo-controlled trial. *Arthritis & Rheumatism.* October 2010;62(10):3077–3087.

Mikita N, Kanazawa N, Yoshimasu T, Ikeda T, Li H-J, Yamamoto Y, et al. The protective effects of ultraviolet A1 irradiation on spontaneous lupus erythematosus-like skin lesions in MRL/lpr mice [Research article]. *Clinical and Developmental Immunology.* 2009. Retrieved October 1, 2011, from www.hindawi.com/journals/cdi/2009/673952/.

Pavel S. Light therapy (with UVA-1) for SLE patients: is it a good or bad idea? [Editorial]. *Rheumatology.* 2006;45:653–655.

Polderman MCA, le Cessie S, Huizinga TWJ, Pavel S. Efficacy of UVA-1 cold light as an adjuvant therapy for systemic lupus erythematosus. *Rheumatology.* 2004;43:1402–1404.

Research. Lupus Foundation of America: DC/MD/VA Chapter. Retrieved October 1, 2011, from www.lupus.org/webmodules/webarticlesnet/templates/gwashington_research.aspx?articleid=908&zone=144.

Schwartzman JS, Gross R, Putterman C. Management of lupus in 2010: how close are the biologics? *Journal of Musculoskeletal Medicine.* November 2010;27(11):427–440.

U.S. National Institutes of Health. Search for clinical trials. Retrieved October 1, 2011, from www.clinicaltrials.gov/ct2/search.

Vasudevan AR, Ginzler EM. Established and novel treatments for lupus: agents in clinical trials are targeting various immunological processes. *Journal of Musculoskeletal Medicine.* August 2009;26(8):291–300.

Wallace D, Petri M, Strand V, Killgallen B, Barry A, et al. Epratuzumab demonstrates clinically meaningful improvements in patients with moderate to severe systemic lupus erythematosus (SLE): results from EMBLEM, a phase IIB study. *Annals of Rheumatic Diseases.* 2010;69:558.

Wofsy D. Trials and tribulations in systemic lupus erythematosus. *Bulletin of the NYU Hospital for Joint Diseases.* 2010;68(3):175–178.

York NR, Jacobe HT. UVA1 phototherapy: a review of mechanism and therapeutic application [Review]. *International Society of Dermatology.* 2010;49:623–630.


CHAPTER 38

Ayán C, Martín V. Systemic lupus erythematosus and exercise. *Lupus.* 2007;16:5–9.

Birmingham DJ, Nagaraja HN, Rovin BH, Spetie L, Zhao Y, Li X, et al. Fluctuations in self-perceived stress and increased risk of flare in patients with lupus nephritis carrying the serotonin receptor 1A-1019 G allele. *Arthritis & Rheumatism.* October 2006;54(10):3291–3299.

Canadian Centre for Occupational Health and Safety. Ultraviolet radiation. Retrieved October 1, 2011, from www.ccohs.ca/oshanswers/phys_agents/ultravioletradiation.html.

Chandrasekhara S, Jayachandran NV, Rajasekhar L, Thomas J, Narsimulu G. The prevalence and associations of sleep disturbances in patients with systemic lupus erythematosus [Original article]. *Modern Rheumatology.* 2009; 19(4):407–415.

de Boer IH, Levin G, Robinson-Cohen C, Biggs ML, Hoofnagle AN, et al. Serum 25-hydroxyvitamin D concentration and risk for major clinical disease events in a community-based population of older adults: a cohort study. *Annals of Internal Medicine.* May 2012;156(9):627–634.

Dennis J, Krewski D, Côté F-S, Fafard E, Little J, Ghadirian P. Breast cancer risk in relation to alcohol consumption and BRCA gene mutations—a case-only study of gene-environment interaction. *The Breast Journal.* 2011;17(5):477–484.

Elkan A-C, Anania C, Gustafsson T, Jogestrand T, Hafström I, Frostegård J. Diet and fatty acid pattern among patients with SLE: associations with disease activity, blood lipids and atherosclerosis. *Lupus.* 2012;21:1405–1411.

Ford ES, Zhao G, Tsai J, Li C. Low-risk lifestyle behaviors and all-cause mortality: findings from the National Health and Nutrition Examination Survey III Mortality Study. *American Journal of Public Health.* October 2011;101(10):1922–1929.

Formica MK, Palmer JR, Rosenberg L, McAlindon TE. Smoking alcohol consumption, and risk of systemic lupus erythematosus in the Black Women's Health Study. *Journal of Rheumatology.* June 2003;30(6):1222–1226.

Ghaussy NO, Sibbitt Jr WL, Qualls CR. Cigarette smoking, alcohol consumption, and the risk of systemic lupus erythematosus: a case-control study. *Journal of Rheumatology.* November 2001;28(11):2449–2453.

Hardy CJ, Palmer BP, Muir KR, Sutton AJ, Powell RJ. Smoking history, alcohol consumption, and systemic lupus erythematosus: a case-control study. *Annals of the Rheumatic Diseases.* 1998;57:451–455.

Hassan N, Clarke AE, Da Costa D, Pineau CA, Bernatsky S. Sleep disturbance in lupus patients. *International Journal of Clinical Rheumatology.* 2009;4(6):641–643.

Kiyohara C, Washio M, Horiuchi T, Asami Y, Saburo I, et al. Cigarette smoking, alcohol consumption, and risk of systemic lupus erythematosus: a case-control study in a Japanese population. *Journal of Rheumatology*. 2012;39:1363–1370.

Klein LR, Elmets CA, Callen JP. Photoexacerbation of cutaneous lupus erythematosus due to ultraviolet A emissions from a photocopier. *Arthritis & Rheumatism*. August 1995;38(8):1152–1156.

Klein RS, Sayre RM, Dowdy JC, Werth VP. The risk of ultraviolet radiation exposure from indoor lamps in lupus erythematosus. *Autoimmunity Reviews*. February 2009;8(4):320–324.

Kozora E, Ellison MC, West S. Life stress and coping styles related to cognition in systemic lupus erythematosus [Research article]. *Stress and Health*. December 2009;25(5):413–422.

LeBlanc ES, Perrin N, Johnson JD, Ballatore A, Hillier T. Over-the-counter and compounded vitamin D: is potency what we expect? *Journal of the American Medical Association Internal Medicine* (Online First). February 2013. Retrieved February 24, 2013, from archinte .jamanetwork.com/article.aspx?articleID=1570096&utm_source=Silverchair+Information +Systems&utm_medium=email&utm_campaign=ArchivesofInternalMedicine%3AOnline First02%2F11%2F2013.

Leiba A, Amital H, Gershwin MD, Shoenfeld Y. Diet and lupus. *Lupus*. 2001;10:246–248.

National Institutes of Health. Sun safety: Save your skin! *The Lupus Newslink* [Brochure].

Okereke OI, Rosner BA, Kim DH, Kang JH, Cook NR, et al. Dietary fat types and 4-year cognitive change in community-dwelling older women. *Annals of Neurology*. July 2012;72(1):124–134.

Peralta-Ramírez MI, Coín-Mejías MÁ, Jiménez-Alonso J, Ortego-Ceneno N, Callejas-Rubio JL, Caracuel-Romero A, et al. Stress as a predictor of cognitive functioning in lupus [Paper]. *Lupus*. 2006;15:858–864.

Petri M. Diet and systemic lupus erythematosus: from mouse and monkey to woman? [Editorial]. *Lupus*. 2001;10:775–777.

Rodriguez D. Healthy Living: 7 ways to zap stress before it strikes. *Everyday Health*. Retrieved on October 1, 2011, from www.everydayhealth.com/healthy-living/ways-to-avoid-stress .aspx?xid=nl_EverydayHealthEmotionalHealth_20101103.

Wang J, Pan H-F, Ye D-Q, Su H, Li X-P. Moderate alcohol drinking might be protective for systemic lupus erythematosus: a systematic review and meta-analysis. *Clinical Rheumatology*. 2008;27(12):1557–1563.

Wojcik E. Sun rules: 5 facts to know about summer sun safety. *Lupus Now*. Summer 2011;6–7.

CHAPTER 39

Aron-Maor A, Shoenfeld Y. Alternative therapies in rheumatic diseases—pros and cons. *Lupus*. 2001;10:453–456.

Astin JA, Harkness E, Ernst E. The efficacy of "distant healing": a systematic review of randomized trials. *Annals of Internal Medicine*. 2000;132(11):903–910.

Bhatt BD, Zuckerman MJ, Foland JA, Polly SM, Marwah RK. Disseminated *Salmonella arizonae* infection associated with rattlesnake meat ingestion. *American Journal of Gastroenterology*. 1989;84:433–435.

Birocco N, Guillame C, Storto S, Ritorto G, Catino C, Gir N, et al. The effects of Reiki therapy on pain and anxiety in patients attending a day oncology and infusion services unit. *American Journal of Hospice and Palliative Medicine*. October 2011. Retrieved October 26, 2011, from www.ajh.sagepub.com/content/early/2011/09/08/1049909111420859.abstract.

Bonakdar ZS, Jahanshahifar L, Jahanshahifar F, Gholamrezaei A. Vitamin D deficiency and its association with disease activity in new cases of systemic lupus erythematosus. *Lupus.* 2011;20:1155–1160.

Casner PR, Zuckerman MJ. *Salmonella arizonae* in patients with AIDS along the U.S.-Mexican Border. *New England Journal of Medicine.* 323(3):198–199.

Chen YS, Hu XE. Auriculo-acupuncture in 15 cases of discoid lupus erythematosus. *Journal of Traditional Chinese Medicine.* 1985;5(4):261–262.

Chou C-T. Alternative therapies: what role do they have in the management of lupus? *Lupus.* 2010;19:1425–1429.

Dongping L. Clinical observation of integrated traditional Chinese medicine and western medicine therapy on the treatment of lupus nephritis. In [*Journal of Shanxi College of Traditional Chinese Medicine*]. 2008. Retrieved on October 26, 2011, from www.en.cnki.com .cn/Article_en/CJFDTOTAL-SHAN200801016.htm.

Ernst E. Chiropractic treatment for fibromyalgia: a systematic review. *Clinical Rheumatology.* 2009;28(10):1175–1178.

Greco CM, Kao AH, Maksimowicz-McKinnon K, Glick RM, Houze M, Sereika SM, et al. Acupuncture for systemic lupus erythematosus: a pilot RCT feasibility and safety study. *Lupus.* 2008;17:1108–1116.

Gunathunga MW, Wijeratne LS, Dissanayake AS, Ruwanchinthani A, Perera KD. Effect of an insight meditation programme on the disease outcome of patients with rheumatoid and related arthritis. *Ceylon Medical Journal.* 2010;55(suppl 1):46.

Jimenez-Caliani A, Jimenez-Jorge S, Molinero P, Rubio A, Guerrero JM, Osuna C. Treatment with testosterone or estradiol in melatonin treated females and males MRL/MpJ-Faslpr mice induces negative effects in developing systemic lupus erythematosus. *Journal of Pineal Research.* September 2008;45(2):204–211.

Kirkpatric RA. Witchcraft and lupus erythematosus. *Journal of the American Medical Association.* 1981;245(19):1937.

Kirkpatric RA. Witchcraft and lupus erythematosus [Letters]. *Journal of the American Medical Association.* 1982;247(2):176.

Kraus A, Guerra-Bautista G, Alarcon-Segovia D. *Salmonella arizonae* arthritis and septicemia associated with rattlesnake ingestion by patients with connective tissue disease: a dangerous complication of folk medicine. *Journal of Rheumatology.* 1991;18:1328–1331.

Lautenschlager J. [Acupuncture in treatment of inflammatory rheumatic diseases.] *Zeitschrift für Rheumatologie.* 1997;56(1):8–20.

Lee MS, Shin BC, Ernst E. Acupuncture for rheumatoid arthritis: a systematic review. *Rheumatology* (Oxford). 2008;47(12):1747–1753.

Maestroni GJ, Otsa K, Cutolo M. Melatonin treatment does not improve rheumatoid arthritis. *British Journal of Clinical Pharmacology.* May 2008;65(5):797–798.

Matthews DA. Prayer and spirituality. *Rheumatic Disease Clinics of North America.* 2000;26(1):177–187.

Nainis N, Paice JA, Ratner J, Wirth JH, Lai J, Shott S. Relieving symptoms in cancer: innovative use of art therapy. *Journal of Pain and Symptom Management.* 2006;31(2):162–169. ·

Nevarrete-Navarrete N, Peralta- Ramírez MI, Sabio-Sánchez JM, Coín MÁ, Robles-Ortega H, Hidalgo-Tenorio C, et al. Efficacy of cognitive behavioural therapy for the treatment of chronic stress in patients with lupus erythematosus: a randomized controlled trial. *Psychotherapy and Psychosomatics.* 2010;79:107–115.

Petri M. Diet and systemic lupus erythematosus: from mouse and monkey to woman? *Lupus.* 2001;10:775–777.

Posadzki P, Alotaibi A, Ernst E. Adverse effects of homeopathy: a systematic review of published case reports and case series. *International Journal of Clinical Practice*. December 2012;66(12):1178–1188.

Richmond SJ, Brown S, Campion PD, Porter AJL, Moffett JAK, Jackson DA, et al. Therapeutic effects of magnetic and copper bracelets in osteoarthritis: a randomized placebo-controlled crossover trial. *Complementary Therapies in Medicine*. 2009;17(5–6):249–256.

Rosenzweig S. Complementary and alternative medicine (CAM). 2009. In: *The Merck Manual: Home Health Handbook*. Retrieved October 26, 2011, from www.merckmanuals.com/home/special_subjects/complementary_and_alternative_medicine_cam/overview_of_complementary_and_alternative_medicine.html.

Schnitzer TJ, Truitt K, Fleischmann R, Dalgin P, Block J, Zeng Q, et al. The safety profile, tolerability, and effective dose range of rofecoxib in the treatment of rheumatoid arthritis. *Clinical Therapeutics*. October 1999;21(10):1688–1702.

Stefanescu M, Matache C, Onu A, Tanaseanu S, Dragomir C, Constantinescu I, et al. Pycnogenol efficacy in the treatment of systemic lupus erythematosus patients. *Phytotherapy Research*. December 2001;15(8):698–704.

Sun S-F, Su J-H, Ye R-G. Integrated traditional Chinese medicine and western medicine therapy for lupus nephritis: a meta-analyses of randomized and controlled trials. [*China Journal of Modern Medicine*]. 2004. Retrieved October 26, 2011, from www.en.cnki.com.cn/Article_en/CJFDTOTAL-ZXDY200417005.htm.

Tao X, Lipsky PE. The Chinese anti-inflammatory and immunosuppressive herbal remedy Tripterygium wilfordii Hook F. *Rheumatic Disease Clinics of North America*. 2000; 26(1):29–50.

Vickers AJ, Cronin AM, Maschino AC, Lewith G, MacPherson H, et al. Acupuncture for chronic pain: individual patient data meta-analysis. *Archives of Internal Medicine*. October 2012;172(19):1444–1453.

Wallace DJ, ed. *The Sjögren's Book*. New York: Oxford University Press; 2012.

Yang X, Liu X. Effect of Chinese herbal medicine combined with western medicine on active systemic lupus erythematosus: an observation of 72 cases. [*Journal of New Chinese Medicine*]. 2008. Retrieved on October 26, 2011, from www.en.cnki.com.cn/Article_en/CJFDTOTAL-REND200803032.htm.

Zautra AJ, Davis MC, Reich JW, Nicassario P, Tennen H, Finnan P, et al. Comparison of cognitive behavioral and mindfulness meditation interventions on adaptation to rheumatoid arthritis for patients with and without history of recurrent depression. *Journal of Consulting and Clinical Psychology*. June 2008;76(3):408–421.

Zhou L-l, Wei W, Si J-F, Yuan D-P. Regulatory effect of melatonin on cytokine disturbances in the pristine-induced lupus mice: mediators of Inflammation. Vol. 2010, Article ID 951210, 7 pages, 2010. doi:10.1155/2010/951210. Retrieved July 4, 2011, from www.hindawi.com/journals/mi/2010/951210/cta/.

CHAPTER 41

Alijotas-Reig J. Treatment of refractory obstetric antiphospholipid syndrome: the state of the art and new trends in the therapeutic management. *Lupus*. January 2013;22(1):6–17.

American Academy of Pediatrics. Maternal medication usually compatible with breastfeeding. Retrieved September 25, 2011, from www.aappolicy.aappublications.org/cgi/content-nw/full/pediatrics;108/3/776/T6.

Bellver J, Pellicer A. Ovarian stimulation for ovulation induction and in vitro fertilization in patients with systemic lupus erythematosus and antiphospholipid syndrome. *Fertility and Sterility*. December 2009;92(6):1803–1810.

Jancin B. Managing rheumatologic diseases in pregnancy. *Rheumatology News*. April 2010;9(4):28.

Lockshin MD, Kim M, Laskin CA, Guerra M, Branch DW, et al. Prediction of adverse pregnancy outcome by the presence of lupus anticoagulant, but not anticardiolipin antibody, in patients with antiphospholipid antibodies. *Arthritis & Rheumatism*. July 2012;64(7):3211–2318.

Østensen M, Khamashta M, Lockshin M, Parke A, Brucato A, Carp H, et al. Anti-inflammatory and immunosuppressive drugs and reproduction [Review]. *Arthritis Research & Therapy*. May 2006;8:209–227.

Petri M. The Hopkins Lupus Pregnancy Center: ten key issues in management. *Rheumatic Disease Clinics of North America*. May 2007;33(2):227–235.

Petri M. *Lupus and Pregnancy*. Retrieved October 9, 2011, from The Johns Hopkins Lupus Center website, www.hopkinslupus.org/lupus-info/lifestyle-additional-information/lupus-pregnancy/.

Pullen LC. The state-of-the-art of rheumatology: lupus and pregnancy. *The Rheumatologist*. June 2012:43.

Wechsler B, Huong du LT, Vautheir-Broues D, et al. Hormone stimulation and replacement therapy in women with rheumatic disease. *Scandinavian Journal of Rheumatology*. 1998;27(S107):53–59.

CHAPTER 42

Bihari M. Pre-existing conditions—understanding exclusions and creditable coverage. About .com Guide. April 15, 2010.

Birken EG. The ten best part-time jobs with benefits. In: *PT Money Personal Finance*. Retrieved October 23, 2011, from www.ptmoney.com/the-ten-best-part-time-jobs-with-benefits/.

Celeste R. Top 10 part-time jobs with benefits. November 9, 2010. Retrieved October 23, 2011, from www.jobs.aol.com/articles/2010/11/09/top-10-part-time-jobs-with-benefits/.

Cohen E. No health insurance? Get help here: health insurance in *CNN Health*. February 12, 2009. Retrieved October 23, 2011, from www.articles.cnn.com/2009-02-12/health/ep.health .insurance.help_1_health-insurance-entire-premium-insurance-policy?_s=PM:HEALTH.

Davis M. *How to Get SSI and Social Security Disability*. Lincoln, Ne: Writers Club Press; 2000.

HIPAA Pre-Existing Condition Protections. About.com Health Insurance. Retrieved October 23, 2011, from www.healthinsurance.about.com/od/healthinsurancebasics/a/preexisting _conditions_overview.htm.

Insure.com. Health insurance basics. May 14, 2011. Retrieved on October 23, 2011, from www.insure.com/articles/healthinsurance/basics.html.

Koelker, Cynthia J. *101 Ways to Save Money on Health Care: Tips to Help You Spend Smart and Stay Healthy* (Kindle Location 610). September 1, 2010. Plume. Kindle Edition.

Li T, Carls GS, Panopalis P, Wang S, Gibson TB, Goetzel RZ. Long-term medical costs and resource utilization in systemic lupus erythematosus and lupus nephritis: a five-year analysis of a large Medicaid population. *Arthritis & Rheumatism*. June 2009;61(6):755–763.

Matthews J, Berman DM. *Social Security, Medicare and Government Pensions: Get the Most out of Your Retirement and Medical Benefits*. 16th ed. Berkeley, Ca: NOLO; 2011.

Mercadante K. 11 best part-time jobs with health insurance benefits. Retrieved October 23, 2011, from www.moneycrashers.com/part-time-jobs-health-insurance-benefits/.

Miller GE. 5 Part-time jobs with health insurance & benefits. June 21, 2011. Retrieved October 23, 2011, from http://20somethingfinance.com/part-time-jobs-with-health-insurance -benefits/.

Panopalis P, Yazdany J, Gillis JZ, Julian L, Trupin L, Hersh AO, et al. Health care costs and costs associated with changes in work productivity among persons with systemic lupus erythematosus. *Arthritis Care & Research*. December 2008;59(12):1788–1795.

Q1Medicare.com. *2012 Medicare Part D Outlook*. Retrieved October 23, 2011, from www .q1medicare.com/PartD-About-Us-About-Us-About-Us-About.php?utm_source=partd&utm _medium=textlink&utm_campaign=footer.

U.S. Department of Health and Human Services. Find a health center. Retrieved October 23, 2011, from www.findahealthcenter.hrsa.gov/Search_HCC.aspx.

U.S. Department of Labor Bureau of Labor Statistics. American time use survey: charts from the American time use survey. June 22, 2011. Retrieved October 23, 2011, from http://www .bls.gov/tus/charts/.

**CHAPTER 43**

Abrams S. Work disability/SSDI/health insurance [Chat transcript for Ms. Sheri Abrams in Lupus Foundation of America]. Retrieved October 23, 2011, from www.lupus.org/ webmodules/webarticlesnet/templates/new_community.aspx?articleid=2779&zoneid=91.

Batiste LC. Accommodation and compliance series: employees with lupus in Job Accommo- dation Network. Retrieved October 23, 2011, from www.askjan.org/media/Lupus.html.

Davis M. *How to Get SSI and Social Security Disability*. Lincoln, Ne: Writers Club Press; 2000.

DisabilitySecrets.com. Social Security Disability (SSDI & SSI): advice from a disability exam- iner. Retrieved October 23, 2011, from www.disabilitysecrets.com/advice.html.

Kazmierczak & Kazmierczak, LLP. *Ultimate Social Security Disability Guide: SSDI, SSI, How to Win, Information*. 2009. Retrieved October 23, 2011, from http://www .ultimatedisabilityguide.com/.

Law Office of John L. Roberts. The 5 step Social Security disability claims process. Retrieved October 23, 2011, from www.disabilitydecision.com/html/disability-claims-process.html.

Matthews J, Berman DM. *Social Security, Medicare and Government Pensions: Get the Most out of Your Retirement and Medical Benefits*. 16th ed. Berkeley, Ca: NOLO; 2011.

McGrath E. Self-esteem at work. *Psychology Today*. October 1, 2001. Retrieved October 23, 2011, from www.psychologytoday.com/articles/200310/self-esteem-work.

Morton III DA. Social Security Disability: eight reasons you may be denied benefits. Will your claim for SSDI or SSI disability benefits be denied? Retrieved October 23, 2011, from www .nolo.com/legal-encyclopedia/social-security-disability-reasons-denial-32396.html.

Page numbers in **bold** refer to pages containing definitions or main sources of terms.